BICARBONATE	IV, IO	1 mEq/kg	Q10 min	1.5 mEq	3 mEq	5 mEq	10 mEq	15 mEq	20 mEq	30 mEq	50 mEq	70 mEq
Metabolic acidosis with good ventilation Hyperkalemia Tricyclic antdepressant overdose		**Newborn:** 0.5 mEq/mL (= 2 mL/kg) **Adult:** 1 mEq/mL (= 1 mL/kg)										

[a]ETT size (mm) = [16 + Age (yr)]/4.

[b]Approximate distance of insertion = Internal diameter (ID) × 3.

[c]Straight blades generally preferred for neonates and infants.

[d]"LANE" drugs may be given by ETT: Lidocine, atropine, *na*loxone, epinephrine. Dilute medication with normal saline to minimum volume of 3–5 mL. Follow with positive pressure ventilations.

[e]Beware: Standard drug concentrations may vary.

[f]Use 1 : 10,000 concentration of epinephrine via ETT for neonates only. Use high-dose (1 : 1000) epinephrine for ETT dosing beyond the neonatal period.

[g]Low-dose epinephrine (1 : 10,000) 0.1–0.3 mL/kg preferred for neonates for all doses and all routes.

NARCAN: 0.1 mg/kg/dose IM/ET/IV/IO to **max.** of 2 mg/dose. May repeat Q2–3 min.

OXYGEN: 100%

GLUCOSE: If hypoglycemic: 2–4 mL/kg bolus of $D_{25}W$, then constant infusion of glucose at 8 mg/kg/min.

CALCIUM: If hypocalcemic, hyperkalemic, or Ca channel blocker toxic: 100 mg/kg 10% Ca gluconate, or 20 mg/kg 10% Ca chloride.

DEFIBRILLATION: 2 J/kg. If ineffective, increase to 4 J/kg and repeat twice rapidly.

CARDIOVERSION: Initial: 0.5 J/kg. If ineffective, increase to 1 J/kg and repeat.

ADENOSINE: 0.1 mg/kg rapid IV push. May double and repeat.
Max. dose: 12 mg

AMIODARONE: 5 mg/kg rapid IV push for pulseless VT/VF. Same dose over 20–60 min. for perfusing arrhythmias.

LIDOCAINE: 1 mg/kg IV. If successful, begin lidocaine infusion.

IV INFUSIONS

$$6 \times \frac{\text{Desired dose (mcg/kg/min)}}{\text{Desired rate (mL/hr)}} \times \text{Wt (kg)} = \frac{\text{mg drug}}{\text{100 mL fluid}}$$

Medication	Usual Dose (mcg/kg/min)	Dilution in 100 mL D_5W	IV Infusion Rate
Dopamine	2–20	6 mg/kg	1 mL/hr = 1 mcg/kg/min
Dobutamine	2.5–15	6 mg/kg	1 mL/hr = 1 mcg/kg/min
Epinephrine	0.1–1	0.6 mg/kg	1 mL/hr = 0.1 mcg/kg/mir
Lidocaine	20–50	6 mg/kg	1 mL/hr = 1 mcg/kg/min
Prostaglandin E_1	0.05–0.1	0.3 mg/kg	1 mL/hr = 0.05 mcg/kg/m
Terbutaline	0.1–0.4	0.6 mg/kg	1 mL/hr = 0.1 mcg/kg/min

seventeenth
EDITION

THE HARRIET LANE HANDBOOK

A Manual for Pediatric House Officers

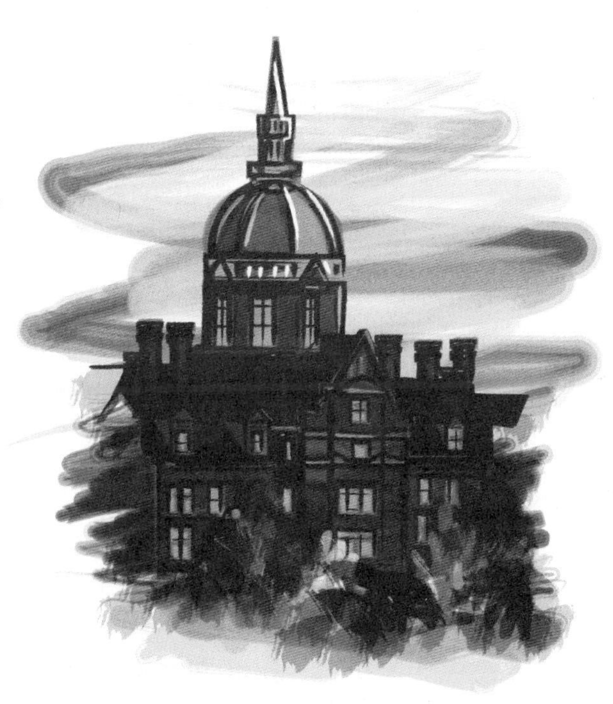

seventeenth
EDITION

THE HARRIET LANE HANDBOOK

A Manual for Pediatric House Officers

The Harriet Lane Service
Children's Medical and Surgical Center of
The Johns Hopkins Hospital

EDITORS
Jason Robertson, MD
Nicole Shilkofski, MD

with 120 illustrations and 50 color plates

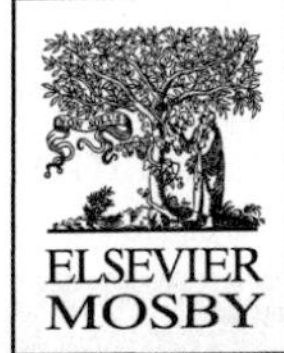

ELSEVIER
MOSBY

1600 John F. Kennedy Blvd.
Ste. 1800
Philadelphia, Pennsylvania 19103-2899

THE HARRIET LANE HANDBOOK 17/e

ISBN: 0-323-02917-5
International Edition 0-8089-2320-X

Notice

Knowledge and best practice in this field are constantly changing. As new research and experience broaden our knowledge, changes in practice, treatment and drug therapy may become necessary or appropriate. Readers are advised to check the most current information provided (i) on procedures featured or (ii) by the manufacturer of each product to be administered, to verify the recomended dose or formula, the method and duration of administration, and contraindications. It is the responsibility of the practitioner, relying on their own experience and knowledge of the patient, to make diagnoses, to determine dosages and the best treatment for each individual patient, and to take all appropriate safety precautions. To the fullest extent of the law, neither the Publisher nor the Editors assumes any liability for any injury and/or damage to persons or property arising out or related to any use of the material contained in this book.

Previous editions copyrighted 2002, 2000, 1996, 1993, 1991, 1987, 1984, 1981, 1978, 1975, 1972, 1969 by Mosby, Inc.

Library of Congress Cataloging-in-Publication Data

The Harriet Lane handbook: a manual for pediatric house officers / the Harriet Lane Service, Children's Medical and Surgical Center of the Johns Hopkins Hospital.–17th ed. / editors, Jason Robertson, Nicole Shilkofski.
p. cm.
ISBN-13: 978-0-323-02917-9 ISBN-10: 0-323-02917-5
1. Pediatrics–Handbooks, manuals, etc. I. Robertson, Jason. II. Shilkofski, Nicole. III. Johns Hopkins Hospital. Children's Medical and Surgical Center.

RJ48.H35 2005
618.92—dc22 2004059296

Editors: Dolores Meloni, Theresa Dudas
Developmental Editor: Jennifer Ehlers
Publishing Services Manager: Joan Sinclair
Project Manager: Mary Stermel
Designer: Karen O'Keefe Owens
Marketing Manager: Michael Passante

Printed in the United States of America

Last digit is the print number: 9 8 7 6 5 4 3 2

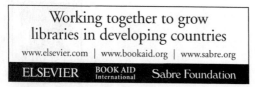

To our parents and families

Annmarie and Joseph Shilkofski,
who have been inspiring me from the day I was born as
my first and most formative teachers

Wade and Patricia Robertson,
for their unwavering support and guidance,

Leila Robertson,
my wonderful wife, for her sacrifice, patience, and love, and

Jocelyn and Ethan, two gifts
who brighten my days with smiles.

Our patients and their parents

Who continue to entrust us with their most prized possession—
their health

Our role model, teacher, and friend

Julia McMillan

And to

George Dover
Chairman of Pediatrics
The Johns Hopkins Hospital
Devoted advocate for residents, children, and their families

Preface

"To study the phenomena of disease without books is to sail an uncharted sea, while to study books without patients is not to go to sea at all."
—Sir William Osler

In 1950, Dr. Harrison Spencer of the Harriet Lane Home for Children first spoke of creating a manual of information for the housestaff. The goal was to have essential medical information collected in a single source that would be easily accessible to the residents. Three years later, the first edition was distributed to house officers. Since that time *The Harriet Lane Handbook* has been revised repeatedly, always by house officers, and always for the reasons outlined by Dr. Jerry Winkelstein in his preface to the sixth edition:

"The content of *The Harriet Lane Handbook* has been determined by the pediatric house officers who have used it in the past. Because of rapid changes in pediatric procedures and practice, they have found it necessary to once again revise its content but not its purpose." That purpose is the same today as when Dr. Winkelstein described it:

"The Handbook is still intended as a convenient, readily accessible synthesis of information useful to the pediatric house officer and pediatric practitioner."

The reality of a handbook written "by house officers for house officers" continues in its current revision cycle every three years. Holding the sixth and seventeenth editions side by side, it's hard to ignore that time has added considerable heft around the middle of the Handbook. Although the steadily increasing size perhaps reflects the exponentially increasing amount of medical knowledge and an expanding formulary, its editors have always tried to keep it to a "pocketable" size.

As the house officers undertook this edition of *The Harriet Lane Handbook*, they were animated by the goal of improving the usefulness of the book. As a result, this edition features a new approach to presenting information. When amenable, text has been translated into tables and boxes to enhance the accessibility of material. This format was employed throughout the text where possible, but nowhere more strikingly than in Fluids and Electrolytes. Incorporating solicited feedback from house officers and practicing pediatricians, this chapter was significantly reworked, with the end result being what we hope is an easy-to-follow approach to fluid management in the dehydrated patient. Surgical diagnoses and issues critical to general pediatrics, previously without a home in the absence of a Surgery chapter, have been inserted into their relevant chapters: bilious emesis in the neonate is now in Neonatology. A resident's search for diagnostic criteria for systemic lupus led to the creation of a brief but useful Rheumatology chapter with some key reference data. Finally, the Pediatric Acute Care section of the handbook has been retooled and reorganized to reflect changes in pediatric critical care. Sections such as ventilatory management that would be most useful to house officers rotating through intensive care units have been consolidated into Chapter 4.

The tireless efforts of the senior residents are, as always, the heart of the book. They exhibited the same level of dedication and vision for their chapters as they show in caring for their patients. Each of the residents' faculty advisors was instrumental in guiding the residents in a critical reappraisal of their chapters. We are extremely grateful to both groups for contributing time from their already busy schedules and for their considerable efforts on their chapters:

Resident	**Chapter Title**	**Faculty Advisor**
M. Denisse Mueller, MD	Emergency Management	Allen R. Walker, MD
Jennifer Lee, MD	Poisonings	Jennifer Schuette, MD
Nicole Shilkofski, MD	Procedures	Ivor Berkowitz, MD
Heather D. Johnson, MD	Trauma, Burns, and Common Critical Care Emergencies	Z. Leah Harris, MD
Tracey Clark, MD	Adolescent Medicine	Hoover Adger, MD, MPH
Kelly K. Gajewski, MD	Cardiology	W. Reid Thompson, MD William Ravekes, MD
Kristen Schwindt Brown, MD	Dermatology	Bernard Cohen, MD
Renay Walker Chung, MD	Development and Behavior	Mary Leppert, MBBCh
David Salikof, MD	Endocrinology	David Cooke, MD
Brian Stone, MD	Fluids and Electrolytes	Michael Barone, MD
Kurlen S.E. Payton, MD	Gastroenterology	Maria Oliva-Hemker, MD
Ai Sakonju, MD Jennifer Huffman, MD	Genetics	Ada Hamosh, MD, MPH
Marissa Brunetti, MD Joanna Cohen, MD	Hematology	James F. Casella, MD
Adam Gower, MD	Immunology and Allergy	Jerry Winkelstein, MD Robert Wood, MD
Megan E. Partridge, MD	Immunoprophylaxis	Mathuram Santosham, MD, MPH
Kabuiya Kimani, MD	Microbiology and Infectious Disease	George Siberry, MD, MPH

Theodora Stavroudis, MD	Neonatology	Susan Aucott, MD
Stephanie O. Omokaro, MD	Nephrology	Susan Furth, MD, MPH
Jennifer Huffman, MD	Neurology	Thomas Crawford, MD
Ai Sakonju, MD		Tyler Reimschisel, MD
Kristin N. Fiorino, MD	Nutrition and Growth	Benjamin Caballero, MD, PhD
Jeanne Cox, MS, RD		
Jason Yustein, MD, PhD	Oncology	Kenneth Cohen, MD
Anthony Caterina, MD		
Celia E. Loughlin, MD	Pulmonology	Gerald Loughlin, MD
Alexander M. Kowal, MD	Radiology	James Crowe, MD Melissa Spevak, MD
Susan McFarland, MD	Rheumatology	Edward Sills, MD
Jason Robertson, MD	Blood Chemistries and Body Fluids	
Jason Robertson, MD	Biostatistics and Evidence-Based Medicine	
Jason Robertson, MD Nicole Shilkofski, MD Carlton Lee, PharmD, MPH	Drug Doses	
Kamie Yang, MD	Analgesia and Sedation	Myron Yaster, MD
Jason Robertson, MD Nicole Shilkofski, MD	Formulary Adjunct	Carlton Lee, PharmD, MPH
Jason Robertson, MD Nicole Shilkofski, MD	Drugs in Renal Failure	Carlton Lee, PharmD, MPH

The Handbook is and always will be a work perpetually in progress. The current edition is as much the work of its previous editors as it is ours: Drs. Harrison Spencer, Henry Seidel, Herbert Swick, William Friedman, Robert Haslam, Jerry Winkelstein, Dennis Headings, Kenneth Schuberth, Basil Zitelli, Jeffrey Biller, Andrew Yeager, Cynthia Cole, Mary Greene, Peter Rowe, Kevin Johnson, Michael Barone, George Siberry, Rob Iannone, Christian Nechyba, and Veronica L. Gunn. As we review the list of previous editors, we are struck by their continuing legacy in our training and by their commitment to the education of the next generation of house officers. We view several of the previous editors as mentors, and are indebted to them not only for their work on The Handbook, but for their example in our lives and careers, particularly Peter Rowe, George Siberry, and Mike Barone.

A project of this size cannot be undertaken without a large group of dedicated and special people. We owe special thanks to Megan Brown and Kathy Miller, who helped us navigate the uncharted waters of overnight shipping and file-zipping (and *un*-zipping). Thanks also to Wayne Reisig for countless literature searches on our behalf. The formulary continues to thrive thanks in large part to the unflagging efforts of Carlton Lee. Heartfelt thanks to Jeanne Cox for her tireless commitment to the nutrition chapter (and for nurturing interns through their first TPN orders in the NICU). Dr. George Dover provides visionary leadership for our department and we have benefited from his guidance both personally and professionally. He continues to challenge us all to strive for excellence in the care of children. Two of our role models in excellent patient care, Dr. Janet Serwint and Dr. Fred Heldrich, have been instrumental in guiding our development as pediatricians. Finally, we count ourselves fortunate to have Dr. Julia McMillan as our mentor and friend. We can think of no greater privilege than to be her colleagues and can pay her no greater compliment than to emulate her as pediatricians.

Despite the effort that goes into producing a book such as The Handbook, we nonetheless are again reminded of the words of Sir William Osler about the importance of learning first from our patients: "Medicine is learned by the bedside and not in the classroom. Let not your conceptions of disease come from words heard in the lecture room or read from the book. See, and then reason and compare and control. But see first." We would like to thank all the residents on the Harriet Lane Housestaff for the privilege of "seeing" with you. We are confident you will shine wherever you choose to tread.

Residents	**Interns**
Naseem Amarasingham	Kristin Barañano
Margaret Brewinski	Bianca Bell
Jason Custer	Shazia Bhombal
Joshua Dishon	Renee Boynton-Jarrett
Yoav Dori	Aaron Chambers
Doran Fink	Carmen Coombs
Anne Gaddy	Brian Costello
Patrick Grohar	Joan Dunlop
Pamela Guerrerio	Michelle Dunn
Anthony Guerrerio	Kari Gillenwater
Erum Aftab Hartung	Deanna Green
Raquel Hernandez	Jared Hershenson
Taryn Holman (PL-3)	Rachel Johnson
Erin Kish	Corinne Keet

Sarah Kline
Andrew Krakowski
Sapna Kudchadkar
Christina Lehane
Mark Lindsay
Justin Lockman
Maya Lodish
Cecilia Melendres
Michael Nemergut
Devang Pastakia
Rachel Plotnick
Rachel Rau
Jesse Sturm
Krishna Upadhya
Jill Whitehurst (PL-3)
Patrick Wilson
Joyce Zmuda
Heather Larkin
Rachel Lestz
Doug Mah
Michael McCrory
Mary Niu
Chris Park
Sarah Polk
Laura Santos
Perry Sheffield
David Shook
Arethusa Stevens
Pranita Tamma
Sabrina Vineberg

Jason Robertson
Nicole Shilkofski

Contents

PART I

Pediatric Acute Care

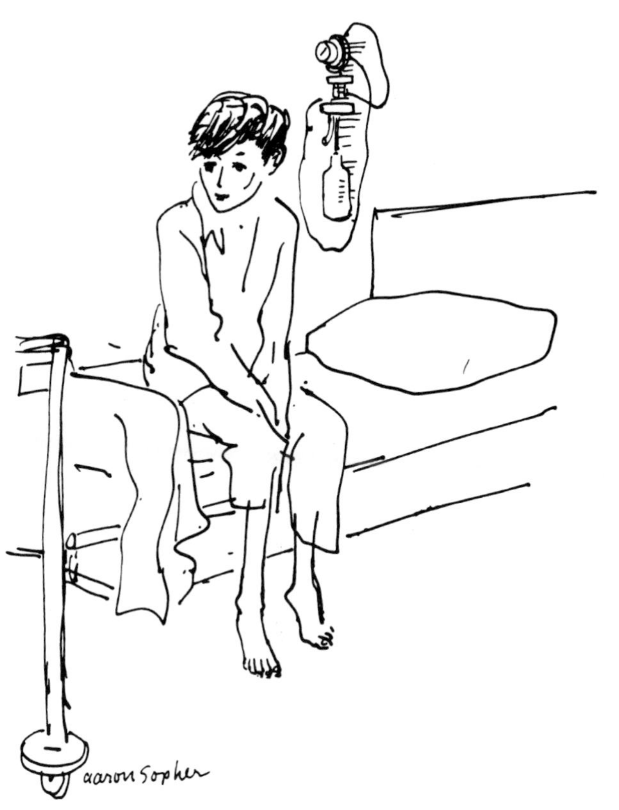

Emergency Management

M. Denisse Mueller, MD

1

I. AIRWAY[1-5]

A. ASSESSMENT

1. Position the child supine on a flat, hard surface.
2. Open airway: Establish an open airway with the head-tilt/chin-lift maneuver. If neck injury is suspected, jaw thrust with cervical spine (C-spine) immobilization should be used.
3. Obstruction: Rule out foreign body, anatomic, or other obstruction.

B. MANAGEMENT

1. Equipment:

a. Oral airway in an unconscious patient.
  (1) Size: With flange at teeth, tip reaches angle of jaw.
  (2) Length ranges from 4 to 10 cm.

b. Nasopharyngeal airway in a conscious patient:
  (1) Rarely provokes vomiting or laryngospasm.
  (2) Size: Length equals tip of nose to angle of jaw. Check the outer diameter so that the airway does not blanch the alae nasi.
  (3) Diameter: 12 to 36 French (F).
  (4) A shortened tracheal tube may be used.

c. Laryngeal mask airway (LMA) is an option for a secure airway in an unconscious patient that does not require laryngoscopy or tracheal intubation. It allows spontaneous or assisted respiration but does not prevent aspiration. It may be useful in patients with abnormal anatomy, difficult airway, or head and neck trauma.

2. **Intubation:** Sedation and paralysis are recommended for intubation except in newborns and in some patients who are unconscious or in cardiorespiratory arrest.

a. Indications: Obstruction (functional or anatomic), prolonged ventilatory assistance or control, respiratory insufficiency, loss of protective airway reflexes, or route for approved medications.

b. Equipment (see table on inside front cover):
  (1) Endotracheal tube (ETT): The following equation should be used to determine the size of the ETT to be used:

$$(\text{Age} + 16)/4 = \text{internal diameter of ETT tube (mm)}$$

Have one ETT 0.5 mm smaller and one ETT 0.5 mm larger than the estimated size.

An uncuffed ETT should be used in patients < 8 years old. The depth of insertion (in centimeters; at the teeth or lips) is about three times the ETT size.

Resuscitation tapes based on length may be used to estimate ETT size.

(2) Laryngoscope blade and handle with a functioning light: Generally, a straight blade can be used in all patients. A curved blade may be easier to use in patients >2 years old.
(3) Bag and mask should be attached to 100% oxygen.
(4) ETT stylets should not extend beyond the distal end of the ETT.
(5) Suction: Use a large-bore (Yankauer) suction catheter or 14F to 18F suction catheter.
(6) Nasogastric (or orogastric) tube: Size from nose to angle of jaw to xiphoid process.
(7) Monitoring equipment: Electrocardiography (ECG), pulse oximetry, blood pressure (BP) monitoring, capnometry (end-tidal CO_2 monitoring).
(8) Tape to secure the tube.
(9) Consider an LMA for difficult airway.

c. Procedure: Attempts should not exceed 30 seconds.
(1) Preoxygenate with 100% O_2. Assist ventilation with positive-pressure ventilation only if the patient's effort is inadequate.
(2) Administer intubation medications (Table 1-1 and Fig. 1-1).
(3) Apply cricoid pressure to prevent aspiration (Sellick maneuver) during bag-valve-mask ventilation and intubation.

TABLE 1-1

RAPID-SEQUENCE INTUBATION MEDICATIONS

Drug	Dose (IV) (mg/kg)	Comments
ADJUNCTS (FIRST)		
Atropine (*vagolytic*)	0.01–0.02 Min: 0.1 mg Max: 1 mg	Vagolytic, prevents bradycardia and reduces oral secretions, may increase HR
Lidocaine (optional anesthetic)	1–2	Blunts ICP spike, cough reflex, and CV effects of intubation; controls ventricular dysrhythmias
SEDATIVE-HYPNOTIC (SECOND)		
Thiopental	1–7	May cause hypotension; myocardial depression (barbiturate); decreases ICP and cerebral blood flow; use low dose in hypovolemia (1–2 mg/kg); may increase oral secretions, cause bronchospasm and laryngospasm; contraindicated in status asthmaticus
or		
Ketamine	1–3	May increase ICP, BP, HR, and oral secretions (general anesthetic); causes bronchodilation, emergence delirium; give with atropine; contraindicated in eye injuries

TABLE 1-1
RAPID-SEQUENCE INTUBATION MEDICATIONS—*cont'd*

Drug	Dose (IV) (mg/kg)	Comments
or		
Midazolam (benzodiazepine)	0.05–0.1	May cause decreased BP and HR and respiratory depression; amnestic properties; benzodiazepines reversible with flumazenil (seizure warning applies)
or		
Fentanyl (opiate)	1–5 mcg/kg	Fewest hemodynamic effects of all opiates; chest wall rigidity with high-dose or rapid administration; opiates reversible with naloxone (seizure warning applies); don't use with MAO inhibitors
or		
Etomidate (imidazole/ hypnotic)	0.2–0.3	Does not cause hypotension or increased ICP. Caution in patients with adrenal suppression; may cause further suppression
PARALYTICS (THIRD)*		
Rocuronium	0.6–1.2	Onset 30–60 sec, duration 30–60 min; coadministration with sedative; may reverse in 30 min with atropine and neostigmine; minimal effect on HR or BP; precipitates when in contact with other drugs, so flush line before and after use
or		
Vecuronium	0.1–0.2	Onset 70–120 sec, duration 30–90 min; minimal effect on BP or HR; may reverse in 30–45 min with atropine and neostigmine
or		
Succinylcholine	1–2	Onset 30–60 sec, duration 3–10 min; increases ICP, irreversible; contraindicated in burns, massive trauma, neuromuscular disease, eye injuries, malignant hyperthermia, and pseudocholinesterase deficiency. *Risk*: Lethal hyperkalemia in undiagnosed muscular dystrophy

BP, Blood pressure; CV, cardiovascular; HR, heart rate; ICP, intracranial pressure; MAO, monoamine oxidase.
*Nondepolarizing neuromuscular blockers, except succinylcholine, which is depolarizing.

(4) With patient lying supine on a firm surface, head midline and slightly extended, open mouth with right thumb and index finger using scissoring technique.
(5) Hold laryngoscope blade in left hand. Insert blade into right side of mouth, sweeping tongue to the left out of line of vision.

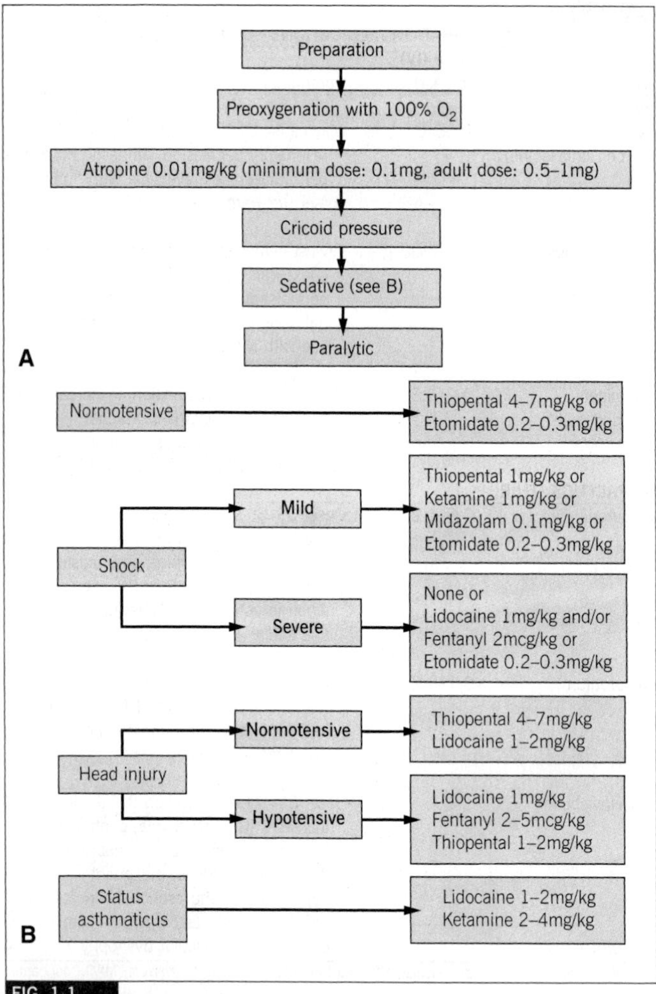

FIG. 1-1

A, Treatment algorithm for intubation. *B*, Sedation options. *(Modified from Nichols DG, et al. (eds): Golden Hour: The Handbook of Advanced Pediatric Life Support. St. Louis, Mosby, 1996.)*

(6) Advance blade to epiglottis. With straight blade, lift laryngoscope straight up, directly lifting the epiglottis until vocal cords are visible. With curved blade, the tip of the blade rests in the vallecula (between the base of the tongue and epiglottis). Lift straight up to elevate the epiglottis and visualize the vocal cords.

(7) While maintaining direct visualization, pass the ETT from the right corner of the mouth through the cords. The double black marker on the tube should be at the level of the vocal cords.

(8) Verify ETT placement: observe chest wall movement, auscultation in both axillae and epigastrium, capnography or colorimetric capnometer, end-tidal CO_2 detection (there will be a false-negative response if there is no effective pulmonary circulation), water vapor in the tube, improvement in oxygen saturation, chest radiograph.

(9) Only when ETT placement is verified should cricoid pressure be removed.

(10) Securely tape ETT in place, noting depth of insertion (cm) at teeth or lips.

C. RAPID-SEQUENCE INTUBATION MEDICATIONS

Note *Titrate drug doses to achieve desired effect (see Fig. 1-1 and Table 1-1).*

II. BREATHING[1–3]

A. ASSESSMENT

After the airway is established, evaluate air exchange. Examine for evidence of abnormal chest wall dynamics, such as tension pneumothorax, or central problems such as apnea. Once intubated, deterioration may be caused by (DOPE): **d**isplacement of the ETT, **o**bstruction, **p**neumothorax, or **e**quipment failure.

B. MANAGEMENT

Positive-pressure ventilation (application of 100% oxygen is never contraindicated in resuscitation situations).

1. **Mouth-to-mouth or mouth-to-nose** breathing is used in situations in which no supplies are available. Provide two slow breaths (1 to 1.5 sec/breath) initially, then 20 breaths/min (30 breaths/min in infants). For newborns, apply 1 breath for every 3 chest compressions. In infants and children <8 years old, apply 1 breath for every 5 chest compressions. For children ≥8 years of age, apply 2 breaths for every 15 chest compressions in cardiopulmonary resuscitation (CPR).
2. **Bag-mask ventilation** is used at a rate of 20 breaths/min (30 breaths/min in infants). Assess chest expansion and breath sounds. Decompress stomach with orogastric (OG) or nasogastric (NG) tube with prolonged bag-mask ventilation.
3. **Endotracheal intubation:**

See prior section.

III. CIRCULATION[1,2,4]

A. ASSESSMENT

1. **Rate:** Assess for bradycardia, tachycardia, or absent heart rate. Generally, bradycardia is <100 beats/min in a newborn and

<60 beats/min in an infant or child; tachycardia of >240 beats/min suggests cardiac dysrhythmia rather than sinus tachycardia.

2. **Rhythm:** Assess sinus versus abnormal rhythm.
3. **Assess pulses (central and peripheral) and capillary refill (assuming extremity is warm):** <2 sec is normal, 2 to 5 sec is delayed, and >5 sec is markedly delayed, suggesting shock. Decreased or altered mental status may be a sign of inadequate perfusion.
4. **BP:** Measuring blood pressure is one of the least sensitive measures of adequate circulation in children.

$$\text{Hypotension} = \text{systolic BP} < [70 + (2 \times \text{age in years})]$$

B. MANAGEMENT (Table 1-2)

1. **Chest compressions.**
2. **Fluid resuscitation with poor perfusion and shock:**

a. If peripheral intravenous (IV) access is not obtained in 90 seconds or after two attempts, *or* if patient is in cardiorespiratory arrest and access predicted to be difficult, place an intraosseous (IO) needle (see Chapter 3). If still unsuccessful, consider central venous access.

b. Initial fluid should be lactated Ringer (LR) or normal saline (NS). Administer a bolus with 20 mL/kg over 5 to 15 minutes. Reassess. If there is no improvement, consider a repeat bolus with 20 mL/kg of the same fluid. Reassess. If replacement requires more than 40 to 60 mL/kg, or if there is acute blood loss, consider colloids: 5% albumin, plasma, or packed red blood cells (RBCs) at 10–15 mL/kg.

c. If cardiogenic etiology is suspected, fluid resuscitation may worsen clinical status. Consider a smaller fluid bolus of 5 to 10 mL/kg.

3. **Pharmacotherapy: See inside front and back covers for guidelines for drugs to be considered in cardiac arrest and arrhythmia algorithms.**

Note *Consider early administration of antibiotics or corticosteroids if clinically indicated.*

TABLE 1-2

MANAGEMENT OF CIRCULATION

	Location*	Rate (per min)	Compressions: Ventilation
Infants	1 fingerbreadth below intermammary line	>100	5 : 1
Children (<8 yr)	2 fingerbreadth below intermammary line	100	5 : 1
Older children (>8 yr)	Lower half of stemum	100	15 : 2

*Depth of compressions should be one third to one half anteroposterior (AP) diameter of the chest and should produce palpable pulses.

IV. ALLERGIC EMERGENCIES (ANAPHYLAXIS)[4]

A. DEFINITION

Anaphylaxis is the clinical syndrome of immediate hypersensitivity. It is characterized by cardiovascular collapse, respiratory compromise, and cutaneous and gastrointestinal (GI) symptoms (e.g., urticaria, emesis).

B. INITIAL MANAGEMENT

1. **ABCs:** Establish airway if necessary. Assess breathing: Supply with 100% oxygen with respiratory support as needed. Assess circulation and establish IV access. Place patient on cardiac monitor.
2. **Epinephrine:** Give epinephrine, 0.01 mL/kg (1:1000) subcutaneously (SC) or IM (maximum dose 0.5 mL). Repeat every 15 minutes as needed.

Note *Some studies suggest that the IM route is superior because of slowed absorption when the drug is given SC.[10] The site of choice is the lateral aspect of the thigh due to its vascularity.*

3. **Albuterol:** Give nebulized albuterol, 0.05 to 0.15 mg/kg in 3 mL NS (quick estimate: 2.5 mg for <30 kg, 5 mg for >30 kg) every 15 min as needed.
4. **Administer a histamine-1 receptor antagonist** such as diphenhydramine, 1 to 2 mg/kg through intramuscular (IM), IV, or oral (PO) routes (maximum dose, 50 mg). Also, consider a histamine-2 receptor antagonist.
5. **Corticosteroids** help prevent the late phase of the allergic response. Administer methylprednisolone in a 2 mg/kg IV bolus, then 2 mg/kg per day IV or IM divided every 6 hours, or prednisone, 2 mg/kg PO in a bolus once daily. Observe for 6 to 24 hours for late-phase symptoms depending on clinical condition and stability.
6. **Patient should be discharged with an Epi-Pen** (>30 kg), Epi-Pen Junior (<30 kg), or comparable injectable epinephrine product with specific instructions on appropriate usage.

C. HYPOTENSION

1. **Trendelenburg position:** Put patient's head at 30-degree angle below feet.
2. **NS:** Administer 20 mL/kg IV NS or LR over 5 to 15 minutes. Repeat bolus as necessary.
3. **Epinephrine:** 0.1 mL/kg (1:10,000) may be given IV over 2 to 5 minutes while an epinephrine or dopamine infusion is being prepared. (See infusion table inside front cover for details of preparation and dosages.)

V. RESPIRATORY EMERGENCIES[4]

The hallmark of upper airway obstruction is inspiratory stridor, whereas lower airway obstruction is characterized by cough, wheeze, and a prolonged expiratory phase.

A. ASTHMA

1. **Assessment:** Assess heart rate (HR), respiratory rate (RR), O_2 saturation, peak expiratory flow rate, use of accessory muscles, pulsus paradoxus (>20 mmHg difference in systolic BP for inspiratory versus expiratory phase), dyspnea, alertness, color.
2. **Initial management:**
   a. Oxygen to keep saturation >95%.
   b. Inhaled β-agonists: Nebulized albuterol, 0.05 to 0.15 mg/kg/dose every 20 minutes (or continuously depending on clinical condition) to effect. Albuterol may be given by metered-dose inhaler (MDI) with aerochamber to a cooperative patient.
   c. Additional nebulized bronchodilators include ipratropium bromide, 0.25 to 0.5 mg, nebulized with albuterol (as above). Benefit has only been demonstrated for moderate to severe exacerbations.
   d. If there is very poor air movement, or the patient is unable to cooperate with a nebulizer, give epinephrine, 0.01 mL/kg SC (1:1000; maximum dose, 0.5 mL) every 15 min up to three doses, or terbutaline, 0.01 mg/kg SC (maximum dose, 0.4 mg) every 15 minutes up to two doses.
   e. Start corticosteroids if there is no response after one nebulized treatment or if patient is steroid dependent, has had a recent emergency department visit or previous admission to an intensive care unit (ICU). Prednisone or prednisolone, 2 mg/kg PO every 24 hr; or (if severe) methylprednisolone, 2 mg/kg IV/IM bolus, then 2 mg/kg/day divided every 6 hours. Parenteral steroids have not been proved to routinely provide more rapid onset of action or greater clinical effect than oral steroids in children with mild to moderate asthma.
3. **Further management if incomplete or poor response:** Consider obtaining an arterial blood gas (ABG) value if breath sounds are minimal.
   a. Continue nebulization therapy every 20 to 30 minutes, and space interval as tolerated.
   b. Administer magnesium sulfate, 25 to 75 mg/kg/dose IV or IM (maximum, 2 g) infused over 20 minutes every 4 to 6 hours up to three to four doses. Many clinicians suggest the higher end of this dosing range (75 mg/kg/dose), although further dosing studies are needed. Do not use in hypotension or renal failure.
   c. Administer terbutaline, 2 to 10 mcg/kg IV load, followed by continuous infusion at 0.1 to 0.4 mcg/kg/min titrated to effect (see table inside front cover). Monitor 12 lead ECG, electrolytes, urinalysis, and cardiac enzymes.
   d. A helium (≥70%) and oxygen mixture may be of some benefit in the critically ill patient but is more useful in upper airway edema. Avoid use in the severely hypoxic patient.
   e. Although aminophylline may be considered, it is no longer considered a preferred mode of therapy for status asthmaticus (see Formulary for dosage information).

4. **Intubation** of those with acute asthma is dangerous and should be reserved for impending respiratory arrest. Indications include deteriorating mental status, severe cyanosis, and respiratory or cardiac arrest. Premedicate with lidocaine, midazolam, and ketamine (see Fig. 1-1 and Table 1-1). Consider using an inhaled anesthetic.

B. UPPER AIRWAY OBSTRUCTION

Upper airway obstruction is most commonly caused by foreign-body aspiration or infection.

1. **Epiglottitis** is a true emergency. Any manipulation, including aggressive physical examination, attempt to visualize the epiglottis, venipuncture, or IV placement, may precipitate complete obstruction. If epiglottitis is suspected, definitive airway placement should precede all diagnostic procedures. A prototypic "epiglottitis protocol" may include the following:

a. Unobtrusively give O_2 (blow-by). Place patient on NPO status. Pulse oximetry may be used if it does not upset the patient.
b. Have parent accompany child to allay anxiety.
c. Have physician accompany patient at all times.
d. Summon "epiglottitis team" (most senior pediatrician, anesthesiologist, and otolaryngologist in hospital).
e. Management options:
   (1) If patient is unstable (unresponsive, cyanotic, bradycardic), emergently intubate.
   (2) If patient is stable with high suspicion, escort patient with team to operating room for endoscopy and intubation under general anesthesia.
   (3) If patient is stable with moderate or low suspicion, obtain lateral neck radiographic examination to confirm. An epiglottitis team must accompany the patient at all times.
f. After airway is secured, obtain cultures of blood and epiglottic surface. Begin antibiotics to cover *Haemophilus influenzae* type B, *Streptococcus pneumoniae*, group A streptococci, *Staphylococcus aureus*. Epiglottitis may be caused by thermal injury.

2. **Croup (laryngotracheobronchitis):**

a. Mild (no stridor at rest): Treat with cool mist therapy, minimal disturbance, hydration, and antipyretics. Consider steroids (see below).
b. Moderate to severe:
   (1) Mist or humidified oxygen mask near child's face may be used, although the efficacy of mist therapy is not established. A mist tent may increase a child's anxiety and decrease the physician's ability to observe the patient.
   (2) Administer racemic epinephrine (2.25), 0.05 mL/kg/dose (maximum dose, 0.5 mL) in 3 mL NS *over 15 minutes*, no more than every 1 to 2 hours, or nebulized epinephrine, 0.5 mL/kg of 1:1000 (1 mg/mL) in 3 mL NS (maximum dose, 2.5 mL for ≤4

years old, 5 mL for >4 years old). Observe for a minimum of 2 to 4 hours if discharge is planned after administering nebulized epinephrine. Hospitalize if more than one nebulization is required.

(3) Administer dexamethasone, 0.3 to 0.6 mg/kg IM or PO once. Prednisolone or prednisone may be adequate but should be administered for several days because of the shorter half-life of these steroid preparations.

(4) Nebulized budesonide (2 mg) has been shown to be effective in mild to moderate croup and is *equivalent to oral dexamethasone*.

(5) A helium-oxygen mixture may decrease the work of breathing by decreasing resistance to turbulent gas flow through a narrowed airway. Inspired helium concentration must be ≥70% to be effective.

c. If a child fails to respond as expected to therapy, consider airway radiography, computed tomography (CT), or evaluation by otolaryngology or anesthesiology. Consider retropharyngeal abscess, bacterial tracheitis, subglottic stenosis, subglottic hemangioma, epiglottitis, or foreign body.

3. **Foreign-body aspiration** occurs most often in children <5 years old. It frequently involves hot dogs, candy, peanuts, grapes, balloons, and other small objects. A high index of suspicion, witnessed event, and history of choking are most important for diagnosis.

a. If the patient is stable (i.e., forcefully coughing, well oxygenated), removal of the foreign body by bronchoscopy or laryngoscopy should be attempted in a controlled environment.

b. If the patient is unable to speak, moves air poorly, or is cyanotic, intervene immediately.

(1) Infant: Place infant over arm or rest on lap. Give five back blows between the scapulae. If unsuccessful, turn infant over and give five chest thrusts, *one per second* (in the same location as external chest compressions). Use tongue-jaw lift to open mouth. Remove object only if visualized. Attempt to ventilate if unconscious. Repeat sequence as often as necessary.

(2) Child: Perform five abdominal thrusts (Heimlich maneuver) from behind a sitting or standing child or straddled over a child lying supine. Direct thrusts upward in the midline and not to either side of the abdomen.

(3) After back, chest, and/or abdominal thrusts, open mouth and remove foreign body if visualized. Blind finger sweeps are not recommended. Magill forceps may allow removal of foreign bodies in the posterior pharynx.

(4) If the patient is unconscious, remove the foreign body using Magill forceps if needed after direct visualization or laryngoscopy. If there is complete airway obstruction, consider percutaneous (needle) cricothyrotomy (Fig. 1-2)[2] if attempts to ventilate by bag-valve mask or ETT are unsuccessful.

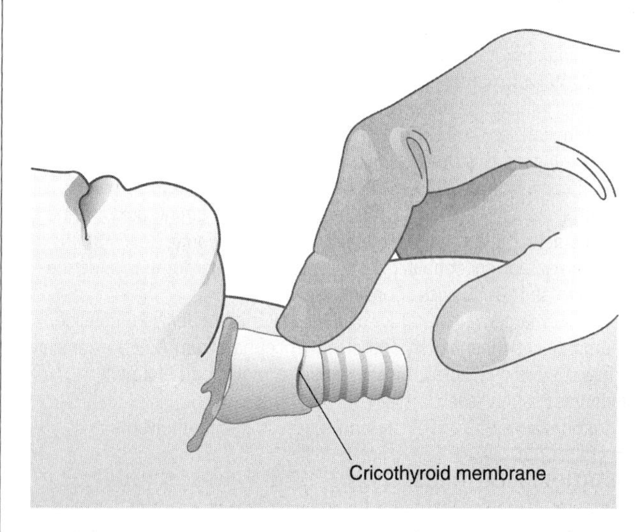

FIG. 1-2

Percutaneous (needle) cricothyrotomy. Extend neck, attach a 3-mL syringe to a 14- to 18-gauge IV catheter, and introduce catheter through the cricothyroid membrane (inferior to the thyroid cartilage, superior to the cricoid cartilage). Aspirate air to confirm position. Remove the syringe and needle, attach the catheter to an adaptor from a 3.0-mm endotracheal tube, which can then be used for positive-pressure oxygenation. *(Modified from Dieckmann RA, Fiser DH, Selbst SM: Illustrated Textbook of Pediatric Emergency and Critical Care Procedures. St. Louis, Mosby, 1997.)*

VI. NEUROLOGIC EMERGENCIES

A. COMA[6,7]

1. Assessment:

a. History: Obtain history of trauma, ingestion, infection, fasting, drug use, diabetes, seizure, or other neurologic disorder.

b. Examination: Assess HR, BP, respiratory pattern, Glasgow Coma Scale (GCS), temperature, pupillary response, funduscopy, rash, abnormal posturing, and focal neurologic signs.

2. Management: "ABC DON'T"

a. **A**irway (with C-spine immobilization), **b**reathing, **c**irculation, **D**extro stick, **o**xygen, **n**aloxone, **t**hiamine.

(1) Naloxone, 0.1 mg/kg IV, IM, SC, or ETT (maximum dose, 2 mg). Repeat as necessary, keeping in mind short half-life of naloxone.

(2) Thiamine, 100 mg IV (before starting glucose). Consider in adolescents for deficiencies secondary to alcoholism or eating disorders.

(3) $D_{25}W$, 2 to 4 mL/kg IV bolus if hypoglycemia is present.

b. Laboratory tests: Consider complete blood count (CBC), electrolytes, liver function tests (LFTs), NH_3, lactate, toxicology screen (serum and urine), blood gas, serum osmolality, prothrombin time (PT), partial thromboplastin time (PTT), and blood and urine culture. If patient is an infant or toddler, consider assessment of plasma amino acids, urine organic acids, and other appropriate metabolic workup.

c. If meningitis or encephalitis is suspected, consider lumbar puncture (LP) and start antibiotics. Consider acyclovir.

d. Request emergent head CT scan after ABCs are stabilized; consider neurosurgical consultation and electroencephalogram (EEG) if indicated.

e. If ingestion is suspected, airway must be protected before GI decontamination (see Chapter 2).

f. Monitor Glasgow Coma Scale and reassess frequently (Table 1-3).

B. STATUS EPILEPTICUS[8,9]

See Chapter 19 for nonacute evaluation and management of seizures.

1. **Assessment:** Common causes of childhood seizures include fever, subtherapeutic anticonvulsant levels, central nervous system (CNS)

TABLE 1-3

COMA SCALES

Glasgow Coma Scale		Modified Coma Scale for Infants	
Activity	Best Response	Activity	Best Response
EYE OPENING			
Spontaneous	4	Spontaneous	4
To speech	3	To speech	3
To pain	2	To pain	2
None	1	None	1
VERBAL			
Oriented	5	Coos, babbles	5
Confused	4	Irritable	4
Inappropriate words	3	Cries to pain	3
Nonspecific sounds	2	Moans to pain	2
None	1	None	1
MOTOR			
Follows commands	6	Normal spontaneous movements	6
Localizes pain	5	Withdraws to touch	5
Withdraws to pain	4	Withdraws to pain	4
Abnormal flexion	3	Abnormal flexion	3
Abnormal extension	2	Abnormal extension	2
None	1	None	1

Data from Jennet B, Teasdale G: Lancet 1977;1:878; and James HE: Pediatr Ann 1986;15:16.

infections, trauma, toxic ingestion, and metabolic abnormalities. Less common causes include vascular, neoplastic, and endocrine diseases.

2. **Acute management of seizures** (Table 1-4). If CNS infection is suspected, give antibiotics and/or acyclovir early.
3. **Diagnostic workup:** When stable, workup may include CT or magnetic resonance imaging (MRI), EEG, and LP.

TABLE 1-4

ACUTE MANAGEMENT OF SEIZURES

Time (min)	Intervention
0–5	Stabilize the patient Assess airway, breathing, circulation, and vital signs Administer oxygen Obtain intravenous access or intraosseous access Correct hypoglycemia if present (dextrose 25% 2–4 mL/kg). In adolescents, give thiamine (100 mg) first Obtain laboratory studies: Consider glucose, electrolytes, calcium, magnesium, BUN, creatinine, and LFTs, CBC, toxicology screen, anticonvulsant levels, blood culture (if infection is suspected) Initial screening history and physical examination
5–15	Begin pharmacotherapy Lorazepam (Ativan), 0.05–0.1 mg/kg IV, up to 4–6 mg *or* Diazepam (Valium), 0.2–0.5 mg/kg IV (0.5 mg/kg rectally) up to 6–10 mg May repeat lorazepam or diazepam 5–10 min after initial dose
15–35	If seizure persists, load with: Phenytoin* 15–20 mg/kg IV at rate not to exceed 1 mg/kg/min via central line *or* Fosphenytoin† 15–20 mg PE/kg IV/IM at 3 mg PE/kg/min via peripheral IV live (maximum 150 mg PE/min). If given IM, may require multiple dosing sites *or* Phenobarbital 15–20 mg/kg IV at rate not to exceed 1 mg/kg/min
45	If seizure persists: Load with phenobarbital if phenytoin was previously used Additional phenytoin or fosphenytoin 5 mg/kg over 12 hr for goal serum level of 10 mg/L Additional phenobarbital 5 mg/kg/dose every 15–30 min (maximum total dose of 30 mg/kg; be prepared to support respirations) Consider IV valproate, especially for partial status epilepticus
60	If seizure persists,‡ consider pentobarbital, midazolam, or general anesthesia in intensive care unit. Avoid paralytics

*Phenytoin may be contraindicated for seizures secondary to alcohol withdrawal or most ingestions (see Chapter 2).
†Fosphenytoin dosed as phenytoin equivalent (PE).
‡Pyridoxine 100 mg IV in infant with persistent initial seizure.
BUN, blood urea nitrogen; CBC, complete blood count; CT, computed tomography; EEG, electroencephalogram.
Modified from Fischer P: Child Adol Psychiatr Clin North Am 1995;4:461.

REFERENCES

1. American Heart Association: Pediatric advanced life support. Circulation 2000;102(8):291.
2. Emergency Cardiac Care Committee, American Heart Association: Pediatric advanced life support. JAMA 1992;268:2262.
3. Bledsoe GH, Schexnayder SM: Pediatric rapid sequence intubation. Pediatr Emerg Care 2004;20:339.
4. Crain EF, Gersel JC: Clinical Manual of Emergency Pediatrics. New York, McGraw-Hill, 2003.
5. Nichols DG, et al. (eds): Golden Hour: The Handbook of Advanced Pediatric Life Support. St. Louis, Mosby, 1996.
6. Jennet B, Teasdale G: Aspects of coma after severe head injury. Lancet 1977;1:878.
7. James HE: Neurologic evaluation and support in the child with an acute brain insult. Pediatr Ann 1986;15:16.
8. Fischer P: Seizure disorders. Child Adol Psychiatr Clin North Am 1995;4:461.
9. Wheless JW: Treatment of status epilepticus in children. Pediatr Ann 2004;33:377.
10. Lieberman P: Use of epinephrine in the treatment of anaphylaxis. Curr Opin Allerg and Clin Immunol 2003;3:313.

Poisonings

Jennifer Lee, MD

2

I. HISTORY

A. INTERVIEWS

1. **Obtain exposure history** from multiple family members and/or friends who may know different details about potential ingestions or exposures.
2. **Important data:** Product name, active ingredients, inactive ingredients, possible contaminants, expiration date, concentration, dose, history of past poisonings, route of exposure, timing and number of exposures (acute, chronic, or repeated ingestion), symptoms and time of onset, prior treatments or decontamination efforts.[1,2]
2. **Environmental information:** Medications and chemicals accessible in the house or garage, recent travel, restaurant dining, other clues to the identity of the ingested agent (plants with missing leaves, open containers, spilled tablets), household members taking medications, herbs, or other complementary medicines.[2]

B. SUBSTANCE IDENTIFICATION

1. Whenever possible, identify the exact name of the substance ingested and its constituents.[1]
2. Consult local poison control center. If the patient ingested a low-toxicity product, ensure that the patient does not have any signs of toxicity, only one substance was ingested, and appropriate follow-up is arranged.

C. QUANTITY OF SUBSTANCE INGESTED

Attempt to estimate a missing volume of liquid or the number of missing pills from a container.

II. PHYSICAL EXAMINATION AND LABORATORY FINDINGS

A. SUBSTANCES WITH DELAYED ONSET OF SYMPTOMS OR DELAYED TOXICITY[1]

Enteric-coated formulations, sustained-release preparations, acetaminophen, calcium-channel blockers, lithium, theophylline.

B. TOXIDROMES AND CLINICAL SIGNS

See Tables 2-1 and 2-2.

C. TOXICOLOGY SCREENS

1. Most toxicology screens include analgesics, amphetamines, antidepressants, barbiturates, cocaine, ethanol, and opiates. If a

Text continues on p. 27

TABLE 2-1
TOXIDROMES

	Vital Signs	Neurologic	Skin, Mucous Membranes	Gastrointestinal	Genitourinary	Other
ADRENERGIC						
Amphetamines, cocaine, sympathomimetics.	↑ or ↔ RR ↑ HR ↑ T ↑ BP	Alert, agitated, dilated and reactive pupils, hyperreflexic, tremulous, delirium, psychosis, seizures.	Diaphoretic, wet mucous membranes.	Hyperactive bowel sounds, emesis, abdominal pain.	Increased urination.	
ANTICHOLINERGIC						
Antihistamines, atropine, belladonna alkaloids (deadly nightshade), jimsonweed, some mushrooms, phenothiazines, scopolamine, tricyclic antidepressants.	↔ RR ↑ HR ↑ T ↔ or ↑ BP	Depressed mental status, confused, psychosis, paranoid ideation, delirium, ataxia, agitation, seizure, coma, extrapyramidal symptoms, dilated and sluggish pupils, normal DTRs, seizures.	Dry skin, flushing, dry mucous membranes, decreased sweating.	Hypoactive bowel sounds, ileus.	Urinary retention.	Respiratory failure, arrhythmias, thirst. “Mad as a hatter, red as a beet, blind as a bat, hot has a hare, dry as a bone.”

ANTICHOLINESTERASE (CHOLINERGIC)						
Black widow spider bites, some mushrooms, organophosphate nerve agents, organophosphate and carbamate pesticides, tobacco.	↑ or ↔ RR ↓ or ↑ HR ↔ T ↔ BP	Confused, depressed mental status, coma, pupillary constriction, normal DTRs or hyporeflexic, seizures, muscle fasciculations, weakness, paralysis.	Diaphoretic, wet mucous membranes, salivation, lacrimation.	Hyperactive bowel sounds, diarrhea, cramping, emesis.	Increased urination. *SLUDGE:* salivation, lacrimation, urination, defecation, gastric cramping, emesis.	Respiratory failure, bronchospasm. *DUMBELS:* diarrhea, urination, miosis, bronchospasm, emesis, lacrimation, salivation.
BARBITURATES—SEE SEDATIVE-HYPNOTIC						
CLONIDINE—SEE OPIOID						
EXTRAPYRAMIDAL						
Haloperidol, metoclopramide, phenothiazines.		Tremor, rigidity, opisthotonos, torticollis, dysphonia, oculogyric crisis.				
HYPERMETABOLIC						
Chlorophenoxy herbicides, some phenols, salicylates.	↑ RR ↑ HR ↑ T	Seizure, restlessness.				Metabolic acidosis.

TABLE 2-1
TOXIDROMES—*cont'd*

	Vital Signs	Neurologic	Skin, Mucous Membranes	Gastrointestinal	Genitourinary	Other
OPIOID, NARCOTIC						
Meperidine, heroin, propoxyphene.	↓ RR ↔ or ↓ HR ↔ or ↓ T ↔ or ↓ BP	Confusion, lethargy, euphoria, somnolence, seizures, ataxia, coma, pupillary constriction, normal or hyporeflexic.	Normal skin and mucous membranes.	Decreased bowel sounds, constipation.	Normal urinary ability.	Pulmonary edema.
SALICYLATES						
	↑ RR ↑ T	Lethargy, seizures.		Emesis.		
SEDATIVE-HYPNOTIC						
	↓ RR ↔ or ↓ HR ↔ or ↓ T	Depressed mental status, CNS depression, normal pupils, normal or hyporeflexic.	Normal skin and mucous membranes.	Normal bowel sounds.	Normal urinary ability.	

SYMPATHOMIMETIC						
Aminophylline, amphetamines, caffeine, cocaine, ephedrine, phenylpropranolamine.	↑ RR ↑ T ↑ BP	Excitation, psychosis, seizure, pupil dilation.				
THEOPHYLLINE						
	↑ RR ↑ HR ↓ BP	Agitation, tremor, seizures.		Emesis.		
WITHDRAWAL						
Cessation of alcohol, barbiturates, benzodiazepines, or narcotics.	↑ HR	Restlessness, hallucinations, anxiety, hyperalgesia, mydriasis.	Lacrimation, "goose bumps," sweating.	Abdominal cramps, diarrhea.		Yawning, rhinorrhea.

RR, respiratory rate; HR, heart rate; T, temperature; BP, blood pressure; DTR, deep tendon reflex.
Data from references 2, 4, 6, 9, and 20.

TABLE 2-2

CLINICAL DIAGNOSTIC AIDS

Clinical Sign	Intoxicant
VITAL SIGNS	
Hypothermia	Alcohols, antidepressants, barbiturates, carbamazepine, clonidine, ethanol, hypoglycemics, narcotics, phenothiazines, sedative-hypnotics.
Hyperpyrexia	Amphetamines, anticholinergics, antihistamines, atropinics, β-blockers, cocaine, iron, isoniazid, monoamine oxidase inhibitors (MAOIs), phencyclidine, phenothiazines, quinine, salicylates (salicylates consistently cause hyperpyrexia in children), sympathomimetics, theophylline, thyroid hormone, tricyclic antidepressants.
Variable thermal dysregulation	Cyclic antidepressants.
Bradypnea	Acetone, alcohol, bartiturates (late), clonidine (with apnea), ethanol, ibuprofen, narcotics, nicotine, sedative hypnotics.
Tachypnea (secondary to toxin-induced metabolic acidosis, noncardiogenic pulmonary edema, or direct pulmonary insult)	Amphetamines, barbiturates (early), carbon monoxide, methanol, salicylates. Direct pulmonary insult: hydrocarbons, organophosphates, salicylates.
Bradycardia	Alcohols, β-blockers, calcium-channel blockers, clonidine, cyanide, digoxin, narcotics, nicotine, organophosphates, plants (lily of the valley, foxglove, oleander), sedative-hypnotics.
Tachycardia	Alcohol, amphetamines, anticholinergics, antihistamines, atropine, cocaine, cyclic antidepressants, cyanide, low-dose iron, phencyclidine, propoxyphene, salicylates, sympathomimetics, theophylline, tricyclic antidepressants.

Hypotension	Barbiturates, cellular asphyxiants (methemoglobinemia, cyanide, carbon monoxide), clonidine, iron, narcotics, opiates, phenothiazine, sedative-hypnotics, tricyclic antidepressants. *Profound hypotension:* ace inhibitors, β-blockers, calcium-channel blockers, cyclic antidepressants, digoxin, imidazolines, nitrites, quinidine, propoxyphene, theophylline.
Hypertension	Amphetamines, anticholinergics, antihistamines, atropinics, clonidine, cocaine, cyclic antidepressants (early after ingestion), diet pills, ephedrine, MAOIs, nicotine, over-the-counter cold remedies, phencyclidine, phenylpropanolamine, pressors, sympathomimetics, tricyclic antidepressants. *Delayed hypertension:* thyroid supplements.
Hypoxia (often with subsequent nervous system effects)	Oxidizing agents.
NEUROMUSCULAR	
Timing of nervous system instability	*Insidious onset:* acetaminophen, benzocaine, opioids. *Abrupt onset:* Lidocaine, monocyclic or tricyclic antidepressants, phenothiazines, theophylline. *Transient instability:* hydrocarbons.
Delayed-onset CNS depression	Atropine, diphenoxylate.
Alternating depression and excitation of nervous system	Clonidine, imidazolines, phencyclidine.
Ataxia	Alcohol, anticonvulsants, barbiturates, carbon monoxide, heavy metals, hydrocarbons, organic solvents, sedative-hypnotics.

TABLE 2-2

CLINICAL DIAGNOSTIC AIDS—*cont'd*

Clinical Sign	Intoxicant
Chvostek, Trousseau signs	Ethylene glycol, hydrofluoric acid–induced hypocalcemia.
Coma	Alcohols, anesthetics, anticholinergics (antihistamines, antidepressants, phenothiazines, atropinics, over-the-counter sleep preparations), anticonvulsants, barbiturates, benzodiazepines, bromide, carbon monoxide, chloral hydrate, clonidine, cyanide, cyclic antidepressants, γ-hydroxybutyrate (GHB), hydrocarbons, hypoglycemics, inhalants, insulin, lithium, narcotics, organophosphate insecticides, phenothiazines, salicylates, sedative-hypnotics, tetrahydrozoline, theophylline.
Delirium, psychosis	Alcohol, anticholinergics (including cold remedies), cocaine, heavy metals, heroin, LSD, marijuana, mescaline, methaqualone, peyote, phencyclidine, phenothiazines, steroids, sympathomimetics.
Miosis	Barbiturates, clonidine, ethanol, narcotics, organophosphates, phencyclidine, phenothiazines, plants (muscarinic mushrooms).
Mydriasis	Amphetamines, antidepressants, antihistamines, atropinics, barbiturates (if comatose), botulism, cocaine, glutethimide, LSD, marijuana, methanol, phencyclidine.
Nystagmus	Barbiturates, carbamazepine, diphenylhydantoin, ethanol, glutethimide, MAOIs, phencyclidine (both vertical and horizontal), sedative-hypnotics, tagretol.
Ocular pH testing	Alkali or acid caustic agents.
Paralysis	Botulism, heavy metals, paralytic shellfish poisoning, plants (poison hemlock).
Seizures	Alcohols, ammonium fluoride, amphetamines, anticholinergics, antidepressants, antihistamines, atropine, β-blockers, boric acid, caffeine, camphor, carbamates, carbamazepine, carbon monoxide, chlorinated insecticides, cocaine, cyclic antidepressants, diethyltoluamide, Dilantin, Ergotrate, ethanol, γ-hydroxybutyrate (GHB), Gyromitra mushrooms, hydrocarbons, hypoglycemics, ibuprofen, imidazolines, isoniazid, lead, lidocaine, lindane, lithium, lysergic acid, meperidine, nicotine, opioids, organophosphate insecticides, phencyclidine, phenothiazines, phenylpropanolamine, physostigmine, plants (water hemlock), propoxyphene, salicylates, strychnine, theophylline.

CARDIOVASCULAR	
Hypoperfusion	Calcium-channel blockers, iron.
Wide QRS complex on 12–lead ECG	Tricyclic antidepressants.
Latent dysrhythmia	Cyclic antidepressants.
ELECTROLYTES	
Anion gap metabolic acidosis*	Carbon monoxide, cyanide, ethanol, ethylene glycol, iron, isoniazid, lactate, methanol, metformin, paraldehyde, phenformin, salicylates.
Electrolyte disturbances	Salicylates, theophylline.
Hypoglycemia	Alcohols, β-blockers, hypoglycemic medications, salicylates. *Delayed hypoglycemia:* Sulfonylureas.
GENITOURINARY	
Urine oxalate crystals	Ethylene glycol.
Positive urine fluorescence under Wood's lamp (on filter paper)	Ethylene glycol.
Urine turns purple-brown when 1–2 drops of 10% ferric chloride solution put into 2 mL of urine	Phenothiazines, salicylates.

Note: Toxins that cause respiratory alkalosis in adults generally do not cause respiratory alkalosis in children because children have smaller respiratory reserve and quicker diaphragm fatigue.

TABLE 2-2

CLINICAL DIAGNOSTIC AIDS—*cont'd*

Clinical Sign	Intoxicant
HEMATOLOGY	
Chocolate brown-colored blood	Methemoglobinemia.
Methemoglobinemia	Aniline dyes, benzocaine-containing teething products, dapsone, naphthalene, nitrites, Pyridium.
Serum osmolar gap	Acetone, ethanol, ethylene, glycol, isopropyl alcohol, methanol.
	Calculated osmolarity = (2 × serum Na) + BUN/2.8 + glucose/18. Normal osmolarity is 290 mOsm/kg.
SKIN	
Cyanosis unresponsive to oxygen	*Cyanotic but asymptomatic indicates methemoglobinemia.*
	Aniline dyes, benzocaine, nitrites, nitrobenzene, phenazopyridine, phenacetin.
Flushing	Alcohols, antihistamines, atropinics, boric acid, carbon monoxide, cyanide.
Jaundice	Acetaminophen, carbon tetrachloride, heavy metals (iron, phosphorus, arsenic), naphthalene, phenothiazines, plants (mushrooms, fava beans).
pH testing	Alkali or acid caustic agents.
ODORS	
Acetone	Acetone, isopropyl alcohol, phenol, salicylates.
Alcohol	Ethanol.
Bitter almond	Cyanide.
Garlic	Heavy metal (arsenic, phosphorus, thallium), organophosphates.
Hydrocarbons	Hydrocarbons (gasoline, turpentine, etc.).
Oil of wintergreen	Salicylates.
RADIOLOGY	
Small opacities on radiograph	Halogenated toxins, heavy metals, iron, lithium, densely packaged products.

Data from references 1, 2, 4, and 6.

particular type of ingestion is suspected, verify that the agent is included in the toxicology test.[2]

2. When obtaining a blood or urine toxicology test, consider measuring both aspirin and acetaminophen levels because these are common analgesic ingredients in many medications.[2]
3. **Medications that may cause false-positive tricyclic antidepressant (TCA) toxicity tests:** Antihistamines (diphenhydramine), some antipsychotic medications (thioridazine), cyclobenzaprine (muscle relaxant). Distinguish between these drugs with gas chromatographic-mass spectrometric testing.[3]
4. **Drugs not detected by routine toxicology screens[4]:**
   a. **Coma inducing:** Bromide, carbon monoxide, chloral hydrate, clonidine, cyanide, organophosphates, tetrahydrozoline (in over-the-counter eye drops).
   b. **Hypotension inducing:** Colchicines, cyanide, iron.
   c. **Hypotension and bradycardia:** β-Blockers, calcium-channel blockers, clonidine, digitalis.

III. ACUTE MANAGEMENT

Assess ABCs: Ensure adequate airway, ventilation, circulatory support, and intravenous (IV) access. Do not give emetic medications initially.[5] Contact local poison control center.

A. SKIN DECONTAMINATION

Indicated if patient was exposed to concentrated lipid-soluble toxins.[1]

B. EYE FLUSHING[6]

Flush ocular exposures for a minimum of 15 minutes before re-evaluating. Remove contact lenses.

C. GASTROINTESTINAL (GI) DECONTAMINATION

1. **Airway protection is extremely important when attempting GI decontamination because of the risk for aspiration.** If the patient does not have an adequate gag reflex or has altered mental status, intubation is necessary before decontamination efforts.
2. **Orogastric lavage[1,5,7]:**
   a. **Indications:** TCAs, calcium-channel blockers, toxins not bound by charcoal (iron, lithium, alcohols), substances that delay gastric emptying, substances that form a concretion.
   b. **Contraindications:** Ingestion of corrosive substances or hydrocarbons, altered mental status, unprotected airway.
   c. Place patient in Trendelenburg position (head lower than feet), left-lateral decubitus, and pass the largest-bore nasogastric tube possible (16- to 28-French [Fr] tube in a child, at least a 36-Fr tube in an adolescent). Confirm tube placement. First, attempt aspiration. Then, administer normal saline, 50–100 mL in young children or

150–200 mL in adolescents. Withdraw the fluid by aspiration or gravity drainage. Repeat until lavaged fluid is clear.

d. Clear effluent does not ensure that all gastric toxins have been retrieved.

e. **Most effective within 60 minutes of most ingestions.**

f. **Risks:** Mechanical trauma to oropharynx or esophagus, aspiration, and deoxygenation.

3. **Activated charcoal[1,4–8]:**

a. **Indications:** Use repeated doses of charcoal for ingestions with enterohepatic circulation. Good evidence for use in carbamazepine, barbiturates, dapsone, quinine, and theophylline ingestions. Some evidence for use with digoxin and phenytoin ingestions. Little evidence for use with salicylates.[5]

b. **Contraindications:** Adynamic ileus, mechanical bowel obstruction, altered mental status with an unprotected airway, caustic ingestion, hydrocarbon ingestion, ingestion of foreign body.

c. **Complications:** Bowel obstruction, bowel perforation, pulmonary aspiration, hypernatremia, hypermagnesemia. Overall, complications from multiple-dose activated charcoal administration are infrequent.[8]

d. Can give activated charcoal after gastric lavage or alone. It is more effective if the charcoal is given within 1 hour of ingestion.

e. **Dosing:** Activated charcoal 1g/kg PO or per nasogastric tube every 1–6 hours. For adolescents or adults, give 50–100 g.

f. Activated charcoal poorly adsorbs most electrolytes, iron, lithium, mineral acids, mineral bases, alcohols, cyanides, most solvents, and most water-soluble compounds (hydrocarbons).

4. **Whole-bowel irrigation[5,6]:**

a. **Indications:** Sustained release or enteric coated preparation; substances not bound by charcoal; substances with a long GI transit time or long absorption time; when large pieces of pills have passed beyond the pylorus on radiographic examination.

b. **Contraindications:** Altered mental status with unprotected airway, caustic ingestion, hydrocarbon ingestion, ingestion of foreign body, ileus, bowel perforation.

c. Administer 30 mL/kg/hr of osmotically balanced polyethylene glycol electrolyte solution (GoLYTELY, NuLYTELY) to induce liquid stool. Alternatively, can give up to 500 mL/hr. Continue until rectal effluent is clear. Slow administration and antiemetic medications may be necessary to reduce bloating, nausea, and emesis.

5. **Syrup of ipecac[4,6,7,9]:**

a. ***Not recommended for routine management of poisonings.***

b. Contains alkaloids emetine and cephaline (locally and centrally acting emetic alkaloids).

c. **Indications:** Early and life-threatening ingestion; toxin is in the stomach, and there is no expected decline in mental status; an oral antidote or more effective technique of elimination is not necessary; toxin does not adsorb to charcoal; ingested substance has delayed toxicity.

d. **Contraindications:** Unprotected airway, altered mental status, elevated intracranial pressure, caustic ingestion, hydrocarbon ingestion, ingestion of foreign body, patient younger than 6 months, uncontrolled hypertension.
e. **Dosage:** child 6 mo–1 yr: 5–10 mL preceded or followed by 120–240 mL of water; 1–12 yr: 15 mL preceded or followed by 120–240 mL of water; >12 yr: 15–30 mL, followed by 240 mL of water. Can give one additional dose if patient does not have emesis within 20–30 minutes of administration.
f. **Most effective if administered within 60 minutes of ingestion.** At best, syrup of ipecac removes approximately one third of the stomach contents. Emesis occurs 20–30 minutes after administration.
g. May be useful if patient ingested a toxin with potential for high morbidity within the past 60 minutes.
h. **Risks:** Ipecac-induced drowsiness, aspiration, exacerbation of cardiac arrhythmias from excessive vagal stimulation.[2]

6. **Cathartics[4,7,15]:**
a. Generally not recommended for treatment of poisonings. Cathartics include sorbitol, magnesium sulfate, and magnesium citrate.
b. Mineral oil and stimulant cathartics (castor oil) may increase absorption of some toxins.
c. If going to give cathartics with activated charcoal, do not give cathartic more frequently than after every three doses of charcoal.
d. High risk for dehydration and electrolyte imbalance.

7. **Simple dilution[4]:**
a. **Indications:** Toxin that causes only local irritation or corrosion.
b. **Contraindications:** Drug ingestions. Dilution techniques may increase absorption by dissolving the ingested tablets or capsules and induce more rapid transit of the drug into the lower GI tract.
c. May use water or milk as a diluent.

D. ENHANCED ELIMINATION

1. **Urinary alkalinization with forced diuresis[1,4]:**
a. **Indications:** To enhance renal excretion of weakly acidic drugs (alkalinization of the urine increases the proportion of ionized drug in the renal tubules that is excreted); salicylates, isoniazid, dichlorophenoxyacetic acid, phenobarbital, chlorpropamide, chlorophenoxy herbicides.
b. **Maintain urine pH 7.5–7.8.**
c. **Dosing:** 0.6 × weight (kg) × 5 mEq = mEq of sodium bicarbonate to be given over the next 4 hours. Administer in intravenous fluid drip containing glucose and KCl.
d. **Alternate dosing:** Sodium bicarbonate, 1–2 mEq/kg IV over 1–2 hours.

e. Monitor amount of sodium and total fluids administered, particularly in patients at risk for pulmonary edema or congestive heart failure.
f. **Correct hypokalemia:** Hypokalemia reduces the ability to alkalinize the urine.

2. **Urinary acidification is not recommended.** Urinary acidification exacerbates metabolic acidosis and increases myoglobin deposition in the renal tubules during rhabdomyolysis. Also, the ammonium chloride used to acidify the urine can result in dangerous acidosis and hyperammonemia.[3]

E. ACTIVE REMOVAL

Hemodialysis and hemofiltration: Consult poison control center and a pediatric nephrologist.

F. MEDICATION INGESTIONS

See Table 2-3.

G. DRUGS OF ABUSE

1. **See Table 2-4.** Drugs obtained from unreliable sources may contain a combination of illegal, prescription, and over-the-counter drugs.
2. Consider mixed drug toxicity even when there is a history of single illicit drug use.
3. **General treatment:**

a. For chemical restraint, give diazepam, midazolam, or haloperidol. (See Formulary for dosing.) Of note, haloperidol decreases ability to dissipate heat and lowers the seizure threshold.
b. Consider GI decontamination.

H. ANTIDOTES

See Table 2-5.

IV. INHALATIONAL INJURIES

A. PHYSICAL EXAMINATION

1. Symptoms may be delayed after the inhalational injury occurs. Symptoms that may predict acute inhalational injury include cough, facial burns, inflamed nares, stridor, sputum production, wheezing, and altered mental status.[10]

Text continues on p. 65

TABLE 2-3

MEDICATION INGESTIONS

Ingestion	Signs and Symptoms	Management
Acetaminophen[4,6,20–25] (see Fig. 2-1) a. Paracetamol, APAP. b. Most children ingest pediatric liquid Tylenol, which contains low doses of acetaminophen, and severe toxicity is rare. Chronic overdose is more likely to be detrimental than acute ingestions. Rectal administration can also lead to toxicity. c. Take special precautions in children who are malnourished or taking cytochrome P450 enzyme–inducing drugs. (Acetaminophen becomes toxic after being metabolized by the cytochrome P450 enzyme	**Phase 1 (first 24 hr after ingestion):** malaise, anorexia, emesis, diaphoresis. Patients may take more acetaminophen in attempts to relieve these symptoms. **Generally, symptoms develop within 14 hr after the toxic ingestion level is reached.** If lethargy develops during the first phase, consider coingestion of other substances. Phase 2 (second 24 hr): hepatomegaly, right upper quadrant pain, hyperbilirubinemia, elevated liver function tests, elevated prothrombin time, oliguria. Symptoms may improve during the	1. No intervention is indicated if the ingestion was less than 140–150 mg/kg and the patient is asymptomatic. 2. If the patient is younger than 7 yr, ingestion was less than 200 mg/kg, the ingestion was not of a sustained release form, and reliable follow-up is arranged, can monitor the patient at home without further intervention. 3. **Measure acetaminophen level at least 4 hr after ingestion.** Samples taken before 4 hr are unreliable because of continued absorption and changing drug distribution. **Levels best predict hepatic toxicity if obtained within 4–10 hr of the ingestion.** Plasma levels are not reliable when measured 15 hr or more after ingestion. a. If an extended-release preparation was taken, recheck the acetaminophen level 8 hr after ingestion. 4. **To determine whether treatment is indicated, compare the measured concentration to the nomogram (Fig. 2-1).** Use the lower treatment threshold (25th percentile of the plasma concentration at which treatment should be started), especially if the patient is in a high-risk group. 5. **Start treatment immediately** (without waiting for plasma levels) if the patient ingested staggered overdoses, if the patient presents more than 6–8 hr after the ingestion, if there are severe symptoms, or if baseline laboratory values suggest hepatotoxicity. a. If the patient presents more than 24 hr after ingestion or if there is a history of chronic or subacute overdose, or if more than 150 mg/kg/day was

TABLE 2-3
MEDICATION INGESTIONS—*cont'd*

Ingestion	Signs and Symptoms	Management
system.) Drugs that increase susceptibility to acetaminophen toxicity: carbamazepine, dexamethasone, doxorubicin, ethanol, isoniazid, phenobarbital, rifampin. Prolonged fasting, diabetes mellitus, chronic malnutrition, concomitant viral infection, family history of hepatotoxic reaction to acetaminophen, and obesity also increase susceptibility. d. **Hepatotoxicity occurs with ingestions greater than 200 mg/kg. Liver damage occurs approximately 18–24 hours after ingestion.** Severe toxicity may occur in adolescents	first 1–4 days after ingestion. **Phase 3 (2–5 days):** encephalopathy, cardiomyopathy, anorexia, emesis, hepatic failure and necrosis, hypoglycemia, coagulopathy, renal failure, malaise. **Phase 4 (7–8 days):** recovery or fatal hepatic failure. The end point of liver damage is reached during this phase.	ingested for 1 or more days or, if the plasma acetaminophen level exceeds 10 μg/mL, begin treatment immediately. 6. **Obtain baseline electrolytes, creatinine, liver functions, coagulation parameters, and urinalysis before initiating therapy.** a. If baseline labs are within normal limits, recheck labs in 48 hr. If the liver functions remain within normal limits, hepatic damage is unlikely to occur. b. ALT > 1000 IU/L is a marker of severe liver injury, but levels are not prognostic. c. Serial prothrombin times (INR) can be used to monitor residual liver functions. 7. **Gastric emptying** procedures are most effective with extended-release preparations. Immediate release forms of acetaminophen are rapidly absorbed. 8. **Activated charcoal** is most useful within 1–2 hr of ingestion. 9. **Administer *N*-acetylcysteine (NAC).** NAC given within 8 hr of ingestion decreases the likelihood of hepatic damage. Administering NAC within 16 hr of ingestion decreases the severity of hepatic damage. a. Empty the stomach of activated charcoal before giving NAC because activated charcoal binds NAC. However, some studies suggest that charcoal insignificantly affects NAC absorption if they are given one hour apart. b. **Dosing: 140 mg/kg PO loading dose, then 70 mg/kg every 4 hr for a total of 17 doses.** Repeat the dose if the patient vomits within 1 hr of administration. If the patient presents more than 6–8 hr after ingestion,

with ingestions of 10 g or more.		consider increasing the loading dose by 40% or repeating the loading dose if charcoal was given within the last 2 hr. c. Can decrease infusion rate if the patient's symptoms are mild. d. Use antiemetics (metoclopramide, ondansetron) as necessary. Administer NAC via nasogastric or nasoduodenal tube if the patient is unable to tolerate oral NAC. Can also dilute NAC to 5% in water, soda, or juice. e. Monitor CBC, liver and renal function tests. f. Risks of NAC: renal tubular damage. g. If patient cannot tolerate enteral therapy or if enteral therapy is contraindicated (GI bleed, bowel obstruction), give NAC loading dose **150 mg/kg diluted in 200 mL 5% dextrose IV administered over 15 minutes. Then, maintenance dosing 50 mg/kg diluted in 500 mL 5% dextrose IV administered over 4 hr, followed by 100 mg/kg diluted in 1000 mL 5% dextrose IV administered over 16 hr.** Contact the local Poison Control Center and hospital pharmacy for further instructions.
Anticholinergics[4,6] See also individual medications. (antidepressants, antihistamines, antispasmodics, phenothiazines)	Paradoxical CNS excitation. See Table 2-1, *Anticholinergic*. Symptoms may develop 12–24 hr after ingestion secondary to decreased GI motility with subsequent delayed absorption. Elimination half-life is 8–55 hr.	1. GI decontamination up to 12–24 hr after ingestion. If patient presents within 8 hr of ingestion, consider gastric-emptying procedures. Give activated charcoal. Since the drug–charcoal complex is excreted in feces, may consider also giving a cathartic. 2. Benzodiazepines for sedation. 3. Treat arrhythmias and seizures according to standard protocols. 4. **Physostigmine.** See Table 2-5, *Antidotes*. Administer physostigmine only if the patient has a normal ECG. Due to the toxicity of physostigmine, the risks and benefits must be carefully considered. a. To treat the muscarinic side effects of physostigmine, give atropine IV at one half of the dose of physostigmine. Have atropine readily available during treatment.

TABLE 2-3
MEDICATION INGESTIONS—*cont'd*

Ingestion	Signs and Symptoms	Management
		b. Treat physostigmine-related seizures with benzodiazepines. c. Monitor the patient closely during infusion. d. Risks of physostigmine: seizure, bradycardia, hypotension, bronchospasm. The risks of seizure and asystole increase when physostigmine is given too rapidly or in too large dosing. e. **Do not give physostigmine** if the patient ingested a drug that affects cardiac conduction (e.g., tricyclic antidepressants).
Antidepressants[4,23,26–27] a. See *anticholinergics.* b. **Tricyclic antidepressants (TCAs):** amitriptyline, clomipramine, desipramine, doxepin, imipramine, nortriptyline, protryptyline, trimipramine.	See Table 2-1, *Anticholinergic.* Hypotension, fatal cardiac arrhythmias. **TCAs:** seizures, arrhythmias (V-tach, V-fib), cardiac conduction delays, hypotension, significantly decreased GI motility. **MAOIs:** CNS	1. **Administer activated charcoal.** Antidepressants have a large volume of distribution and cannot be eliminated through extracorporeal means. 2. Obtain 12–lead ECG and start continuous **cardiac monitoring.** **TCA overdose:** 1. In addition to activated charcoal, **gastric lavage** up to 12 hr postingestion. TCAs significantly decrease GI motility. 2. **Administer sodium bicarbonate 1–2 mEq/kg bolus while doing continuous cardiac monitoring.** Then, start sodium bicarbonate infusion to maintain serum pH 7.45–7.55. Give additional boluses of sodium bicarbonate if the QRS interval widens.

1. Ingestion of 35 mg/kg or more may be fatal.

c. **SSRIs:** amoxapine, citalopram, clomipramine, fluoxetine, fluvoxamine, nefazodone, paroxetine, sertraline, venlafaxine.
   1. Coingestion of paroxetine with TCAs delays TCA metabolism and increases TCA toxicity.

d. **MAOIs:**
   1. Cause irreversible inhibition of monoamine oxidase.
   2. A single ingestion of 6 mg/kg or more can be fatal.
   3. MAOIs interact with foods that contain biogenic amines (tyramine) and medications to cause severe toxicity.

hyperstimulation, seizures, muscle rigidity, hyperpyrexia, blood pressure instability, rhabdomyolysis.

Coingest MAOIs and foods or drugs with biogenic amines (wine, cheese, soy sauce, decongestants): cerebrovascular accident, seizure, severe hypertension.

Coingest MAOIs with sympathomimetic or serotonergic drugs dextromethorphan (in over-the-counter cough and cold remedies), analgesics (meperidine), psychotropic drugs (clomipramine), SSRIs: serotonin syndrome.

SSRIs: CNS depression, seizures, coma, agitation,

3. Treat arrhythmias with sodium bicarbonate 1–2 mEq/kg IV boluses (first-line treatment). May also use lidocaine, atenolol, propranolol, phenytoin, or magnesium sulfate. Give lidocaine for ventricular arrhythmias. May need to cardiovert. Do not give quinidine or procainamide (class Ia and Ic antiarrhythmics will exacerbate heart block).
4. **Norepinephrine** infusion and intravenous fluids with bicarbonate to treat hypotension. May need to change to dopamine if arrhythmias occur. **Glucagon** may also be helpful to stabilize blood pressure.
5. Monitor electrolytes. Bicarbonate infusion may induce hypokalemia which worsens arrhythmias.
6. **Do not give physostigmine or flumazenil.** Physostigmine worsens cardiac conduction defects and lowers the seizure threshold.
7. Treat seizure with **benzodiazepines** first. Then, give barbiturates if necessary. Do not give phenytoin (may induce ventricular arrhythmias).
8. TCAs have long half-lives and slow elimination rates. Prolonged course of treatment may be necessary.
9. Do not base therapeutic decision making on serum TCA levels.

MAOI overdose:
1. Admit to hospital for at least 24 hr of observation.
2. Treat hypertension with short-acting antihypertensive drug (nitroprusside). Give IV fluids and vasopressors for hypotension. If there is blood pressure lability, monitor in an intensive care setting.
3. Dantrolene and cooling measures to treat hyperpyrexia. Hyperpyrexia is associated with increased muscle rigidity and rhabdomyolysis.
4. Monitor for rhabdomyolysis (elevated creatine kinase, myoglobinuria).

TABLE 2-3

MEDICATION INGESTIONS—*cont'd*

Ingestion	Signs and Symptoms	Management
e. **Serotonin syndrome** occurs most commonly in adults taking two or more drugs that increase serotonin exposure (SSRIs, MAOIs, amphetamines). Serotonin syndrome may occur in children who coingested MAOIs and SSRIs.	tremor, drowsiness, nystagmus, delirium, arrhythmias, hypertension, emesis, hepatic toxicity. **Serotonin syndrome:** autonomic dysfunction, seizures, muscle rigidity, myoclonus, hyperpyrexia, tachycardia, fatal cardiac arrhythmias, blood pressure instability, circulatory collapse, rhabdomyolysis, flushing.	5. Treat severe muscle rigidity and hyperthermia with benzodiazepines and neuromuscular blockade. **Serotonin syndrome:** 1. Supportive care. 2. Diazepam for seizures. 3. External cooling measures, sedatives, paralysis, and/or mechanical ventilation for hyperthermia. 4. Symptoms usually resolve within 72 hr of ingestion.

Antihistamines[3,4,6,26] a. Astemizole, cetirizine, fexophenadine, loratadine, terfenadine, b. See *anticholinergics*: chlorpheniramine, diphenhydramine, orphenadrine. c. Antihistamines are in cough syrups, sedatives, antinauseants, drugs to prevent motion sickness, cold preparations, and sleep aids.	See Table 2-1, *Anticholinergic.* Paradoxical CNS stimulation, hyperactivity, tremors, dizziness, coma, hypotension, arrhythmias, cardiorespiratory arrest, muscle weakness. **Terfenadine, astemizole:** prolonged QT interval, ventricular tachyarrhythmias.	1. **Obtain 12–lead ECG.** 2. **To treat arrhythmia:** *First line:* sodium bicarbonate for QT prolongation. *Second line:* magnesium sulfate, propranolol, isoprenaline, flecainide. 3. **Continuous ECG** monitoring for symptomatic patients and for patients who ingested terfenadine or astemizole. 4. **Give benzodiazepines** for seizures and delirium. Do not give phenothiazine-based sedatives or phenytoin. 5. **Activated charcoal** up to 4 hr postingestion. Whole bowel irrigation for ingestion of sustained-release preparations. 6. **Physostigmine** to treat anticholinergic toxidrome. See *Anticholinergics* and Table 2-5, *Antidotes.* 7. Cooling measures and sedation for hyperpyrexia. 8. Observe patient for at least 4 hr postingestion. If patient ingested terfenadine, astemizole, or a slow-release preparation, must admit the patient to the hospital regardless of whether symptoms are present. 9. May cause false-positive tricyclic antidepressant toxicity test. 10. Hemodialysis or hemoperfusion are not indicated.
Barbiturates Phenobarbital levels are most useful if measured within 1–2 hr after ingestion. a. Amobarbital, pentobarbital, phenobarbital, secobarbital. b. See Table 2-4, *Sedative-Hypnotic*.	See Table 2-4	See Table 2-4

TABLE 2-3

MEDICATION INGESTIONS—*cont'd*

Ingestion	Signs and Symptoms	Management
Benzodiazepines[26,28] a. Adult sedatives, anxiolytics. b. Alprazolam, chlorazepate, chlordiazepoxide, clonazepam, diazepam, flurazepam, lorazepam, midazolam, oxazepam, temazepam, triazolam.	Coma, dysarthria, ataxia, drowsiness, hallucinations, confusion, agitation, bradycardia, hypotension, respiratory depression.	1. **Administer activated charcoal** if treating within 1 hr of ingestion and consciousness is not impaired. 2. **Supportive therapy.** 3. **Flumazenil** (competitive benzodiazepine antagonist) is indicated when the patient cannot protect the airway, is in respiratory distress, or has circulatory compromise. See Table 2-5, *Antidotes*. There is risk for seizures in patients treated for epilepsy with benzodiazepines or in coingestion of epileptogenic substances (TCAs, theophylline, chloral hydrate, isoniazid, carbamazepine). 4. Can detect in serum and urine.
β-Blockers[4–6,28] a. Atenolol, esmolol, labetalol, metoprolol, nadolol, propranolol, timolol. b. Overdoses most commonly occur with propranolol.	Coma, seizure, altered mental status, hallucinations, cardiac arrhythmia (AV node blockade, accelerated junctional rhythms), decreased myocardial contractility, bradycardia, hypotension, respiratory depression, bronchospasm in patients with RAD, hypoglycemia.	1. **Aggressive GI decontamination** with gastric lavage and activated charcoal. Whole-bowel irrigation for ingestion of sustained release preparations. 2. **Obtain serial 12–lead ECGs** to evaluate for conduction delays. 3. **Glucagon** has inotropic and vasopressor effects. Administer normal saline or D_5W during glucagon treatment. See Table 2-5, *Antidotes*. 4. **Atropine, IV fluids, and pressors** for hypotension or myocardial depression. However, these measures are often ineffective. Aggressive resuscitation efforts may be required, including high-dose epinephrine. 5. Pacemaker, aortic balloon pump, cardiopulmonary bypass. 6. Hemodialysis and hemoperfusion are not useful.

Calcium-channel blocker[4,6,28,29] a. Amlodipine, bepridil, diltiazem, isradipine, nicardipine, nifedipine, nimodipine, verapamil. b. Overdoses most commonly occur with verapamil.	Seizure, coma, dysarthria, lethargy, confusion, decreased myocardial contractility, cardiac arrhythmia, profound bradycardia, reflex tachycardia, profound hypotension, peripheral vasodilation, apnea, pulmonary edema, bowel infarction, lactic acidosis, hyperglycemia, mild hyperkalemia, flushing, peripheral cyanosis. **Nifedipine:** seizures. **Bepridel:** prolonged QT interval, torsades de pointes. Symptoms may develop hours after ingestion. Most morbidity occurs with sustained-release (SR) verapamil or diltiazem.	1. **Do not induce emesis.** Vagal stimulus may exacerbate heart block. 2. **Aggressive GI decontamination** with gastric lavage and activated charcoal. Do whole-bowel irrigation for ingestion of sustained-release preparations. 3. Observe patients who ingested regular-release preparations for at least 3–6 hr post-ingestion (even if the patient is asymptomatic). Observe patients with larger ingestion amounts for 24 hr. 4. **Obtain serial 12–lead ECGs** to evaluate for conduction delays. 5. **Glucagon** has inotropic and vasopressor effects. Administer normal saline or D_5W during glucagon treatment. See Table 2-5, *Antidotes*. 6. **Atropine, IV fluids, and pressors** for hypotension or myocardial depression. However, these measures are often ineffective. 7. **Isoproterenol,** for severely impaired cardiac conduction and peripheral vasodilation. 8. **For severe peripheral vasodilation,** norepinephrine, high-dose dopamine, epinephrine, or phenylephrine may be necessary. 9. **If unresponsive to atropine, give calcium salts.** Calcium salts may improve cardiac contractility, but they generally have little effect on conduction abnormalities or peripheral vasodilation. See Table 2-5, *Antidotes*. Calcium infusion may be necessary. a. Do not exceed serum calcium level of 14 mg/dL or double the normal ionized calcium level. 10. If all other therapies fail, can give **insulin and glucose**. Maintain serum glucose approximately 100 mg/dL.

TABLE 2-3
MEDICATION INGESTIONS—*cont'd*

Ingestion	Signs and Symptoms	Management
		11. **For nifedipine ingestion,** treat seizures with lorazepam, diazepam, or calcium. 12. Pacemaker, aortic balloon pump, cardiopulmonary bypass. 13. Hemodialysis and hemoperfusion are not useful.
Carbamazepine[3,25] a. Levels increase when coadministered with cytochrome P450 3A4 inhibitors (cimetidine, diltiazem, erythromycin). b. One of the most common pediatric overdoses.	Coma, seizures, ataxia, motor restlessness, twitching, tremor, athetosis, mydriasis, nystagmus, altered mental status, tachycardia, cardiac conduction abnormalities, hypotension, hypertension, respiratory depression, emesis, delayed gastric emptying.	1. Gastric lavage. 2. Multiple doses of activated charcoal. 3. Hemodialysis and hemoperfusion in massive overdose. 4. Serum carbamazepine level is most useful if obtained 2–4 hr after ingestion. However, serum levels do not correlate with clinical toxicity. May cause false-positive tricyclic antidepressant toxicity test.
Clonidine[4,6] a. Small ingestions cause significant toxicity in children. b. Clonidine is used to treat hypertension, ADHD, and withdrawal from nicotine and opiates.	CNS depression, coma, lethargy, hypothermia, miosis, bradycardia, profound hypotension, respiratory depression. Hypertension rarely occurs. Symptoms occur within 30–60 min of ingestion	1. ABCs. 2. Administer a single dose of activated charcoal. Clonidine is rapidly absorbed and distributed, so GI decontamination is only effective within 2 hr of ingestion. 3. Naloxone for neurologic, cardiovascular, or respiratory symptoms. Give a trial dose of naloxone, 1–2 mg initially. Large amounts (up to 8 mg) may be necessary. If the patient responds to naloxone, continue to give boluses, or start an infusion. See Table 2-5, *Antidotes*.

c. Prescribed adult doses are usually 100–300 μg.	and last 8–24 hr. Ingestion of 10–20 μg/kg causes cardiovascular compromise. Greater than 20 μg/kg causes respiratory depression.	4. Give atropine if bradycardia does not respond to naloxone. 5. Intravenous fluids and vasopressors to treat hypotension.
Digoxin[4,5,19] a. Foxglove and oleander plant ingestions appear similar to digoxin ingestion. b. Chronic ingestions are more likely to be toxic than an acute ingestion. c. Patient with an acute ingestion may clinically appear to have nontoxic digoxin levels and/or have serum levels within normal range. However, complete absorption takes 2–4 hr postingestion. Once peak serum level is achieved, digoxin is rapidly redistributed and serum levels fall.	Seizure, lethargy, headache, disorientation, visual disturbances (blurry, altered color vision, "halos" of color), AV node dissociation and heart block, ventricular or supraventricular escape rhythms, emesis, anorexia, electrolyte imbalances (hyperkalemia). Manifestations of toxicity depends on serum potassium, calcium, and magnesium.	1. **Digoxin levels are most useful if measured 4–6 hr after ingestion.** However, do not base therapeutic decisions on serum digoxin levels even if the levels are low. The complicated pharmacokinetics of digoxin make serum levels unreliable in predicting clinical toxicity. a. Therapeutic serum digoxin concentration (SDC) is less than 2 ng/mL. SDC greater than 4 ng/mL is associated with toxicity. 2. Obtain ECG and start **continuous cardiac monitoring.** Treat arrhythmias according to standard protocols (also see below). 3. Administer **activated charcoal** up to several hours postingestion. Avoid gastric lavage or syrup of ipecac. (Increased vagal tone may precipitate bradydysrhythmias.) 4. Monitor electrolytes (including calcium and magnesium), acid-base status, and SDC. Check urinalysis. 5. **Treat electrolyte disturbances** (especially hyperkalemia) and acid-base imbalance. Treat hyperkalemia with insulin and glucose, sodium bicarbonate, and Kayexelate. Electrolyte imbalances aggravate arrhythmias. 6. **Digoxin-specific antibody fragments (Fab).** See Table 2-6, *Antidotes*. a. Indications: progressing clinical toxicity, life-threatening arrhythmias, arrhythmias associated with hypotension or organ ischemia, arrhythmias

TABLE 2-3

MEDICATION INGESTIONS—*cont'd*

Ingestion	Signs and Symptoms	Management
d. Impaired renal function, quinidine, amiodarone, hypokalemia, hypomagnesemia, and low thyroxine increase digoxin toxicity.		that do not improve despite conventional treatment, recurring arrhythmias, arrhythmias that require electric cardioversion or pacing, or serum potassium 5.5 mEq/L or greater in acute poisoning. b. Digoxin–antibody complex is renally excreted. c. After Fab administration, the SDC increases secondary to diffusion into the intravascular compartment of antibody-bound, inactive digoxin. d. Adverse reactions: allergic reaction, rebound hypokalemia, congestive heart failure (secondary to the sudden decrease in digoxin's inotropic effect). 7. **Bradyarrhythmias:** Fab is first-line therapy. If Fab is not immediately available, give atropine, 0.02 mg/kg, minimum 0.1 mg. Alternatively, may give dopamine, epinephrine, or isoproterenol. **Phenytoin** may reverse digoxin-induced AV block. Start cardiac pacing if the arrhythmia does not improve and until Fab is available. a. For asystole and PEA, treat with epinephrine and atropine according to PALS protocols. Consider giving sodium bicarbonate early because of the likelihood of hyperkalemia. 8. **Life-threatening tachyarrhythmias:** Fab is first-line therapy. If Fab is not immediately available, follow standard PALS protocols. May require overdrive cardiac pacing. 9. **Supraventricular tachyarrhythmias** generally do not require treatment. For patients with underlying congestive heart failure, give β-blockers or calcium-channel blockers to control the ventricular rate. Use short-acting agents, such as esmolol or diltiazem.

		10. **If there is AV block, do not give propranolol, procainamide, isoproterenol, or disopyramide.** 11. Hemofiltration, hemodialysis, and hemoperfusion are not useful.
Hypoglycemics[4,6] a. Sulfonylureas: chlorpropamide, glipizide, glyburide. b. Biguanides: metformin.	Status epilepticus, fatigue, dizziness, agitation, confusion, tachycardia, cardiovascular compromise, poor feeding, diaphoresis. Hypoglycemia may be delayed 16–24 hr after ingestion. **Biguanides:** metabolic acidosis. Hypoglycemia may not occur.	1. Hospitalize for 24 hr of observation, even if the patient is asymptomatic. 2. Serial glucose checks. 3. Repeat doses of activated charcoal for ingestion of sulfonylureas, particularly if the patient presents within 1–2 hr of ingestion. Glipizide undergoes enterohepatic recirculation. 4. Urinary alkalinization enhances excretion of chlorpropamide. 5. Hypertonic glucose (10–20% solution, $D_{25}W$, $D_{50}W$) boluses as needed to treat hypoglycemia. Encourage eating. Glucose infusion may be necessary for several days. As the hypoglycemia improves, gradually taper the glucose infusion. Maintain blood glucose greater than 80 mg/dL. 6. Diazoxide, 3–5 mg/kg IV infusion over 30 min to treat hypotension. Give repeat doses of diazoxide, 3–5 mg/kg IV every 4–6 hr as needed. Diazoxide may also improve hypoglycemia. 7. Octreotide, 1–10 μg/kg to treat refractory hypoglycemia.
Iron[4,20,26] a. Ingestion of elemental, prenatal, or multivitamin preparations may cause iron toxicity. b. Iron ingestion is one of the most common poisonings among children.	**Phase 1** (first 6 hr after ingestion): encephalopathy, coma, shock, abdominal pain, emesis, GI hemorrhage, diarrhea, hyperglycemia, metabolic acidosis, leukocytosis.	1. If the patient is asymptomatic and consumed less than 30 mg/kg of elemental iron, no treatment beyond observation is necessary. Children who remain asymptomatic 6 hr after ingestion are unlikely to develop systemic toxicity. 2. **Hospitalize patients who consumed more than 30 mg/kg elemental iron.** 3. If severe signs of toxicity (emesis, diarrhea, GI bleed, hypotension, or coma): do GI decontamination, immediately obtain abdominal radiograph, electrolytes, BUN, liver function tests, CBC, and serum iron levels, and start desferoxamine. Type and cross-match blood type.

TABLE 2-3
MEDICATION INGESTIONS—*cont'd*

Ingestion	Signs and Symptoms	Management
c. Excess free iron is a mitochondrial poison, particularly in hepatocytes. d. Serum iron level less than 350 µg/dL usually does not cause symptoms. Levels 350–500 µg/dL cause phase I toxicity. Levels greater than 500 µg/dL cause phase 3 toxicity.	**Phase 2:** symptoms improve 6–72 hr postingestion. **Phase 3** (6–48 hr after ingestion): Coma, seizure, shock, cyanosis, abdominal pain, emesis, hepatic dysfunction and necrosis, metabolic acidosis, coagulopathy, hypoglycemia. **Phase 4** (4–6 wk after ingestion): GI tract strictures, pyloric stenosis, acute bowel obstruction. Multiorgan failure signs develop 12–48 hr after ingestion. Fulminant hepatic failure is the most common.	4. If the patient does not have severe symptomatology, consider gastric decontamination, obtain an abdominal x-ray, check serum iron level 4 hr after ingestion, and check labs for anion gap acidosis. a. If there is radiopaque material on the abdominal x-ray (indicative of significant iron absorption), an anion gap acidosis, serum iron level greater than 500 µg/dL, or symptoms develop, start desferoxamine and GI decontamination. b. If the abdominal x-ray is normal, the patient is not acidotic, serum iron level is less than 500 µg/dL, and the patient is asymptomatic, observe the patient for 6 hr and discharge home if remains asymptomatic. Start desferoxamine if symptoms or acidosis develop. 5. Generally, **serum iron levels** obtained after 6 hr are misleading because the liver has already cleared most of the free iron. If a sustained iron preparation was consumed, also obtain levels 8 hr postingestion. a. **Serum iron less than 55 µmol/L**: no further treatment necessary (except GI evacuation as indicated by radiograph). b. **Serum iron, 55–90 µmol/L:** observe for at least 24 hr. If patient remains asymptomatic after 24 hr, no further intervention is necessary. c. **Serum iron greater than 90 µmol/L:** administer IV desferoxamine (See Table 2-5). 6. If unable to obtain quantitative serum iron levels, monitor electrolytes and CBC. Metabolic acidosis correlates with toxicity. TIBC is not a useful measurement. a. Can also do a **desferoxamine challenge test:** administer deferoxamine, 50 mg/kg IM (maximum: 1 g). Vin rose–colored urine indicates elevated serum iron.

		7. **GI evacuation.** Do whole-bowel irrigation (WBI) if iron tablets are visible on radiograph. 8. **Desferoxamine should be started immediately if there are signs of organ failure.** a. Obtain serum iron level before starting desferoxamine, but do not delay starting therapy if unable to obtain levels quickly. b. See Table 2-5, *Antidotes*. c. Chelate complex is excreted in the urine ("vin rose"–colored urine). Can remove the chelate complex via hemodialysis if renal function is impaired. d. Continue treatment until symptoms resolve and the urine discoloration clears for 24 hr. 9. Vigorous hydration. Maintain adequate urine output.
NSAIDs[21] a. Diclofenac, ibuprofen, mefanamic acid, phenylbutazone.	**Ibuprofen:** bradycardia, hepatic dysfunction. **Phenylbutazone, mefanamic acid:** CNS depression, headache, dizziness, tinnitus, vision change, hypothermia, tachycardia, prolonged QT interval, hypotension, respiratory failure, GI irritation, electrolyte disturbances, metabolic acidosis.	1. Administer activated charcoal if the patient consumed more than 100 mg/kg of regular ibuprofen. a. Give activated charcoal if child consumed more than 25 mg/kg of mefanamic acid. b. Give repeat doses of charcoal if phenylbutazone was consumed. 2. Observe asymptomatic patients for 4 hr postingestion. a. If mefanamic acid or sustained release NSAID was ingested, observe for 12 hr. 3. Diazepam to treat seizures.

TABLE 2-3
MEDICATION INGESTIONS—*cont'd*

Ingestion	Signs and Symptoms	Management
	Mefanamic acid: seizures. **Phenylbutazone:** arrhythmias, liver failure, marrow suppression.	
Opioids See Table 2-4, *Opioids*.		
Phenothiazines, butyrophenone[4] a. Tranquilizers. b. Chlorpromazine, fluphenazine, haloperidol, perphenazine, prochlorperazine, promethazine, thioridazine, trifluoperazine.	See Table 2-1, *Anticholinergic*. Risk neuroleptic malignant syndrome. Symptoms may occur 6–24 hr after ingestion. Psychotic reactions are dose dependent and occur 8–40 hrs after ingestion.	1. In moderate to severe overdose, administer activated charcoal if the patient presents within 4–6 hr of ingestion. 2. Continuous cardiorespiratory monitoring. 3. Vasopressors to treat hypotension. 4. Nitroprusside to treat hypertension. (Hypertension is a rare complication.) 5. See *Tricyclic Antidepressants* for treatment of arrhythmias. 6. External cooling and sedation for hyperthermia. 7. For dystonic reactions, give diphenhydramine, 1–2 mg/kg, maximum 50 mg, slowly over 2–5 min. For adults, give 25–50 mg. Repeat this dose in 15–20 min if there is no clinical response. a. Alternatively, can give benztropine. See Table 2-5, *Antidotes*. b. Continue PO therapy every 6 hr for 24–48 hr to prevent recurrence of dystonia. 8. Severe hyperthemia and muscle rigidity may require neuromuscular paralysis with or without benzodiazepines.

Phenytoin[19]	Coma, ataxia, weakness, headache, hypotonia, tremor, dysarthria, choreoathetosis, seizure, diplopia, blurry vision, nystagmus, hyper- or hyporeflexia, lethargy, fever, confusion, euphoria, hallucinations, irritability, arrhythmias, emesis, hyperglycemia, hypernatremia, Stevens-Johnson syndrome.	1. ABCs. 2. After 6–8 hr of observation, if the patient has no signs of toxicity and phenytoin levels are not elevated or increasing, can discharge to home. 3. Gastric lavage if patient presents early, ingested a large amount, and is intubated. 4. Monitor serial phenytoin concentrations for delayed absorption, which may occur for days. Follow free phenytoin levels, particularly in cases of hypoalbuminemia or coingestion of medications that displace phenytoin from albumin. 5. Repeat doses of activated charcoal every 2–6 hr until toxicity resolves and phenytoin levels are decreasing. 6. Cardiac monitoring is required if coingestion is suspected. For phenytoin ingestion alone, cardiac monitoring is not necessary. 7. Treat seizures with diazepam, lorazepam, or phenobarbital. See Formulary for dosing. 8. Intravenous dextrose for hypoglycemia. 9. Give thiamine, 100 mg IV or IM, because Wernicke encephalopathy clinically mimics phenytoin toxicity. 10. For bradycardia, give atropine 0.02 mg/kg IV (minimum dose 0.1 mg; maximum dose 1–2 mg). 11. Extracorporal elimination is not useful.

TABLE 2-3

MEDICATION INGESTIONS—*cont'd*

Ingestion	Signs and Symptoms	Management
Salicylates[4,21] **(Fig. 2-2)** a. Aspirin, methyl salicylate, nonaspirin salicylate. b. Salicylates are also present in cough and cold powders, topical preparations (oil of wintergreen), creams, Pepto Bismol, and wart and callus treatments. c. Children's aspirin tablets are 81 mg. Adults tablets are 325 mg.	Coma, cerebral edema, dizziness, lethargy. dysarthria, seizure, tinnitus, impaired hearing, hyperpyrexia, respiratory stimulation, pulmonary edema, hepatic dysfunction, hyperglycemia, hypokalemia, hyponatremia, hypernatremia, metabolic acidosis (lactic and ketoacidosis), renal failure, coagulopathy CNS excitement or respiratory depression and coma.	1. Asymptomatic children who consumed less than 120 mg/kg of aspirin do not require specific treatment. a. **Ingestion of 150–300 mg/kg:** mild symptoms (GI upset, tachypnea, tinnitus). Serum salicylate level 30–50 mg/dL. b. **Ingestion of 300–500 mg/kg:** moderate toxicity (agitation, fever, diaphoresis). Serum salicylate level, 50–100 mg/dL. c. **Ingestion of more than 500 mg/kg:** severe toxicity (seizure, coma, dysarthria, pulmonary edema, cardiorespiratory arrest). Serum salicylate level exceeds 100 mg/dL. d. In chronic salicylism, symptoms of severe toxicity may occur at lower ingestion and serum salicylate levels. 2. Carefully weigh risks (bezoar formation) and benefits of **GI decontamination** in patients who present within 4–6 hr of ingestion. For patients who present more than 6 hr after ingestion, in cases of chronic salicylism, or if salicylate levels continue to rise 6 hr after ingestion, multiple doses of activated charcoal should still be given because charcoal enhances postabsorptive salicylate elimination (GI dialysis).

Typical ABG shows metabolic acidosis with respiratory alkalosis. Respiratory acidosis quickly develops because children lack the respiratory capacity to hyperventilate to attain or sustain respiratory alkalosis.

Hypoglycemia occurs in chronic salicylism.

   a. If a large number of tablets were consumed, gastric lavage is indicated up to 4 hr postingestion.
   b. WBI if enteric-coated formulation was ingested.
3. Obtain ECG.
4. Monitor electrolytes (including calcium), liver and renal functions, glucose, PT, PTT, and ABG. Anion gap metabolic acidosis is often present. Monitor urine pH and specific gravity.
5. Check **plasma salicylate level** 4 hr postingestion. Then, to monitor for ongoing absorption, check levels every 3 hr until levels begin to decline. Check levels 6–12 hr after ingestion of sustained-released formulation. **Nomogram is helpful (Figure 2-2), but clinical symptomatology should dominate therapeutic decision making. Plasma levels may not correlate with clinical toxicity.**
6. **Aggressively treat dehydration.** Dehydration increases plasma salicylate concentration which may cause renal failure. Give intravenous fluids with 5% dextrose, potassium, and 50–100 mEq/L sodium bicarbonate at 10–15 mL/kg/h or twice maintenance IV fluid rate to initiate fluid resuscitation. Alkalinization increases salicylate excretion and decreases entry into the CNS.
   a. Goal urine output is 2 mL/kg/hr. Monitor for pulmonary edema.
   b. Monitor calcium homeostasis while giving bicarbonate.
7. Give additional **bicarbonate** boluses for severe acidosis.

TABLE 2-3
MEDICATION INGESTIONS—*cont'd*

Ingestion	Signs and Symptoms	Management
		8. **Urinary alkalinization** is indicated if the patient has symptoms other than emesis or when there is evidence of metabolic disturbance. Metabolic disturbances most often occur when plasma salicylate concentration exceeds 400 mg/L. a. Maintain urine pH greater than 7.5 by administering $NaHCO_3$ in maintenance intravenous fluids. b. Monitor for hypokalemia secondary to alkalinization. It is difficult to alkalinize the urine if the patient is hypokalemic. 9. Do a combination of urine alkalinization and repeat charcoal administration until symptoms resolve and salicylate concentration is less than 30–40 mg/dL. 10. Forced diuresis is not recommended. 11. **Hemodialysis** is indicated if the patient has unresponsive acidosis, electrolyte disturbances, seizures, coma, renal failure, progressive deterioration despite treatment, plasma salicylate level 100 mg/dL or greater after acute ingestion or 60 mg/dL or greater in chronic salicylism. Hemodialysis does not restore metabolic and fluid homeostasis.
Valproate[27] a. Divalproex, Depakote.	Coma, somnolence, cardiac conduction delays.	1. Multiple doses of activated charcoal. 2. There are case reports of using naloxone to treat CNS depression. 3. Hemodialysis or hemoperfusion in massive overdose.

TABLE 2-4
DRUGS OF ABUSE

Drug	Acute Signs and Symptoms	Management of Acute Use
Amphetamines, stimulants[4,32,33] a. Administration: enteral, nasal insufflation, intravenous. b. Methamphetamine: "ice, crank, crystal meth, speed." c. Amphetamine: "hearts, speed." d. See *Cocaine* and *Ecstasy*. e. Dextroamphetamine. f. Ephedrine: "Ma Huang, herbal ecstasy." g. Methylphenidate: Ritalin, "white dragon, Ciba-19." h. Phenylpropanolamine: Propagest, "BT 72s, co-pilot." i. Caffeine, pseudoephedrine.	Seizure, coma, tremors, dizziness, weakness, stereotypy, hyperreflexia, dilated and reactive pupils, hyperthermia, confusion, hallucinations, irritability, delusions, hyperacute sensorium, paranoid ideation, delirium, euphoria, increased confidence, panic, suicidal or homicidal ideation, insomnia, increased concentration, pressured speech, impulsivity, violence, hyperactivity, tachycardia, reflex bradycardia, angina, dysrhythmias, hypertensive crises, cardiovascular collapse, anorexia, emesis, diarrhea, bladder sphincter contraction, rhabdomyolysis, diaphoresis, flushing, dry mouth, exhaustion.	1. GI decontamination with activated charcoal. 2. Give benzodiazepines or haloperidol for agitation and seizures. 3. To treat hypertension unresponsive to benzodiazepines, give hydralazine or sodium nitroprusside IV. 4. Maintain adequate urine output for renal excretion of amphetamines. 5. Treat rhabdomyolysis with IV fluids and urinary alkalinization. 6. Treat hyperpyrexia with external cooling measures, intravenous fluids and sedation, if necessary. 7. Detectable in blood or urine up to 48 hr after last use.

TABLE 2-4
DRUGS OF ABUSE—*con'd*

Drug	Acute Signs and Symptoms	Management of Acute Use
Barbiturates See *Sedative-hypnotic.*		
Cocaine[4,5,19,33,34] a. Administration: nasal insufflation, intravenous, ingestion (rare). Ingested cocaine is the least toxic. b. "Crack, freebase" (smokable form), "coke." c. Inhibits reuptake of dopamine and norepinephrine. Chronic use depletes dopamine and other neurotransmitters. d. Half-life through oral or nasal route is approximately 1 hr. e. Users may coingest cholinesterase inhibitors, cytochrome P450 inhibitors (organophosphate insecticides, cimetidine) or phenytoin to increase cocaine's effect.	Seizure, coma, insomnia, cerebrovascular accident, pressured speech, muscle rigidity, tremors, hyperreflexia, hyperthermia ("coke fever"), dilated pupils, agitation, euphoria, decreased sense of fatigue, paranoid delusions, hallucinations, aggression, tachycardia, bradycardia (small doses), tachyarrhythmias, myocardial ischemia, hypertensive crises, cardiovascular collapse, pneumomediastinum, tachypnea, hemoptysis, bronchospasm, pneumothorax, renal failure, rhabdomyolysis, diaphoresis, chills, nasal mucosa irritation or ulceration, flushing. **Infants:** dystonic posturing, seizure, hyperactivity, altered mental status. **Withdrawal:** depression, cravings. Symptoms peak 2–3 days after last use.	1. ABCs. Monitor vital signs and rectal temperature closely. 2. Treat seizures with benzodiazepines. 3. May also give benzodiazepines for tachycardia, hypertension, or agitation. Benzodiazepines are associated with decreased mortality from cocaine use. 4. For hypertensive crisis, liberally administer benzodiazepines and a short-acting antihypertensive drug, such as nitroprusside. Given the high risk for CVA and myocardial ischemia, treat hypertension quickly and aggressively. 5. Treat arrhythmias according to standard protocols. Tachyarrhythmias may be intractable and fatal. 6. Obtain serial ECGs and cardiac enzymes to monitor for cardiac ischemia. 7. Treat hyperthermia with external cooling, IV fluids, and sedation. 8. Obtain head CT to evaluate for CVA. 9. Aggressive diuresis if myoglobinuria or rhabdomyolysis. 10. If suspect "body packing/stuffing" (ingestion of cocaine bags), do GI decontamination with multiple doses of activated charcoal and WBI. Rupture of the bag can be catastrophic. Do not attempt gastric emptying or endoscopic removal because of the high risk for bag rupture.

		11. Admit to intensive care unit if patient has severe symptoms or if ingested more than 1 g. 12. Metabolites are detectable in blood up to 2–3 days after last use. Can also be detected in urine up to 3 days after last use.
Ecstasy[4,35] a. 3, 4–methylenedioxy-methamphetamine (MDMA). b. Administration: tablet, powder, intranasal, smoke. c. Ketamine, Ma Huang, GBL, and GHB are sometimes called "ecstasy." d. "Hug drug, love drug, E, XTC, X, Adam." e. Ecstasy is a derivative of amphetamine and a type of hallucinogen. See *Amphetamines* and *Hallucinogens*.	Three stages: 1. Disorientation. 2. Tingling, spasmodic jerking. 3. Distortion, illusions, overly sociable. Cerebrovascular accident, tremor, tics, ataxia, nystagmus, insomnia, malignant hyperthermia, mydriasis, depression, confusion, anxiolysis, agitation, tachycardia, hypertension, nausea, liver failure, dilutional hyponatremia, trismus (tightening of jaw muscles), bruxism (jaw-clenching), diaphoresis, severe dehydration, DIC, rhabdomyolysis. Withdrawal/rebound: generalized fatigue, myalgias, poor concentration, confusion, anxiety, depression, insomnia for 1–2 days after use.	1. Aggressively treat hyperthermia with external cooling, acetaminophen, and benzodiazepines. Consider paralysis with intubation to reduce muscular thermogenesis in severe cases. 2. Treat hypertension with sedation. May also use nitroprusside and calcium-channel blockers. Do not give β-blockers (risk unopposed α-induced hypertension). 3. Manage cardiac arrhythmias using standard protocols. 4. Administer activated charcoal if recently ingested. 5. Urinary alkalinization or acidification is not indicated. Alkalinization reduces rate of ecstasy excretion. Acidification may cause myoglobin precipitation in renal tubules. 6. **Usually not detectable in urine screens.** In high concentrations, ecstasy may cross-react with amphetamines. Can detect via gas chromatography, mass spectrometry. Ecstasy is present in urine up to 16 hours after use.

TABLE 2-4

DRUGS OF ABUSE—*con'd*

Drug	Acute Signs and Symptoms	Management of Acute Use
Ethanol[4,6,23,32–34,36] a. One mL of pure ethanol is 0.8 g of ethanol. b. Beer contains 5% ethanol. Ingestion of approximately 10–15 mL/kg of beer causes serious toxicity. Wine contains 14% ethanol. Approximately 4–6 mL/kg of wine causes serious toxicity. 80–proof liquor contains 40% ethanol. Approximately 1–2 mL/kg of 80–proof liquor causes significant toxicity. c. Without active removal techniques, ethanol is eliminated from the body at 10–25 mg/dL/hr. d. Benzodiazepines are often coingested to heighten the effect of ethanol.	Inebriation, ataxia, coma, arrhythmia (atrial fibrillation most common), hypotension, respiratory depression, emesis, hypoglycemia, hypokalemia. Fatal blood alcohol level is approximately 0.3% . A single ingestion of 0.5 g/kg of ethanol (approximately 1.5 mL/kg) may cause significant intoxication in young children. Ethanol may decrease symptoms from coingested CNS stimulants or exacerbate effects of CNS depressants. **Infants, toddlers:** Blood ethanol greater than 50–100 mg/dL may cause coma, hypothermia, hypoglycemia, metabolic acidosis.	1. ABCs. Secure the airway. 2. Measure serum electrolytes, glucose, and ethanol levels. a. Blood ethanol levels cannot be predicted by clinical symptoms. b. In adolescents, greater than 500 mg/dL may be lethal. c. Can estimate blood ethanol level by calculating the osmolar gap: Gap = measured serum osmolality – [(2 × serum Na) + BUN (mg/dL)/2.8 + serum glucose (mg/dL)/18.] 3. Monitor and correct hypoglycemia and electrolyte imbalances. 4. Intravenous fluids. Monitor fluid status for cerebral edema. 5. Treat hypoglycemic seizures with anticonvulsants and glucose. 6. Warming techniques to increase core temperature. 7. If patient presents within 1–2 hr of ingestion, consider GI decontamination. Ethanol is rapidly absorbed from the GI tract and is not adsorbed by activated charcoal. In adolescents, though, do administer activated charcoal because of the high risk for drug coingestion. 8. Consider hemodialysis if blood ethanol level exceeds 450 mg/dL, in cases of impaired hepatic function, or if severe symptomatology.

		9. Obtain broad-spectrum toxicology test to evaluate for coingestion of other drugs. 10. No clear benefit has been demonstrated from use of flumazenil, naloxone, or fructose.
Gamma Hydroxybutyrate (GHB), Gamma Hydroxybutyrolactone (GBL)[4,33,34] a. GBL is a precursor to GHB. b. Colorless, odorless, and tasteless powder and liquid forms c. "Date rape drug, Georgia home boy, liquid ecstasy, soap, easy lay." d. Popular at rave parties. e. Also used for anabolic and growth hormone–stimulating effects to increase muscle mass.	Seizure, coma, CNS depression, sedation, tremor, nystagmus, miosis, ataxia, hypothermia, euphoria, increased libido, insomnia, confusion, aggression, bradycardia, hypotension, respiratory failure, emesis, muscle cramps. Sudden-onset coma is most common presentation. Coma usually lasts 1–2 hr. Patients are often delirious and vomiting upon emerging from the coma. Onset of action is within 15 min. Peak concentration is attained in 20–60 min, and half-life is approximately 30 min. Effects last 6–8 hr. Toxicity prolonged with coingestion of alcohol. **Withdrawal:** feelings of "doom."	1. ABCs. Administer 100% oxygen, and secure the airway. Despite poor gag reflex, patient may be very responsive to airway stimulation during intubation attempts. 2. Supportive care. 3. Atropine to treat bradycardia. 4. GI lavage and charcoal are not indicated because GHB is rapidly absorbed by GI mucosa. 5. Drug is rapidly metabolized into carbon dioxide and exhaled. **Small amount is excreted in the urine but is not detectable on routine urine toxicology tests.** May test for GHB precursors via gas chromatography and mass spectrometry.

TABLE 2-4

DRUGS OF ABUSE—*con'd*

Drug	Acute Signs and Symptoms	Management of Acute Use
Hallucinogens[4,32,33,37] a. Psychadelics. b. Mescaline: peyote cactus, "Aztec, blue cap." c. Psilocybin: "magic mushrooms, Aztec, purple passion." d. Lysergic acid diethylamide: LSD, "acid, blotter." e. Phencyclidine: PCP. f. Methylenedioxy-methamphetamine (MDMA): "Ecstasy, Adam." See *Ecstasy*. g. Dimethyltryptamine, diethyltryptamine. h. Half-life is 1–3 days.	Psychosis, disinhibition, euphoria, anxiety, paranoid thought disorder, mood lability, time and visual distortions, visual hallucinations, depersonalization, hyperreflexia, hyperthermia, dilated pupils, tachycardia, hypertension, facial flushing. **LSD:** "flashbacks" (exaggerations or distortions of real auditory and visual stimuli), psychosis with hyperalertness, change in body image, delusions with grandiosity, hallucinations, visual perception distortion (LSD directly affects the visual system), perception that time passes slowly, paresthesias, weakness, drowsy, dizziness. **PCP:** seizures, cyclic coma, ataxia, dysarthria, blank stare, normal or small pupils, nystagmus, muscle rigidity, dystonia, tardive dyskinesia, athetosis, extreme hyperactivity, aggression, analgesia, psychosis, violence, amnesia, bronchospasm, hypoglycemia, urinary retention, diaphoresis.	1. Benzodiazepines for seizures. 2. Benzodiazepines or haloperidol for anxiety and agitation. 3. Put patient in a quiet environment. Provide reassurance. 4. GI decontamination if suspect coingestion. 5. Monitor uric acid, CPK, creatinine, and SGOT/SGPT for signs of rhabdomyolysis and renal failure. Avoid physical restraints if possible. Can chemically restrain the patient with benzodiazepines or haloperidol. 6. Some hallucinogens are detectable in urine and blood. Ecstasy is only detectable if ingested in large amounts and will cross-react with amphetamines. Use EMIT (enzyme-multiple immunoassay technique) to test for PCP. Level of hallucinogens detected in the urine does not correlate with clinical toxicity. May also detect through examination of gastric contents.

Ketamine[32,35] a. Dissociative. b. Inhibits catecholamine reuptake. c. "Ketalar, K-hole, vitamin K."	Nystagmus, analgesia, anxiety, sedation, amnesia, disordered thought, hallucination, moderate tachycardia, moderate hypertension, emesis, rhabdomyolysis.	1. Treat agitation or emergence reactions with benzodiazepines. 2. Monitor electrolytes and creatinine given risk for rhabdomyolysis. 3. Keep patient in calm, quiet environment. 4. Maintain hydration status in case of rhabdomyolysis. 5. Once patient returns to baseline mental status and vital signs are stable (about 2 hr after presentation), can discharge home. 6. **Not detected by routine toxicology screens.** Can detect via high-performance liquid chromatography.
Marijuana[4,19,32,33] a. Cannabis group. b. Smoking is three-fold more potent than enteral use. c. "Delta-9-THC, hash-ish, hash oil, pot, reefer, smoke, hemp, grass, nickel bags." d. May be "laced" with PCP, cocaine, or other drugs. Users may coingest phenytoin to increase marijuana's effect.	Ataxia, dysarthria, euphoria, drowsy, anxiety, clear sensorium, time-space distortion (temporal disintegration), delusions, paranoia, relaxation, confusion, depersonalization, impaired memory, vivid visual imagery, increased sense of hearing, injected conjunctiva, pupils unchanged, tachycardia, hypertension, orthostatic hypotension, respiratory distress with airway obstruction, increased appetite, dry mucous membranes. Symptoms begin 30–60 min after ingestion. Peak effects occur up to 2–3 hr after ingestion. Hallucinations and violence are rare.	1. To treat adolescents with psychotic reactions or acute toxic delirium, give diazepam. 2. Symptoms generally improve after 4–6 hr of observation. 3. Cannabinoids are detectable in the urine up to 3 days after single use, 5 days after use 3 times per week, and 10 days after use 6 times per week. **To treat withdrawal:** 1. Trazodone to treat disabling insomnia.

TABLE 2-4

DRUGS OF ABUSE—*con'd*

Drug	Acute Signs and Symptoms	Management of Acute Use
	Infants, toddlers: lethargy, coma. **Withdrawal:** flu-like illness, cravings. Symptoms peak 4–5 days after last use and slowly resolve over 2 wk.	
Opioids[4,6,28,32,33,37] a. Codeine, fentanyl, heroin, hydromorphone, meperidine, methadone, morphine, opiate–analgesic combinations, opium, oxycodone, pentazocine, propoxyphene. b. Routes: oral, intranasal, subcutaneous, intramuscular, intravenous. Opium and heroin freebase can be smoked. c. Fentanyl: duragesic, "STP, six pack." d. Heroin: "China cat, skag." e. Methadone: "orange barrel, dolphin." f. Morphine: "morph." g. Opium: "dust, yen shee." h. Propoxyphene: Darvon, "lily." i. Pentazocine: Talwin, "T's." j. Oxycodone-Aspirin: Percodan, "perks."	Seizures, coma, stupor, analgesia, emotional lability, anxiolysis, drowsy, sedation, pinpoint pupils, hypothermia, hyporeflexia, hypotension, respiratory depression, apnea, cyanosis, pulmonary edema, emesis, decreased pancreatic secretions, decreased gastric HCl secretion, biliary colic, decreased GI motility, constipation, colonic spasm, increased anal sphincter tone, clammy skin, miosis, anaphylactoid reaction with histamine release. **Intravenous use:** septic emboli, endocarditis, abscesses, localized skin infections. **Meperidine:** seizures, dilated pupils. **Propoxyphene:** seizures, arrhythmias. **Withdrawal:** insomnia, agitation, irritability, piloerection.	1. ABCs. 2. **Naloxone. See Table 2-5, *Antidotes*.** Naloxone may induce abstinence syndrome. In patients with opiate dependence, start naloxone, 0.2–0.4 mg and titrate upward slowly. 3. Give methadone to prevent severe withdrawal. Ideally, start methadone dosing once or twice a day before withdrawal symptoms occur. Methadone is less euphoric and has longer elimination half-life compared with other opiates. 4. Thin-layer chromatography and radioimmunoassay techniques detect opiate metabolites for up to 3 days after last use in the urine. May also be detected in serum.

Sedative-Hypnotics[4,32,33,37] a. Barbiturates: Secobarbital, Seconal, "ace, yellow jackets." b. Meprobamate: Miltown, "bams." c. Methaqualone: Parest, Somnafae, "Soapers, 714." d. Methyprylon: "Roach 19, Easter bunny." e. Rohypnol: "Rib, date pill." f. Benzodiazepines: flunitrazepam ("date rape drug"). Often used to heighten the effect of alcohol and other drugs. g. Chlordiazepoxide, diazepam, flurazepam, meprobamate. h. Half-lives range from 5–100 hr. i. Sometimes used to relieve cocaine-induced anxiety.	Coma, dysarthria, headache, ataxia, vertigo, drowsiness, lateral nystagmus, sluggish pupillary response, normal or small pupillary size, impaired memory and judgment, confusion, delirium, impulsivity, euphoria, emotional lability, irritability, short attention span, cardiovascular collapse, bradypnea, hypotension, respiratory compromise, pulmonary edema. Symptoms are similar to ethanol intoxication. **Withdrawal:** seizure, increased REM sleep, tremors, insomnia, apathy, weakness, agitation, anxiety, cravings, flu-like illness. Symptoms peak 4–5 days after last use and slowly resolve over 2 wk.	1. ABCs. Cardiovascular collapse may occur in cases of coingestion. Monitor in an intensive care unit. Consider ECG monitoring. 2. GI decontamination with repeat doses of activated charcoal. Can consider giving a cathartic. 3. Urinary alkalinization increases excretion of phenobarbital. 4. Consider hemodialysis or charcoal hemoperfusion in severe toxicity. 5. Flumazenil. See Table 2-5, *Antidotes*. 6. Do toxicology screen for other substances of abuse. Severe poisonings are rare with only benzodiazepine use.

TABLE 2-5

ANTIDOTES (NOTE: CONTACT LOCAL POISON CONTROL CENTER FOR MOST CURRENT RECOMMENDATIONS)

Indication	Antidote	Administration	Adverse Effects
Acetaminophen	*N*-acetylcysteine (NAC, Mucomyst)	140 mg/kg PO loading dose, followed by 70 mg/kg every 4 hr for 17 doses. Administer in water, soda, or fruit juice. See Table 2-3, *Acetaminophen*. *IV Alternative*: Loading dose, 150 mg/kg diluted in 200 mL 5% dextrose IV administered over 15 min. Maintenance dosing, 50 mg/kg diluted in 500 mL 5% dextrose IV administered over 4 hr, followed by 100 mg/kg diluted in 1000 mL 5% dextrose IV administered over 16 hr.	Emesis, renal tubule acidosis.
Alcohols	Calcium gluconate	0.6 mL/kg of calcium gluconate 10% IV slowly until symptoms resolve and serum calcium normalizes.	
Alcohols (ethylene glycol, methanol)	Ethanol 10%	Indicated if serum methanol or ethylene glycol level is 20 mg/dL or greater.	Emesis, sedation.
Alcohols (ethylene glycol, methanol)	Fomepizole (4–methylpyrazole, Antizol)	15 mg/kg IV infusion over 30 min, then 10 mg/kg every 12 hr for 4 doses. Then, 15 mg/kg every 12 hr until methanol or ethylene glycol level is less than 20 mg/dL. Maintain adequate urine output. Increase frequency of dosing to every 4 hr if also dialyzing.	
Anticholinesterase	Atropine	*Child*: 0.05–0.1 mg/kg IM, IV, or ET. *Adult*: 2–5 mg. Dilute in 1–2 mL of normal saline for endotracheal tube administration. Repeat dose every 10–30 min as needed to obtain atropinization (cleared bronchial secretions, pulmonary rales, and oral secretions).	Tachycardia, dry mouth, blurred vision, urinary retention.

Antihistamines, other anticholinergic agents	Physostigmine (Antilirium)	Do not give physostigmine if patient coingested any substance that affects cardiac conduction (e.g., tricyclic antidepressants). *Child*: 0.5 mg IV over 3–5 min. *Adult*: 1–2 mg IV over 5 min. *Alternate dosing*: 0.02 mg/kg IV, infuse over 3–5 mins. May repeat every 10–15 min up to a maximum total of 2 mg (4 mg in adults) to establish the minimum effective dose. Then, give minimal effective dose every 30–60 minutes for recurring symptoms over the next 6–8 hr. See Table 2-3, *Antihistamines*, *Anticholinergic drugs*. Have atropine readily available to treat side effects. Dosing for IV atropine is one half the dose of physostigmine given.	Seizure, headache, bradycardia, asystole, bronchospasm, emesis, cholinergic crisis, hypotension. Increased risk for seizure or asystole if administered too rapidly.
Benzodiazepines	Flumazenil (Romazicon)	0.01–0.02 mg/kg IV, maximum cumulative dose 1 mg. *Note*: Do not use for antidepressant or unknown ingestion. May not reverse respiratory depression. Risk seizures in patients with seizure disorder or in coingestion of epileptogenic substance.	Emesis, facial flushing, agitation, headache, dizziness, seizure, transient hypotension.
β-Blockers	Glucagon	*Child*: 0.05–0.15 mg/kg IV bolus, then 0.05–0.1 mg/kg/hr infusion. *Alternate dosing*: 50 μg/kg IV. *Adult*: 3–5 mg IV bolus. Repeat dose 2–3 times to a maximum of 10 mg total. Then, 1–5 mg/hr infusion.	Hyperglycemia, emesis.
Calcium-channel blockers	Calcium	*Child*: CaCl 10% 0.2 mL/kg, or calcium gluconate 10% 0.6 mL/kg IV. *Adult*: CaCl 10% 10 mL, or calcium gluconate 10% 30 mL. Give 2–3 repeat doses PRN.	

TABLE 2-5
ANTIDOTES—*cont'd*

Indication	Antidote	Administration	Adverse Effects
Calcium-channel blockers	Glucagon	See β-*Blockers*.	
Carbon monoxide	Hyperbaric oxygen	100% oxygen via non-rebreather mask or ventilator.	
Cyanide	Cyanide antidote kit	1. **Amyl nitrite**: 1 crushable ampule inhalation. Inhale for 15–30 sec every 60 sec pending administration of sodium nitrite. 2. **If hemoglobin level is known for a child:** **(Sodium nitrite 3% IV solution. Sodium thiosulfate 25% IV solution.)** Hgb = 8 g: Na nitrite 6.6 mg/kg (0.22 mL/kg); Na thiosulfate 1.1 mL/kg. Hgb = 10 g: Na nitrite 8.7 mg/kg (0.27 mL/kg); Na thiosulfate 1.35 mL/kg. Hgb = 12 g: 10 mg/kg (0.33 mL/kg); Na thiosulfate 1.65 mL/kg. Hgb = 14 g: 11.6 mg/kg (0.39 mL/kg); Na thiosulfate 1.95 mL/kg. 3. **If hemoglobin level is not known for a child:** **Sodium nitrite**: 0.33 mL/kg IV of 3% solution. **Sodium thiosulfate**:1.6 mL (400 mg)/kg IV of 25% solution repeated every 30–60 min to maximum of 50 mL. Administer immediately after sodium nitrite. 4. **Adult dosing:** **Sodium nitrite**: *Adult*: 300 mg (10 mL of 3% solution) IV over 2–4 min. **Sodium thiosulfate**: *Adult*: 12.5 g IV (2.5–5 mL/min of 25% solution).	Methemoglobinemia

Digitalis glycosides (synthetic or natural)	Digoxin-specific Fab antibodies (Digibind)	One vial IV binds 0.6 mg of digitalis glycoside. See Table 2-4, *Digoxin*.	Allergic reaction, rebound hypokalemia, congestive heart failure.
Iron	Desferoxamine (Desferal)	5–15 mg/kg/h (maximum 360 mg/kg or 6 g in 24 hr or 50 mg/kg/24 hr) IV. *Alternate dosing*: 90 mg/kg/dose IM every 8 hr (maximum 6 g in 24 hr). Infuse slowly. Use higher doses for severe symptoms (hypotension) and decrease as symptoms resolve. Continue chelation until serum iron level returns to normal range, metabolic acidosis resolves, the patient clinically improves, and urine returns to normal color.	Hypotension.
Methemoglobinemia	Methylene blue[11]	0.1–0.2 mL/kg IV of 1% solution (1–2 mg/kg), infuse over 5–10 minutes, every 30–60 min for severe cyanosis or methemoglobin >30% . Maximum, 7 mg/kg. If the offending drug has long half-life (e.g., dapsone), give 0.1 mg/kg/hr infusion. Contraindicated in G6PD deficiency.	Emesis, retrosternal chest pain, tachycardia, hypertension, anxiety, green-blue urine, oxidative hemolysis, headache, dizziness, factitious cyanosis.
Opioids	Naloxone (Narcan): serum half-life is 1 hr. Duration of action is 1–4 hr.	0.01–0.1 mg/kg IV. Repeat as needed. (Can start with 0.01 mg/kg. If no effect, then give 0.1 mg/kg.) *Alternate dosing*: 1–2 mg for all patients older than neonate. *Respiratory depression*: 2 mg IV, ET, or sublingual. Repeat every 2 minutes up to total of 10 mg in adolescents or adults. *No respiratory depression*: initial dose of 1 mg.	Opioid withdrawal syndrome, seizure, ventricular irritability, hypertension, pulmonary edema.

TABLE 2-5
ANTIDOTES—*cont'd*

Indication	Antidote	Administration	Adverse Effects
Pesticides (carbamate, organophosphate)	Atropine	See *Anticholinesterase*.	
Pesticides (carbamate, organophosphate)	Pralidoxime (2–PAM, Protopam)	*Child*: for patients younger than 12 years, give 25–50 mg/kg in 250 mL saline infusion over 30 min. For patients older than 12 years, give 1–2 g IV over 10 min. *Adult*: 1–2 g. Repeat in 1 hr PRN, then every 6–12 hr PRN for 24–48 hr. Infuse slowly. Alternatively, can give continuous infusion of 10–20 mg/kg/hr (up to 500 mg/hr) for 24 hours.	Nausea, dizziness, headache, tachycardia, muscle rigidity, bronchospasm.
Phenothiazines	Diphenhydramine (Benadryl)	5 mg/kg/24 hr IV or PO divided every 8 hr. Maximum, 300 mg/24 hr. *Alternate dosing*: 1–2 mg/kg/dose IM or IV.	Sedation, ataxia, paradoxical agitation.
Phenothiazines—acute dystonic reaction	Benztropine (Cogentin)	*Child*: 0.02 mg/kg (maximum 1 mg) IV or IM. Use in patients younger than 3 years only in life-threatening situations. *Adult*: 1–2 mg IV or IM.	Sedation, blurred vision, dry mouth, tachycardia.
Warfarin, "superwarfarin" rat poison	Vitamin K	*Child*: 1–5 mg IV, IM, SC, or PO. *Adult*: 10 mg.	

Data from references 4, 9, 11, 19, and 20.

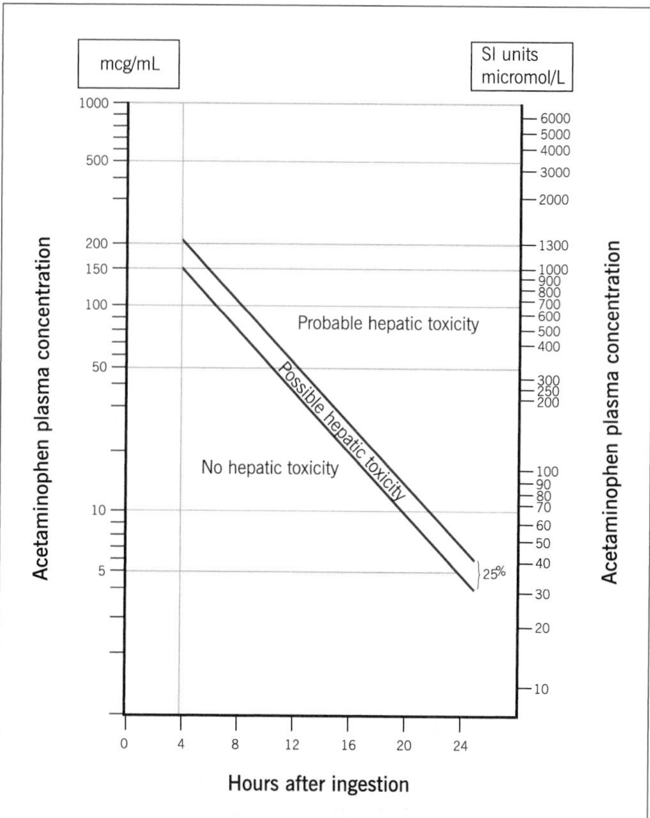

FIG. 2-1

Semilogarithmic plot of plasma acetaminophen levels versus time. *(From Jones AL: J Toxicology 1998;36:277–285)*

Note: This nomogram is valid for use after acute ingestions of acetaminophen. The need for treatment cannot be extrapolated based on a level before 4 hours. In chronic overdose, toxicity can be seen with much lower plasma levels.

2. Tissue asphyxiants cause headache, dizziness, chest pain, and emesis.

B. MANAGEMENT[10]

1. **Assess stability of the airway.** Intubate if there are signs of airway edema. Upper airway obstruction progresses rapidly in the setting of thermal or chemical burns to the face, nares, or oropharynx.

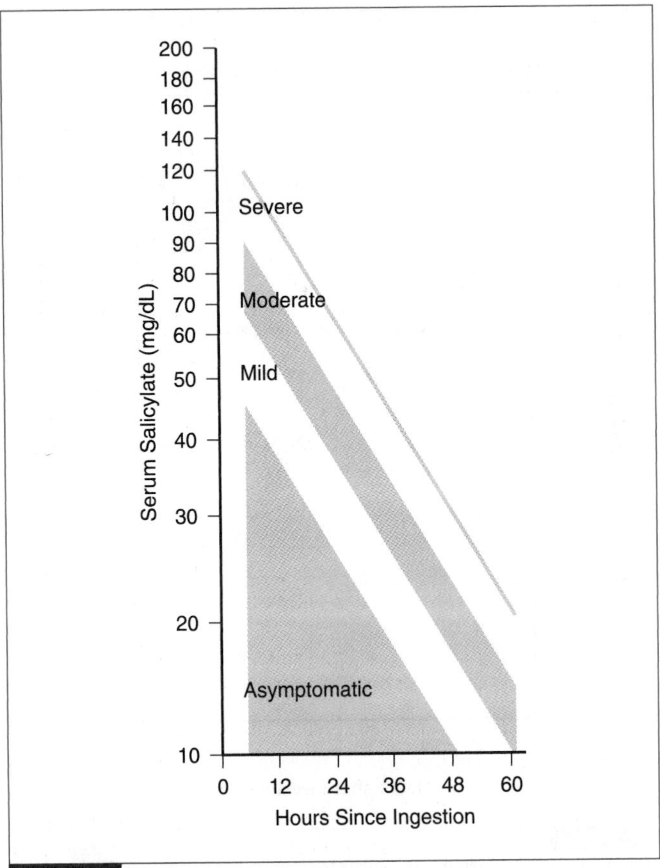

FIG. 2-2

The Done nomogram for estimating severity of salicylate poisoning using serum salicylate levels. *(From Temple AR: Acute and chronic effects of aspirin toxicity and their treatment. Arch Intern Med 1981;141:366.)*

2. Administer supplemental oxygen through a non-rebreather mask.

a. Can give aerosolized bronchodilators. Do not give corticosteroids.

b. Methods to evaluate the severity of airway injury include chest radiography, arterial blood gases with co-oximetry, serial peak expiratory flow rates, and bedside spirometry. These initially may be normal.

c. Use co-oximetry instead of pulse oximetry to measure oxyhemoglobin. Pulse oximetry cannot distinguish between carboxyhemoglobin or methemoglobin and oxyhemoglobin.

3. **Obtain 12-lead electrocardiogram (ECG)** to evaluate for myocardial ischemia or infarction.
4. **Send blood and urine toxicology tests.** Multiple agents may be involved in the inhalational injury.
5. **Observe for at least 24 hours.**

V. CARBON MONOXIDE POISONING[11,12,13]

A. CARBON MONOXIDE

Carbon monoxide (CO) is a colorless, odorless, and tasteless toxic gas.

B. ENVIRONMENTAL EXPOSURES

1. Garages, campers, tents, other confined spaces, gas furnaces, gas heaters, gas ovens, gas clothes dryers, other fuel-powered equipment, wood and coal heating, fireplaces, charcoal grills, automobiles, generators, lawn mowers, snow blowers, leaf blowers, paint remover or thinner with methylene chloride.
2. Increased incidence of CO poisoning occurs during electricity shortages or when families are not able to afford electric heating.
3. Multiple household members may have similar symptoms.
4. In fires, consider exposure to cyanide as well.

C. AFFINITY FOR HEMOGLOBIN

1. CO affinity for hemoglobin is approximately 240-fold greater than oxygen.
2. Leftward shift of the oxyhemoglobin dissociation curve results in decreased oxygen delivery to tissues. Organs with high metabolic rates and high oxygen demand are most affected.

D. PHYSICAL EXAMINATION

1. Headache, dizziness, seizure, syncope, confusion, loss of consciousness, fatigue, irritability, emotional lability, irrational behavior, weakness, poor motor coordination, drowsiness, chest pain, respiratory distress, tachypnea, emesis, diarrhea, hyponatremia, lactic acidosis, skin pallor, dyspnea on exertion, palpitations, myalgias, flu-like illness.
2. Risk for cerebral edema, coma, permanent ocular toxicity, cardiac ischemia, severe respiratory depression, pulmonary edema, muscle necrosis, myoglobinuria, renal failure.
3. Symptoms may not correlate with carboxyhemoglobin (COHb) levels in the blood.
4. Cherry-red mucosal membranes and retinal hemorrhages are late and rare findings.

E. MANAGEMENT

1. **Secure the airway and avoid hypercapnia.**

a. For a conscious patient, administer 100% oxygen via non-rebreather face mask at a flow rate of 10 L/min until COHb is less than 10% and symptoms resolve.

b. Intubate and mechanically ventilate in cases of severe respiratory compromise, cardiovascular instability, altered alertness, nervous system dysfunction, or coma.

c. Pulse oximetry is not accurate.

2. **Measure carboxyhemoglobin levels in the blood.**

a. In general, patients are symptomatic when COHb exceeds 15%. Toxicity occurs at levels greater than 20%. If COHb is more than 40%, severe neurologic effects may occur. Levels greater than 50% result in irreversible central nervous system (CNS) damage.

b. Elimination half-life of COHb is approximately 4–6 hours when breathing room air and approximately 1 hour when breathing 100% oxygen.

3. **Obtain ECG and chest radiograph** to evaluate for myocardial ischemia, pneumonitis, atelectasis, or pulmonary edema.

4. **Hyperbaric oxygen therapy decreases the half-life of COHb.** It should be considered in patients with high levels of COHb or serious clinical toxicity, although specific indications are controversial.

VI. METHEMOGLOBINEMIA

Methemoglobinemia forms when deoxygenated heme is oxidized to Fe^{3+}, which has decreased oxygen-carrying capacity and increased oxygen affinity (resulting in decreased oxygen release to tissues).

A. ETIOLOGIES

1. Congenital hemoglobinopathy, genetic deficiency of enzymes that reduce methemoglobin.

2. Oxidative hemoglobin injury in ill infants, such as during a diarrheal illness.

3. Oxidative injury secondary to poisoning, drugs, or environmental exposure.

a. Aniline dyes, chloroquine, dapsone, fertilizers containing nitrogens, local anesthetics, high doses of methylene blue, metoclopramide, naphthalene, nitrates, nitrites, rifampin, toluidine, contaminated well water.

b. Routine urine toxicology tests generally do not detect the etiology of methemoglobinemia.

B. PHYSICAL EXAMINATION AND DIAGNOSIS

1. Clinical toxicity is more apparent in acute-onset methemoglobinemia—CNS depression, cardiac instability, hemolysis, tissue ischemia. Metabolic acidosis may or may not occur.

2. Cyanosis unresponsive to oxygen therapy but with normal arterial oxygen tension on arterial blood gas. Cyanosis occurs with 1.5 g/dL of methemoglobin or when 10% or more of the hemoglobin is methemoglobin.

3. Arterial blood has chocolate-brown color and does not turn red upon exposure to air.
4. Pulse oximetry underestimates oxygen saturation in low levels of methemoglobin and overestimates oxygen saturation in high levels of methemoglobin.

C. MANAGEMENT

1. Remove the offending agent.
2. ABCs. Administer 100% oxygen. Note that pulse oximetry is not accurate.
3. Offer supportive care.
4. Skin decontamination.
5. Activated charcoal if suspect oxidant ingestion.
6. Co-oximetry analysis of the blood to confirm and quantify methemoglobinemia. Estimate the oxygen-carrying capacity based on the percentage of methemoglobin and the total amount of hemoglobin.
7. Monitor serial ECGs for signs of myocardial ischemia.
8. Obtain electrolytes, blood urea nitrogen (BUN), creatinine, arterial blood gas, complete blood count (CBC) with differential, blood smear to evaluate for hemolysis, and urinalysis.
9. Correct electrolyte, fluid, and acid-base imbalances.
10. **Methylene blue** is indicated for severe tissue hypoxia (beyond cyanotic discoloration), CNS depression, cardiovascular instability, coexisting medical condition that decreases tolerance for low oxygen delivery to tissues, and methemoglobin level greater than 30%. See Table 2-5.

a. Methylene blue is contraindicated in patients with glucose-6-phosphate dehydrogenase (G6PD) deficiency.
b. After giving one dose of methylene blue, reassess the patient's clinical status, and recheck the current methemoglobin level before giving a repeat dose.
c. Methylene blue causes factitious cyanosis and alters accuracy of pulse oximetry.

11. For comatose patients, give IV glucose and naloxone.
12. Ascorbic acid slowly reduces the amount of methemoglobin.
13. If the patient has G6PD deficiency, consider hyperbaric oxygen therapy or exchange transfusion. Do not administer methylene blue.

REFERENCES

1. Bryant S, Singer J: Management of toxic exposure in children. Emerg Med Clin North Am 2003;21(1):101–119.
2. Woolf AD: Poisoning by unknown agents. Pediatr Rev 1999;20(5):166–170.
3. Matos ME, Burns MM, Shannon MW: False-positive tricyclic antidepressant drug screen results leading to the diagnosis of carbamazepine intoxication. Pediatrics 2000;105(5):e66.

4. Osterhoudt KC, Shannon M, Henretig FM: Toxicologic emergencies. In Fleisher GR, Ludwig S (eds): Textbook of Pediatric Emergency Medicine, 4th ed. Philadelphia, Lippincott Williams & Wilkins, 2000.
5. Riordan M, Rylance G, Berry K: Poisoning in children 1: General management. Arch Dis Child 2002;87:392–396.
6. Abruzzi G, Stork CM: Pediatric toxicologic concerns. Emerg Med Clin North Am 2002;20(1):223–247.
7. Simpson WM, Schuman SH: Recognition and management of acute pesticide poisoning. Am Fam Physician 2002;65(8):1599–1604.
8. Dorrington CL, Johnson DW, Brant R: The frequency of complications associated with the use of multiple-dose activated charcoal. Ann Emerg Med 2003;41(3):370–377.
9. Rodgers GC, Matyunas NJ: Poisonings: Drugs, chemicals, and plants. In Behrman RE, Kliegman R, Jenson HB (eds): Nelson Textbook of Pediatrics, 16th ed. Philadelphia, WB Saunders, 2000.
10. Miller K, Chang A: Acute inhalation injury. Emerg Med Clin North Am 2003;21(2):533–557.
11. Etzel RA: Indoor air pollutants in homes and schools. Pediatr Clinic North Am 2001;48(5):1153–1165.
12. Foster M, Goodwin SR, Williams C, Loeffler J: Recurrent acute life-threatening events and lactic acidosis caused by chronic carbon monoxide poisoning in an infant. Pediatrics 1999;104(3):e34.
13. Winter PM, Miller JN: Carbon monoxide poisoning. JAMA 1976;236:1502–1504.
14. Ratnapalan S, Potylitsina Y, Tan LH, et al: Measuring a toddler's mouthful: Toxicologic considerations. J Pediatr 2003;142:729–730.
15. Casavant MJ. Fomepizole in the treatment of poisoning. Pediatrics 2001;107(1):e170.
16. Bandle HPR, Davis SH, Hopkins NE: Lipoid pneumonia: a silent complication of mineral oil aspiration. Pediatrics 1999;103(2):e19.
17. Piomelli S: Childhood lead poisoning. Pediatr Clin North Am 2002;49(6):1285–1304.
18. Davoli CT, Golstein GW: Childhood lead poisoning. In Johnson RT, Griffin JW, McArthur JC (eds): Current Therapy in Neurologic Disease, 6th ed. St. Louis, Mosby, 2001.
19. Ford MD, Delaney KA, Ling LL, Erickson T (eds): Clinical Toxicology, 1st ed. Philadelphia, WB Saunders, 2001.
20. Johnson KB, Oski FA: Oski's Essential Pediatrics. Philadelphia, Lippincott Williams & Wilkins, 1997.
21. Riordan M, Rylance G, Berry K: Poisoning in children 2: Painkillers. Arch Dis Child 2002;87:297–399.
22. Mohler CR, Nordt SP, Williams SR, et al: Prospective evaluation of mild to moderate pediatric acetaminophen exposure. Ann Emerg Med 2000;35(3):239–244.
23. McGuigan ME: Poisoning potpourri. Pediatr Rev 2001;22(9):295–302.
24. American Academy of Pediatrics Committee on Drugs: Acetaminophen toxicity in children. Pediatrics 2001;108(4):1020–1024.
25. McClain CJ, Holtzman J, Allen J, et al: Clinical features of acetaminophen toxicity. J Clin Gastroenterol 1988;10:76–80.
26. Riordan M, Rylance G, Berry K: Poisoning in children 3: Common medicines. Arch Dis Child 2002;87:400–402.

27. Goldberg JF: Psychiatric emergencies: new drugs in psychiatry. Emerg Med Clin North Am 2000;18(2):211–231.
28. Marx J: Resuscitation pharmacology. In Marx J, Hockberger R, Walls R (eds): Rosen's Emergency Medicine: Concepts and Clinical Practice, 5th ed. St. Louis, Mosby, 2002.
29. Belson MG, Gorman SE, Sullivan K, Geller RJ: Calcium channel blocker ingestions in children. Am J Emerg Med 2000;18(5):581–586.
30. Gunn VL, Taha SH, Liebelt EL, Serwint JR: Toxicity of over-the-counter cough and cold medications. Pediatrics 2001;108(3):e52.
31. Meyer RJ, Flynn JT, Brophy PD, et al: Hemodialysis followed by continuous hemofiltration for treatment of lithium intoxication in children. Am J Kidney Dis 2001;37(5):1044–1047.
32. Giannini AJ: An approach to drug abuse, intoxication and withdrawal. Am Fam Physician 2000;61(9):2763–2774.
33. Kaul P, Coupey SM: Clinical evaluation of substance abuse. Pediatr Rev 2002;23(3):85–94.
34. Dias PJ: Adolescent substance abuse: assessment in the office. Pediatr Clin North Am 2002;49(2):269–300.
35. Koesters SC, Rogers PD, Rajasingham CR: MDMA ("ecstasy") and other "club drugs": The new epidemic. Pediatr Clin North Am 2002;49(2):415–433.
36. Riordan M, Rylance G, Berry K: Poisoning in children 4: Household products, plants, and mushrooms. Arch Dis Child 2002;87:403–406.
37. Hogan MJ: Diagnosis and treatment of teen drug use. Med Clin North Am 2000;84(4):927–966.
38. Keriotis AA, Upadhyaya HP: Inhalant dependence and withdrawal symptoms. J Am Acad Child Adolesc Psychiatry 2000;39(6):679–680.
39. Scalley RD, Ferguson DR, Piccaro JC, et al: Treatment of ethylene glycol poisoning. Am Fam Physician 2002;66(5):807–812.
40. Brown MJ, Shannon MW, Woolf A, Boyer EW: Childhood methanol ingestion treated with fomepizole and hemodialysis. Pediatrics 2001;108(4):e77.
41. Boyer EW, Mejia M, Woolf A, Shannon M: Severe ethylene glycol ingestion treated without hemodialysis. Pediatrics 2001;107(1):172–173.

Procedures

Nicole Shilkofski, MD

3

I. GENERAL GUIDELINES

A. CONSENT

1. It is crucial to obtain informed consent from the parent or guardian before performing any procedure by explaining the procedure, the indications, any risks involved, and any alternatives. Obtaining consent for life-saving emergency procedures is unnecessary.

B. RISKS

1. All invasive procedures involve pain and risk for infection and bleeding. Specific complications are listed by procedure.
2. Sedation and analgesia should be planned in advance, and the risks of such explained to the parent and/or patient as applicable. In general, 1% lidocaine buffered with sodium bicarbonate is adequate for local analgesia.
3. Universal precautions should be followed for all patient contact that exposes the health care provider to blood, amniotic fluid, pericardial or pleural fluid, synovial fluid, cerebrospinal fluid, semen, or vaginal secretions.
4. Proper sterile technique is crucial to achieve good wound closure, decrease transmittable diseases, and prevent wound contamination.

II. BLOOD SAMPLING AND VASCULAR ACCESS

A. HEELSTICK AND FINGERSTICK

1. **Indications:** Blood sampling in infants for laboratory studies unaffected by hemolysis.
2. **Complications:** Infection, bleeding, osteomyelitis.
3. **Procedure:**

a. Warm heel or finger.

b. Clean with alcohol.

(1) Puncture heel using a lancet on the lateral part of the heel, avoiding the posterior area.

(2) Puncture finger using a lancet on the palmar lateral surface of the finger near the tip.

c. Wipe away the first drop of blood, then collect the sample using a capillary tube or container.

d. Alternate between squeezing blood from the leg toward the heel (or from the hand toward the finger) and then releasing the pressure for several seconds.

B. INTRAVENOUS PLACEMENT AND ACCESS SITES

1. **Indications:** To obtain access to peripheral venous circulation to deliver fluid, medications, or blood products.

2. Complications:

a. Thrombosis.

b. Infection.

3. Procedure:

a. Choose intravenous (IV) placement site and prepare with alcohol.

b. Apply tourniquet and then insert IV catheter, bevel up, at angle almost parallel to the skin, advancing until "flash" of blood is seen in the catheter hub. Advance the plastic catheter only, remove the needle, and secure the catheter.

c. After removing tourniquet, attach T connector filled with saline to the catheter, flush with several mL of normal saline (NS) to ensure patency of the IV line.

C. EXTERNAL JUGULAR PUNCTURE[1]

1. **Indications:** Blood sampling in patients with inadequate peripheral vascular access or during resuscitation.
2. **Complications:** Infection, bleeding, pneumothorax.
3. **Procedure** (Fig. 3-1):

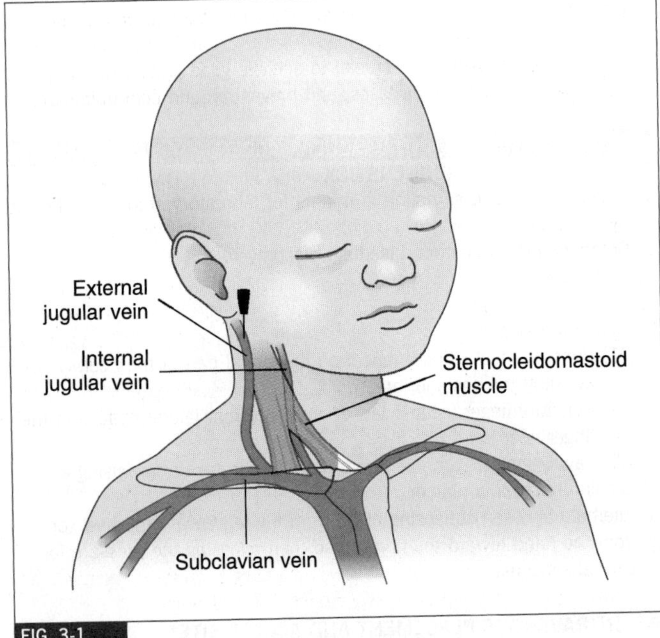

FIG. 3-1

External jugular cannulation. *(From Dieckmann R, Selbst S: Pediatric Emergency and Critical Care Procedures. St. Louis, Mosby, 1997.)*

a. Restrain infant securely. Place infant with head turned away from side of blood sampling. Position with towel roll under shoulders or with head over side of bed to extend neck and accentuate the posterior margin of the sternocleidomastoid muscle on the side of the venipuncture.
b. Prepare area with povidone-iodine or chlorhexidine and alcohol in a sterile fashion.
c. The external jugular vein will distend if its most proximal segment is occluded or if the child cries. The vein runs from the angle of the mandible to the posterior border of the lower third of the sternocleidomastoid muscle.
d. With continuous negative suction on the syringe, insert the needle at about a 30-degree angle to the skin. Continue as with any peripheral venipuncture.
e. Apply a sterile dressing, and put pressure on the puncture site for 5 minutes.

D. FEMORAL ARTERY AND FEMORAL VEIN PUNCTURE[1,2]

1. **Indications:** Venous or arterial blood sampling in patients with inadequate vascular access or during resuscitation.
2. **Contraindications:** Femoral puncture is particularly hazardous in neonates and is not recommended in this age group. There is also a risk in children for trauma to the femoral head and joint capsule. Avoid femoral punctures in children who have thrombocytopenia or coagulation disorders and in those who are scheduled for cardiac catheterization.
3. **Complications:** Infection, bleeding, hematoma of femoral triangle, thrombosis of vessel, osteomyelitis, and septic arthritis of hip.
4. **Procedure** (Fig. 3-2)**:**

a. Hold child securely in frog-leg position with the hips flexed and abducted. It may help to place a roll under the hips.
b. Prepare area in sterile fashion.
c. Locate femoral pulse just distal to the inguinal crease (**note that vein is medial to pulse**). Insert needle 2 cm distal to the inguinal ligament and 0.5 to 0.75 cm into the groin. Aspirate while maneuvering the needle until blood is obtained. Right femoral vein is easier to cannulate than left owing to straighter path to inferior vena cava.
d. Apply direct pressure for minimum of 5 minutes.

E. RADIAL ARTERY PUNCTURE AND CATHETERIZATION[1,2]

1. **Indications:** Arterial blood sampling or frequent blood gases and continuous blood pressure monitoring in an intensive care setting.
2. **Complications:** Infection, bleeding, occlusion of artery by hematoma or thrombosis, ischemia if ulnar circulation is inadequate.
3. **Procedure:**

a. Before procedure, test adequacy of ulnar blood flow with the Allen test. Clench the hand while simultaneously compressing ulnar and radial

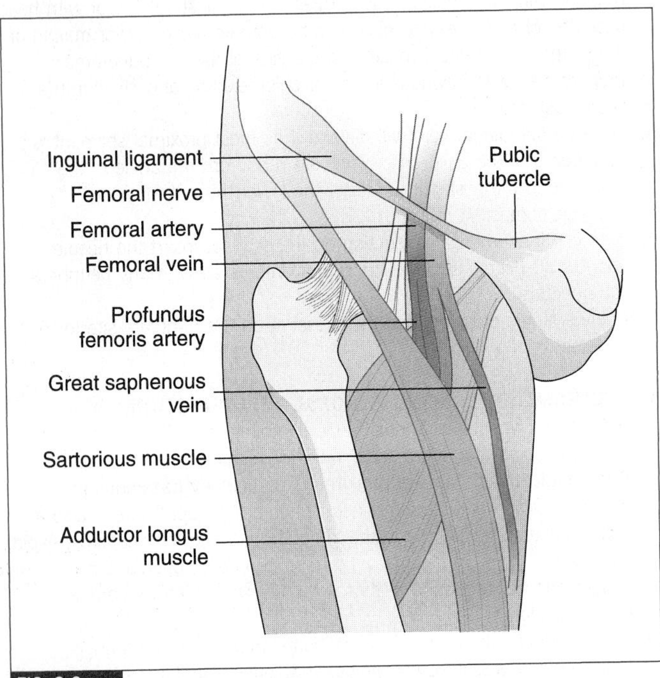

FIG. 3-2

Femoral artery and vein anatomy. *(From Dieckmann R, Selbst S: Pediatric Emergency and Critical Care Procedures. St. Louis, Mosby, 1997.)*

arteries. The hand will blanch. Release pressure from the ulnar artery, and observe the flushing response. Procedure is safe to perform if entire hand flushes.

b. Locate the radial pulse. It is optional to infiltrate the area over the point of maximal impulse with lidocaine. Avoid infusion into the vessel by aspirating before infusing. Prepare the site in sterile fashion.
   (1) Puncture: Insert butterfly needle attached to a syringe at a 30- to 60-degree angle over the point of maximal impulse; blood should flow freely into the syringe in a pulsatile fashion; suction may be required for plastic tubes. Once the sample is obtained, apply firm, constant pressure for 5 minutes and then place a pressure dressing on the puncture site.
   (2) Catheter placement: Secure the patient's hand to an arm board. Leave the fingers exposed to observe any color changes. Prepare

the wrist with sterile technique and infiltrate over the point of maximal impulse with 1% lidocaine. Make a small skin puncture over the point of maximal impulse with a needle, then discard the needle. Insert an IV catheter with its needle through the puncture site at a 30-degree angle to the horizontal; pass the needle and catheter through the artery to transfix it, then withdraw the needle. Very slowly, withdraw the catheter until free flow of blood is noted. Then advance the catheter and secure in place using sutures or tape. Seldinger technique using a guidewire can also be used. Apply a sterile dressing. Infuse heparinized isotonic fluid (per protocol) at 1 mL/hr. A pressure transducer may be attached to monitor blood pressure.

Note *Do not infuse any medications, blood products, or hypotonic or hypertonic solutions through an arterial line.*

F. POSTERIOR TIBIAL AND DORSALIS PEDIS ARTERY PUNCTURE[2]

1. **Indications:** Arterial blood sampling when radial artery puncture is unsuccessful or inaccessible.
2. **Complications:** Infection, bleeding, ischemia if inadequate circulation.
3. **Procedure (see section II.E for technique):**
   a. Posterior tibial artery: Puncture the artery posterior to the medial malleolus while holding the foot in dorsiflexion.
   b. Dorsalis pedis artery: Puncture the artery at the dorsal midfoot between the first and second toes while holding the foot in plantar flexion.

G. CENTRAL VENOUS CATHETER PLACEMENT[1,3]

1. **Indications:** To obtain emergency access to central venous circulation, to monitor central venous pressure, to deliver high-concentration parenteral nutrition or prolonged IV therapy, or to infuse blood products or large volumes of fluid.
2. **Complications:** Infection, bleeding, arterial or venous perforation, pneumothorax, hemothorax, thrombosis, catheter fragment in circulation, air embolism.
3. **Access sites:**
   a. External jugular vein.
   b. Subclavian vein.
   c. Internal jugular vein.
   d. Femoral vein.

Note *Femoral vein catheterization is contraindicated in severe abdominal trauma, and internal jugular catheterization is contraindicated in patients with elevated intracranial pressure (ICP).*

4. **Procedure: Seldinger technique.**

a. Secure patient, prepare site, and drape in sterile fashion.
b. Insert needle, applying negative pressure to locate vessel.
c. When there is blood return, insert a guidewire through the needle into the vein. Watch cardiac monitor for ectopy.
d. Remove the needle, holding the guidewire firmly.
e. Slip a catheter that has been preflushed with sterile saline over the wire into the vein in a twisting motion. The entry site may be enlarged with a small skin incision or dilator. Pass the entire catheter over the wire until the hub is at the skin surface. Slowly remove the wire, secure the catheter by suture, and attach IV infusion.
f. Apply a sterile dressing over the site.
g. For neck vessels, obtain a chest radiograph to rule out pneumothorax.

5. **Approach:**

a. **External jugular (see Fig. 3-1):** Place patient in 15- to 20-degree Trendelenburg position. Turn the head 45 degrees to the contralateral side. Enter the vein at the point where it crosses the sternocleidomastoid muscle.
b. **Internal jugular:** Place patient in 15- to 20-degree Trendelenburg position. Hyperextend the neck to tense the sternocleidomastoid muscle, and turn head away from the site of line placement. Palpate the sternal and clavicular heads of the muscle and enter at the apex of the triangle formed. An alternative landmark for puncture is halfway between the sternal notch and tip of the mastoid process. Insert the needle at a 30-degree angle to the skin, and aim toward the ipsilateral nipple. When blood flow is obtained, continue with Seldinger technique. Right side is preferable because of straight course to right atrium, absence of thoracic duct, and lower pleural dome on right side.
c. **Subclavian vein (Fig. 3-3):** Position the child in the Trendelenburg position with a towel roll under the thoracic spine to hyperextend the back. Aim the needle under the distal third of the clavicle toward the sternal notch. When blood flow is obtained, continue with Seldinger technique.

   Note *This is the least common site for central lines because of the increased risk for complications.*

d. **Femoral vein (Fig. 3-4):** Hold the child securely with the hip flexed and abducted. Locate the femoral pulse just distal to the inguinal crease. In infants, vein is 5 to 6 mm *medial* to arterial pulse. In adolescents, vein is usually 10 to 15 mm *medial* to the pulse. Place the thumb of the nondominant hand on the femoral artery. Insert the needle medial to the thumb. The needle should enter the skin 2 to 3 cm distal to the inguinal ligament at a 30-degree angle to avoid entering the abdomen. When blood flow is obtained, continue with Seldinger technique.

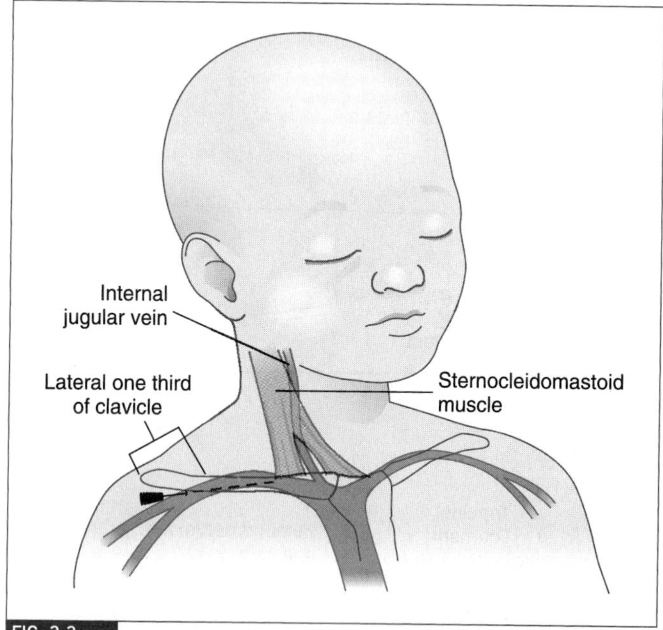

FIG. 3-3

Subclavian vein cannulation. *(From Dieckmann R, Selbst S: Pediatric Emergency and Critical Care Procedures. St. Louis, Mosby, 1997.)*

H. INTRAOSSEOUS (IO) INFUSION[1,2] (Fig. 3-5)

1. **Indications:** Obtain emergency access in children during life-threatening situations. This is very useful during cardiopulmonary arrest, shock, burns, and life-threatening status epilepticus. IO line can be used to infuse medications, blood products, or fluids. The IO needle should be removed once adequate vascular access has been established.
2. **Complications:**
   a. Complications are rare, particularly with correct technique. Frequency of complications increases with prolonged infusions.
   b. Extravasation of fluid from incomplete cortex penetration, infection, bleeding, osteomyelitis, compartment syndrome, fat embolism, fracture, epiphyseal injury.
3. **Sites of entry (in order of preference):**
   a. Anteromedial surface of the proximal tibia, 2 cm below and 1 to 2 cm medial to the tibial tuberosity on the flat part of the bone (see Fig. 3-5).
   b. Distal femur 3 cm above the lateral condyle in the midline.

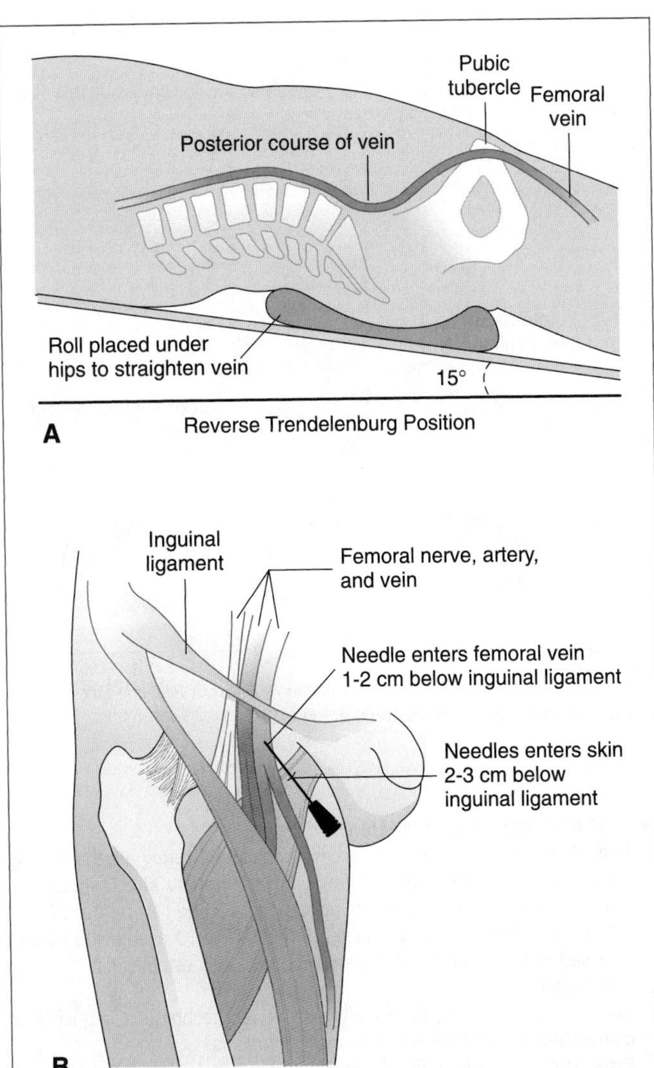

FIG. 3-4

Femoral vein cannulation. *(From Dieckmann R, Selbst S: Pediatric Emergency and Critical Care Procedures. St. Louis, Mosby, 1997.)*

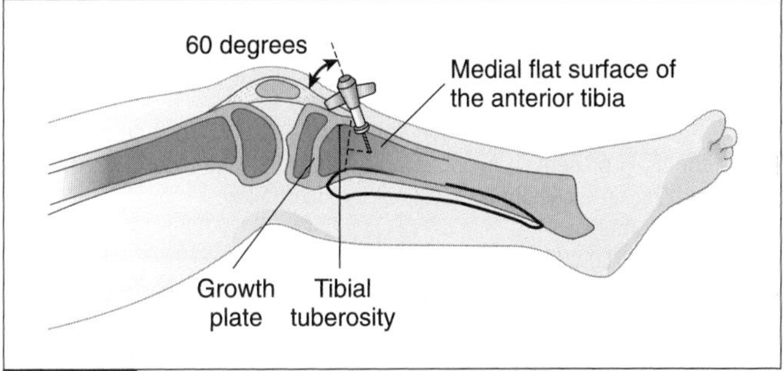

FIG. 3-5

Intraosseous needle placement using standard anterior tibial approach. The insertion point is in the midline on the medial flat surface of the anterior tibia, 1 to 3 cm (2 fingerbreadths) below the tibial tuberosity. *(From Dieckmann R, Selbst S: Pediatric Emergency and Critical Care Procedures. St. Louis, Mosby, 1997.)*

c. Medial surface of the distal tibia 1 to 2 cm above the medial malleolus (may be a more effective site in older children).
d. Anterosuperior iliac spine at an angle of 90 degrees to the long axis of the body.

4. Procedure:

a. Prepare the selected site in sterile fashion if situation allows.
b. If the child is conscious, anesthetize the puncture site down to the periosteum with 1% lidocaine (optional in emergency situations).
c. Insert a 15- to 18-gauge IO needle perpendicular to the skin at angle away from epiphyseal plate and advance to the periosteum. With a boring rotary motion, penetrate through the cortex until there is a decrease in resistance, indicating that you have reached the marrow. The needle should stand firmly without support. Secure the needle carefully.
d. Remove the stylet, and attempt to aspirate marrow. (Note that it is not necessary to aspirate marrow.) Flush with 10 to 20 mL heparinized normal saline (NS). Observe for fluid extravasation. Marrow can be sent for determination of glucose levels, chemistries, blood type and cross-match, hemoglobin, blood gas analysis, and cultures.
e. Attach standard IV tubing. Any crystalloid, blood product, or drug that may be infused into a peripheral vein may also be infused into the IO space, but an increased pressure (through pressure bag or push) is needed for infusion. There is a high risk for obstruction if continuous high-pressure fluids are not flushed through the IO needle.

I. UMBILICAL ARTERY (UA) AND VEIN (UV) CATHETERIZATION[1]

1. **Indications:** Vascular access (via UV), blood pressure (via UA), and blood gas (via UA) monitoring in critically ill neonates.

2. **Complications:** Infection, bleeding, hemorrhage, perforation of vessel; thrombosis with distal embolization; ischemia or infarction of lower extremities, bowel, or kidney; arrhythmia if the catheter is in the heart; air embolus.
3. **Caution:** UA catheterization should never be performed if omphalitis or peritonitis is present. It is contraindicated in the presence of possible necrotizing enterocolitis or intestinal hypoperfusion.
4. **Line placement:**

a. Arterial line: Low line versus high line.

(1) **Low line:** The tip of the catheter should lie just above the aortic bifurcation between L3 and L5. This avoids renal and mesenteric arteries near L1, perhaps decreasing the incidence of thrombosis or ischemia.

(2) **High line:** The tip of the catheter should be above the diaphragm between T6 and T9. A high line may be recommended in infants weighing less than 750 g, in whom a low line could easily slip out.

b. UV catheters should be placed in the inferior vena cava above the level of the ductus venosus and the hepatic veins and below the level of the right atrium.

c. Catheter length: Determine the length of catheter required using either a standardized graph or the regression formula. Add length for the height of the umbilical stump.

(1) **Standardized graph:** Determine the shoulder-umbilical length by measuring the perpendicular line dropped from the tip of the shoulder to the level of the umbilicus. Use the graph in **Figure 3-6** to determine the arterial catheter length, and the graph in **Figure 3-7** to determine venous catheter length.

(2) **Birth weight (BW) regression formula:**

$$\text{Low line: UA catheter length (cm)} = \text{BW (kg)} + 7.$$

$$\text{High line: UA catheter length (cm)} = [3 \times \text{BW (kg)}] + 9.$$

$$\text{UV catheter length (cm)} = [0.5 \times \text{high line UA (cm)}] + 1.$$

Note *Formula may not be appropriate for small-for-gestational-age (SGA) or large-for-gestational-age (LGA) infants.*

5. **Procedure for UA line (Fig. 3-8):**

a. Determine the length of the catheter to be inserted for either high (T6 to T9) or low (L3 to L5) position.

b. Restrain the infant. Prepare and drape the umbilical cord and adjacent skin using sterile technique. Maintaining the infant's temperature is critical.

c. Flush the catheter with a sterile saline solution before insertion.

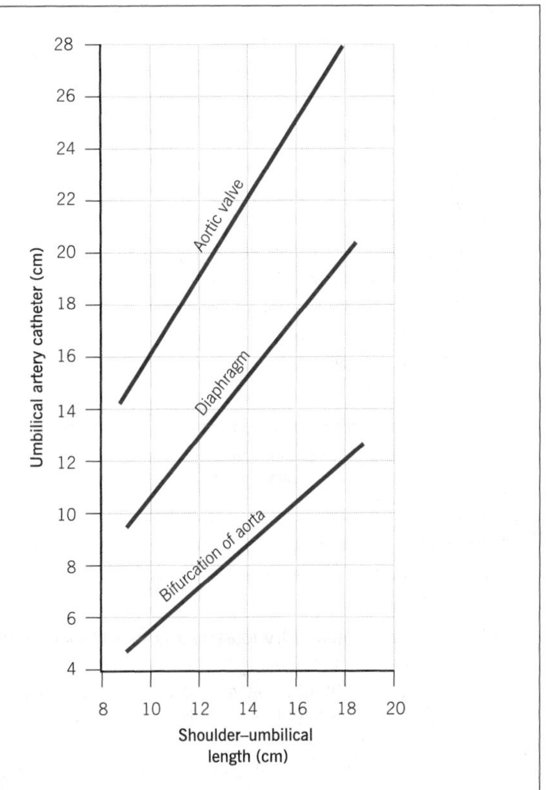

FIG. 3-6
Umbilical artery catheter length.

d. Place sterile umbilical tape around the base of the cord. Cut through the cord horizontally about 1.5 to 2.0 cm from the skin; tighten the umbilical tape to prevent bleeding.
e. Identify the one large, thin-walled umbilical vein and two smaller, thick-walled arteries. Use one tip of open, curved forceps to probe and dilate one artery gently; use both points of closed forceps, and dilate artery by allowing forceps to open gently.
f. Grasp the catheter 1 cm from its tip with toothless forceps, and insert the catheter into the lumen of the artery. Aim the tip toward the feet, and gently advance the catheter to the desired distance. Do not force. If

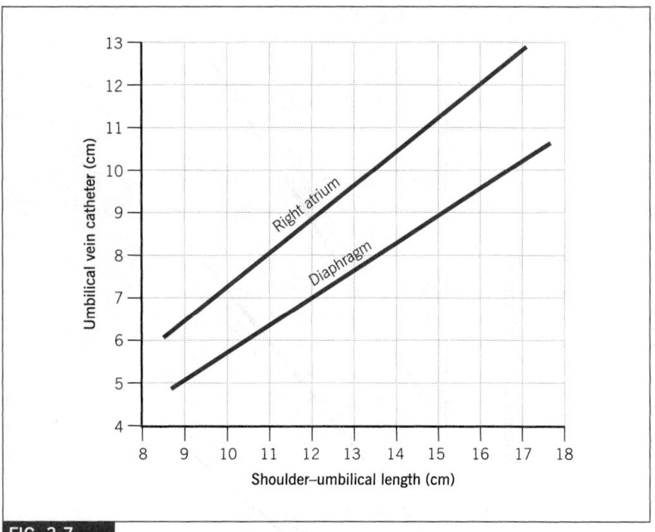

FIG. 3-7
Umbilical vein catheter length.

resistance is encountered, try loosening umbilical tape; applying steady, gentle pressure; or manipulating the angle of the umbilical cord to skin. Often the catheter cannot be advanced because of creation of a "false luminal tract." There should be good blood return when the catheter enters the iliac artery.

g. Confirm the position of the catheter tip radiologically. Secure the catheter with a suture through the cord, a marker tape, and a tape bridge. The catheter may be pulled back but not advanced once the sterile field is broken.
h. Observe for complications: Blanching or cyanosis of lower extremities, perforation, thrombosis, embolism, or infection. If any complications occur, the catheter should be removed.

Note *There are no definitive guidelines on feeding with a UA catheter in place. There is concern (up to 24 hours after removal) that the UA catheter or thrombus may interfere with intestinal perfusion. A risk-to-benefit assessment should be individualized. Use isotonic fluids, which contain 0.5 U/mL of heparin. Never use hypo-osmolar fluids in the UA.*

6. Procedure for UV line (see Fig. 3-8):

a. Follow steps A–D for UA catheter placement. However, determine catheter length using Figure 3-7.

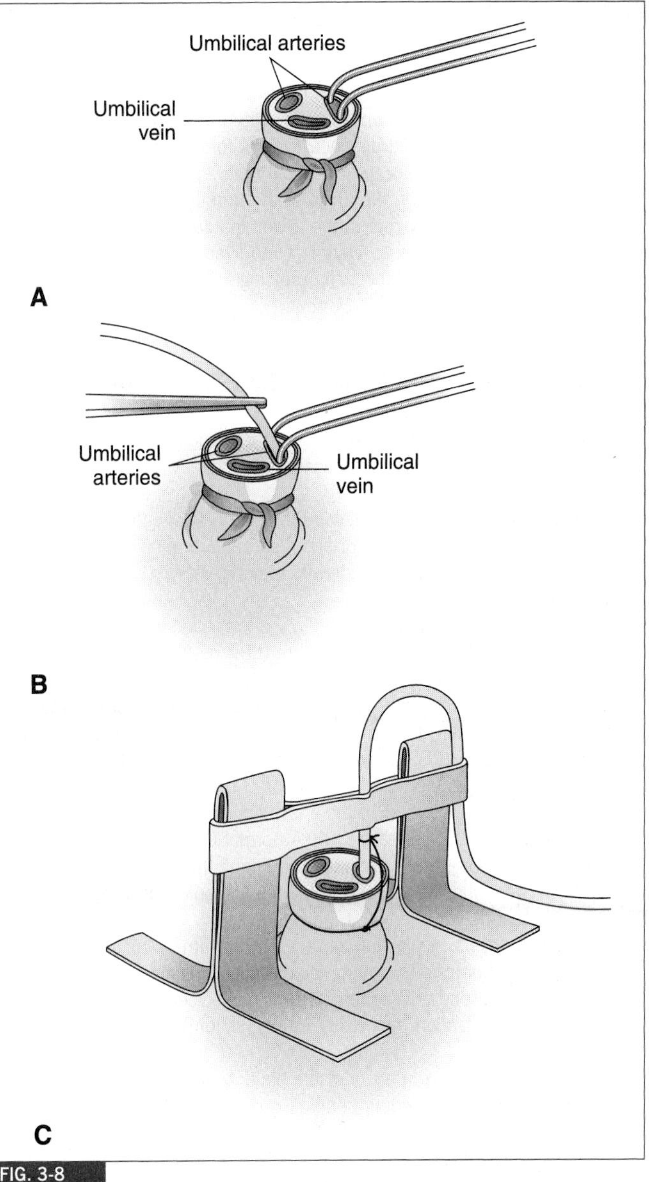

FIG. 3-8

Placement of umbilical arterial catheter. *A*, Dilating the lumen of umbilical artery. *B*, Insertion of umbilical artery catheter. *C*, Securing the catheter to the abdominal wall using a "bridge" method of taping. *(From Dieckmann R, Selbst S: Pediatric Emergency and Critical Care Procedures. St. Louis, Mosby, 1997.)*

b. Isolate the thin-walled umbilical vein, clear thrombi with forceps, and insert catheter, aiming the tip toward the right shoulder. Gently advance the catheter to the desired distance. Do not force. If resistance is encountered, try loosening the umbilical tape; applying steady, gentle pressure; or manipulating the angle of the umbilical cord to skin. Resistance is commonly met at the abdominal wall and again at the portal system. Do not infuse anything into liver.

c. Confirm position of the catheter tip radiologically. Secure catheter as described in step G for UA placement.

III. BODY FLUID SAMPLING

A. LUMBAR PUNCTURE[1,2]

1. **Indications:** Examination of spinal fluid for suspected infection or malignancy, instillation of intrathecal chemotherapy, or measurement of opening pressure.
2. **Complications:** Local pain, infection, bleeding, spinal fluid leak, hematoma, spinal headache, or acquired epidermal spinal cord tumor (caused by implantation of epidermal material into spinal canal if no stylet is used on skin entry).
3. **Cautions and contraindications:**

a. **Increased ICP:** Before lumbar puncture (LP), perform funduscopic examination. The presence of papilledema, retinal hemorrhage, or clinical suspicion of increased ICP may be contraindications to the procedure. A sudden drop in intraspinal pressure by rapid release of cerebrospinal fluid (CSF) may cause fatal herniation. If LP is to be performed, proceed with extreme caution. Computed tomography (CT) may be indicated before LP if there is suspected intracranial bleeding, focal mass lesion, or increased ICP. A normal CT scan does not rule out increased ICP but usually excludes conditions that may put the patient at risk for herniation. Decision to obtain CT should not delay appropriate antibiotic therapy if indicated.

b. **Bleeding diathesis:** A platelet count >50,000/mm^3 is desirable before LP, and correction of any clotting factor deficiencies can minimize the risk for bleeding and subsequent cord or nerve root compression.

c. Overlying skin infection may result in inoculation of CSF with organisms.

d. LP should be deferred in an unstable patient, and appropriate therapy should be initiated, including antibiotics if indicated.

4. **Procedure:**

a. Apply local anesthetic cream if sufficient time is available.

b. Position the child in either the sitting position (Fig. 3-9) or lateral recumbent position (Fig. 3-10), with hips, knees, and neck flexed. Do not compromise a small infant's cardiorespiratory status by positioning.

c. Locate the desired intervertebral space (either L3-4 or L4-5) by drawing an imaginary line between the top of the iliac crests.

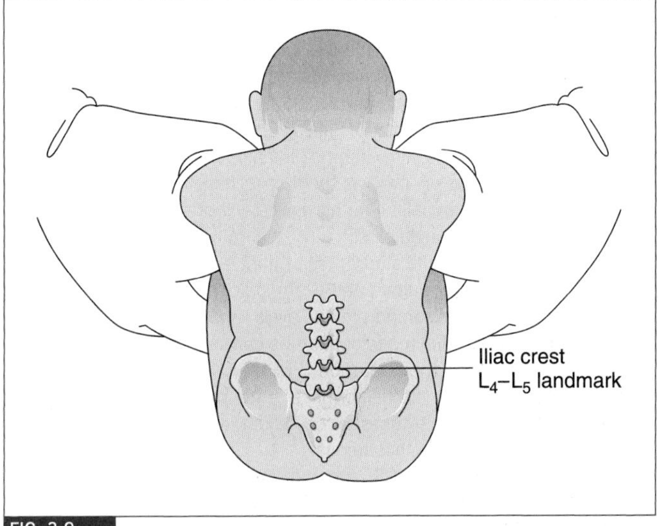

FIG. 3-9

Lumbar puncture site in the sitting position. *(From Dieckmann R, Selbst S: Pediatric Emergency and Critical Care Procedures. St. Louis, Mosby, 1997.)*

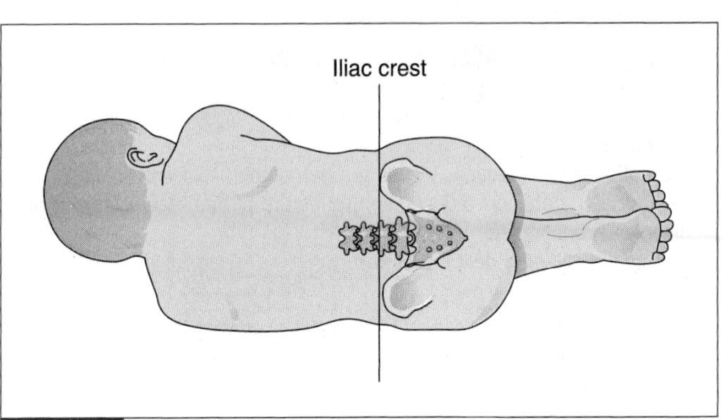

FIG. 3-10

Lumbar puncture site in lateral (recumbent) position. *(From Dieckmann R, Selbst S: Pediatric Emergency and Critical Care Procedures. St. Louis, Mosby, 1997.)*

d. Prepare the skin in sterile fashion. Drape conservatively so that it is possible to monitor the infant. Use a 20- to 22-gauge spinal needle with stylet (1.5-inch for children younger than 12 years of age, 3.5 inches for children 12 years and older). A smaller-gauge needle will decrease the incidence of spinal headache and CSF leak.

e. The overlying skin and interspinous tissue can be anesthetized with 1% lidocaine using a 25-gauge needle.
f. Puncture the skin in the midline just caudad to the palpated spinous process, angling slightly cephalad toward the umbilicus. Advance several millimeters at a time and withdraw the stylet frequently to check for CSF flow. The needle may be advanced without the stylet once it is completely through the skin. In small infants, one may *not* feel a change in resistance or "pop" as the dura is penetrated.
g. If resistance is met initially (you hit bone), withdraw needle to the skin surface and redirect angle slightly.
h. Send CSF for appropriate studies (see Chapter 25 for normal values). Send the first tube for culture and Gram stain, the second tube for measurement of glucose and protein levels, and the last tube for cell count and differential. An additional tube can be collected for viral cultures, polymerase chain reaction (PCR), or CSF metabolic studies if indicated. If subarachnoid hemorrhage or traumatic tap is suspected, send the first and fourth tubes for cell count, and ask the laboratory to examine the CSF for xanthochromia.
i. Accurate measurement of CSF pressure can be made only with the patient lying quietly on his or her side in an unflexed position. It is not a reliable measurement in the sitting position. Once free flow of spinal fluid is obtained, attach the manometer and measure CSF pressure. Opening pressure is recorded as level at which CSF is steady.

B. CHEST TUBE PLACEMENT AND THORACENTESIS[1,3]

1. **Indications:** Evacuation of a pneumothorax, hemothorax, chylothorax, large pleural effusion, or empyema for diagnostic or therapeutic purposes.
2. **Complications:** Infection; bleeding; pneumothorax; hemothorax; pulmonary contusion or laceration; puncture of diaphragm, spleen or liver; or bronchopleural fistula.
3. **Procedure: Needle decompression.**

Note *For tension pneumothoraces, it is imperative to attempt decompression quickly by inserting a large-bore needle (14 to 22 gauge, based on size) in the anterior second intercostal space in the mid-clavicular line. Insert needle over superior aspect of rib margin to avoid vascular structures.*

a. When the pleural space is entered, attach catheter to a three-way stopcock and syringe, and aspirate air.
b. Subsequent insertion of a chest tube is still necessary.

4. **Procedure (Fig. 3-11): Chest tube insertion (see inside front cover for chest tube sizes):**

a. Position child supine or with affected side up with arm restrained over the head.

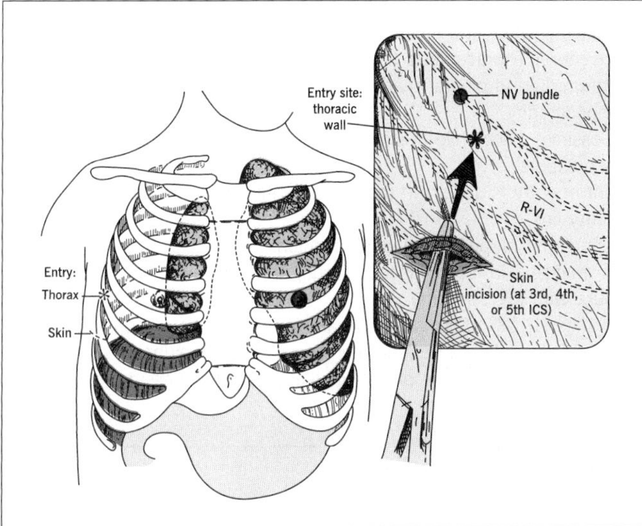

FIG. 3-11

Technique for insertion of chest tube. ICS, intercostal space; NV neurovascular; R-VI, sixth rib. *(Modified from Fleisher G, Ludwig S: Pediatric Emergency Medicine, 3rd ed. Baltimore, Williams & Wilkins, 2000.)*

b. Point of entry is the third to fifth intercostal space in the mid to anterior axillary line, usually at the level of the nipple (avoid breast tissue).
c. Prepare and drape in sterile fashion.
d. Patient may require sedation (see Formulary). Locally anesthetize skin, subcutaneous tissue, periosteum of rib, chest wall muscles, and pleura with 1% lidocaine.
e. Make sterile 1- to 3-cm incision one intercostal space below desired insertion point, and bluntly dissect with a hemostat through tissue layers until the superior portion of the rib is reached, avoiding the neurovascular bundle on the inferior portion of the rib.
f. Push the hemostat over the top of the rib, through the pleura, and into the pleural space. Enter the pleural space cautiously and not deeper than 1 cm. Spread hemostat to open, place chest tube in clamp, and guide through entry site to desired distance.
g. For a pneumothorax, insert the tube anteriorly toward the apex. For a pleural effusion, direct the tube inferiorly and posteriorly.
h. Secure the tube with pursestring sutures in which the suture is first tied at the skin, then wrapped around the tube once and tied at the tube.
i. Attach to a drainage system with –20 to –30 cm H_2O pressure.

j. Apply a sterile occlusive dressing.
k. Confirm position and function with chest radiograph.

5. Procedure: Thoracentesis (Fig. 3-12).

a. Confirm fluid in pleural space by clinical examination and radiographs or sonography.
b. If possible, place child in sitting position leaning over table; otherwise place supine.
c. Point of entry is usually in the seventh intercostal space and posterior axillary line.
d. Prepare and drape area in sterile fashion.
e. Anesthetize skin, subcutaneous tissue, rib periosteum, chest wall, and pleura with 1% lidocaine.
f. Advance an 18- to 22-gauge IV catheter or large-bore needle attached to a syringe onto the rib, and then "walk" over the superior aspect into the pleural space, while providing steady negative pressure; often a

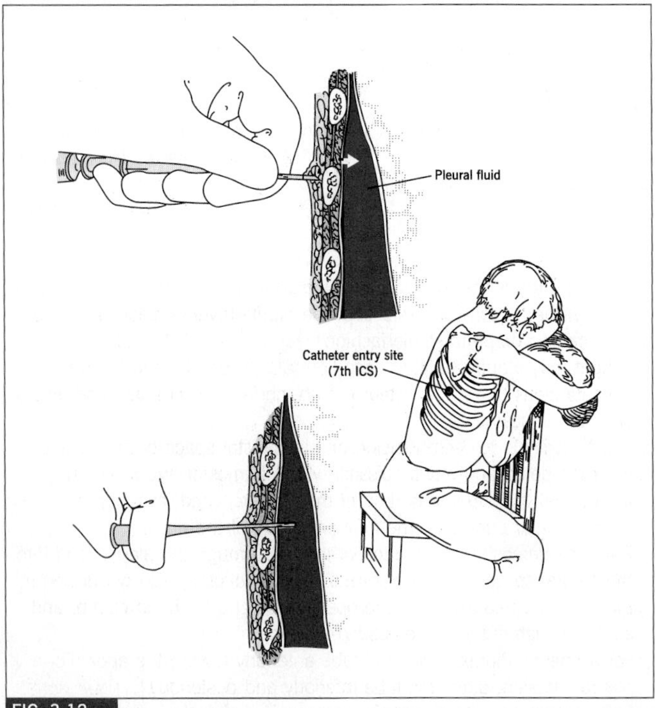

FIG. 3-12

Thoracentesis. ICS, intercostal space. *(Modified from Fleisher G, Ludwig S: Pediatric Emergency Medicine, 3rd ed. Baltimore, Williams & Wilkins, 2000.)*

popping sensation is generated. Be careful not to advance too far into the pleural cavity. If an IV or pigtail catheter (with guidewire) is used, the soft catheter may be advanced into the pleural space aiming downward.

g. Attach syringe and stopcock device to remove fluid for diagnostic studies and symptomatic relief (see Chapter 25 for evaluation of pleural fluid.)
h. After removing needle or catheter, place an occlusive dressing over the site and obtain a chest radiograph to rule out pneumothorax.

C. PERICARDIOCENTESIS[1,3]

1. **Indications:** To obtain pericardial fluid in cardiac tamponade emergently for diagnostic or therapeutic purposes.
2. **Complications:** Bleeding, infection, puncture of cardiac chamber, cardiac dysrhythmia, hemopericardium or pneumopericardium, pneumothorax, hemothorax, cardiac arrest, death.
3. **Procedure** (Fig. 3-13)**:**

a. Unless contraindicated, provide sedation and/or analgesia for the patient. Monitor electrocardiogram (ECG).
b. Place patient at a 30-degree angle (reverse Trendelenburg). Have patient secured.
c. Sterilely prepare and drape puncture site. A drape across the upper chest is unnecessary and may obscure important landmarks.
d. Anesthetize the puncture site with 1% lidocaine.
e. Insert an 18- or 20-gauge needle just to the left of the xiphoid process, 1 cm inferior to the bottom rib at about a 45-degree angle to the skin.
f. While gently aspirating, advance needle toward the patient's left shoulder until pericardial fluid is obtained.
g. Upon entering the pericardial space, clamp the needle at the skin edge with hemostat to prevent further penetration. Attach a 30-mL syringe with a stopcock.
h. Gently and slowly remove the fluid. Rapid withdrawal of the pericardial fluid can result in shock or myocardial insufficiency.
i. Send fluid for appropriate laboratory studies (see Chapter 25).
j. In nonemergent conditions, this is best performed under two-dimensional echocardiographic guidance.

D. PARACENTESIS[2]

1. **Indications:** Percutaneous removal of intraperitoneal fluid for diagnostic or therapeutic purposes.
2. **Complications:** Bleeding, infection, puncture of viscera.
3. **Cautions:**

a. Do not remove a large amount of fluid too rapidly because hypovolemia and hypotension may result from rapid fluid shifts.
b. Avoid scars from previous surgery; localized bowel adhesions increase the chances of entering a viscus in these areas.

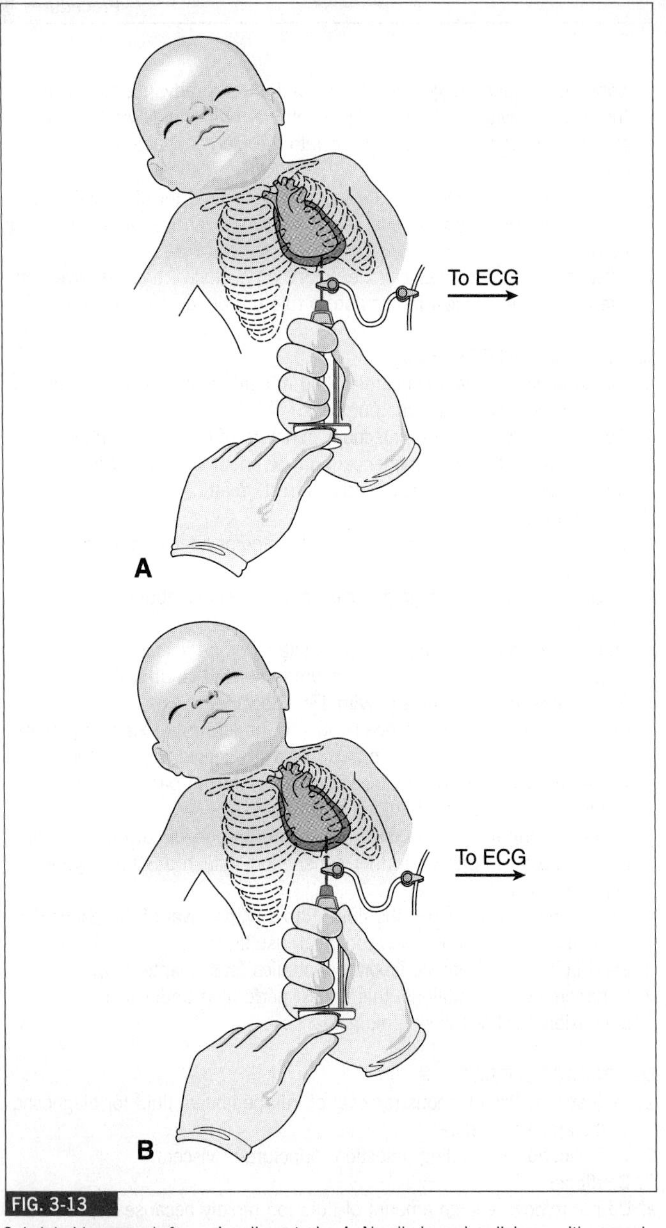

FIG. 3-13

Subxiphoid approach for pericardiocentesis. *A*, Needle in pericardial sac with normal electrocardiogram (ECG). *B*, Needle in heart with current of injury pattern on ECG. *(From Dieckmann R, Selbst S: Pediatric Emergency and Critical Care Procedures. St. Louis, Mosby, 1997.)*

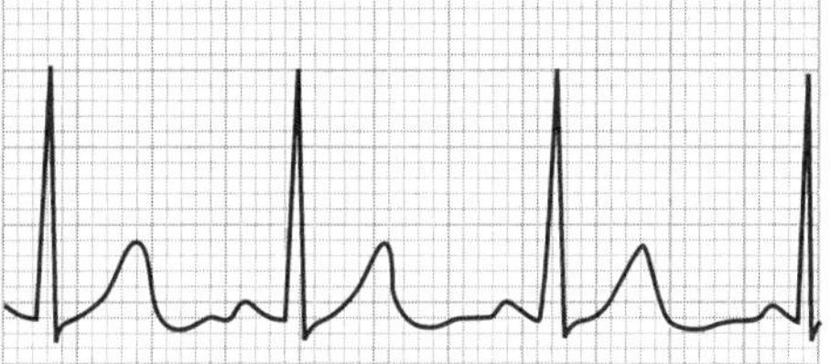

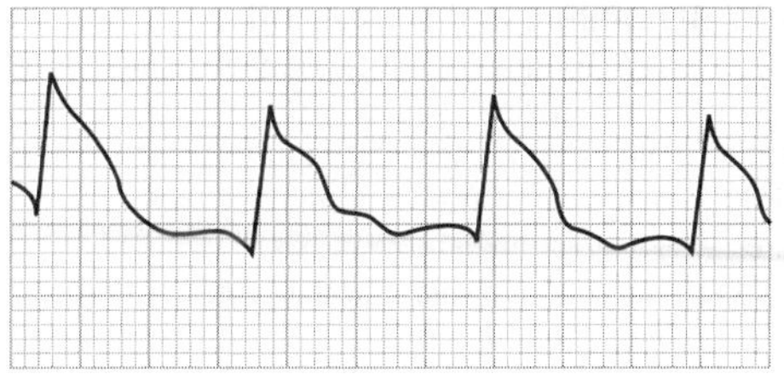

FIG. 3-13—cont'd

c. The bladder should be empty to avoid perforation.
d. Never perform paracentesis through an area of cellulitis.

4. **Procedure:**

a. Prepare and drape the abdomen as for a surgical procedure. Anesthetize the puncture site.
b. With the patient in semisupine, sitting, or lateral decubitus position, insert a 16- to 22-gauge IV catheter attached to a syringe in midline 2 cm below the umbilicus; in neonates, insert just lateral to the rectus muscle in the right or left lower quadrants, a few centimeters above the inguinal ligament.
c. Aiming cephalad, insert the needle at a 45-degree angle while one hand pulls the skin caudally until entering the peritoneal cavity. This creates a Z tract when the skin is released and the needle removed. Apply continuous negative pressure.
d. Once fluid appears in the syringe, remove introducer needle and leave catheter in place. Attach a stopcock and aspirate slowly until an adequate amount of fluid has been obtained for studies or symptomatic relief.
e. If, on entering the peritoneal cavity, air is aspirated, withdraw the needle immediately. Aspirated air indicates entrance into a hollow viscus. (In general, penetration of a hollow viscus during paracentesis does not lead to complications.) Repeat paracentesis with sterile equipment.
f. Send fluid for appropriate laboratory studies (see Chapter 25).

E. URINARY BLADDER CATHETERIZATION[2]

1. **Indications:** To obtain urine for urinalysis and culture sterilely and to accurately monitor hydration status.
2. **Complications:** Hematuria, infection, trauma to urethra or bladder, intravesical knot of catheter (rarely occurs).
3. **Procedure:**

a. Infant/child should not have voided within 1 hour of procedure.

Note *Catheterization is contraindicated in pelvic fractures, known trauma to the urethra, or blood at the meatus.*

b. Prepare the urethral opening using sterile technique.
c. In boys, apply gentle traction to the penis to straighten the urethra.
d. Gently insert a lubricated catheter into the urethra. Slowly advance the catheter until resistance is met at the external sphincter. Continued pressure will overcome this resistance, and the catheter will enter the bladder. In girls, the urethral orifice may be difficult to visualize, but it is usually immediately anterior to the vaginal orifice. Only a few centimeters of advancement is required to reach the bladder in girls. In boys, insert a few centimeters longer than the shaft of the penis.

e. Carefully remove the catheter once the specimen is obtained, and cleanse skin of iodine.
f. If indwelling Foley catheter is inserted, inflate balloon with sterile water as indicated on bulb, then connect catheter to drainage tubing attached to urine drainage bag. Secure catheter tubing to inner thigh.

F. SUPRAPUBIC BLADDER ASPIRATION[1]

1. **Indications:** To obtain urine for urinalysis and culture sterilely in children less than 2 years of age (avoid in children with genitourinary tract anomalies, coagulopathy, or intestinal obstruction). Bypasses distal urethra, thereby minimizing risk for contamination.
2. **Complications:** Infection (cellulitis), hematuria (usually microscopic), intestinal perforation.
3. **Procedure** (Fig. 3-14):

a. Anterior rectal pressure in girls or gentle penile pressure in boys may be used to prevent urination during the procedure. Child should not have voided within 1 hour of procedure.
b. Restrain the infant in the supine, frog-leg position. Prepare suprapubic area in sterile fashion.
c. The site for puncture is 1 to 2 cm above the symphysis pubis in the midline. Use a syringe with a 22-gauge, 1-inch needle, and puncture at a 10- to 20-degree angle to the perpendicular, aiming slightly caudad.
d. Exert suction gently as the needle is advanced until urine enters syringe. The needle should not be advanced more than 1 inch. Aspirate the urine with gentle suction.
e. Cleanse skin of iodine.

G. SOFT TISSUE ASPIRATION[5]

1. **Indications:** Cellulitis that is unresponsive to initial standard therapy, recurrent cellulitis or abscesses, immunocompromised patients in whom organism recovery is necessary and may affect antimicrobial therapy.
2. **Complications:** Pain, infection, bleeding.
3. **Procedure:**

a. Select site to aspirate at *point of maximal inflammation* (more likely to increase recovery of causative agent than leading edge of erythema or center).[5]
b. Clean area in sterile fashion.
c. Local anesthesia with 1% lidocaine is optional.
d. Fill tuberculin syringe with 0.1 to 0.2 mL of *nonbacteriostatic* sterile saline and attach to needle.
e. Using 18- or 20-gauge needle (22-gauge for facial cellulitis), advance to appropriate depth and apply negative pressure while withdrawing needle.

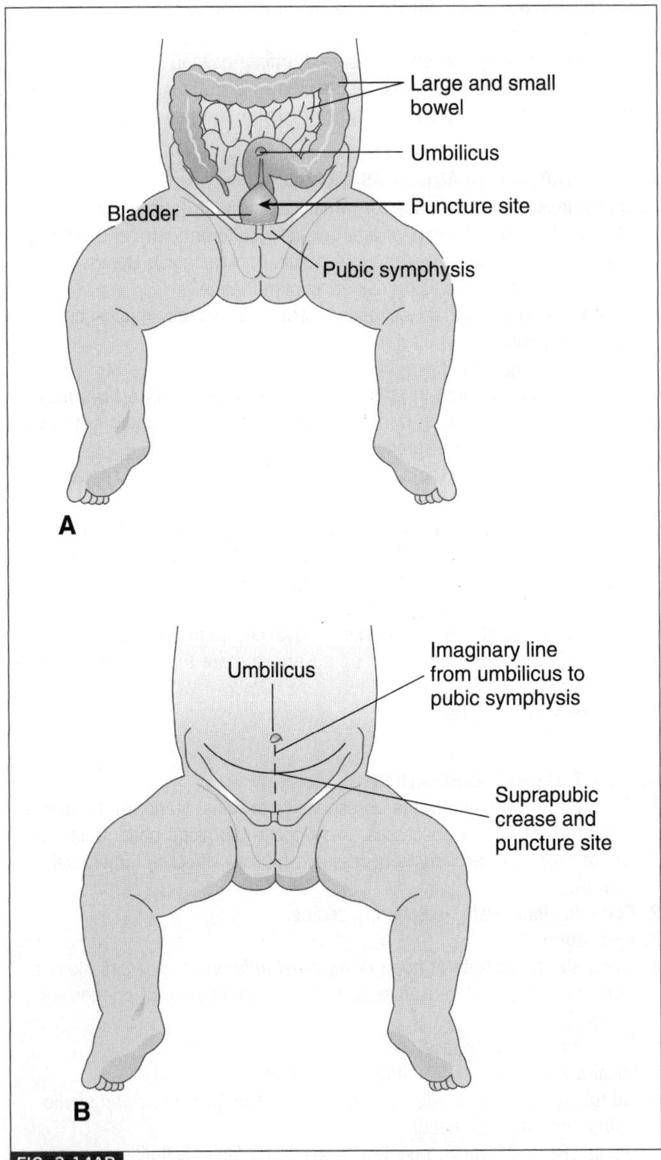

FIG. 3-14AB
Landmarks for suprapubic bladder aspiration. *(From Dieckmann R, Selbst S: Pediatric Emergency and Critical Care Procedures. St. Louis, Mosby, 1997.)*

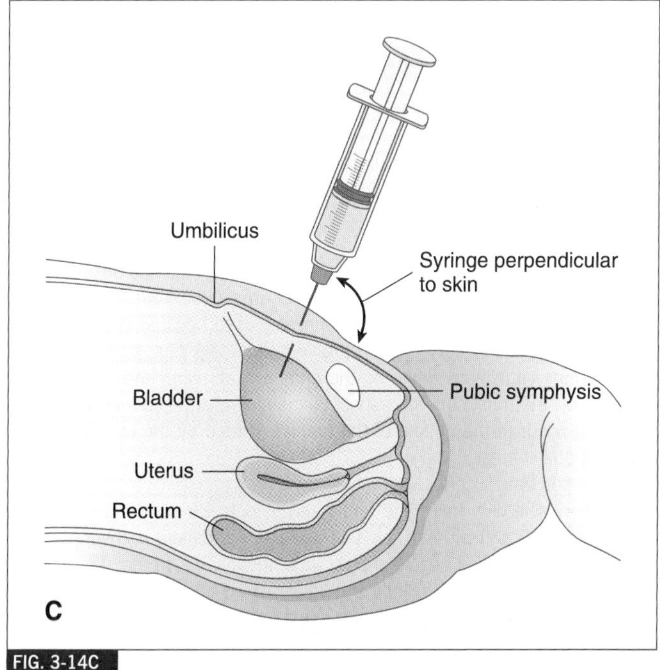

FIG. 3-14C

f. Send fluid from aspiration for Gram stain and cultures. If no fluid is obtained, you can streak needle on agar plate. Consider AFB and fungal stains in immunocompromised patients.

IV. IMMUNIZATION AND MEDICATION ADMINISTRATION[2]

A. SUBCUTANEOUS INJECTIONS

1. **Indications:** Immunizations and other medications.
2. **Complications:** Bleeding, infection, allergic reaction, lipohypertrophy or lipoatrophy after repeated injections.
3. **Procedure:**

a. Locate injection site: Upper outer arm or outer aspect of upper thigh.
b. Clean skin with alcohol.
c. Insert 0.5-inch, 25- or 27-gauge needle into the subcutaneous layer at a 45-degree angle to the skin. Aspirate for blood, then inject medication.

B. INTRAMUSCULAR INJECTIONS

1. **Indications:** Immunizations and other medications.
2. **Complications:** Bleeding, infection, allergic reaction, nerve injury.
3. **Cautions:**
   a. Avoid intramuscular (IM) injections in a child with a bleeding disorder or thrombocytopenia.
   b. Maximum volume to be injected is 0.5 mL in a small infant, 1 mL in an older infant, 2 mL in a school-aged child, and 3 mL in an adolescent.
4. **Procedure:**
   a. Locate injection site: Anterolateral upper thigh (vastus lateralis muscle) in smaller child, or outer aspect of upper arm (deltoid) in older one. The dorsal gluteal region is less commonly used because of risk for nerve or vascular injury. To find the ventral gluteal site, form a triangle by placing your index finger on the anterior iliac spine and your middle finger on the most superior aspect of the iliac crest. The injection should occur in the middle of the triangle formed by the two fingers and the iliac crest.
   b. Clean skin with alcohol.
   c. Pinch muscle with free hand and insert 1-inch, 23- or 25-gauge needle until the hub is flush with the skin surface. For deltoid and ventral gluteal muscles, the needle should be perpendicular to the skin. For the anterolateral thigh, the needle should be 45 degrees to the long axis of the thigh. Aspirate for blood, then inject medication.

V. BASIC LACERATION REPAIR[1]

A. SUTURING

1. **Techniques** (Fig. 3-15):
   a. Simple interrupted.
   b. Horizontal mattress: Provides eversion of wound edges.
   c. Vertical mattress: For added strength in areas of thick skin or areas of skin movement; provides eversion of wound edges.
   d. Running intradermal: For cosmetic closures.
2. **Procedure:**

Note *Lacerations of the face, lips, hands, genitalia, mouth, or periorbital area may require consultation with a specialist. Ideally, lacerations at increased risk for infection (areas with poor blood supply, contaminated/crush injury) should be sutured within 6 hours of injury. Clean wounds in cosmetically important areas may be closed up to 24 hours after injury in the absence of significant contamination or devitalization. In general, bite wounds should not be sutured except in areas of high cosmetic importance (face). The longer sutures are left in place, the greater the scarring and potential for infection. Sutures in cosmetically sensitive areas should be removed as soon as possible. Sutures in high-tension areas, such as extensor surfaces, should stay in longer* (Table 3-1).

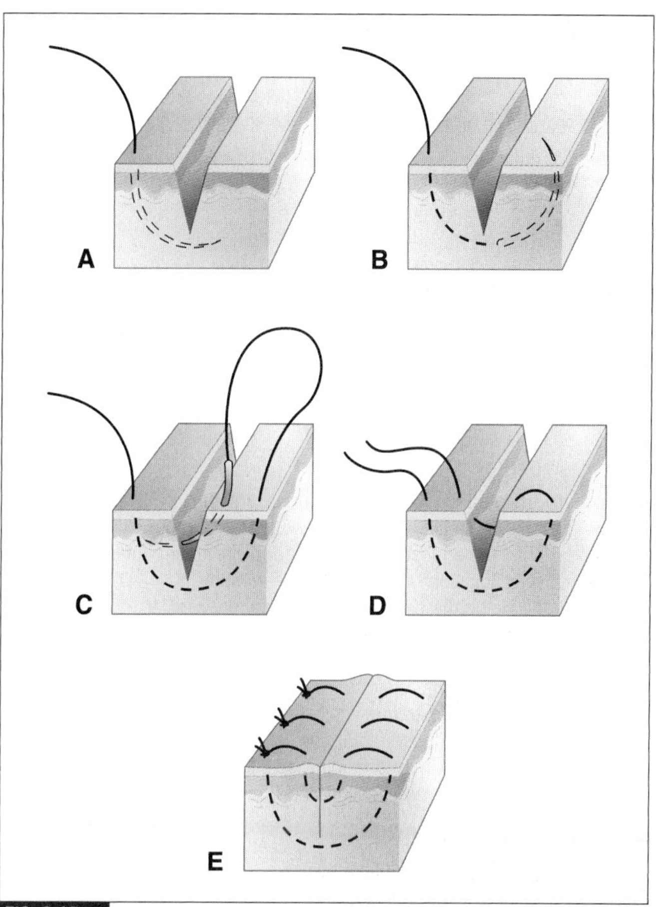

FIG. 3-15

A-E, The vertical mattress suture. After initial placement of a simple interrupted stitch with a larger bite, make a backhand pass across the wound, taking small, superficial bites. When the knot is tied, the edges of the laceration should evert slightly. *(From Dieckmann R, Selbst S: Pediatric Emergency and Critical Care Procedures. St. Louis, Mosby, 1997.)*

a. Prepare child for procedure with appropriate sedation, analgesia, and restraint.
b. Anesthetize the wound with topical anesthetic or with lidocaine-bicarbonate by injecting the anesthetic into the subcutaneous tissues (see Formulary).

TABLE 3-1

GUIDELINES FOR SUTURE MATERIAL, SIZE, AND REMOVAL

Body Region	Monofilament* (for Superficial Lacerations)	Absorbable† (for Deep Lacerations)	Duration (days)
Scalp	5–0 or 4–0	4–0	5–7
Face	6–0	5–0	3–5
Eyelid	7–0 or 6–0	—	3–5
Eyebrow	6–0 or 5–0	5–0	3–5
Trunk	5–0 or 4–0	3–0	5–7
Extremities	5–0 or 4–0	4–0	7
Joint surface	4–0	—	10–14
Hand	5–0	5–0	7
Foot sole	4–0 or 3–0	4–0	7–10

*Examples of monofilament nonabsorbable sutures: nylon, polypropylene.

†Examples of absorbable sutures: polyglycolic acid and polyglactin 910 (Vicryl).

c. Forcefully irrigate the wound with copious amounts of sterile NS. Use at least 250 mL for smaller, superficial wounds and more for larger wounds. This is the most important step in preventing infection. Avoid high-pressure irrigation of deep puncture wounds.
d. Prepare and drape the patient for a sterile procedure.
e. Debride the wound when indicated. Probe for foreign bodies as indicated. Consider obtaining a radiograph if a radiopaque foreign body was involved in the injury.
f. Select suture type for percutaneous closure (see Table 3-1).
g. When suturing is complete, apply topical antibiotic and sterile dressing. If laceration is in proximity of a joint, splinting of the affected area to limit mobility often speeds healing and prevents wound separation.
h. Check wounds at 48 to 72 hours in cases in which wounds are of questionable viability, if wound was packed, or for patients prescribed prophylactic antibiotics. Change dressing at check.
i. For hand lacerations, close skin only; do not use subcutaneous stitches. Elevate and immobilize the hand.
j. Consider the child's need for tetanus prophylaxis.

VI. MUSCULOSKELETAL

A. BASIC SPLINTING[1]

1. **Indications:** To provide short-term stabilization of limb injuries.
2. **Complications:** Pressure sores, dermatitis, neurovascular impairment.
3. **Procedure:**

a. Determine style of splint needed.
b. Measure and cut fiberglass or plaster to appropriate length. If using plaster, upper-extremity splints require 8 to 10 layers, and lower-extremity splints require 12 to 14 layers.

c. Pad extremity with cotton Webril, taking care to overlap each turn by 50%. In prepackaged fiberglass splints, additional padding is not generally required. Bony prominences may require additional padding. Place cotton between digits if they are in a splint.
d. Immerse plaster slabs into room-temperature water until bubbling stops. Smooth out wet plaster slab, avoiding any wrinkles.
   Warning: Plaster becomes hot after drying.
e. Position splint over extremity and wrap externally with gauze. When dry, an elastic wrap can be added.
f. Alternatively, wet one side of fiberglass until saturated. Roll or fold to remove excess water. Mold splint as indicated. *Note*: Using warm water will decrease drying time. This may result in inadequate time to mold splint. Turn edge of the splint back on itself to produce a smooth surface. Take care to cover the sharp edges of fiberglass. When dry, wrap with elastic bandage.
g. Use crutches or slings as indicated.
h. The need for orthopedic referral should be individually assessed.

B. LONG ARM POSTERIOR SPLINT (Fig. 3-16)

1. **Indications:** Immobilization of elbow and forearm injuries.

C. SUGAR TONG FOREARM SPLINT (Fig. 3-17)

1. **Indications:** For distal radius and wrist fractures, to immobilize the elbow and minimize pronation and supination.

D. ULNAR GUTTER SPLINT

1. **Indications:** Nonrotated fourth or fifth (boxer) metacarpal metaphyseal fracture with less than 20 degrees of angulation, uncomplicated fourth and fifth phalangeal fracture.

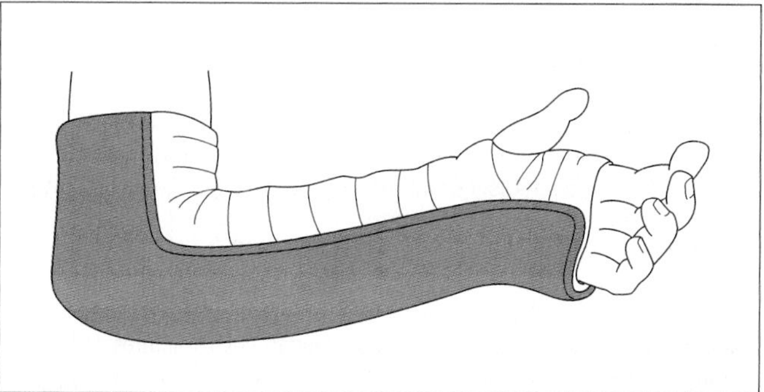

FIG. 3-16
Long arm posterior splint.

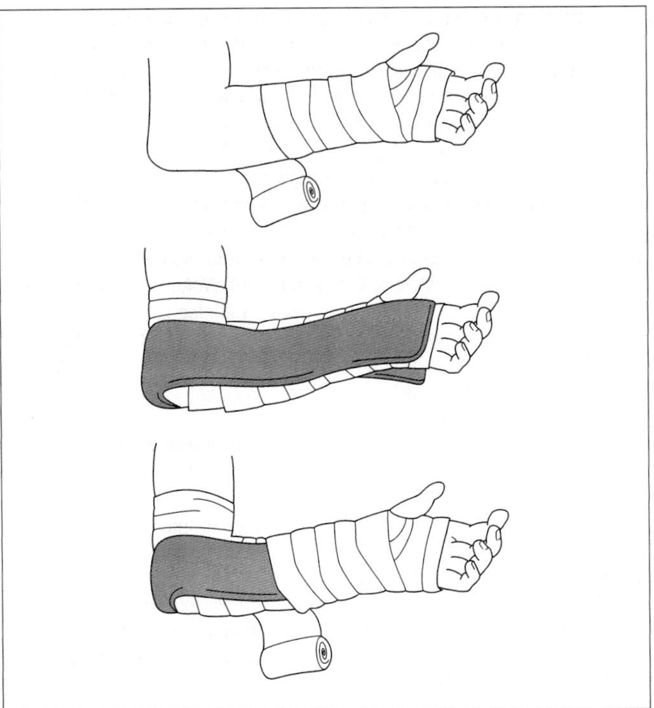

FIG. 3-17
Sugar tong forearm splint.

2. Assess for malrotation, displacement (especially Salter I–type fracture), angulation, and joint stability before splinting.
3. **Procedure:** Elbow in neutral position, wrist in neutral position, metacarpophalangeal (MP) joint at 70 degrees, interphalangeal (IP) joint at 20 degrees. Apply splint in U shape from the tip of the fifth digit to 3 cm distal to the volar crease of the elbow. The splint should be wide enough to enclose the fourth and fifth digits.

E. THUMB SPICA SPLINT

1. **Indications:** Nonrotated, nonangulated, nonarticular fractures of the thumb metacarpal or phalanx, ulnar collateral ligament injury (gamekeeper's or skier's thumb), scaphoid fracture or suspected scaphoid fracture (pain in anatomic snuff box).

2. **Procedure:** Wrist in slight dorsiflexion, thumb in some flexion and abduction, IP joint in slight flexion. Apply splint in U shape from tip of thumb to mid-forearm. Mold the splint along the long axis of the thumb so that thumb position is maintained. This will result in a spiral configuration along the forearm.

F. VOLAR SPLINT

1. **Indications:** Wrist immobilization.
2. **Procedure:** Wrist in slight dorsiflexion. Apply splint on palmar surface from the MP joint to 2 to 3 cm distal to the volar crease of the elbow. It is useful to curve the splint to allow the MP joint to rest at an 80- to 90-degree angle.

G. POSTERIOR ANKLE SPLINT

1. **Indications:** Immobilization of ankle sprains and fractures of the foot, ankle, and distal fibula.
2. **Procedure:** Measure leg for appropriate length of plaster. The splint should extend to base of toes and the upper portion of the calf. A sugar tong (stirrup) splint can be added to increase stability for ankle fractures.

H. RADIAL HEAD SUBLUXATION REDUCTION (NURSEMAID'S ELBOW)

1. **Presentation:** Commonly occurs in children ages 1 to 4 years with a history of inability to use an arm after it was pulled. The child presents with the affected arm held at the side in pronation with elbow slightly flexed.
2. **Caution:** Rule out a fracture clinically before doing procedure. Consider radiograph if mechanism of injury or history is atypical.
3. **Procedure:**

a. Support the elbow with one hand, and place your thumb laterally over the radial head at the elbow. With your other hand, grasp the child's hand in a handshake position.
b. Quickly and deliberately supinate and externally rotate the forearm, and simultaneously flex the elbow. Alternatively, hyperpronation alone may be used. You may feel a click as reduction occurs.
c. Most children will begin to use the arm within 15 minutes, some immediately after reduction. If reduction occurs after a prolonged period of subluxation, it may take the child longer to recover use of the arm. In this case, the arm should be immobilized with a posterior splint.
d. If procedure is unsuccessful, consider obtaining a radiograph. Maneuver may be repeated if needed.

REFERENCES

1. Fleisher G, Ludwig S: Pediatric Emergency Medicine, 3rd ed. Baltimore: Williams & Wilkins; 2000.

2. Dieckmann R, Fiser D, Selbst S: Illustrated Textbook of Pediatric Emergency and Critical Care Procedures. St. Louis, Mosby, 1997.
3. Nichols DG, et al: Golden Hour: The Handbook of Advanced Pediatric Life Support. St. Louis, Mosby, 1996.
4. Barone MA, Rowe PC: Pediatric procedures. In Oski's Pediatrics: Principles and Practice, 3rd ed. Baltimore, Lippincott Williams & Wilkins, 1999.
5. Howe PM, et al: Etiologic diagnosis of cellulitis: Comparison of aspirates obtained from the leading edge and the point of maximal inflammation. Pediatr Infect Dis J 1987;6(7):685.

Trauma, Burns, and Common Critical Care Emergencies

Heather D. Johnson, MD

4

I. TRAUMA: OVERVIEW[1]

A. PRIMARY SURVEY

The primary survey includes assessment of the ABCs: **a**irway, **b**reathing, and **c**irculation. See Chapter 1 for a complete algorithm.

B. SECONDARY SURVEY

Procedures included in a secondary survey are listed in Table 4-1.

C. "AMPLE" HISTORY

Obtain an AMPLE history: **a**llergies, **m**edications, **p**ast illnesses, **l**ast meal, **e**vents preceding injury.

II. SPECIFIC TRAUMATIC INJURIES

A. CLOSED HEAD TRAUMA—MINOR[2]

1. **Introduction:** See section VI.B. for treatment of severe closed head trauma [CHT]. Head injury can be caused by penetrating trauma, blunt force, rotational acceleration, or acceleration-deceleration injury. CHT may result in depressed or nondepressed skull fracture, epidural hematoma, subdural hematoma, cerebral contusion, brain edema, increased intracranial pressure (ICP), brain herniation, concussion (mild to moderate diffuse brain injury), and/or coma (diffuse axonal injury [DAI]). CHT not warranting intensive care or surgical management can be termed minor CHT and should be managed according to the following principles.
2. **Evaluation:**

a. Initial assessment: Follow basic trauma principles, including assessment of ABCs and cervical spine immobilization.

b. Physical examination:

(1) Evaluate patient using Glasgow Coma Scale (GCS) (see Chapter 1).

(2) Obtain vital signs (look for Cushing triad with hypertension, bradycardia, and abnormal respiratory pattern).

(3) Perform secondary survey with careful neurologic evaluation (see Table 4-1).

(4) If severe symptoms are present, or if CHT is not minor, follow procedures for emergency management of increased ICP and coma (see section VI.B.).

c. Associated symptoms: Loss of consciousness (LOC), amnesia (before, during, or after the event), mental status change, behavior change, seizure activity, vomiting, headache, gait disturbance, visual change,

TABLE 4-1

SECONDARY SURVEY

Remove all of patient's clothing, and perform a thorough head-to-toe examination, with special emphasis on the following. Remember to keep the child warm throughout the examination.

Organ System	Secondary Survey
Head	Scalp/skull injury
	Raccoon eyes: Periorbital ecchymoses, which suggests orbital roof fracture
	Battle sign: Ecchymoses behind pinna, which suggests mastoid fracture
	CSF leak from ears/nose or hemotympanum suggests basilar skull fracture
	Pupil size, symmetry, and reactivity: Unilateral dilation of one pupil suggests compression of cranial nerve III (CNIII) and possible impending herniation; bilateral dilation of pupils is ominous and suggests bilateral CNIII compression or severe anoxia and ischemia
	Corneal reflex
	Funduscopic examination for papilledema as evidence of increased ICP
	Hyphema
Neck	Cervical spine tenderness, deformity, injury
	Trachea midline
	Subcutaneous emphysema
Chest	Clavicle deformity, tenderness
	Breath sounds, heart sounds
	Chest wall symmetry, paradoxical movement, rib deformity/fracture
	Petechiae over chest/head suggest traumatic asphyxia
Abdomen	Serial examinations to evaluate tenderness, distention, ecchymosis
	Shoulder pain suggests referred subdiaphragmatic process
	Orogastric aspirates with blood or bile suggest intra-abdominal injury
	Splenic laceration suggested by left upper quadrant rib tenderness, flank pain, and/or flank ecchymoses
Pelvis	Tenderness, symmetry, deformity, stability
Genitourinary	Laceration, ecchymoses, hematoma, bleeding
	Rectal tone, blood, displaced prostate
	Blood at urinary meatus suggests urethral injury; do not catheterize
Back	Log-roll patient to evaluate spine for step-off along spinal column
	Tenderness
	Open or penetrating wound
Extremities	*Neurovascular status:* Pulse, perfusion, pallor, paresthesias, paralysis, pain
	Deformity, crepitus, pain
	Motor/sensory examination
	Compartment syndrome: Pain out of proportion to expected; distal pallor/pulselessness

TABLE 4-1

SECONDARY SURVEY—*cont'd*	
Neurologic	*Quick screen:* **AVPU** (**a**lert, **v**ocal stimulation response, **p**ainful stimulation response, **u**nresponsive).
	Glasgow Coma Scale (see Chapter 1)
Skin	Capillary refill, perfusion
	Lacerations, abrasions
	Contusion:
	Blue-purple: 0–5 days old
	Green: 5–7 days old
	Yellow: 7–10 days old
	Brown: 10–14 days old
	Resolution: 2–4 weeks old

altered level of consciousness, and altered level of activity since time of event.

d. Mechanism of injury:
   (1) Linear forces are less likely to cause LOC; they more commonly lead to skull fractures, intracranial hematoma, or cerebral contusion.
   (2) Rotational forces commonly cause LOC and are occasionally associated with DAI.
   (3) If mechanism of injury is not consistent with sustained injuries, suspect abuse.
e. Medications and illicit drug use: Determining whether a patient takes any medications or uses illicit drugs is helpful in determining the complete etiology of mental status changes.

3. Management:

a. Initial management of minor CHT: Conduct according to basic trauma principles, with attention to ABCs, secondary survey, cervical spine immobilization, and basic radiologic evaluation of cervical spine. Apply basic wound management to any lacerations sustained to the scalp or face.
b. Computed tomography (CT) scan of the head: A CT scan is warranted in the child with documented LOC. In the child with an unwitnessed event, unknown LOC, or no documented LOC, the decision to obtain a head CT scan must be based on the mechanism of injury, severity of known injuries, and persistence of complaints or deficits. Confusion and amnesia can occur without LOC and may not always warrant head CT when present without other concerns or complaints. Noncontrast CT is the preferred study in the emergency setting. See Box 4-1.
c. Observation: All children with significant CHT should be monitored for at least 4 to 6 hours to detect delayed signs or symptoms of intracranial injury. This commonly occurs with epidural bleeds, in which a symptom-free lucid period can precede variable degrees of

BOX 4-1
INDICATIONS FOR IMAGING IN MINOR CLOSED HEAD TRAUMA
CHILDREN ≤1 YEAR OF AGE
Normal neurologic examination, no symptoms, no scalp hematoma: no imaging
Normal neurologic examination, no symptoms, scalp hematoma: skull radiographs
If positive for fracture, follow with CT scan
Abnormal neurologic examination, symptoms: CT scan
CHILDREN >1 YEAR OF AGE
Normal neurologic examination, no symptoms: no imaging
Normal neurologic examination, symptoms: consider CT scan
Abnormal neurologic examination, with or without seizure: CT scan

(Modified from Marx JA: Rosen's Emergency Medicine: Concepts and Clinical Practice, 5th ed. St. Louis, Mosby, 2002.)

acute-onset mental status change. The patient should also be observed for at least 48 hours after CHT. The decision of where (home versus hospital) to continue this observation period can be based on the degree of identified head injury or associated injuries, follow-up and reliability of the caretaker, and persistence of symptoms.

d. Indications for hospitalization:
    (1) Depressed or declining level of consciousness or prolonged unconsciousness (GCS 8–12).
    (2) Neurologic deficit.
    (3) Increasing headache or persistent vomiting.
    (4) Seizures.
    (5) Cerebrospinal fluid (CSF) otorrhea or rhinorrhea, hemotympanum, Battle sign, or raccoon eyes.
    (6) Linear skull fracture crossing the groove of the middle meningeal artery, a venous sinus of the dura, or the foramen magnum.
    (7) Compound skull fracture or fracture into the frontal sinus.
    (8) Depressed skull fracture.
    (9) Bleeding disorder or patient receiving anticoagulation therapy.
    (10) Intoxication or illness obscuring neurologic state.
    (11) Suspected child abuse.

e. If a child is stable for discharge, counsel parents on indications for re-evaluation, including excessive sleepiness, more than two or three episodes of emesis, gait disturbance, severe headache not relieved with standard doses of acetaminophen or ibuprofen, drainage of blood or liquid from nose or ears, visual change, unequal pupil size, and/or seizure activity.

4. Sports-related closed head trauma[3]:

a. CHT occurring during sporting events frequently results in concussion, defined as a trauma-induced alteration in mental status that may or may not involve loss of consciousness.

b. Guidelines for return to play[4]: Depends on grade of injury. Patients are at risk for second impact syndrome and its severe sequelae (cerebral edema and death) for at least several days after injury. Refer to Centers for Disease Control and Prevention (CDC) guidelines: "Summary of Recommendations for Management of Concussion in Sports" at www.cdc.gov/mmwr/PDF/wk/mm4610.pdf.

B. NECK INJURIES[2]

1. Introduction:

a. Infants and toddlers: At risk for subluxation of atlantooccipital joint (skull base to C1) or atlantoaxial joint (C1–C2).

b. School-aged children: At risk for lower cervical spine involvement (C5–C6).

c. Cervical spine injury is more likely to occur in children with an acceleration-deceleration injury such as a motor vehicle crash or fall. Assume cervical spine injury in the child with multiple injuries of any cause. Neurologic recovery after acute spinal cord injury is improved with prompt administration of methylprednisolone.

2. Evaluation:

a. Immobilize cervical spine, then perform careful history and physical examination.

b. Radiographic studies: Obtain posteroanterior (PA) view, lateral view to include seventh cervical vertebra, and odontoid view. Additional flexion and extension views of the cervical spine should be obtained if there is point tenderness, symptoms on palpation, or any suspicion of abnormality on PA or lateral views. Flexion and extension views may be contraindicated if an unstable cervical spine injury is suspected. For details on reading cervical spine films, see Chapter 23. If neurologic symptoms persist despite normal cervical spine and flexion-extension views, magnetic resonance imaging (MRI) is indicated to rule out swelling or intramedullary hemorrhage of the spinal cord.

c. Clinically clear the cervical spine: Patient must be awake and without a distracting injury examiner must palpate posterior neck for localized tenderness. If there is no pain, assess active and passive range of motion. If there is any direct pain over bone, a cervical spine collar should be maintained until further evaluation can definitively rule out injury.

C. BLUNT THORACIC TRAUMA[5]

1. **Internal injuries:** Often, internal injuries present without external signs of trauma secondary to pliable rib cage and mediastinal mobility.
2. **Injury type:** Pulmonary contusion or laceration, pneumothorax or hemothorax, rib or sternal fractures, cardiac, diaphragm, major blood vessel.

3. Evaluation:

a. Careful history and physical examination.

b. Laboratory studies: Pulse oximetry, complete blood count (CBC); consider assessment of arterial blood gas (ABG) values if patient is in severe distress, and type and cross-match if patient is unstable.

c. Obtain a chest radiograph and chest CT with intravenous (IV) contrast if patient is stable.

4. Emergent treatment:

a. Tension pneumothorax: Presents as severe respiratory distress, distended neck veins, contralateral tracheal deviation, diminished breath sounds, and compromised systemic perfusion by obstruction of venous return. Perform needle decompression followed by chest tube placement directed to the lung apex (see Chapter 3).

b. Open pneumothorax: An open pneumothorax, also known as a sucking chest wound, is rare but allows free flow of air between atmosphere and hemithorax. Cover defect with an occlusive dressing (i.e., petroleum jelly gauze), give positive-pressure ventilation, and insert chest tube (see Chapter 3).

c. Hemothorax: Provide fluid resuscitation followed by placement of a chest tube directed posteriorly and inferiorly.

D. BLUNT ABDOMINAL TRAUMA[5]

1. **Anatomic risk factors** in children include: small, pliable rib cages; solid organs proportionally larger than those of adults; and underdeveloped abdominal muscles.
2. **Serious injuries** in children from blunt abdominal trauma include: splenic contusion or laceration, liver contusion or laceration, renal injury, gastrointestinal (GI) tract or duodenal hematoma, genitourinary (GU) tract injury, pancreatic injury, and disruption of major blood vessels.
3. **Evaluation:**

a. Careful history and physical examination.

b. Laboratory studies: Consider serial CBCs (to guide emergence of imaging and surgery), electrolytes, liver function tests (LFTs), amylase, lipase, urinalysis, and microscopy; type and cross-match if patient is unstable.

c. Consider abdominal CT scan with IV contrast (routine oral contrast is not indicated secondary to high false-negative rate for hollow viscus injury).

d. Consider focused abdominal ultrasound or diagnostic peritoneal lavage (DPL) when coexisting injuries (e.g., neurologic or significant orthopedic) prevent CT scan. If DPL is used, the open method is preferred in small children, with warmed isotonic saline lavage (10–15 mL/kg).

4. **If significant abdominal trauma is suspected** or diagnosed, a pediatric surgeon should be consulted.

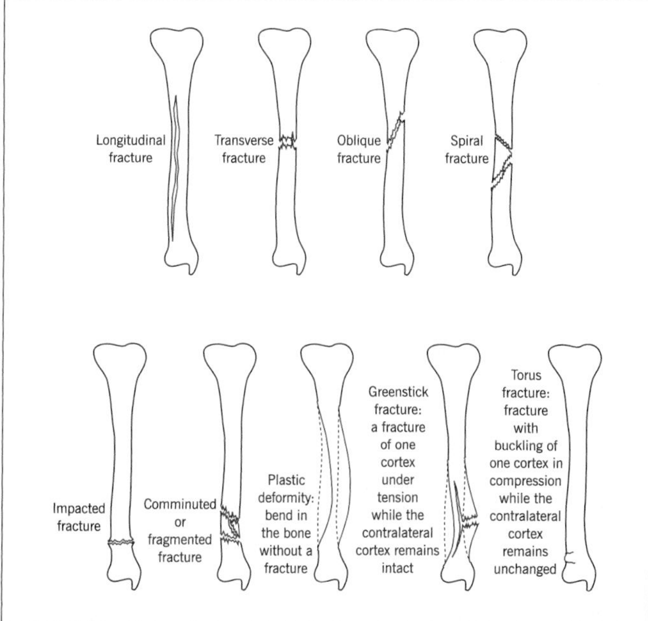

FIG. 4-1

Fracture patterns unique to children. *(Modified from Ogden JA: Skeletal Injury in the Child, 3rd ed. Philadelphia, WB Saunders, 2000.)*

E. ORTHOPEDIC/LONG BONE TRAUMA[6]

1. **Fractures:** Some fracture patterns are unique to children (Fig. 4-1); growth-plate injuries are classified by the Salter-Harris classification (Table 4-2). Ligaments are stronger than bones or growth plates in children; thus, dislocations and sprains are relatively uncommon, whereas growth-plate disruption and bone avulsion are more common. For basic splinting techniques, see Chapter 3.
2. **Compartment syndrome:**[1,7] Elevated muscle compartment venous pressure (enclosed by surrounding fascia) secondary to hemorrhage and cellular swelling from ischemia or trauma impair blood flow and oxygenation, resulting in nerve and muscle damage.

a. Can be seen in open or closed fractures, crush injuries, burns, and necrotizing fasciitis; most common with tibial fractures but also occurs with displaced forearm and supracondylar humerus fractures. Chronic compartment syndrome is occasionally seen in athletes.

b. Severe, unremitting pain exacerbated by passive motion of the fingers or toes; swollen extremity that is tense to palpation.

TABLE 4-2

SALTER-HARRIS CLASSIFICATION OF GROWTH-PLATE INJURY

Class I	Class II	Class III	Class IV	Class V
Fracture along growth plate	Fracture along growth plate with metaphyseal extension	Fracture along growth plate with epiphyseal extension	Fracture across growth plate, including metaphysis and epiphysis	Crush injury to growth plate without obvious fracture

I II III IV V

c. 6 Ps: **P**ain (earliest symptom), **P**allor, **P**aresthesias, **P**oikilothermia, **P**aralysis (late finding), **P**ulselessness (late finding).
d. Studies: Reading of intracompartmental pressure (normal = 10 mmHg; 20–30 mm Hg usually produces clinical symptoms).
e. Management: Emergent (within 6 hours of symptom onset) surgical fasciotomy (absolutely indicated if pressure ≥30 mmHg).
f. Can cause rhabdomyolysis. Follow urinalysis, creatinine kinase, and electrolytes (risk for hyperkalemia). Consider saline resuscitation, urine alkalinization (to keep urine pH >6.5) and mannitol, 250 to 500 mg/kg, if laboratory studies show evidence of rhabdomyolysis.
g. Outcome: Determined by duration of increased pressure.
   (1) <6 hours: Good outcome after fasciotomy in 95% of cases.
   (2) >12 hours: Good outcome after fasciotomy in 6% of cases.

III. ANIMAL BITES[2]

A. WOUND CONSIDERATIONS

1. Special considerations:

a. Deep bites: Possibility of foreign body or fracture—consider radiographs (especially hand or scalp).
b. Periorbital bites: Possibility of corneal abrasion, lacrimal duct involvement, or other ocular damage—consider ophthalmologic evaluation.
c. Hand: Prone to infection—follow for development of osteomyelitis.
d. Nose: Evaluate for cartilage injury.

TABLE 4-3
ANIMAL BITES

Animal	Common Organism(s)	Special Considerations
Dog	*Staphylococcus aureus* *Pasteurella multocida*	Crush injury
Cat	*P. multocida*	Deep puncture wound Often associated with fulminant infection Slow to respond to treatment
Human	*Streptococcus viridans* *S. aureus* Anaerobes *Eikenella corrodens*	Consider child abuse Assess risk for hepatitis B, HIV, and HSV transmission
Rodent	*Streptobacillus moniliformis* *Spirillum minus*	Low incidence of secondary infection Rat-bite fever—occurs rarely

2. High Infection Risk:

a. Puncture wounds.
b. Hand or foot wounds.
c. Cat or human bites.
d. Wounds in asplenic or immunocompromised patients.
e. Wounds with care delayed beyond 12 hours.

3. Animal species (Table 4-3).

B. MANAGEMENT

1. Wound hygiene:

a. Irrigate with copious amounts of sterile saline using high-pressure syringe irrigation. Do not irrigate puncture wounds.
b. Debride devitalized tissue.
c. Explore for foreign bodies. Consider surgical debridement and exploration for extensive wounds, wounds involving metacarpophalangeal joint, and cranial bites by a large animal.
d. Cultures only if evidence of infection is present.

2. Closure:

a. Avoid closing wounds of high infection risk (list above).
b. Wounds that involve tendons, joints, deep fascial layers, or major vasculature should be evaluated by a plastic or hand surgeon and, if indicated, closed in the operating room.
c. Suturing: When indicated, closure should be done with a minimal number of simple, interrupted, nylon sutures and loose approximation of wound edges. Deep sutures should be avoided.
   (1) Head and neck: The head and neck can usually be safely sutured (with the exceptions noted above) after copious irrigation and wound debridement if within 6 to 8 hours of injury and with no signs of infection. Facial wounds often require primary closure for cosmetic reasons; infection risk is lower given the good vascular supply.

(2) Extremities: In large hand wounds, the subcutaneous dead space should be closed with minimal absorbable sutures, with delayed cutaneous closure in 3 to 5 days if there is no evidence of infection.

3. **Antibiotics:** Prophylactic antibiotics are only indicated for wounds at risk for infection, as listed above. See Chapter 16 for appropriate antibiotic choices.
4. **Rabies and tetanus prophylaxis:** See Chapter 15.
5. **Disposition:**

a. Outpatient care: Careful follow-up of all bite wounds, especially those requiring surgical closure, should be obtained within 24 to 48 hours. Extremity wounds, especially the hands, should be immobilized in position of function and kept elevated. Wound should be kept clean and dry.

b. Inpatient care: Consider hospitalization for observation and parenteral antibiotics for significant human bites, immunocompromised or asplenic hosts, established deep or severe infections, bites associated with systemic complaints, bites with significant functional or cosmetic morbidity, and/or unreliable follow-up or care by the parent/guardian.

6. **The infected wound:** Drainage and debridement are required for wounds that subsequently become infected. Gram stain and culture should be performed before start or change of antibiotics. If deep tissue layers or structures are involved, exploration and debridement under general anesthesia may be indicated.

IV. BURNS[2,8]

A. EVALUATION OF PEDIATRIC BURNS (Tables 4-4 and 4-5)

Note *The extent and severity of burn injury may change over the first few days after injury; therefore, be cautious in discussing prognosis with the victim or victim's family.*

B. BURN MAPPING

1. **Burn assessment chart:** Use chart (Fig. 4-2) to map areas of second- and third-degree burns.
2. **Calculate total body surface area (BSA) burned:** based only on percentage of second- and third-degree burns.

C. EMERGENT MANAGEMENT OF PEDIATRIC BURNS

1. **Acute stabilization:** Special considerations of basic trauma principles.

a. Airway:

(1) Intubation: For greater than 20% to 25% BSA burned. For pulmonary toilet or if there is evidence of inhalational injury. Neuromuscular blockade with succinylcholine for intubation is appropriate for patients less than 48 hours postburn, but it is contraindicated after this time frame because of the risk for worsening hyperkalemia. (See also Chapter 1.)

TABLE 4-4

THERMAL INJURY

Type of Burn	Description/Comment
Flame	Most common type of burn; when clothing burns, the exposure to heat is prolonged, and the severity of the burn is worse.
Scald/contact	Mortality is similar to that in flame burns when total BSA involved is equivalent; see text for description of patterns of scald injury and burns suspicious of intentional injury.
Chemical	Tissue damaged by protein coagulation or liquefaction rather than hyperthermic activity.
Electrical	Injury is often extensive, involving skeletal muscle and other tissues in addition to the skin damage. Extent of damage may not be initially apparent. The tissues that have the least resistance are the most heat sensitive. Bone has the greatest resistance, nerve tissue the least. Cardiac arrest may occur from passage of the current through the heart.
Inhalation	Present in 30% of victims of major flame burns and should be considered when there is evidence of fire in enclosed space: singed nares, facial burns, charred lips, carbonaceous secretions, posterior pharynx edema, hoarseness, cough, or wheezing. Inhalation injury increases mortality.
Cold injury/frostbite	Freezing results in direct tissue injury. Toes, fingers, ears, and nose are commonly involved. Initial treatment includes rewarming in tepid (105°–110°F) water for 20–40 min. Excision of tissue should not be done until complete demarcation of nonviable tissue has occurred.

TABLE 4–5

BURN DEGREE

Burn Depth/Degree	Description/Comment
First degree	Only epidermis involved; painful and erythematous.
Second degree	Epidermis and dermis involved, but dermal appendages spared. Superficial second-degree burns are blistered and painful. Any blistering qualifies as a second-degree burn. Deep second-degree burns may be white and painless, require grafting, and progress to full-thickness burns with wound infection.
Third degree	Full-thickness burns involving epidermis and all of the dermis, including dermal appendages; leathery and painless; require grafting.

(2) Inhalation injury: All patients with large burns and/or closed space burns should be assumed to have carbon monoxide (CO) poisoning until examination and evaluation of blood carboxyhemoglobin is undertaken (see Chapter 2). Humidified 100% O_2 should be administered during initial assessment.

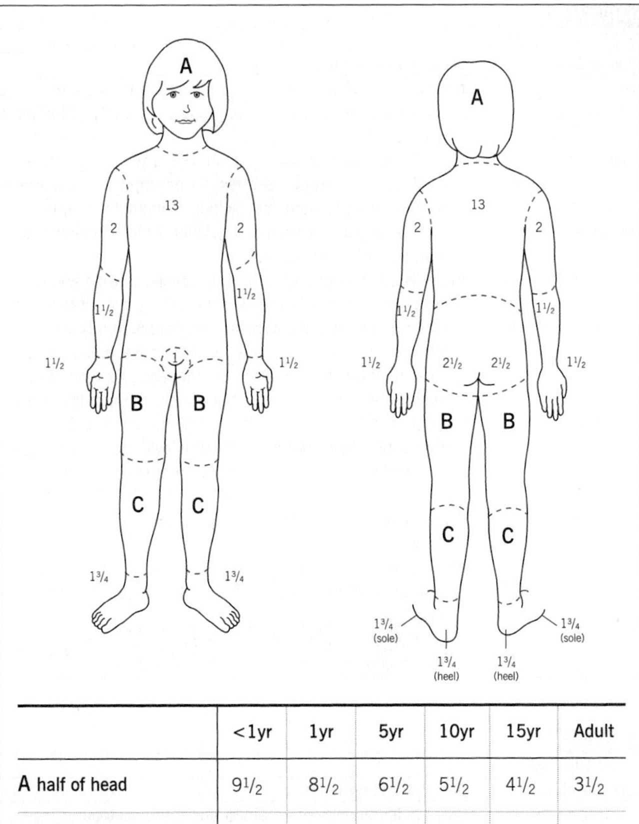

	<1yr	1yr	5yr	10yr	15yr	Adult
A half of head	9 1/2	8 1/2	6 1/2	5 1/2	4 1/2	3 1/2
B half of thigh	2 3/4	3 1/4	4	4 1/4	4 1/2	4 3/4
C half of leg	2 1/2	2 1/2	2 3/4	3	3 1/4	3 1/2

FIG. 4-2

Burn assessment chart. All numbers are percentages. *(From Barkin RM, Rosen P: Emergency Pediatrics: A Guide to Ambulatory Care, 6th ed. St. Louis, Mosby, 2003.)*

((2) continued) Delivery of 100% O_2 counteracts the effects of CO and speeds its clearance. Carboxyhemoglobin absorbs light at the same wavelength as oxyhemoglobin; thus, oxygen saturation, as determined by pulse oximetry, is not altered; a PaO_2 level must be obtained.

(3) Cyanide poisoning: through inhalation of combustible materials, can produce almond-scented breath and may cause profound positive anion gap metabolic acidosis (see Chapter 2).

b. Breathing:
   (1) Monitor pulmonary status with serial ABGs and chest radiographs as indicated.
   (2) Increasing tachypnea may be seen in patients with pulmonary insufficiency caused by acute asphyxia and CO toxicity, upper airway obstruction secondary to edema, or overwhelming parenchymal damage.

c. Circulation/initial fluid resuscitation: Start IV fluid resuscitation of infants with burns greater than 10% of BSA, children with burns greater than 15% BSA, or children with evidence of smoke inhalation. Consider a bolus of 20 mL/kg lactated Ringer (LR) or NS solutions. Further fluid resuscitation should maintain a urine output of 0.5 to 2 mL/kg/hr.

d. Secondary survey: Consider associated traumatic injuries. Electrical injury can produce deep tissue damage, intravascular thrombosis, cardiac and respiratory arrest, fractures secondary to muscle contraction, and cardiac arrhythmias. Look for exit site for electrical injury.

e. Laboratory evaluation: Consider CBC, type and cross-match, carboxyhemoglobin, coagulation studies, chemistry panel, ABGs, and chest radiograph (may not show changes for 24–72 hours).

f. GI: Place nasogastric tube for decompression; patient should receive nothing by mouth (NPO); begin stress ulcer prophylaxis with histamine-2 (H_2) receptor blockers and/or antacids.

g. Obtain bladder decompression and monitor urine output with Foley catheter.

h. Cardiac: Consider electrocardiogram (ECG).

i. Eye: Carefully examine patient for burns or abrasions to eyes, with referral to ophthalmology if suspected. Use topical ophthalmic antibiotics if abrasions are present.

j. Special considerations:
   (1) Tetanus immunoprophylaxis (see Chapter 15).
   (2) Temperature management: Cooling decreases the severity of the burn if administered within 30 minutes of injury; it also helps to relieve pain. If burn is less than 10% of BSA, apply clean towels soaked in cold water to help prevent burn progression. If burns are more than 10% of BSA, apply clean, dry towels to burn to avoid hypothermia.
   (3) Chemical burns: It is important to wash away or neutralize the chemical. Except in rare circumstances, the most efficacious first aid for chemical burns is lavaging with copious volumes of water for about 20 minutes.
   (4) Analgesia: IV analgesia is often necessary to treat pain. Do not attribute combativeness or anxiety to pain until adequate perfusion,

TABLE 4-6

TOPICAL ANTIBACTERIAL AGENTS

Agent	Action	Side Effects	Use
Silver sulfadiazine (Silvadene)	Broad antibacterial, painless, fair eschar penetration	Sulfonamide sensitivity, occasional leukopenia, contraindicated in pregnancy	Q12 hr; cover with light dressings; leave face and chest open
Bacitracin ointment	Limited antibacterial action, poor eschar penetration, transparent, easy to apply	Rapid development of resistance; conjunctivitis develops if ointment comes into contact with eye	Q12 hr; apply to small areas; acceptable with facial burns
Mafenide (Sulfamylon)	Excellent antibacterial for gram-positive and gram-negative bacteria, and *Clostridium*; rapid eschar penetration	Painful, sulfonamide sensitivity, carbonic anhydrase inhibition may lead to acidosis	Q12 hr; cover with light dressings; leave face, chest, abdomen open

oxygenation, and ventilation are established. Consider narcotic therapy for pain management (see Formulary).

D. TRIAGE AND FURTHER MANAGEMENT OF PEDIATRIC BURNS

1. Outpatient management:

a. Considerations: If burn is less than 10% of an infant's BSA, or less than 15% of a child's BSA and involves no full-thickness areas, patient may be treated as an outpatient.

b. Management:

(1) Cleanse with warm saline or mild soap and water. Debride open wounds and necrotic tissue.

(2) Apply topical antibacterial agent (Table 4-6).

(3) Prophylactic oral antibiotics are not indicated.

(4) Daily follow-up is recommended.

(5) Have patient cleanse burn at home twice daily with mild soap (taking special care to remove previously applied antibacterial agent), followed by application of an antibacterial agent and sterile dressing, as above. Once epithelialization has begun, dressing may be changed once daily.

(6) Pain management.

2. **Inpatient management:**
a. Indications:
   (1) BSA >10% with full-thickness areas, or >15%. For 20% to 30%, transfer to burn center.
   (2) Electrical or chemical burns.
   (3) Burns of critical areas, such as face, hands, feet, perineum, or joints.
   (4) Burns suspicious of abuse or unsafe home environment.
   (5) Patient with underlying chronic illness.
   (6) Evidence of smoke inhalation, cyanide poisoning, or CO poisoning.
   (7) Circumferential, full-thickness injury.
b. Fluid therapy: Figure 4-3.
   (1) Consider central venous access for burns greater than 25% BSA.
   (2) Use the Parkland formula as a guideline to estimate fluid need. Requirements decrease after first 24 hours by 25% to 50%. Determine concentrations and rates by monitoring weight, serum electrolytes, urine output, nasogastric losses, and so forth.
   (3) Consider adding colloid after 18 to 24 hours (albumin, 1 g/kg/day) to maintain serum albumin >2 g/dL.
   (4) Withhold potassium generally for the first 48 hours because of a large release of potassium from damaged tissues. To manage electrolytes most effectively, monitor urine electrolytes twice weekly and replace urine losses accordingly.
3. **Prevention of burns:** Measures include child-proofing the home, installing smoke detectors, and turning hot-water tap temperature down to 49° to 52°C (<120° F). It takes 2 minutes of immersion at 52°C to cause a full-thickness burn, compared with 5 seconds of immersion at 60°C.

V. CHILD ABUSE

A. INTRODUCTION

Involve the medical professional, social worker, and community agencies such as emergency medical service providers, police, social services, and prosecutors.

B. MANAGEMENT[2,9]

The medical professional should suspect, diagnose, treat, report, and document all cases of child abuse, neglect, or maltreatment.

1. **Suspect:** Be suspicious whenever there is inconsistent or inadequate history of injury, inappropriate parental response to the situation, delay in seeking medical attention, discrepancy between mechanism of injury and physical examination findings, evidence of neglect or failure to thrive, evidence of disturbed emotions or expressions in a child, prior history of suspicious events, or parental substance abuse.

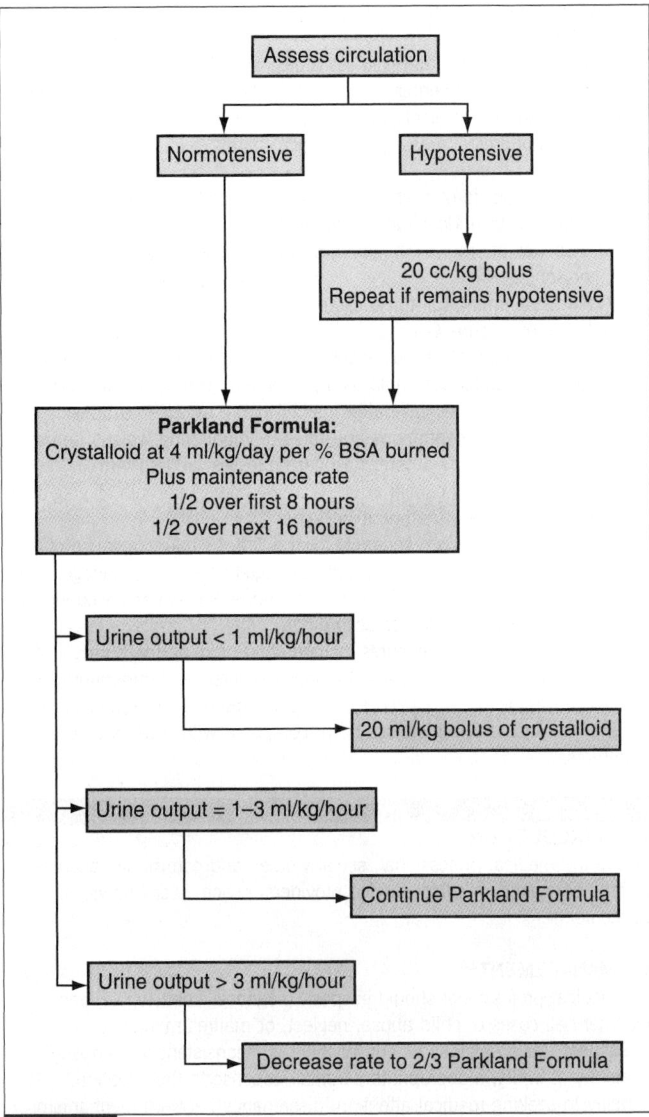

FIG. 4-3

Fluid management of life-threatening burns. *(Modified from Nichols DG, Yaster M, Lappe D, et al. (eds): Golden Hour: The Handbook of Pediatric Advanced Life Support. St. Louis, Mosby, 1996.)*

2. **Diagnose:** Characteristic or concerning injuries.

a. Bruises: Shape, color, and dating of bruises are important (see Table 4-1); correlate with history. Be suspicious of bruises in protected areas (chest, abdomen, back, buttocks). Looped marks or railroad track marks may indicate injury from cords, belts, and ropes.

b. Bites: Shape, size, and location are important; correlate with history and dental anatomy of questioned perpetrator. Intercanine distances of more than 3 cm are suggestive of human bites; they generally crush more than lacerate.

c. Burns: Absence of splash marks and/or clearly demarcated edges are suggestive of nonaccidental injury. Stocking glove patterns, symmetrically burned buttocks and/or lower legs, spared inguinal creases, and symmetric involvement of palms or soles all suggest intentional injury.

d. Hemorrhage: Hemorrhages throughout the retina are virtually pathognomonic of abuse and always warrant evaluation for head trauma. Duodenal hematoma, causing eventual upper GI obstruction secondary to blunt trauma, is suspicious for intentional injury.

e. Skeletal injury: Correlate mechanism of injury with physical finding; rule out any underlying bony pathology.

(1) Long bones: Classic fracture of abuse is the epiphyseal/metaphyseal chip fracture, seen as the "bucket handle" or "corner" fracture at the end of long bones, secondary to jerking or shaking of a child's limb. Spiral fractures of the femur and humerus may be suspicious of abuse, especially if no history of rotational force is given as mechanism of injury. However, spiral fractures of the tibia in a toddler (i.e., "toddler's fracture") are commonly caused by minor accidental trauma.

(2) Ribs: Nonaccidental rib fractures are usually nondisplaced and often are posterior, near the attachment to the spine; they may not be readily visible on acute plain-film radiographs. Pleural thickening, pleural fluid, and contusion may suggest an undetected rib fracture. Fractures are secondary to direct blows or severe squeezing of the rib cage. Closed-chest compressions from cardiopulmonary resuscitation do not appear to cause rib fractures in children.

(3) Skull: Fractures suggestive of force greater than that sustained with minor household trauma are suspicious for abuse; these include fractures more than 3 mm wide, complex fractures, bilateral fractures, and nonparietal fractures.

f. Genital injury: Vaginal bleeding in the prepubertal female, or injury to external genitalia, especially the posterior region, is suspicious for abuse. The hymen should be examined for irregularity outside the realm of normal variation. ***Note:*** **A normal examination does not rule out abuse.** The anus should be evaluated for bruising, laceration, hemorrhoids, scars that extend beyond the anal verge, absence of anal wink, and evidence of infection, such as genital warts. Circumferential hematoma of the anal sphincter is associated with forced penetration. When recent (within 72 hours) sexual abuse is suspected, defer interview and detailed GU examination whenever possible until a multidisciplinary forensic team with expertise in the clinical and laboratory evaluation of sexual abuse can be involved. Avoid collection of laboratory specimens without input from this team.

g. Shaken-baby syndrome: Classically presents with retinal hemorrhages, long bone or rib fractures, and central nervous system (CNS) dysfunction, such as seizure, apnea, or lethargy secondary to intracranial injury. Shaken-baby syndrome is usually found in children < 12 months of age but has been reported in children as old as 5 years of age.

3. **Useful studies:**

a. Skeletal surveys (see Chapter 23 for components) are suggested to evaluate suspicious bony trauma in any child; these studies are mandatory for children <2 years of age.

b. Bone scan may be indicated to identify early or difficult-to-detect fractures.

c. CT scan of the head is unreliable for detection of skull fractures but useful in detecting intracranial pathology secondary to trauma.

d. MRI may identify lesions not detected by CT scan (e.g., posterior fossa injury and diffuse axonal injury). MRI also provides more useful information about the dating of injuries identified.

e. Ophthalmologic evaluation for retinal hemorrhages is necessary in suspected shaken-baby syndrome: dilated, indirect ophthalmoscopy performed by an ophthalmologist.

f. In the setting of intracranial hemorrhage, send laboratory studies to evaluate for coagulopathy: platelet count, prothrombin time (PT), partial thromboplastin time (PTT).

4. **Treat:** Refer to basic principles of trauma management. Special attention should be paid to "stabilizing" the existing and immediate environment of the child (utilizing available social and protective services) to protect the child from incurring further injury during the workup.

5. **Report:** All health care providers are required by law to report suspected maltreatment of a child to the local police and/or welfare agency. Suspicion, supported by objective evidence, is criterion for reporting and should first be discussed with not only the rest of the involved medical team but also the family. The professional who makes such reports is immune from any civil or criminal liability.

6. **Document:** Write legibly, carefully documenting the following: reported and suspected history and mechanisms of injury; any history given by the victim in his or her own words (use quotation marks); information

provided by other providers or services; and physical examination findings, including drawings of injuries and details of dimensions, color, shape, and texture. Always consider early utilization of police crime laboratory photography to document injuries.

VI. COMMON CRITICAL CARE EMERGENCIES

A. ACUTE HYPERTENSION[10]

1. Assessment:

a. The width of the bladder in the blood pressure (BP) cuff should be at least two thirds the length of the upper arm and completely encircle the upper arm. Inadequate bladder size can result in a falsely elevated reading.

b. Patients with BP over the 95th percentile require further evaluation.

c. *Hypertensive urgency*, much more common in children, is significant elevation in BP without accompanying end-organ damage. Symptoms include headache, blurred vision, and nausea. *Hypertensive emergency* is defined as elevation of both systolic and diastolic BP with acute end-organ damage (e.g., cerebral infarction, pulmonary edema, renal failure, hypertensive encephalopathy, seizures, and cerebral hemorrhage). It is important to note that the clinical differentiation between hypertensive urgencies and hypertensive emergencies depends on end-organ damage rather than BP measurement.

d. Evaluate for underlying etiology: Medication or ingestion, cardiovascular, renovascular, renal parenchymal, endocrine, or CNS. Rule out hypertension secondary to elevated intracranial pressure (ICP) before lowering BP.

e. A physical examination should include measurement of four-extremity BP, funduscopy (papilledema, hemorrhage, exudate), visual acuity, thyroid examination, evidence for congestive heart failure (tachycardia, gallop rhythm, hepatomegaly, edema), abdominal examination (mass, bruit), thorough neurologic examination, evidence of virilization, or cushingoid effect.

f. Initial diagnostic evaluation should include urinalysis, blood urea nitrogen (BUN), creatinine, electrolytes, chest radiograph, and ECG. Consider obtaining renin level before beginning antihypertensive therapy. Consider a toxicology screen, thyroid and adrenal testing, urine catecholamines, abdominal ultrasound, renal Doppler ultrasound, and CT of the head as indicated.

2. Management:

a. Hypertensive emergency: IV line, monitor, possible arterial line for continuous BP monitoring. Seek consultation with a nephrologist or cardiologist. The goal is to lower BP promptly but gradually to preserve cerebral autoregulation. The mean arterial pressure (MAP) (where MAP $= 1/3$ systolic BP $+ 2/3$ diastolic BP) should be lowered by one third of the planned reduction over 6 hours, an additional one third over the next 24 to 36 hours, and the final one third over the next 48 hours.

After elevated ICP is ruled out, do not delay treatment because of diagnostic evaluation (Table 4-7).

b. Hypertensive urgency: Aim to lower MAP by 20% over 1 hour and return to baseline levels over 24 to 48 hours. An oral route may be adequate. Observe in the emergency department for 4 to 6 hours. Close follow-up is mandatory. Many other medications are available; the two listed in Table 4-8 have been used with success. Note that use of sublingual nifedipine is not recommended because this agent can result in a precipitous, uncontrolled fall in BP.

B. INCREASED INTRACRANIAL PRESSURE[11]

See Chapter 19 for evaluation and management of hydrocephalus.

1. **Assessment:**

a. History: Obtain history regarding trauma, vomiting, fever, headache, neck pain, unsteadiness, seizure or other neurologic conditions, visual change, gaze preference, and change in mental status. In infants, look for irritability, poor feeding, lethargy, and bulging fontanel.

b. Examination: Assess for Cushing response (hypertension, bradycardia, abnormal respiratory pattern), neck stiffness, photophobia, pupillary response, cranial nerve dysfunction (especially paralysis of upward gaze or of abduction), papilledema, absence of venous pulsations on eye grounds, neurologic deficit, abnormal posturing, and abnormal mental status examination.

2. **Management:** Do not lower BP if elevated ICP is suspected. Cervical spine immobilization is necessary if trauma is suspected.

a. Stable child (not comatose, stable vital signs, no focal findings): Apply cardiac monitor. Elevate head of the bed 30 degrees. Obtain CBC, electrolyte and glucose levels, and blood culture as indicated. Request an urgent head CT scan and emergent neurosurgical consultation and management. Give antibiotics early if meningitis is suspected.

b. Unstable child: Request emergent neurosurgical consultation and management.

   (1) Elevate head of the bed 30 degrees.

   (2) Use normal saline or hyperosmolar solutions for maintenance fluids.

   (3) 3% NaCl, 2 to 5 mL/kg, or mannitol, 0.25 g/kg IV, for temporary reduction of ICP. May increase mannitol gradually to a 0.5 g/kg/dose if needed, although a lower dose of mannitol is generally recommended because high-dose mannitol can produce significant hypotension.

   (4) Reserve hyperventilation for acute management; keep Pco_2 at 30 to 35 mmHg. Provide controlled neuroprotective intubation as outlined in Figure 1-1 and Table 1-1 (consider lidocaine, atropine, thiopental, rocuronium; avoid ketamine). Continue paralysis and sedation.

   (5) Request emergent head CT scan and a shunt series of radiographs if patient has a ventriculoperitoneal (VP) shunt. Lumbar puncture

TABLE 4-7

MEDICATIONS FOR HYPERTENSIVE EMERGENCY*

Drug	Onset (Route)	Duration	Interval to Repeat or Increase Dose	Comments
Diazoxide (arteriole vasodilator)	1–5 min (IV)	Variable (2–12 hr)	15–30 min	May cause edema, hyperglycemia
Hydralazine (arteriole vasodilator)	5–20 min (IV)	2–6 hr	4–6 hr	May cause reflex tachycardia, prolonged hypotension, nausea
INFUSIONS				
Nitroprusside (arteriole and venous vasodilator)	<30 sec (IV)	Very short	30–60 min	Requires ICU setting; follow thiocyanate level
Labetalol (α-, β-blocker)	1–5 min (IV)	Variable, about 6 hr	10 min	May require ICU setting
Nicardipine (calcium channel blocker)	1 min (IV)	3 hr	15 min	May cause edema, headache, nausea, vomiting

*See Formulary for dosing.
ICU, intensive care unit.

TABLE 4-8

MEDICATIONS FOR HYPERTENSIVE URGENCY*

Drug	Onset (Route)	Duration	Interval to Repeat	Comments
Enalaprilat	15 min (IV)	12–24 hr	8–24 hr	May cause hyperkalemia, hypoglycemia
Minoxidil	30 min (PO)	2–5 days	4–8 hr	Contraindicated in pheochromocytoma

*See Formulary for dosing.

PO, Per os.

(LP) is contraindicated because of herniation risk. Do not delay antibiotics if meningitis is suspected. In space-occupying lesions (tumors, abscesses), consider dexamethasone to reduce cerebral edema in consultation with neurosurgeon. Consider epinephrine or phenylephrine infusion to maintain and keep systemic pressure above ICP.

Cerebral perfusion pressure (CPP) = MAP – ICP

(6) Prevent hyperthermia. Goal body temperature <37.5°C.

(7) Avoid hypotension, hypoxia, hypercarbia, and hypovolemia.

C. MECHANICAL VENTILATION

1. Types of ventilatory support:

a. Volume limited:

(1) Delivers a preset tidal volume to a patient regardless of pressure required.

(2) Risk for barotrauma reduced by pressure alarms and pressure pop-off valves that limit peak inspiratory pressure (PIP).

b. Pressure limited:

(1) Gas flow is delivered to the patient until a preset pressure is reached and then held for the set inspiratory time (reduces the risk for barotrauma).

(2) Useful for neonatal and infant ventilatory support (<10 kg) in which the volume of gas being delivered is small in relation to the volume of compressible air in the ventilator circuit, which makes reliable delivery of a set tidal volume difficult.

c. High-frequency ventilation[12]:

(1) High-frequency oscillatory ventilation (HFOV):

(a) High-amplitude and high-frequency pressure waveform generated in the ventilator circuit. Tidal volumes are less than dead space. Bias gas flow provides fresh gas at ventilator and maintains airway pressure.

(b) Minimizes barotrauma and oxygen toxicities.

(c) Patient must be euvolemic secondary to risk for decreased venous return.

(2) High-frequency jet ventilation:

(a) Used simultaneously with a conventional ventilator.

(b) A jet injector port delivers short bursts of inspiratory gas.

(c) Adequate gas exchange can be achieved at low airway pressures providing maintenance of lung volume and minimal risk for barotrauma.

2. Ventilator parameters:

a. Peak Inflating Pressure (PIP): Attained during the respiratory cycle.

b. Positive end-expiratory pressure (PEEP): Airway pressure maintained between inspiratory and expiratory phases (prevents alveolar collapse during expiration, decreasing work of reinflation and improving gas exchange).

c. Rate (intermittent mandatory ventilation) or frequency (Hz): Number of mechanical breaths delivered per minute or rate of oscillations in HFOV.

d. Inspired oxygen concentration (FiO_2): Fraction of oxygen present in inspired gas.

e. Inspiratory time (Ti): Length of time spent in the inspiratory phase of the respiratory cycle.

f. Tidal volume (TV): Volume of gas delivered during inspiration.

g. Power (ΔP): Amplitude of the pressure waveform in HFOV.

h. Mean airway pressure (MAP): Average pressure over entire respiratory cycle.

3. Modes of operation:

a. Intermittent mandatory ventilation (IMV): A preset number of breaths are delivered each minute. The patient can take breaths on his or her own, but the ventilator may cycle on during a patient breath.

b. Synchronized IMV (SIMV): Similar to IMV, but the ventilator synchronizes delivered breaths with inspiratory effort and allows the patient to finish expiration before cycling on. More comfortable for patient than IMV.

c. Assist control (AC or AMV): Every inspiratory effort by the patient triggers a ventilator-delivered breath at the set tidal volume. Ventilator-initiated breaths are delivered when the spontaneous rate falls below the backup rate.

d. Pressure support ventilation (PSV): Inspiratory effort opens a valve allowing airflow at a preset positive pressure. Patient determines rate and inspiratory time. May be used in combination with other modes of operation. Determine effectiveness of ventilation by monitoring tidal volumes.

e. Noninvasive positive-pressure ventilation (NIPPV): Respiratory support provided through face mask.

(1) Continuous positive airway pressure (CPAP): Delivers airflow (with set FiO_2) to maintain a set airway pressure.

(2) Bilevel positive airway pressure (BiPAP): Delivers airflow to maintain set pressures for inspiration and expiration.

4. Initial ventilator settings:

a. Volume limited:

(1) Rate: Approximately normal range for age (see Table 22-1).

(2) Tidal volume: Approximately 8 to 10 mL/kg.

(3) Inspiratory time: Generally use inspiration-to-expiration (I/E) ratio of 1:2. More prolonged expiratory phases are required for obstructive diseases to avoid air trapping.

(4) FiO_2: Selected to maintain targeted oxygen saturation and Pao_2.

b. Pressure limited:

(1) Rate: Approximately normal range for age (see Table 22-1).

(2) PEEP: Start with 3 to 5 cm H_2O and increase as clinically indicated. (Monitor for decreases in cardiac output with increasing PEEP.)

(3) PIP: Set at pressure required to produce adequate chest wall movement (approximate this using hand-bagging and manometer).

(4) FiO_2: Selected to maintain targeted oxygen saturation and Pao_2.

c. High-frequency oscillatory ventilator

(1) Frequency: 10 to 15 Hz for neonates, 5 to 8 Hz for children.

(2) Power: Select to achieve adequate chest wall movement.

(3) MAP: 1 to 4 cm H_2O higher than settings on a conventional ventilator.

(4) FiO_2: Selected to maintain targeted oxygen saturation and Pao_2.

d. High-frequency jet ventilator:

(1) PIP: Increase 2 cm H_2O over conventional ventilator setting.

(2) Inspiratory time: Set at 0.02 seconds.

(3) Frequency: In neonates, set at 420 cycles per second.

5. Further ventilator management:

a. Follow patient closely with pulse oximetry, end-tidal carbon dioxide measurements, and clinical assessment. Confirm findings with blood gases, and adjust ventilator parameters as indicated (Table 4-9).

TABLE 4-9

EFFECTS OF VENTILATOR SETTING CHANGES

	Typical Effects on Blood Gases	
Ventilator Setting Changes	$Paco_2$	Pao_2
↑ PIP	↓	↑
↑ PEEP	↑	↑
↑ Rate (IMV)	↓	Minimal ↑
↑ I : E ratio	No change	↑
↑ FiO_2	No change	↑
↑ Flow	Minimal ↓	Minimal ↑
↑ Power (in HFOV)	↓	No change
↑ MAP (in HFOV)	Minimal ↓	↑

Modified from Carlo WA, Chatbum RL: Neonatal Respiratory Care, 2nd ed. St Louis, Mosby, 1988.

b. In cases of adult respiratory distress syndrome (ARDS) or other condition of poor compliance or air leaks, permissive hypercapnia and tidal volumes of 5 mL/kg should be used to avoid barotrauma in patients.

c. Parameters for initiating high-frequency ventilation:
   (1) Oxygenation Index (OI) >40 (see D. below for calculation of OI).
   (2) Inability to provide adequate oxygenation or ventilation with conventional ventilator.

d. Parameters predictive of successful extubation:
   (1) $Paco_2$ appropriate for patient.
   (2) PIP generally 14 to 16 cm H_2O.
   (3) PEEP 2 to 3 cm H_2O (infants) or 5 cm H_2O (children).
   (4) IMV 2 to 4 breaths per minute (infants); children may wean to CPAP or pressure support.
   (5) FiO_2 <40% (maintaining Pao_2 >70).
   (6) Adequate air leak around endotracheal tube in cases of airway edema or stenosis.
   (7) Maximum negative inspiratory pressure (NIF) >20 to 25 cm H_2O.
   (8) Minimal secretions.

D. CRITICAL CARE REFERENCE DATA

1. Minute ventilation (V_E):

$$V_E = \text{Respiratory rate} \times \text{tidal volume (TV)}$$

a. $V_E \times Paco_2$ = constant (for volume-limited ventilation)

b. Normal TV = 10 to 15 mL/kg

2. Alveolar gas equation:

$$P_{AO_2} = Pio_2 - (P_{ACO_2}/R)$$

$$Pio_2 = Fio_2 \times (P_B - 47\ \text{mmHg})$$

a. PiO_2 = Partial pressure of inspired O_2 minus 150 mmHg at sea level on room air.

b. R = Respiratory exchange quotient (CO_2 produced/O_2 consumed) = 0.8.

c. P_{ACO_2} = Partial pressure of alveolar CO_2 minus partial pressure of arterial CO_2 ($Paco_2$).

d. P_B = Atmospheric pressure = 760 mmHg at sea level. Adjust for high-altitude environment.

e. Water vapor pressure = 47 mmHg.

f. P_{AO_2} = Partial pressure of O_2 in the alveoli.

3. Alveolar-arterial oxygen gradient (A-a gradient):

$$\text{A-a gradient} = P_{AO_2} - Pao_2$$

a. Obtain ABG measuring P_{AO_2} and P_{ACO_2} with patient on 100% FiO_2 for at least 15 minutes.

b. Calculate the P_{AO_2} (see above) and then the A-a gradient.

c. The larger the gradient, the more serious the respiratory compromise. A normal gradient is 20 to 65 mmHg on 100% O_2, or 5 to 20 mmHg on room air.

4. Oxygen content (CAO_2):

O_2 content of sample (mL/dL) =
(O_2 capacity × O_2 saturation [as decimal]) + dissolved O_2

a. O_2 capacity = hemoglobin (g/dL) × 1.34.
b. Dissolved O_2 = Po_2 (of sample) × 0.003.
c. Hemoglobin carries more than 99% of O_2 in blood under standard conditions.

5. Arteriovenous O_2 difference ($AVDo_2$)

$$AVDo_2 = Cao_2 - Cvo_2 = \text{arterial } O_2 \text{ content} - \text{mixed venous } O_2 \text{ content}$$

a. Usually done after placing patient on 100% Fio_2 for 15 minutes.
b. Obtain ABG and mixed venous blood sample (best obtained from pulmonary artery catheter), and measure O_2 saturation in each sample.
c. Calculate arterial and mixed venous oxygen contents (see section 4 above) and then $AVDo_2$ (normal, 5 mL/100 dL).
d. Used in the calculation of O_2 extraction ratio.

6. O_2 extraction ratio:

$$O_2 \text{ extraction} = (AVDo_2/Cao_2) \times 100$$
Normal range, 28% to 33%.

a. Calculate $AVDO_2$ and O_2 contents (see above).
b. Extraction ratios are indicative of the adequacy of O_2 delivery to tissues, with increasing extraction ratios suggesting that metabolic needs may be outpacing the oxygen content being delivered.[13]

7. Oxygenation Index (OI):

$$OI = \frac{\text{mean airway pressure (cm } H_2O) \times FiO_2 \times 100}{PaO_2}$$

OI > 35 for 5 to 6 hours is one criterion for ECMO (extracorporeal membrane oxygen) support.

8. Intrapulmonary shunt fraction (Qs/Qt):

$$\frac{Qs}{Qt} = \frac{(A - a \text{ gradient}) \times 0.003}{(AVDO_2) + (A - a \text{ gradient} \times 0.003)}$$

where Qt is cardiac output and Qs is flow across right-to-left shunt.
a. Formula assumes blood gases obtained on 100% Fio_2.
b. Represents the mismatch of ventilation and perfusion and is normally <5%.
c. A rising shunt fraction (usually >15%–20%) is indicative of progressive respiratory failure.

REFERENCES

1. Marx JA: Rosen's Emergency Medicine: Concepts and Clinical Practice, 5th ed. St. Louis, Mosby, 2002.
2. Fleisher GR, Ludwig S (eds): Textbook of Pediatric Emergency Medicine, 4th ed. Philadelphia, Lippincott Williams & Wilkins, 2000.
3. Proctor M, Cantu R: Head and neck injuries in young athletes. Clin Sports Med 2000;19(4):693–714.
4. Kelly JP, Rosenberg JH: Diagnosis and management of concussion in sports. Neurology 1997;48(3):575–580.
5. Sachez J, Paidas C: Childhood trauma: Now and in the new millennium. Surg Clin North Am 1999;79(6):1503–1535.
6. Ogden JA: Skeletal Injury in the Child, 3rd ed. Philadelphia, WB Saunders, 2000.
7. Mabee JR, Bostwick TL: Pathophysiology and mechanisms of compartment syndrome. Orthop Rev 1993;22(2):175–181.
8. Barkin RM, Rosen P: Emergency Pediatrics: A Guide to Ambulatory Care, 6th ed. St. Louis, Mosby, 2003.
9. Lane WE: Diagnosis and management of physical abuse in children. Clin Fam Pract 2003;5(2).
10. Nichols DG, Yaster M, Lappe D, et al. (eds): Golden Hour: The Handbook of Advanced Pediatric Life Support. St. Louis, Mosby, 1996.
11. James HE: Neurologic evaluation and support in the child with an acute brain insult. Pediatr Ann 1986;15:16.
12. Charney J: Pediatric ventilation outside the operating room. Anesthesiol Clin North Am 2001;19(2):399.
13. Rogers M: Textbook of Pediatric Intensive Care, 3rd ed. Baltimore, Williams & Wilkins, 1996.

PART II

Diagnostic and Therapeutic Information

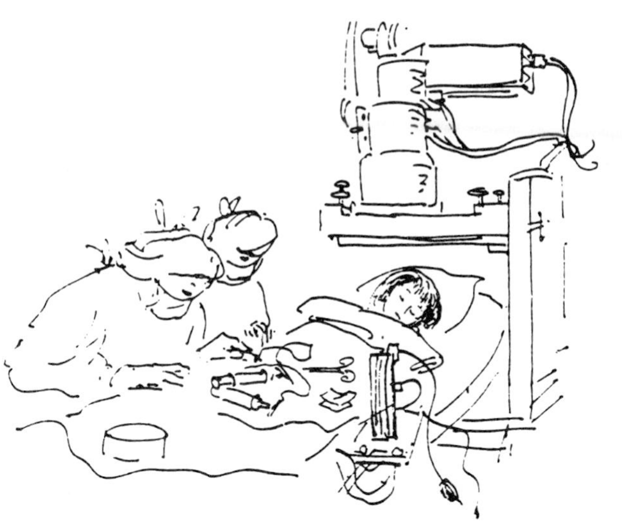

Adolescent Medicine

Tracey Clark, MD

5

I. ADOLESCENT HEALTH MAINTENANCE (Table 5-1)

A. CHIEF COMPLAINT[1]

Hidden agenda: adolescents often present with chief complaints that are not the true concern or motivation for the visit. Gentle but persistent questioning ("Is there anything else?") often leads to the actual reason for the visit.

B. MEDICAL HISTORY[2,3]

Medical history includes any information regarding immunizations, chronic illness, trauma or injury (fractures, burns, head injury, fights, sports-related injury), medications (including hormonal contraception, over-the-counter drugs, nutritional supplements, and complementary and alternative medicines), recent dental care, hospitalizations, or surgeries.

C. FAMILY HISTORY[2,3]

Family history includes any information regarding psychiatric disorders, suicide, alcoholism or substance abuse, and chronic medical conditions or familial risk factors (hypertension, diabetes, cholesterol, heart attack, stroke, cancer, asthma, tuberculosis [TB], human immunodeficiency virus [HIV]).

D. REVIEW OF SYSTEMS (AREAS OF EMPHASIS WITH AN ADOLESCENT)[2,3]

1. **Nutrition:** Dietary habits, including skipped meals, special diets, purging methods, recent weight gain or loss.
2. **Skin:** Acne, moles, rashes, warts.
3. **Genitourinary:** Dysuria, urgency, frequency, discharge, bleeding.
4. **Menstrual:** Menarche, frequency, duration, pain, menometrorrhagia.

E. PSYCHOSOCIAL AND MEDICOSOCIAL HISTORY (HEADSS)[2–4]

1. **Home:** Household composition; family dynamics and relationships; living and sleeping arrangements; guns in the home; recent changes.
2. **Education:** School attendance, absences, suspensions; ever failed a grade; grades as compared with previous years; attitude toward school; favorite, most difficult, best subjects; special educational needs; goals for the future, including vocational or technical school, college, career.
3. **Activities:** Friendships with same or opposite sex, age of friends, best friend, dating, recreational activities, physical activity and exercise, sports participation, hobbies and interests, job, weapon carrying, fighting.

TABLE 5-1

COMPARISONS AMONG RECOMMENDATIONS FOR ADOLESCENT PREVENTIVE SERVICES

Subject	AAFP	AAP	AMA	BF	USPSTF
Immunizations					
ACIP recommendations	Yes	Yes	Yes	Yes	Yes
Health guidance for teens					
Normal development[a,b]	Yes	Yes	Yes	Yes	No
Injury prevention[a,c]	Yes	Yes	Yes	Yes	Yes
Nutrition[a]	Yes	Yes	Yes	Yes	Yes
Physical activity[a]	Yes	Yes	Yes	Yes	Yes
Dental health[a]	Yes	Yes	No	Yes	Yes
Breast or testicular self-examination[a]	Yes	Yes	No	Yes	No
Skin protection[a]	Yes	Yes	Yes	Yes	Yes
Health guidance for parents[a]	No	Yes	Yes	Yes	No
Screening/counseling[d]					
Obesity[a]	Yes	Yes	Yes	Yes	Yes
Contraception[e]	Yes	Yes	Yes	Yes	Yes
Tobacco use[a]	Yes	Yes	Yes	Yes	Yes
Alcohol use[a]	Yes	Yes	Yes	Yes	Yes
Substance use[a]	Yes	Yes	Yes	Yes	Yes
Hypertension[a]	Yes	Yes	Yes	Yes	Yes
Depression/suicide[a]	No	Yes	Yes	Yes	No
Eating disorders[a]	No	Yes	Yes	Yes	No
School problems[a]	No	Yes	Yes	Yes	No
Abuse[a]	No	Yes	Yes	Yes	No[f]
Hearing[a]	Yes	Yes	No	Yes	No
Vision[a]	No	Yes	No	Yes	No
Tests					
Tuberculosis[e]	Yes	Yes	Yes	Yes	Yes
Papanicolaou test[e]	Yes	Yes	Yes	Yes	Yes
Human immunodeficiency virus infection[e]	Yes	Yes	Yes	Yes	Yes
Sexually transmitted diseases[e]	Yes	Yes	Yes	Yes	Yes
Cholesterol[e]	Yes	Yes	Yes	Yes	No
Urinalysis[a]	No	Yes	No	No	No
Hematocrit[a]	No	Yes	No	No	No
Periodicity of visits	Tailored	Annual	Annual	Annual	Tailored
Target age range (yr)[g]	13–18	11–21	11–21	11–21	11–24

[a]Procedure is recommended for all adolescents/parents.

[b]This includes providing adolescents with information on normal physical, psychosocial, and sexual development.

[c]This includes activities such as promoting the use of safety belts and safety helmets, placement of home fire alarms, and reducing the risk for injury from firearms and violence. Organizations differ in the activities they include for injury prevention.

[d]The AAP recommends "development/behavioral assessment."

[e]Procedure is recommended for selected adolescents who are at high risk for the medical problem.

[f]Child abuse is not addressed as a separate screening topic, but is included in the general screening for family violence.

[g]The AAP, AMA, and BF make a distinction among developmental stages of adolescence.

AAFP, American Academy of Family Physicians; AAP, American Academy of Pediatrics; ACIP, Advisory Committee on Immunization Practices; AMA, American Medical Association; BF, Bright Futures; USPSTF, U.S. Preventive Services Task Force.

From Elster AB: Comparison of recommendations for adolescent clinical preventive services developed by national organizations. Arch Pediatr Adolesc Med 1998;152:193.

4. **Drugs:** Personal use of tobacco, alcohol, illicit drugs, anabolic steroids; peer substance use; family substance use and attitudes; driving while intoxicated or with someone who was intoxicated; negative consequences of substance use. If personal use, administer CAGE questionnaire: *Have you ever felt the need to* ***C****ut down; have others* ***A****nnoyed you by commenting on your use; have you ever felt* ***G****uilty about your use or about something you said or did while using; have you ever needed an* ***E****ye-opener (alcohol first thing in morning)?* Any affirmative answer on CAGE indicates high risk for alcoholism or dependence and requires further assessment.
5. **Sexuality:** Sexual feelings toward opposite or same sex; sexual intercourse or types of sexual practices—age at first intercourse, number of lifetime and current partners, age of partners, recent change in partners; contraception and sexually transmitted disease (STD) prevention; history of STD, prior pregnancies, abortions, ever fathered a child; history of nonconsensual intimate physical contact or sex; sex for money or drugs.
6. **Suicide/depression:** Feelings about self, both positive and negative; history of depression or other mental health problems; current or prior suicidal thoughts; prior suicide attempts; sleep problems: difficulty getting to sleep, early waking; changes in appetite or weight; anhedonia; irritability; anxiety.

F. PHYSICAL EXAMINATION (MOST PERTINENT ASPECTS)[2,3]

1. **Height, weight (calculate body mass index [BMI]), and blood pressure with percentiles.**
2. **Dentition and gums (smokeless tobacco use, enamel erosion from induced vomiting).**
3. **Skin:** Acne (type and distribution of lesions), scars, piercings, tattoos.
4. **Thyroid.**
5. **Spine:** scoliosis (see section V)
6. **Breasts:** Tanner stage (Fig. 5-1), masses (females); gynecomastia (males).
7. **External genitalia:**
   a. Visual inspection (human papillomavirus [HPV], ulcers, rashes, pubic lice, trauma, discharge).
   b. Pubic hair distribution: Tanner stage (Figs. 5-2 and 5-3).
   c. Testicular examination: Tanner stage (Table 5-3), masses (hydrocele, varicocele, hernia).
8. **Pelvic examination:** Any age female who is sexually active or has a gynecologic complaint; suggest a screening Papanicolaou (Pap) smear to all females aged 18 to 21 years.

G. LABORATORY TESTS[2,3]

1. **Purified protein derivative (PPD):** If high risk for tuberculosis, see Chapter 16 for screening recommendations.

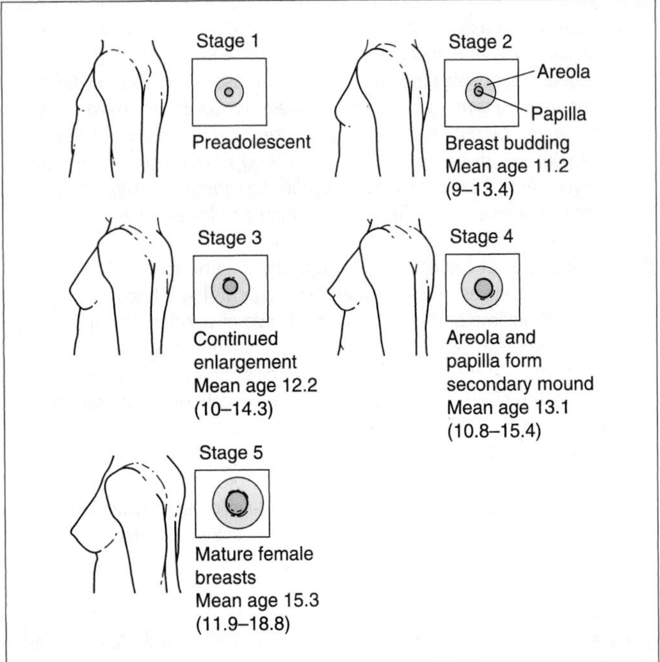

FIG. 5-1

Tanner stages of breast development in females. *(Modified from Johnson TR, Moore WM, Jeffries JE: Children are different: Developmental physiology, 2nd ed. Columbus, OH, Ross Laboratories, 1978. Mean age and range [2 standard deviations around mean] from Joffe A: Introduction to adolescent medicine. In McMillan JA, DeAngelis CD, Feigan RD, Warshaw J [eds]: Oski's Pediatrics Principles and Practice, 3rd ed. Philadelphia, Lippincott Williams & Wilkins, 1999, p 531.)*

2. **Hemoglobin and hematocrit:** Once during puberty for males; at least once after menarche for females.
3. **Urinalysis and microscopic evaluation:** first encounter or end of puberty, pyuria indication for further evaluation for urinary tract infection (UTI) and, in males, chlamydia.
4. **Sexually active adolescents:**

a. Serologic tests: Syphilis and HIV annually.

b. Males: First-part voided urinalysis and leukocyte esterase screen with positive results confirmed by detection tests for gonorrhea and chlamydia (i.e., cultures, ligase chain reaction [LCR], polymerase chain reaction [PCR]).

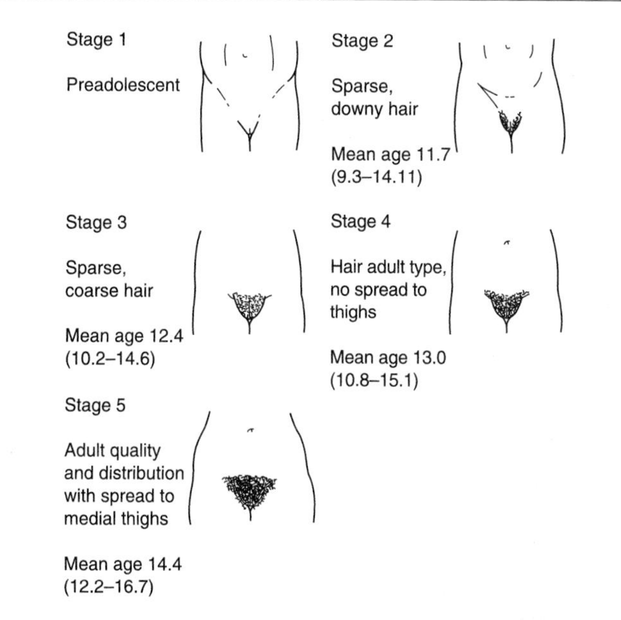

FIG. 5-2

Pubic hair development in females. *(Modified from Neinstein LS, Kaufman FR: Normal Physical Growth and Development. In Neinstein LS [ed]: Adolescent Healthcare: A Practical Guide, 4th ed. Philadelphia: Lippincott Williams & Wilkins, 2002, p 28. Age range [2 standard deviations around mean] from Joffe A: Introduction to adolescent medicine. In McMillan JA, DeAngelis CD, Feigan RD, Warshaw J [eds]: Oski's Pediatrics Principles and Practice, 3rd ed. Philadelphia, Lippincott Williams & Wilkins, 1999, p 531.)*

c. Females: Detection tests for gonorrhea and chlamydia (i.e., cultures, LCR, PCR), wet preparation, potassium hydroxide (KOH), cervical Gram stain, Pap smear, mid-vaginal pH.

5. **Cholesterol:** Once during puberty or if personal or familial risk factors.

H. IMMUNIZATIONS[2,3,5]

See Chapter 15 for dosing, route, formulation, and schedules.

1. **Tetanus and diphtheria (Td):** Booster at age 11 to 12 years and every 10 years thereafter.
2. **Measles:** Two doses of live attenuated vaccine are required after the first birthday. Use measles, mumps, rubella (MMR) vaccine if not

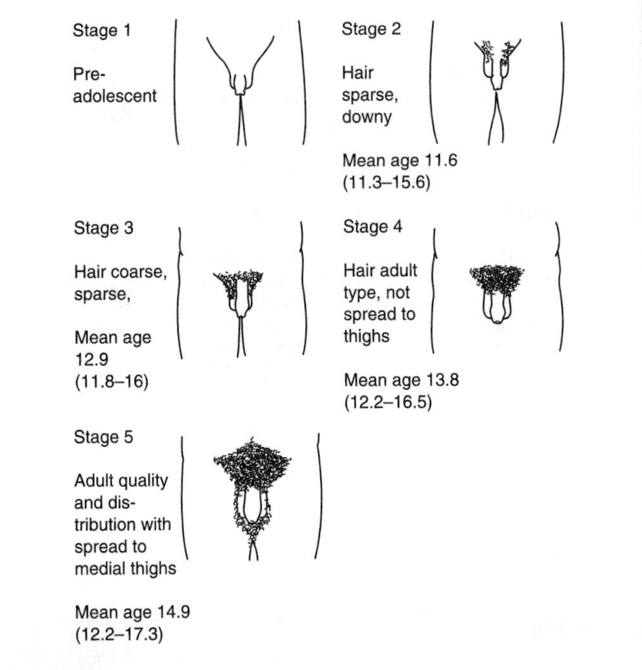

FIG. 5-3

Pubic hair development in males. *(Data from Neinstein LS, Kaufman FR: Normal physical growth and development. In Neinstein LS [ed]: Adolescent Healthcare: A Practical Guide, 4th ed. Philadelphia, Lippincott Williams & Wilkins, 2002, p 30. Age range [2 standard deviations around mean] from Joffe A: Introduction to adolescent medicine. In McMillan JA, DeAngelis CD, Feigan RD, Warshaw J [eds]: Oski's Pediatrics Principles and Practice, 3rd ed. Philadelphia, Lippincott Williams & Wilkins, 1999, p 531.)*

previously immunized for mumps or rubella. Assess pregnancy status; do not administer rubella vaccine to any woman anticipating pregnancy within 90 days.

3. **Hepatitis B vaccine (HBV):** Recommended for all adolescents if not previously vaccinated using the three-dose regimen recommended by the Advisory Committee on Immunization Practices (ACIP) and the American Academy of Pediatrics (AAP).
4. **Varicella vaccine:** Recommended if not previously vaccinated and no personal history of disease. One dose if younger than 13 years of age; 2 doses 4 to 8 weeks apart if older than 13 years.

TABLE 5-2

PSYCHOSOCIAL DEVELOPMENT OF ADOLESCENTS

Task	Early Adolescence	Middle Adolescence	Late Adolescence
Independence	Less interest in parental activities Wide mood swings	Peak of parental conflicts	Reacceptance of parental advice and values
Body image	Preoccupation with self and pubertal changes Uncertainty about appearance	General acceptance of body Concern over making body more attractive	Acceptance of pubertal changes
Peers	Intense relationships with same-sex friend	Peek of peer involvement Conformity with peer values Increased sexual activity and experimentation	Peer group less important More time spent in sharing intimate relationships
Identity	Increased cognition Increased fantasy world Idealistic vocational goals Increased need for privacy Lack of impulse control	Increased scope of feelings Increased intellectual ability Feeling of omnipotence Risk-taking behavior	Practical, realistic vocational goals Refinement of moral, religious, and sexual values Ability to compromise and to set limits

5. **Meningococcal:** Routine vaccination of nonmilitary personnel not currently recommended. However, college freshmen, especially living in residence halls and dormitories, have modestly increased risk. Therefore, vaccine should be discussed with students and their parents to make individualized decisions.

I. ANTICIPATORY GUIDANCE

See Table 5-1.

II. PUBERTAL EVENTS AND TANNER STAGE DIAGRAMS[2]

A. PSYCHOSOCIAL DEVELOPMENT (see Table 5-2)

B. TEMPORAL RELATIONSHIP OF THE BIOLOGIC EVENTS OF ADOLESCENCE (see Figs. 5-1 to 5-3 and Table 5-3) (AGE LIMITS FOR THE EVENTS AND STAGES ARE APPROXIMATIONS AND MAY DIFFER FROM THOSE USED BY OTHER AUTHORS)

1. **Precocious puberty** is the onset of secondary sexual characteristics before age 8 years in girls and 9 years in boys.
2. **Delayed puberty** is the lack of secondary sexual development by age 13 years in girls and 14 years in boys.
3. **Mean peak height velocity:**

a. Girls: 12.1 years (±2 standard deviations;10.4 to 13.9 years).
b. Boys: 14.1 years (±2 standard deviations;12.2 to 15.9 years).

III. CONTRACEPTIVE INFORMATION

A. METHODS OF CONTRACEPTION (Table 5-4)

B. COMBINED HORMONAL CONTRACEPTIVES (ESTROGEN AND PROGESTERONE)

1. **Contraindications**[6] (developed for oral contraceptive pill [OCP] but apply to any contraceptive containing estrogen).

TABLE 5-3

GENITAL DEVELOPMENT (MALE)

Stage	Comment (±2 standard deviation around mean age)
1	Preadolescent: testes, scrotum, and penis about same size and proportion as in early childhood
2	Enlargement of scrotum and testes; skin of scrotum reddens and changes in texture; little or no enlargement of penis; mean age 11.4 yr (9.5–13.8 yr)
3	Enlargement of penis, first mainly in length; further growth of testes and scrotum; mean age 12.9 yr (10.8–14.9 yr)
4	Increased size of penis with growth in breadth and development of glans; further enlargement of testes and scrotum and increased darkening of scrotal skin; mean age 13.77 yr (11.7–15.8 yr)
5	Genitalia adult in size and shape; mean age 14.9 yr (13–17.3 yr)

Data from Joffe A: Introduction to adolescent medicine. In McMillan JA, DeAngelis CD, Feigan RD, Warshaw J (eds): Oski's Pediatrics Principles and Practice, 3rd ed. Philadelphia, Lippincott Williams & Wilkins, 1999, pp 530–531.

TABLE 5-4
METHODS OF CONTRACEPTION

Method	Typical Use Failure Rate (%)	Benefits	Risk/Disadvantage
COMBINED HORMONAL			
Oral Transdermal Injectable Vaginal Ring	2.5–6.0 0.7–1.3* 0.1 0.7–1.8†	Intercourse independent; rapid reversibility; daily, weekly, or monthly dosing options; decreased risk for dysmenorrhea, rheumatoid arthritis, iron-deficiency anemia, ovarian and uterine cancers, ovarian cysts, acne, eptopic pregnancy, benign breast disorders	Thromboembolic phenomena, cerebrocascular accident, hypertension, worsening of migraines, nausea, weight gain, breast tenderness, breakthrough bleeding, amenorrhea, depression, not a barrier to STD
PROGESTIN ONLY			
DMPA Progestin pill Implant	0.3 3.0–10.0 0.09	Intercourse independent, can be used while breast-feeding, no estrogen, decreased risk for ovarian/endometrial cancer; no drug interactions; pill and implant have rapid reversibility	Menstrual irregularity/ammeorrhea, weight gain, reversible osteopenia, mood changes, breast tenderness, headaches, not a barrier to STD, DMPA delayed return to fertility
IUD			
CopperT380A Levonorgestrel IUS	0.7 0.1	Decreased ectopic pregnancy, intercourse independent, rapidly reversible, discreet	Practitioner placement/removal required, only appropriate for low risk (parous and monogamous), no STD protection, may increase PID, actinomyces colonization, or infection, increased menstrual bleeding and cramping (CopperT380A only), expulsion, perforation, or embedment

TABLE 5-4

METHODS OF CONTRACEPTION—cont'd

Method	Typical Use Failure Rate (%)	Benefits	Risk/Disadvantage
BARRIER			
Condom	12.0	No major risks, low cost, nonprescription, male involved, protects against STD and cervical cancer	Decreased sensation, use with each act of coitus, requires male cooperation
Diaphragm with contraceptive cream or jelly	16.0–18.0	Most effective female barrier method, reduced risk for STD, may be placed in anticipation, single insertion for multiple acts of intercourse	Professional fitting and prescription only; requires motivation, preparation, and access; messy, allergies, increased risk for UTI, small risk for toxic shock syndrome
Female condom	21.0–26.0	May be inserted up to 8 hr before coitus	Complex and difficult to place, low efficacy, lack of STD reduction evidence, expensive, use with each act of coitus, associated noise
OTHER			
Withdrawal	19.0		
Spermicide	40.0		
NO METHOD			
	85.0		

Note: The following methods are generally not recommended for adolescents[12]: progesterone only pill, intrauterine devices, diaphragm, cervical cap, female condom, withdrawal, spermicide, natural family planning.

*http://www.contraceptiononline.org/slides/slide01.cfm?tk=5&dpg=21

†http://www.contraceptiononline.org/slides/slide01.cfm?tk=7&dpg=9

DMPA, depomedroxyprogesterone acetate; IUD, intrauterine device; STD, sexually transmitted disease; UTI, urinary tract infection.

Data from Neinstein LS, Nelson AL: Contraception. In Neinstein LS (ed): Adolescent Healthcare: A Practical Guide, 4th ed. Lippincott Williams & Wilkins, 2002, p 836.

a. Refrain from providing (World Health Organization [WHO] category 4): History of thrombophlebitis or thromboembolic disease, stroke, ischemic (coronary) heart disease, complicated structural heart disease, breast cancer, estrogen-dependent neoplasia, pregnancy, lactation for less than 6 weeks, liver disease (including liver cancer, benign hepatic adenoma, active viral hepatitis, severe cirrhosis), diabetes for more than 20 years or with complications, headaches with focal neurologic symptoms, major surgery with prolonged immobilization, any surgery on the legs, hypertension with pressures higher than 160/100 mmHg or with vascular disease.

b. Exercise caution (WHO category 3): Postpartum for less than 21 days, lactation for 6 weeks to 6 months, undiagnosed abnormal vaginal or uterine bleeding, use of drugs that affect liver enzymes, gallbladder disease.

c. Advantages generally outweigh disadvantages (WHO category 2): Major surgery without prolonged immobilization, sickle cell disease, moderate hypertension (140–159/100–109 mmHg), undiagnosed breast mass, headaches without focal neurologic symptoms, diabetes without complications, mental retardation, drug or alcohol abuse, severe psychiatric disorders, family history of hyperlipidemia or myocardial infarction before age 50 years.

2. Serious complications (ACHES)[6]:

a. **A**bdominal pain (pelvic vein or mesenteric vein thrombosis, pancreatitis),

b. **C**hest pain (pulmonary embolism),

c. **H**eadaches (thrombotic or hemorrhagic stroke, retinal vein thrombosis),

d. **E**ye symptoms (thrombotic or hemorrhagic stroke, retinal vein thrombosis),

e. **S**evere leg pain (thrombophlebitis of the lower extremity).

3. OCP instructions[7]:

a. Take 1 pill each day, preferably at the same time of day.

b. Take the **first** pill on the first to the seventh day (first day is preferred, Sunday start most common) after the beginning of your menstrual period.

c. Some pill packs have 28 pills; others have 21 pills. When the 28-day pack is empty, immediately start taking pills from a new pack. When the 21-day pack is empty, wait 1 week (7 days) and then begin taking pills from a new pack.

d. If you **vomit** within 30 minutes of taking a pill, take another pill or use a backup method if you have sex during the next 7 days.

e. If you forget to take 1 pill, take it as soon as you remember, even if it means taking 2 pills in 1 day.

f. If you forget to take 2 or more pills, take 2 pills every day until you are back on schedule. Use a backup method (e.g., condoms) or do not have sex for 7 days.

g. If you miss 2 or more menstrual periods, come to the clinic for a pregnancy test.
h. Need backup method for first month.
i. No STD protection; therefore, a barrier method should be used in addition to the pill.

4. Transdermal (patch) instructions[8]:
a. Apply within 5 days of the onset of menses anywhere on trunk or upper extremities except breasts.
b. Replace every 7 days for 3 weeks.
c. Allow 7 days without patch for menses, then restart cycle.
d. Rotate location of application to avoid skin irritation.
e. If patch falls off, put on new patch as soon as possible and use backup method of contraception.

5. Combination monthly injection instructions[8,9]:
a. First injection during first 5 days of menstrual cycle or 7 days after first- or second-trimester abortion or 21 to 29 days postpartum if not breast-feeding.
b. Reinjection 23 to 33 days after prior injection.
c. Return to clinic for pregnancy test if you have missed two periods.

6. Vaginal ring instructions[8,10]:
a. Ring placed in vagina for 3 weeks.
b. Ring removed for 1 week for withdrawal bleeding.
c. New ring placed in vagina for 3 weeks.
d. If ring is expelled, rinse with water and reinsert; backup contraception is needed if ring is out for more than 3 hours.

7. Follow-up recommendations[11]:
a. Pelvic examination at baseline or during first 3 to 6 months of use, then annually.
b. Two or three follow-up visits per year to monitor patient compliance, blood pressure, and side effects.

C. LONG-ACTING PROGESTIN METHODS

1. **Contraindications[12]:** Active thrombophlebitic or thromboembolic disorders, undiagnosed abnormal genital bleeding, pregnancy, acute liver disease, carcinoma of the breast, history of intracranial hypertension, hypersensitivity to components.
2. **Not contraindicated[12,13]:** postpartum, breast-feeding, history of thrombosis, hypertriglyceridemia, tobacco abuse, hypertension, migraine, systemic lupus, hepatic disease, sickle cell (reduces sickling), seizure disorder.
3. **Depomedroxyprogesterone acetate (DMPA) injection instructions[12]:**

a. Initial injection first 5 days after onset of menses.
b. Reinjection every 11 to 13 weeks.
c. Reinjection after 13 weeks or initial injection after first 5 days of cycle (Fig. 5-4).

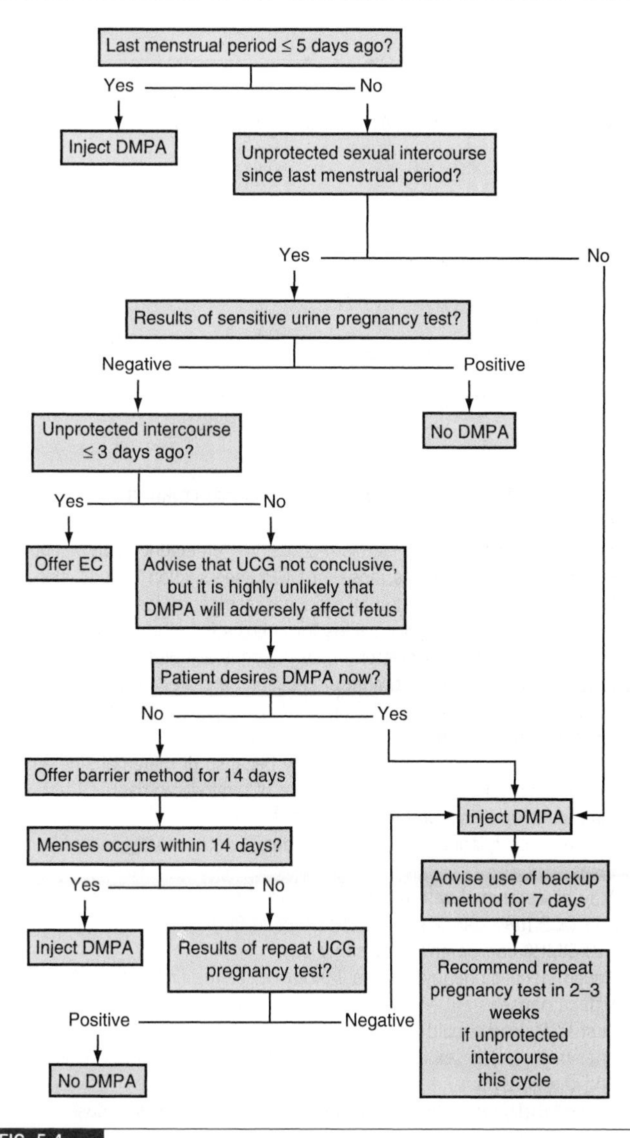

FIG. 5-4

Depomedroxyprogesterone acetate (DMPA) use algorithm for initial or late injection. *(Data from Nelson AL, Neinstein LS: Long acting progestins. In Neinstein LS [ed]: Adolescent Healthcare: A Practical Guide, 4th ed. Philadelphia, Lippincott Williams & Wilkins, 2002, p 93.)*

TABLE 5-5
EMERGENCY CONTRACEPTIVE PILL

Trade Name	Ethinyl Estradiol per Dose (mg)	Levonorgestrel per Dose (mg)	Pills per Dose
Plan B*	0	0.75	1 white
Preven*	0.1	0.5	2 blue
Ovral	0.1	0.5	2 white
Lo-Ovral	0.12	0.6	4 white
Nordette	0.12	0.6	4 light-orange
Levlen	0.12	0.6	4 light-orange
Triphasil	0.12	0.5	4 yellow
Trilevlen	0.12	0.5	4 yellow
Alesse	0.1	0.5	5 pink

*Manufactured solely for the purpose of emergency contraception.
Modified from Brill SR, Rosenfeld WD: Med Clin North Am, Adolesc Med 2000;84:12.

D. EMERGENCY CONTRACEPTIVE PILL (ECP) (Table 5-5)

1. Contraindications[14]:

a. The contraindications for estrogen-containing emergency contraception regimens are the same as those for OCPs (see section III.B.1), but use over time has shown that such stringent restrictions for single use are not necessary. History of previous thrombosis is not a contraindication for single use, but progesterone-only methods are preferred.
b. Progesterone-only regimen contraindications are pregnancy, undiagnosed abnormal genital bleeding, or hypersensitivity to a component of the product.
c. ECP is contraindicated with pregnancy because of maternal side effects without offsetting benefits; no evidence of teratogenic risk.

2. Guidelines and instructions for use[14,15]:

a. Advance prescription should be considered with sexually active teens.
b. May be combined with other ongoing methods of birth control.
   (1) OCP may start 24 hours after second ECP dose.
   (2) DMPA can be given the same day.
c. Recommend diphenhydramine 1 hour before the first dose of ECP to reduce nausea.
d. First ECP dose should be taken as soon as possible, within 72 hours after unprotected sex. There is a linear relationship between efficacy and the time from intercourse to treatment.
e. Second ECP dose should be taken 12 hours after the first dose.
f. Pregnancy test may be administered before taking an ECP, but the dose should not be delayed for this because efficacy diminishes over time to dosing.
g. Take the opportunity to discuss proper use of regular birth control for the future.

h. No absolute limit of ECP frequency during a cycle if there is need, but women using ECP frequently should be advised of other, more effective methods of birth control.
i. Perform pregnancy test if there is no menstrual period within 3 weeks of ECP treatment.

IV. VAGINAL INFECTIONS, GENITAL ULCERS, AND WARTS

See Chapter 16 for discussion of infection with chlamydia, gonorrhea, pelvic inflammatory disease (PID), and HIV and for further discussion of syphilis. See Part IV, Formulary, for additional information and comments regarding specific medications. After diagnosis of an STD, encourage the patient to refrain from intercourse until full therapy is complete, the partner is treated, and all visible lesions are resolved.

A. DIAGNOSTIC FEATURES AND MANAGEMENT OF VAGINAL INFECTION (Table 5-6)

B. DIAGNOSTIC FEATURES AND MANAGEMENT OF GENITAL ULCERS AND WARTS (Table 5-7)

V. SCOLIOSIS[16]

Refer to Figure 5-5 for routine screening for scoliosis. Many curves that are detected on screening are nonprogressive or too slight to be significant.

A. ASSESSMENT

1. **Radiographic determination of the Cobb angle** (Fig. 5-6)**:** if there is clinical suspicion of significant scoliosis on screening, use erect thoracoabdominal spinal view.
2. **Bone scan with or without magnetic resonance imaging (MRI):** if pain is worse at night, progressive, well localized, or otherwise suspicious, obtain bone scan or MRI to look for tumor, infection, or fracture.
3. **MRI:** obtain if patient is younger than 10 years of age or if "opposite" curves are present (i.e., left-sided thoracic or right-sided lumbar).

B. TREATMENT

Treatment plan is determined according to the Cobb angle and skeletal maturity, which is assessed by grading the ossification of the iliac crest or can be estimated in females; skeletal maturity is reached 18 months after menarche.

1. **Skeletally immature:**

a. <10 Degrees: obtain a single follow-up radiograph in 4 to 6 months to ensure there has been no significant progression of the scoliosis.
b. 10 to 20 Degrees: obtain follow-up radiographs every 4 to 6 months while still growing.
c. 20 to 40 Degrees: bracing is required.

Text continues on p. 154

TABLE 5-6
DIAGNOSTIC FEATURES AND MANAGEMENT OF VAGINAL INFECTIONS

	Normal Vaginal Examination	Yeast Vaginitis	Trichomoniasis	Bacterial Vaginosis
Etiology	Uninfected; *Lactobacillus* predominant	*Candida albicans* and other yeasts	*Trichomonas vaginalis*	Associated with *Gardnerella vaginalis*, various anaerobic bacteria, and mycoplasma
Typical symptoms	None	Vulvar itching and/or irritation, increased discharge	Malodorous purulent discharge, vulvar itching	Malodorous, slightly increased discharge
DISCHARGE				
Amount	Variable; usually scant	Scant to moderate	Profuse	Moderate
Color*	Clear or white	White	Yellow-green	Usually white or gray
Consistency	Nonhomogeneous, floccular	Clumped; adherent plaques	Homogeneous	Homogeneous, low viscosity; smoothly coating vaginal walls
Inflammation of vulvar or vaginal epithelium	No	Yes	Yes	No
pH of vaginal fluid†	Usually <4.5	Usually <4.5	Usually >5.0	Usually >4.5
Amine ("fishy") odor with 10% KOH	None	None	May be present	Present

Microscopy[‡]	Normal epithelial cells; *Lactobacillus* predominates	Leukocytes, epithelial cells, yeast, mycelia, or pseudomycelia in 40%–80% of cases	Leukocytes; motile trichomonads seen in 50%–70% of symptomatic patients, less often in the absence of symptoms	Clue cells, few leukocytes; *Lactobacillus* outnumbered by profuse mixed flora, nearly always including *G. vaginalis* plus anaerobic species, on Gram stain
Usual treatment	None	Single dose of oral fluconazole, or miconazole or clotrimazole vaginal suppository	Metronidazole, single dose or 7–dy course	Oral or topical metronidazole or oral clindamycin
Usual management of sex partners	None	None; topical treatment if candidal dermatitis of penis is present	Treatment recommended	Examine for sexually transmitted disease, routine treatment not recommended

Note: Gram stain is also excellent for detecting yeasts and pseudomycelia and for distinguishing normal flora from the mixed flora seen in bacterial vaginosis, but it is less sensitive than the saline preparation for detection of *T. vaginalis*. Refer to Formulary for dosing information.

*Color of discharge is determined by examining vaginal discharge against the white background of a swab.

[†]pH determination is not useful if blood is present.

[‡]To detect fungal elements, vaginal fluid is digested with 10% KOH before microscopic examination; to examine for other features, fluid is mixed (1 : 1) with physiologic saline.

From Holmes KK, et al: Sexually Transmitted Diseases. New York: McGraw-Hill; 1990 and Centers for Disease Control and Prevention: Guidelines for treatment of sexually transmitted diseases. MMWR 1998;47(RR-1):1–118.

TABLE 5-7

DIAGNOSTIC FEATURES AND MANAGEMENT OF GENITAL ULCERS AND WARTS

Infection	Clinical Presentation	Presumptive Diagnosis	Definitive Diagnosis	Treatment/Management of Sex Partners
Genital herpes	Grouped vesicles, painful shallow ulcers; tender inguinal adenopathy	Tzanck smear looking for multinucleated giant cells	Viral culture	No known cure. Prompt initiation of therapy shortens duration of first episode. For severe recurrent disease, initiate therapy at start of prodrome or within 1 day of onset of lesions. See formulary for dosing of acyclovir, famciclovir, or valacyclovir. Transmission can occur during asymptomatic periods.
Primary syphilis	Indurated, well defined, usually single painless ulcer or "chancre"; nontender inguinal adenopathy	Nontreponemal serologic test: VDRL, RPR, or STS	Treponemal serologic test: FTA-ABS or MHA-TP; darkfield microscopy or direct fluorescent antibody tests of lesion exudates or tissue	Parenteral penicillin G is preferred treatment; preparation(s), dosage, and length of treatment depend on stage and clinical manifestations (see Chapter 16). All sexual contracts of persons with acquired syphilis should be evaluated. Contacts within the previous 3 months may be falsely seronegative; presumptive treatment recommended.
HPV infection (genital warts)	Single or multiple soft, fleshy, papillary or sessile, painless growth around the anus, vulvovaginal area, penis, urethra, or perineum; no inguinal adenopathy	Typical clinical presentation	Papanicolaou smear revealing typical cytologic changes	Treatment does not eradicate infection. *Goal:* Removal of exophytic warts. Exclude cervical dysplasia before treatment. Patient-administered therapies include podofilox and imiquimod cream. Clinician-applied therapies include podophyllin 10%–25% in compound tincture of benzoin, bichloroacetic or trichloroacetic acid, and surgical removal. Podofilox, imiquimod, and podophyllin are contraindicated in pregnancy. Period of communicability is unknown.

Note: Chancroid, lymphogranuloma venereum (LGV), and granuloma inguinale should be considered in the differential diagnosis of genital ulcers if the clinical presentation is atypical and testing for herpes and syphilis are negative.

FTA-ABS, Fluorescent treponemal antibody absorbed; HPV, human papilloma virus; MHA-TP, microhemagglutination assay for antibody to *T. pallidum*; RPR, rapid plasma reagin; STS, serologic test for syphilis; VDRL, Venereal Disease Research Laboratory.

Modified from Centers for Disease Control and Prevention: Guidelines for treatment of sexually transmitted diseases. MMWR 1998;47(RR-1):1–118 and Adger H: Sexually transmitted diseases. In Oski FA, et al (eds): Principles and Practice of Pediatrics. Philadelphia, Lippincott, Williams & Wilkins; 1999.

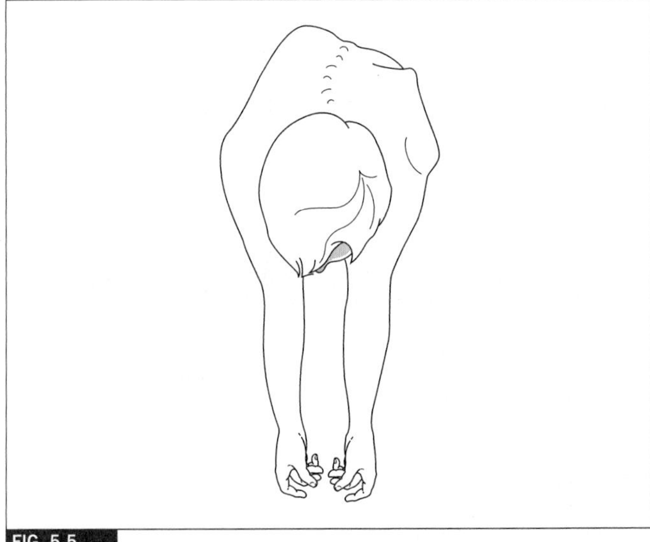

FIG. 5-5
Forward bending test. This emphasizes any asymmetry of the paraspinous muscles and rib cage.

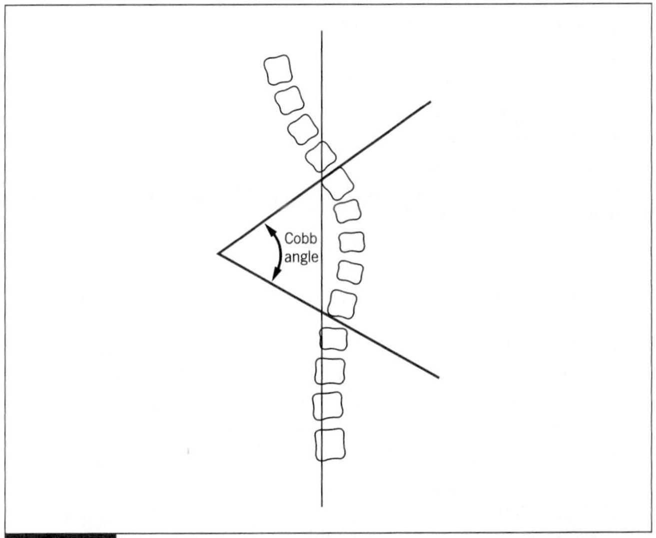

FIG. 5-6
Cobb angle. This is measured using the superior and inferior end plates of the most tilted vertebrae at the end of each curve.

d. >40 Degrees: surgical correction is necessary.

2. **Skeletally mature:**

a. <40 Degrees: no further evaluation or intervention is indicated.

b. >40 Degrees: surgical correction is required.

3. **Orthopedic referral** is indicated if the patient is skeletally immature with a curve >20 degrees or skeletally mature with a curve >40 degrees, or in the presence of suspicious pain or neurologic symptoms.

VI. RECOMMENDED COMPONENTS OF THE PREPARTICIPATION PHYSICAL EVALUATION (PPE)[17,18]

A. MEDICAL HISTORY

The medical history should include information regarding illnesses or injuries since the last examination or PPE; chronic conditions and medications; hospitalizations or surgeries; medications used by athletes (including those they may be taking to enhance performance); use of any special equipment or protective devices during sports participation; allergies, particularly those associated with anaphylaxis or respiratory compromise and those provoked by exercise; immunization status, including hepatitis B, MMR, tetanus, and varicella.

B. REVIEW OF SYSTEMS AND PHYSICAL EXAMINATION ITEMS

Examination items are in italics.

1. **Height and weight.**
2. **Vision:** Visual problems, corrective lenses; *visual acuity, pupil equality.*
3. **Cardiac:** History of congenital heart disease; symptoms of syncope, dizziness, or chest pain during exercise; history of high blood pressure or heart murmurs; family history of heart disease; previous history of disqualification or limited participation in sports because of a cardiac problem; *blood pressure, heart rate and rhythm, pulses (including radial/femoral lag), auscultation for heart sounds, murmurs—both standing and supine.*
4. **Respiratory:** Asthma, coughing, wheezing, or dyspnea during exercise.
5. **Abdomen:** Organomegaly and single kidney are contraindications for contact sports.
6. **Genitourinary:** Age at menarche, last menstrual period, regularity of menstrual periods, number of periods in the last year, longest interval between periods, dysmenorrhea; *palpation of the abdomen, palpation of the testicles, examination of the inguinal canals.*
7. **Orthopedic:** Previous injuries that have limited sports participation; injuries that have been associated with pain, swelling, or the need for medical intervention; screening orthopedic examination (Fig. 5-7).
8. **Neurology:** History of a significant head injury or concussion; numbness or tingling in the extremities; severe headaches; seizure disorder.

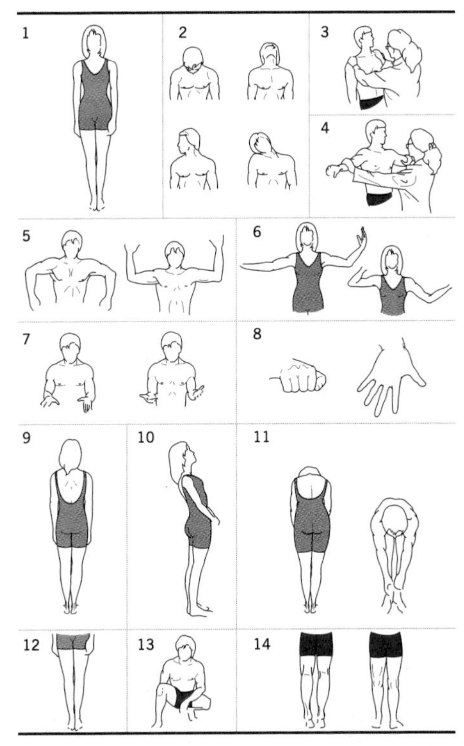

FIG. 5-7

Screening orthopedic examination. The general musculoskeletal screening examination consists of the following: (1) inspection, athlete standing, facing examiner (symmetry of trunk, upper extremities); (2) forward flexion, extension, rotation, lateral flexion of neck (range of motion, cervical spine); (3) resisted shoulder shrug (strength, trapezius); (4) resisted shoulder abduction (strength, deltoid); (5) internal and external rotation of shoulder (range of motion, glenohumeral joint); (6) extension and flexion of elbow (range of motion, elbow); (7) pronation and supination of elbow (range of motion, elbow and wrist); (8) clenching of fist, then spreading of fingers (range of motion, hand and fingers); (9) inspection, athlete facing away from examiner (symmetry of trunk, upper extremities); (10) back extension, knees straight (spondylolysis and spondylolisthesis); (11) back flexion with knees straight, facing toward and away from examiner (range of motion, thoracic and lumbosacral spine; spine curvature; hamstring flexibility); (12) inspection of lower extremities, contraction of quadriceps muscles (alignment symmetry); (13) "duck walk" four steps (motion of hips, knees, and ankles; strength; balance); (14) standing on toes, then on heels (symmetry, calf; strength; balance). *(Modified from American Academy of Family Physicians: Preparticipation Physical Examination, 2nd ed. Kansas City, MO, American Academy of Family Physicians, 1997.)*

9. **Skin:** Rashes; *evidence of contagious infections (e.g., varicella or impetigo).*
10. **Psychosocial:** Weight control and body image; stresses at home or in school; use or abuse of drugs and alcohol; *attention to signs of eating disorders, including oral ulcerations, eroded tooth enamel, edema, lanugo hair, calluses or ulcerations on knuckles.*

REFERENCES

1. Woods ER, Neinstein LS: Office visit, interview techniques and recommendations to parents. In Neinstein LS (ed): Adolescent Healthcare: A Practical Guide, 4th ed. Philadelphia, Lippincott Williams & Wilkins, 2002, p 64.
2. Joffe A: Introduction to adolescent medicine. In McMillan JA, DeAngelis CD, Feigan RD, Warshaw J (eds): Oski's Pediatrics Principles and Practice, 3rd ed. Philadelphia, Lippincott Williams & Wilkins, 1999, pp 528, 531, 535.
3. Rosen DS, Neinstein LS: Preventive healthcare for adolescents. In Neinstein LS (ed): Adolescent Healthcare: A Practical Guide, 4th ed. Philadelphia, Lippincott Williams & Wilkins, 2002, pp 82, 98–99,107–109, 117.
4. Fishman M, Bruner A, Adger H: Substance abuse among children and adolescents. Pediatr Rev 1997;18:397–398.
5. Centers for Disease Control and Prevention: Immunization of adolescents: recommendation of the Advisory Committee on Immunization Practices, the American Academy of Pediatrics, the American Academy of Family Physicians, and the American Medical Association. MMWR 1996;45(No. RR-13):5,10–11.
6. Hatcher RA, Trussel J, Stuart F, et al: Contraceptive Technology, 17th ed. New York: Ardent Media, 1998, pp 420–424.
7. http://www.reproline.jhu.edu/english/6read/6multi/pg/ci3.htm
8. Nelson AL, Neinstein LS: Combination hormonal contraceptives. In Neinstein LS (ed): Adolescent Healthcare: A Practical Guide, 4th ed. Philadelphia, Lippincott Williams & Wilkins, 2002, pp 875–876, 878.
9. http://www.reproline.jhu.edu/english/6read/6multi/pg/ci4.htm
10. http://www.fpnotebook.com/GYN89.htm
11. Wilson MD: Adolescent pregnancy and contraception. In McMillan JA, DeAngelis CD, Feigan RD, Warshaw J (eds): Oski's Pediatrics Principles and Practice, 3rd ed. Philadelphia, Lippincott Williams & Wilkins, 1999, pp 544–546.
12. Nelson AL, Neinstein LS: Long acting progestins. In Neinstein LS (ed): Adolescent Healthcare: A Practical Guide, 4th ed. Philadelphia, Lippincott Williams & Wilkins, 2002, pp 922–923, 926, 932.
13. http://www.fpnotebook.com/GYN126.htm
14. Nelson AL, Neinstein LS: Emergency contraception. In Neinstein LS (ed): Adolescent Healthcare: A Practical Guide, 4th ed. Philadelphia, Lippincott Williams & Wilkins, 2002, pp 913–916.
15. Brill SR, Rosenfeld WD: Contraception. Med Clin North Am 2000;84:919–920.
16. Kautz SM, Skaggs DL: Getting an angle on spinal deformities. Contemp Pediatr 1998;15:114–123.
17. Andrews JS: Making the most of the sports physical. Contemp Pediatr 1997;14:188.
18. Hergenroeder AC, Neinstein LS: Guidelines in sports medicine. In Neinstein LS (ed): Adolescent Healthcare: A Practical Guide, 4th ed. Philadelphia, Lippincott Williams & Wilkins, 2002, pp 382–383, 386, 391.

19. Nelson AL, Neinstein LS: Combination hormonal contraceptives. In Neinstein LS (ed): Adolescent Healthcare: A Practical Guide, 4th ed. Philadelphia, Lippincott Williams & Wilkins, 2002, pp 862–872.
20. Nelson AL, Neinstein LS: Intrauterine devices. In Neinstein LS (ed): Adolescent Healthcare: A Practical Guide, 4th ed. Philadelphia, Lippincott Williams & Wilkins, 2002, pp 884–887.
21. Nelson AL, Neinstein LS: Long acting progestins. In Neinstein LS (ed): Adolescent Healthcare: A Practical Guide, 4th ed. Philadelphia, Lippincott Williams & Wilkins, 2002.

Cardiology

Kelly K. Gajewski, MD

6

I. WEBSITES

www.americanheart.org (Open the Heart and Stroke Encyclopedia)
www.cincinnatichildrens.org/heartcenter/encyclopedia/
www.pted.org
www.murmurlab.org

II. THE CARDIAC CYCLE (FIG. 6-1)

III. PHYSICAL EXAMINATION

A. PRESSURE

1. **Pulse pressure = systolic pressure − diastolic pressure.**

See Box 6-1 (pulse pressure differential diagnosis).

2. **Mean arterial pressure (MAP) = diastolic pressure + (pulse pressure/3). In preterm infants and newborns, generally a normal MAP = gestational age in weeks + 5.**

See Figure 6-2. (Please see also Zubrow AB, et al: J Perinatol 1995;15:470, for more neonatal blood pressure norms.)

3. **Blood pressure**

a. Four limb blood pressure measurements can be used to assess for coarctation of the aorta; pressure must be measured in both the right and left arms because of the possibility of an aberrant right subclavian artery.

b. Pulsus paradoxus is an exaggeration of the normal drop in systolic blood pressure (SBP) seen with inspiration. Determine the SBP at the end of exhalation and then during inhalation; if the difference in SBP is greater than 10 mmHg, consider pericardial effusion, tamponade, pericarditis, severe asthma, or restrictive cardiomyopathies.

c. See Figures 6-3 and 6-4[1,2] and Tables 6-1 and 6-2 for blood pressure norms.

B. HEART SOUNDS

1. **S1 is best heard at the apex or left lower sternal border (LLSB).**
2. **S2, heard best at the left upper sternal border (LUSB), has a normal physiologic split that increases with inspiration.**
3. **S3 is heard best at the apex or LLSB.**
4. **S4 is heard at the apex.**

See Box 6-2 for abnormal heart sounds.[3]

C. SYSTOLIC AND DIASTOLIC SOUNDS

1. **An ejection click sounds like splitting of the S1 but is most audible at the apex, in contrast to the commonly heard, normal finding of a split S1, which is best heard at the LLSB.** The ejection click is associated

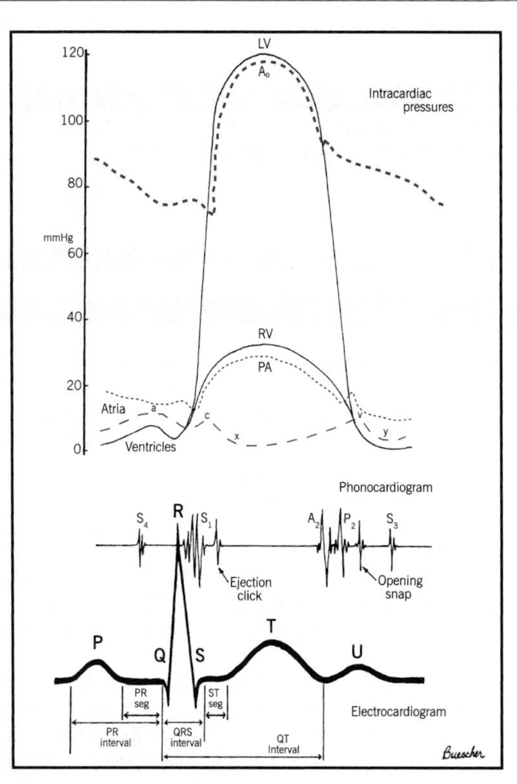

FIG. 6-1
The cardiac cycle.

BOX 6-1

PULSE PRESSURE DIFFERENTIAL DIAGNOSIS

WIDE PULSE PRESSURE (>40 MMHG)	NARROW PULSE PRESSURE (<25 MMHG)
Thyrotoxicosis	*Pericarditis*
Arteriovenous (AV) fistula	*Pericardial effusion*
Patent ductus arteriosus (PDA)	*Pericardial tamponade*
Aortic insufficiency	*Aortic stenosis (AS)*
	Significant tachycardia

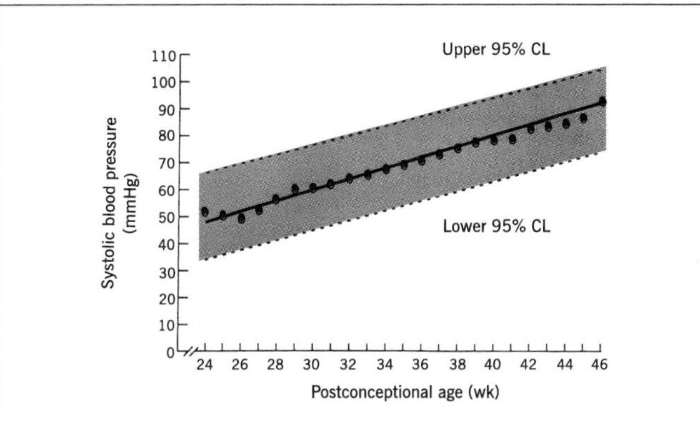

FIG. 6-2

Linear regression of mean systolic blood pressure on postconceptional age (gestational age in weeks plus weeks after delivery). *(Data from Zubrow AB, et al: J Perinatol 1995;15:470.)*

BOX 6-2

SUMMARY OF ABNORMAL HEART SOUNDS

ABNORMAL SPLITTING

Widely Split S1
Ebstein's anomaly
RBBB

Widely Split and Fixed S2
RV volume overload (e.g., ASD, PAPVR)
Abnormal pulmonary valve (e.g., PS)
Electrical delay (e.g., RBBB)
Early aortic closure (e.g., MR)
Occasional normal child

Narrowly Split S2
Pulmonary hypertension
AS
LBBB
Occasional normal child

Single S2
Pulmonary hypertension
One semilunar valve (e.g., pulmonary atresia, aortic atresia, truncus arteriosus)
P2 not audible (e.g., TGA, TOF, severe PS)
Severe AS
Occasional normal child

Paradoxically Split S2
Severe AS
LBBB, Wolff-Parkinson-White syndrome (type B)

Continued

Abnormal Intensity of P2
Increased P2 (e.g., pulmonary hypertension)
Decreased P2 (e.g., severe PS, TOF, TS)
S3
Occasionally heard in healthy children or adults
Dilated ventricles (large VSD, CHF)
S4
Always pathologic
Decreased ventricular compliance

AS, aortic stenosis; ASD, atrial septal defect; LBBB, left bundle-branch block; MR, mitral regurgitation; PAPVR, partial anomalous pulmonary venous return; PS, pulmonary stenosis; RBBB, right bundle-branch block; TGA, transposition of the great arteries; TOF, tetralogy of Fallot; TS, tricuspid stenosis.

Modified from Park MK: Pediatric Cardiology for Practitioners, 3rd ed. St. Louis, Mosby, 1996.

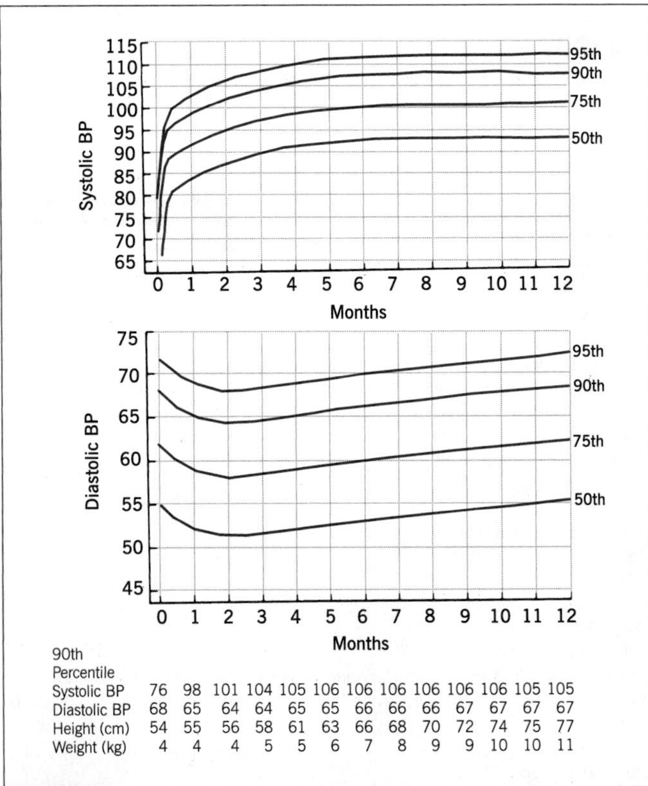

90th Percentile													
Systolic BP	76	98	101	104	105	106	106	106	106	106	106	105	105
Diastolic BP	68	65	64	64	65	65	66	66	66	67	67	67	67
Height (cm)	54	55	56	58	61	63	66	68	70	72	74	75	77
Weight (kg)	4	4	4	5	5	6	7	8	9	9	10	10	11

FIG. 6-3

Age-specific percentile of blood pressure (BP) measurements in girls from birth to 12 months of age; Korotkoff phase IV (K4) used for diastolic BP. *(From Horan MJ, et al: Pediatrics 1987;79(1):1–25.)*

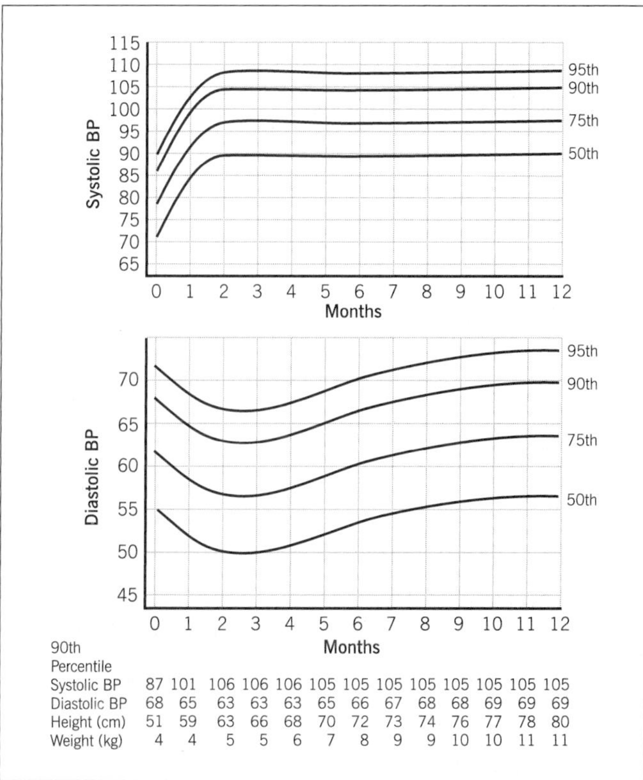

90th Percentile													
Systolic BP	87	101	106	106	106	105	105	105	105	105	105	105	105
Diastolic BP	68	65	63	63	63	65	66	67	68	68	69	69	69
Height (cm)	51	59	63	66	68	70	72	73	74	76	77	78	80
Weight (kg)	4	4	5	5	6	7	8	9	9	10	10	11	11

FIG. 6-4

Age-specific percentiles of blood pressure (BP) measurements in boys from birth to 12 months of age; Korotkoff phase IV (K4) used for diastolic BP. *(From Horan MJ, et al: Pediatrics 1987;79(1):1–25.)*

with stenosis of the semilunar valves and large great arteries (e.g., systemic hypertension; pulmonary hypertension; idiopathic dilation of the pulmonary artery [PA]; tetralogy of Fallot [TOF], in which the aorta is dilated; and persistent truncus arteriosus).

2. **A midsystolic click with or without a late systolic murmur is heard near the apex in mitral valve prolapse (MVP).**
3. **Diastolic opening snap is audible at the apex or LLSB in mitral stenosis.**

Text continues on p. 168

TABLE 6-1

BLOOD PRESSURE LEVELS FOR THE 90TH AND 95TH PERCENTILES OF BLOOD PRESSURE FOR *GIRLS* AGED 1–17 YEARS BY PERCENTILES OF HEIGHT

	Height* →	Systolic BP (SBP) (mmHg) by Percentile of Height							Diastolic BP (DBP) (mmHg) by Percentile of Height						
Age (yr)	BP[†]↓	5%	10%	25%	50%	75%	90%	95%	5%	10%	25%	50%	75%	90%	95%
1	90th	97	98	99	100	102	103	104	53	53	53	54	55	56	56
	95th	101	102	103	104	105	107	107	57	57	57	58	59	60	60
2	90th	99	99	100	102	103	104	105	57	57	58	58	59	60	61
	95th	102	103	104	105	107	108	109	61	61	62	62	63	64	65
3	90th	100	100	102	103	104	105	106	61	61	61	62	63	63	64
	95th	104	104	105	107	108	109	110	65	65	65	66	67	67	68
4	90th	101	102	103	104	106	107	108	63	63	64	65	65	66	67
	95th	105	106	107	108	109	111	111	67	67	68	69	69	70	71
5	90th	103	103	104	106	107	108	109	65	66	66	67	68	68	69
	95th	107	107	108	110	111	112	113	69	70	70	71	72	72	73
6	90th	104	105	106	107	109	110	111	67	67	68	69	69	70	71
	95th	108	109	110	111	112	114	114	71	71	72	73	73	74	75
7	90th	106	107	108	109	110	112	112	69	69	69	70	71	72	72
	95th	110	110	112	113	114	115	116	73	73	73	74	75	76	76
8	90th	108	109	110	111	112	113	114	70	70	71	71	72	73	74
	95th	112	112	113	115	116	117	118	74	74	75	75	76	77	78

9	90th	110	110	112	113	114	115	116	71	72	72	73	74	74	75
	95th	114	114	115	117	118	119	120	75	76	76	77	78	78	79
10	90th	112	112	114	115	116	117	118	73	73	73	74	75	76	76
	95th	116	116	117	119	120	121	122	77	77	77	78	79	80	80
11	90th	114	114	116	117	118	119	120	74	74	75	75	76	77	77
	95th	118	118	119	121	122	123	124	78	78	79	79	80	81	81
12	90th	116	116	118	119	120	121	122	75	75	76	76	77	78	78
	95th	120	120	121	123	124	125	126	79	79	80	80	81	82	82
13	90th	118	118	119	121	122	123	124	76	76	77	78	78	79	80
	95th	121	122	123	125	126	127	128	80	80	81	82	82	83	84
14	90th	119	120	121	122	124	125	126	77	77	78	79	79	80	81
	95th	123	124	125	126	128	129	130	81	81	82	83	83	84	85
15	90th	121	121	122	124	125	126	127	78	78	79	79	80	81	82
	95th	124	125	126	128	129	130	131	82	82	83	83	84	85	86
16	90th	122	122	123	125	126	127	128	79	79	79	80	81	82	82
	95th	125	126	127	128	130	131	132	83	83	83	84	85	86	86
17	90th	122	123	124	125	126	128	128	79	79	79	80	81	82	82
	95th	126	126	127	129	130	131	132	83	83	83	84	85	86	86

*Height percentile determined by standard growth curves.

†Blood pressure percentile determined by a single measurement.

TABLE 6-2

BLOOD PRESSURE LEVELS FOR THE 90TH AND 95TH PERCENTILES OF BLOOD PRESSURE FOR *BOYS* AGED 1–17 YEARS BY PERCENTILES OF HEIGHT

	Height* →	Systolic BP (SBP) (mmHg) by Percentile of Height							Diastolic BP (DBP) (mmHg) by Percentile of Height						
Age (yr)	BP†↓	5%	10%	25%	50%	75%	90%	95%	5%	10%	25%	50%	75%	90%	95%
1	90th	94	95	97	98	100	102	102	50	51	52	53	54	54	55
	95th	98	99	101	102	104	106	106	55	55	56	57	58	59	59
2	90th	98	99	100	102	104	105	106	55	55	56	57	58	59	59
	95th	101	102	104	106	108	109	110	59	59	60	61	62	63	63
3	90th	100	101	103	105	107	108	109	59	59	60	61	62	63	63
	95th	104	105	107	109	111	112	113	63	63	64	65	66	67	67
4	90th	102	103	105	107	109	110	111	62	62	63	64	65	66	66
	95th	106	107	109	111	113	114	115	66	67	67	68	69	70	71
5	90th	104	105	106	108	110	112	112	65	65	66	67	68	69	69
	95th	108	109	110	112	114	115	116	69	70	70	71	72	73	74
6	90th	105	106	108	110	111	113	114	67	68	69	70	70	71	72
	95th	109	110	112	114	115	117	117	72	72	73	74	75	76	76
7	90th	106	107	109	111	113	114	115	69	70	71	72	72	73	74
	95th	110	111	113	115	116	118	119	74	74	75	76	77	78	78
8	90th	107	108	110	112	114	115	116	71	71	72	73	74	75	75
	95th	111	112	114	116	118	119	120	75	76	76	77	78	79	80

9	90th	109	110	112	113	115	117	117	72	73	73	74	75	76	77
	95th	113	114	116	117	119	121	121	76	77	78	79	80	80	81
10	90th	110	112	113	115	117	118	119	73	74	74	75	76	77	78
	95th	114	115	117	119	121	122	123	77	78	79	80	80	81	82
11	90th	112	113	115	117	119	120	121	74	74	75	76	77	78	78
	95th	116	117	119	121	123	124	125	78	79	79	80	81	82	83
12	90th	115	116	117	119	121	123	123	75	75	76	77	78	78	79
	95th	119	120	121	123	125	126	127	79	79	80	81	82	83	83
13	90th	117	118	120	122	124	125	126	75	76	76	77	78	79	80
	95th	121	122	124	126	128	129	130	79	80	81	82	83	83	84
14	90th	120	121	123	125	126	128	128	76	76	77	78	79	80	80
	95th	124	125	127	128	130	132	132	80	81	81	82	83	84	85
15	90th	123	124	125	127	129	131	131	77	77	78	79	80	81	81
	95th	127	128	129	131	133	134	135	81	82	83	83	84	85	86
16	90th	125	126	128	130	132	133	134	79	79	80	81	82	82	83
	95th	129	130	132	134	136	137	138	83	83	84	85	86	87	87
17	90th	128	129	131	133	134	136	136	81	81	82	83	84	85	85
	95th	132	133	135	136	138	140	140	85	85	86	87	88	89	89

*Height percentile determined by standard growth curves.

†Blood pressure percentile determined by a single measurement.

D. MURMURS[4]

1. **Benign heart murmurs** are caused by a disturbance of the laminar flow of blood, frequently produced as the diameter of the blood's pathway decreases and the velocity increases. More than 80% of children have innocent murmurs sometime during childhood, most commonly beginning at 3 to 4 years of age. Innocent murmurs are accentuated in high-output states, especially with fever and anemia, and are associated with normal electrocardiogram (ECG) and radiographic findings. However, note that an ECG and a chest radiograph are not routinely useful or cost-effective screening tools for distinguishing benign from pathologic murmurs. Clinical characteristics of these murmurs are summarized in Table 6-3.[3] When one or more of the following are present, the murmur is likely to be pathologic and require cardiac consultation:
   - Symptoms
   - Cyanosis
   - Systolic murmur that is loud (grade 3/6 or with a thrill), harsh, and long in duration

TABLE 6-3

COMMON INNOCENT HEART MURMURS

Type (Timing)	Description of Murmur	Age Group
Classic vibratory murmur (Still's murmur; systolic)	Maximal at MLSB or between LLSB and apex Grade 2–3/6 in intensity Low-frequency vibratory, twanging string, groaning, squeaking, or musical	3–6 yr; occasionally in infancy
Pulmonary ejection murmur (systolic)	Maximal at ULSB Early to mid-systolic Grade 1–3/6 in intensity Blowing in quality	8–14 yr
Pulmonary flow murmur of newborn (systolic)	Maximal at ULSB Transmits well to left and right chest, axillae, and back Grade 1–2/6 in intensity	Premature and full-term newborns Usually disappears by 3–6 mo
Venous hum (continuous)	Maximal at right (or left) supraclavicular and infraclavicular areas Grade 1–3/6 in intensity Inaudible in supine position Intensity changes with rotation of head and disappears with compression of jugular vein	3–6 yr
Carotid bruit (systolic)	Right supraclavicular area over carotids Grade 2–3/6 in intensity Occasional thrill over carotid	Any age

LLSB, lower left sternal border; MLSB, middle left sternal border; ULSB, upper left sternal border.
From Park MK: Pediatric cardiology for practitioners, 3rd ed. St. Louis, Mosby, 1996.

Diastolic murmur
Abnormal heart sounds
Presence of a click
Abnormally strong or weak pulses

2. Systolic murmurs (Fig. 6-5).
3. Diastolic murmurs (see Fig. 6-5).

IV. LIPID MONITORING RECOMMENDATIONS: PREVENTION OF ATHEROSCLEROTIC DISEASE (AMERICAN ACADEMY OF PEDIATRICS [AAP] RECOMMENDATIONS)

A. SCREENING OF CHILDREN AND ADOLESCENTS

1. Those whose parents or grandparents, at ≤55 years of age, were found to have coronary atherosclerosis.

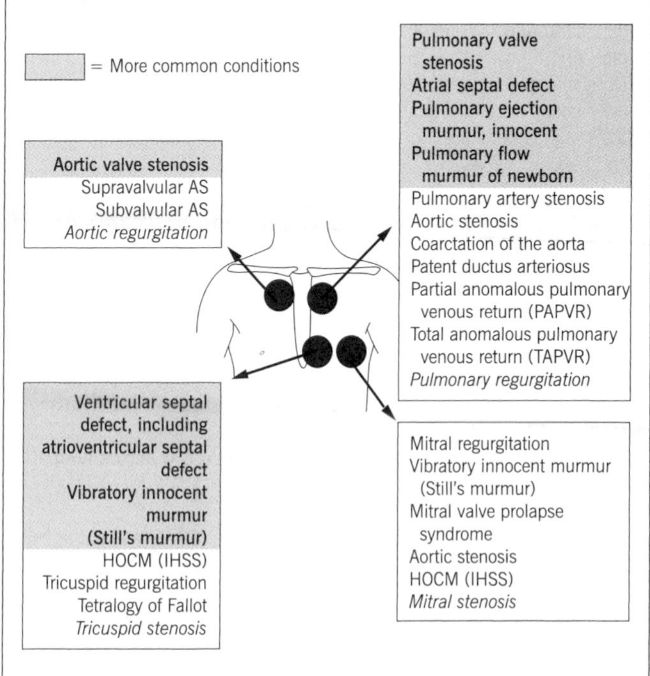

FIG. 6-5

The location at which various murmurs may be heard. Diastolic murmurs are in italics. AS, aortic stenosis; HOCM, hypertrophic obstructive cardiomyopathy; IHSS, idiopathic hypertrophic subaortic stenosis. *(From Park MK: Pediatric Cardiology for Practitioners, 3rd ed. St. Louis, Mosby, 1996.)*

2. Those whose parents or grandparents, at ≤55 years of age, had a documented myocardial infarction, angina pectoris, peripheral vascular disease, cerebrovascular disease, or sudden cardiac death.
3. Those whose parent has an elevated blood cholesterol level (240 mg/dL or higher).
4. Those whose parental history is unobtainable, particularly for those with other risk factors, such as smoking, diets high in saturated fats and cholesterol, or obesity.

B. GOALS FOR LIPID LEVELS IN CHILDHOOD (Figs. 6-6 and 6-7)

C. MANAGEMENT OF HYPERLIPIDEMIA

1. **For normal and borderline low-density lipoprotein (LDL) levels:** education and risk factor intervention, including diet, smoking cessation, and an exercise program. For borderline levels, re-evaluate in 1 year.
2. **For high LDL levels:** Examine for secondary causes (liver, thyroid, renal disorders) and familial disorders. Then initiate low-fat, low-cholesterol diet, and re-evaluate in 3 months.
3. Drug therapy should only be considered in children >10 years of age after failure of an adequate trial of diet therapy (6–12 months). Bile acid sequestrants are the recommended drugs for treatment in children.

V. ELECTROCARDIOGRAPHY

A. BASIC ELECTROCARDIOGRAPHY PRINCIPLES

1. **Lead placement** (Fig. 6-8).
2. **ECG complexes (see Fig. 6-1).**
   a. P wave: Represents atrial depolarization.
   b. QRS complex: Represents ventricular depolarization.
   c. T wave: Represents ventricular repolarization.
   d. U wave: May follow T wave, representing late phases of ventricular repolarization.
3. **Systematic approach for evaluating ECGs** (Table 6-4 shows normal **ECG parameters)**[3,5]**:**
   a. Rate.
      (1) Standardization: Paper speed is 25 mm/sec. One small square = 1 mm = 0.04 sec. One large square = 5 mm = 0.2 sec. Amplitude standard: 10 mm = 1 mV.
      (2) Calculation: Heart rate (beats per minute) = 60 divided by the average R-R interval in seconds, or 1500 divided by the R-R interval in millimeters.
   b. Rhythm.
      (1) Sinus rhythm: Every QRS complex is preceded by a P wave, normal PR interval (the PR interval may be prolonged, as in first-degree atrioventricular [AV] block), and normal P-wave axis (upright P in lead I and aVF).

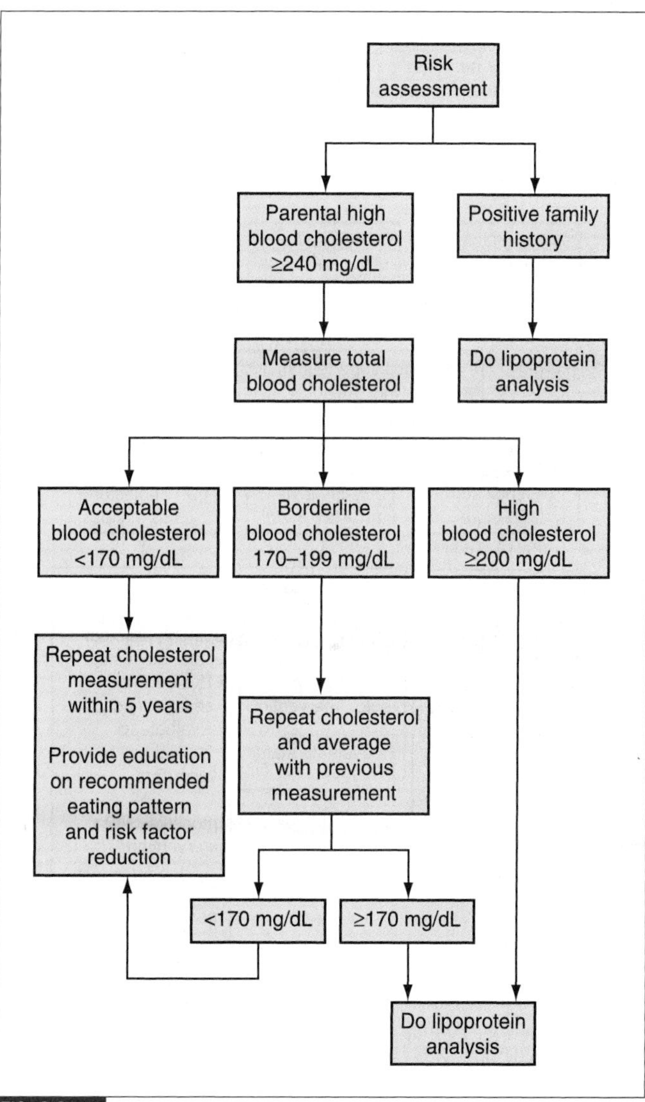

FIG. 6-6
Cholesterol flow chart.

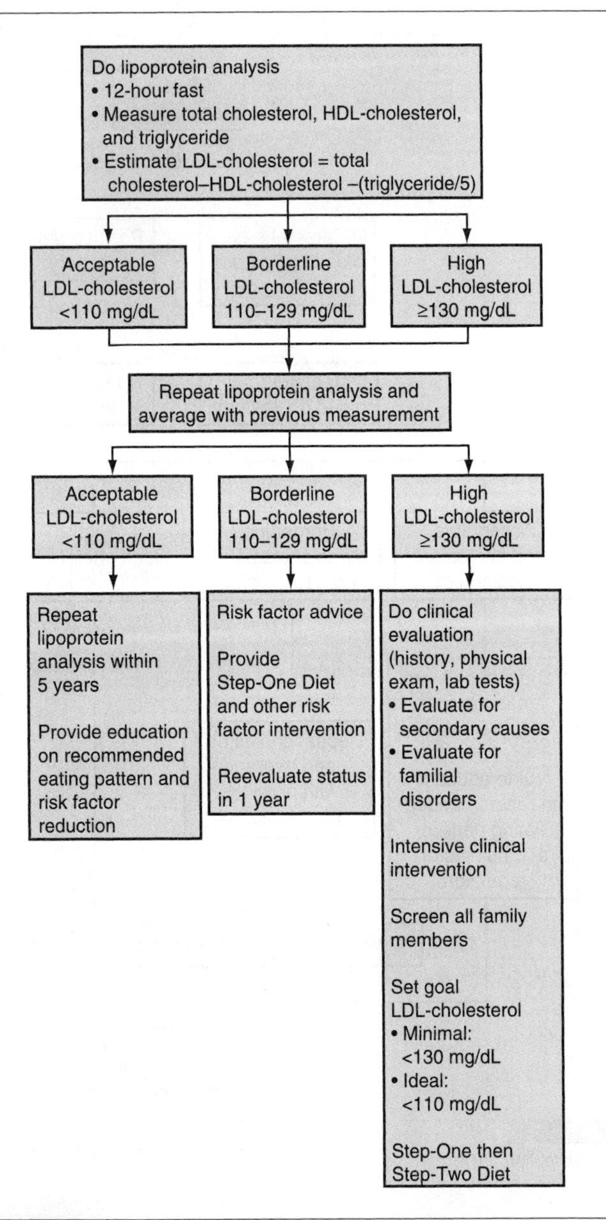

FIG. 6-7

Lipoprotein analysis flow chart.

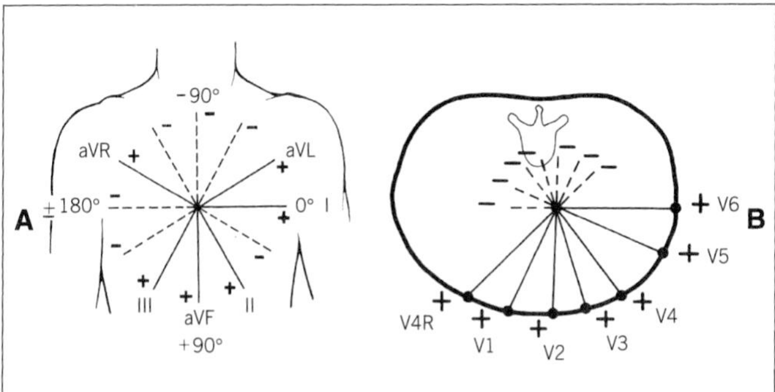

FIG. 6-8

A, Hexaxial reference system. *B*, Horizontal reference system. *(Modified from Park MK, Guntheroth WG: How to Read Pediatric ECGs, 3rd ed. St. Louis, Mosby, 1992.)*

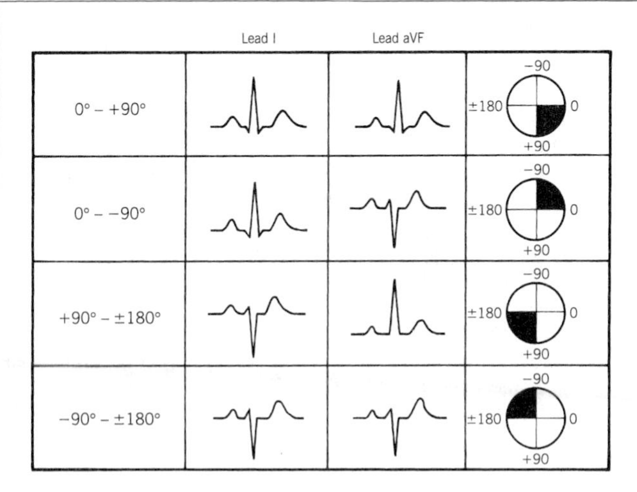

FIG. 6-9

Locating quadrants of mean QRS axis from leads 1 and aVF. *(From Park MK, Guntheroth WG: How to Read Pediatric ECGs, 3rd ed. St. Louis, Mosby, 1992.)*

(2) There is normal respiratory variation of the R-R interval without morphologic changes of the P wave or QRS complex.

c. Axis: Determine quadrant and compare with age-matched normal values (Fig. 6-9; see Table 6-4).

d. Intervals: (PR, QRS, QT_c). See Table 6-4 for normal PR and QRS intervals. The QT_c is calculated as

TABLE 6-4
NORMAL PEDIATRIC ECG PARAMETERS

					Lead V_1			Lead V_6		
Age	Heart Rate (bpm)	QRS Axis*	PR Interval (sec)*	QRS Duration (sec)†	R Wave Amplitude (mm)†	S Wave Amplitude (mm)†	R/S Ratio	R Wave Amplitude (mm)†	S Wave Amplitude (mm)†	R/S Ratio
0–7 days	95–160 (125)	+30 to 180 (110)	0.08–0.12 (0.10)	0.05 (0.07)	13.3 (25.5)	7.7 (18.8)	2.5	4.8 (11.8)	3.2 (9.6)	2.2
1–3 wk	105–180 (145)	+30 to 180 (110)	0.08–0.12 (0.10)	0.05 (0.07)	10.6 (20.8)	4.2 (10.8)	2.9	7.6 (16.4)	3.4 (9.8)	3.3
1–6 mo	110–180 (145)	+10 to +125 (+70)	0.08–0.13 (0.11)	0.05 (0.07)	9.7 (19)	5.4 (15)	2.3	12.4 (22)	2.8 (8.3)	5.6
6–12 mo	110–170 (135)	+10 to +125 (+60)	0.10–0.14 (0.12)	0.05 (0.07)	9.4 (20.3)	6.4 (18.1)	1.6	12.6 (22.7)	2.1 (7.2)	7.6
1–3 yr	90–150 (120)	+10 to +125 (+60)	0.10–0.14 (0.12)	0.06 (0.07)	8.5 (18)	9 (21)	1.2	14 (23.3)	1.7 (6)	10
4–5 yr	65–135 (110)	0 to +110 (+60)	0.11–0.15 (0.13)	0.07 (0.08)	7.6 (16)	11 (22.5)	0.8	15.6 (25)	1.4 (4.7)	11.2
6–8 yr	60–130 (100)	–15 to +110 (+60)	0.12–0.16 (0.14)	0.07 (0.08)	6 (13)	12 (24.5)	0.6	16.3 (26)	1.1 (3.9)	13
9–11 yr	60–110 (85)	–15 to +110 (+60)	0.12–0.17 (0.14)	0.07 (0.09)	5.4 (12.1)	11.9 (25.4)	0.5	16.3 (25.4)	1.0 (3.9)	14.3
12–16 yr	60–110 (85)	–15 to +110 (+60)	0.12–0.17 (0.15)	0.07 (0.10)	4.1 (9.9)	10.8 (21.2)	0.5	14.3 (23)	0.8 (3.7)	14.7
>16 yr	60–100 (80)	–15 to +110 (+60)	0.12–0.20 (0.15)	0.08 (0.10)	3 (9)	10 (20)	0.3	10 (20)	0.8 (3.7)	12

*Normal range and (mean).
†Mean and (98th percentile).
New data compiled from Park MK: Pediatric cardiology for practitioners, 3rd ed. St Louis, Mosby, 1996 and Davignon A, et al: Pediatr Cardiol 1979;1:123–131.

TABLE 6-5

NORMAL T-WAVE AXIS

Age	V1, V2	AVF	I, V5, V6
Birth–1 day	±	+	±
1–4 days	±	+	+
4 days to adolescent	–	+	+
Adolescent to adult	+	+	+

+, T wave positive; –, T wave negative; ±, T wave normally either positive or negative.

$$QT_c = QT\ (sec)\ m/MrR\text{-}R\ (sec)$$

The R-R interval should extend from the R wave in the QRS complex in which you are measuring QT to the preceding R wave. Normal values for QT_c are as follows:

(1) 0.440 sec is 97th percentile for infants 3 to 4 days old[6]

(2) ≤0.45 sec in infants <6 months old

(3) ≤0.44 sec in children

(4) ≤0.44 sec in adults

e. P-wave size and shape: Normal P wave should be <0.10 sec in children, <0.08 sec in infants, with amplitude <30 mV (3 mm in height, with normal standardization).

f. R-wave progression: There is generally a normal increase in R-wave size and decrease in S-wave size from leads V1 to V6 (with dominant S waves in right precordial leads and dominant R waves in left precordial leads), representing dominance of left ventricular forces. However, newborns and infants have a normal dominance of the right ventricle.

g. Q waves: Normal Q waves are usually <0.04 second (1 mm) in duration and <25% of the total QRS amplitude. Q waves are <5 mm deep in left precordial leads and aVF and ≤8 mm deep in lead III for children <3 years of age.

h. ST-segment and T-wave evaluation: ST-segment elevation or depression >1 mm in limb leads and >2 mm in precordial leads is consistent with myocardial ischemia or injury. Tall, peaked T waves may be seen in hyperkalemia. Flat or low T waves may be seen in hypokalemia, hypothyroidism, normal newborn, and myocardial and pericardial ischemia and inflammation (Table 6-5 and Fig. 6-10).

i. Hypertrophy.

(1) Atrial: Figure 6-11.

(2) Ventricular: Diagnosed by QRS axis, voltage, and R/S ratio (Box 6-3; see also Table 6-4).

B. ECG ABNORMALITIES

1. Nonventricular arrhythmias (Table 6-6).[7]

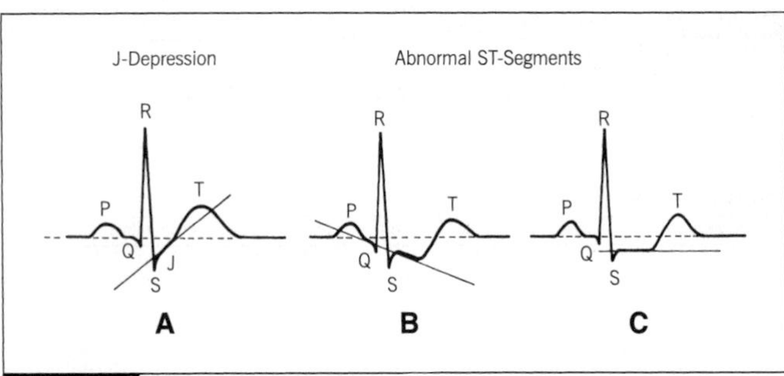

FIG. 6-10

Nonpathologic (nonischemic) and pathologic (ischemic) ST and T changes. *A*, Characteristic nonischemic ST-segment alteration called J depression; note that the ST slope is upward. *B* and *C*, Ischemic or pathologic ST-segment alterations. *B*, Downward slope of the ST segment. *C*, Horizontal segment is sustained. *(From Park MK, Guntheroth WG: How to Read Pediatric ECGs, 3rd ed. St. Louis, Mosby; 1992.)*

RAE	LAE	CAE
>3mm	>0.10 >0.10 V_1	

FIG. 6-11

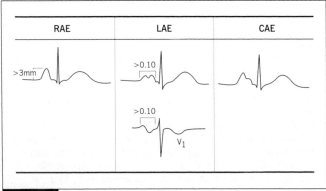

Criteria for atrial enlargement. CAE, combined atrial enlargement; LAE, left atrial enlargement; RAE, right atrial enlargement. *(From Park MK: Pediatric Cardiology for Practitioners, 3rd ed. St. Louis, Mosby, 1996.)*

BOX 6-3

VENTRICULAR HYPERTROPHY CRITERIA

RIGHT VENTRICULAR HYPERTROPHY (RVH) CRITERIA

Must have at least one of the following:

- Increased right and anterior QRS voltage (with normal QRS duration):
  - R in lead V1, >98th percentile for age
  - S in lead V6, >98th percentile for age
  - Upright T wave in lead V1 after 3 days of age to adolescence

Supplemental criteria

- Presence of q wave in V1 (qR or qRs pattern)
- Right axis deviation (RAD) for patient's age
- Right ventricle (RV) strain (associated with inverted T wave in V1 with tall R wave)

LEFT VENTRICULAR HYPERTROPHY (LVH) CRITERIA

Increased QRS voltage in left leads (with normal QRS duration):

- R in lead V6 (and I, aVL, V5), >98th percentile for age
- S in lead V1, >98th percentile for age

Supplemental criteria

- Left axis deviation (LAD) for patient's age
- Volume overload (associated with Q wave >5 mm and tall T waves in V5 or V6)
- Left ventricle (LV) strain (associated with inverted T wave in leads V6, I, or aVF)

TABLE 6-6

NONVENTRICULAR ARRHYTHMIAS

Name/Description	Cause	Treatment
SINUS		
Tachycardia		
Normal sinus rhythm with HR >95th percentile for age (usually less than 230 beats/min)	Hypovolemia, shock, anemia, sepsis, fever, anxiety, CHF, PE, myocardial disease, drugs (e.g., β-agonists, aminophylline, atropine)	Address underlying cause
Bradycardia		
Normal sinus rhythm with HR <5th percentile for age	Normal (especially in athletic individuals), increased ICP, hypoxia, hyperkalemia, hypercalcemia, vagal stimulation, hypothyroidism, hypothermia, drugs (e.g., digoxin, β-blockers), long QT syndrome	Address underlying cause; if symptomatic, refer to inside back cover for bradycardia algorithm

continued

TABLE 6-6

NONVENTRICULAR ARRHYTHMIAS—*cont'd*

Name/Description	Cause	Treatment
SUPRAVENTRICULAR		
Abnormal rhythm resulting from ectopic focus in atria or AV node, or from accessory conduction pathways. Characterized by varying P-wave shape and abnormal P-wave axis. QRS morphology usually normal. See Fig. 6-12.[7]		
Premature Atrial Contraction		
Narrow QRS. Ectopic focus in atria or in AV node. Abnormal P wave and normal QRS	Digitalis toxicity, medications (e.g., caffeine, theophylline, sympathomimetics)	Treat digitalis toxicity, otherwise no treatment needed
Atrial Flutter		
Atrial rate between 250 and 350 beats/min, yielding characteristic sawtooth or flutter pattern (no discrete P waves) with variable ventricular response rate and normal QRS complex	Dilated atria, previous intraatrial surgery, valvular or ischemic heart disease, digitalis toxicity	Digoxin ± β-blockers, synchronized cardioversion or overdrive pacing; treat underlying cause (consult cardiologist)
Atrial Fibrillation		
Ectopic atrial foci with atrial rate between 350 and 600 beats/min, yielding characteristic fibrillatory pattern (no discrete P waves) and irregularly irregular ventricular response rate of about 110–150 beats/min with normal QRS complex	See above	See Atrial Flutter, may need anticoagulation pretreatment
SVT		
Sudden run of three or more premature supraventricular beats at >230 beats/min, with narrow QRS complex and abnormal P wave. Either sustained (>30 sec) or unsustained. *I. AV Reentrant:* Presence of accessory bypass pathway, in conjunction with AV node, establishes cyclic pattern of signal reentry,	Most commonly idiopathic but may be seen in congenial heart disease (e.g., Ebstein's anomaly, transposition)	Vagal maneuvers, adenosine; if unstable, need immediate synchronized cardioversion (0.5 j/kg up to 1 j/kg). Consult cardiologist. See "Tachycardia with Poor Perfusion" and "Tachycardia with Adequate Perfusion" algorithms in back of handbook.

TABLE 6-6
NONVENTRICULAR ARRHYTHMIAS—*cont'd*

Name/Description	Cause	Treatment
independent of SA node. Most common cause of nonsinus tachycardia in children (see Wolff-Parkinson-White syndrome). *II. AV nodal/junctional:* Cyclical reentrant pattern resulting from dual AV node pathways. Simultaneous depolarization of atria and ventricles yields invisible P wave or retrograde P wave *III. Ectopic atrial:* Rapid firing of ectopic focus in atrium.		
Nodal Escape/Junctional Rhythm Abnormal rhythm driven by AV node impulse, giving normal QRS complex and invisible P wave (buried in preceding QRS or T wave) or retrograde P wave (negative in lead II, positive in aVR)		

AV, atrioventricular; CHF, congestive heart failure; HR, heart rate; ICP, intracranial pressure; PE, pulmonary embolism; SA, sinoatrial; SVT, supraventricular tachycardia.

2. **Ventricular arrhythmias (Table 6-7):** Abnormal rhythm resulting from ectopic focus in ventricles. Characterized by wide QRS complex, T wave in opposite direction to QRS, random relation of QRS to P wave (i.e., AV dissociation); see Figures 6-12 and 6-13.
3. **Nonventricular conduction disturbances (Table 6-8 and Fig. 6-14).**[8]
4. **Ventricular conduction disturbance (Table 6-9):** Abnormal transmission of electrical impulse through ventricles leading to prolongation of QRS complex (≥0.08 second for infants, ≥0.10 second for adults).

C. MYOCARDIAL INFARCTION IN CHILDREN

1. **Etiology:** Myocardial infarction (MI) in children is rare but could occur in children with anomalous origin of a left coronary artery, Kawasaki disease, congenital heart disease (presurgical and postsurgical), and dilated cardiomyopathy. It is rarely seen in children with hypertension, lupus, myocarditis, cocaine ingestion, and use of adrenergic drugs (e.g., β-agonists used for asthma).

TABLE 6-7

VENTRICULAR ARRHYTHMIAS

Name/Description	Cause	Treatment
PVC		
Ectopic ventricular focus causing early depolarization. Abnormally wide QRS complex appears prematurely, usually with full compensatory pause. May be unifocal or multifocal. **Bigeminy** is alternating normal and abnormal QRS complexes; **trigeminy** is two normal QRS complexes followed by an abnormal one. A **couplet** is two consecutive PVCs.	Myocarditis, myocardial injury, cardiomyopathy, long QT syndrome, congenital and acquired heart disease, drugs (e.g., digitalis, catecholamines, theophylline, caffeine, anesthetics), MVP, anxiety, hypokalemia, hypoxia, hypomagnesemia	More worrisome if associated with underlying heart disease, if worse with activity, if symptomatic, or if they are multiform (especially couplets). Address underlying cause, rule out structural heart disease.
VENTRICULAR TACHYCARDIA		
Series of three or more PVCs at rapid rate (120–250 beats/min), with wide QRS complex and dissociated, retrograde, or no P wave.	See above (70% have abnormal cardiac anatomy)	See "Tachycardia with Poor Perfusion" and "Tachycardia with Adequate Perfusion" algorithms in back of handbook.
VENTRICULAR FIBRILLATION		
Depolarization of ventricles in uncoordinated, asynchronous pattern, yielding abnormal QRS complexes of varying size and morphology with irregular, rapid rate. Rare in children.	Myocarditis, MI, postoperative state, digitalis or quinidine toxicity, catecholamines, severe hypoxia, electrolyte disturbances	Requires immediate defibrillation. See algorithm for "Asystole and Pulseless Arrest" inside back cover.

MI, Myocardial infarction; MVP, mitral valve prolapse; PVC, premature ventricular contraction.

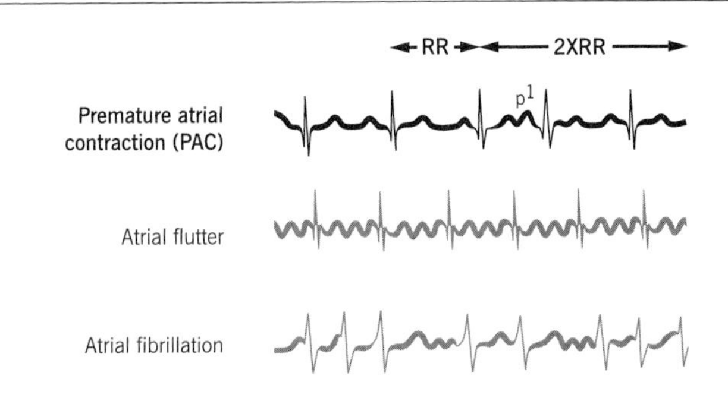

FIG. 6-12

Supraventricular arrhythmias. p^1, Premature atrial contraction. *(From Garson A Jr: The electrocardiogram in infants and children: A systematic approach. Philadelphia, Lea & Febiger, 1983.)*

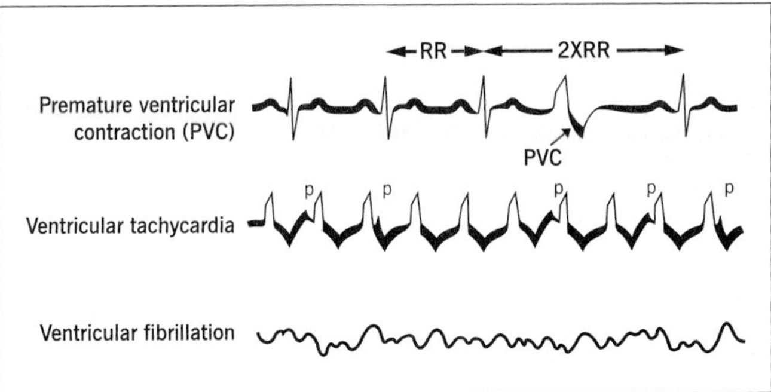

FIG. 6-13

Ventricular arrhythmias. P, P wave.

TABLE 6-8

NONVENTRICULAR CONDUCTION DISTURBANCES

Name/Description*	Cause	Treatment
FIRST-DEGREE HEART BLOCK		
Abnormal but asymptomatic delay in conduction through AV node, yielding prolongation of PR interval	Acute rheumatic fever, tickborne (i.e., Lyme) disease, connective tissue disease, congenital heart disease, cardiomyopathy, digitalis toxicity, postoperative state and normal children	None necessary except address the underlying cause
SECOND-DEGREE HEART BLOCK: MOBITZ TYPE I (WENCKEBACH)		
Progressive lengthening of PR interval until a QRS is not conducted and ventricular contraction does not occur. Does not usually progress to complete heart block.	Myocarditis, cardiomyopathy, congenital heart disease, postoperative state, MI, toxicity (digitalis, β-blocker), normal children	Address underlying cause
SECOND-DEGREE HEART BLOCK: MOBITZ TYPE II		
Paroxysmal skipped ventricular conduction without lengthening of the PR interval. Block is at the level of the bundle of His and may progress to complete heart block.	Same as for Mobitz Type I (not found in normal children)	Address underlying cause, may need pacemaker
THIRD-DEGREE (COMPLETE) HEART BLOCK		
Complete dissociation of atrial and ventricular conduction. P wave and PR interval regular; RR interval regular and much slower (driven by junctional or ectopic ventricular pacemaker with intrinsic rate of 30–50 beats/min). Width of QRS will be narrow with junctioinal pacemaker, wide with ventricular pacemaker.	Congenital, maternal lupus or other connective tissue disease, structural heart disease, or acquired (acute rheumatic fever, myocarditis, Lyme carditis, postoperative, cardiomyopathy, MI, drug overdose)	If bradycardic, consider pacing and see "Bradycardia" algorithm on inside back cover.

AV, atrioventricular; MI, myocardial infarction.

*Higher AV block: Conduction of atrial impulse at regular intervals, yielding 2:1 block (two atrial impulses for each ventricular response), 3:1 block, etc.

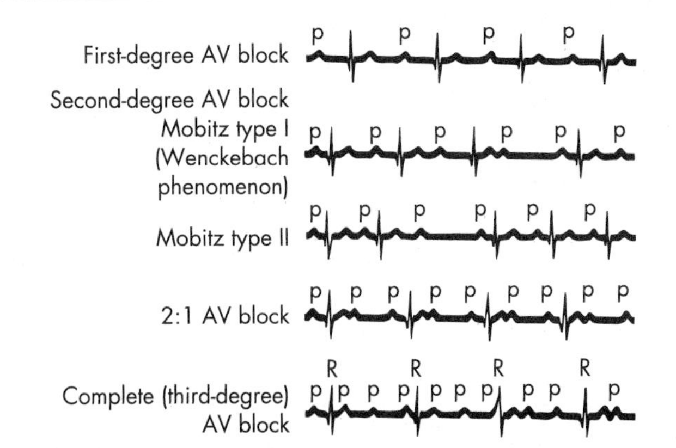

FIG. 6-14
Conduction blocks. P, P wave; R, QRS complex. *(From Park MK, Guntheroth WG: How to Read Pediatric ECGs, 3rd ed. St. Louis, Mosby, 1992.)*

2. Frequent ECG findings in children with acute MI[9]

a. New-onset wide Q waves (>0.035 sec), with or without Q-wave notching, seen within first few hours (and persistent over several years).
b. ST-segment elevation (>2 mm), seen within first few hours.
c. Diphasic T waves, seen within first few days (becoming sharply inverted, then normalizing over time).
d. Prolonged QT_c interval (>0.44 sec) with accompanying abnormal Q waves.
e. Deep, wide Q waves in leads I, aVL, or V6, without Q waves in II, III, aVF, suggestive of anomalous origin of the left coronary artery.

3. Other criteria:

a. An elevated creatinine kinase (CK)/MB fraction, although this is not specific for detection of acute MI in children.
b. Cardiac troponin I is likely to be a more sensitive indicator of early myocardial damage in children.[10] It becomes elevated within hours of cardiac injury, persists for 4 to 7 days, and is specific for cardiac injury.

D. ECG FINDINGS SECONDARY TO ELECTROLYTE DISTURBANCES, MEDICATIONS, AND SYSTEMIC ILLNESSES

1. Digitalis

a. Digitalis effect: Associated with shortened QT_c interval, ST depression ("scooped" or "sagging"), mildly prolonged PR interval, and flattened T wave.

TABLE 6-9
VENTRICULAR CONDUCTION DISTURBANCES

Name/Description	Criteria	Causes/Treatment
RIGHT BUNDLE-BRANCH BLOCK (RBBB)		
Delayed right bundle conduction prolongs RV depolarization time, leading to wide QRS	1. RAD 2. Long QRS with terminal slurred R′ (M-shaped RSR′ or RR′) in V1, V2, aVR 3. Wide and slurred S wave in leads I and V6	ASD, surgery with right ventriculostomy, Ebstein's anomaly, coarctation in infants <6 mo, endocardial cushion defect, and partial anomalous pulmonary venous return; occasionally occurs in normal children
LEFT BUNDLE-BRANCH BLOCK (LBBB)		
Delayed left bundle conduction prolongs septal and LV depolarization time, leading to wide QRS with loss of usual septal signal; there is still a predominance of left ventricle forces. Rare in children.	1. Wide negative QS complex in lead V1 with loss of septal R wave 2. Entirely positive wide R or RR′ complex in lead V6 with loss of septal Q wave	Hypertension, ischemic or valvular heart disease, cardiomyopathy
WOLFF-PARKINSON-WHITE (WPW)		
Atrial impulse transmitted via anomalous conduction pathway to ventricles, by passing AV node and normal ventricular conduction system. Leads to premature and prolonged depolarization of ventricles. Bypass pathway is a predisposing condition for SVT.	1. Shortened PR interval 2. Delta wave 3. Wide QRS	Acute management of SVT if necessary as previously described; consider ablation of accessory pathway if recurrent SVT

ASD, atrial septal defect; AV, atrioventricular; LV, left ventricle; RAD, right axis deviation; RV, right ventricle; SVT, supraventricular tachycardia.

b. Digitalis toxicity: Primarily arrhythmias (bradycardia, supraventricular tachycardia [SVT], ectopic atrial tachycardia, ventricular tachycardia, AV block).

2. Other conditions

See Table 6-10.[7,11]

E. LONG QT SYNDROME

1. **Diagnosis:** QTc >0.44 seconds in absence of other underlying causes (electrolyte disturbances, prematurity). The diagnosis may be supported by associated bradycardia, second-degree AV block, multiform premature ventricular contractions (PVCs), ventricular tachycardia, or abnormal T-wave morphologies. In some cases, patients may have a family history of long QT with unexplained syncope, seizure, or cardiac arrest without prolongation of QTc on ECG. Treadmill exercise test will usually prolong the QT and will sometimes incite arrhythmias.
2. **Complications:** Long QT is associated with the development of arrhythmias (torsades de pointes), syncope, and sudden death.
3. **Management:** Patients are most often managed with β-blockers but occasionally require cardiac sympathetic denervation, demand cardiac pacemakers, or internal cardiac defibrillators.

VI. IMAGING

A. CHEST RADIOGRAPH

1. Evaluate the heart:

a. Size: The cardiac shadow should be less than 50% of the thoracic width, which is the maximal width between inner margins of the ribs, as measured on a posteroanterior radiograph during inspiration.

b. Shape: The shape of the heart can aid in the diagnosis of chamber/vessel enlargement and some congenital heart disease (CHD) (Fig. 6-15).

c. Situs (levocardia, mesocardia, dextrocardia).

2. Evaluate the lung fields.

a. Decreased pulmonary blood flow is seen in pulmonary or tricuspid stenosis/atresia, TOF, pulmonary hypertension ("peripheral pruning").

b. Increased pulmonary blood flow can be seen as increased pulmonary vascular markings (PVMs) with redistribution from bases to apices of lungs and extension to lateral lung fields (Tables 6-11 and 6-12).

c. Venous congestion, or congestive heart failure (CHF), causes increased PVMs centrally, interstitial and alveolar pulmonary edema (air bronchograms), septal lines, and pleural effusions (see Tables 6-11 and 6-12).

3. **Evaluate the airway:** The trachea usually bends slightly to the right above the carina in normal patients with a left-sided aortic arch. A

Text continues on p. 192

TABLE 6-10

SYSTEMIC EFFECTS ON ELECTROCARDIOGRAM

	Short QT	Long QT-U	Prolonged QRS	ST-T Changes	Sinus Tachycardia	Sinus Bradycardia	AV Block	Ventricular Tachycardia	Miscellaneous
CHEMISTRY									
Hyperkalemia			X	X			X	X	Low-voltage Ps; peaked Ts
Hypokalemia		X	X	X					
Hypercalcemia	X					X	X	X	
Hypocalcemia		X			X		X		
Hypermagnesemia							X		
Hypomagnesemia		X							
DRUGS									
Digitalis	X			X		T	X	T	
Phenothiazines		T						T	
Phenytoin	X								
Propranolol	X					X	X		
Quinidine		X	X			T	T	T	
Tricyclics		T	T	T	T		T		
Verapamil						X	X		
Imipramine							T	T	Atrial flutter

MISCELLANEOUS								
CNS injury	X		X	X	X	X		
Freidreich's ataxia			X	X				Atrial flutter
Duchenne's muscular dystrophy			X	X				Atrial flutter
Myotonic dystrophy		X	X	X		X		
Collagen vascular disease			X			X	X	
Hypothyroidism					X			Low voltage
Hyperthyroidism		X	X	X		X		
Other diseases	Romano-Ward	Lyme disease				Holt-Oram, maternal lupus		

CNS, central nervous system; T, present only with drug toxicity; X, present.

From Garson A Jr. The Electrocardiogram in Infants and Children: A Systematic Approach. Philadelphia, Lea & Febiger, 1983 and Walsh EP: In Fyler DC, Nadas A (eds): Pediatric Cardiology. Philadelphia, Hanley & Belfus, 1992.

TABLE 6-11

ACYANOTIC CONGENITAL HEART DISEASE

Lesion Type	Examination Findings	ECG Findings	Chest Radiograph Findings
Ventricular septal defect (VSD) 20%–25% of CHD	2–5/6 holosystolic murmur loudest at the LLSB A systolic thrill may be felt at the LLSB ± Apical diastolic rumble with large shunt S2 may be narrow and P2 may be increased with large VSD and pulmonary hypertension	*Small VSD:* Normal *Medium VSD:* LVH ± LAE *Large VSD:* BVH ± LAE, pure RVH	May show cardiomegaly and increased PVMs dependent on the amount of left to right shunting
Atrial septal defect (ASD)	Wide, fixed split S2 with a grade 2–3/6 SEM at the LUSB May have mid-diastolic rumble at LLSB	*Small ASD:* Normal *Hemodynamically significant ASD:* RAD and mild RVH or RBBB with an RSR′ in V1	May show cardiomegaly with increased PVMs if hemodynamically significant lesion
Patent ductus arteriosus (PDA) 5%–10% of CHD in term infants; 40%–60% in preterm infants weighing <1500 g	1–4/6 continuous "machinery" murmur loudest at the LUSB	*Small–moderate PDA:* Normal or LVH *Large PDA:* BVH	May have cardiomegaly and increased PVMs depending on size of shunt (see p. 390 for treatment)
Atrioventricular septal defects 30%–60% occur in Down syndrome	Hyperactive precordium with systolic thrill at LLSB and loud S2. There may be a grade 3–4/6 holosystolic regurgitant murmur along LLSB. May hear systolic murmur of MR at apex. May hear mid-diastolic rumble at LLSB or at apex. Gallop rhythm may be present.	Superior QRS axis RVH and LVH may be present	Cardiomegaly with increased PVMs

Pulmonary stenosis (PS)	Ejection click at LUSB with valvular PS. Click intensity will vary with respiration, decreasing with inspiration and increasing with expiration. S2 may split widely with P2 diminished in intensity. SEM (2–5/6) ± thrill at LUSB with radiation to the back and sides.	*Mild PS:* Normal *Moderate PS:* RAD and RVH *Severe PS:* RAE and RVH with strain	Normal heart size with normal to decreased PVMs
Aortic stenosis (AS)	Systolic thrill at RUSB, suprasternal notch, or over carotids. Ejection click, which does not vary with respiration, if valvular AS. Harsh SEM (2–4/6) at second RICS or third LICS with radiation to neck and apex. May have early diastolic decrescendo murmur as a result of AR. Narrow pulse pressure if severe stenosis.	*Mild AS:* Normal *Moderate–severe AS:* LVH ± strain	Usually normal
Coarctation of the aorta 8%–10% of CHD with male/female ratio of 2:1. May present as (1) infant in CHF; (2) child with HTN; (3) child with murmur	2–3/6 SEM at LUSB with radiation to the left interscapular area. Bicuspid valve is often associated and thus may have systolic ejection click at the apex and RUSB. BP in lower extremities will be lower than in upper extremities. Pulse oximetry discrepancy of >5% between upper and lower extremities is also suggestive of coarctation.	*In infancy:* RVH or RBBB *In older children:* LVH	Marked cardiomegaly and pulmonary venous congestion. Rib notching from collateral circulation not seen in infants because collaterals not yet established; usually seen after 5 years of age.

AR, aortic regurgitation; BP, blood pressure; BVH, biventricular hypertrophy; CHD, congenital heart disease; CHF, congestive heart failure; HTN, hypertension; LAE, left atrial enlargement; LICS, left intercostal space; LLSB, left lower sternal border; LUSB, left upper sternal border; LVH, left ventricular hypertrophy; MR, mitral regurgitation; PVM, pulmonary vascular markings; RAD, right axis deviation; RAE, right atrial enlargement; RICS, right intercostal space; RBBB, right bundle-branch block; RUSB, right upper sternal border; RVH, right ventricular hypertrophy; SEM, systolic ejection murmur.

TABLE 6-12

CYANOTIC CONGENITAL HEART DISEASE

Lesion	Examination Findings	ECG Findings	Chest Radiograph Findings
Tetralogy of Fallot: 1. Large VSD 2. RVOT obstruction 3. RVH 4. Overriding aorta The degree of RVOT obstruction will determine whether there is clinical cyanosis. If there is only mild PS, there will be a left to right shunt, and the child will be acyanotic. Increased obstruction leads to increased right to left shunting across the VSD and cyanosis.	Loud systolic ejection murmur at middle and upper LSB and a loud, single S2. May also have a thrill at the middle and lower LSB. *Tet spells:* Occur in young infants. As RVOT obstruction increases or systemic resistance decreases, right to left shunting across the VSD occurs. May present with tachypnea, increasing cyanosis, and decreasing murmur. See Table 6–15 for treatment.	RAD and RVH	Boot-shaped heart with normal heart size ± decreased PVMs
Transposition of great arteries	Nonspecific findings. Extreme cyanosis. S2 will be single and loud. May have murmur from associated VSD or PS, but if not present, there may not be a murmur	Because RV acts as systemic ventricle, patient will have RAD and RVH. Upright T wave in V1 after 3 days old may be only abnormality.	Classic finding is "egg on a string" with cardiomegaly. Increased PVMs may also be present.
Tricuspid atresia Absent tricuspid valve and hypoplastic RV and PA. Must have ASD, PDA, or VSD for survival.	Single S2. A grade 2–3/6 systolic regurgitation murmur at the LLSB is present if there is a VSD. Occasionally, there is a PDA murmur.	Superior QRS axis. RAE or CAE, and LVH	Normal or slightly enlarged heart size. May have boot-shaped heart.

Total anomalous pulmonary venous return Pulmonary veins drain into RA or other location besides LA. Must have ASD or PFO for survival: 1. *Supracardiac* (most common): Common pulmonary vein into SVC 2. *Cardiac:* Pulmonary vein into coronary sinus or RA 3. *Subdiaphragmatic:* Common pulmonary vein into IVC, portal vein, ductus venosus or hepatic vein 4. *Mixed type*	Hyperactive RV impulse, quadruple rhythm, S2 fixed and widely split, 2–3/6 SEM at LUSB and mid-diastolic rumble at LLSB.	RAD, RVH (RSR′ in V1). May see RAE.	Cardiomegaly and increased PVMs. Classic is the "snowman in a snowstorm" finding, but this is rarely seen until after 4 months of age.
OTHER			
Cyanotic CHDs that occur at a frequency of <1% each include pulmonary atresia, Ebstein's anomaly, truncus arteriosus, single ventricle, and double outlet right ventricle.			

ASD, atrial septal defect; CAE, common atrial enlargement; IVC, inferior vena cava; LA, left atrium; LLSB, left lower sternal border; LSB, left upper sternal border; LUSB, left upper sternal border; LVH, left ventricular hypertrophy; PA, pulmonary artery; PDA, patent ductus arteriosus; PFO, patent foramen ovale; PVM, pulmonary vascular markings; PS, pulmonary stenosis; RA, right atrium; RAD, right axis deviation; RAE, right atrial enlargement; RV, right ventricle; RVH, right ventricular hypertrophy; RVOT, right ventricular outflow tract; SEM, systolic ejection murmur; SVC, superior vena cava; VSD, ventral septal defect.

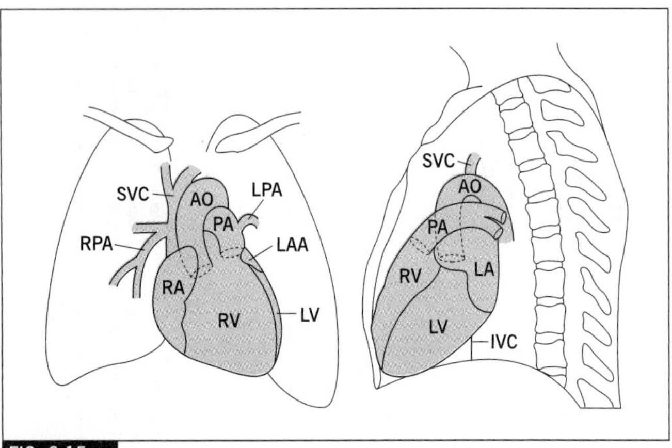

FIG. 6-15

Radiologic contours of the heart. AO, Aorta; IVC, inferior vena cava; LA, left atrium; LAA, left atrial appendage; LPA, left pulmonary artery; LV, left ventricle; PA, pulmonary artery; RA, right atrium; RPA, right pulmonary artery; RV, right ventricle; SVC, superior vena cava.

perfectly straight or left-bending trachea suggests a right aortic arch, which may be associated with other defects (TOF, truncus arteriosus, vascular rings, chromosome 22 microdeletion).

4. **Skeletal anomalies:**
   a. Rib notching (e.g., from collateral vessels in patients >5 years of age with coarctation of the aorta).
   b. Sternal abnormalities (e.g., Holt-Oram syndrome; pectus excavatum in Marfan, Ehlers-Danlos, and Noonan syndromes).
   c. Vertebral anomalies (e.g., VATER/VACTERL syndrome: Vertebral anomalies, Anal atresia, Tracheoesophageal fistula, Radial and Renal, Cardiac, and Limb anomalies).

Please see Chapter 23 for more information on the chest radiograph.

B. ECHOCARDIOGRAPHY

1. **Approach**
   a. Transthoracic echocardiography (TTE) does not require general anesthesia, is simpler to perform than transesophageal echocardiography (TEE), but does have limitations in some patients (e.g., uncooperative, obese, or those with suspected valvular endocarditis).
   b. TEE uses an ultrasound transducer on the end of a modified endoscope to view the heart from the esophagus and stomach, allowing for

better imaging of the aorta and atria. It allows for better imaging in obese and intraoperative patients. TEE is also useful for visualizing valvular anatomy, including valvular vegetations.

2. **Shortening fraction:** Very reliable index of left ventricle (LV) function. Normal values range from approximately 30% to 45%, depending on age.[12]

VII. CONGENITAL HEART DISEASE

Table 6-13 shows common genetic syndromes associated with cardiac lesions.

A. ACYANOTIC LESIONS (see Table 6-11)

B. CYANOTIC LESIONS (see Table 6-12)

An oxygen challenge test is used to evaluate the etiology of cyanosis in neonates. Obtain baseline arterial blood gas (ABG) with saturation at $FiO_2 = 0.21$, then place infant in an oxygen hood at $FiO_2 = 1$ for a minimum of 10 minutes, and repeat ABG. Pulse oximetry will not be useful for following the change in oxygenation once the saturations reach 100% (approximately $PaO_2 > 90$) (Table 6-14).[13–16] Table 6-15 shows acute management of hypercyanotic spells in TOF.

C. SURGERIES AND OTHER INTERVENTIONS

1. **Atrial septostomy:** Atrial septostomy creates an intra-atrial opening to allow for mixing or shunting between atria (i.e., for transposition of the great arteries [TGA], tricuspid atresia, mitral atresia). This is most commonly performed percutaneously with a balloon-tipped catheter (Rashkind procedure), in patients with TGA and a small patent foramen ovale, to improve mixing of systemic and pulmonary venous return.
2. **Palliative systemic-to-pulmonary artery shunts,** such as the **Blalock-Taussig shunt,** use systemic arterial flow to increase pulmonary blood flow in cardiac lesions with impaired pulmonary perfusion (e.g., TOF, hypoplastic right heart, tricuspid atresia, pulmonary stenosis [PS]) **(Fig. 6-16).**
3. **Palliative cava-to-pulmonary artery shunts** use systemic venous flow to increase pulmonary blood flow (usually performed outside of the neonatal period in infants with lower pulmonary vascular resistance) as an intermediate step to a **Fontan procedure (see Fig. 6-16).** This is **called a** unidirectional or bidirectional Glenn shunt.
4. **Repair of TGA:**
   a. Atrial inversion (Mustard or Senning) (rarely performed today).
   b. Arterial switch (of Jatene).
5. **Fontan:** Anastomosis of the superior vena cava (SVC) to the right pulmonary artery (RPA) (Glenn shunt), together with anastomosis of the right artery (RA) and/or inferior vena cava (IVC) to pulmonary arteries via conduits; separates systemic and pulmonary circulations in

TABLE 6-13
COMMON GENETIC SYNDROMES ASSOCIATED WITH CARDIAC DEFECTS

Syndrome	Dominant Cardiac Defect
CHARGE	Ventricular, atrioventricular, and ASDs
DiGeorge	Aortic arch anomalies, tetralogy of Fallot
Down	Atrioventricular septal defects, VSD
Marfan	Aortic root dissection, mitral valve prolapse
Noonan	Pulmonic stenosis, ASD
Turner	Coarctation of the aorta, bicuspid aortic valve
Williams	Supravalvular aortic stenosis

ASD, atrial septal defect; CHARGE, a syndrome of associated defects, including coloboma of the eye, heart anomaly, choanal atresia, retardation, and genital and ear anomalies; VSD, ventricular septal defect.
From Pelech AN: Pediatr Clin North Am 1999;46(2):167–168.

TABLE 6-14
INTERPRETATION OF OXYGEN CHALLENGE TEST

	$FiO_2 = 0.21$ PaO_2 (% Saturation)		$FiO_2 = 1.00$ PaO_2 (% Saturation)	$PaCO_2$
Normal	70 (95)		>200 (100)	35
Pulmonary disease	50 (85)		>150 (100)	50
Neurologic disease	50 (85)		>150 (100)	50
Methemoglobinemia	70 (85)		>200 (85)	35
Cardiac disease				
Separate circulation*	<40 (<75)		<50 (<85)	35
Restricted PBF†	<40 (<75)		<50 (<85)	35
Complete mixing without restricted PBF‡	50 (85)		<150 (<100)	35
Persistent pulmonary hypertension	Preductal	Postductal		
PFO (no R to L shunt)	70 (95)	<40 (<75)	Variable	35–50
PFO (with R to L shunt)	<40 (<75)	<40 (<75)	Variable	35–50

*D-Transposition of the great arteries (D-TGA) with intact ventricular septum.
†Tricuspid atresia with pulmonary stenosis or atresia; pulmonary atresia or critical pulmonary stenosis with intact ventricular septum; or tetralogy of Fallot.
‡Truncus, total anomalous pulmonary venous return, single ventricle, hypoplastic left heart, D-TGA with ventricular septal defect, tricuspid atresia without pulmonary stenosis or atresia.
PBF, Pulmonary blood flow; PFO, patent foramen ovale.
From Lees MH: J Pediatr 1970;77:484; Kitterman JA: Pediatr Rev 1982;4:13; and Jones RW, et al: Arch Dis Child 1976;51:667.

patients with functionally single ventricles (tricuspid atresia, hypoplastic left heart syndrome).

6. **Norwood: Used for hypoplastic left heart syndrome.**
   a. Stage 1: Anastomosis of the proximal main pulmonary artery (MPA) to the aorta, with aortic arch reconstruction and transection and

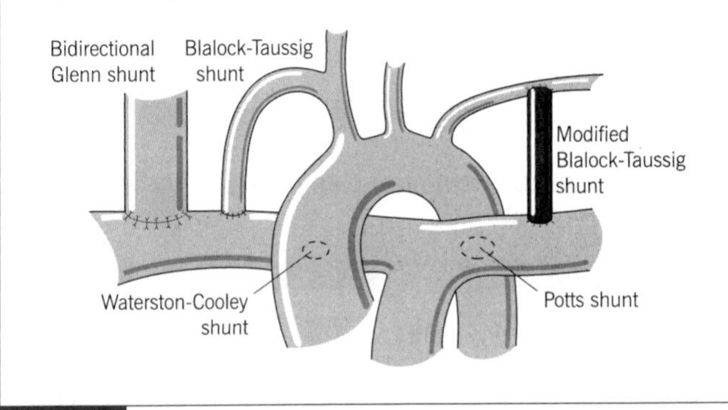

FIG. 6-16

Schematic diagram of cardiac shunts.

TABLE 6-15

TREATMENT OPTIONS FOR "TET SPELLS"

Treatment	Rationale
Oxygen	Reduces hypoxemia (limited value)
Calm child, encourage knee-chest position	Decreases venous return and increases systemic resistance
Propranolol	Negative inotropic effect on infundibular myocardium; may block drop in systemic vascular resistance (0.15–0.25 mg/kg slow IV push)
Morphine	Decreases venous return, depresses respiratory center, relaxes infundibulum (morphine sulfate 0.1–0.2 mg/kg SC or IM). Do not try to establish IV access initially. Use the SC route.
Phenylephrine	Increases systemic vascular resistance (0.02 mg/kg IV)
Methoxamine	Increases systemic vascular resistance
Sodium bicarbonate	Reduces metabolic acidosis (1 mEq/kg IV)
Correct anemia	Increases delivery of oxygen to tissues
Correct pathologic tachyarrhythmias	May abort hypoxic spell
Infuse glucose	Avoids hypoglycemia from increased utilization and depletion of glycogen stores

IM, intramuscular; IV, intravenous; SC, subcutaneous.

patch closure of the distal MPA; a modified right Blalock-Taussig shunt (subclavian artery to RPA) to provide pulmonary blood flow; alternatively, an RV to PA conduit can be used for pulmonary blood flow. An atrial septal defect (ASD) is created to allow for adequate left to right flow.

b. Stage 2: Bidirectional Glenn shunt to reduce volume overload of single right ventricle and modified Fontan procedure to correct cyanosis.
7. **Ross:** Pulmonary root autograft for aortic stenosis; autologous pulmonary valve replaces aortic valve, and aortic or pulmonary allograft replaces pulmonary valve.

D. EXERCISE RECOMMENDATIONS FOR CONGENITAL HEART DISEASE (Table 6-16)[17]

VIII. ACQUIRED HEART DISEASE

A. ENDOCARDITIS

1. **Common causative organisms:** About 70% of causes of endocarditis are streptococcal species (*Streptococcus viridans, enterococci*); 20% are staphylococcal species (*Staphylococcus aureus, Staphylococcus epidermidis*); 10% are other organisms (*Haemophilus influenzae,* Gram-negative bacteria, fungi).
2. **Clinical findings:** New heart murmur, fever, splenomegaly, petechiae, Osler nodes (tender nodules at fingertips), Janeway lesions (painless hemorrhagic areas on palms or soles), splinter hemorrhages, and Roth spots (retinal hemorrhages).

B. BACTERIAL ENDOCARDITIS PROPHYLAXIS

See Tables 6-17, 6-18, and 6-19 and Boxes 6-4 and 6-5.[16]

C. MYOCARDIAL DISEASE

1. **Dilated cardiomyopathy is the end result of myocardial damage, leading to atrial and ventricular dilation with decreased contractile function of the ventricles.**

a. Etiology: Infectious, toxic (alcohol, doxorubicin), metabolic (hypothyroidism, muscular dystrophy), immunologic, collagen vascular disease.
b. Symptoms: Fatigue, weakness, shortness of breath.
c. Examination: Look for signs of CHF, including tachycardia, tachypnea, rales, cold extremities, jugular venous distention, hepatomegaly, peripheral edema, S3 gallop, and displacement of point of maximal impulse (PMI) to the left and inferiorly.
d. Chest radiograph: Generalized cardiomegaly, pulmonary congestion.
e. ECG: Sinus tachycardia, left ventricular hypertrophy (LVH), possible atrial enlargement, arrhythmias, conduction disturbances, ST-segment and T-wave changes.
f. Echocardiography: Enlarged ventricles (increased end-diastolic and end-systolic dimensions) with little or no wall thickening; decreased shortening fraction.
g. Treatment: Management of CHF (digoxin, diuretics, vasodilation, rest). Consider anticoagulants to decrease risk for thrombus formation.

Text continues on p. 201

TABLE 6-16

EXERCISE RECOMMENDATIONS FOR CONGENITAL HEART DISEASE AND SPORTS ALLOWED FOR SOME SPECIFIC CARDIAC LESIONS

Diagnosis	Sports Allowed
Small ASD or VSD	All
Mild aortic stenosis	All
MVP (without other risk factors)	All
Moderate aortic stenosis	IA, IB, IIA
Mild LV dysfunction	IA, IB, IC
Moderate LV dysfunction	IA only
Hypertrophic cardiomyopathy	None (or IA only)
Severe aortic stenosis	None
Long QT syndrome	None

	Low Dynamic (A)	Moderate Dynamic (B)	High Dynamic (C)
I. Low static	Billiards Bowling Cricket Curling Golf Riflery	Baseball Softball Table tennis Tennis (doubles) Volleyball	Badminton Cross-country skiing Field hockey* Orienteering Race walking Racquetball Running (long distance) Soccer* Squash Tennis (singles)
II. Moderate static	Archery Auto racing*,† Diving*,† Equestrian*,† Motorcycling*,†	Fencing Field events (jumping) Figure skating* Football (American)* Rodeoing*,† Rugby* Running (sprint) Surfing*,† Synchronized swimming†	Basketball* Ice hockey* Cross-country skiing (skating technique) Football (Australian)* Lacrosse* Running (middle distance) Swimming Team handball
III. High static	Bobsledding*,† Field events (throwing) Gymnastics*,† Karate/judo* Luge*,† Sailing Rock climbing*,† Waterskiing*,† Weight lifting*,† Windsurfing*,†	Body building*,† Downhill skiing*,† Wrestling*	Boxing* Canoeing/kayaking Cycling*,† Decathlon Rowing Speed skating

*Danger of bodily collision.

†Increased risk if syncope occurs.

From 26th Bethesda Conference, 1994 and Washington RL, et al: Medical conditions affecting sports participation. Pediatrics 2001;107(5):1205–1209.

TABLE 6-17
PROCEDURES AND ENDOCARDITIS PROPHYLAXIS

	Prophylaxis Recommended	Prophylaxis Not Recommended
Respiratory tract	Tonsillectomy, adenoidectomy, or both	Endotracheal intubation
	Surgical operations that involve respiratory mucosa	Bronchoscopy with a flexible bronchoscope, with or without biopsy*
	Bronchoscopy with a rigid bronchoscope	Tympanostomy tube insertion
Gastrointestinal tract†	Sclerotherapy for esophageal varices	Transesophageal echocardiography*
	Esophageal stricture dilation	Endoscopy with or without gastrointestinal biopsy*
	Endoscopic retrograde cholangiography with biliary obstruction	
	Biliary tract surgery	
	Surgical operations that involve intestinal mucosa	
Genitourinary tract	Prostatic surgery	Vaginal hysterectomy*
	Cystoscopy	Vaginal delivery*
	Urethral dilation	Cesarean section
		In uninfected tissue:
		Urethral catheterization
		Uterine dilation and curettage
		Therapeutic abortion
		Sterilization procedures
		Insertion or removal of intrauterine devices
Other		Cardiac catheterization, including balloon angioplasty
		Implanted cardiac pacemakers, implanted defibrillators, and coronary stents
		Incision or biopsy of surgically scrubbed skin
		Circumcision

*Prophylaxis is optional for high-risk patients.
†Prophylaxis is recommended for high-risk patients; optional for medium-risk patients.
From American Academy of Pediatrics: 2000 Red Book: Report of the Committee on Infectious Diseases, 25th ed. Elk Grove Village, IL, The Academy; 2000.

TABLE 6-18

PROPHYLACTIC REGIMENS FOR DENTAL, ORAL, RESPIRATORY TRACT, OR ESOPHAGEAL PROCEDURES

Situation	Agent	Regimen*
Standard general prophylaxis	Amoxicillin	Adults: 2 g; children: 50 mg/kg orally 1 hr before procedure
Unable to take oral medications	Ampicillin	Adults: 2 g intramuscularly (IM) or intravenously (IV); children: 50 mg/kg IM or IV within 30 min before procedure
Allergic to penicillin	Clindamycin	Adults: 600 mg; children: 20 mg/kg orally 1 hr before procedure
	or	
	Cephalexin† or cefadroxil†	Adults: 2 g; children: 50 mg/kg orally 1 hr before procedure
	or	
	Azithromycin or clarithromycin	Adults: 500 mg; children: 15 mg/kg orally 1 hr before procedure
Allergic to penicillin and unable to take oral medications	Clindamycin	Adults: 600 mg; children: 20 mg/kg IV within 30 min before procedure
	or	
	Cefazolin†	Adults: 1 g; children: 25 mg/kg IM or IV within 30 min before procedure

*Total children's dose should not exceed adult dose.

†Cephalosporins should not be used for persons with immediate-type hypersensitivity reaction to penicillins.

From American Academy of Pediatrics: 2003 Red Book: Report of the Committee on Infectious Diseases, 26th ed. Elk Grove Village, IL, The Academy; 2003.

TABLE 6–19

PROPHYLACTIC REGIMENS FOR GENITOURINARY AND GASTROINTESTINAL TRACT (EXCLUDING ESOPHAGEAL) PROCEDURE

Situation	Agents*	Regimen†
High-risk patients	Ampicillin *plus* Gentamicin	Adults: Ampicillin 2 g intramuscularly (IM) or intravenously (IV) plus gentamicin 1.5 mg/kg (not to exceed 120 mg) within 30 min of starting the procedure; 6 hr later, ampicillin 1 g IM or IV or amoxicillin 1 g orally Children: Ampicillin 50 mg/kg IM or IV (not to exceed 2 g) plus gentamicin 1.5 mg/kg within 30 min of starting the procedure; 6 hr later, ampicillin 25 mg/kg IM or IV or amoxicillin 25 mg/kg orally
High-risk patients allergic to ampicillin or amoxicillin	Vancomycin *plus* Gentamicin	Adults: Vancomycin 1 g IV over 1–2 hr plus gentamicin 1.5 mg/kg IV or IM (not to exceed 120 mg); complete injection/infusion within 30 min of starting the procedure Children: Vancomycin 20 mg/kg IV over 1–2 hr plus gentamicin 1.5 mg/kg IV or IM; complete injection or infusion within 30 min of starting the procedure
Moderate-risk patients	Amoxicillin *or* Ampicillin	Adults: Amoxicillin 2 g orally 1 hr before procedure, or ampicillin 2 g IM or IV within 30 min of starting the procedure Children: Amoxicillin 50 mg/kg orally 1 hr before procedure, or ampicillin 50 mg/kg IM or IV within 30 min of starting the procedure
Moderate-risk patients allergic to ampicillin or amoxicillin	Vancomycin	Adults: Vancomycin 1 g IV over 1–2 hr; complete infusion within 30 min of starting the procedure Children: Vancomycin 20 mg/kg IV over 1–2 hr; complete infusion within 30 min of starting the procedure

*Total children's dose should not exceed adult dose.

†No second dose of vancomycin or gentamicin is recommended.

From American Academy of Pediatrics: 2003 Red Book: Report of the Committee on Infectious Diseases, 26th ed. Elk Grove Village, IL, The Academy; 2003.

BOX 6-4

CARDIAC CONDITIONS ASSOCIATED WITH ENDOCARDITIS

PROPHYLAXIS RECOMMENDED

High Risk

Prosthetic cardiac valves, including bioprosthetic and homograft valves

Previous bacterial endocarditis

Complex cyanotic congenital heart disease (e.g., single ventricle states, transposition of the great arteries, tetralogy of Fallot)

Surgically constructed systemic pulmonary shunts or conduits

Moderate Risk

Most other congenital cardiac malformations (other than those in the high-risk and negligible-risk categories)

Acquired valvular dysfunction (e.g., rheumatic heart disease)

Hypertrophic cardiomyopathy

Mitral valve prolapse with valvular regurgitation and/or thickened leaflets†

PROPHYLAXIS NOT RECOMMENDED

Negligible Risk*

Isolated secundum atrial septal defect

Surgical repair of atrial septal defect, ventricular septal defect, or patent ductus arteriosus (without residua and beyond 6 mo of age)

Previous coronary artery bypass graft surgery

Mitral valve prolapse without valvular regurgitation†

Physiologic, functional, or innocent heart murmurs†

Previous Kawasaki disease without valvular dysfunction

Previous rheumatic fever without valvular dysfunction

Cardiac pacemakers (intravascular and epicardial) and implanted defibrillators

*No greater risk than the general population.

†For further information, see Dajani AS, et al: JAMA 1997;277:1794–1801.

From American Academy of Pediatrics: 2003 Red Book: Report of the Committee on Infectious Diseases, 26th ed. Elk Grove Village, IL, The Academy, 2003.

2. **Hypertrophic cardiomyopathy is an abnormality of myocardial cells leading to significant ventricular hypertrophy, particularly of the LV, with small to normal ventricular dimensions. Contractile function is increased, but filling is impaired secondary to stiff ventricles. The most common type is asymmetric septal hypertrophy, also called idiopathic hypertrophic subaortic stenosis (IHSS), with varying degrees of obstruction. There is a 4% to 6% incidence of sudden death in children and adolescents.**

a. Etiology: Genetic (autosomal dominant, 60% of cases) or sporadic (40% of cases).
b. Symptoms: Easy fatigability, anginal pain, shortness of breath, occasional palpitations.
c. Examination: Usually found in adolescents or young adults, signs include left ventricular heave, sharp upstroke of arterial pulse, murmur

BOX 6-5

DENTAL PROCEDURES AND ENDOCARDITIS PROPHYLAXIS

Prophylaxis Recommended*

Dental extractions

Periodontal procedures, including surgery, scaling and root planing, probing, and routine maintenance

Dental implant placement and reimplantation of avulsed teeth

Endodontic (root canal) instrumentation or surgery only beyond the apex

Subgingival placement of antibiotic fibers or strips

Initial placement of orthodontic bands but not brackets

Intraligamentary local anesthetic injections

Prophylactic cleaning of teeth or implants during which bleeding is anticipated

Prophylaxis Not Recommended

Restorative dentistry† (operative and prosthodontic) with or without retraction cord‡

Local anesthetic injections (nonintraligamentary)

Intracanal endodontic treatment; postplacement and buildup

Placement of rubber dams

Postoperative suture removal

Placement of removable prosthodontic or orthodontic appliances

Taking of oral impressions

Fluoride treatments

Taking of oral radiographs

Orthodontic appliance adjustment

Shedding of primary teeth

*Prophylaxis is recommended for patients with high- and moderate-risk cardiac conditions.
†This includes restoration of decayed teeth (filling cavities) and replacement of missing teeth.
‡Clinical judgment may indicate antibiotic use in selected circumstances that may create significant bleeding.
From American Academy of Pediatrics: 2003 Red Book: Report of the Committee on Infectious Diseases, 26th ed. Elk Grove Village, IL, The Academy; 2003.

of mitral regurgitation, mid-systolic ejection murmur along left mid-sternal border (LMSB) that increases in intensity in the standing position (in patients with mid-cavity LV obstruction).

d. Chest radiograph shows a globular-shaped heart with LV enlargement.
e. ECG indicates LVH, prominent Q waves (septal hypertrophy), ST-segment and T-wave changes, arrhythmias.
f. Echocardiography shows extent and location of hypertrophy, obstruction, increased contractility.
g. Treatment includes moderate restriction of physical activity, administration of negative inotropes (β-blocker, calcium-channel blocker) to help improve filling, and subacute bacterial endocarditis (SBE) prophylaxis. If at increased risk for sudden death, may consider implantable defibrillator. If symptomatic with subaortic obstruction, may benefit from myectomy.

3. Restrictive cardiomyopathy: Myocardial or endocardial disease (usually infiltrative or fibrotic) resulting in stiff ventricular walls, with restriction of diastolic filling but normal contractile function. Results in atrial enlargement. Very rare in children.

4. Myocarditis: Inflammation of myocardial tissue.

a. Etiology: Viral (coxsackievirus, echovirus, poliomyelitis, mumps, rubella, cytomegalovirus [CMV], human immunodeficiency virus [HIV], arbovirus, adenovirus, influenza); bacterial, rickettsial, fungal, or parasitic infection; immune-mediated disease (Kawasaki disease, acute rheumatic fever); collagen vascular disease; toxin-induced condition.

b. Symptoms: Nonspecific and inconsistent, depending on severity of disease. Variably see anorexia, lethargy, emesis, lightheadedness, cold extremities, shortness of breath.

c. Examination: Look for signs of CHF (tachycardia, tachypnea, jugular venous distention, rales, gallop, hepatomegaly); occasionally, a soft, systolic murmur or arrhythmias may be noted.

d. Chest radiograph: Shows variable cardiomegaly and pulmonary edema.

e. ECG: Indicates low QRS voltages throughout (<5 mm), ST-segment and T-wave changes (e.g., decreased T-wave amplitude), prolongation of QT interval, arrhythmias (especially premature contractions, first- or second-degree AV block).

f. Echocardiography: Indicates enlargement of heart chambers, impaired LV function.

g. Treatment: Bed rest, diuretics, inotropes (dopamine, dobutamine, milrinone), digoxin, gamma globulin (2 g/kg over 24 hours), afterload reducer (e.g., angiotensin-converting enzyme [ACE] inhibitor), possibly steroids. May require heart transplantation if no improvement (about 20% to 25% of cases).

D. PERICARDIAL DISEASE

1. Pericarditis: Inflammation of visceral and parietal layers of pericardium.

a. Etiology: Viral or idiopathic (especially echovirus, coxsackievirus B), tuberculous, bacterial, uremic, neoplastic, collagen vascular, post-MI or postpericardiotomy, radiation induced, drug induced (e.g., procainamide, hydralazine).

b. Symptoms: Chest pain (retrosternal or precordial, radiating to back or shoulder, pleuritic in nature, alleviated by leaning forward, aggravated by supine position), dyspnea.

c. Examination: Pericardial friction rub, distant heart sounds, fever, tachypnea.

d. ECG: Diffuse ST-segment elevation in almost all leads (representing inflammation of adjacent myocardium); PR-segment depression.

e. Treatment: Often self-limited. Treat underlying condition, and provide symptomatic treatment with rest, analgesia, and anti-inflammatory drugs.

2. Pericardial effusion: Accumulation of excess fluid in pericardial sac.

a. Etiology: Associated with acute pericarditis (exudative fluid) or serous effusion resulting from increased capillary hydrostatic pressure (e.g., CHF), decreased plasma oncotic pressure (e.g., hypoproteinemia), and increased capillary permeability (transudative fluid).

b. Symptoms: Can present with no symptoms, dull ache in left chest, abdominal pain, or symptoms of cardiac tamponade, discussed below.

c. Examination: Muffled distant heart sounds, dullness to percussion of posterior left chest (secondary to atelectasis from large pericardial sac), hemodynamic signs of cardiac compression (see section VIII.D.3.c).

d. Chest radiograph: Globular, symmetric cardiomegaly.

e. ECG: Decreased voltage of QRS complexes, electrical alternans (variation of QRS axis with each beat secondary to swinging of heart within pericardial fluid).

f. Echocardiography: Fluid within pericardial cavity visualized by M-mode and two-dimensional echocardiography.

g. Treatment: Address underlying condition. Observe if asymptomatic; use pericardiocentesis if there is sudden increase in volume or hemodynamic compromise. Nonsteroidal anti-inflammatory drugs (NSAIDs) or steroids may be of benefit, depending on etiology.

3. Cardiac tamponade: Accumulation of pericardial fluid under high pressure, causing compression of cardiac chambers, limiting filling, and decreasing stroke volume and cardiac output.

a. Etiology: As above for pericardial effusion. Most commonly associated with neoplasm, uremia, viral infection, and acute hemorrhage.

b. Symptoms: Dyspnea, fatigue, cold extremities.

c. Examination: Jugular venous distention, hepatomegaly, peripheral edema, tachypnea, rales (from increased systemic and pulmonary venous pressure), hypotension, tachycardia, pulsus paradoxus (decrease in systolic blood pressure by >10 mmHg with each inspiration), decreased capillary refill (from decreased stroke volume and cardiac output), quiet precordium, and muffled heart sounds.

d. ECG: Sinus tachycardia, decreased voltage, electrical alternans.

e. Echocardiography: Right ventricle (RV) collapse in early diastole, right atrial/left atrial (RA/LA) collapse in end diastole and early systole.

f. Treatment: Pericardiocentesis with temporary catheter left in place if necessary (see Chapter 2), pericardial window or stripping if it is a recurrent condition.

E. KAWASAKI DISEASE

Kawasaki disease is the leading cause of acquired heart disease in children in developed countries. It is seen almost exclusively in children younger than 8 years of age. Patients present with acute febrile vasculitis, which may lead to long-term cardiac complications from vasculitis of coronary arteries. The numbers of cases peaks in winter and spring.

1. Etiology: Unknown. Thought to be immune-regulated, in response to infectious agents or environmental toxins.
2. Diagnosis: Based on clinical criteria. These include high fever lasting 5 days or more, plus at least four of the following five criteria:
   a. Bilateral bulbar conjunctival injection without exudate.
   b. Erythematous mouth and pharynx, strawberry tongue, or red, cracked lips.
   c. Polymorphous exanthem (may be morbilliform, maculopapular, or scarlatiniform).
   d. Swelling of hands and feet, with erythema of palms and soles.
   e. Cervical lymphadenopathy (>1.5 cm in diameter), usually single and unilateral.

Note *Atypical Kawasaki disease, more often seen in infants, consists of fever with fewer than four of the above criteria but findings of coronary artery abnormalities.*

3. **Other clinical findings:** Often associated with extreme irritability, abdominal pain, diarrhea, vomiting. Also seen are anterior uveitis (80%), arthritis and arthralgias (35%), aseptic meningitis (25%), pericardial effusion or arrhythmias (20%), gallbladder hydrops (<10%), carditis (<5%), and perineal rash with desquamation.
4. **Laboratory findings:** Leukocytosis with left shift, neutrophils with vacuoles or toxic granules, elevated C-reactive protein (CRP) or erythrocyte sedimentation rate (ESR) (seen acutely), thrombocytosis (after first week, peaking at 2 weeks), normocytic and normochromic anemia, sterile pyuria (70%), increased liver function tests (LFTs) (40%).
5. **Subacute phase (11 to 25 days after onset of illness):** Resolution of fever, rash, and lymphadenopathy. Often, desquamation of fingertips or toes and thrombocytosis occur.
6. **Cardiovascular complications:** If untreated, 15% to 25% develop coronary artery aneurysms and dilation in this phase (peak prevalence occurs about 2 to 4 weeks after onset of disease; rarely appears after 6 weeks) and are at risk for coronary thrombosis acutely and coronary stenosis chronically. Carditis; aortic, mitral, and tricuspid regurgitation; pericardial effusion; CHF; MI; LV dysfunction; and ECG changes may also occur.
7. **Convalescent phase:** ESR, CRP, and platelet count return to normal. Those with coronary artery abnormalities are at increased risk for MI, arrhythmias, and sudden death.
8. **Management**[17] **(Table 6-20)**
   a. Intravenous immune globulin (IVIG) has been shown to reduce incidence of coronary artery dilation to <3% and decrease duration of fever if given in the first 10 days of illness. Current recommended regimen is a single dose of IVIG, 2 g/kg over 10 to 12 hours.

TABLE 6-20

GUIDELINES FOR TREATMENT AND FOLLOW-UP OF CHILDREN WITH KAWASAKI DISEASE

Risk Level	Pharmacologic Therapy	Physical Activity	Follow-up and Diagnostic Testing	Invasive Testing
I (no coronary artery changes at any stage of illness)	None beyond initial 6–8 weeks	No restrictions beyond initial 6–8 weeks	None beyond first year unless cardiac disease suspected	None recommended
II (transient coronary artery ectasia that disappears during acute illness)	None beyond initial 6–8 weeks	No restrictions beyond initial 6–8 weeks	None beyond first year unless cardiac disease suspected; physician may see patient at 3– to 5–year intervals	None recommended
III (small to medium solitary coronary artery aneurysm)	3–5 mg/kg aspirin per day, at least until abnormalities resolve	For patients in first decade of life, no restriction beyond initial 6–8 weeks; for patients in second decade, physical activity guided by stress testing every other year; competitive contact athletics with endurance training discouraged	Annual follow-up with echocardiogram ± electrocardiogram in first decade of life	Angiography, if stress testing or echocardiography suggests stenosis

IV (one or more giant coronary artery aneurysms or multiple small to medium aneurysms, without obstruction)	Long-term aspirin (3–5 mg/kg/day) ± warfarin	For patients in first decade of life, no restriction beyond initial 6–8 weeks; for patients in second decade, annual stress testing guides recommendations; strenuous athletics are strongly discouraged; if stress test rules out ischemia, noncontact recreational sports allowed	Annual follow-up with echocardiogram ± electrocardiogram ± chest x-ray ± additional electrocardiogram at 6–mo intervals; for patients in first decade of life, pharmacologic stress testing should be considered	Angiography, if stress testing or echocardiography suggests stenosis; elective catheterization may be done in certain circumstances
V (coronary artery obstruction)	Long-term aspirin (3–5 mg/kg/day) ± warfarin; use of calcium-channel blockers should be considered to reduce myocardial oxygen consumption	Contact sports, isometrics, and weight training should be avoided; other physical activity recommendations guided by outcome of stress testing or myocardial perfusion scan	Echocardiogram and electrocardiogram at 6–mo intervals and annual Holter and stress testing	Angiography recommended for some patients to aid in selecting therapeutic options; repeat angiography with new-onset or worsening ischemia

b. Aspirin is recommended for both its anti-inflammatory and its antiplatelet effects. Some recommend initial high-dose aspirin (80 to 100 mg/kg/day divided in four doses) until fever resolves. Then continue with 3 to 5 mg/kg/day every 24 hours for 6 to 8 weeks or until platelet count and ESR are normal (if there are no coronary artery abnormalities) or indefinitely if coronary artery abnormalities persist. Others recommend starting with low-dose aspirin (3 to 5 mg/kg/day) and continuing as above.
c. Dipyridamole, 4 mg/kg divided in three doses, is sometimes used as alternative to aspirin.
d. Follow-up: Serial echocardiography is recommended to assess coronary arteries and LV function (at time of diagnosis, at 2 to 4 weeks, at 6 to 8 weeks, and at 6 to 12 months). More frequent intervals and long-term follow-up are recommended if abnormalities are seen on echocardiography (see Table 6-20).

F. RHEUMATIC HEART DISEASE

1. **Etiology:** Believed to be immunologically mediated delayed sequela of group A streptococcal pharyngitis.
2. **Clinical Findings:** History of streptococcal pharyngitis 1 to 5 weeks before onset of symptoms. Often with pallor, malaise, easy fatigability.
3. **Diagnosis:** Jones criteria (Box 6-6).
4. **Management:** Penicillin, bed rest, salicylates, supportive management of CHF (if present) with diuretics, digoxin, morphine.

BOX 6-6

GUIDELINES FOR THE DIAGNOSIS OF INITIAL ATTACK OF RHEUMATIC FEVER

Major Manifestations	Minor Manifestations
Carditis	*Clinical findings*
Polyarthritis	Arthralgia
Chorea	Fever
Erythema marginatum	*Laboratory findings*
Subcutaneous nodule	Elevated acute phase reactants (erythrocyte sedimentation rate, C-reactive protein)
	Prolonged PR interval

Plus

Supporting evidence of antecedent group A streptococcal infection

Positive throat culture or rapid streptococcal antigen test

Elevated or rising streptococcal antibody titer

If supported by evidence of preceding group A streptococcal infection, the presence of two major manifestations or of one major and two minor manifestations indicates a high probability of acute rheumatic fever.

REFERENCES

1. Zubrow AB, et al: Determinants of blood pressure in infants admitted to neonatal intensive care units: A prospective multicenter study. Philadelphia Neonatal Blood Pressure Study Group. J Perinatol 1995;15:470.
2. Horan MJ, et al: Report of the second task force on blood pressure control in children. Pediatrics 1987;79(1):1–25.
3. Park MK: Pediatric Cardiology for Practitioners, 3rd ed. St. Louis, Mosby, 1996.
4. Sapin SO: Recognizing normal heart murmurs: a logic-based mnemonic. Pediatrics, 1997;99(4):616–619.
5. Davignon A, et al: Normal ECG standards for infants and children. Pediatr Cardiol 1979;1:123–131.
6. Schwartz PJ, et al: Prolongation of the QT interval and the sudden infant death syndrome. N Engl J Med 1998;338:1709–1714.
7. Garson A Jr: The Electrocardiogram in Infants and Children: A Systematic Approach. Philadelphia, Lea & Febiger, 1983.
8. Park MK, Guntheroth WG: How to Read Pediatric ECGs, 3rd ed. St. Louis, Mosby, 1992.
9. Towbin JA, Bricker JT, Garson A Jr: Electrocardiographic criteria for diagnosis of acute myocardial infarction in childhood. Am J Cardiol 1992;69:1545.
10. Hirsch R, et al: Cardiac troponin I in pediatrics: Normal values and potential use in assessment of cardiac injury. J Pediatr 1997;130:872–877.
11. Walsh EP: In Fyler DC, Nadas A (eds): Pediatric Cardiology. Philadelphia, Hanley & Belfus, 1992.
12. Colon SD, et al: Developmental modulation of myocardial mechanics: Age- and growth-related alterations in afterload and contractility. J Am Coll Cardiol 1992;19:619.
13. Lees MH: Cyanosis of the newborn infant: recognition and clinical evaluation. J Pediatr 1970;77:484.
14. Kitterman JA: Cyanosis in the newborn infant. Pediatr Rev 1982;4:13–24.
15. Jones RW, et al: Arterial oxygen tension and response to oxygen breathing in differential diagnosis of heart disease in infancy. Arch Dis Child 1976;51:667.
16. American Academy of Pediatrics: 2003 Red Book: Report of the Committee on Infectious Diseases, 26th ed. Elk Grove Village, IL, The Academy, 2003.
17. Dajani AS, et al: Guidelines for the long-term management of patients with Kawasaki disease: Report from the Committee on Rheumatic Fever, Endocarditis, and Kawasaki Disease, Council on Cardiovascular Disease in the Young, American Heart Association. Circulation 1994;89:916.

Dermatology

Kristen Schwindt Brown, MD

7

I. WEBSITE

www.med.jhu.edu/peds/dermatlas

Please refer to the Color Plates section after p. 230 for photographic examples of rashes.

II. EVALUATION AND CLINICAL DESCRIPTION OF SKIN FINDINGS

A. PRIMARY SKIN LESIONS (Fig. 7-1A)

Macule/patch: small flat lesion with altered color (<0.5 cm)/large macule (>0.5 cm)

Papule/plaque: elevated, well-circumscribed lesion (<0.5 cm)/large papule (>0.5 cm)

Nodule/tumor: mass located in dermis or subcutaneous fat (may be solid or soft)/large nodule

Vesicle/bulla: blister with transparent fluid/large vesicle

Wheal: erythematous, well-circumscribed, raised, edematous lesion that appears/disappears quickly

B. SECONDARY SKIN LESIONS (Fig. 7-1B)

Scale: a small, thin plate of horny epithelium

Pustule: a well-circumscribed elevated lesion filled with pus

Crust: exudative mass consisting of blood, scale, and pus from skin erosions or ruptured vesicles/papules

Ulcer: erosion of dermis and cutis with clearly defined edges

Scar: formation of new connective tissue after damage to epidermis and cutis leaving permanent change in skin

Excoriation: surface marks often linear secondary to scratching

Fissure: linear skin crack with inflammation and pain

III. HEMANGIOMAS

A. PATHOGENESIS

Hemangiomas have a phase of rapid proliferation followed by spontaneous involution. During the proliferative phase, densely packed endothelial cells form small capillaries; subsequent vessels develop from existing vasculature.

B. CLINICAL MANIFESTATIONS

1. **Appearance:**

a. Newborns may demonstrate pale macules with thread-like telangiectasias.

b. The most recognizable form is a bright red, slightly elevated, noncompressible plaque. Frequently, both superficial and deep

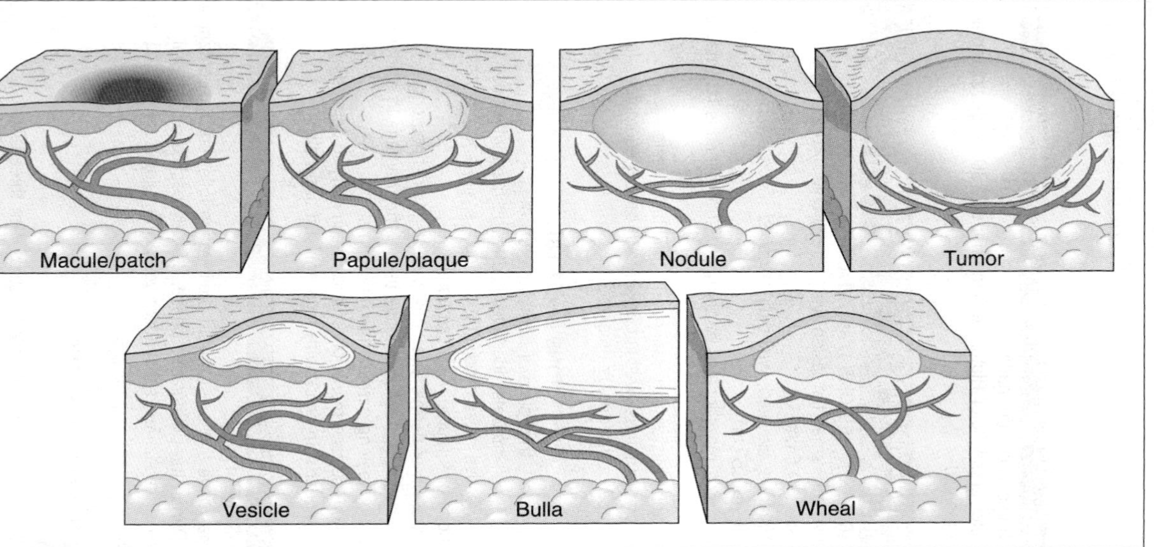

FIG. 7-1A
Pattern diagnosis. *A*, Primary skin lesions. *B*, Secondary skin lesions. *(From Cohen BA: Pediatric Dermatology, 2nd ed. St. Louis, Mosby, 1999, p 5.)*

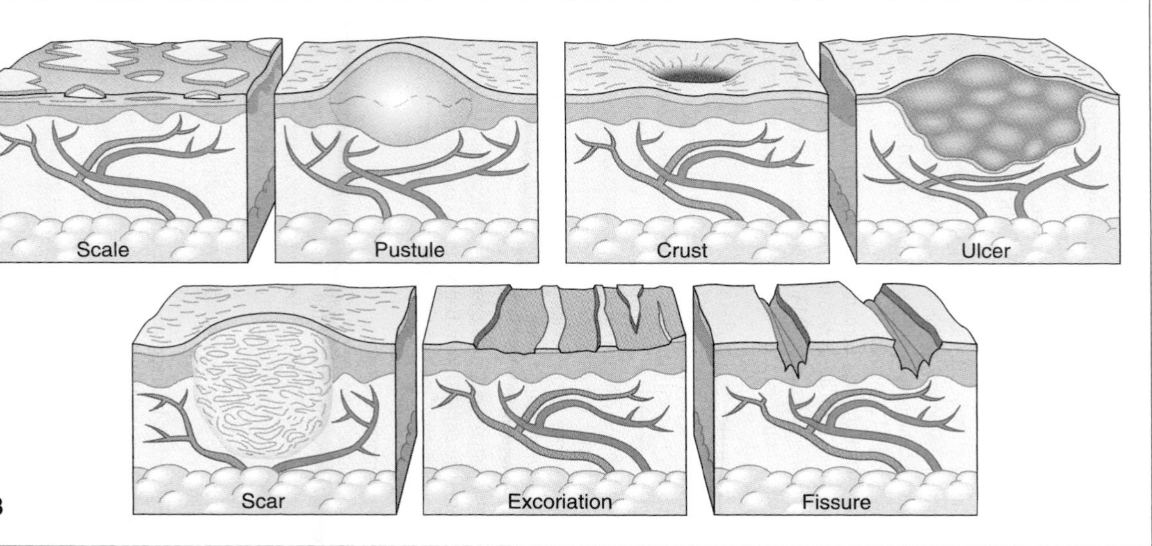

FIG. 7-1B

components are present, with deep components appearing bluish in color.

c. Size can range from a few millimeters to several centimeters.

2. **Incidence:** Hemangiomas are the most common soft tissue tumors in infancy, with increased incidence in premature infants, and are three times more likely in girls than boys. Notably, about 5% to 10% of 1-year-olds have these lesions.
3. **Natural history:** About 20% of hemangiomas are present at birth, with the remainder developing within the first 4 weeks of life. The most rapid growth phase occurs between 2 and 4 months, with regression beginning at 6 to 12 months.
4. **Diagnosis:** Although most hemangiomas are diagnosed clinically, imaging techniques (e.g., ultrasound, computed tomography [CT], magnetic resonance imaging [MRI]) can be used to differentiate hemangiomas from vascular malformations or neoplastic processes.

C. COMPLICATIONS

1. **Ulceration** is the most common complication and may result in severe pain, infection, hemorrhage, or scarring; ulceration results from necrosis of superficial components. Hemorrhage and superinfection may also occur. Hemorrhage, although alarming in appearance, is usually minimal and can be controlled by direct pressure. Superinfection may lead to cellulitis, osteomyelitis, or septicemia.
2. **Kasabach-Merritt phenomenon,** a complication of rapidly enlarging, usually deep lesions, is characterized by anemia, thrombocytopenia, and coagulopathy, requiring aggressive medical management. These lesions are differentiated from benign hemangiomas by their deep red-blue appearance, marked firmness, and a different histologic appearance.
3. **Regionally important lesions:**

a. Periorbital lesions: Hemangiomas in the periorbital region may cause amblyopia from obstruction of the visual axis or astigmatism from insidious compression of the globe or extension into the retrobulbar space. They require careful observation and evaluation by an ophthalmologist.

b. External auditory canal lesions may result in otitis or conductive hearing loss.

c. Multiple cutaneous hemangiomas and large facial hemangiomas are associated with visceral hemangiomas and may warrant abdominal ultrasound to look for organ involvement (i.e., liver hemangiomas). A high occurrence of hemangiomas in the cervical-tracheal region (Phaces syndrome)[17] may be associated with abnormalities of the urogenital system.[1]

d. Visceral hemangiomas are often characterized by high-flow patterns and may result in high-output cardiac failure and anemia. Large facial hemangiomas are also associated with posterior fossa vascular malformations and thus should have neuroimaging with special attention to the posterior fossa.

e. Airway hemangiomas are often located in the subglottic region and may cause hoarseness and stridor. Infants with cutaneous lesions in a beard distribution (chin, lips, mandibular region, and neck) are at greatest risk for airway involvement.

f. Lumbosacral hemangiomas that span the midline are associated with spinal malformations, dysraphism, and anomalies of the anorectal and urogenital regions. An ultrasound of the L-5 spine in infants younger than 6 months of age is an effective noninvasive screening study.

D. MANAGEMENT

1. **Because most hemangiomas require no intervention,** the decision to treat should be based on location and depth of the lesion, age of the patient, and likelihood of complication. Photo documentation is used to follow the growth and regression process.
2. **Systemic corticosteroids** are the mainstay of therapy for lesions that require intervention to prevent subsequent complication (i.e., periorbital or subglottic lesions). Usually, doses of 2 to 3 mg/kg/day of prednisone or prednisolone are used. One third of lesions demonstrate dramatic shrinkage, one third demonstrate stabilization of growth, and one third show no response.
3. **Laser ablation.**
4. **Interferon.**
5. **Embolization** can be used to treat cutaneous hemangiomas that have not responded to medical therapy.
6. **Surgical excision.**[2]

IV. WARTS

A. PATHOGENESIS

Warts are caused by more than 60 types of the human papillomavirus (HPV). The virus enters the skin through breaks in the epithelium, causing hyperplasia of the squamous epithelium.

B. MORPHOLOGY

1. **Common warts:** The lesions of common warts are skin-colored, rough, minimally scaly papules and nodules found on the exposed surfaces of the hands, face, arms, and legs. Lesions can be solitary or multiple, a few millimeters to several centimeters in diameter, and may form large plaques or a confluent, linear pattern secondary to autoinoculation.
2. **Flat warts** occur over the hands, arms, and face, and are usually less than 2 mm wide. They often present in clusters.
3. **Plantar warts** are found on the soles of the feet as sometimes painful but often asymptomatic, inward-growing, hyperkeratotic plaques and

papules. Trauma on weight-bearing surfaces results in small black dots ("seeds" from thrombosed vessels on the surface of the wart).

4. **Anogenital warts.**

See Chapter 5.

C. TREATMENT (Table 7-1)

1. **Spontaneous resolution** occurs in more than 75% of warts in otherwise healthy individuals within 3 years.
2. **Keratolytics (i.e., topical salicylates)** work by removing excess scale within and around warts and by triggering an inflammatory reaction. This is particularly effective in combination with adhesive tape occlusion; however, a response may take 4 to 6 months.
3. **Destructive techniques** depend on destruction of wart and surrounding normal skin and should be used only with the consent of the patient.

a. Cryotherapy results in necrosis and blister formation. Treatment may produce scarring, and warts may recur.

b. Caustic agents can be applied after warts have been shaved but require application for several weeks or months.

c. Cantharidin is a topical vesicant that causes the formation of intraepidermal blisters. Recurrence risk is high, and blister formation can be difficult to control.

d. Electrocautery and CO_2 laser ablation require local or general anesthesia. These can be particularly useful for treating large lesions on the trunk and extremities and discrete plantar warts. Both can leave scars, and recurrence is well documented. Open wounds and prolonged healing pose significant problems in weight bearing.

TABLE 7-1

WART THERAPY

Treatment	Advantages	Disadvantages
Keratolytics (lactic acid, salicylic acid, tretinoin	Available without prescription, home therapy, low cost, low risk, little pain	Slow response, irritation
DESTRUCTIVE AGENTS		
Cryotherapy	Quick office procedure, relatively low cost	Pain, scarring, recurrence
Caustics (topical acids)	Home or office therapy, relatively low cost	Irritation, recurrence, systemic toxicity (podophyllin)
Cantharidin (vesicant)	Occasionally effective	High risk for recurrence, prominent pigmentary changes
Electrocautery and laser	Usually effective	Pain, scarring, recurrence, requires anesthesia moderate cost

From Cohen BA: Contemp Pediatr 1997;2:128–149.

e. Intradermal bleomycin has also been used.
f. Destructive options for therapy are often not good choices in the treatment of young children.

4. **Immunotherapy:**

a. Immunotherapy involves contact sensitization with a potent allergen initially, followed by the application of a low concentration of the allergen in cream form to the wart site. Intralesional injection of antigens has also been recently used.
b. Cimetidine can be used in doses of 30 to 40 mg/kg/day divided into two doses for 2 months; however, it may be no better than placebo.[3]

As with molluscum contagiosum (discussed subsequently), recalcitrant or widespread lesions should be screened for immunodeficiency (congenital and acquired).

V. MOLLUSCUM CONTAGIOSUM

A. MORPHOLOGY (Color Plate 1)

Molluscum contagiosum, caused by the pox virus, consists of dome-shaped, often umbilicated, translucent to white papules that range from 1 mm to 1 cm, with a tiny keratotic core at the center. Lesions are often surrounded by scaling and erythema that resemble eczema. They may appear inflamed and secondarily infected when undergoing spontaneous involution. These lesions often occur in children on the trunk, axillary region, face, and diaper regions, often spreading by autoinoculation. In teens, lesions may occur in the genital area as a sexually transmitted disease.

B. TREATMENT

Lesions are benign and self-limited. Treatment, with the consent of the child, is directed toward symptomatic lesions because destruction of the individual lesions may lead to scarring and recurrences of new papules are common despite treatment.

1. Use a small curette with gentle pressure to débride the lesion. This treatment is the least likely to cause scarring.
2. Liquid nitrogen may be an option in older children.
3. Topical preparations of salicylic-lactic acid combinations, cantharidin, and retinoic acid may also be used.[4]

VI. ATOPIC DERMATITIS (ECZEMA)

A. PATHOPHYSIOLOGY (Color Plates 2–5)

Atopic dermatitis involves a genetic predisposition and elevated immunoglobulin E (IgE) levels, which suggests an abnormal response to triggering agents, resulting in the release of histamine, prostaglandins, and cytokines. Inflammation causes itching and subsequent scratching, which produces the clinical lesions of eczema.

B. EPIDEMIOLOGY

1. Atopic dermatitis affects 5% to 7% of children, with the peak prevalence between 6 months and 8 to 10 years of age.
2. About 95% of children with atopic dermatitis have asthma or allergic rhinitis.

C. CLINICAL PRESENTATIONS (Box 7-1)

Acute changes include erythema, vesicles, crusting, and secondary infection. Chronic changes include lichenification, scaling, and postinflammatory hypopigmentation or hyperpigmentation.

1. **Infantile form:** Extensor surfaces are more affected than flexors. Truncal, facial, and scalp involvement are common, with sparing of the diaper area.
2. **Early to middle childhood:** Flexural surfaces are more severely involved.
3. **Late childhood and adolescence:** Lesions tend to be restricted to skin creases and hand dermatitis.

BOX 7-1
IDENTIFYING CHARACTERISTIC OF ATOPIC DERMATITIS
Major Criteria (Seen in All Patients)
Pruritus
Typical morphology and distribution of lesions
Facial and extensor involvement in infants
Flexural lichenification in older children and adults
Tendency toward chronic or chronically relapsing dermatitis
Common Findings (At Least 2)
Personal or family history of atopic disease (asthma, allergic rhinitis, atopic dermatitis)
Immediate skin test reactivity
White dermatographism and/or delayed blanch to cholinergic agents
Anterior subcapsular cataracts
Associated Findings (At Least 4)
Xerosis/ichthyosis/hyperlinear palms and soles
Pityriasis alba
Keratosis pilaris
Facial pallor/infraorbital darkening
Dennie-Morgan infraorbital fold
Elevated serum IgE
Tendency toward nonspecific hand dermatitis
Tendency toward repeated cutaneous infections

From Cohen BA: Contemp Pediatr 1992;7:64–81.

D. TREATMENT

1. **Chronic disease:** Bland lubricants, including petroleum jelly, Aquaphor, Eucerin, and vegetable shortening, are the mainstays of therapy but may need to be more elegant for older patients. Lubricants should be used two to three times per day and immediately after bathing or swimming. Bathing time should be short (no more than 5 minutes), and the skin should be patted dry, not rubbed, before application of lubricant.
2. **Topical steroids:**
 a. Low- and medium-potency steroid creams should be used once or twice per day in the most severely affected areas for eczema flares and for generally no more than 7 days. Severe flares may require a longer duration of therapy followed by a taper to lower-potency steroids. Even with low-potency steroids, special care is required in areas in which the skin is thin, such as the diaper area, groin, armpits, under the breasts, around the neck, and on the face. High-potency topical steroids should generally be used in consultation with a dermatologist.
 b. Topical steroids can be applied at the same time as lubricants and can be mixed with lubricants when weaning from the topical steroid.
3. **Systemic steroids should generally be avoided.** They may be used for short periods of uncontrolled eczema flares or for severe disease requiring hospitalization.
4. **Antihistamines** may be used when hives cause scratching, thus exacerbating underlying eczema. Sedating antihistamines (i.e., diphenhydramine, hydroxyzine) are more effective for pruritus because there is no evidence that nonsedating antihistamines are effective in controlling itching. Cetirizine is the most effective of the nonsedating antihistamines.
5. **Protective clothing should be worn.**
6. **Topical tacrolimus** (formally known as FK506, currently marketed with brand name Protopic 0.03% and 0.1% ointment) and pimecrolimus (marketed as Elidel 1% cream) are both topical immunomodulators that may be used as an alternative to topical steroids. Neither agent causes skin atrophy,[5] allowing for safe alternatives for recalcitrant facial eczema, as well as possibly preventing the need for topical steroids. Both agents can be used safely on patients >2 years of age.[6,7]

E. COMPLICATIONS

1. **For weeping or blistering lesions with no evidence of infection,** cold-water compresses three or four times per day or tepid baths followed by bland lubricant application may be used.
2. **Bacterial infection, usually staphylococcal and sometimes streptococcal,** must be recognized quickly. Localized infections can

be treated with topical antibiotics, whereas more serious infections require systemic antibiotics.[8]

3. **Eczema herpeticum** must be treated systemically with acyclovir.

VII. ACNE VULGARIS

A. PATHOPHYSIOLOGY

Acne is the result of the obstruction of sebaceous follicles, located primarily on the face and trunk, by excessive amounts of sebum and desquamated epithelial cells. The resident anaerobic organism, *Propionibacterium acnes*, proliferates and produces chemotactic and inflammatory mediators that lead to inflammation.

1. **Noninflammatory open comedones, or "blackheads."**
2. **Noninflammatory closed comedones, or "whiteheads."**
3. **Inflammatory papules, pustules, nodules, or cysts.**

B. TREATMENT (Table 7-2)

1. **Gentle, nonabrasive cleaning is best.** Vigorous scrubbing, abrasive cleaners, and mechanical devices can promote the development of inflammatory lesions.
2. **Dietary factors play no role in sebum production.**
3. **Comedonal acne:** The treatment goal for noninflammatory acne is first prevention and second to minimize the formation of new comedones and colonization with *P. acnes.* This type of acne is most common in the preadolescent and early adolescent years.

a. Topical tretinoin or Adapalene and benzoyl peroxide (either or both) are the treatments of choice. Salicylic acid and topical antibiotics may also be used.

b. Topical cream or gel should be applied sparingly once daily, starting with a low concentration and increasing concentration if local irritation does not occur. It may take several weeks for desired clinical results to become apparent.

c. Continue therapy until it is clear that new lesions are not developing.

4. **Mild inflammatory acne:** Scattered small papules or pustules develop, with a minimum of comedones. Proliferation of *P. acnes* occurs at this stage. This often occurs in the early teens and in adult women in their 20s.

a. Most patients improve after a 2- to 4-week course of topical antibiotics applied twice daily, topical benzoyl peroxide, or a combination of the two.

b. Treatment should be continued until no new lesions develop and then should be slowly tapered.

5. **Inflammatory acne** is a generalized eruption of papules and pustules on the face and trunk. A few patients have a more destructive type of inflammation associated with large, deep inflammatory nodules.

a. A topical retinoid plus a topical and/or systemic antibiotic should be used, depending on the severity of the lesions, for 4 to 6 weeks.

TABLE 7-2

TOPICAL AND SYSTEMIC ANTIBIOTICS USED TO TREAT ACNE

Antibiotic	Characteristics
TOPICAL	
Erythromycin	*P. acnes* very sensitive; least lipophilic
Clindamycin	*P. acnes* very sensitive; more lipophilic than erythromycin, but less than benzoyl peroxide
Benzoyl peroxide plus erythromycin	*P. acnes* very sensitive; most lipophilic topical agent; less irritating than benzoyl peroxide alone
Benzoyl peroxide plus clindamycin	Similar to above
Azelaic acid	*P. acnes* sensitive; minimal lipophilia; can reduce abnormal desquamation
Metronidazole	*P. acnes* not sensitive; has antiinflammatory properties
Benzoyl peroxide plus glycolic acid	Glycolic acid may enhance penetration and reduce abnormal desquamation
SYSTEMIC	
Tetracycline	*P. acnes* sensitive; inexpensive; usually needs to be taken two to four times a day; compliance can be a problem because of need to take on an empty stomach
Erythromycin	*P. acnes* very sensitive; resistance emerging; gastrointestinal upset common; inexpensive
Doxycycline	Lipophilic; *P. acnes* very sensitive; resistance not yet seen; photosensitivity can occur; more expensive than tetracycline and erythromycin
Minocycline	Lipophilic; *P. acnes* very sensitive; resistance not yet seen; no photosensitivity; abnormal pigmentation in oral mucosa and skin; vertigo-like symptoms; most expensive
Trimethoprim-sulfamethoxazole	Lipophilic; *P. acnes* very sensitive; severe erythema multiforme and toxic epidermal necrolysis limit use
Clindamycin	*P. acnes* very sensitive; somewhat lipophilic; pseudomembranous colitis limits use

From Leyden JJ. N Engl J Med 1997;16:1156–1162.

b. Systemic antibiotics may be used with a topical antibiotic. In general, the dose of the antibiotic should not be reduced for 2 to 4 months.

c. Patients with nodular, cystic lesions may not respond to systemic antibiotics and may require systemic isotretinoin. This should be used in consultation with a dermatologist such that labs may be followed secondary to risk for leukocytosis, to screen for depression, and to ensure that two forms of effective and reliable contraception for women are in place secondary to the medication's teratogenic effects. In addition, use in patients with acute promyelocytic leukemia (APL) is extremely dangerous and can lead to retinoic acid–APL syndrome characterized by respiratory distress, fever, weight gain, and effusions of the heart and lungs.[9]

d. Women with persistent acne unresponsive to antibiotics and topical tretinoin may respond to therapy with oral contraceptives after appropriate gynecologic and endocrine evaluation, especially for polycystic ovarian syndrome and other androgen excess conditions.[10]

VIII. COMMON CAUSES OF HAIR LOSS IN CHILDREN

A. TINEA CAPITIS (Color Plate 6)

1. Epidemiology:

a. *Trichophyton tonsurans* accounts for greater than 90% of tinea capitis in North America. It is an anthropophilic organism with no known natural reservoir. The fungus persists for long periods on fomites, such as hairbrushes, combs, furniture, stuffed toys, and clothing.

b. Most patients are between 1 and 10 years of age, but infection may occur at any age.

c. The incidence is highest in African American children and second highest in Hispanic youths. This predisposition in African American children is not completely understood, but it may be the result of the character of the hair follicle, tight braiding, or the use of pomades.

2. Clinical presentation:

a. Classic tinea capitis presents as one or more round to oval patches of partial to complete alopecia, with varying degrees of erythema. Scale is present, and the border is slightly raised and more erythematous than the central area.

b. A kerion is an inflammatory presentation of tinea capitis. It presents as a boggy, tender, edematous plaque or cluster of nodules with erythema. It is usually solitary and is frequently accompanied by cervical or occipital adenopathy and papular morbilliform eruption classified as an "id" reaction.

c. The seborrheic dermatitis–like pattern (most common) may produce minimal or no alopecia and show diffuse scaling over the scalp, with pruritus.

d. Follicular pustules with crusting and scaling scattered over the scalp is a pattern seen predominantly in African American children with tight braiding and constant pomade use. It often resembles bacterial folliculitis, but bacterial culture is negative.

3. Diagnosis: The presumptive clinical diagnosis of tinea capitis may be confirmed by either direct microscopic examination or culture of scale (may be collected with a toothbrush on a culture plate or on a moistened culturette swab).

4. Treatment:

a. Successful treatment requires oral therapy; griseofulvin is the agent of choice. It is best taken with fatty food to promote absorption (see Formulary for dosage information). Standard references suggest 4 to 6 weeks of therapy, although 8 to 12 weeks may be required for eradication. Patients should be reevaluated monthly, and repeat culture may be obtained 2 weeks *before* therapy is discontinued to document cure. Patients will often develop an eczema-like rash associated with the fungal infection, known as an id reaction. This is not a drug reaction, and griseofulvin therapy should be continued.

b. Kerions (Color Plate 7) should be treated with prednisone or prednisolone (0.5 mg/kg/day for 10 to 14 days) if no contraindication exists in addition to standard griseofulvin therapy.
c. The use of sporicidal shampoos in addition to oral therapy promotes rapid elimination of spores, thus decreasing the contagion risk to family members and schoolmates. The use of selenium sulfide 2.5% shampoo twice weekly is recommended.[11] Ketoconazole 1% and 2% shampoo is also available for this purpose.

B. ALOPECIA AREATA

Alopecia areata is a common condition characterized by the sudden onset of asymptomatic, noninflammatory, round, bald patches located on any hair-bearing part of the body, most commonly the scalp (Color Plate 8).

1. **Alopecia areata is best differentiated by the absence of hair follicles in the bald spot.** There is also a lack of scaly erythema, pustules, and crusts.
2. **Although the course is irregular and unpredictable, most patients develop good regrowth of hair within 1 or 2 years.**
3. **Treatments include topical corticosteroids, topical minoxidil, tar preparations, anthralin, topical sensitizers, and ultraviolet light therapy.**[12] Systemic steroids should generally not be used because they do not alter prognosis. In adolescents and adults, hair loss often resolves over months to years, but in younger children, the prognosis is more guarded.

C. TELOGEN EFFLUVIUM

Telogen effluvium is a form of alopecia characterized by diffuse hair loss that is usually not clinically obvious to anyone but the patient and parent.

1. **Growing hair follicles respond to physiologic and pathologic stress (e.g., high fever, severe influenza, infection, surgery, drugs, pregnancy, hypothyroidism) by regressing to the resting, or telogen, state.**
2. **Telogen effluvium usually occurs 3 to 5 months after the stressor and is self-limited.**

D. TRACTION ALOPECIA

Traction alopecia is often a result of hairstyles that apply tension for long periods of time (Color Plate 9).

1. **Traction alopecia is characterized by noninflammatory linear areas of hair loss at the margins of the hairline, part line, or scattered regions, depending on hair styling procedures used.**
2. **Treatment is avoidance of styling products or styles resulting in traction.**

E. HAIR PULLING

Hair pulling is a benign, self-limited activity common in young children.

F. TRICHOTILLOMANIA

Trichotillomania is a type of alopecia caused by the compulsion to pull out one's own hair, resulting in irregular areas of incomplete hair loss, mainly on the scalp, but the eyebrows and eyelashes may also be involved.

1. **The clinical appearance is characterized by areas of hair loss within which are short, broken hair shafts of varying lengths.**
2. **Most cases spontaneously resolve, but in severe cases a psychiatric evaluation may be warranted.**

IX. COMMON NEONATAL DERMATOLOGIC PROBLEMS

A. ERYTHEMA TOXICUM NEONATORUM (ET)

ET is the most common rash (pustular) in infants and is described as a papular rash (2–3 mm in diameter at first), often evolving into vesicles. Rash occurs in neonates, most often on the second or third days of life (but can emerge as late as 2–3 weeks). Lesions may be clustered and usually resolve in 5–7 days from emergence; recurrences, however, may occur. Vesicular fluid is significant for the presence of eosinophils; treatment is supportive only because rash is self-limited (Color Plate 10).

B. TRANSIENT NEONATAL PUSTULAR MELANOSIS

This disease occurs in 4% of infants, especially infants with darker skin tones, and is usually present at birth. This vesicular rash is described as 2 to 5 mm pustules with a hyperpigmented, nonerythematous base, which over time develops a central crust and leaves a hyperpigmented macule with concurrent scale. This rash, as the name implies, is self-limiting (Color Plates 11 and 12).

C. MILIARIA

Noted commonly on the nose, these (often erythematous) lesions occur secondary to obstruction of eccrine sweat ducts. Miliaria may also occur as small papules and pustules secondary to obstruction of these ducts in the mid-epidermis (also known as "prickly heat"). These lesions occur often after the first week of life in areas of high heat production and occlusion by clothes or coverings; course is self-limiting and can be hastened by removal of tight wraps or clothing (Color Plate 13).

D. MILIA

These common (up to 50% occurrence) lesions are 1 to 3 mm papules (white to yellow in color), occurring mostly on the upper body and face of newborns, usually within the first month of life. These papules can persist for several months and are epidermal inclusion cysts requiring no treatment (Color Plate 14).

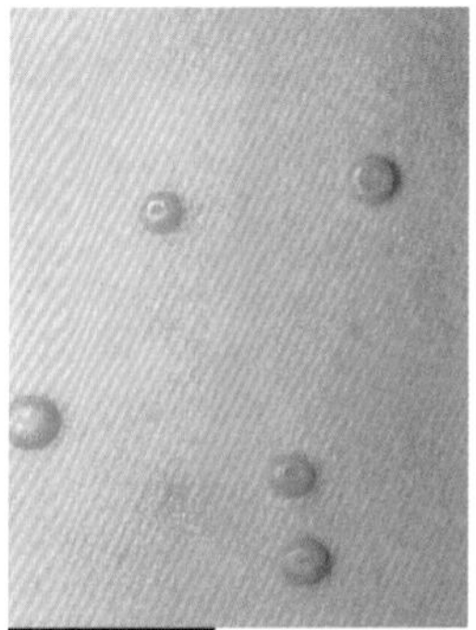

PLATE 1

Molluscum contagiosum. *(From Cohen BA: Atlas of Pediatric Dermatology. St. Louis, Mosby, 1993.)*

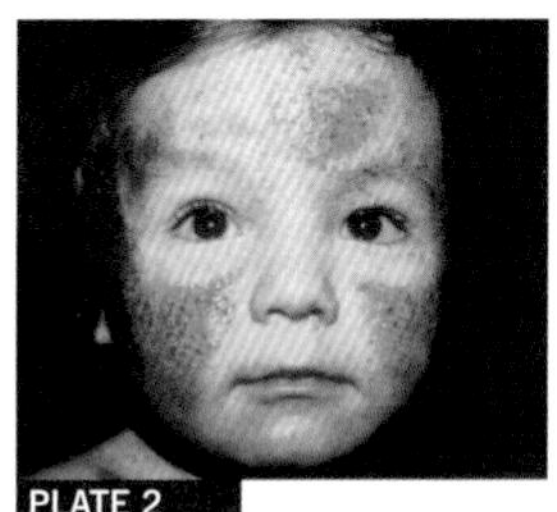

PLATE 2

Infantile eczema. *(From Cohen BA: Atlas of Pediatric Dermatology. St. Louis, Mosby, 1993.)*

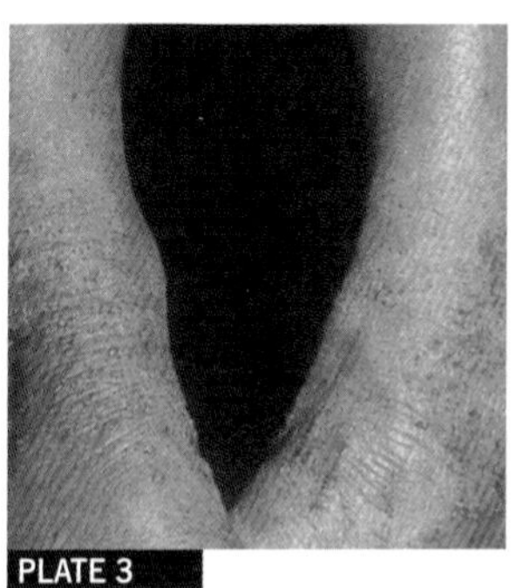

PLATE 3

Childhood eczyma. *(From Cohen BA: Atlas of Pediatric Dermatology. St. Louis, Mosby, 1993.)*

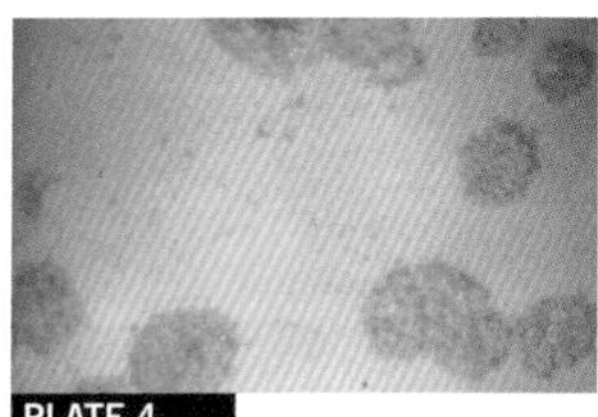

PLATE 4

Nummular eczyma. *(From Cohen BA: Atlas of Pediatric Dermatology. St. Louis, Mosby, 1993.)*

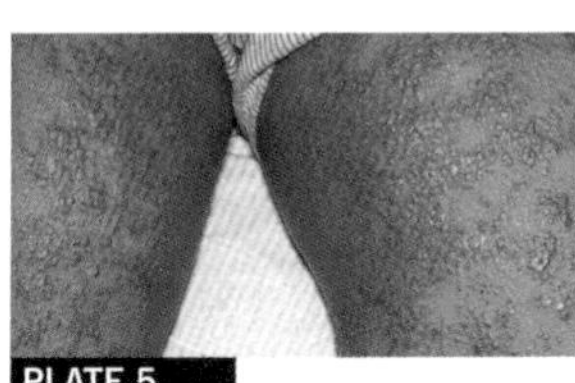

PLATE 5

Follicular eczema. *(From Cohen BA: Atlas of Pediatric Dermatology. St. Louis, Mosby, 1993.)*

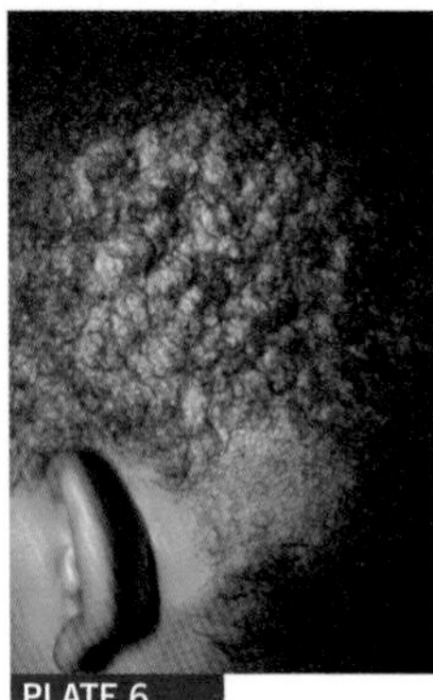

PLATE 6

"Black Dot" tinea capitis. *(From Cohen BA: www.med.jhu.edu/peds/dermatlas, 2001.)*

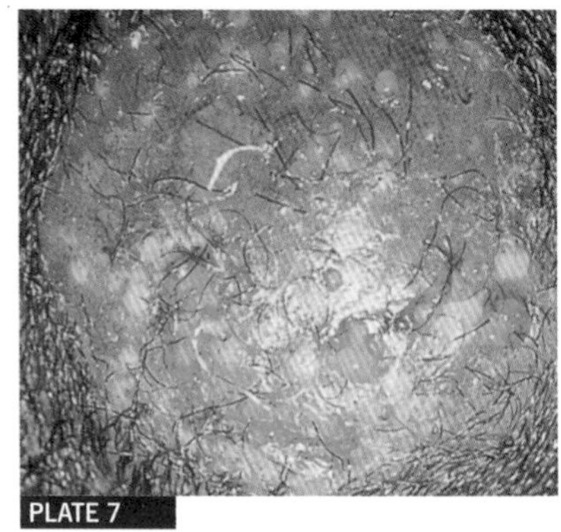

PLATE 7

Kerion. *(From Cohen BA: Atlas of Pediatric Dermatology. St. Louis, Mosby, 1993.)*

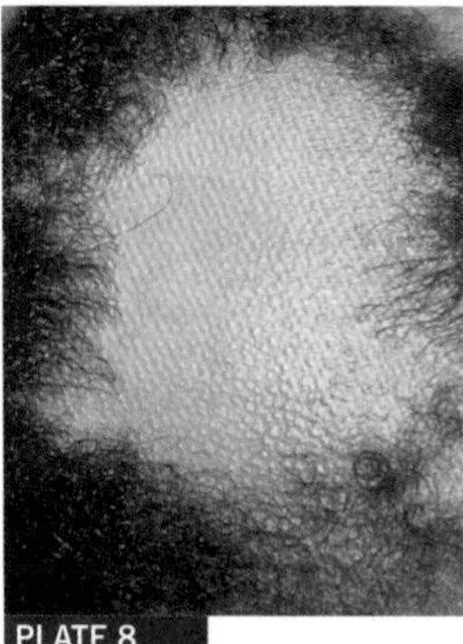

PLATE 8

Alopecia areata. *(From Cohen BA: Atlas of Pediatric Dermatology. St. Louis, Mosby, 1993.)*

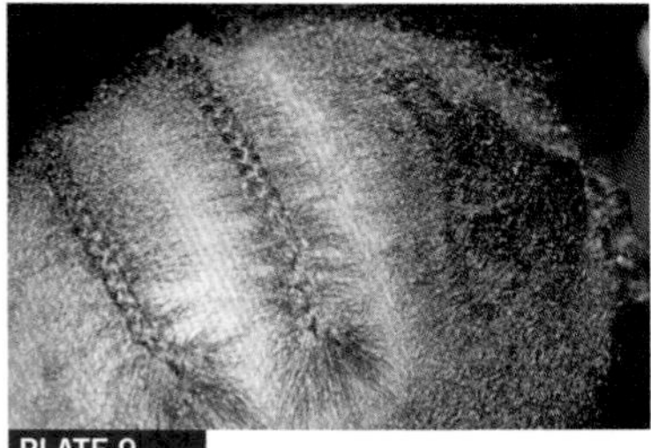

PLATE 9

Traction alopecia. *(From Cohen BA: Atlas of Pediatric Dermatology. St. Louis, Mosby, 1993.)*

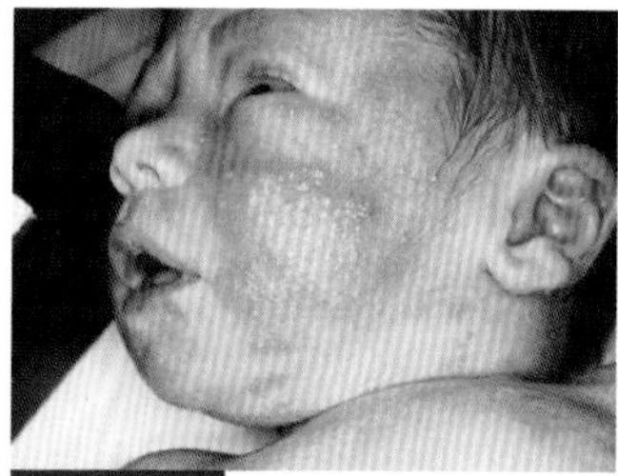

PLATE 10

Erythema toxicum. *(From Cohen BA: www.med.jhu.edu/peds/dermatlas, 2001.)*

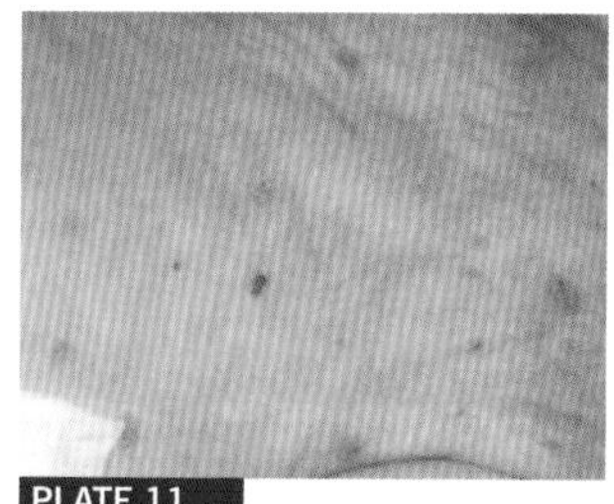

PLATE 11

Neonatal pustular melanosis. *(From Cohen BA: Atlas of Pediatric Dermatology. St. Louis, Mosby, 1993.)*

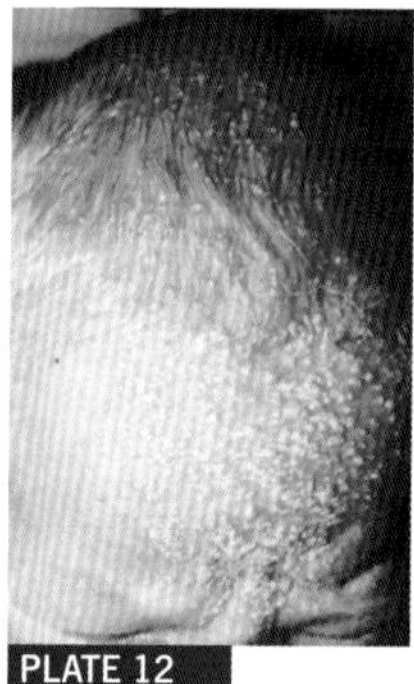

PLATE 12

Transient neonatal pustular melanosis. *(From Cohen BA: Pediatric Dermatology, 2nd ed. St. Louis, Mosby, 1999.)*

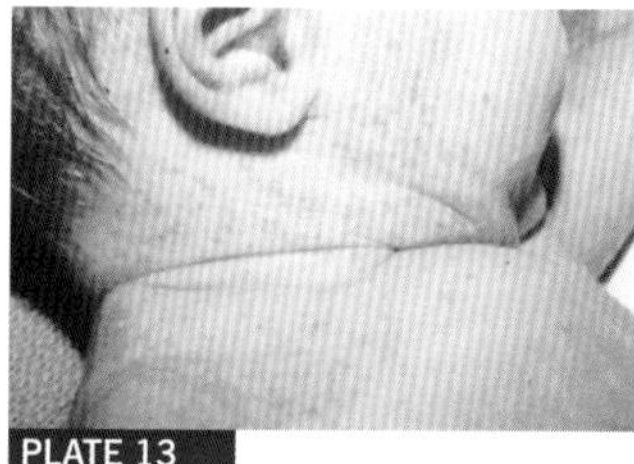

PLATE 13

Miliaria rubra. *(From Cohen BA: Pediatric Dermatology, 2nd ed. St. Louis, Mosby, 1999.)*

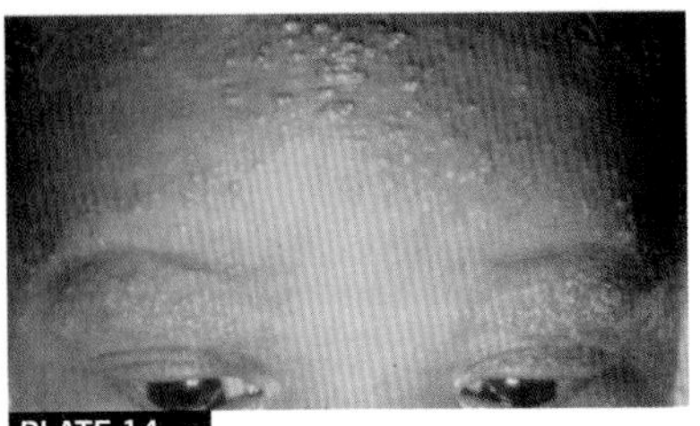

PLATE 14
Milia. *(From Cohen BA: Atlas of Pediatric Dermatology. St. Louis, Mosby, 1993.)*

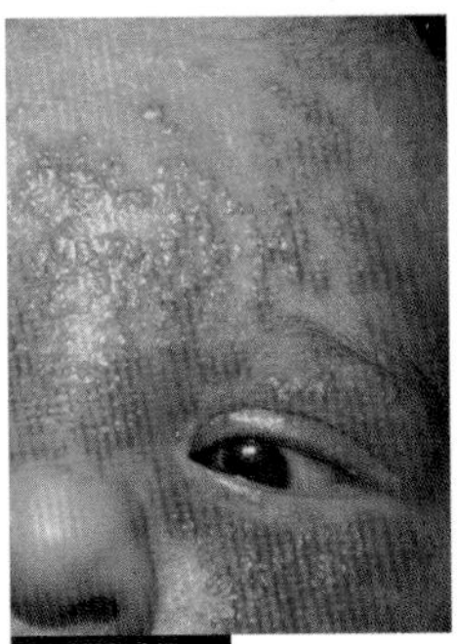

PLATE 15
Neonatal acne. *(From Cohen BA: Atlas of Pediatric Dermatology. St. Louis, Mosby, 1993.)*

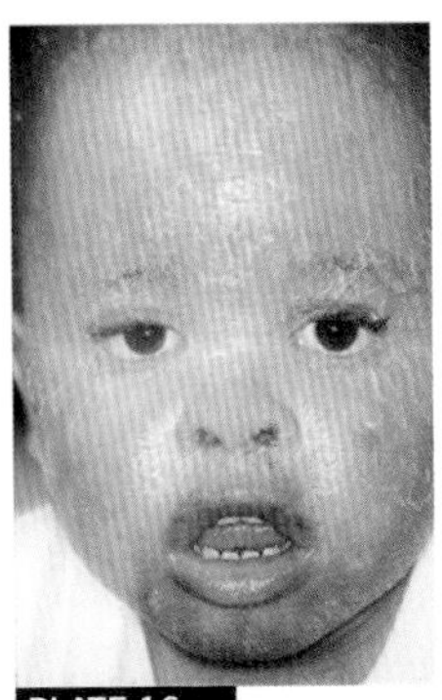

PLATE 16
Congenital ichthyosiform erythroderma. *(From Cohen BA: Pediatric Dermatology, 2nd ed. St. Louis, Mosby, 1999.)*

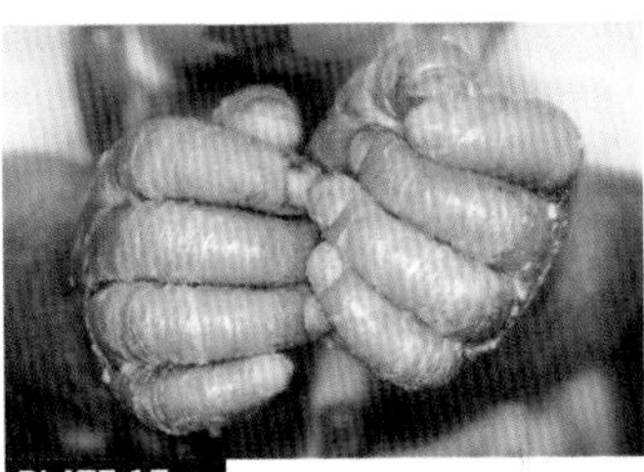

PLATE 17
Congenital ichthyosiform erythroderma. *(From Cohen BA: Pediatric Dermatology, 2nd ed. St. Louis, Mosby, 1999.)*

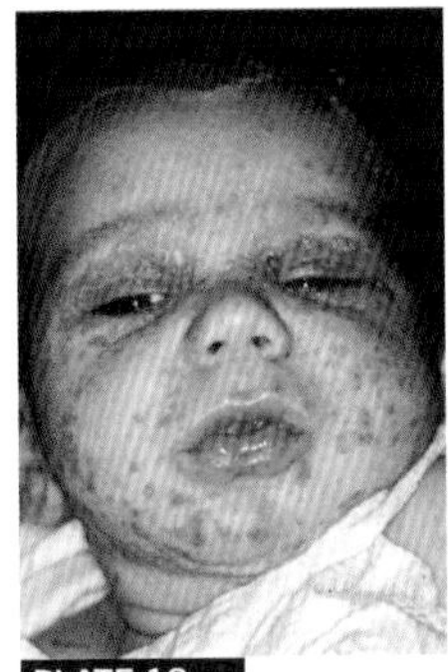

PLATE 18
Seborrheic dermatitis. *(From Cohen BA: Pediatric Dermatology, 2nd ed. St. Louis, Mosby, 1999.)*

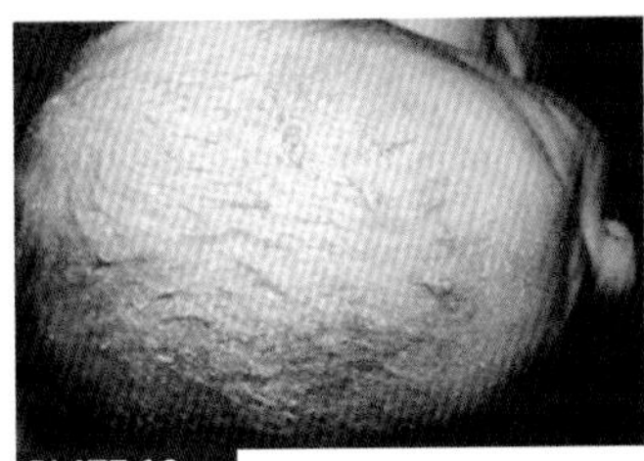

PLATE 19
Seborrheic dermatitis. *(From Cohen BA: Pediatric Dermatology, 2nd ed. St. Louis, Mosby, 1999.)*

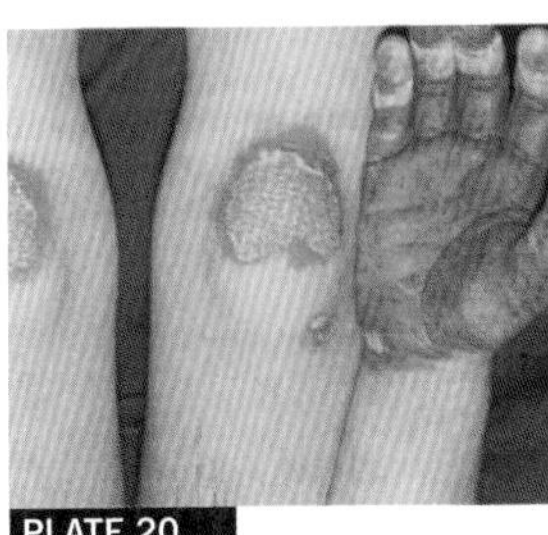

PLATE 20
Psoriasis. *(From Cohen BA: Atlas of Pediatric Dermatology. St. Louis, Mosby, 1993.)*

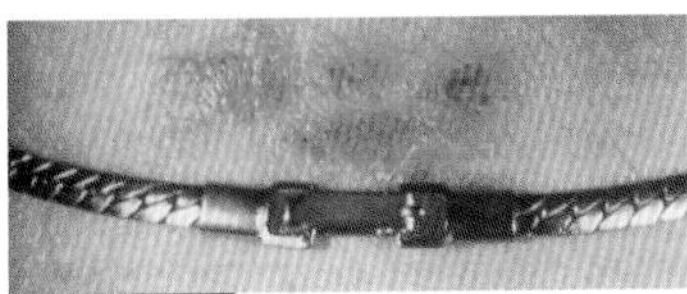

PLATE 21
Allergic contact dermatitis. *(From Cohen BA: Atlas of Pediatric Dermatology. St. Louis, Mosby, 1993.)*

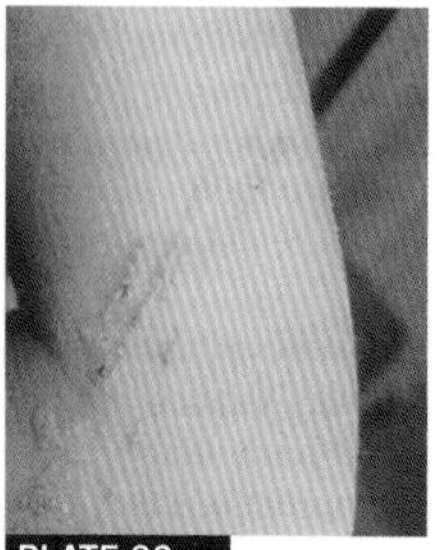

PLATE 22

Poison ivy. *(From Cohen BA: Atlas of Pediatric Dermatology. St. Louis, Mosby, 1993.)*

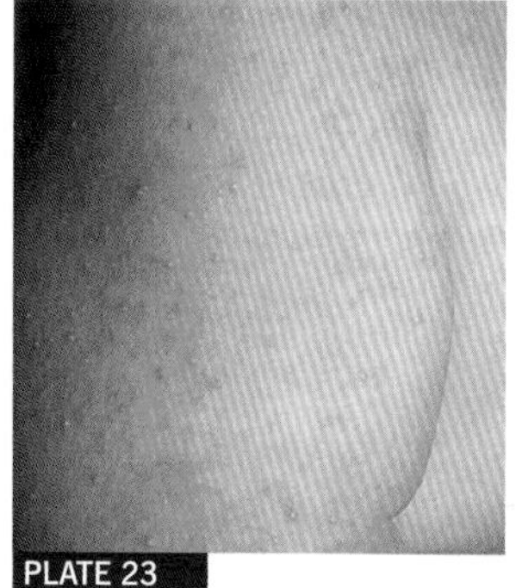

PLATE 23

Keratosis pilaris. *(From Cohen BA: Atlas of Pediatric Dermatology. St. Louis, Mosby, 1993.)*

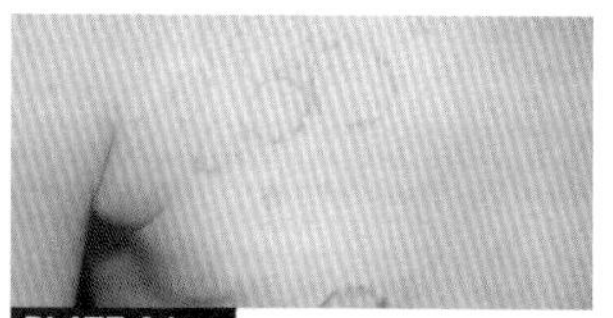

PLATE 24

Tinea corporis. *(From Cohen BA: Atlas of Pediatric Dermatology. St. Louis, Mosby, 1993.)*

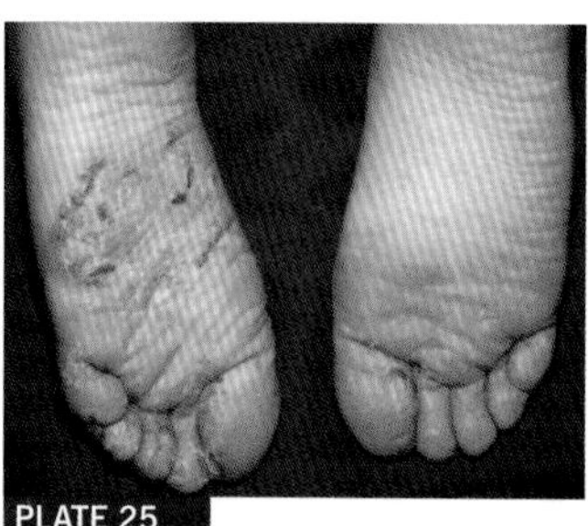

PLATE 25

Tinea pedis. *(From Cohen BA: www.med.jhu.edu/peds/dermatlas, 2001.)*

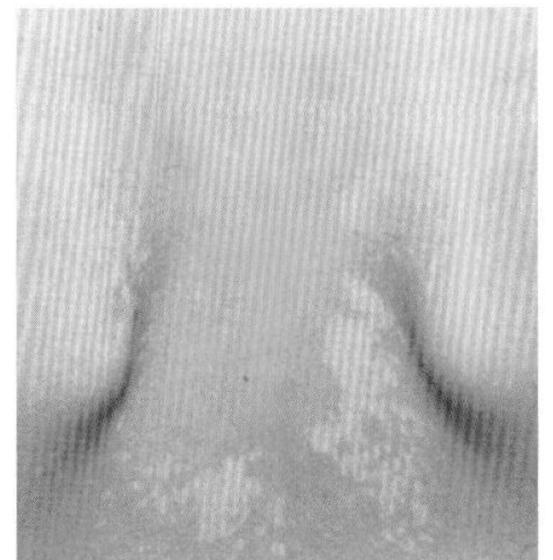

PLATE 26

Tinea versicolor. *(From Cohen BA: Atlas of Pediatric Dermatology. St. Louis, Mosby, 1993.)*

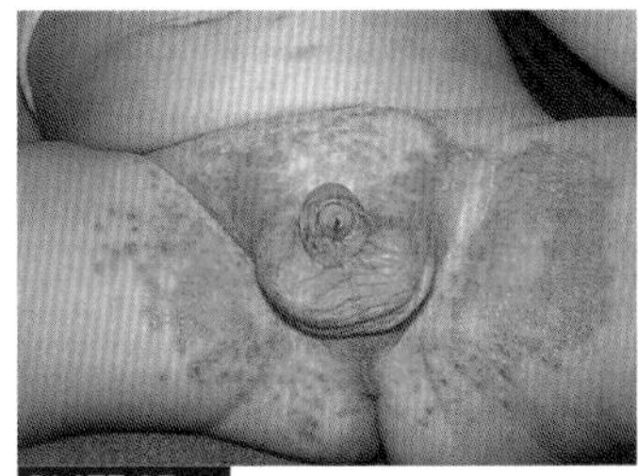

PLATE 27

Diaper candidiasis. *(From Cohen BA: Atlas of Pediatric Dermatology. St. Louis, Mosby, 1993.)*

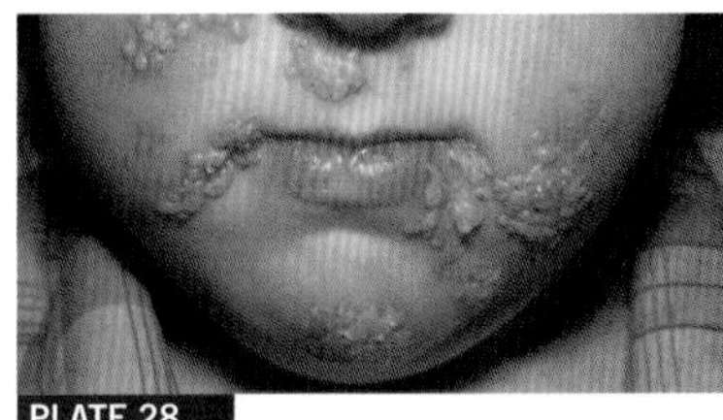

PLATE 28

Herpetic gingivostomatitis. *(From Cohen BA: Atlas of Pediatric Dermatology. St. Louis, Mosby, 1993.)*

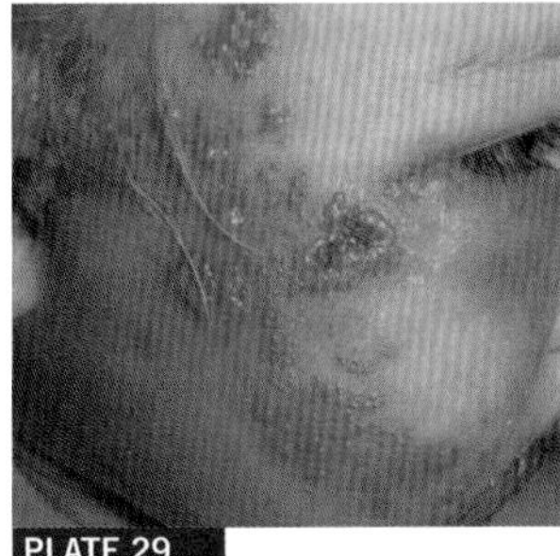

PLATE 29

Herpes zoster. *(From Cohen BA: Atlas of Pediatric Dermatology. St. Louis, Mosby, 1993.)*

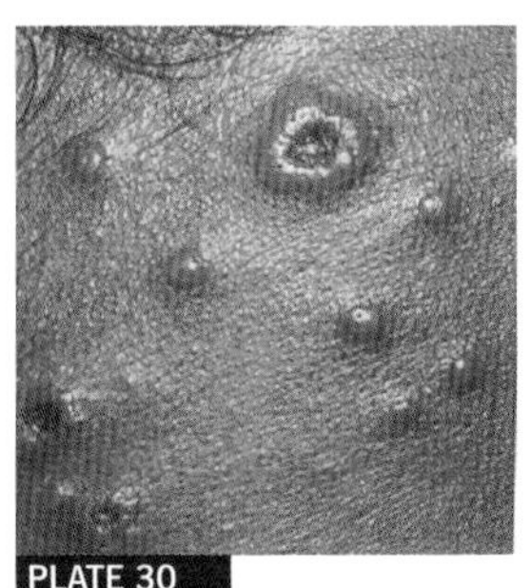

PLATE 30

Varicella. *(From Cohen BA: Atlas of Pediatric Dermatology. St. Louis, Mosby, 1993.)*

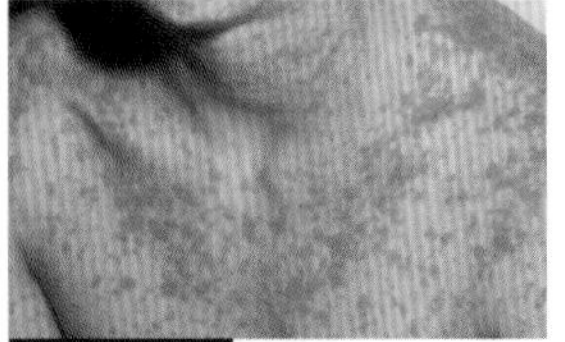

PLATE 31

Measles. *(From Cohen BA: Atlas of Pediatric Dermatology. St. Louis, Mosby, 1993.)*

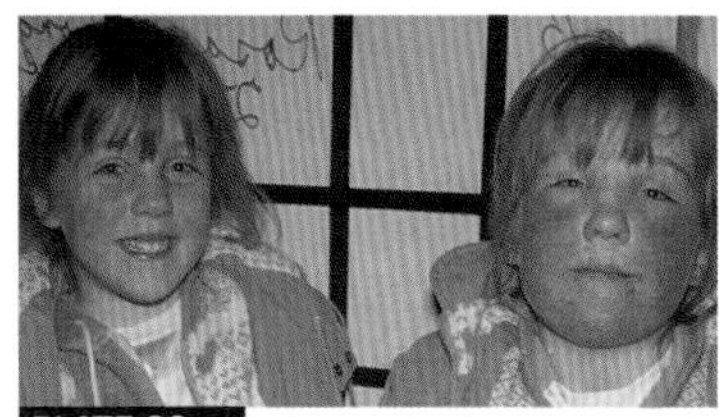

PLATE 32

Fifth disease. *(From Cohen BA: Atlas of Pediatric Dermatology. St. Louis, Mosby, 1993.)*

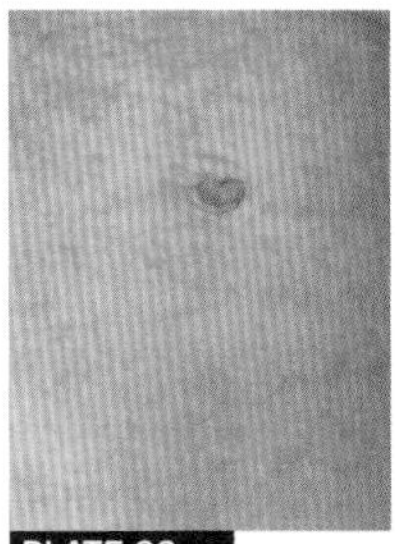

PLATE 33

Roseola. *(From Cohen BA: Atlas of Pediatric Dermatology. St. Louis, Mosby, 1993.)*

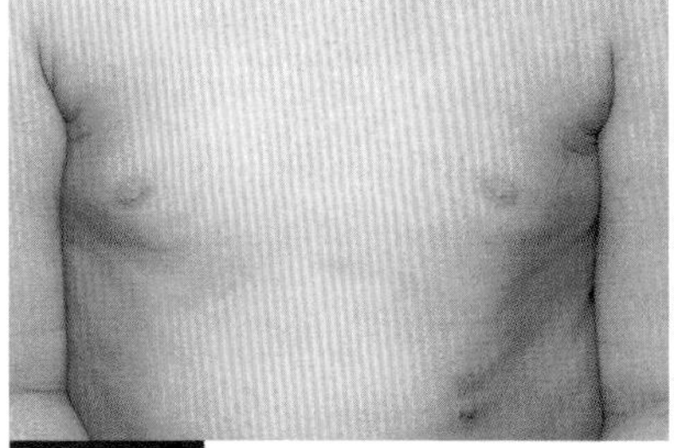

PLATE 34

Scarlet fever. *(From Cohen BA: Atlas of Pediatric Dermatology. St. Louis, Mosby, 1993.)*

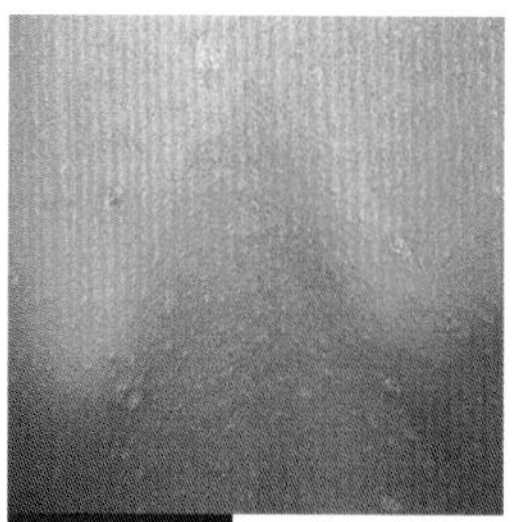

PLATE 35
Pityriasis rosea. *(From Cohen BA: Atlas of Pediatric Dermatology. St. Louis, Mosby, 1993.)*

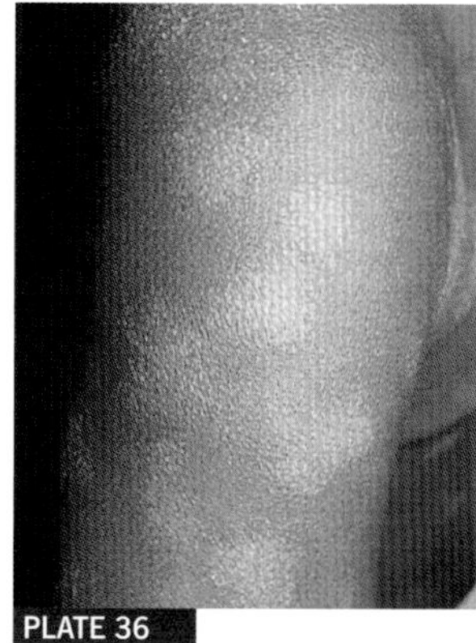

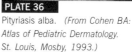

PLATE 36
Pityriasis alba. *(From Cohen BA: Atlas of Pediatric Dermatology. St. Louis, Mosby, 1993.)*

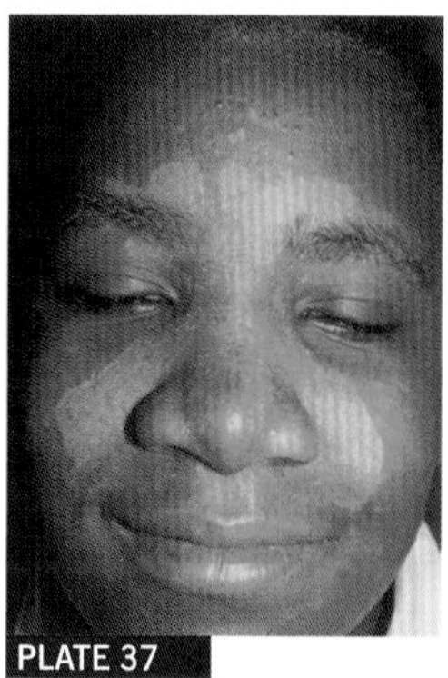

PLATE 37
Seborrheic dermatitis. *(From Cohen BA: Atlas of Pediatric Dermatology. St. Louis, Mosby, 1993.)*

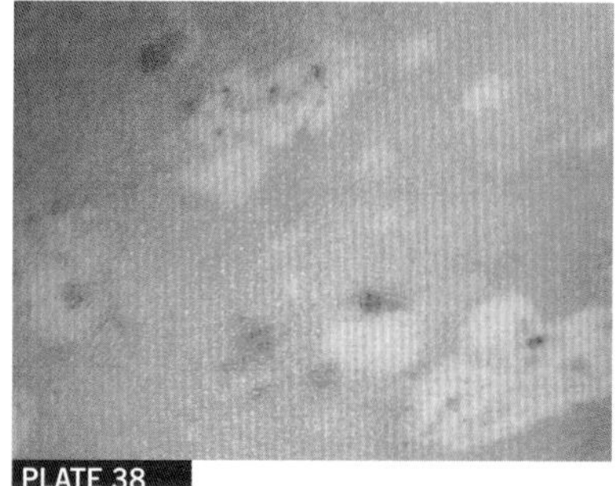

PLATE 38
Post-inflammatory hyperpigmentation. *(From Cohen BA: Atlas of Pediatric Dermatology. St. Louis, Mosby, 1993.)*

TABLE 7-3
ICHTHYOSES

Variant	Inheritance	Incidence	Clinical Feature	Onset	Histology	Molecular/biochemical Marker
Congenital ichthyosiform erythroderma	Autosomal recessive	1/100,000 to 1/50,000	Collodion baby Fine white scale on trunk, face, and scalp Large scale on legs Variable erythroderma Variable scarring, alopecia, nail dystrophy	Birth	$\Uparrow$ Stratum corneum $\Uparrow$ Granular layer	Accelerated epidermal turnover
Lamellar ichthyosis	Autosomal recessive	1/100,000	Collodion baby Generalized, large, dark, plate-like scale Ectropion, eclabium Mild palmar–plantar hyperkeratosis	Birth	$\Uparrow\Uparrow$ Stratum corneum	Normal epidermal turnover
Epidermolytic hyperkeratosis	Autosomal dominant (sporadic)	Rare	Widespread blisters at birth $\Uparrow$ Erythema, $\Uparrow$ scale with $\Uparrow$ age Marked scale in intertriginous areas, palms, soles Foul odor, bacterial overgrowth	Birth	Epidermocytic hyperkeratosis	Accelerated epidermal turnover Mutations in K1 or K10 keratin genes

TABLE 7-3
ICHTHYOSES—*cont'd*

Variant	Inheritance	Incidence	Clinical Feature	Onset	Histology	Molecular/biochemical Marker
Ichthyosis vulgaris	Autosomal dominant (variable expression)	1/250 (may be much higher)	Generalized mild scales Spares flexures Improves with age	After 3 mo	⇑ Stratum corneum ⇓ Granular layer	Normal epidermal turnover Defect in profilaggrin expression)
X-linked ichthyosis	X-linked recessive	1/6000 to 1/2000 males	Large "dirty" scales on trunk, extremities Spares flexures Variable in female carriers Corneal opacities on Descemet's membrane Cryptorchidism Placental sulfatase deficiency syndrome Contiguous gene syndromes	Within first 3 mo	⇑ Stratum corneum	⇓ Corticosteroid sulfatase in amniocytes, fibroblasts, leukocytes, keratinocytes Corticosteroid sulfatase gene defect

Data from Cohen BA: Pediatric Dermatology, 2nd ed. St. Louis, Mosby, 1999.

TABLE 7-4
ICHTHYOSIS SYNDROMES

Syndrome/Disease	Biochemical Marker	Associated Defects
Netherton syndrome		Hair shaft anomaly, ichthyosis linearis circumflexa
Refsum disease	⇓ Phytanic oxidase ⇑ Phytanic acid	Retinitis pigmentosa, chronic polyneuritis with deafness, flaccid paralysis, ataxia
Rud syndrome		Mental retardation, seizures, dwarfism, sexual infantilism
Sjögren = Larsson syndrome	⇓ Fatty alcohol oxidoreductase	Spastic paralysis, mental retardation, seizures, glistening dots on retina, dental–bone dysplasia
Conradi disease	Peroxisome deficiency, X linked	Chondrodysplasia punctata, alopecia, skeletal anomalies, cataracts, dysmorphic facies, ichthyosiform erythroderma
KID (keratitis, ichthyosis, deafness		Fixed keratotic plaques, keratoderma, atypical ichthyosis with prominent keratoses on extremities and head, neurosensory deafness, keratoconjunctivitis

Data from Cohen BA: Pediatric Dermatology, 2nd ed. St. Louis, Mosby, 1999.

E. NEONATAL ACNE

Often present at birth, these common (occurring in up to 20% of infants), open or closed comedones are thought to be triggered by maternal and endogenous androgens. No treatment is necessary because these lesions are self-limiting (Color Plate 15).

F. ICHTHYOSIS

This disease constitutes a group of scaling disorders consisting of five major variants: congenital ichthyosiform erythroderma, lamellar ichthyosis, epidermolytic hyperkeratosis, ichthyosis vulgaris, and X-linked ichthyosis (Table 7-3). There are also six separate ichthyotic syndromes of which these lesions are a feature (Table 7-4; Color Plates 16 and 17).

G. SEBORRHEIC DERMATITIS (CRADLE CAP)

This skin rash is characterized by a greasy yellow scale occurring most frequently in the scalp, diaper area, and intertriginous regions and may persist until 1 year of age. Affected areas may also have fissuring, weeping, and maceration, although these infants remain otherwise healthy and largely asymptomatic. Specific etiology is unknown. Treatment is unnecessary, though antiseborrheic shampoos (salicylic acid) as well as low-potency corticosteroids may shorten the course (Color Plates 18 and 19).

H. MONGOLIAN SPOTS

These skin macules, seen especially in Asian, black, and other dark-skin-toned infants, are common and are seen most often on the buttocks and legs. Resolution is spontaneous, usually within the first year of life.[13]

REFERENCES

1. Faranoff AA: Neonatal-Perinatal Medicine: Diseases of the Fetus and Infant, 7th ed. St. Louis, Mosby, 2002.
2. Drolet BA, Esterly NB, Frieden IJ: Hemangiomas and children. Primary Care 1999;3:173–181.
3. Cohen BA: Warts and children: Can they be separated? Contemp Pediatr 1997;2:128–149.
4. Gellia SE: Warts and molluscum contagiosum in children. Pediatr Ann 1987;1:69–76.
5. Rikkers SM, Holland GN, Drayton GE, et al: Topical tacrolimus treatment of atopic eyelid disease. Am J Ophthalmol 2003;135:297.
6. Boguniewicz M, Fiedler VC, Raimer S, et al, for the Pediatric Tacrolimus Study Group: A randomized, vehicle-controlled trial of tacrolimus ointment for treatment of atopic dermatitis in children. J Allergy Clin Immunol 1998;102:637.
7. Reitamo S, Van Leent EJ, Ho V, et al: Efficacy and safety of tacrolimus ointment compared with that of hydrocortisone acetate ointment in children with atopic dermatitis. J Allergy Clin Immunol 2002;109:539.
8. Cohen BA: Atopic dermatitis: Breaking the itch-scratch cycle. Contemp Pediatr 1992;7:64–81.

9. Mosby's Drug Consult. St. Louis, Mosby, 2004.
10. Leyden JJ: Therapy for acne vulgaris. N Engl J Med 1997;16:1156–1162.
11. Smith ML: Tinea capitis. Pediatr Ann 1996;25:101–105.
12. Cohen BA: Pediatric Dermatology, 2nd ed. London, Mosby, 1999.
13. Behrman RE: Nelson Textbook of Pediatrics, 17th ed. Philadelphia, Elsevier, 2003.
14. Wollenberg A, Sharma S, von Bubnoff D, et al: Topical tacrolimus (FK506) leads to profound phenotypic and functional alterations of epidermal antigen-presenting dendritic cells in atopic dermatitis. J Allergy Clin Immunol 2001;107:519.
15. Eichenfield LF, Lucky AW, Boguniewicz M, et al: Safety and efficacy of pimecrolimus (ASM 981) cream 1% in the treatment of mild and moderate atopic dermatitis in children and adolescents. J Am Acad Dermatol 2002;46:495.
16. Wahn U, Bos JD, Goodfield M, et al: Efficacy and safety of pimecrolimus cream in the long-term management of atopic dermatitis in children. Pediatrics 2002;110:e2.
17. Bhattacharya JJ, Luo CB, Alvarez H, et al: PHACES Syndrome: a review of eight previously unreported cases with late arterial occlusions. Neurobiology 2004;46:227–233.

Development and Behavior

Renay Walker Chung, MD

I. WEBSITES

www.chadd.org (ADHD)
www.dbpeds.org/handouts
www.disability.gov
www.ninds.nih.gov (cerebral palsy)
www.ldanatl.org (Learning Disabilities Association of America)
Arclink (MR)

II. INTRODUCTION

Developmental disabilities are a group of interrelated, nonprogressive, neurologic disorders occurring in childhood. This chapter focuses on screening and assessment of neurodevelopment to identify possible developmental disability.

A. DEVELOPMENT

Development can be divided into five major streams or skill areas: visual-motor, language (the cognitive streams), motor, social, and adaptive. Each stream has a spectrum of normal and abnormal presentation. Abnormal development in one stream increases the risk for deficit in another stream and should alert the examiner to consider a careful assessment of all streams. A developmental diagnosis is a functional description and classification that does not specify an etiology or medical diagnosis.

All of developmental assessment is based on the premise that milestone acquisition occurs at a specific rate and in a very orderly and sequential manner. When development is not progressing normally, the pattern of abnormal development usually includes delay, deviancy, or dissociation.

III. DEFINITIONS[1]

A. DEVELOPMENTAL QUOTIENT (DQ)

Developmental quotient is a calculation that reflects the rate of development in any given stream. The DQ represents the percentage of normal development present at the time of testing.

The developmental quotient (DQ) can be calculated for any given stream as follows:

$$DQ = (\text{developmental age/chronologic age}) \times 100$$

Two separate developmental assessments over time are more predictive than a single assessment.

B. DELAY

Delay is defined as performance significantly below average (DQ <75) in a given area of skill. Delay may occur in a single stream or several streams.

C. DEVIANCY

Deviancy is defined as atypical development within a single stream, such as developmental milestones occurring out of sequence. Deviancy does not necessarily imply abnormality but should alert one to the possibility that problems may exist. Examples: An infant who crawls before sitting, or an infant with early development of hand preference.

D. DISSOCIATION

Dissociation is defined as a substantial difference in the rate of development between two or more streams. Example: Cognitive-motor difference in some children with mental retardation or cerebral palsy.

IV. DISORDERS

A. MENTAL RETARDATION (MR)

MR is characterized by significantly below-average intellectual functioning (IQ <70–75) existing concurrently with related limitation in two or more of the following adaptive skill areas: communication, self-care, home living, social skills, community use, self-direction, health and safety, functional academics, leisure, and work (Table 8-1). MR manifests itself before age 18 years. Formal psychometric testing is needed to make the diagnosis of MR. Patients should be referred for diagnosis, review of potential etiology, and guidance if the DQ for any given stream is <70 or if there is significant learning difficulty.

B. COMMUNICATION DISORDERS

Communication disorders can be subdivided into expressive language disorders, mixed receptive-expressive language disorders, pragmatic language disorders, phonologic disorders, and stuttering. Developmental language disorders can be characterized by deficits of comprehension, interpretation, production, or use of language. Differential diagnosis includes hearing loss, specific language disability, expressive language disorder, mixed expressive-receptive language disorder, selective mutism, and autism (or another pervasive developmental disorder).

C. LEARNING DISABILITIES (LDs)

LDs are a heterogeneous group of disorders that manifest as significant difficulties in one or more of the following seven areas (as defined by the federal government): basic reading skills, reading comprehension, oral expression, listening comprehension, written expression, mathematical calculation, and mathematical reasoning. Specific learning disabilities are diagnosed when the individual's achievement on standardized tests in a given area is substantially below that expected for age, schooling, and level of intelligence.[2]

D. CEREBRAL PALSY (CP)

Cerebral palsy is a disorder of movement and posture resulting from a permanent, nonprogressive lesion of the immature brain. Manifestations,

TABLE 8-1
MENTAL RETARDATION

Level	IQ	Academic Potential	Daily Living	Work	Expected Mental Age as an Adult (yr)	Intensity of Support
Borderline	70–80	Educable to about the 6th grade	Fully independent	Employable; may need training to be competitive	—	Intermittent
Mild	50–69	Reading and writing to 4th–5th grade or less	Relatively independent with some training	Employable, often need training	9–11	Intermittent
Moderate	35–49	Limited reading to 1st or 2nd grade	Dress without help, use toilet, prepare food	Likely to need sheltered employment	5–8	Limited
Severe	20–34	Very unlikely to read or write	Can be toilet trained, dress with help, may be able to sign name	Sheltered employment	3–5	Extensive
Profound	<20	None	Occasionally can be toilet trained, dress with help, often nonverbal	Very limited	Below 3	Pervasive

From American Association on Mental Retardation. Mental retardation: definition, classification and systems of supports, 9th ed. Washington, DC: AAMR; 1992.

TABLE 8-2

CLINICAL CLASSIFICATION OF CEREBRAL PALSY

Type	Pattern of Involvement
I. SPASTIC (INCREASED TONE, CLASPED KNIFE, CLONUS, FURTHER CLASSIFIED BY DISTRIBUTION)	
Hemiplegia	Ipsilateral arm and leg; arm worse than leg
Diplegia	Legs primarily effected
Quadriplegia	All four extremities impaired; legs worse than arms
Double hemiplegia	All four extremities; arms notably worse than legs
Monoplegia	One extremity, usually upper; probably reflects a mild hemiplegia
Triplegia	One upper extremity and both lower; probably represents a hemiplegia plus a diplegia or incomplete quadriplegia
II. EXTRAPYRAMIDAL (LEAD PIPE OR CANDLE WAX RIGIDITY, VARIABLE TONE, +/– CLONUS)	
Choreoathetosis, rigidity, dystonia	Complex movement/tone disorders reflecting basal ganglia pathology
Ataxia, tremor	Movement and tone disorders reflecting cerebellar origin
Hypotonia	Usually related to diffuse, often severe, cerebral and/or cerebellar cortical damage

From Capute AJ, Accardo PJ (eds): Cerebral Palsy: Developmental Disabilities in Infancy and Childhood, 2nd ed. Baltimore, Paul H. Brookes, 1996.

however, may change with brain growth and development. A child with significant motor impairment can be identified at any age. The diagnosis of CP should be made before age 12 months; however, the mean age of diagnosis is 13 months. CP is classified in terms of physiologic and topographic characteristics as well as severity (Table 8-2). Classification of cerebral palsy is important because different classifications often have very different etiologies and associated deficits.

E. ATTENTION DEFICIT/HYPERACTIVITY DISORDER (ADHD) (Table 8-3)

ADHD is a neurobehavioral disorder characterized by inattention, distractibility, impulsivity, and hyperactivity, all behaviors that are more frequent and severe than typically observed in children of the same developmental age. Symptoms must persist for at least 6 months, occur before age 7 years, and be evident in two or more settings. The differential diagnosis is broad. Proper diagnosis, evaluation, and treatment are paramount to ensuring cognitive, academic, behavioral, emotional, and social function.

F. AUTISM SPECTRUM DISORDERS

The autism spectrum disorders include autism, Rett disorder, childhood disintegrative disorder, Asperger disorder, and pervasive developmental

TABLE 8-3

PHARMACOTHERAPY FOR ADHD*

Medication	Duration of Action	Side Effects
Methylphenidate (Ritalin, Methylin, Concerta)	8 hr	Anorexia, appetite disturbance, sleep disturbance, weight loss, headache, irritability, nervousness, decreased linear growth, transient tics in 15%–30% of population
Dextroamphetamine (Dexedrine)	5–6 hr	Same as above
Amphetamine-dextroamphetamine (Adderall)	8 hr	Same as above
Pemoline	12 hr	Hepatotoxicity, drug dependence, appetite disturbance, sleep disturbance, seizures, tics
Nonstimulant atomoxetine (Strattera)	5 hr (may vary as elimination is through CYP2D6)	Weight loss, abdominal pain, decreased appetite, nausea, vomiting, dyspepsia, headache, irritability, tachycardia

*See Formulary for dosage.

disorder, not otherwise specified (NOS). See the American Psychiatric Association's *Diagnostic and Statistical Manual of Mental Disorders*, 4th edition[3] (DSM-IV) for diagnostic criteria.

1. **Autism:** The essential features of autism are impaired social interaction and communication and a restricted group of activities and interests, with stereotyped behaviors, rituals, or mannerisms. Autism is also characterized by uneven skill development, often deficient in certain areas and normal to exaggerated in others. Onset of abnormal functioning occurs before age 3 years. Of note, 75% of autistic children function in the mentally retarded range. See DSM-IV for full diagnostic criteria.
2. **Rett disorder:** Characterized by normal development in the first 6 months of life and usually described in females. Affected individuals exhibit symptoms of autism, receptive and expressive language delay, psychomotor retardation, decreased head growth, breathing abnormalities, seizures, and poor coordination of gait and trunk movements.
3. **Asperger disorder:** Characterized by impairment in social interactions and restricted repetitive patterns of behavior. More common in boys. Those affected fail to develop peer relationships and display an i nability to express pleasure in the happiness of others. Otherwise, there is no general delay in language, cognition, or attainment of self-help skills.

4. Pervasive developmental disorder NOS.
5. Childhood disintegrative disorder.

V. MEDICAL EVALUATION OF DEVELOPMENTAL DISORDERS

A. HISTORY

A thorough past medical history should include assessment of risk.

1. **Prenatal and birth:** Toxins, trauma, prematurity, infection.
2. **Past medical problems or trauma:** Infection, medication.
3. **Developmental history:** Inquire about loss of skills and all streams.
4. **Behavioral history:** Social skills, eye contact, affection, hyperactivity, impulsivity, inattention, distractibility, perseveration, stereotypies, peculiar habits.
5. **Educational history:** Need for special services, retention, established educational plans.
   a. Services needed as a toddler.
   b. Review of report card.
6. **Family history of developmental problems, late talkers or walkers, trouble with education, ADHD, seizures, tics.**

B. PHYSICAL EXAMINATION

1. **General:** Height, weight, head circumference, cardiac murmurs, midline defects.
2. **Review for dysmorphic features.**
3. **Age-directed neurologic examination:** primitive reflexes, postural reactions (Tables 8-4 and 8-5).
   a. Neurologic examination in motor age equivalent younger than 1 year of age.
   b. Standard neurologic examination and soft signs in older children.

C. DEVELOPMENTAL TESTING

1. **Age-appropriate cognitive, learning, language, visual, motor, and behavioral evaluation** (Table 8-6).

D. INTERVENTION

1. **Liaison between family and school.**
2. **Advocate for and monitor appropriately.**
3. **Medical workup when indicated.**
4. **Medication intervention (especially in ADHD and autism).**

VI. DEVELOPMENTAL SCREENING AND EVALUATION

A. DEVELOPMENTAL MILESTONES (Table 8-7)

B. DENVER DEVELOPMENT ASSESSMENT (DENVER II) (see Foldout)

1. **The Denver II is a tool for screening the apparently normal child between the ages of 0 and 6 years;** its use is suggested at every

Text continues on p. 242

TABLE 8-4
POSTURAL REACTIONS

Postural Reaction	Age of Appearance	Description	Importance
Head righting	6 wk–3 mo	Lifts chin from tabletop in prone position	Necessary for adequate head control and sitting
Landau response	2–3 mo	Extension of head, then trunk and legs when held prone	Early measure of developing trunk control
Derotational righting	4–5 mo	Following passive or active head turning, the body rotates to following the direction of the head	Prerequisite to independent rolling
Anterior propping	4–5 mo	Arm extension anteriorly in supported sitting	Necessary for tripod sitting
Parachute	5–6 mo	Arm extension when falling	Facial protection when falling
Lateral propping	6–7 mo	Arm extension laterally in protective response	Allows independent sitting
Posterior propping	8–10 mo	Arm extension posteriorly	Allows pivoting in sitting

Modified from Milani-Comparetti A, Gidoni EA: Dev Med Child Neurol 1967;9:631; Capute AJ: Pediatr Ann 1986;15:217; Capute AJ, et al: Dev Med Child Neurol 1984;26:375; and Palmer FB, Capute AJ: Developmental disabilities. In Oski FA (ed): Principles and Practice of Pediatrics. Philadelphia, JB Lippincott, 1994.

TABLE 8-5
PRIMITIVE REFLEXES

Primitive Reflexes	Elicitation	Response	Timing
Moro reflex (MR, "embrace" response) of fingers, wrists, and elbows	*Supine*: Sudden neck extension; allow head to fall back about 3 cm	Extension, adduction, and then abduction of UEs, with semiflexion	Present at birth, disappears by 3–6 mo
Galant reflex (GR)	*Prone suspension*: Stroking paravertebral area from thoracic to sacral region	Produces truncal incurvature with concavity toward stimulated side	Present at birth, disappears by 2–6 mo
Asymmetric tonic neck reflex (ATNR, "fencer" response)	*Supine*: Rotate head laterally about 45–90 degrees	Relative extension of limbs on chin side and flexion on occiput side	Present at birth, disappears by 4–9 mo
Symmetric tonic neck reflex (STNR, "cat" reflex)	*Sitting*: Head extension/flexion	Extension of UEs and flexion of LEs/flexion of UEs and LE extension	Appear at 5 mo; not present in most normal children; disappears by 8–9 mo
Tonic labyrinthine supine (TLS)	*Supine*: Extension of the neck (alters relation of the labyrinths)	Tonic extension of trunk and LEs, shoulder retraction and adduction, usually with elbow flexion	Present at birth, disappears by 6–9 mo
Tonic labyrinthine prone (TLP)	*Prone*: Flexion of the neck	Active flexion of trunk with protraction of shoulders	Present at birth, disappears by 6–9 mo

Positive support reflex (PSR)	Vertical suspension; bouncing hallucal areas on firm surface	*Neonatal*: Momentary LE extension followed by flexion	Present at birth; disappears by 2–4 mo
		Mature: Extension of LEs and support of body weight	Appears by 6 mo
Stepping reflex (SR, walking reflex)	Vertical suspension; hallucal stimulation	Stepping gait	Disappears by 2–3 mo
Crossed extension reflex (CER)	Prone; hallucal stimulation of an LE in full extension	Initial flexion, adduction, then extension of contralateral limb	Present at birth; disappears by 9 mo
Plantar grasp	Stimulation of hallucal areas	Plantar flexion grasp	Present at birth; disappears by 9 mo
Palmar grasp	Stimulation of palm	Palmar grasp	Present at birth; disappears by 9 mo
Lower extremity placing (LEP)	Vertical suspension; rubbing tibia or dorsum of foot against edge of tabletop	Initial flexion, then extension, then placing of LE on tabletop	Appears at 1 day
Upper extremity placing (UEP)	Rubbing lateral surface of forearm along edge of tabletop from elbow to wrist to dorsal hand	Flexion, extension, then placing of hand on tabletop	Appears at 3 mo
Downward thrust (DT)	Vertical suspension; thrust LEs downward	Full extension of LEs	Appears at 3 mo

UE, Upper extremity; LE, lower extremity.

TABLE 8-6

AGE-APPROPRIATE BEHAVIORAL ISSUES IN INFANCY AND EARLY CHILDHOOD

Age	Behavioral Issue	Symptoms	Guidance
1–3 mo	Colic	Paroxysms of fussiness/crying, 3+ hours per day, 3+ days per week, may pull knees up to chest, pass flatus	Crying usually peaks at 6 weeks and resolves by 3–4 months. Prevent overstimulation; swaddle infant; use white noise, swing, or car rides to soothe. Avoid medication and formula changes. Encourage breaks for the primary caregiver.
3–4 mo	Trained night feeding	Night awakening	Comfort quietly, avoid reinforcing behavior (i.e., avoid night feeds). Do not play at night. Introducing cereal or solid food does not reduce awakening. Develop a consistent bedtime routine. Place baby in bed while drowsy and not fully asleep.
9 mo	Stranger anxiety/ separation anxiety	Distress when separated from parent or approached by a stranger	Use a transitional object, such as a special toy or blanket; use routine or ritual to separate from parent; may continue until 24 months but can reduce intensity.
	Developmental night waking	Separation anxiety at night	Keep lights off. Avoid picking child up or feeding. May reassure verbally at regular intervals or place a transitional object in crib.
12 mo	Aggression	Biting, hitting, kicking in frustration	Say "no" with negative facial cues. Begin time out (1 min/yr of age). No eye contact or interaction, place in a nonstimulating location. May restrain child gently until cooperation is achieved.
	Need for limit setting	Exploration of environment, danger of injury	Avoid punishing exploration or poor judgment. Emphasize child-proofing and distraction.
18 mo	Temper tantrums	Occur with frustration, attention-seeking rage, negativity/refusal	Try to determine cause and react appropriately (i.e., help child who is frustrated, ignore attention-seeking behavior). Make sure child is in a safe location.

24 mo	Toilet training	*Child needs to demonstrate readiness*: shows interest, neurologic maturity (i.e., recognizes urge to urinate or defecate), ability to walk to bathroom and undress self, desire to please/imitate parents, increasing periods of daytime dryness.	Age range for toilet training is usually 2 to 4 yr. Give guidance early; may introduce potty seat but avoid pressure or punishment for accidents. Wait until the child is ready. Expect some periods of regression, especially with stressors.
24–36 mo	New sibling	Regression, aggressive behavior	Allow for special time with parent, 10–20 min daily of one-on-one time exclusively devoted to the older sibling(s). Child chooses activity with parent. No interruptions. May not be taken away as punishment.
36 mo	Nightmare	Awakens crying, may or may not complain of bad dream	Reassure child, explain that they had a bad dream. Leave bedroom door open, use a nightlight, demonstrate there are no monsters under the bed. Discuss dream the following day. Avoid scary movies or television shows.
	Night terrors	Agitation, screaming 1–2 hr after going to bed. Child may have eyes open but not respond to parent. May occur at same time each night.	May be familial, not volitional. *Prevention*: For several nights, awaken child 15 min before terrors occur. Avoid over-tiredness. *Acute*: Be calm, speak in soft, soothing, repetitive tones, help child return to sleep. Protect child against injury.

From Dixon SD, Stein MT: Encounters with children: Pediatric behavior and development. St. Louis, Mosby, 2000; Schmitt BD: Instructions for Pediatric Patients, 2nd ed. Philadelphia, WB Saunders, 1999; and Howard BJ: Audio Digest Pediatrics 2000;46(2).

TABLE 8-7

DEVELOPMENTAL MILESTONES

Age	Gross Motor	Visual-Motor/Problem Solving
1 mo	Raises head from prone position	*Birth*: Visually fixes *1 mo*: Has tight grasp, follows to midline
2 mo	Holds head in midline, lifts chest off table	No longer clenches fists tightly, follows object past midline
3 mo	Supports on forearms in prone position, holds head up steadily	Holds hands open at rest, follows in circular fashion, responds to visual threat
4 mo	Rolls over, supports on wrists, and shifts weight	Reaches with arms in unison, brings hands to midline
6 mo	Sits unsupported, puts feet in mouth in supine position	Unilateral reach, uses raking grasp, transfers objects
9 mo	Pivots when sitting, crawls well, pulls to stand, cruises	Uses immature pincer grasp, probes with forefinger, holds bottle, throws objects
12 mo	Walks alone	Uses mature pincer grasp, can make a crayon mark, releases voluntarily
15 mo	Creeps up stairs, walks backwards independently	Scribbles in imitation, builds tower of two blocks in imitation
18 mo	Runs, throws objects from standing without falling	Scribbles spontaneously, builds tower of 3 blocks, turns 2–3 pages at a time
24 mo	Walks up and down steps without help	Imitates stroke with pencil, builds tower of 7 blocks, turns pages one at a time, removes shoes, pants, etc.
3 yr	Can alternate feet when going up steps, pedals tricycle	Copies a circle, undresses completely, dresses partially, dries hands if reminded, unbuttons
4 yr	Hops, skips, alternates feet going down steps	Copies a square, buttons clothing, dresses self completely, catches ball
5 yr	Skips alternating feet, jumps over low obstacles	Copies triangle, ties shoes, spreads with knife

From Capute AJ, Biehl RF: Pediatr Clin North Am 1973;20:3; Capute AJ, Accardo PJ: Clin Pediatr 1978;17:847; and Capute AJ, et al: Am J Dis Child 1986;140:694. Rounded norms from Capute AJ, et al: Dev Med Child Neurol 1986;28:762.

well-child visit. This screen allows the practitioner to identify those children who may have developmental delay. These children should be further evaluated for the purpose of definitive diagnosis. The test screens the child in four areas: personal-social, fine motor, gross motor, and language.

2. **Age calculation:** For children born before 38 weeks' gestation, age should be corrected for prematurity, up to 2 years of age.

Language	Social/Adaptive
Alerts to sound	Regards face
Smiles socially (after being stroked or talked to)	Recognizes parent
Coos (produces long vowel sounds in musical fashion)	Reaches for familiar people or objects, anticipates feeding
Laughs, orients to voice	Enjoys looking around
Babbles, ah-goo, razz, lateral orientation to bell	Recognizes that someone is a stranger
Says "mama, dada" indiscriminately, gestures, waves bye-bye, understands "no"	Starts exploring environment, plays gesture games (e.g., pat-a-cake)
Uses two words other than mama/dada or proper nouns, jargoning (runs several unintelligible words together with tone or inflection), one-step command with gesture	Imitates actions, comes when called, cooperates with dressing
Uses 4–6 words, follows one-step command without gesture	*15–18 mo*: Uses spoon and cup
Mature jargoning (includes intelligible words), 7–10 word vocabulary, knows 5 body parts	Copies parent in tasks (sweeping, dusting), plays in company of other children
Uses pronouns (I, you, me) inappropriately, follows two-step commands, has a 50-word vocabulary, uses two-word sentences	Parallel play
Uses minimum of 250 words, 3-word sentences, uses plurals, knows all pronouns, repeats two digits	Group play, shares toys, takes turns, plays well with others, knows full name, age, gender
Knows colors, says song or poem from memory, asks questions	Tells "tall tales," plays cooperatively with a group of children
Prints first name, asks what a word means	Plays competitive games, abides by rules, likes to help in household tasks

3. **Scoring:** Note that items that can be passed by report of caregiver are denoted with a letter R. Each item that intersects or is just adjacent to the age line should be scored. Items should be scored as pass, fail, no opportunity, or refused to cooperate. Assess each item as follows:

a. Advanced: Child passes item that falls completely to the right of age line.

b. Normal: Child passes, fails, or refuses item on which the age line falls between the 25th and 75th percentiles.
c. Caution: Child fails or refuses item on which the age line falls between the 75th and 90th percentiles.
d. Delayed: Child fails or refuses item that falls completely to the left of age line.

4. **Assessment:** A child fails a Denver screen if he or she has two or more delays noted. Re-evaluate the child in 3 months if there is one delay and/or two or more cautions. A child passes the screen with no delays and a maximum of one caution. Additionally, some children may be termed untestable if there are a significant number of refusals or no opportunity test items. Indications for referral are a failed test or a classification of untestable on two consecutive screenings.

C. CAT/CLAMS (CAPUTE SCALES) (TABLE 8-8)

1. **The Capute Scales are an assessment tool that gives quantitative developmental quotients for visual-motor/problem-solving and language abilities.** The CLAMS (Clinical Linguistic and Auditory Milestone Scale) was developed for the assessment of language milestones from birth to 36 months of age. The CAT (Clinical Adaptive Test) consists of problem-solving items for ages from birth to 36 months, adapted from standardized infant psychological tests.
2. **Scoring:** Scoring is done by calculating the basal age as the highest age group in which a child accomplishes all of the test tasks correctly. The age equivalent is then determined by adding the decimal number (recorded in parentheses) next to each correctly scored item passed at age groups beyond the basal age to the basal age itself. Each of these age equivalents (language and visual motor) is then divided by the child's chronologic age and multiplied by 100 to determine a developmental quotient. Again, DQ <70 constitutes delay and warrants referral.

D. EVALUATION OF VISUAL-MOTOR AND PROBLEM-SOLVING SKILLS

For these tests, it is important to observe how they are done and to evaluate the final product.

1. **Goodenough-Harris Draw-a-Person Test**

a. Procedure: Give the child a pencil and a sheet of blank paper. Instruct the child to "draw a person; draw the best person you can." Supply encouragement if needed (e.g., "draw a whole person"); however, do not suggest specific supplementation or changes.
b. Scoring: Ask the child to describe or explain the drawing to you. Give the child one point for each detail present using the guide in Box 8-1 (maximum score: 51) and compare to norms for age.

TABLE 8-8
CLAMS/CAT*

Age (mo)	CLAMS	Yes	No	CAT	Yes	No
1	1. Alerts to sound (0.5)[†]	—	—	1. Visually fixates momentarily upon red ring (0.5)	—	—
	2. Soothes when picked up (0.5)	—	—	2. Chin off table in prone position (0.5)	—	—
2	1. Social smile (1.0)[†]	—	—	1. Visually follows ring horizontally and vertically (0.5)	—	—
		—	—	2. Chest off table prone (0.5)	—	—
3	1. Cooing (1.0)	—	—	1. Visually follows ring in circle (0.3)	—	—
				2. Supports on forearms in prone position (0.3)	—	—
				3. Visual threat (0.3)	—	—
4	1. Orients to voice (0.5)[†]	—	—	1. Unfisted (0.3)	—	—
	2. Laughs aloud (0.5)	—	—	2. Manipulates fingers (0.3)	—	—
		—	—	3. Supports on wrists in prone position (0.3)	—	—
5	1. Orients toward bell laterally (0.3)[†]	—	—	1. Pulls down rings (0.3)	—	—
	2. Ah-goo (0.3)	—	—	2. Transfers (0.3)	—	—
	3. Razzing (0.3)	—	—	3. Regards pellet (0.3)	—	—
6	1. Babbling (1.0)	—	—	1. Obtains cube (0.3)	—	—
				2. Lifts cup (0.3)	—	—
				3. Radial rake (0.3)	—	—

(continued)

TABLE 8-8

CLAMS/CAT*—*cont'd*

Age (mo)	CLAMS	Yes	No	CAT	Yes	No
7	1. Orients toward bell (1.0)[†] (upwardly/indirectly 90°)	—	—	1. Attempts pellet (0.3)	—	—
				2. Pulls out peg (0.3)	—	—
				3. Inspects ring (0.3)	—	—
8	1. Says "dada" inappropriately (0.5)	—	—	1. Pulls on ring by string (0.3)	—	—
	2. Says "mama" inappropriately (0.5)	—	—	2. Secures pellet (0.3)	—	—
				3. Inspects bell (0.3)	—	—
9	1. Orients toward bell (upward directly 180°) (0.5)[†]	—	—	1. Three-finger scissor grasp (0.3)	—	—
	2. Gesture language (0.5)	—	—	2. Rings bell (0.3)	—	—
				3. Over the edge for toy (0.3)	—	—
10	1. Understands "no" (0.3)	—	—	1. Combine cube-cup (0.3)	—	—
	2. Uses "dada" appropriately (0.3)	—	—	2. Uncovers bell (0.3)	—	—
	3. Uses "mama" appropriately (0.3)	—	—	3. Fingers pegboard (0.3)	—	—
11	1. One word (other than "mama" and "dada" (1.0)	—	—	1. Mature overhand pincer movement (0.5)	—	—
				2. Solves cube under cup (0.5)	—	—
12	1. One-step command with gesture (0.5)	—	—	1. Release one cube in cup (0.5)	—	—
	2. Two-word vocabulary (0.5)	—	—	2. Makes crayon mark (0.5)	—	—
14	1. Three-word vocabulary (1.0)	—	—	1. Solves glass frustration (0.6)	—	—
	2. Immature jargoning (1.0)	—	—	2. Out-in with peg (0.6)	—	—
				3. Solves pellet-bottle with demonstration (0.6)	—	—
16	1. Four- to six-word vocabulary (1.0)	—	—	1. Solves pellet-bottle spontaneously (0.6)	—	—
	2. One-step command without gesture (1.0)	—	—	2. Round block on form board (0.6)	—	—
				3. Scribbles in imitation (0.6)	—	—

18	1. Mature jargoning (0.5)	—	—	1. 10 cubes in cup (0.5)	—	—
	2. 7–10 word vocabulary (0.5)	—	—	2. Solves round hole in form board reversed (0.5)	—	—
	3. Points to one picture (0.5)†	—	—	3. Spontaneous scribbling with crayon (0.5)	—	—
	4. Knows body parts (0.5)	—	—	4. Pegboard completed spontaneously (0.5)	—	—
21	1. 20–word vocabulary (1.0)	—	—	1. Obtains object with stick (1.0)	—	—
	2. Two-word phrases (1.0)	—	—	2. Solves square in form board (1.0)	—	—
	3. Points to two pictures (1.0)†	—	—	3. Tower of three cubes (1.0)	—	—
24	1. 50–word vocabulary (1.0)	—	—	1. Attempts to fold paper (0.7)	—	—
	2. Two-step command (1.0)	—	—	2. Horizontal four-cube train (0.7)	—	—
	3. Two-word sentences (1.0)	—	—	3. Imitates stroke with pencil (0.7)	—	—
				4. Completes form board (0.7)	—	—
30	1. Uses pronouns appropriately (1.5)	—	—	1. Horizontal-vertical stroke with pencil (1.5)	—	—
	2. Concept of one (1.5)†	—	—	2. Form board reversed (1.5)	—	—
	3. Points to 7 pictures (1.5)†	—	—	3. Folds paper with definite crease (1.5)	—	—
	4. Two digits forward (1.5)†	—	—	4. Train with chimney (1.5)	—	—
36	1. 250–word vocabulary (1.5)	—	—	1. Three-cube bridge (1.5)	—	—
	2. Three-word sentence (1.5)	—	—	2. Draws circle (1.5)	—	—
	3. Three digits forward (1.5)†	—	—	3. Names one color (1.5)	—	—
	4. Follows two prepositional commands (1.5)†	—	—	4. Draws a person with head plus one other part of body (1.5)	—	—

*See p. 244 for instructions.

†Indicates CLAMS item that must be demonstrated for examiner to receive credit.

BOX 8-1

GOODENOUGH-HARRIS SCORING

General:	☐ Head Present ☐ Legs present ☐ Arms present
Trunk:	☐ Present ☐ Length greater than breadth ☐ Shoulders
Arms/legs:	☐ Attached to trunk ☐ At correct point
Neck:	☐ Present ☐ Outline of neck continuous with head, trunk, or both
Face:	☐ Eyes ☐ Nose ☐ Mouth ☐ Nose and mouth in two dimensions ☐ Nostrils
Hair:	☐ Present ☐ On more than circumference; nontransparent
Clothing:	☐ Present ☐ Two articles; nontransparent ☐ Entire drawing (sleeves and trousers) nontransparent ☐ Four articles ☐ Costume complete
Fingers:	☐ Present ☐ Correct number ☐ Two dimensions; length, breadth ☐ Thumb opposition ☐ Hand distinct from fingers and arm
Joints:	☐ Elbow, shoulder, or both ☐ Knee, hip, or both
Proportion:	☐ *Head*: 10% to 50% of trunk area ☐ *Arms*: Approximately same length as trunk ☐ *Legs:* 1–2 times trunk length; width less than trunk width ☐ *Feet*: To leg length ☐ Arms and legs in two dimensions ☐ Heel
Motor coordination:	☐ Lines firm and well connected ☐ Firmly drawn with correct joining ☐ Head outline ☐ Trunk outline ☐ Outline of arms and legs ☐ Features
Ears:	☐ Present ☐ Correct position and proportion
Eye detail:	☐ Brow or lashes ☐ Pupil ☐ Proportion ☐ Glance directed front in profile drawing
Chin:	☐ Present; forehead ☐ Projection
Profile:	☐ Not more than one error ☐ Correct

TABLE 8-9

GOODENOUGH AGE NORMS

Age (yr)	3	4	5	6	7	8	9	10	11	12	13
Points	2	6	10	14	18	22	26	30	34	38	42

From Taylor E. Psychological appraisal of children with cerebral defects. Boston: Harvard University; 1961.

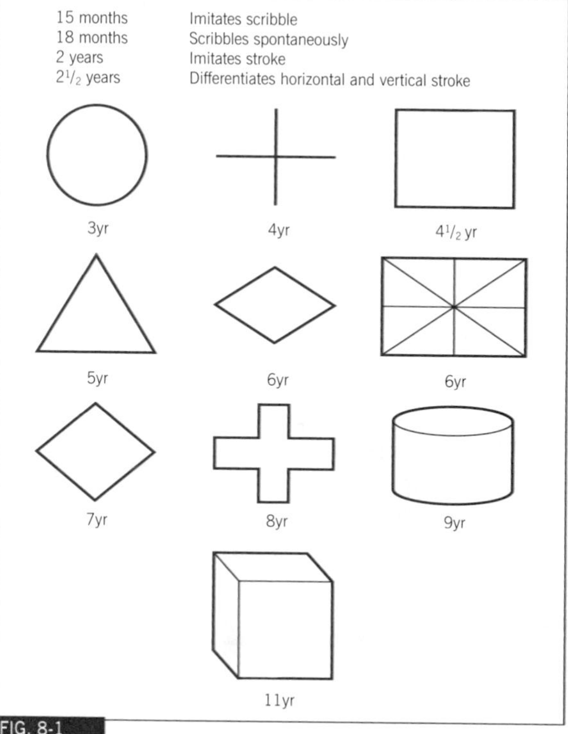

FIG. 8-1

Gesell figures. *(From Illingsworth RS: The development of the infant and young child, normal and abnormal, 5th ed. Baltimore, Williams & Wilkins, 1972; Cattel P: The measurement of intelligence of infants and young children. New York, The Psychological Corporation, 1960.)*

2. **Gesell figures (Fig. 8-1):** When using Gesell figures, the examiner is not supposed to demonstrate the drawing of the figures for the patient.
3. **Gesell block skills:** The structures in Figure 8-2 should be demonstrated for the child. Figure 8-2 includes the developmental age at which each structure can usually be accomplished.

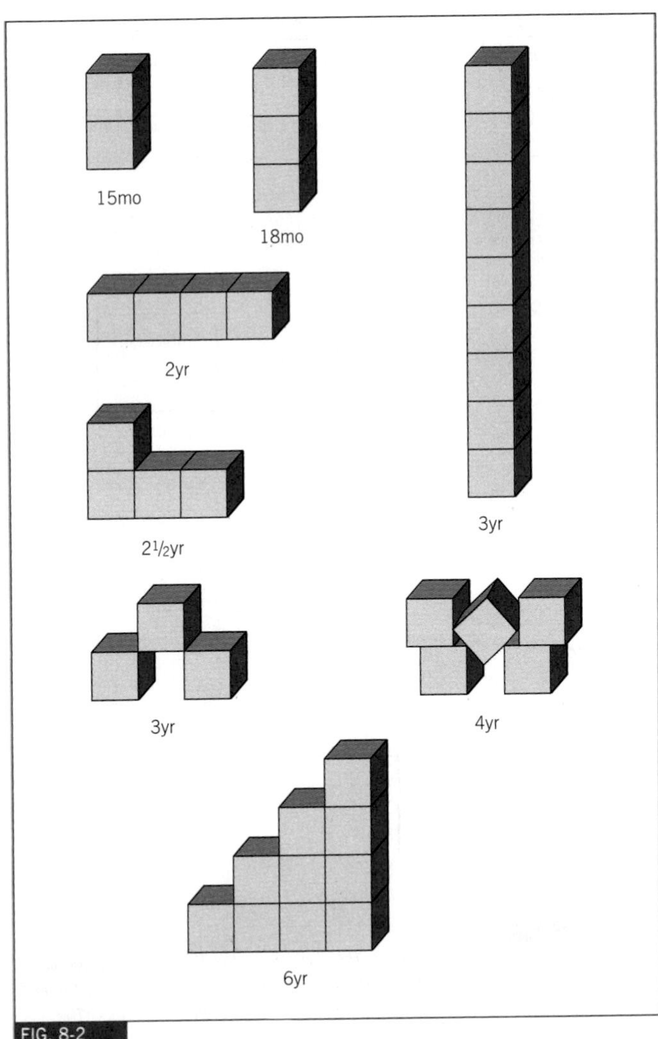

FIG. 8-2

Block skills. *(From Capute AJ, Accardo PJ: The pediatrician and the developmentally disabled child: A clinical textbook on mental retardation. Baltimore, University Press, 1979.)*

TABLE 8-10
APPROPRIATE SCREENING IN EACH DEVELOPMENTAL STREAM BY AGE*

Age	Cognitive		Motor	Behavior
	Visual Motor	Language		
Infants and toddlers	CAT, Denver II	CLAMS, Denver II	Milestones, Denver II, neurologic examination, primitive reflexes	Temperament, social skills, activity level, Denver II
Preschool age	Draw-a-person, Gesell figures, block skills, Denver II	Articulation, comprehension (example: following commands), expression (example: estimate of vocabulary), Denver II	Milestones, neurologic examination, Denver II	Child behavior checklist, ADHD checklist, Denver II
School age	Draw-a-person, Gesell figures, handwriting	Reading, decoding comprehension, listening, written language	Coordination, neurologic examination, soft neurologic signs	Child behavior checklist, ADHD checklist

*If significant delays are noted, referral to a developmental pediatrician or psychologist is indicated.

E. DEVELOPMENTAL SCREENING

1. **Appropriate screening tests vary with age (Table 8-9).** Significant delays on screening merit referral for formal testing.
2. **In assessing for delay, an individual DQ can be calculated for any given developmental stream;** if the quotient is <70%, a diagnosis of delay can be made and warrants further evaluation or referral. For example, a 13-month-old child who does not yet walk alone but is able to walk when led with two hands held (i.e., a 10-month level of motor development) has a DQ of 10/13 = 77% and is not considered delayed.

REFERENCES

1. Capute AJ, Shapiro BK, Palmer FB: Spectrum of developmental disabilities: Continuum of motor dysfunction. Orthop Clin North Am 1981;12:15–21.
2. Shapiro BK, Gallico RP: Learning disabilities. Pediatr Clin North Am 1993;40: 491–505.
3. American Psychiatric Association: Diagnostic and Statistical Manual of Mental Disorders, 4th ed. Washington, DC, The Association, 1994.
4. Capute AJ, Accardo PJ (eds): Cerebral palsy: Developmental disabilities in infancy and childhood, 2nd ed, vol 2. Baltimore, Paul H Brookes, 1996.
5. Strattera Package Insert, Eli Lilly and Company, November 2002.

Endocrinology

David Salikof, MD

9

I. DIABETES

A. DIABETIC KETOACIDOSIS

Diabetic ketoacidosis (DKA) is defined by hyperglycemia, ketonemia, ketonuria, and metabolic acidosis (pH <7.30, bicarbonate <15 mEq/L).

1. **Assessment**

a. History: In a *known* diabetic child, determine the usual insulin regimen, last dose, history of infection, or inciting event. In a *suspected* diabetic child, determine whether there is a history of polydipsia, polyuria, polyphagia, weight loss, vomiting, or abdominal pain.

b. Examination: Assess for dehydration, Kussmaul respirations, fruity breath, a change in mental status, and current weight.

c. Laboratory tests: See Figure 9-1 for a management algorithm. In addition, consider assessing the hemoglobin A1c level in a known diabetic as an index of chronic hyperglycemia (normal values are 4.5% to 6.1%); in a new-onset diabetic, consider islet cell antibodies, insulin antibodies, thyroid antibodies, and thyroid function tests.

2. **Management:** See Figures 9-1 and 9-2. Because the fluid and electrolyte requirements of patients in DKA may vary greatly, the following guidelines should be taken as a starting point for therapy that must be individualized based on the dynamics of the patient. Cerebral edema is the most important complication of DKA; overaggressive hydration and overly rapid correction of hyperglycemia should be avoided because they may play a role in its development. Remember that pH is a good indicator of insulin deficiency, and if acidosis is not resolving, the patient may need more insulin, whereas the degree of hyperglycemia is often a reflection of hydration status. Be cautious because initial insulin administration will cause a transient worsening of acidosis as potassium is driven into the cells in exchange for hydrogen ions.

B. DIAGNOSTIC CRITERIA

Under the American Diabetes Association guidelines,[1] one of three criteria must be met to make the diagnosis of diabetes mellitus:

Symptoms of diabetes (polyuria, polydipsia, and weight loss) *and*

A random blood glucose ≥200 mg/dL *or*

A fasting blood glucose (no caloric intake for at least 8 hours) ≥126 mg/dL *or*

An oral glucose tolerance test (OGTT) with a 2-hour postload blood glucose of ≥200 mg/dL (See section VI.A. for more information on OGTT.)

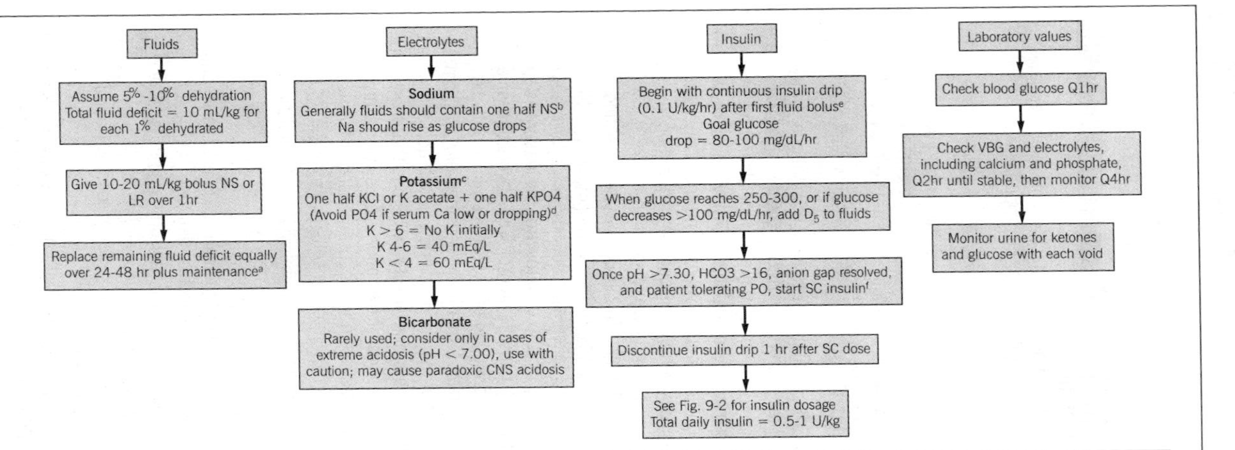

[a]If urine output is high, include in maintenance until osmotic diuresis slows; therefore maintenance = urine output + insensible losses (one third of standard maintenance calculations).
[b]Some DKA protocols recommend using NS rather than half NS during part of the replacement period in an effort to further decrease risk of cerebral edema.
[c]Patients with DKA are total body K^+ depleted and are at risk for severe hypokalemia during DKA therapy. However, serum K^+ levels may be normal or elevated as a result of the shift of K^+ to the extracellular compartment in the setting of acidosis.
[d]Phosphate is depleted in DKA and will drop further with insulin therapy. Consider replacing half of K as KPO4 for first 8hr, then all as KCl. Excessive phosphate may induce hypocalcemic tetany.
[e]Lower dose insulin infusions can be considered in very young patients.
[f]Some protocols recommend also waiting for urine ketones to decrease or clear before starting SC insulin.

FIG. 9-1

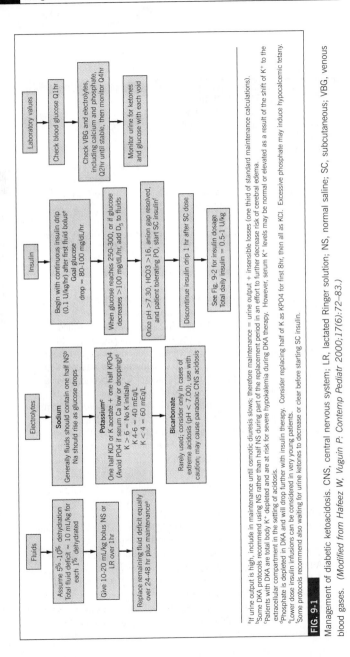

Management of diabetic ketoacidosis. CNS, central nervous system; LR, lactated Ringer solution; NS, normal saline; SC, subcutaneous; VBG, venous blood gases. *(Modified from Hafeez W, Vuguin P: Contemp Pediatr 2000;17(6):72–83.)*

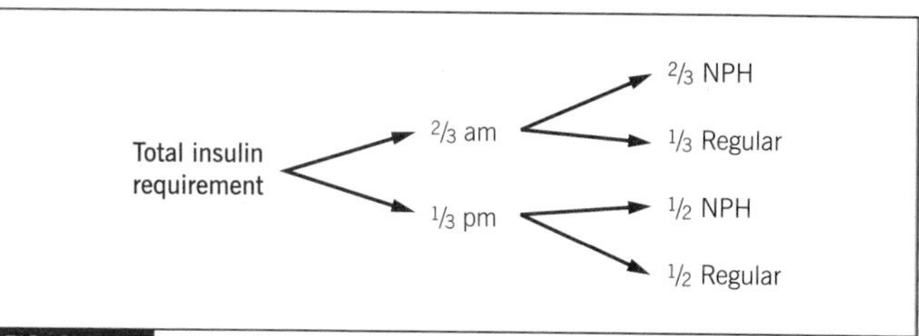

FIG. 9-2

Conversion to daily insulin dosage. NPH, neutral protamine Hagedorn.

C. TYPE II DIABETES MELLITUS

1. **There is an increasing prevalence of type II diabetes mellitus among children, especially among African Americans, Hispanics, and Native Americans;** *this increase is related to an increased prevalence of childhood obesity.*
2. **An abnormality in glucose levels is caused by insulin resistance and an insulin secretory defect.**
3. **It can present in ketoacidosis** (chronic high glucose impairs β-cell function and increases peripheral insulin resistance).
4. **Consider screening by measuring fasting blood glucose levels among children who are overweight (body mass index [BMI] >85th percentile for age and gender)** ***and*** **have two of the following risk factors:**

   Family history of type II diabetes in a first- or second-degree relative

   Race/ethnicity of African American, Native American, Hispanic, or Asian or Pacific Islander

   Signs associated with insulin resistance (acanthosis nigricans, hypertension, dyslipidemia, polycystic ovarian disease)
5. **Screening, if done, should begin at age 10 years or onset of puberty (whichever occurs first) and repeated every 2 years.**[2]
6. **Primary treatment is with diet and exercise,** although pharmacologic agents are often necessary for those who fail conservative management or are symptomatic at presentation. No validated treatment protocols currently exist in children. Metformin has been used for patients with serum glucose levels <350 mg/dL without ketones (see Formulary for additional details).

   There has been no reported experience in adolescents with acarbose, the newer insulin-sensitizing drugs (i.e., rosiglitazone and pioglitazone), or sulfonylureas. Because of concerns of liver toxicity, the thiazolidinediones are contraindicated in adolescents.
7. **Managing children with diabetes involves close monitoring of daily blood glucose as well as following hemoglobin A1c levels.**[3] Frequent eye exams and screening for hypertension, hyperlipidemia, and proteinuria are also important.[4]

TABLE 9-1

THYROID FUNCTION TESTS: INTERPRETATION

	TSH	T_4	Free T_4
Primary hyperthyroidism	L	H	High N to H
Primary hypothyroidism	H	L	L
Hypothalamic/pituitary hypothyroidism	L, N, H*	L	L
TBG deficiency	N	L	N
Euthyroid sick syndrome	L, N, H*	L	L to low N
TSH adenoma or pituitary resistance	N to H	H	H
Compensated hypothyroidism†	H	N	N

*Can be normal, slightly low, or slightly high.

†Treatment may not be necessary.

H, High; L, low; N, normal; T_4, thyroxine; TBG, thyroxine-binding globulin; TSH, thyroid-stimulating hormone.

II. THYROID AND PARATHYROID FUNCTION[5-8]

A. THYROID TESTS

1. **Interpretation of thyroid function tests (see Table 9-1).**
2. **Thyroid scan:** Used to assess thyroid clearance and to study structure and function of the thyroid. Localizes ectopic thyroid tissue and hyperfunctioning and nonfunctioning thyroid nodules.
3. **Technetium uptake:** Measures uptake of technetium by thyroid gland; levels are increased in hyperthyroidism and decreased in thyroxine-binding globulin (TBG) deficiency and in hypothyroidism (except dyshormonogenesis, when it may be increased).

B. HYPOTHYROIDISM (Table 9-2)

C. HYPERTHYROIDISM (Table 9-3)

D. HYPERPARATHYROIDISM AND HYPOPARATHYROIDISM (Table 9-4)

E. MULTIPLE ENDOCRINE NEOPLASIA SYNDROMES (MEN) (Table 9-5)

III. ADRENAL AND PITUITARY FUNCTION[9-11]

A. ADRENAL INSUFFICIENCY

Most common causes are congenital adrenal hyperplasia (CAH) and long-term glucocorticoid treatment. Other causes include Addison disease and hypothalamic or pituitary disease secondary to tumors, surgery, radiation therapy, or congenital defects.

1. **Congenital adrenal hyperplasia[10,11]:**

a. Group of autosomal recessive disorders characterized by a defect in one of the enzymes required in the synthesis of cortisol from cholesterol. Cortisol deficiency results in oversecretion of adrenocorticotropic hormone (ACTH) and hyperplasia of the adrenal cortex.

b. CAH is the most common cause of ambiguous genitalia in females.

c. 21-Hydroxylase deficiency accounts for 90 of cases.

Text continues on p. 263

TABLE 9-2

HYPOTHYROIDISM

Disease and Clinical Symptoms	Onset	Etiology	Evaluation	Management	Follow-up
PRIMARY/CONGENITAL					
Large fontanelles, lethargy, constipation, hoarse cry, hypotonia, hypothermia, and jaundice	Symptoms usually develop within the first 2 weeks of life and are almost always present by 6 weeks. However, if the cause is other than absence of the thyroid gland, some infants may be relatively asymptomatic. They are still at risk for developmental delay.	Deficiency of thyrotropin-releasing hormone (TRH), thyrotropin (TSH) *or* The most common cause is a defect of fetal thyroid development (athyrosis). Other causes include a mutation in the TSH receptor and thyroid dyshormonogensis.	↓ T_4 ↓ or ↑ TSH	Replacement with L-thyroxine should begin as soon as diagnosis is confirmed, usually by newborn screens. Goal of therapy is to achieve T_4 levels in the upper half of normal range. If hypothyroidism is due to a primary cause, TSH should be kept <5. Be aware that a minority of infants maintain a persistently high TSH despite correction of the T_4 level.	Monitor T_4 and TSH levels at the end of weeks 1 and 2 of therapy. If levels are adequate, follow every 1–3 months during the first 12 months.

continued

TABLE 9-2

HYPOTHYROIDISM—*cont'd*

Disease and Clinical Symptoms	Onset	Etiology	Evaluation	Management	Follow-up
ACQUIRED					
Deceleration of growth is often the first manifestation. Other signs may include coarse, brittle hair; dry, scaly skin; and delayed tooth eruption.	Can occur as early as the first 2 years of life	Hashimoto thyroiditis Head/neck radiation	↓ T_4, ↑ TSH The presence of antithyroglobulin and antimicrosomal antibodies suggests Hashimoto thyroiditis.	Replacement with L-thyroxine.	As above. After 2 years, monitoring levels every 6 to 12 months should be adequate as dose changes become less frequent.

Thyroid hormone levels in premature infants are lower than those seen in full-term infants. Further, the TSH surge seen at approximately 24 hours of age in full-term babies does not appear in preterm infants. In this population, lower levels are associated with increased illness, but the effect of replacement therapy remains controversial.

TABLE 9-3

HYPERTHYROIDISM

Disease and Clinical Symptoms	Onset	Etiology	Evaluation	Management	Follow-up
Hyperactivity, irritability, altered mood, insomnia, heat intolerance, increased sweating, pruritus, tachycardia, palpitations, fatigue, weakness, weight loss despite increased appetite, increased stool frequency, oligomenorrhea or amenorrhea, fine tremor, hyperreflexia, hair loss	Prevalence increases with age beginning in adolescence. Has a 4 : 1 female-to-male predilection.	The most common cause in childhood is Graves disease (see below). Other causes include subacute thyroiditis, factitious hyperthyroidism (intake of exogenous hormone), and rarely a TSH-secreting pituitary tumor. Pituitary resistance to thyroid hormone demonstrates a compensatory rise in T_4, but TSH remains within the normal range.	↓ TSH* ↑ T_4, T_3 Further tests include assessment of TSH receptor stimulating antibody, antithyroglobulin and antimicrosomal antibodies, free T_4, and free T_3.	Treat with Propothiouracil (PTU) or methimazole, which inhibit formation of thyroid hormone. Radioactive iodine (^{131}I) is an option for refractory cases.	Follow symptoms and level of T_4 and TSH.

continued

TABLE 9-3

HYPERTHYROIDISM—*cont'd*

Disease and Clinical Symptoms	Onset	Etiology	Evaluation	Management	Follow-up
Graves disease: Diffuse goiter, a feeling of grittiness and discomfort in the eye, retrobulbar pressure or pain, eyelid lag or retraction, periorbital edema, chemosis, scleral injection, exophthalmos, extraocular muscle dysfunction, localized dermopathy, and lymphoid hyperplasia	Peak incidence between 11 and 15 years of age. There is a 5 : 1 female-to-male ratio. Most children with Graves disease have a family history of some form of autoimmune thyroid disease.	Autoimmune	↑ T_4, T_3 ↓ TSH	As above	
Thyroid storm: Acute in onset. Manifested by hyperthermia, tachycardia, and restlessness.			↑ T_4, T_3 ↓ TSH	Propranolol is used to suppress signs and symptoms of thyrotoxicosis. Potassium iodide may also be used for	

Untreated, this may progress to delirium, coma, and death.				acute hyperthyroid management. Long-term management may include radiation therapy.	
Neonatal thyrotoxicosis: Microcephaly, frontal bossing, intrauterine growth retardation (IUGR), tachycardia, systolic hypertension leading to widened pulse pressure, irritability, failure to thrive, exophthalmos, goiter, flushing, vomiting, diarrhea, jaundice, thrombocytopenia, and cardiac failure or arrhythmias	Ranges from immediate to delayed for weeks	Seen exclusively in infants born to mothers with Graves disease. Caused by transplacental passage of maternal thyroid-stimulating immunoglobulin (TSI). Occasionally, mothers are unaware that they have Graves disease. Also, note that if a mother has received definitive treatment (thyroidectomy or radition therapy), the possible passage of TSI remains.	↑ T_4, T_3 ↓ TSH	As above Digoxin may be indicated for heart failure.	Disease usually resolves by 6 months of age.

*With the rare case of a TSH-secreting tumor, the patient does not have hyperthyroidism if the TSH is not suppressed, regardless of the levels of T_3 and T_4.

TABLE 9-4

HYPOPARATHYROIDISM AND HYPERPARATHYROIDISM

Disease and Clinical Symptoms	Onset	Etiology	Evaluation	Management	Follow-up
HYPOPARATHYROIDISM					
Clinical manifestations range from asymptomatic or mild muscle cramps to hypocalcemic tetany, prolonged QTc, and convulsions.		Hypoparathyroidism results from a decrease in parathyroid hormone (PTH) Pseudohypoparathyroidism results from PTH resistance and is distinguished by normal or elevated PTH.	↓ PTH ↓ Serum Ca^{2+} ↑ Serum phos Nml/↓ alk phos ↓ 1,25-OH vitamin D_3	Calcium supplementation for documented hypocalcemia Vitamin D supplementation with calcitriol	Carefully monitor serum calcium and phosphorous during therapy. Also, monitor urine calcium levels to avoid hypercalciuria.
HYPERPARATHYROIDISM					
Causes hypercalcemia from increased bone and renal resorption and increased intestinal absorption of calcium via increased activated vitamin D. Symptoms of hypercalcemia include vomiting, constipation, abdominal pain, weakness, paresthesias, malaise, and bone pain.	Uncommon in childhood	Associated with multiple endocrine neoplasia syndromes. (see Table 9-5) Secondary hyperparathyroidism is more common and develops in response to hypocalcemic states, such as renal failure or rickets. The distinguishing lab finding in secondary hyperparathyroidism is normal to somewhat decreased calcium levels.	↑ PTH ↑ Serum Ca^{2+} ↓ Serum phos NmL/↑ alk phos	Hydration is the mainstay of treatment by enhancing calciuria. Furosemide may be used with caution if hydration is adequate. Hydrocortisone, 1 mg/kg q6hr, reduces intestinal absorption of calcium. Calcitonin transiently opposes bone resorption. In severe hypercalcemia, bisphosphates may be considered. Surgical removal of parathyroid glands.	Beware of hypoparathyroidism following surgical removal of the parathyroid gland.

TABLE 9-5
MULTIPLE ENDOCRINE NEOPLASIA (MEN) SYNDROMES

MEN I: An autosomal dominant condition characterized by hyperplasia of the endocrine pancreas (which usually secretes gastrin, insulin), the anterior pituitary (prolactin, growth hormone, corticotrophin or non–hormone secreting), and the parathyroid glands. This syndrome is classified as the presence of two of three of the above benign tumors. Hyperparathyroidism is the most common presenting sign. Although asymptomatic cases require no treatment, proton pump inhibitors are the mainstay for gastrinomas, and surgery is the treatment of choice for parathyroid tumors. Any tumors in the head of the pancreas also should be removed.

MEN IIa: An autosomal dominant condition characterized by hyperplasia or carcinoma of thyroid C cells in association with pheochromocytoma and primary parathyroid hyperplasia. C-cell hyperplasia or tumors usually appear earlier than pheochromocytoma, and hypercalcemia is a late manifestation indicating hyperparathyroidism.

MEN IIb: An autosomal dominant syndrome characterized by the occurrence of multiple neuromas in combination with medullary thyroid carcinoma and pheochromocytoma. The neuromas most often occur on mucosal surfaces. Feeding difficulties, poor sucking, diarrhea, constipation, and failure to thrive may begin in infancy or early childhood, many years before the appearance of neuromas or endocrine symptoms.

For the MEN II family, genetic testing is recommended for all family members. For those who test positive, prophylactic thyroidectomy universally is advised owing to the aggressiveness of medullary thyroid tumors. The ideal age for surgery remains unclear. Recommended ages range from infancy up into adolescence, with most experts concurring that thyroid removal in early childhood (5 years) is reasonable.

d. The enzymatic defect results in impaired synthesis of adrenal steroids beyond the enzymatic block and overproduction of the precursors before the block. Two major classifications consist of:
   (1) Classic (complete enzyme deficiency):
      (a) Occurs with or without salt loss.
      (b) Adrenal insufficiency occurs under basal conditions.
      (c) Adrenal crisis in untreated patients occurs at 1 to 2 weeks of life, with signs and symptoms of adrenal insufficiency rarely occurring before 3 to 4 days of life. (Non–salt-losing forms have a less severe risk for adrenal crisis owing to preservation of mineralocorticoid synthesis.)
      (d) Diagnosis is based on elevated 17-hydroxyprogesterone (17-OHP) levels.
      (e) Levels of testosterone in girls and androstenedione in boys and girls are also elevated.
   (2) Nonclassic or simple virilizing form (partial enzyme deficiency):
      (a) Adrenal insufficiency tends to occur only under stress and manifests as androgen excess after infancy (precocious

pubarche, irregular menses, hirsutism, acne, advanced skeletal maturation).

(b) Morning 17-OHP levels may be elevated, but diagnosis may require an ACTH stimulation test (see section VI.B.). A significant rise in the 17-OHP level 60 minutes after ACTH injection is diagnostic. Cortisol response will be decreased.

(3) For infants with ambiguous genitalia a karyotype is an essential feature of the evaluation.

(a) For apparent male infants presenting with classic CAH, a karyotype should be evaluated to rule out the possibility of a severely masculinized female infant.

2. Daily management of adrenal insufficiency:

a. Glucocorticoid maintenance:

(1) Physiologic glucocorticoid production is approximately 9 to 12 mg/m^2/day. See Formulary Adjunct for forms of steroids used in physiologic replacement.

(2) For congenital adrenal hyperplasia, 12.5 mg/m^2/day of hydrocortisone through intravenous (IV) or intramuscular (IM) route or 25 mg/m^2/day orally (PO) is recommended for daily maintenance to allow for suppression of the ACTH axis.

(3) For pure adrenal insufficiency, daily oral dosing of 9 to 12 mg/m^2/day of hydrocortisone is often sufficient and helps decrease the toxic effects seen at higher doses.

(4) Doses often are titrated to preserve normal skeletal growth and rate of skeletal maturation. In addition, doses are adjusted to prevent inappropriate adrenergic effects.

b. Mineralocorticoid maintenance:

(1) These patients should have ready access to salt.

(2) For salt-losing forms of adrenal insufficiency, 0.1 to 0.2 mg/day of oral fludrocortisone acetate once daily is recommended. For patients who cannot take the oral form, IV hydrocortisone at 50 mg/m^2/day will supply a maintenance amount of mineralocorticoid activity. (Note that synthetic steroids such as prednisone and dexamethasone do not supply appropriate mineralocorticoid effects.)

(3) Infants also require 1 to 2 g (17–34 mEq) of sodium supplementation per day.

(4) Always monitor blood pressure and electrolytes when supplementing mineralocorticoids.

c. Stress dose glucocorticoids:

(1) The dose of glucocorticoids should increase in patients with fever or other illness.

(2) The stress dose is 25 to 50 mg/m^2/day of hydrocortisone IV/IM (as a continuous drip or divided every 3 to 6 hours) or 75 mg/m^2/day PO divided every 6 to 8 hours.

(3) For surgery or severe illness, hydrocortisone doses of 50 to 100 mg/m^2/day IV may be indicated.

3. Acute adrenal crisis:
a. Crises are often precipitated by any acute illness, trauma, surgery, or exposure to excess heat.
b. Characterized by emesis, diarrhea, dehydration, hypotension, metabolic acidosis, and shock.
c. Lab values often demonstrate hypoglycemia, hyponatremia, and hyperkalemia. In addition, serum cortisol and aldosterone are decreased, and ACTH and renin are elevated. In infants with CAH, 17-OHP is increased.
   (1) These studies are useful to perform before steroid administration to confirm the diagnosis, but treatment should not be delayed.
d. Management includes rapid volume expansion to support blood pressure, sufficient dextrose to maintain blood glucose, close monitoring of electrolytes, and corticosteroid administration.
   (1) Give 50 mg/m^2 of hydrocortisone by IV bolus (rapid estimate: infants = 25 mg; children = 50 to 100 mg), followed by 50 mg/m^2/24 hours by continuous drip (preferable) or divided every 3 to 4 hours.
   (2) *Hydrocortisone and cortisone are the only glucocorticoids that provide the necessary mineralocorticoid effects.*

B. SYNDROME OF INAPPROPRIATE ANTIDIURETIC HORMONE SECRETION[12] (Table 9-6)

C. DIABETES INSIPIDUS (DI)[12] (Table 9-7)

IV. GROWTH AND SEXUAL DEVELOPMENT[13-18]

A. GROWTH

1. **Target height range is calculated as mid-parental stature ± 2 SD (1 SD = 2 inches).**
a. Mid-parental stature for boys is (paternal height + maternal height + 5 inches)/2.
b. Mid-parental stature for girls is (paternal height + maternal height − 5 inches)/2.
2. **Short stature (Fig. 9-3)[13,14]:**
a. Differential diagnosis: It is important to differentiate constitutional growth delay (CGD) and familial short stature (FSS) from pathologic causes of short stature. FSS is characterized by slow growth rate during the first 2 to 3 years of life followed by a low-normal growth velocity. Children with CGD follow similar growth charts to those with FSS; however, a delay in the onset of puberty and skeletal maturation allow for a period of catch-up growth. Family history of delayed puberty is often present. *Pathology is suggested by a child who is not tracking toward his or her target height or by a child with an abnormal growth velocity.* Deceleration of linear growth in a well-nourished child is typical of growth hormone deficiency, hypothyroidism, or glucocorticoid excess. Initial decline in weight followed by decreased height velocity is

TABLE 9-6

SYNDROME OF INAPPROPRIATE ANTIDIURETIC HORMONE SECRETION (SIADH)

Disease and Clinical Symptoms	Etiology	Evaluation	Management
The hallmark is hyponatremia ($Na^+ < 135$) with inappropriately concentrated urine in the setting of euvolemia or mild hypervolemia	Associated with many conditions, including central nervous system (CNS) trauma, CNS infection, pneumonia, and CNS surgery.	↓ Serum Na^+ and Cl^- with nl HCO_3^- Hypouricemia Inappropriately concentrated urine	Hyponatremia should be corrected slowly with fluid restriction. A reasonable goal is a 10% rise in Na^+ per 24 hr *In the setting of coma or seizures,* more rapid Na^+ correction should be undertaken by treating with hypertonic saline. The goal is to acutely raise the serum [Na^+] to ~120–125. Definitive therapy is to identify and treat the underlying cause.

TABLE 9-7

DIABETES INSIPIDUS (DI)[12]

Characterized by an impaired ability to concentrate urine. The water-deprivation test (see section VI.C.) is diagnostic of DI, and the vasopressin test (see section VI.D.) is used to differentiate between central and nephrogenic DI. Infants with DI may present with failure to thrive, vomiting, constipation, and unexplained fevers, and more severe cases show signs of severe dehydration, hypovolemic shock, and convulsions.

LABORATORY FINDINGS

Low urine specific gravity (<1.005)
Low urine osmolarity (50–200)
Low vasopressin (<0.5 pg/mL)

Central DI	Nephrogenic DI
Caused by vasopressin deficiency and is associated with CNS injury, including trauma and tumors.	Caused by renal tubular resistance to vasopressin and can be genetic or acquired.
Management consists of DDAVP (desmopressin acetate) in nasal spray, IV, PO, or subcutaneous preparation. Titrate the DDAVP dosage to urine output, aiming for at least 1-hour period of diuresis per day that is sufficient to stimulate thirst.	Provision of free water and a diet that is low in salt is the cornerstone of therapy in nephrogenic DI.
Electrolytes must be monitored closely.	
Infants are often not treated with DDAVP because of difficulties monitoring their input and output. Rather, they are treated with increased free water and salt restriction.	

Following trauma to axons of vasopressin containing neurons, a temporary or permanent DI may result. Due to the initial edema occurring in the area of the hypothalamus and pituitary, a short-lived period (2–5 days) of DI is observed. This is succeeded by a stage of SIADH, as dying neurons release vasopressin. The final stage results in permanent DI, if a significant number of neurons were injured.

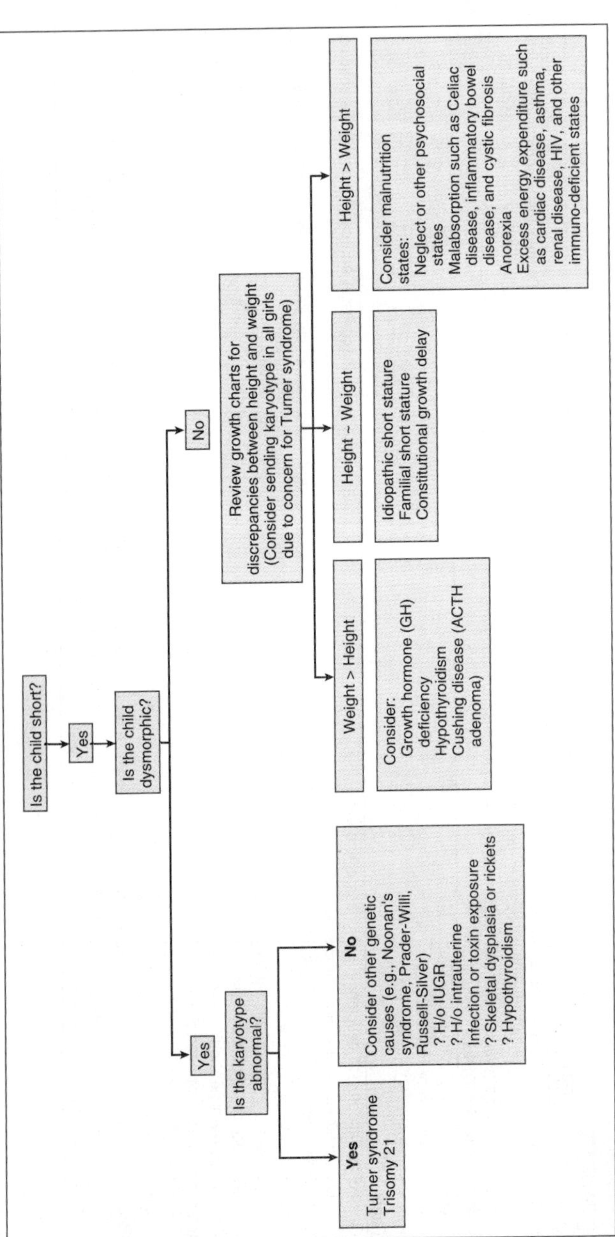

FIG. 9-3 Differential diagnosis of short stature.

suggestive of systemic illness, malnutrition, or other psychosocial factors. Dysmorphic features may indicate a chromosomal abnormality (trisomy 21 or Turner syndrome) or other specific syndrome. Disproportionate features or skeletal abnormalities are consistent with skeletal dysplasias or metabolic bone disease.

b. Initial evaluation: Begin with a thorough history, physical examination, evaluation of growth curves and pubertal stage. Initial screening tests include complete blood count (CBC), liver function tests (LFTs), electrolytes, erythrocyte sedimentation rate (ESR), and urinalysis (including pH and specific gravity). Also consider thyroid function tests, serum insulin-like growth factor-1 (IGF-1) and IGF binding protein (IGFBP-3), stool fat for malabsorption syndromes, antiendomysial and antigliadin antibodies for celiac disease, bone age (radiograph of left wrist and hand), and karyotype. Bone age is delayed in CGD but consistent with chronologic age in FSS. Consider a skeletal survey in a patient with disproportionate features.

B. SEXUAL DEVELOPMENT[15–18]

1. **Delayed puberty** is defined as no signs of pubertal development by 13 years in girls and 14 years in boys, or an arrest in pubertal maturation. There are two major categories:

a. Hypergonadotropic hypogonadism (high luteinizing hormone [LH] and follicle-stimulating hormone [FSH]) is secondary to primary gonadal failure. Common causes are tumor, chemotherapy, radiation therapy, and autoimmune glandular failure. Other causes include androgen insensitivity, history of inflammation (e.g., mumps), history of bilateral torsion, Turner's syndrome and Klinefelter's syndrome. Karyotype should be obtained for initial evaluation.

b. Hypogonadotropic hypogonadism (low or normal LH and FSH) is secondary to constitutional delay or a central gonadotropin deficiency. Kallman syndrome is the most common cause of isolated gonadotropin deficiency. Other causes include CNS tumors, hypopituitarism, Prader-Willi syndrome, and chronic disease. Anorexia nervosa and hypothyroidism also should be considered.

c. Initial evaluation should include LH and FSH. Bone age and thyroid studies should also be obtained. A gonadotropin-releasing hormone (GnRH) stimulation test can be obtained to rule out hypogonadotropic hypogonadism.

2. **Precocious puberty** is traditionally defined as any sign of secondary sexual maturation before 8 years in girls and 9 years in boys. More recent data suggest early puberty may not warrant extensive evaluation or intervention if it occurs after 6 years in African American girls or after 7 years in Caucasian girls.

a. Central, true, isosexual, *or* complete precocious puberty (CPP) refers to GnRH-dependent puberty and involves activation of the hypothalamic-pituitary-gonadal axis. Most common causes are CNS lesions (congenital anomalies, tumors, trauma, infections) and idiopathic. Pathologic etiologies are more commonly seen in boys.

b. Peripheral *or* pseudoprecocious puberty refers to GnRH-independent puberty and involves adrenal, gonadal, ectopic, or exogenous sources of hormone production. Most common causes are CAH, adrenal tumors, McCune-Albright syndrome, gonadal tumors, human chorionic gonadotropin (hCG)-producing tumors, and exogenous sex hormones. Hypothyroidism can also cause GnRH-independent precocity.

c. Initial evaluation: Begin with a complete history, physical examination, and evaluation of growth curves. Penile length is disproportionately greater than testicular size in pseudoprecocious puberty, whereas testicular volume is disproportionately greater than penile size in normal puberty and in CPP. Growth rate in precocious puberty is usually more rapid than along a single height percentile. Patients with suspected precocious puberty should have a bone age study to confirm the diagnosis. Bone age is generally more than 2 years in advance of chronologic age in long-standing precocious puberty because of the action of sex hormones. Further studies should include basal and/or GnRH-stimulated LH levels (see section VI.F.), estradiol measurement in girls, testosterone levels in boys, 17-OHP levels, dehydroepiandrosterone (DHEA) levels, and urinary 17-ketosteroids (see section VI.G.). A magnetic resonance imaging (MRI) scan of the brain to identify CNS lesions should be obtained in any patient suspected of having CPP.

3. **Ambiguous genitalia:**

a. Clinical findings in a neonate that indicate possible ambiguous genitalia include anogenital ratio >0.5 (distance between anus and posterior fourchette divided by distance between anus and base of clitoris), phallus length <2.2 cm (mean newborn length – 2 SD), clitoromegaly (length >1 cm), nonpalpable gonads in an apparent male, and hypospadias associated with separation of scrotal sacs or undescended testis.

b. Etiology: The most common cause of ambiguous genitalia is CAH. Other causes include testicular regression syndrome, androgen insensitivity, testosterone biosynthesis disorders, and chromosomal abnormalities.

c. Diagnosis: based on karyotype, measurement of gonadotropins (LH, FSH), adrenal steroids (cortisol, 17-OHP, and ACTH stimulation test), testosterone precursors (DHEA, androstenedione), testosterone, dihydrotestosterone (DHT), and hCG stimulation test (see section VI.I.).

d. Cryptorchidism occurs in 3% of term male infants. About 50% of cryptorchid testicles descend by 3 months of age, and 80% drop by 12 months. Neoplasm occurs in 48.9% of individuals with untreated cryptorchidism, and 25% of those tumors occur in the contralateral testis. Rule out virilized female with a karyotype. An hCG stimulation test can be used to differentiate cryptorchidism from anorchia (see section VI.I.). Treatment is removal of trapped testicle at 1 year of life.

V. NORMAL VALUES (Tables 9-8 to 9-27)

Normal values may differ among laboratories because of variation in technique and in type of radioimmunoassay used. Unless otherwise noted, the values below are reference ranges from the Johns Hopkins Hospital Laboratories or from SmithKline Beecham clinical laboratories in Baltimore, Maryland.

TABLE 9-8
GONADOTROPINS

Age	FSH (mIU/mL)	LH (mIU/mL)
Prepubertal children	0.0–2.8	0.0–1.6
Men	1.4–14.4	1–10.2
Women, follicular phase	3.7–12.9	0.9–14

Normal infants have a transient rise in FSH (follicle-stimulating hormone) and LH (luteinizing hormone) to pubertal levels or higher within the first 3 mo, which then declines to prepubertal values by the end of the first year.

TABLE 9-9
TESTOSTERONE

Age	Testosterone, Serum Total (ng/dL)	Testosterone, Unbound (pg/mL)
Prepubertal children	10–20	0.15–0.6
Men	275–875	52–280
Women	23–75	1.1–6.3
Pregnancy	35–195	

TABLE 9-10
DIHYDROTESTOSTERONE (DHT)

Age	Males (ng/dL)	Females (ng/dL)
Cord blood	<2–8	<2–5
1–6 mo	12–85	<5
Prepubertal	<5	<5
Tanner stage II–III	3–33	5–19
Tanner stage IV–V	22–75	3–30

TABLE 9-11
ESTRADIOL

Age	pg/mL
Prepubertal children	<25
Men	6–44
Women	
Luteal phase	26–165
Follicular phase	None detected–266
Midcycle	118–355
Adult women on OCP	None detected–102

Normal infants have an elevated estradiol at birth, which decreases to prepubertal values during the first week of life. Estradiol levels increase again between 1 and 2 mo of age and return to prepubertal values by 6–12 mo of age.

TABLE 9-12
ANDROSTENEDIONE, SERUM

Age	Males (ng/dL)	Females (ng/dL)
Preterm infants		
26–28 wk to day 4 of life	92–892	92–892
31–35 wk to day 4 of life	80–446	80–446
Full-term infants		
1–7 day	20–290	20–290
1–12 mo	6–68	6–68
Prepubertal children	8–50	8–50
Tanner II	31–65	42–100
Tanner III	50–100	80–190
Tanner IV	48–140	77–225
Tanner V	65–210	80–240
Adults	78–205	85–275

TABLE 9-13
DEHYDROEPIANDROSTERONE (DHEA)

Age	DHEA (ng/dL)	DHEA Sulfate (mcg/dL)
Prepubertal children	25 ± 8	2.3–15
Men	643 ± 112	223 ± 93
Women	516 ± 106	138 ± 51

Adapted from Bertrand J, Rappaport R, et al: Pediatric Endocrinology, 2nd ed. Baltimore, Williams and Wilkins, 1993.

VI. TESTS AND PROCEDURES

A. ORAL GLUCOSE TOLERANCE TEST (OGTT)

1. **Pretest preparation:** A calorically adequate diet is required for 3 days before the test, with 50 of total calories taken as carbohydrate.
2. **Delay test 2 weeks after illness.** *Discontinue all hyperglycemic and hypoglycemic agents (e.g., salicylates, diuretics, oral contraceptives, phenytoin).*
3. **Give 1.75 g/kg (maximum of 75 g) of glucose orally after a 12-hour fast, allowing up to 5 minutes for ingestion.** Mix glucose with water and lemon juice as a 20 dilution. Quiet activity is permissible during the OGTT. Draw blood samples at 0, 30, 60, 120, 180, and 240 minutes after ingestion.
4. **Interpretation:** 2-hour blood glucose <140 mg/dL = normal; 140 to 199 mg/dL = impaired glucose tolerance; ≥200 mg/dL = diabetes mellitus.

TABLE 9-14

17-HYDROXYPROGESTERONE, SERUM

Age	Baseline (ng/dL)	60 min after ACTH Stimulation (ng/dL)
Premature infants (31–35 wk)	≤360	N/A
Term infants, 1st wk of life	≤63	N/A
1–5 days	80–420	N/A
<1 yr	11–170	85–465
1–5 yr	4 – 115	50–350
6–12 yr	7 – 69	75–220
Male, Tanner stages II–III	12–130	69–310
Female, Tanner stages II–III	18–220	80–420
Male, Tanner stages IV–V	51–190	105–230
Female, Tanner stages IV–V	36–200	80–225
Adult male	50–250	42–250
Adult female, premenopausal		
Follicular phase	20–100	42–250
Midcycle peak	100–250	
Luteal phase	100–500	

8 AM level is most accurate given diurnal variation. Levels are normally increased in newborns for the first few days of life. Be aware that infant serum contains substances that may cross-react in the assay for 17-hydroxyprogesterone and artificially elevate the level, unless they are separated by chromatography. Before interpreting results on infants, be sure that the laboratory has prepared samples appropriately.

TABLE 9-15

CORTISOL, SERUM WITH ACTH STIMULATION TEST

Condition	mcg/dL
Any gender/any age/pre-ACTH, 8 AM	5.7–16.6
1 hr post-ACTH	16–36

TABLE 9-16

CORTISOL, URINE

Age	mcg/g Creatinine	mcg/24 hr
Prepubertal children	7–25	3–9
Men	7–45	11–84
Women	9–32	10–34

TABLE 9-17

17-KETOSTEROIDS, URINE

Age	mg/24 hr
<1 mo	<2.0
1 mo–5 yr	<0.5
6–8 yr	1.0–2.0
Men	9–22
Women	5–15

TABLE 9-18

17-HYDROXYCORTICOSTEROIDS, URINE

Children (body weight variable)	3 ± 1 mg/m²/24 hr
Men	3–9 mg/24 hr
Women	2–8 mg/24 hr

TABLE 9-19

CATECHOLAMINES, URINE

Compound	Amount/24 hr Urine Collection
Dopamine	100–440 mcg
Epinephrine	<15 mcg
Norepinephrine	15–86 mcg
Metanephrines	<0.4 mg
Normetanephrines	<0.9 mg
Homovanillic acid (HVA)	0 – 10 mg
Vanillyl mandelic acid (VMA)	2 – 10 mg

Catecholamines are elevated in a variety of tumors including neuroblastoma, ganglioneuroma, ganglioblastoma, and pheochromocytoma.

TABLE 9-20

CATECHOLAMINES, SERUM

Compound	Supine (μg)	Sitting (μg)
Dopamine	<87	<87
Epinephrine	<50	<60
Norepinephrine	110–410	120–680

TABLE 9-21

INSULIN-LIKE GROWTH FACTOR 1 (IGF-1)

Age	Males (ng/mL)	Females (ng/mL)
2 mo–6 yr	17–248	17–248
6–9 yr	88–474	88–474
9–12 yr	110–565	117–771
12–16 yr	202–957	261–1096
16–26 yr	182–780	182–780
>26 yr	123–463	123–463

A clearly normal IGF-1 level argues against growth hormone (GH) deficiency, although in young children, there is considerable overlap between normals and those with GH deficiency.

TABLE 9-22

INSULIN-LIKE GROWTH FACTOR-BINDING PROTEIN (IGF-BP3)

Age (yr)	Males (mg/L)	Females (mg/L)
0–2	0.94–1.76	0.66–2.51
2–4	1.12–2.33	0.84–3.77
4–6	1.16–3.13	1.32–3.60
6–8	1.32–3.38	1.21–4.66
8–10	1.35–3.94	1.58–3.99
10–12	1.53–5.02	1.93–6.46
12–14	1.73–5.11	1.78–6.08
14–16	1.90–6.40	2.02–5.44
16–18	1.70–6.04	1.88–5.29
18–20	1.52–6.01	1.63–6.02
20–22	1.79–5.41	1.82–5.35
Adult (continues to vary with age)	1.15–5.18	1.19–5.69

Levels below the 5th percentile suggest a GH deficiency. This test may have greater discrimination than the IGF-1 test in younger patients.

TABLE 9-23

VITAMIN D

Compound	Value
25-Hydroxy-vitamin D	ng/mL
Newborns	8–21
Children	17–54
Adults	10–55
1,25-Dihydroxy-vitamin D	pg/mL
Newborns	8–72
Children	15–90
Adults	24–64

Note that 1,25-dihydroxy-vitamin D is the physiologically active form; however, 25-hydroxyvitamin D is the value to monitor for vitamin D deficiency, since this approximates body stores of vitamin D.

B. ACTH STIMULATION TEST

1. **The ACTH stimulation** test measures the ability of the adrenal gland to produce cortisol in response to ACTH. It is most useful in diagnosis of adrenal insufficiency.
2. **Method:** For patients older than 2 years of age, give 250 micrograms (mcg) ACTH. For those less than 2 years of age, give 125 mcg. The doses are given intravenously over 2 minutes, and cortisol levels are measured at 0, 30, and 60 minutes.
3. **Interpretation:** With a normal pituitary-adrenal axis, there is a rise in serum cortisol after ACTH administration (see Table 9-15 for values). With ACTH deficiency or prolonged adrenal suppression, there is no rise in cortisol after a single ACTH dose. A blunted cortisol response is indicative of CAH. A lack of response after 3 consecutive days of ACTH stimulation is pathognomonic of Addison disease.

TABLE 9-24

ROUTINE STUDIES (THYROID)

Test	Age	Normal	Comments
T_4 RIA (mcg/dL)	Cord	6.6–17.5	Measures total T_4 by radioimmunoassay
	1–3 d	11.0–21.5	
	1–4 wk	8.2–16.6	
	1–12 mo	7.2–15.6	
	1–5 yr	7.3–15.0	
	6–10 yr	6.4–13.3	
	11–15 yr	5.6–11.7	
	16–20 yr	4.2–11.8	
	21–50 yr	4.3–12.5	
Free T_4 (ng/dL)	1–10 d	0.6–2.0	Metabolically active form; the normal range for free T_4 is very assay dependent
	>10 d	0.7–1.7	
T_3 RIA (ng/dL)	Cord	14–86	Measures T_3 by RIA
	1–3 d	100–380	
	1–4 wk	99–310	
	1–12 mo	102–264	
	1–5 yr	105–269	
	6–10 yr	94–241	
	11–15 yr	83–213	
	16–20 yr	80–210	
	21–50 yr	70–204	
TSH (mIU/mL)	Cord	<2.5–17.4	TSH surge peaks from 80–90 mIU/mL in term newborn by 30 min after birth. Values after 1 wk are within adult normal range. Elevated values suggest primary hypothyroidism, whereas suppressed values are the best indicator of hyperthyroidism.
	1–3 d	<2.5–13.3	
	1–4 wk	0.6–10.0	
	1–12 mo	0.6–6.3	
	1–15 yr	0.6–6.3	
	16–50 yr	0.2–7.6	
TBG (mg/dL)	Cord	0.7–4.7	
	1–3 d	—	
	1–4 wk	0.5–4.5	
	1–12 mo	1.6–3.6	
	1–5 yr	1.3–2.8	
	6–20 yr	1.4–2.6	
	21–50 yr	1.2–2.4	

RIA, radioimmunoassay; RU, resin uptake; T_3 triiodothyronine; T_4, thyroxine; TBG, thyroxine-binding globulin; TSH, thyroid-stimulating hormone.

From Fisher DA: The thyroid. In Rudolf AM (ed): Pediatrics. Norwalk, CT, Appleton & Lange; 1991 and LaFranchi SH: Pediatr Clin North Am 1979;26(1):33–51.

C. WATER DEPRIVATION TEST

1. **The water deprivation test** determines ability to concentrate urine and is useful in the diagnosis of DI. It requires careful supervision because dehydration and hypernatremia may occur.
2. **Method:** Begin the test after a 24-hour period of adequate hydration and stable weight. Obtain a baseline weight after bladder emptying.

TABLE 9-25

SERUM T_4 (μg/dL) IN PRETERM AND TERM INFANTS

	Birthweight		
Age (days)	VLBW	LBW	Term
1–3	7.9 ± 3.3	11.4 ± 2.5	12 ± 1.9
4–6	6.5 ± 2.9	9.9 ± 2.5	11 ± 2.5
7–10	6.3 ± 3.0	9.5 ± 2.3	
11–14	5.7 ± 2.8	9.2 ± 2.1	
15–28	7.0 ± 2.5	9.1 ± 2.3	
29–56	7.8 ± 2.5	9.3 ± 3.3	

LBW, Low birth weight: 1500–2499 g; Term: 2500–5528 g; VLBW, very low birth weight: 400–1499 g.

From Frank JE et al. J Pediatr 1996;128(4):548–555.

TABLE 9-26

MEAN STRETCHED PENILE LENGTH (cm)

Age	Mean ± SD	–2.5 SD
Birth		
30 wk gestation	2.5 ± 0.4	1.5
34 wk gestation	3.0 ± 0.4	2.0
Full term	3.5 ± 0.4	2.5
0–5 mo	3.9 ± 0.8	1.9
6–12 mo	4.3 ± 0.8	2.3
1–2 yr	4.7 ± 0.8	2.6
2–3 yr	5.1 ± 0.9	2.9
3–4 yr	5.5 ± 0.9	3.3
4–5 yr	5.7 ± 0.9	3.5
5–6 yr	6.0 ± 0.9	3.8
6–7 yr	6.1 ± 0.9	3.9
7–8 yr	6.2 ± 1.0	3.7
8–9 yr	6.3 ± 1.0	3.8
9–10 yr	6.3 ± 1.0	3.8
10–11 yr	6.4 ± 1.1	3.7
Adult	13.3 ± 1.6	9.3

Measured from pubic ramus to tip of glans while traction is applied along length of phallus to point of increased resistance.

SD, standard deviation.

From Feldman KW, Smith DW: J Pediatr 1975;86:395; and Lee PA, et al: Johns Hopkins Med J 1980;146:156–163.

Restrict fluids for 7 hours. Measure body weight and urinary specific gravity and volume hourly. Check serum Na^+ and urine and serum osmolality every 2 hours. Hematocrit and blood urea nitrogen (BUN) levels may also be obtained at these times but are not critical. Monitor carefully to ensure that fluids are not ingested during the test. Terminate the test if weight loss approaches 5%.

TABLE 9-27
TESTICULAR SIZE

Tanner Stage (Genital)	Length (cm) (Mean ± SD)	Volume (mL)
I	2.0 ± 0.5	2
II	2.7 ± 0.7	5
III	3.4 ± 0.8	10
IV	4.1 ± 1.0	20
V	5.0 ± 0.5	29

Testicular volume of >4 mL or a long axis >2.5 cm is evidence that pubertal testicular growth has begun.
SD, standard deviation.

3. **Interpretation:**
   a. Normal individuals and those with psychogenic DI who are water deprived will concentrate their urine to 500 to 1400 mOsm/L, and plasma osmolality will be 288 to 291 mOsm/L. Urinary specific gravity rises to at least 1.010, urinary–to–plasma osmolality ratio is >2, urine volume decreases significantly, and there should be no appreciable weight loss.
   b. In patients with central or nephrogenic DI, specific gravity remains <1.005. Urine osmolality remains <150 mOsm/L, with no significant reduction of urine volume. A weight loss of up to 5% usually occurs. At the end of the test, a serum osmolality >290 mOsm/L, Na^+ >150 mEq/L, and a rise of BUN and hematocrit provide evidence that the patient did not receive water.

D. VASOPRESSIN TEST

1. **A vasopressin test** is used for differentiation between central (antidiuretic hormone [ADH]-deficient) and nephrogenic DI.
2. **Method:** Vasopressin is given subcutaneously, preferably at the end of the water deprivation test. Urine output, urine specific gravity, and water intake are monitored.
3. **Interpretation:** Patients with central DI concentrate their urine (>1.010) and demonstrate a reduction of urine volume and decreased fluid intake in response to exogenous vasopressin. Patients with nephrogenic DI have no significant change in fluid intake or urine volume or specific gravity. Continued fluid intake associated with decreased output and increased specific gravity suggests psychogenic DI.

E. DEXAMETHASONE SUPPRESSION TEST (DST)

1. **Dexamethasone suppresses secretion of ACTH** by the normal pituitary, decreasing endogenous production of cortisol and excretion of 17-hydroxycorticosteroids (17-OHCS) and 17-ketosteroids. It is

useful in determining the etiology of glucocorticoid or androgen overproduction.

2. **Method:** Give dexamethasone PO for 3 days (low dose, 1.25 mg/m^2/day; high dose, 3.75 mg/m^2/day divided every 6 hours), and collect 24-hour urine for 17-OHCS.
3. **Interpretation:** In normal patients, low-dose DST causes 17-OHCS to fall to <1 mg/m^2/day. In CAH, 17-OHCS levels are suppressed only by the high-dose DST. 17-OHCS levels are not suppressed even with the high-dose DST in ectopic ACTH production, adrenocortical carcinoma, and some hypothalamic tumors. Incomplete suppression of 17-ketosteroids suggests that the patient has entered puberty. Markedly increased, nonsuppressible 17-ketosteroids suggest the presence of an androgen-producing tumor.

F. GONADOTROPIN-RELEASING HORMONE (GNRH) STIMULATION TEST

1. **The GnRH stimulation test** measures pituitary LH and FSH reserve. It is helpful in the differential diagnosis of precocious or delayed sexual development.
2. **Method:** Give 100 mcg of synthetic GnRH (Factrel) SC, and measure LH and FSH levels at 0 and 40 minutes.
3. **Interpretation:** Prepubertal children should show no or minimal increase in LH and FSH in response to GnRH. A rise of LH into the adult range occurs in central precocious puberty. See Table 9-8 for normal gonadotropin values.

G. URINARY 17-KETOSTEROIDS

1. **Measurement of urinary 17-ketosteroid levels** reveals some end products of androgen metabolism. It is most useful in evaluation of androgen excess.
2. **Method:** Collect and refrigerate 24-hour urine specimen.
3. **Interpretation (see Table 9-17 for normal values):**
   a. Increased in CAH (it may take 1 to 2 weeks for 17-ketosteroids to rise above the normally high newborn levels), virilizing adrenal tumors, androgen-producing gonadal tumors, Cushing syndrome, and stressful illness.
   b. Decreased in Addison disease, anorexia nervosa, and panhypopituitarism.

H. URINARY 17-HYDROXYCORTICOSTEROID (17-OHCS)

1. **17-OHCS measures approximately one third of end products of cortisol metabolism.** It is most useful in evaluation of cortisol excess.
2. **Method:** Collect a 24-hour urine specimen. Refrigerate during collection and process immediately (17-OHCS are destroyed at room temperature).

3. **Interpretation (see Table 9-18 for normal values):**
   a. Increased in Cushing syndrome, stressful illness, obesity, hyperthyroidism, and 11-hydroxylase deficiency.
   b. Decreased in malnutrition, pituitary disorders involving ACTH, Addison disease, administration of exogenous corticosteroids, liver disease, hypothyroidism, and newborn period (as a result of decreased glucuronidation).
   c. Urinary free cortisol (see Table 9-16) can also be measured, eliminating some of the nonspecificity of 17-OHCS measurement. Interpretation is similar to that for 17-OHCS.

I. HUMAN CHORIONIC GONADOTROPIN (HCG) STIMULATION TEST

1. **An hCG test measures capacity for testosterone biosynthesis.** It is useful in differentiation of cryptorchidism (undescended testes) from anorchia (absent testes).
2. **Method:** Give 1000 units of hCG IV or IM for 3 days and measure serum testosterone and dihydrotestosterone on day 0 and day 4.
3. **Interpretation:** Testosterone level >100 ng/dL in response to hCG stimulation is evidence for adequate testosterone biosynthesis. In cryptorchidism, testosterone rises to adult levels after hCG administration; in anorchia, there is no rise.

REFERENCES

1. Report of the Expert Committee on the Diagnosis and Classification of Diabetes Mellitus. Diabetes Care 1999;22(Suppl 1):S5–19.
2. American Diabetes Association: Consensus statement: Type 2 diabetes in children. Diabetes Care 2000;22(12):381.
3. Pinhas-Hamiel O, Zeitler P: Type 2 diabetes: Not just for grownups anymore. Contemp Pediatr 2001;18(1):102–125.
4. American Diabetes Association: Hyperglycemic crises in patients with diabetes mellitus. Diabetes Care 2001;24(1):154–161.
5. Fisher DA: The thyroid. In Rudolf AM (ed): Pediatrics. Norwalk, CT, Appleton & Lange, 1991.
6. LaFranchi SH: Hyperthyroidism. Pediatr Clin North Am 1979;26(1):33–51.
7. Frank JE, et al: Thyroid function in very low birth weight infants: Effects on neonatal hypothyroidism screening. J Pediatr 1996;128(4):548–555.
8. Biswas S: A longitudinal assessment of thyroid hormone concentrations in preterm infants younger than 30 weeks' gestation during the first 2 weeks of life and their relationship to outcome. Pediatrics 2002;109(2):222–227.
9. Orth DN, Kovacs WJ: The adrenal cortex. In Wilson JD (ed): Williams' Textbook of Endocrinology. Philadelphia, WB Saunders, 1998.
10. American Academy of Pediatrics, Section on Endocrinology and Committee on Genetics: Technical report: Congenital adrenal hyperplasia. Pediatrics 2000;106(6):1511–1518.
11. Levine LS: Congenital adrenal hyperplasia. Pediatr Rev 2000;21(5):159–170.
12. Reeves WB, Bichet DG, Andreoli TE: Posterior pituitary and water metabolism. In Wilson JD (ed): Williams' Textbook of Endocrinology. Philadelphia, WB Saunders, 1998.

13. Plotnick L: Growth, growth hormone, and pituitary disorders. In McMillan J (ed): Oski's Pediatrics Principles and Practice. Philadelphia, Lippincott Williams & Wilkins, 1999.
14. MacGillivray MH: The basics for the diagnosis and management of short stature: A pediatric endocrinologist's approach. Pediatr Ann 2000;29(9):570–575.
15. Styne DM: New aspects in the diagnosis and treatment of pubertal disorders. Pediatr Endocrinol 1997;44(2):505–529.
16. Root AW: Precocious puberty. Pediatr Rev 2000;21(1):10–19.
17. Rosen DS, Foster C: Delayed puberty. Pediatr Rev 2001;22(9):309–314.
18. American Academy of Pediatrics, Committee on Genetics, Sections on Endocrinology and Urology: Evaluation of newborn with developmental anomalies of the external genitalia. Pediatrics 2000;106(1):138–142.

Fluids and Electrolytes

Brian Stone, MD

I. MAINTENANCE REQUIREMENTS

Maintenance requirements stem from basal metabolism. Metabolism creates two by-products, heat and solute, that need to be eliminated to maintain homeostasis. Heat dissipation through insensible losses and solute excretion in urine each can be considered as representing 50% of maintenance needs; that is, in the management of children who have anuric renal failure, maintenance fluid needs decrease by 50% because the only fluids that need to be replaced are insensible losses.[1]

10

A. CALORIC EXPENDITURE METHOD

The caloric expenditure method is based on the understanding that water and electrolyte requirements more accurately parallel caloric expenditure than body weight or body surface area (BSA). This method is effective for all ages, types of body habitus, and clinical states.

1. **Determine the child's standard basal calorie (SBC) expenditure as approximated by resting energy expenditure (REE) (see Table 20-1 in Chapter 20).**
2. **Adjust caloric expenditure needs by various factors (e.g., fever, activity) as described in Chapter 20.**
3. **For each 100 calories metabolized in 24 hours, the average patient will need 100 to 120 mL H_2O, 2 to 4 mEq Na^+, and 2 to 3 mEq K^+, as seen in Table 10-1.**

B. HOLLIDAY-SEGAR METHOD (Table 10-2 and Box 10-1)

The Holliday-Segar method estimates caloric expenditure in fixed weight categories; it assumes that for each 100 calories metabolized, 100 mL of H_2O will be required. Specifically, for each 100 kcal expended, about 50 mL of fluid is required to provide for skin, respiratory tract, and basal stool losses, and 55 to 65 mL of fluid is required for the kidneys to excrete an ultrafiltrate of plasma at 300 mOsm/L without having to concentrate the urine. Note: The Holliday-Segar method is not suitable for neonates <14 days old; generally, it overestimates fluid needs in neonates compared with the caloric expenditure method.

C. BODY SURFACE AREA METHOD

The BSA method is based on the assumption that caloric expenditure is related to BSA (Table 10-3). It should not be used for children <10 kg. See page 599 for BSA nomogram and conversion formula.

TABLE 10-1

AVERAGE WATER AND ELECTROLYTE REQUIREMENTS PER 100 CALORIES PER 24 HOURS

Clinical State	H_2O (mL)	Na^+ (mEq)	K^+ (mEq)
Average patient receiving parenteral fluids*	100–120	2–4	2–3
Anuria	45	0	0
Acute CNS infections and inflammation	80–90	2–4	2–3
Diabetes insipidus	Up to 400	Var	Var
Hyperventilation	120–210	2–4	2–3
Heat stress	120–240	Var	Var
High-humidity environment	80–100	2–4	2–3

*Adequate maintenance solution: dextrose 5% to 10% (as needed) in 0.2% NaCl + 20 mEq/L KCl or K acetate.

CNS, central nervous system; Var, variable requirement.

TABLE 10-2

HOLLIDAY-SEGAR METHOD

	Water			Electrolytes
Body Weight	mL/kg/day		mL/kg/hr	(mEq/100 mL H_2O)
First 10 kg	100	÷24 hr/day	~4	Na^+ 3
Second 10 kg	50	÷24 hr/day	~2	Cl^- 2
Each additional kg	20	÷24 hr/day	~1	K^+ 2

TABLE 10-3

STANDARD VALUES FOR USE IN BODY SURFACE AREA METHOD

H_2O	1500 mL/m²/24 hr
Na^+	30–50 mEq/m²/24 hr
K^+	20–40 mEq/m²/24 hr

Data from Finberg L, Kravath RE, Fleishman AR: Water and Electrolytes in Pediatrics. Philadelphia, WB Saunders, 1982; and Hellerstein S: Pediatr Rev 1993;14(3):103–115.

BOX 10-1

HOLLIDAY-SEGAR METHOD

Example: Based on the Holliday-Segar method, determine the correct fluid rate for an 8-year-old child weighing 25 kg:

4 mL/kg/hr (for first 10 kg)	× 10 kg = 40 mL/hr	100 mL/kg/day (for first 10 kg)	× 10 kg = 1000 mL/day
2 mL/kg/hr (for second 10 kg)	× 10 kg = 20 mL/hr	50 mL/kg/day (for second 10 kg)	× 10 kg = 500 mL/day
1 mL/kg/hr (per additional kg)	× 5 kg = 5 mL/hr	20 mL/kg/hr (per additional kg)	× 5 kg = 100 mL/day
	25 kg 65 mL/hr		25 kg 1600 mL/day

Answer: 65 mL/hr

Answer: 1600 mL/day

II. DEFICIT THERAPY

A. CALCULATED ASSESSMENT

The most precise method of assessing fluid deficit is based on preillness weight:

Fluid deficit (L) = preillness weight (kg) – illness weight (kg)

% Dehydration = (preillness weight – illness weight)/preillness weight × 100%

If this is not available, clinical observation may be used, as described subsequently.

B. CLINICAL ASSESSMENT (Table 10-4)

III. GUIDELINES FOR DEHYDRATION CALCULATION

The extracellular fluid space is about 20% of the body's weight (40% in the newborn) and is divided 3:1 between interstitial (15% of body weight) and intravascular (5% of body weight) space.[2]

TABLE 10-4
CLINICAL OBSERVATIONS IN DEHYDRATION*

	Older Child 3% (30 mL/kg)	6% (60 mL/kg)	9% (90 mL/kg)
Examination	**Infant 5% (50 mL/kg)**	**10% (100 mL/kg)**	**15% (150 mL/kg)**
Dehydration	Mild	Moderate	Severe
Skin turgor	Normal	Tenting	None
Skin (touch)	Normal	Dry	Clammy
Buccal mucosa/lips	Moist	Dry	Parched/cracked
Eyes	Normal	Deep set	Sunken
Tears	Present	Reduced	None
Fontanelle	Flat	Soft	Sunken
CNS	Consolable	Irritable	Lethargic/ obtunded
Pulse rate	Normal	Slightly increased	Increased
Pulse quality	Normal	Weak	Feeble/impalpable
Capillary refill	Normal	~2 sec	>3 sec
Urine output	Normal	Decreased	Anuric

*For the same degree of dehydration, clinical symptoms are generally worse for hyponatremic dehydration than for hypernatremic dehydration.

CNS, central nervous system.

Data from Behrman RE, Kliegman RM, Arvin AM: Nelson Textbook of Pediatrics, 16th ed. Philadelphia, WB Saunders, 2000; and Oski FA: Principles and Practice of Pediatrics, 3rd ed. Philadelphia, JB Lippincott, 1999.

A. INTRACELLULAR FLUID (ICF) AND EXTRACELLULAR FLUID (ECF) COMPARTMENTS

1. Normal ICF and ECF composition (Table 10-5).
2. In dehydration, there are variable losses from the extracellular and intracellular compartments. The percentage deficit from these compartments is based on the total duration of illness (Table 10-6).
3. Electrolyte deficit (from ECF and ICF losses):

a. Na^+ deficit is the amount of Na^+ that was lost from the Na^+-containing ECF compartment during the dehydration period (see Table 10-5):

Na^+ deficit (mEq) = fluid deficit (L) × proportion from ECF × Na^+ concentration (mEq/L) in ECF. (Intracellular Na^+ is negligible as a proportion of total; therefore, it can be disregarded.)

b. K^+ deficit is the amount of K^+ that was lost from the K^+-containing ICF compartment during the dehydration period (see Table 10-5):

K^+ deficit (mEq) = fluid deficit (L) × proportion from ICF × K^+ concentration (mEq/L) in ICF. (Extracellular K^+ is negligible as a proportion of total; therefore it can be disregarded.)

B. ELECTROLYTE DEFICITS (IN EXCESS OF ECF/ICF ELECTROLYTE LOSSES)

$$\text{mEq required} = (CD - CP) \times fD \times wt$$

where

CD = concentration desired (mEq/L)

CP = concentration present (mEq/L)

fD = distribution factor as fraction of body weight (L/kg)

1. HCO_3^-: 0.4–0.5.
2. Cl^-: 0.2–0.3.
3. Na^+: 0.6–0.7.

Note *wt = baseline weight before illness (kg).*

TABLE 10-5

INTRACELLULAR AND EXTRACELLULAR FLUID COMPOSITION

	Intracellular (mEq/L)	Extracellular (mEq/L)
Na^+	20	133–145
K^+	150	3–5
Cl^-	—	98–110
HCO_3^-	10	20–25
PO_4^{3-}	110–115	5
Protein	75	10

TABLE 10-6

PERCENTAGE OF DEFICIT FROM EXTRACELLULAR AND INTRACELLULAR COMPARTMENTS

Duration of illness	Deficit from ECF (%)	Deficit from ICF (%)
<3 days	80	20
≥3 days	60	40

C. PROBABLE DEFICITS OF WATER AND ELECTROLYTES IN SEVERE DEHYDRATION (Table 10-7)

D. ONGOING LOSSES IN DEHYDRATION (Tables 10-8, 10-9, and 10-10)

E. DEFICIT CALCULATIONS (Fig. 10-1)

1. Sample calculations (Tables 10-11, 10-12, and 10-13)

IV. SERUM ELECTROLYTE DISTURBANCES

A. POTASSIUM

1. Hypokalemia:

a. Etiologies and laboratory data (Table 10-14).

b. Clinical manifestations: Skeletal muscle weakness or paralysis, ileus, and cardiac dysrhythmias.[3,4] Electrocardiogram (ECG) changes include delayed depolarization, with flat or absent T waves and, in extreme cases, U waves.

c. Laboratory tests to consider:

(1) Blood: Electrolytes, with blood urea nitrogen/creatinine (BUN/Cr), creatine phosphokinase (CPK), glucose, renin, arterial blood gas (ABG), cortisol

(2) Urine: Urinalysis, K^+, Na^+, Cl^-, osmolality, 17-ketosteroids.

(3) Other: ECG.

d. Management: Rapidity of treatment should be proportional to severity of symptoms.

Text continued on p. 295

TABLE 10-7

DEFICITS OF WATER AND ELECTROLYTES IN SEVERE DEHYDRATION

Condition	H_2O (mL/kg)	Na^+ (mEq/kg)	K^+ (mEq/kg)	Cl^- (mEq/kg)
Diarrheal dehydration				
Hyponatremic [Na^+]* <130 mEq/L	100–120	10–15	8–15	10–12
Isotonic [Na^+]* = 130–150 mEq/L	100–120	8–10	8–10	8–10
Hypernatremic [Na^+]* >150 mEq/L	100–120	2–4	0–6	0–3
Pyloric stenosis	100–120	8–10	10–12	10–12
Diabetic ketoacidosis	100	8	6–10	6

*[Na], serum or plasma sodium concentration.

Data from Hellerstein S: Pediatr Rev 1993;14(3):103–115.

TABLE 10-8

ELECTROLYTE COMPOSITION OF VARIOUS BODY FLUIDS*

Fluid	Na^+ (mEq/L)	K^+ (mEq/L)	Cl^- (mEq/L)
Gastric	20–80	5–20	100–150
Pancreatic	120–140	5–15	90–120
Small bowel	100–140	5–15	90–130
Bile	120–140	5–15	80–120
Ileostomy	45–135	3–15	20–115
Diarrhea	10–90	10–80	10–110
Burns*	140	5	110
Sweat			
Normal	10–30	3–10	10–35
Cystic fibrosis	50–130	5–25	50–110

*This table is useful in determining ongoing electrolyte losses in dehydration.

†3–5 g/dL of protein may be lost in fluid from burn wounds.

Data from Behrman RE, Kliegman RM, Arvin AM: Nelson Textbook of Pediatrics, 16th ed. Philadelphia, WB Saunders, 2000.

TABLE 10-9

ORAL REHYDRATION SOLUTIONS

	CHO (g/dL)	Na^+ (mEq/L)	K^+ (mEq/L)	Cl^- (mEq/L)	Base (mEq/L)	mOsm/kg H_2O
Ceralyte	4	70	20	60	30	220
Infalyte	3	50	25	45	30	200
Naturalyte	2.5	45	20	35	48	265
Pedialyte	2.5	45	20	35	30	250
Rehydralyte	2.5	75	20	65	30	310
WHO/UNICEFORS*	2	90	20	80	30	310

*Available from Jianas Bros. Packaging Co., 2533 SW Boulevard, Kansas City, MO 64108.

CHO, carbohydrate.

Data from Snyder J: Semin Pediatr Infect Dis 1994;5:231.

TABLE 10-10

APPROXIMATE ELECTROLYTE COMPOSITION OF COMMONLY CONSUMED FLUIDS (NOT RECOMMENDED FOR ORAL REHYDRATION THERAPY)*

	CHO (g/dL)	Na^+ (mEq/L)	K^+ (mEq/L)	Cl^- (mEq/L)	HCO_3^- (mEq/L)	mOsm/kg H_2O
Apple juice	11.9	0.4	26	—	—	700
Coca-cola	10.9	4.3	0.1	—	13.4	656
Gatorade	5.9	21	2.5	17	—	377
Ginger ale	9	3.5	0.1	—	3.6	565
Milk	4.9	22	36	28	30	260
Orange juice	10.4	0.2	49	—	50	654

*Values vary slightly depending on source.

CHO, carbohydrate.

Data from Behrman RE, Kliegman RM, Arvin AM: Nelson Textbook of Pediatrics, 16th ed. Philadelphia, WB Saunders, 2000.

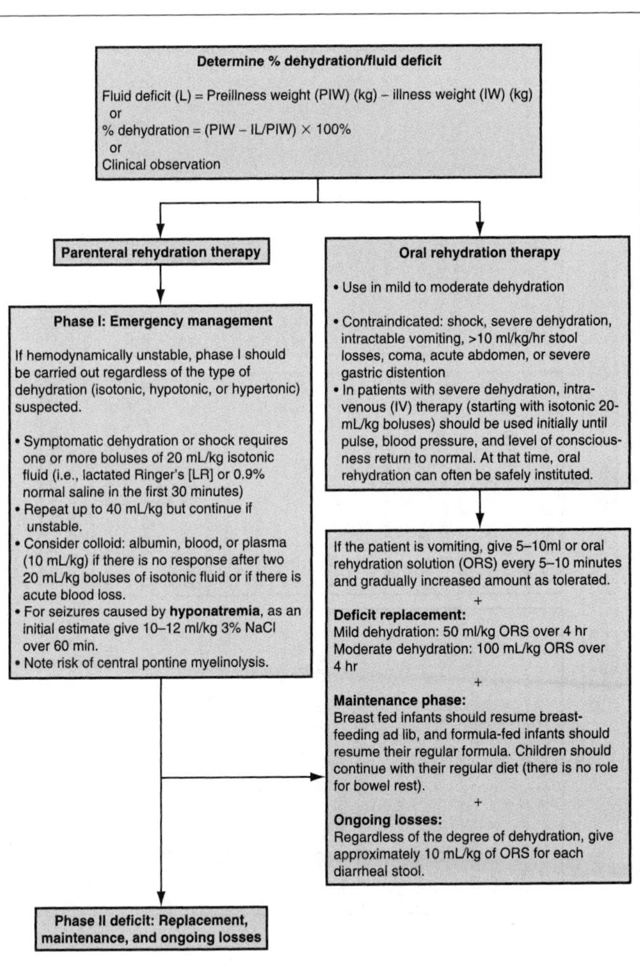

FIG. 10-1A
Algorithm for dehydration correction.

Phase II deficit: Replacement, maintenance, and ongoing losses*

Hyponatremic dehydration:
implies excess Na^+ loss (Na^+ <130 mEq/L)

Replacement:
Fluid deficit (L) = % dehydration x Wt (kg)

Na^+ deficit (mEq) = [Fluid deficit (L)] x [Proportion Na^+ from ECF] x [Na^+ concentration (mEq/L) in ECF]

Excess Na^+ deficit = (CD–CP) x fD x Wt (pre-illness weight in kg):
CD = concentration Na^+ desired (mEq/L)
CP = concentration Na^+ present (mEq/L)
fD = distribution factor as fraction of body weight (L/kg). Example: Na^+: 0.6–0.7

K^+ deficit = [Fluid deficit (L) x [Proportion K^+ from ICF] x [K^+ concentration (mEq/L) in ICF]
+
Maintenance: calculate maintenance fluids and electrolytes using Holliday-Segar Method

Ongoing losses: Use Table 10–8 to estimate ongoing electrolyte losses for various body fluids. Significant losses should be measured and may require replacement every 6–8 hr.

Isonatremic dehydration:
implies proportional losses of Na^+ and free water (FW). (Na^+ 130–149 mEq/L)

Replacement:
Fluid deficit (L) = % dehydration x Wt (kg)

Na^+ deficit (mEq) = [Fluid deficit (L)] x [Proportion Na^+ from ECF] x [Na^+ concentration (mEq/L) in ECF]

K^+ defecit = [Fluid deficit (L)] x [Proportion K^+ from ICF] x [K^+ concentration (mEq/L) in ICF]
+
Maintenance: calculate maintenance fluids and electrolytes using Holliday-Segar Method
+
Ongoing losses: use Table 10–8 to estimate ongoing electrolyte losses for various body fluids. Significant losses should be measured and may require replacement every 6–8 hr.

Hypernatremic dehydration:
implies excess FW loss. Note: The skin may appear thick and doughy, with normal turgor, and children may be excessively irritable on examination. (Na^+ ≥150 mEq/L)

Replacement:
FW deficit (FWD) estimated (L) : 4 ml/kg needed to decrease serum Na^+ by 1 mEq/L OR 3 mL/kg if Na^+ >170 because less FW is required to decrease serum Na^+ at higher concentrations.
Therefore: FWD = [4 mL/kg (or 3 mL/kg)] x weight x [concentration Na^+ present – concentration Na^+ desired]

Solute fluid deficit (SFD) (L) = Total fluid deficit (L) – FWD(L)

Solute Na^+ deficit = SFD x [Proportion Na^+ from ECF] x [Na^+ concentration (mEq/L) in ECF]

Solute K^+ deficit = SFD x [Proportion K^+ from ICF] x [K^+ concentration (mEq/L) in ICF]
+
Maintenance: calculate maintenance fluids and electrolytes using Holliday-Segar Method
+
Ongoing losses: Use Table 10–8 to estimate ongoing electrolyte losses for various body fluids. Significant losses should be measured and may require replacement every 6–8 hr.

* Phase cross-reference Tables 10-5 & 10-6 for calculations.

Give half of the replacement therapy in addition to the maintenance needs over the first 8 hr and the second half over the next 16 hr.

Rapid correction of hyponatremia may be associated with central pontine myelinolysis. Rapid increases in serum Na^+ level should therefore be reserved for symptomatic patients only. In asymptomatic patients, the target rate of rise should not exceed 2–4 mEq/L every 4 hours, or about 10–20 mEq/L in 24 hr.

Note: To calculate volume of 3% NaCl needed to raise the serum Na^+ by 'X' mEq/L: Amount of 3% NaCl (ml) = ['X' mEq/L × body weight (kg) × 0.6 L/kg]/0.513 mEq/mL Where 'X' = (125 mEq/L – actual serum [Na] to initially raise the serum Na^+ rapidly to 125 mEq/L

Give half of the replacement therapy in addition to the maintenance needs over the first 8 hr and the second half over the next 16 hr.

Half of the FW deficit and all of the solute deficit can be replaced over 24 hr. Replace the remainder of the FWD + maintenance during the next 24 hr.

Note: avoid dropping the serum Na^+ > 15 mEq/L per 24 hours to minimize the risk of cerebral edema. Thus for total Na^+ corrections of >30 (i.e., serum Na^+ >175), FW deficit replacement should be spread over >48 hours. Follow serum Na^+ levels at least evey 4 hr initially.

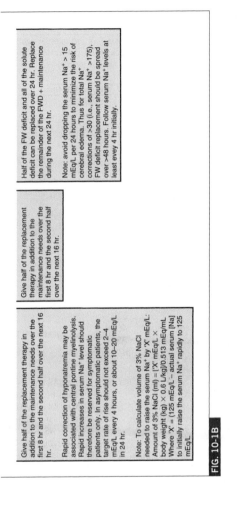

FIG. 10-1B

TABLE 10-11

EXAMPLE OF ISONATREMIC DEHYDRATION

Determine an adequate fluid schedule for a 7-kg (preillness weight) infant who has been ill for ≥3 days and clinically appears 10% dehydrated. Current weight is 6.3 kg. Serum Na^+ = 137. An IV line has just been placed, and no IVF has been administered.

Deficit Replacement		H_2O (mL)	Na^+ (mEq)	K^+ (mEq)
Fluid deficit				
% Dehydration × wt (kg) = 10% × 7 kg × (1000 mL/kg)		700		
Na^+ deficit 0.7 × 0.6 × 145 =			61	
K^+ deficit 0.7 × 0.4 × 150 =				42
Maintenance				
H_2O 7 kg × 100 mL/kg/day =		700		
Na^+ 700 mL/day × 3 mEq/100 mL =			21	
K^+ 700 mL/day × 2 mEq/100 mL =				14
24–hour total		1400	82	56
Fluid Schedule				
First 8 hr	⅓ Maintenance	233	7	5
	+½ Deficit	350	31	21
First 8 hr total		583	38	26
Next 16 hr	⅔ Maintenance	467	14	9
	½ Deficit	350	30	21
Next 16–hr total		817	44	30

Answer

Therefore, first 8 hr:
Rate: 583 mL/8 hr = 73 mL/hr
Na^+: 38 mEq/0.583 L = 65 mEq/L
K^+: 26 mEq/0.583 L = 45 mEq/L
D_5 ½ NS + 40 mEq/L of KCl or K acetate @ ~75 mL/hr × 8 hr

Next 16 hr:
Rate: 817 mL/16 hr = 51 mL/hr
Na^+: 44 mEq/0.817 L = 54 mEq/L
K^+: 30 mEq/0.817 L = 37 mEq/L
D_5 ½ NS + 40 mEq/L of KCl or K acetate @ ~50 mL/hr × 16 hr

In the absence of hypokalemia, 20 to 30 mEq/L of potassium is commonly used and is usually adequate; monitor carefully for hyperkalemia and adequate urine output if high concentrations of potassium are used. Potassium infusion rates should not exceed 1 mEq/kg/hr. If rate exceeds 0.5 mEq/kg/hr, the patient should be placed on a cardiorespiratory monitor.

Note Remember to account for ongoing losses. They should be replaced concurrently ("piggybacked") with a solution that matches the fluid being lost (see Table 10-8).

TABLE 10-12

EXAMPLE OF HYPONATREMIC DEHYDRATION

Determine an adequate fluid schedule for a 7-kg (preillness weight) infant who has been ill for ≥3 days and clinically appears 10% dehydrated. Current weight is 6.3 kg. Serum Na^+ = 115. An IV line has just been placed, and no IVF has been administered.

Deficit Replacement		H_2O (mL)	Na^+ (mEq)	K^+ (mEq)
Fluid deficit				
% Dehydration × wt (kg) = 10% × 7 kg × (1000 mL/kg)		700		
Na^+ deficit 0.7 × 0.6 × 145 =			61	
Excess Na^+ deficit: (135–115) × 0.6 × 7 =			84	
K^+ deficit 0.7 × 0.4 × 150 =				42
Maintenance				
(see Table 10-11 for exact calculations)		700	21	14
24–hour total		1400	166	56
Fluid Schedule				
First 8 hr	⅓ maintenance	233	7	5
	+½ deficit	350	73	21
First 8–hr total		583	80	26
Next 16 hr	⅔ maintenance	467	14	9
	½ deficit	350	72	21
Next 16–hr total		817	86	30

Answer

Therefore, first 8 hr:
Rate: 583 mL/8 hr = 73 mL/hr
Na^+: 80 mEq/0.583 L = 137 mEq/L
K^+: 26 mEq/0.583 L = 45 mEq/L
D_5 NS + 40 mEq/L of KCl or K acetate @ ~75 mL/hr × 8 hr

Next 16 hr:
Rate: 817 mL/16 hr = 51 mL/hr
Na^+: 86 mEq/0.817 L = 105 mEq/L
K^+: 30 mEq/0.817 L = 37 mEq/L
D_5 ½ NS + 40 mEq/L of KCl or K acetate @ ~50 mL/hr × 16 hr

In the absence of hypokalemia, 20 to 30 mEq/L of potassium is commonly used and is usually adequate; monitor carefully for hyperkalemia and adequate urine output if high concentrations of potassium are used. Potassium infusion rates should not exceed 1 mEq/kg/hr. If rate exceeds 0.5 mEq/kg/hr, the patient should be placed on a cardiorespiratory monitor.

Note Remember to account for ongoing losses. They should be replaced concurrently ("piggybacked") with a solution that matches the fluid being lost (see Table 10-8).

TABLE 10-13

EXAMPLE OF HYPERNATREMIC DEHYDRATION

Determine an adequate fluid schedule for a 7-kg (preillness weight) infant who has been ill for ≥3 days and clinically appears between 10% and 15% dehydrated. Current weight is 6.1 kg. Serum Na^+ = 160.

Replacement		H_2O (mL)	Na^+ (mEq)	K^+ (mEq)
Free-water deficit		420		
4 mL/kg × 7 kg × [160–145]				
Solute fluid deficit (SFD)		480		
Total fluid deficit (free water deficit)				
900–420				
Solute Na^+ deficit			42	
0.48 × 0.6 × 145				
Solute K^+ deficit				29
0.48 × 0.4 × 150				
Maintenance				
(see Table 10-11 for exact calculations)		700	21	14
Fluid Schedule				
First 24 hr				
	24–hr maintenance	700	21	14
	+½ Free-water deficit	210		
	Solute fluid and electrolyte deficit	480	42	29
First 24–hr total		1390	63	43
Second 24 hr	24–hr Maintenance	700	21	14
	+½ Free-water deficit	210		
Second 24–hr total		910	21	14

Answer

Therefore, first 24 hr:
Rate: 1390 mL/24 hr = 58 mL/hr
Na^+: 63 mEq/1.39 L = 45 mEq/L
K^+: 43 mEq/1.39 L = 31 mEq/L
D_5 ¼ NS + 30 mEq/L KCl or K acetate @ 58 mL/hr × 24 hr

Second 24 hr:
Rate: 910 mL/24 hr = 38 mL/hr
Na^+: 21 mEq/0.91 L = 23 mEq/L
K^+: 14 mEq/0.91 L = 15 mEq/L
D_5 ¼ NS + 10 mEq/L KCl or K acetate @ 38 mL/hr × 24 hr

Follow serum Na^+ and adjust fluid composition and rate based on clinical response. The second half of the free-water deficit may be replaced subsequently over the next 24 hr, or more rapidly depending on the rate of decline of serum Na^+ (avoid decline of >15 mEq/L in 24 hr).

Note In severe hypernatremic dehydration initial LR/NS resuscitation boluses should be accounted for in order to minimize dropping serum sodium >15 mEq/L per 24 hr to minimize risk of cerebral edema.

TABLE 10-14
CAUSES OF HYPOKALEMIA

Decreased Stores			
	Normal Blood Pressure		
Hypertension	Renal	Extrarenal	Normal Stores
Renovascular disease	RTA	Skin losses	Metabolic alkalosis
Excess renin	Fanconi syndrome	GI losses	Increased insulin
Excess mineralocorticoid	Bartter syndrome	High CHO diet	Leukemia
Cushing syndrome	DKA	Enema abuse	β_2 Catecholamines
	Antibiotics	Laxative abuse	Familial hypokalemic periodic paralysis
	Diuretics	Anorexia nervosa	
	Amphotericin B	Malnutrition	
LABORATORY DATA			
↑ Urine K^+	↑ Urine K^+	↓ Urine K^+	↑ Urine K^+

CHO, carbohydrate; DKA, diabetic ketoacidosis; GI, gastrointestinal; RTA, renal tubular acidosis.

TABLE 10-15
CAUSES OF HYPERKALEMIA

Increased Stores		
Increased Urinary K^+	Decreased Urine K^+	Normal Stores
Transfusion with aged blood	Renal failure	Cell lysis syndrome
Exogenous K^+ (e.g., salt substitutes)	Hypoaldosteronism	Leukocytosis (>100 K/mm^3)
Spitzer syndrome	Aldosterone insensitivity	Thrombocytosis (>750 K/mm^3)
	↓ Insulin	Metabolic acidosis*
	K^+-sparing diuretics	Blood drawing (hemolyzed sample)
	Congential adrenal hyperplasia	Type IV RTA
		Rhabdomyolysis/crush injury
		Malignant hyperthermia
		Theophylline intoxication

*For every 0.1–unit reduction in arterial pH, there is an approximately 0.2–0.4 mEq/L increase in plasma K^+.
RTA, renal tubular acidosis.

(1) Acute: Calculate electrolyte deficiency and replace with potassium acetate or potassium chloride. See Formulary for dosage information. Enteral replacement is safer when feasible, with less risk for iatrogenic hyperkalemia. Follow serum K^+ closely.

(2) Chronic: Calculate daily requirements and replace with potassium chloride or potassium gluconate. See Formulary for dosage information.

2. Hyperkalemia:

a. See Table 10-15 for etiologies of hyperkalemia and Table 10-16 for clinical manifestations.

TABLE 10-16

CLINICAL MANIFESTATIONS OF K^+ DISTURBANCES

Serum K^+ (mEq/L)	ECG Changes	Other Symptoms
~2.5	AV conduction defect, prominent U wave, ventricular dysrhythmia, ST-segment depression	Apathy, weakness, paresthesias
~7.5	Peaked T waves	Weakness, paresthesias
~8.0	Loss of P wave, widening of QRS	—
~9.0	ST-segment depression, further widening of QRS	Tetany
~10	Bradycardia, sine wave QRS-T, first-degree AV block, ventricular dysrhythmias, cardiac arrest	—

AV, atrioventricular; ECG, electrocardiogram.
Data from Feld LG, Kaskel FJ, Schoeneman MJ; Adv Pediatr 1988;35:497–535.

b. Management (Fig. 10-2):
   (1) Rapid temporizing therapy: antagonize the effect of K^+ on membrane potentials, and redistribute K^+ internally into cells.
   (2) Slow, long-term therapy: remove K^+ from the body.

B. SODIUM

1. Hyponatremia:

a. Etiologies (Table 10-17).

b. Factitious etiologies.
   (1) Hyperlipidemia: Na^+ decreased by 0.002 × lipid (mg/dL).
   (2) Hyperproteinemia: Na^+ decreased by 0.25 × [protein (g/dL) – 8].
   (3) Hyperglycemia: Na^+ decreased 1.6 mEq/L for each 100-mg/dL rise in glucose.

c. Hyponatremia secondary to syndrome of inappropriate antidiuretic hormone (SIADH) (Table 10-18).

2. Hypernatremia:

a. Etiologies and management (Table 10-19).

b. Diabetes insipidus (Table 10-20).

C. CALCIUM (Tables 10-21 and 10-22)

D. MAGNESIUM (Tables 10-23 and 10-24)

E. PHOSPHATE (Tables 10-25 and 10-26)

V. ACID–BASE/OSMOLAR GAP DISTURBANCES

A. DEFINITIONS

1. Serum osmolality: Number of particles per liter. Can be calculated as follows:

$$2[Na^+] + \text{glucose (mg/dL)}/18 + \text{BUN (mg/dL)}/2.8$$

a. Normal range: 275 to 295 mOsm/L.

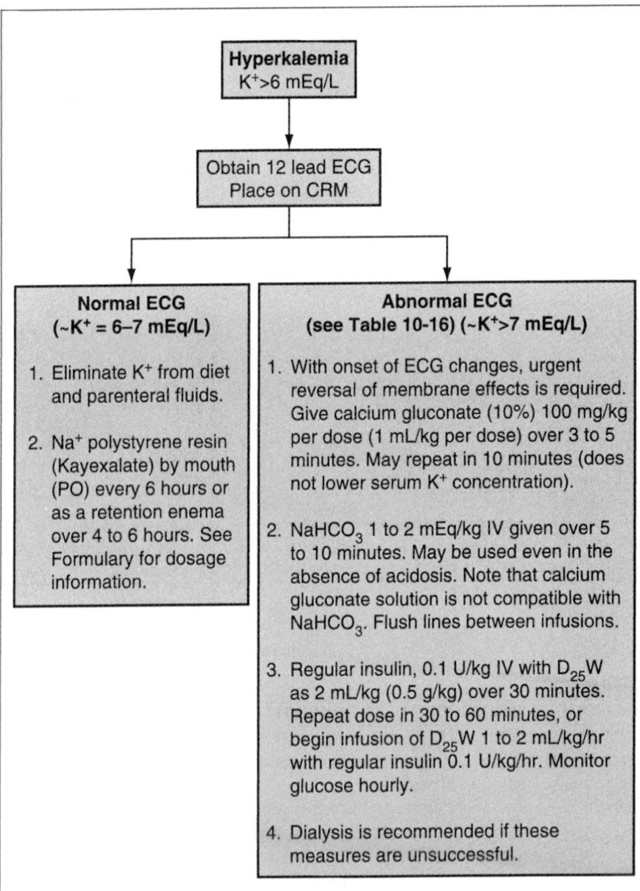

FIG. 10-2

Algorithm for hyperkalemia.

b. Serum osmolar gap = calculated serum osmolality – laboratory measured osmolality.
   (1) May be elevated in some anion gap acidosis, but a markedly elevated osmolar gap in the setting of an anion gap acidosis is highly suggestive of acute methanol or ethylene glycol intoxication.

Text continued on p. 303

TABLE 10-17

HYPONATREMIA*

Decreased Weight		
Renal Losses	Extrarenal Losses	Increased or Normal Weight
CAUSE		
Na^+-losing nephropathy	GI losses	Nephrotic syndrome
Diuretics	Skin losses	Congestive heart failure
Adrenal insufficiency	Third spacing	SIADH
	Cystic fibrosis	Acute/chronic renal failure
		Water intoxication
		Cirrhosis
		Excess salt-free infusions
LABORATORY DATA		
↑ Urine Na^+	↓ Urine Na^+	↓ Urine Na^+†
↑ Urine volume	↓ Urine volume	↓ Urine volume
↓ Specific gravity	↑ Specific gravity	↑ Specific gravity
↓ Urite osmolality	↑ Urine osmolality	↑ Urine osmolality
MANAGEMENT		
Replace losses	Replace losses	Restrict fluids
Treat cause	Treat cause	Treat cause

*Hyperglycemia and hyperlipidemia cause spurlous hyponatremia.

†Urine Na^+ may be appropriate for level of Na^+ intake in patients with SIADH and water intoxication.

GI, gastrointestinal; SIADH, syndrome of inappropriate antidiuretic hormone secretion.

TABLE 10-18

SYNDROME OF INAPPROPRIATE ANTIDIURETIC HORMONE SECRETION (SIADH)

Conditions associated with SIADH	CNS disease or injury (head injury, meningitis, subarachnoid hemorrhage, meningoencephalitis, brain tumors, neurosurgery
Treatment	1. Treat normovolemia with fluid restriction 2. To maintain normovolemia a. Diuretic (e.g., furosemide) b. Administer replacement of insensible fluid losses plus isotonic fluid to replace hourly urine output 3. Use 3% NaCl for partial correction of hyponatremia if patient presents with CNS symptoms (i.e., seizures, obtundation, coma)

Data from Nichols DG, Yaster M, Lappe DG, Buck J: Golden Hour: The Handbook of Advanced Pediatric Life Support. Philadelphia, Elsevier, 1996.

TABLE 10–19

HYPERNATREMIA

Decreased Weight		
Renal Losses	**Extrarenal Losses**	**Increased Weight**
Nephropathy	GI losses	Exogenous Na^+
Diuretic use	Skin losses	Mineralocorticoid excess
Diabetes insipidus	Respiratory*	Hyperaldosteronism
Postobstructive diuresis		
Diuretic phase of ATN		
LABORATORY DATA		
↑ Urine Na^+	↓ Urine Na^+	Relative ↓ Urine Na^+†
↑ Urine volume	↓ Urine volume	Relative ↓ Urine volume
↓ Specific gravity	↑ Specific gravity	Relative ↑ Specific gravity

CLINICAL MANIFESTATIONS

Predominantly neurologic symptoms: lethargy, weakness, altered mental status, irritability, and seizures.[3,4] Additional symptoms may include muscle cramps, depressed deep tendon reflexes, and respiratory failure.

MANAGEMENT

Replace FW losses based on calcuations in text and treat cause. Consider a natriuretic agent if there is increased weight.

*This cause of hypernatremia is usually secondary to free water loss, so that the fractional excretion of sodium may be decreased or normal.

†Exogenous Na^+ administration will cause an increase in the fractional excretion of sodium.

ATN, acute tubular necrosis; FW, free water; GI, gastrointestinal.

TABLE 10–20

DIABETES INSIPIDUS (DI)

CONDITIONS ASSOCIATED WITH DI

Global CNS ischemia or injury
1. Severe head injury
2. Hypoxia
3. Infection
4. Brain tumors
5. Neurosurgery involving the anterior hypothalamus

Renal disease
1. Polycystic kidney
2. Acute tubular necrosis
3. Obstructive uropathy

TREATMENT

1. Hypovolemia should be treated with isotonic fluid (10–20 mL/kg).
2. Administer DDAVP intranasally (see Formulary for dosage information). Wait for mild polyuria before each dose.
3. Vasopressin: see Formulary for dosage information.
   a. Replace insensible fluid losses.

Note Above treatments stop water loss but do not correct any prior deficits created from DI.

Data from Nichols DG, Yaster M, Lappe DG, Buck J: Golden Hour: The Handbook of Advanced Pediatric Life Support. Philadelphia, Elsevier, 1996.

TABLE 10-21

HYPOCALCEMIA

ETIOLOGIES

Hypoparathyroidism (decreased parathyroid hormone [PTH] levels or ineffective PTH response)
Vitamin D deficiency
Hyperphosphatemia (i.e., secondary to excessive use of sodium phosphate enemas)
Pancreatitis
Malabsorption states (malnutrition)
Drug therapy (anticonvulsants, cimetidine, aminoglycosides, Ca^{+}-channel blockers)
Hypomagnesemia/hypermagnesemia
Maternal hyperparathyroidism if patient is a neonate
Calcitriol (activated vitamin D) insuffiency
Tumor lysis syndrome
Ethylene glycol ingestion

CLINICAL MANIFESTATIONS

Tetany
Neuromuscular irritability with weakness
Paresthesias
Fatigue
Cramping
Altered mental status
Seizures
Laryngospasm and cardiac dysrhythmias[3,4]
ECG changes (prolonged QT interval)
Trousseau's sign: carpopedal spasm after aterial occlusion of an extremity for 3 minutes
Chvostek sign: muscle twitching with percussion of facial nerve

LABORATORY DATA

Blood	Urine	Other
Ca^{2+} (total and ionized) phosphate	Ca^{2+}	Chest x-ray (to visualize thymus)
Alkaline phosphatase	Phosphate	Ankle and wrist films (assess for rickets)
Mg^{2+}	Creatinine	
Total protein		
Albumin (a change in serum albumin of 1 g/dL changes total serum Ca^{2+} in the same direction by 0.8 mg/dL)		
Blood urea nitrogen, creatinine		
PTH		
pH (acidosis increases ionized calcium)		
25–OH vitamin D		

MANAGEMENT

Acute symptomatic: Consider use of IV forms, such as calcium gluconate, calcium gluceptate, or calcium chloride (cardiac arrest dose). See Formulary for dosage information. (Symptoms of hypocalcemia that are refractory to Ca^{2+} supplementation may be caused by hypomagnesemia.)

Note Significant hyperphosphatemia should be corrected before correction of hypocalcemia because soft tissue calcification may occur if total $[Ca^{2+}] \times [PO_4^{3-}] > 80$ (see Chapter 9).

Chronic: Consider use of oral supplements of calcium carbonate, calcium gluconate, calcium glubionate, or calcium lactate. See Formulary for dosage information.

TABLE 10-22

HYPERCALCEMIA

ETIOLOGIES

Hyperparathyroidism
Vitamin D intoxication
Excessive exogenous calcium administration
Malignancy
Prolonged immobilization
Diuretics (thiazides)
Williams syndrome
Granulomatous disease (i.e., sarcoidosis)
Hyperthyroidism
Milk-alkali syndrome

CLINICAL MANIFESTATIONS

Weakness
Irritability
Lethargy
Seizures
Coma
Abdominal cramping
Anorexia, nausea, vomiting
Polyuria, polydipsia
Renal calculi
Pancreatitis
ECG changes: shortened QT interval

LABORATORY DATA

Blood	Urine	Other
Ca^{2+} (total and ionized)	Ca^{2+}	ECG
Phosphate	Phosphate	KUB radiograph, renal ultrasound (for renal calculi)[7]
Alkaline phosphatase	Creatinine	
Total protein		
Albumin		
Blood urea nitrogen, creatinine		
PTH		
Vitamin D		

MANAGEMENT

1. Treat the underlying disease.
2. Hydrate to increase urine output and Ca^{2+} excretion. If glomerular filtration rate (GFR) and blood pressure (BP) are stable, give NS with maintenance K^+ at two to three times maintenance rate until Ca^{2+} is normalized.
3. Diuresis with furosemide.
4. Consider hemodialysis for severe or refractory cases.
5. Steroids may be indicated in malignancy, granulomatous disease, and vitamin D toxicity to decrease vitamin D and Ca^{2+} absorption. Consult appropriate specialists before administering steroids for these conditions.
6. For severe or persistently elevated Ca^{2+}, give calcitonin or bisphosphonate in consultation with an endocrinologist.

TABLE 10-23

HYPOMAGNESEMIA

ETIOLOGIES

Increased urinary losses: diuretic use, renal tubular acidosis, hypercalcemia, chronic adrenergic stimulants, chemotherapy

Increased gastrointestinal losses: malabsorption syndromes, severe malnutrition, diarrhea, vomiting, short bowel syndromes, enteric fistulas

Endocrine etiologies: diabetes mellitus, parathyroid hormone (PTH) disorders, hyperaldosterone states

Decreased intake (i.e., prolonged parenteral fluid therapy with Mg^{2+}-free solutions)

CLINICAL MANIFESTATIONS

Anorexia, nausea
Weakness
Malaise
Depression
Nonspecific psychiatric symptoms
Hyperreflexia
Carpopedal spasm
Clonus
Tetany
ECG changes: atrial and ventricular ectopy; torsades de pointes

LABORATORY DATA

Blood	Other
Mg^{2+} Ca^{2+} (total and ionized)	Consider evaluation for renal or gastrointestinal losses or endocrine etiologies outlined above.

MANAGEMENT

Acute: Give magnesium sulfate. See Formulary for dosing and side effects.
Chronic: Magnesium oxide or magnesium sulfate.[7] See Formulary for dosing.

TABLE 10-24

HYPERMAGNESEMIA

ETIOLOGIES

Renal failure

Excessive administration (e.g., eclampsia/pre-eclampsia states, status asthmaticus, cathartics, enemas, administration of magnesium for phosphate binding in renal failure)

CLINICAL MANIFESTATIONS

Depressed deep tendon reflexes
Lethargy
Confusion
Respiratory failure (in extreme cases)

Note Neonates born prematurely after tocolysis with magnesium sulfate are at high risk for respiratory sequelae, but serum magnesium levels tend to normalize within 72 hours.

LABORATORY DATA

Blood

Mg^{2+}
Blood urea nitrogren, creatinine
Ionized and total Ca^{2+}

MANAGEMENT

1. Stop supplemental Mg^{2+}.
2. Diuresis.
3. Give Ca^{2+} supplements such as calcium chloride (use cardiac arrest doses), calcium gluceptate, or calcium gluconate. See Formulary for dosing.
4. Dialysis if life-threatening levels are present.

TABLE 10-25

HYPOPHOSPHATEMIA

ETIOLOGIES

Starvation
Protein-energy malnutrition
Malabsorption syndromes
Intracellular shifts associated with respiratory or metabolic alkalosis
Treatment of diabetic ketoacidosis
Corticosteroid administration
Increased renal losses (i.e., renal tubular defects, diuretic use)
Vitamin D–deficient and vitamin D–resistant rickets
Very-low-birthweight (VLBW) infants when intake does not meet demand

CLINICAL MANIFESTATIONS

Symptomatic only at very low levels (<1 mg/dL) with irritability, paresthesias, confusion, seizures, apnea in VLBW infants, and coma

LABORATORY DATA

Blood	Urine
Phosphate	Ca^{2+}
Ca^{2+} (total and ionized)	Phosphate
Electrolytes including blood urea nitrogen, creatinine (follow for low K^+, Mg^{2+}, Na^+)	Creatinine
	pH
Consider vitamin D, parathyroid hormone	

MANAGEMENT

Insidious onset of symptoms: Give oral potassium phosphate or sodium phosphate. See Formulary for dosing.
Acute onset of symptoms: Give IV potassium phosphate or sodium phosphate. See Formulary for dosing.

TABLE 10-26

HYPERPHOSPHATEMIA

ETIOLOGIES

Hypoparathyroidism (but rarely occurs in the absence of renal insufficiency)
Reduction of GFR to <25% (may occur at smaller reductions of GFR in neonates)
Excessive administration of phosphate (PO, IV, or enemas)
Cytotoxic drugs to treat malignancies

CLINICAL MANIFESTATIONS

Symptoms of the resulting hypocalcemia (see Table 10-21)

LABORATORY DATA

Blood	Urine
Phosphate	Ca^{2+}
Ca^{2+} (ionized and total)	Phosphate
Electrolytes, including blood urea nitrogen, creatinine	Creatinine
Consider CBC, vitamin D, parathyroid hormone, arterial blood gases	Urinalysis

MANAGEMENT

1. Restrict dietary phosphate.
2. Give phosphate binders (calcium carbonate, aluminum hydroxide; use with caution in renal failure). See Formulary for dosing.
3. For cell lysis (with normal renal function), give an NS bolus and IV mannitol. See Chapter 21 for management of tumor lysis syndrome.
4. If patient has poor renal function, consider dialysis.

2. **Anion gap (AG):** represents anions other than bicarbonate and chloride required to balance the positive charge of Na^+. K^+ is considered negligible in AG calculations. Clinically, it is calculated as follows:

$$AG = Na^+ - (Cl^- + HCO_3^-)$$

(Normal: 12 mEq/L ± 2 mEq/L)

3. **Acidosis: pH <7.35.**
a. Respiratory acidosis: occurs when PCO_2 is higher than normal (>45 mmHg)
b. Metabolic acidosis: occurs when arterial bicarbonate level is less than normal (<22 mmol/L)
4. **Alkalosis: pH >7.45.**
a. Respiratory alkalosis: occurs when PCO_2 is lower than normal (<35 mmHg)
b. Metabolic alkalosis: occurs when arterial bicarbonate level is greater than normal (>26 mmol/L)

B. RULES FOR DETERMINING PRIMARY ACID–BASE DISORDERS[5]

1. **Determine the pH:** The body does not fully compensate for primary acid–base disorders; therefore, the primary disturbance will shift the pH away from 7.40. Examine the PCO_2 and HCO_3 to determine whether the primary disturbance is a metabolic acidosis/alkalosis or respiratory acidosis/alkalosis.
2. **Calculate the anion gap:** If the anion gap is ≥20 mmol/L, there is a primary metabolic acidosis regardless of pH or serum bicarbonate concentration. (The body does not generate a large anion gap to compensate for a primary disorder.)
3. **Calculate the excess anion Gap (i.e., "ΔGap" or "Gap–Gap"):**

$$\Delta Gap = [\text{calculated anion gap} - \text{normal anion gap (i.e., 12) mmol/L}] + \text{measured } HCO_3^-$$

a. If the ΔGap is greater than a normal serum bicarbonate concentration (>30 mmol/L), there is an underlying metabolic alkalosis.
b. If the ΔGap is less than a normal bicarbonate concentration (<23 mmol/L), there is an underlying nonanion gap metabolic acidosis *(1 mmol of unmeasured acid titrates 1 mmol of bicarbonate)* *($+\Delta$ anion gap $= -\Delta[HCO_3^-]$)*

C. ETIOLOGY OF ACID–BASE DISTURBANCES (Fig. 10-3)

VI. PARENTERAL FLUID COMPOSITION (Table 10-27)

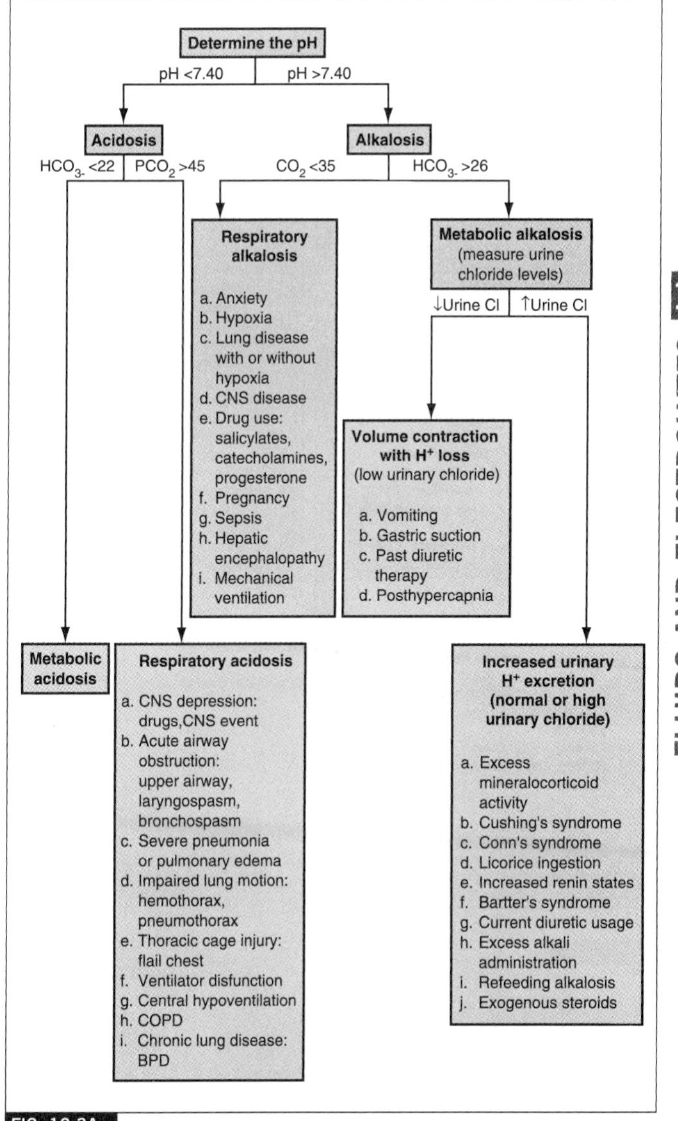

FIG. 10-3A

Etiology of acid–base disturbances.

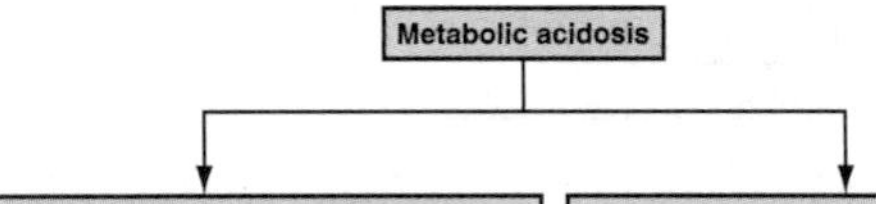

Anion gap metabolic acidosis

1. Increased acid production (noncarbonic acid)
   a. β-hydroxybutyric acid and acetoacetic acid production
      (1) Insulin deficiency (diabetic ketoacidosis)
      (2) Starvation or fasting
   b. Increased lactic acid production
      (1) Tissue hypoxia
      (2) Sepsis
      (3) Exercise
      (4) Ethanol ingestion
      (5) Methanol ingestion[1]
      (6) Ethylene glycol ingestion[1]
      (7) Paraldehyde intoxication
      (8) Systemic diseases (e.g., leukemia, diabetes mellitus, cirrhosis, pancreatitis)
      (9) Inborn errors of metabolism (IEMs) (carbohydrates, urea cycle, amino acids, organic acids)
   c. Increased short-chain fatty acids (acetate, propionate, butyrate, d-lactate) from colonic fermentation
      (1) Viral gastroenteritis
      (2) Other causes of carbohydrate malabsorption
   d. Drugs
      (1) Salicylate intoxication
      (2) NSAID intoxication
      (3) Topiramate
      (4) Metformin
   e. Increased sulfuric acid
      (1) Decreased acid execretion
      (2) Acute and chronic renal failure[7]

[1]Note: A large osmolar-gap acidosis can be seen in both methanol and ethylene glycol intoxication and when present is suggestive of acute intoxication.

Nonanion gap metabolic acidosis (hyperchloremic metabolic acidosis)

1. Gastrointestinal loss of bicarbonate
   a. Diarrhea (secretory)
   b. Fistula or drainage of the small bowel or pancreas
   c. Surgery for necrotizing enterocolitis
   d. Ureteral sigmoidostomy or ileal loop conduit
   e. Ileoileal pouch
   f. Use of anion exchange resins in presence of renal impairment

2. Renal bicarbonate loss
   a. Renal tubular acidosis, especially type II (see Table 18-3)
   b. Early renal failure
   c. Carbonic anhydrase inhibitors
   d. Aldosterone inhibitors

3. Other causes
   a. Administration of HCl, NH_4Cl, arginine, or lysine hydrochloride
   b. Hyperalimentation

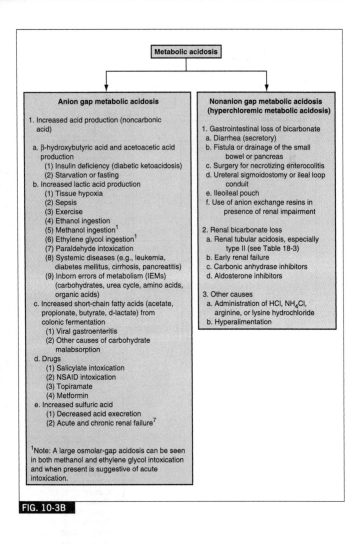

FIG. 10-3B

TABLE 10-27

COMPOSITION OF FREQUENTLY USED PARENTERAL FLUIDS

Liquid	CHO (g/100 mL)	Protein* (g/100 mL)	Cal/L	Na^+ (mEq/L)	K^+ (mEq/L)	Cl^- (mEq/L)	HCO_3^-† (mEq/L)	Ca^{2+} (mEq/L)	mOsm/L
D_5W	5	—	170	—	—	—	—	—	252
$D_{10}W$	10	—	340	—	—	—	—	—	505
NS (0.9% NaCl)	—	—	—	154	—	154	—	—	308
½ NS (0.45% NaCl)	—	—	—	77	—	77	—	—	154
D_5 ¼ NS (0.225% NaCl)	5	—	170	34	—	34	—	—	329
3% NaCl	—	—	—	513	—	513	—	—	1027
8.4% sodium bicarbonate (1 mEq/mL)	—	—	—	1000	—	—	1000	—	2000
Ringer solution	0–10	—	0–340	147	4	155.5	—	≈4	
Lactated Ringer	0–10	—	0–340	130	4	109	28	3	273
Amino acid 8.5% (Travasol)	—	8.5	340	3	—	34	52	—	880
Plasmanate	—	5	200	110	2	50	29	—	
Albumin 25% (salt poor)	—	25	1000	100–160	—	<120	—	—	300
Intralipid‡	2.25	—	1100	2.5	0.5	4.0	—	—	258–284

*Protein or amino acid equivalent.

†Bicarbonate or equivalent (citrate, acetate, lactate).

‡Values are approximate; may vary from lot to lot. Also contains <1.2% egg-phosphatides.

CHO, carbohydrate; HCO_3^-, bicarbonate; NS, normal saline.

REFERENCES

1. Roberts KB: Fluids and electrolytes: Parenteral fluid therapy: Pediatr Rev 2001;22:112.
2. Nichols DG, Yaster M, Lappe DG, Buck J: Golden Hour: The Handbook of Advanced Pediatric Life Support. Philadelphia, Elsevier, 1996.
3. Barkin R: Pediatric Emergency Medicine, 2nd ed. St. Louis, Mosby, 1997.
4. Feld LG, Kaskel FJ, Schoeneman MJ: The approach to fluid and electrolyte therapy in pediatrics. Adv Pediatr 1988;35:497–535.
5. Haber RJ: A practical approach to acid-base disorders. West J Med 1991;155:146–151.
6. Segar WE: Parenteral fluid therapy. Curr Probl Pediatr 1972;3:23–40.
7. Fleisher G, Ludwig S: Textbook of Pediatric Emergency Medicine. Baltimore, Williams & Wilkins, 2000.
8. American Academy of Pediatrics: Practice parameter: The management of acute gastroenteritis in young children. Pediatrics 1996;97:424–431.
9. Saavedra J: Probiotics and infectious diarrhea. Am J Gastroenterol 2000;95: S16–18.
10. Hanna J, Scheinman J, Chan J: The kidney in acid–base balance. Pediatr Clin North Am 1995;42(61):365.

Gastroenterology

Kurlen S. E. Payton, MD

11

I. WEBSITES

www.aap.org (American Academy of Pediatrics)
www.naspghan.org (North American Society for Pediatric Gastroenterology, Hepatology, and Nutrition)
www.acg.gi.org (American College of Gastroenterology)

II. GASTROINTESTINAL EMERGENCIES

A. GASTROINTESTINAL BLEEDING

1. **Initial evaluation (Fig. 11-1):**
   a. Assess airway, breathing, and circulation (ABCs) and hemodynamic stability.
   b. Perform physical examination, looking for evidence of bleeding.
   c. Verify bleeding with rectal examination and/or testing of stool or emesis for occult blood. Obtain baseline laboratory tests. Consider the following laboratory studies: complete blood count (CBC), prothrombin time/partial thromboplastin time (PT/PTT), blood type and cross-match, reticulocyte count, blood smear, blood urea nitrogen/creatinine (BUN/Cr), electrolytes, and a panel to assess for disseminated intravascular coagulation (DIC).
   d. Consider gastric lavage to differentiate upper from lower gastrointestinal (GI) bleeding and to assess for ongoing bleeding.
   e. Provide specific therapy based on assessment and site of bleeding.
   f. Begin initial fluid resuscitation with normal saline (NS) or lactated Ringer (LR) solution. Consider transfusion if there is continued bleeding, symptomatic anemia, and/or a hematocrit level <20%. Initiate intravenous acid suppression therapy, preferably proton pump inhibitor (PPI).
2. **For a differential diagnosis of GI bleeding, see Table 11-1.**

B. ACUTE ABDOMEN[1]

1. **Differential diagnosis:**
   a. GI source: Appendicitis, pancreatitis, intussusception, malrotation with volvulus, inflammatory bowel disease (IBD), gastritis, bowel obstruction, mesenteric lymphadenitis, irritable bowel syndrome, abscess, hepatitis, perforated ulcer, Meckel diverticulitis, cholecystitis, choledocholithiasis, constipation, gastroenteritis.
   b. Renal source: Henoch-Schönlein purpura (HSP), urinary tract infection (UTI), pyelonephritis, nephrolithiasis.
   c. Gynecologic source: Ectopic pregnancy, ovarian cyst/torsion, pelvic inflammatory disease (PID).
   d. Oncologic source: Wilms tumor, neuroblastoma.

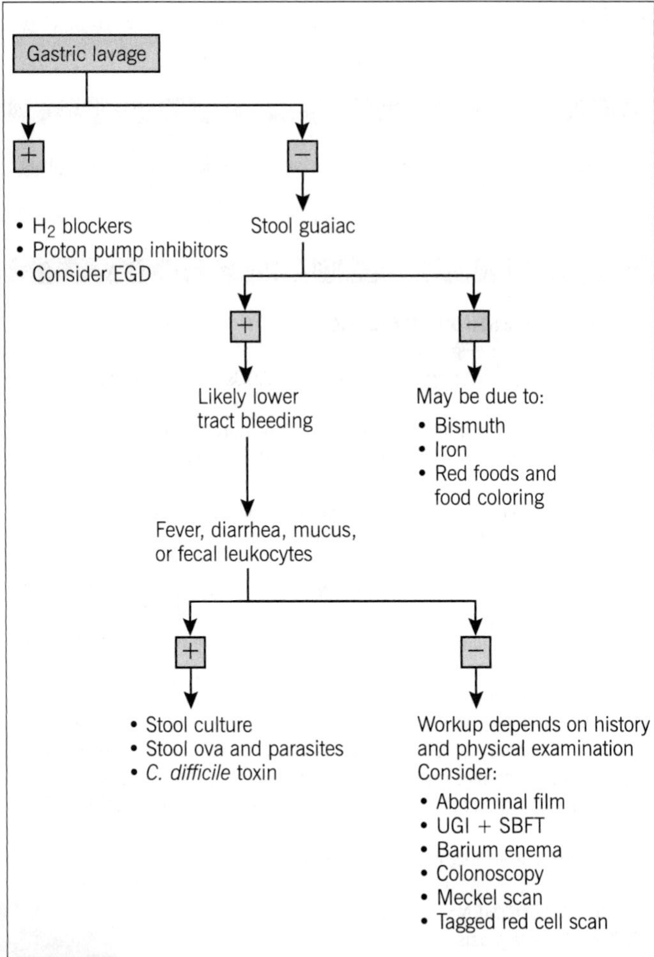

FIG. 11-1

Evaluation of GI bleeding. May use gastrostomy (G tube) if present; use nasogastric tube with caution if esophageal varices suspected. EGD, esophagogastroduodenoscopy; SBFT, small bowel follow through; UGI, upper gastrointestinal.

TABLE 11-1

DIFFERENTIAL DIAGNOSIS OF GI BLEEDING*

	Upper GI Bleed	Lower GI Bleed
Newborns	**Swallowed maternal blood**	**Anal fissure**
	Hemorrhagic gastritis	**Allergic proctocolitis**
	Stress ulcer	**Infectious diarrhea**
	Idiopathic	Hirschsprung disease
	Coagulopathy	Necrotizing enterocolitis
	Gastric outlet obstruction	Volvulus
	Gastric volvufus	Stress ulcer
	Pyloric stenosis	Vascular malformation
	Antral/pyloric webs	GI duplication
Infants	**Epistaxis**	**Anal fissure**
	Gastritis	**Infectious diarrhea**
	Esophagitis	**Allergic proctocolitis**
	Stress ulcer	**Meckel diverticulum**
	Gastric/duodenal ulcer	Intussusception
	Foreign bodies	GI duplication
	Gastric volvulus	Peptic ulcer
	Esophageal varices	Foreign body
Children	**Epistaxis**	**Anal fissure**
	Tonsillitis/sinusitis	**Infectious diarrhea**
	Gastritis	Polyp
	Mallory-Weiss tear	Hemorrhoids
	Gastric/duodenal ulcer	Inflammatory bowel disease
	Medications	Henoch-Schönlein purpura
	Tumors	Meckel diverticulum
	Hematologic disorders	Peptic ulcer
	Esophageal varices	Hemolytic-uremic syndrome
	Munchausen by proxy	Vascular malformations

*In order of frequency, most common in bold.

From Mezoff AG, Preud Homme DL: Contemp Pediatr 1994;11:60–92.

e. Other sources: Pneumonia, sickle cell anemia, diabetic ketoacidosis (DKA), juvenile rheumatoid arthritis (JRA).

2. Diagnosis:

a. History: Course and characterization of pain, diarrhea, melena, hematochezia, fever, last oral intake, menstrual history, vaginal discharge/bleeding, urinary symptoms, and respiratory symptoms. Also, assess past GI history, travel history, and diet.

b. Physical examination:

(1) General: Vital signs, toxicity, rashes, arthritis, jaundice.

(2) Abdominal: Moderate to severe abdominal tenderness on palpation, rebound/guarding, rigidity, masses, change in bowel sounds.

(3) Rectal: Include testing stool for occult blood.

(4) Pelvic: Discharge, masses, adnexal/cervical motion tenderness.

3. **Studies:**
a. Radiology: First obtain plain abdominal radiographs to assess for obstruction, constipation, free air, gallstones, kidney stones, and chest radiographs to check for pneumonia. Then consider abdominal/pelvic ultrasonography, abdominal spiral computed tomography (CT) with contrast (include rectal contrast for appendicitis evaluation), other contrast studies, and endoscopy.
b. Laboratory: Electrolytes, chemistry panel, CBC, liver and kidney function tests, coagulation studies, blood type and screen/cross-match, urinalysis, amylase, lipase, gonorrhea/chlamydia cultures (or ligase chain reaction [LCR] probes), beta-human chorionic gonadotropin (β-hCG), erythrocyte sedimentation rate (ESR), C-reactive protein (CRP).
4. **Management:**
a. Immediate: Patient should be placed on nothing by mouth (NPO) status. Begin rehydration. Consider nasogastric decompression, serial abdominal examinations, surgical/gynecological/GI evaluation as indicated, pain control (may confound examination), and antibiotics as indicated.
b. Definitive: Surgical or endoscopic exploration as warranted.

III. VOMITING

See Table 11-2 for evaluation of vomiting.

IV. GASTROESOPHAGEAL REFLUX DISEASE[2]

Gastroesophageal reflux (GER) is passage of gastric contents into the esophagus, and gastroesophageal reflux disease (GERD) is defined as symptoms or complications of gastroesophageal reflux.
1. **Diagnosis:**
a. History and physical examination: Usually sufficient to reliably diagnose GER, identify complications, and initiate management.
b. Upper GI series: Neither sensitive nor specific for GER. Useful for the evaluation of anatomic abnormalities.
c. Esophageal pH monitoring: Valid and reliable method of measuring acid reflux.
2. **Treatment options:**
a. Diet: Milk-thickening agents (e.g., cereal) may decrease frequency of vomiting. Trial of hypoallergenic formula (e.g., protein hydrolysate) in formula-fed infants.
b. Acid-suppressant therapy: PPIs and histamine-2 receptor antagonists (H_2 RAs) are effective in relieving symptoms and promoting mucosal healing. PPIs are superior to H_2 RAs for this purpose.
c. Prokinetic therapy: No available prokinetic agents have been shown to be effective in the management of GERD in children in pediatric (clinical) trials; however, metoclopramide and low-dose erythromycin can be used.

TABLE 11-2
EVALUATION OF VOMITING

Type	Etiology	Evaluation
Typically bilious	Obstruction Intussusception Malrotation ± volvulus Pancreatitis Intestinal dysmotility Peritoneal adhesions Incarcerated inguinal hernia Intestinal atresia, stenosis Superior mesenteric artery syndrome Incarcerated inguinal hernia	• Review feeding and medication history • NG/OG tube for decompression if GI obstruction is suspected • If bilious and/or hematemesis, consider surgical consultation • Serum electrolytes, CBC • Plain abdominal film with upright or cross-table lateral views of rule out obstruction, free air • Abdominal ultrasound if pyloric stenosis is suspected • Upper GI series to rule out pyloric stenosis, obstruction, anomalies, evaluate GI motility • Neurologic evaluation and imaging • Consider feeding modifications ± medications if GERD is suspected • Avoid antiemetics unless specific, benign etiology is identified
Typically nonbilious	Overfeeding GERD Milk-protein sensitivity Infection Peptic disease Drugs Electrolyte imbalance Eating disorders Necrotizing enterocolitis Metabolic abnormality Pyloric stenosis CNS lesion Esophageal/gastric atresia, stenosis Hirschsprung disease Annular pancreas Web	
Either bilious or nonbilious	Ileus Appendicitis	

Modified from Saavedra J: Gastroenterology. In Seidel H, et al: Primary Care of the Newborn. St. Louis, Mosby, 2001, pp 119–120; Murray K, et al: Vomiting. Pediatr Rev 1998;19(10):337–341.

3. Special considerations:

a. Infant with recurrent vomiting and poor weight gain: If poor weight gain is occurring despite adequate caloric intake, pursue evaluation to determine other potential causes of vomiting. Consider the following laboratory tests: CBC, electrolytes, bicarbonate, BUN/Cr, aminotransferases, ammonia, glucose, urinalysis, urine-reducing substances, and review of newborn screening tests. Upper GI series to evaluate anatomy.
b. GER and asthma: In patients with GER and asthma (or recurrent cough and wheezing as well as recurrent reflux), a 3-month trial of aggressive acid suppressant therapy should be considered. In patients with

persistent asthma without symptoms of GER, esophageal pH monitoring should be considered.

V. CELIAC DISEASE

Immune-mediated small bowel enteropathy caused by gluten sensitivity of the GI tract in genetically predisposed individuals has been found to be much more prevalent in the United States than estimated in the past.

1. **Symptoms:** May have variable presentation. Children may present with diarrhea, vomiting, failure to thrive, malaise, and/or signs and symptoms of hypoproteinemia. Often presents in combination with other autoimmune disorders (e.g., diabetes mellitus).
2. **Diagnosis:** Serologic studies for celiac disease include immunoglobulin A (IgA), endomysial IgA, antitissue transglutaminase, and antigliadin antibody assays. There is wide variation in test sensitivity and specificity between different laboratories. Also, test sensitivity may be affected by the severity of disease. In general, the antiendomysial antibody test is the most accurate, with moderate sensitivity and high specificity. The antitissue transglutaminase assay is more sensitive, yet less specific compared with the endomysial assay. The antigliadin assays are not as accurate diagnostically as the endomysial and antitissue transglutaminase assays. Biopsy of the small bowel should reveal villous flattening, which is reversible with elimination of gluten from diet.
3. **Management:** Gluten-free diet is the mainstay of treatment, with strict adherence necessary for villous recovery.

VI. EVALUATION OF LIVER TESTS

1. **Study results suggestive of liver cell injury:** Aspartate aminotransferase (AST), alanine aminotransferase (ALT), lactate dehydrogenase (LDH).
2. **Study results suggestive of cholestasis:** Increased bilirubin, urobilinogen, γ-glutamyltransferase (GGT), alkaline phosphatase, 5′-nucleotidase, serum bile acids.
3. **Tests of synthetic function:** Albumin, prealbumin, PT, activated partial prothrombin time (aPTT), cholesterol. Elevated NH3 is evidence of decreased ability to detoxify ammonia. See Table 11-3 for evaluation and interpretation of liver tests.

Note *See Chapter 15 for hepatitis immunization recommendations.*

VII. HYPERBILIRUBINEMIA[3,4]

Bilirubin is the product of hemoglobin metabolism. There are two forms: direct (conjugated) and indirect (unconjugated). Hyperbilirubinemia is usually the result of increased hemoglobin load, reduced hepatic uptake, reduced hepatic conjugation, or decreased excretion.

TABLE 11-3

EVALUATION OF LIVER FUNCTION TESTS

Enzyme	Source	Increased	Decreased	Comments
AST/ALT	Liver Heart Skeletal muscle Pancreas RBCs Kidney	Hepatocellular injury Rhabdomyolysis Muscular dystrophy Hemolysis Liver cancer	Vitamin B_6 deficiency Uremia	ALT more specific than AST for liver AST > ALT in hemolysis AST/ALT >2 in 90% of alcohol disorders in adults
Alkaline phosphatase	Liver Osteoblasts Small intestine Kidney Placenta	Hepatocellular injury Bone growth, disease, trauma Pregnancy Familial	Low phosphate Wilson disease Zinc deficiency Hypothyroidism Pernicious anemia	Highest in cholestatic conditions Must be differentiated from bone source
GGT	Bile ducts Renal tubules Pancreas Small intestine Brain	Cholestasis Newborn period Induced by drugs	Estrogen therapy Artificially low in hyperbilirubinemia	Not found in bone Increased in 90% primary liver disease Biliary obstruction Intrahepatic cholestasis Induced by alcohol Specific for hepatobiliary disease in nonpregnant patient
5′-NT	Liver cell membrane Intestine Brain Heart Pancreas	Cholestasis		Specific for hepatobiliary disease in nonpregnant patient
NH_3	Bowel Bacteria Protein metabolism	Hepatic disease secondary to urea cycle dysfunction Hemodialysis Valproic acid therapy Urea cycle enzyme deficiency Organic acidemia and carnitine deficiency		Converted to urea in liver

AST/ALT, aspartate aminotransferase/alanine aminotransterase; GGT, γ-glutamyl transpeptidase; 5′-NT, 5′-nucleotidase; RBCs, red blood cells.

Direct hyperbilirubinemia is defined as direct bilirubin >15% of total or direct bilirubin >2 mg/dL. See Box 11-1 for differential diagnosis of hyperbilirubinemia. Also refer to Chapter 17 for evaluation and treatment of newborn jaundice.

VIII. DIARRHEA

Usual stool output is 10 g/kg/day in children and 200 g/day in adults. Diarrhea is increased water in stool, resulting in increased stool frequency or loose consistency. Chronic diarrhea is diarrhea lasting more than 14 days. Acute diarrhea most commonly has an infectious, usually viral, etiology. A bacterial etiology is more common in bloody diarrhea; it is usually secretory or dysenteric. See Tables 11-4 and 11-5 for general treatment information.

The etiology of diarrhea may be *infectious* or *malabsorptive,* and the mechanism is osmotic or secretory. In *osmotic diarrhea,* stool volume depends on diet and decreases with fasting (fecal Na^+ <60 mOsm/L). In *secretory diarrhea,* stool volume is increased and does not vary with diet (fecal Na^+ >60 mOsm/L).

Oral rehydration therapy (ORT) is almost always successful and should be attempted with an appropriate oral rehydration solution in cases of mild to moderate dehydration. See Chapter 10 for calculation of deficit and maintenance fluid requirements and oral rehydration composition. Breast-feeding should continue, and a regular diet should be restarted as soon as the patient is rehydrated. Parenteral hydration is indicated in severe dehydration, hemodynamic instability, or failure of ORT.

IX. CONSTIPATION AND ENCOPRESIS

Constipation is the failure to evacuate the lower colon regularly and is defined clinically as painful passage of stools with hard consistency. There is a wide variation in normal stooling patterns from several times daily to weekly. Encopresis is the leakage of stool around impaction. This occurs with chronic constipation, in which there is a loss of sensation in the distended rectal vault.

A. DIFFERENTIAL DIAGNOSIS OF NONFUNCTIONAL CONSTIPATION

1. Neurologic (e.g., Hirschsprung disease, spinal pathology, botulism).
2. Obstructive (e.g., anal ring, small left colon, meconium ileus, mass).
3. Endocrine/metabolic (e.g., collagen vascular disease, hypothyroidism).
4. Medicinal (e.g., opiates, iron, tricyclic antidepressants, chemotherapy agents).

B. COMPLICATIONS

1. Abdominal pain.
2. Rectal fissures, ulcers, rectal prolapse.
3. UTI, urinary incontinence, ureteral obstruction.

BOX 11-1

DIFFERENTIAL DIAGNOSIS OF HYPERBILIRUBINEMIA

INDIRECT HYPERBILIRUBINEMIA

Transient Neonatal Jaundice
Physiologic jaundice
Breast-feeding jaundice
Breast milk jaundice
Reabsorption of extravascular blood
Polycythemia

Hemolytic Disorders
Blood group incompatibility
Hemoglobinopathies
Red cell membrane disorders
Microangiopathies
Red cell enzyme deficiencies
Autoimmune disease

Enterohepatic Recirculation
Hirschsprung disease
Cystic fibrosis
Ileal atresia
Pyloric stenosis

Disorders of Bilirubin Metabolism
Crigler-Najjar syndrome
Gilbert syndrome
Hypothyroidism
Hypoxia
Acidosis

Miscellaneous
Sepsis
Dehydration
Hypoalbuminemia
Drugs

DIRECT HYPERBILIRUBINEMIA

Biliary Obstruction
Biliary atresia
Paucity of intrahepatic bile ducts (Alagille)
Choledochal cyst
Inspissated bile syndrome
Fibrosing pancreatitis
Primary sclerosing cholangitis
Gallstones
Neoplasm

Infection
Sepsis
Urinary tract infection
Cholangitis
Liver abscess
Viral hepatitis
Herpes simplex virus
Varicella-zoster virus
Syphilis
Toxoplasmosis
Tuberculosis
Leptospirosis
Histoplasmosis
Toxocariasis

Metabolic Disorders
α_1-Antitrypsin deficiency
Cystic fibrosis
Galactosemia
Galactokinase deficiency
Wilson disease
Hereditary fructose intolerance
Niemann-Pick disease
Glycogen storage disease
Dubin-Johnson syndrome
Rotor syndrome

Chromosomal Abnormalities
Turner syndrome
Trisomy 18
Trisomy 21

Drugs
Aspirin
Acetaminophen
Iron
Isoniazid
Vitamin A
Erythromycin
Sulfonamides
Oxacillin
Rifampin
Ethanol
Steroids
Tetracycline
Methotrexate

Miscellaneous
Neonatal hepatitis syndrome
Parenteral alimentation
Reye syndrome

TABLE 11-4

TREATMENT RECOMMENDATIONS FOR BACTERIAL ENTERIC INFECTIONS

Organism	Clinical Syndrome	Treatment Recommendations	Therapy*
Salmonella	Diarrhea	No treatment, can prolong carriage	
	Invasive disease or: <3 mo of age Malignancy Hemoglobinopathy Immunosuppressed Chronic GI disease Severe colitis	Treatment recommended: length of treatment depends on site of infection; relapses are common, and retreatment recommended	Amoxicillin TMP/SMZ Third-generation cephalosporin
Shigella	Diarrhea or dysentery	Treatment shortens duration of signs and symptoms, eliminates organism from feces, prevents spread of organism	TMP/SMZ
Yersinia	Noninvasive diarrhea	Treatment in normal host does not have established benefit	
	Septicemia and infection other than GI tract	Treatment recommended	TMP/SMZ Third-generation cephalosporin
Campylobacter	Diarrhea or dysentery	Treatment shortens duration of illness; prevents relapse	Erythromycin
Escherichia coli EHEC (0157) (enterohemorrhagic)†	HUS	Antimicrobial therapy does not appear to prevent progression to HUS and routine antibiotics are discouraged	
EPEC (enteropathogenic)	Diarrhea	Nonabsorbable oral antibiotics	Gentamycin/neomycin
	Chronic carriage	Absorbable oral antibiotics	TMP/SMZ
ETEC (enterotoxigenic)	Diarrhea	Disease usually self-limited, and no treatment recommended	
EIEC (enteroinvasive)	Diarrhea	Treatment recommended	

*Definitive therapy should be based on culture sensitivities.

†From Wong S, et al: N Engl J Med 2000;342(26):1930–1936.

HUS, hemolytic-uremic syndrome; TMP/SMZ, trimethoprim/sulfamethoxazole.

TABLE 11-5
TREATMENT OF PARASITIC ENTERIC INFECTIONS

Orgainsm	Clinical Syndrome	Treatment Recommendations	Antiparasitic
Giardia lamblia	Asymptomatic carriage	No treatment unless household member with: Pregnancy Cystic fibrosis Hypogammaglobulinemia	Metronidazole
	Diarrhea	Symptomatic disease should be treated	Metronidazole Furazolidone
Amebae	Asymptomatic	Treatment recommended for all infection	Paromomycin
	Diarrhea/dysentery	Treatment recommended for all infection	Metronidazole followed by iodoquinol
	Extraintestinal		

4. **Stasis syndrome with bacterial overgrowth.**
5. **Social isolation.**

C. TREATMENT OF FUNCTIONAL CONSTIPATION: LONG-TERM BEHAVIORAL MODIFICATION ALONG WITH MEDICATION

The goal of treatment of functional constipation is weaning of medication once normal colorectal sensation and stooling patterns have been established. The three stages of treatment are as follows:

1. **Disimpaction (2–5 days):** This may be accomplished with oral and/or rectal medication. Enemas may be attempted at home once daily for 2 to 5 days. Prolonged use of hypertonic phosphate enemas may result in hypophosphatemia and hypocalcemia. Refractory constipation may require colonic lavage with isotonic polyethylene glycol-electrolyte solution (see Formulary for dosage). This can be given orally at home or via nasogastric (NG) tube in the hospital.

a. Enema (see Formulary for dosage):
   (1) Mineral oil.
   (2) Hypertonic phosphate.
   (3) Milk and molasses, 50:50 mix up to 6-oz maximum.

b. Oral/nasogastric (see Formulary for dosage):
   (1) Sodium phosphate oral solution (Fleet Phospho-Soda).
   (2) Magnesium citrate.
   (3) Polyethylene glycol: Also available for outpatient use (MiraLax): In adults, dissolve 17 g in 8 oz water once daily for up to 2 weeks.
   (4) Mineral oil: Use with caution in patients younger than 1 year of age and in those with neurologic impairment because of risk for aspiration.

2. **Sustained evacuation (usually 3–12 months):** This stage restores normal colorectal tone and requires habitual toilet use with positive rewards and behavioral therapy. Initial diet should be low in fiber, with a transition to a high-fiber diet once disimpaction has occurred. Medications include lubricants, hyperosmolar sugars, and stimulants. These medications can also be used for mild constipation. See Formulary for specific dosages. Generic names of medications follow:
a. Fiber supplements: Barley malt, cellulose, psyllium, polycarbophil.
b. Lubricants: Mineral oil, surfactant.
c. Hyperosmolar sugars: Fructose/sorbitol (prune juice); lactulose (do not use in patients younger than 6 months).
d. Laxatives and stool softeners: Magnesium hydroxide, senna, diphenylmethane, docusate sodium, bisacodyl, glycerin.
3. **Gradual weaning from medications.**

X. MISCELLANEOUS TESTS

A. OCCULT BLOOD

1. **Purpose:** To screen for the presence of blood through detection of heme in stool.
2. **Method:** Smear a small amount of stool on the test areas of an occult blood test card and allow to air dry. Apply developer as directed.
3. **Interpretation:** A blue color resembling that of the control indicates the presence of heme. Brisk transit of ingested red meat and inorganic iron may yield a false-positive result. Screening for the presence of blood in gastric aspirates or vomitus should be performed using Gastroccult, not stool Hemoccult, cards.

B. TESTS FOR FAT MALABSORPTION: QUANTITATIVE FECAL FAT

1. **Purpose:** To screen for fat malabsorption by quantitating fecal fat excretion.
2. **Method:** Patient should be on a normal diet (35% fat) with the amount of calories and fat ingested recorded for 2 days before the test and during the test itself. Collect and freeze all stools passed within 72 hours, and send to the laboratory for determination of total fecal fatty acid content.
3. **Interpretation:**
a. Total fecal fatty acid excretion of >5 g fat per 24 hours may suggest malabsorption.

Note *Results will vary with amount of fat ingested, and normal values have not been established for children <2 years old.*

b. The coefficient of absorption (CA) is a more accurate indicator of malabsorption and does not vary with fat intake: CA = (grams of fat ingested – grams of fat excreted)/(grams of fat ingested) × 100.

Note *Quantitative fecal fat is recommended over qualitative methods (e.g., staining with Sudan III), which depend on spot checks and are thus unreliable for diagnosing fat malabsorption.*

REFERENCES

1. Moir CR: Abdominal pain in infants and children. Mayo Clin Proc 1996;71:(10)984–989.
2. Rudolph CD, et al: Guidelines for evaluation and treatment of gastroesophageal reflux in infants and children: Recommendations of the North American Society for Pediatric Gastroenterology and Nutrition. J Pediatr Gastroenterol Nutr 2001;S1–S31.
3. Provisional Committee for Quality Improvement and Subcommittee on Hyperbilirubinemia Practice Parameter: Management of hyperbilirubinemia in the healthy term newborn. Pediatrics 1994;94:558–565.
4. Gartner L: Neonatal jaundice. Pediatr Rev 1994;15(11)422–431.

Genetics

Ai Sakonju, MD and Jennifer Huffman, MD

When evaluating any child for a genetic disorder, one of the most valuable tools is the three-generation pedigree. For each family member, note age, gender, and medical status or cause of death. Specifically ask about family history of neonatal or childhood deaths, mental retardation, developmental delay, birth defects, seizure disorders, known genetic disorders, ethnicity, consanguinity, infertility, miscarriages, and stillbirths.

12

I. WEBSITES

http://genes-r-us.uthscsa.edu/resources.htm

www.ncbi.nlm.nih.gov/omim (Online Mendelian Inheritance in Man [OMIM] website for free text searches of patient findings and diagnostic differentials)

www.genetests.org (online list of genetic diagnostic tests, genetics clinics, and a glossary of terms)

II. MANAGEMENT OF GENETIC DISEASES WITH ACUTE PRESENTATION: INBORN ERRORS OF METABOLISM[1–5]

Inborn errors of metabolism (IEMs) may present any time from the neonatal period to adulthood. Although these disorders are often thought of as rare, when considered collectively, they represent significant treatable causes of morbidity and mortality.

A. PRESENTATIONS

1. **Neonatal onset:** Often presents with anorexia, lethargy, vomiting, and/or seizures. Symptoms often develop at 24 to 72 hours of age. One in five sick full-term neonates with no risk factors for infection will have metabolic disease.
2. **Late onset (>28 days old):** Some IEMs characteristically present late, whereas others present beyond the newborn period if the defect is partial.

a. Typical symptoms: Vomiting, respiratory distress, and changes in mental status, including confusion, lethargy, irritability, aggressive behavior, hallucinations, seizures, and coma.

b. Symptoms are usually brought on by intercurrent illness, prolonged fast, dietary indiscretion, or any process causing increased catabolism.

B. EVALUATION OF SUSPECTED METABOLIC DISEASE

1. For laboratory tests recommended to detect IEMs, see Box 12-1. For sample collection requirements, see Table 12-1.
2. If the initial evaluation is suspicious for metabolic disease, obtain further testing as listed in Box 12-1 and consult a geneticist. *Early diagnosis and appropriate therapy are essential for preventing irreversible brain damage and death.*

BOX 12-1

LABORATORY TESTS FOR INBORN ERRORS OF METABOLISM

Initial Tests

Complete blood count with differential
Serum electrolytes (calculate anion gap)
Blood glucose
Aspartate aminotransferase (AST)
Alanine aminotransferase (ALT)
Total and direct bilirubin
Blood gas
Plasma ammonium
Plasma lactate
Urine dipstick: pH, ketones, glucose, protein, bilirubin
Urine odor (see Table 12-2)
Urine-reducing substances (Clinitest tablet [Ames Co.], identifies all reducing substances in urine; see Box 12-2)
Acylcarnitine profile

Further Testing If Workup Is Suspicious

Plasma amino acids
Quantitative plasma carnitine
Urine organic acids
If lactate level is elevated, serum pyruvate and repeat lactate level.

BOX 12-2

DISORDERS ASSOCIATED WITH A POSITIVE URINE-REDUCING SUBSTANCES TEST

Galactose: Galactosemia, galactokinase deficiency, severe liver disease
Fructose: Hereditary fructose intolerance, essential fructosuria
Glucose: Diabetes mellitus, renal tubular defects
p-Hydroxyphenylpyruvic acid: Tyrosinemia
Xylose: Pentosuria

C. DIFFERENTIAL DIAGNOSIS

1. Differential diagnosis of hyperammonemia (Fig. 12-1).
2. Differential diagnosis of hypoglycemia (see section II.E).
3. Abnormal urine odors (Table 12-2).
4. Positive urine reducing substances (Box 12-2).

D. GENERAL ACUTE MANAGEMENT OF INBORN ERRORS OF METABOLISM

1. **Stop dietary sources of protein.**
2. **Start intravenous (IV) fluids:** D_{10} at 1.5 to 2 times maintenance dose delivers 10 to 15 mg/kg/min of glucose to stop catabolism.

TABLE 12-1

SAMPLE COLLECTION

Specimen	Volume (mL)	Tube*	Handling
Plasma ammonium	1–3	Green or purple top (check with your lab)	On ice; immediate transport to laboratory; levels rise rapidly on standing
Plasma amino acids†	1–3	Green top	On ice; if must store, spin down, separate plasma, and freeze
Plasma carnitine	1–3	Green top	On ice
Acylcarnitine profile	Saturate newborn screen filter paper with blood		Dry and mail to reference laboratory
Lactate	3	Gray top	On ice
Karyotype	3	Green top	Room temperature
Very-long-chain fatty acids	3	Purple top	Room temperature
White blood cells for enzymes/DNA	3	Purple top	Room temperaure
Urine organic acids	5–10	—	Deliver immediately or freeze
Urine amino acids	5–10	—	Deliver immediately or freeze
Skin biopsy		Tissue culture medium or patient's plasma	Refrigerate; do not freeze

*Additives in tubes: purple, K3EDTA; green, lithium heparin; gray, potassium oxalate and sodium fluoride.
†Obtain after a 3–hour fast.

TABLE 12-2

UNUSUAL URINE ODORS

Disease	Odor
ACUTE DISEASE	
Maple syrup urine disease	Maple syrup, burned sugar
Isovaleric acidemia	Cheesy or sweaty feet
Multiple carboxylase deficiency	Cat urine
3-OH,3-methyl glutaryl-CoA lyase deficiency	Cat urine
NONACUTE DISEASE	
Phenylketonuria	Musty
Hypermethioninemia	Rancid butter, rotten cabbage
Trimethylaminuria	Fishy

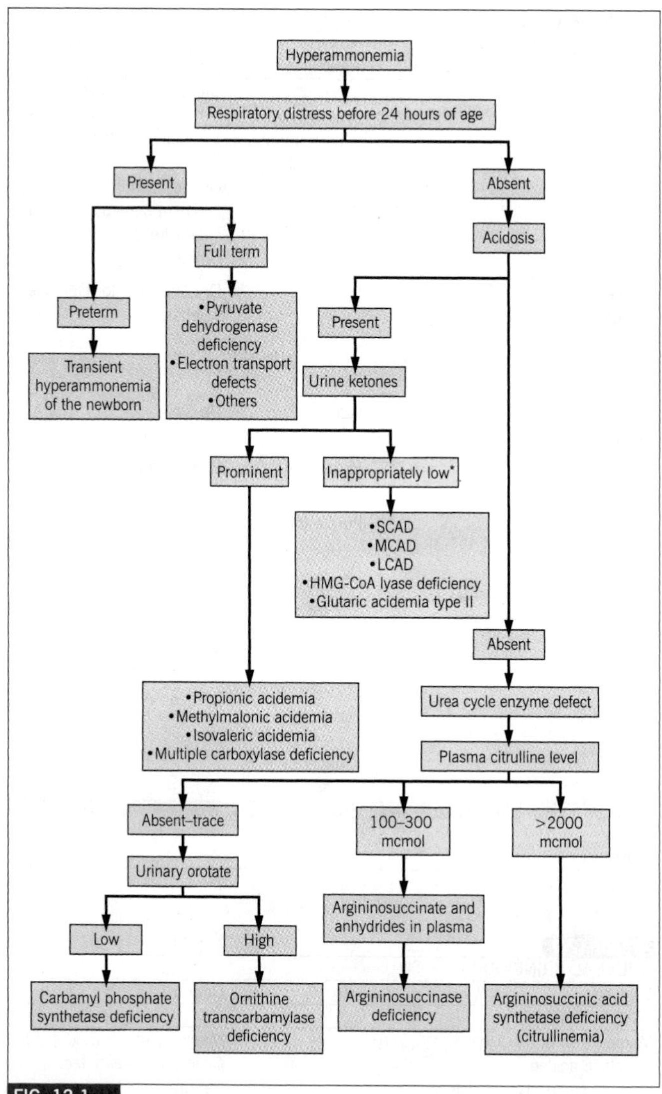

FIG. 12-1

Differential diagnosis of hyperammonemia. HMG-CoA, hydroxymethylglutaryl-CoA; LCAD, long-chain acyl-CoA dehydrogenase; MCAD, medium-chain acyl-CoA dehydrogenase; SCAD, short-chain acyl-CoA dehydrogenase.

*Indicates inappropriately low urinary ketones in setting of symptomatic hypoglycemia.

(A catabolic state results in an endogenous protein load.) Add Na^+/K^+ based on the degree of dehydration and electrolyte levels. In severe dehydration, give a normal saline (NS) bolus in addition to D_{10} at 1.5 to 2 times the maintenance dose to stop catabolism.

3. Provide HCO_3^- replacement for severe acidosis (pH <7.1) only.
4. In cases of hyperammonemia, the following experimental drugs may be used. They should only be used in consultation with a geneticist because overdoses may be lethal: sodium benzoate 250 mg/kg (5.5 g/m^2) IV; sodium phenylacetate 250 mg/kg (5.5 g/m^2) IV; and arginine-HCl (10% solution) 6 mL/kg (12 g/m^2) IV. Give these doses as a bolus over 90 minutes. Repeat the same doses over 24 hours as a maintenance dose. Ondansetron may be used to decrease nausea and vomiting associated with these drugs. (Benzoate and phenylacetate are substrates for alternate pathways of nitrogen excretion; arginine supplementation allows continued operation of the urea cycle in defects in which the block is proximal to arginine.)
5. If the patient's condition is unresponsive to above management, hemodialysis should be initiated. Hemodialysis is often required in neonates because of their inherently catabolic state. Exchange transfusion should not be used.
6. Long-term therapy will likely include protein restriction, citrulline supplementation, and oral sodium phenylbutyrate (Buphenyl).

E. HYPOGLYCEMIA

A glucose concentration <40 mg/dL typically is considered hypoglycemia. Potential causes include endocrine disorders or IEMs, including defects in gluconeogenesis, glycogen breakdown (glycogen storage diseases), and fatty acid oxidation, or toxic impairment of gluconeogenesis (organic acidemias).

1. **History questions:** What is the patient's age? What is the relationship between the hypoglycemia and caloric intake? (Does it occur postprandially or after prolonged fasting, or is it constant?) Is the patient septic? Does the patient have hepatomegaly?
2. **Laboratory evaluation** (ideally, collect samples before glucose administration): Complete metabolic panel, including liver function tests (LFTs), insulin, cortisol, growth hormone, acylcarnitine profile, and urinary ketones. Hypoglycemia with inappropriately low urinary ketones is the hallmark of fatty acid oxidation disorders. Consult a geneticist to help interpret laboratory results and further guide the workup.

III. NONACUTE MANAGEMENT OF GENETIC DISEASES

A. NEWBORN METABOLIC SCREEN

All states screen for phenylketonuria and hypothyroidism; for a list of screening tests and number of states that use each test, see website:

http://genes-r-us.uthscsa.edu/resources.htm. **A normal newborn screen does not imply that there are no genetic abnormalities.**

1. **Timing:**
   a. Screen after at least 24 hours of normal protein and lactose feeding. Formula-fed infants may not have a diagnostic abnormality before 36 hours of age. Breast-fed infants may not have a diagnostic abnormality before 48 to 72 hours of age.
   b. Recommendations from the American Academy of Pediatrics:
      (1) Screen all infants before hospital discharge. For normal term infants, screen as close as possible to hospital discharge.
      (2) All infants should be screened by 7 days of age. If first screen is before 24 hours of age, rescreen by 14 days of age.

Note *Many geneticists recommend rescreening at 14 days of age if the first screen is before 48 hours of age.*

B. DEGENERATIVE DISORDERS

Note *Many are progressive neurodegenerative disorders; an exhaustive list is beyond the scope of this chapter.*

1. **Lysosomal disorders:** Lysosomal disorders (e.g., the mucopolysaccharidoses) include neurodegeneration with systemic storage resulting from lysosomal enzyme defects (e.g., Hurler, Hunter, Scheie, Sanfilippo, and Sly syndromes).
   a. **Presentation:** Hepatosplenomegaly, corneal clouding (except Hunter syndrome), dysostosis multiplex, coarse features, neurologic deterioration.
   b. **Laboratory findings:** Inclusion bodies on peripheral blood smear, positive urine mucopolysaccharide (MPS) spot; characteristic findings on eye examination and skeletal survey.
   c. **Definitive diagnosis:** Assay of skin fibroblasts for specific lysosomal hydrolases.
   d. **Therapy:** Experimental therapy with exogenous enzyme; bone marrow transplantation may provide some enzyme activity but cannot reverse brain damage.
2. **Peroxisomal disorders:** Peroxisomal disorders include Refsum syndrome, X-linked adrenoleukodystrophy (ALD), Zellweger syndrome, and others.
   a. **Presentation:** Seizures, loss of milestones, loss of white matter on magnetic resonance imaging (MRI) scans. There is progressive neurodegeneration and eventually death.
   b. **Laboratory findings:** Elevated very-long-chain fatty acids, pipecolic acid, phytanic acid, and plasmalogens.
   c. **Definitive diagnosis:** Enzyme assays in cultured skin fibroblasts and microscopy of peroxisomes.

d. **Therapy:** Treat adrenal insufficiency if present; provide vitamin K. Research protocols include dietary lipid therapy, bone marrow transplantation, and immunosuppression.

IV. DYSMORPHOLOGY

The suspicion for many syndromes and chromosomal anomalies is often raised by major or minor anomalies noted on physical examination. The most common anomalies and commonly used diagnostic tests are listed here. More complete information can be found in reference works by Hall and colleagues[6] and Jones.[7] In addition to well-known syndromes, many rare genetic disorders are listed in reference works.[7,8]

A. PHYSICAL EXAMINATION

1. **Head:** Hypotelorism; hypertelorism (for inner and outer canthal distance charts, see Jones[7]); abnormal palpebral fissure length and angle[6] or epicanthal folds; long, short, or flat philtrum; ear pits or tags; low-set or posteriorly rotated ears; micrognathia; retrognathia.
2. **Skeletal:** Fifth-digit clinodactyly, syndactyly, polydactyly. Rhizomelic shortening (shortening of proximal long bones) is typical of conditions such as achondroplasia. Proportionate dwarfism is characteristic of growth hormone deficiency. The upper-to-lower segment ratio is low in Marfan syndrome.

B. STRUCTURAL DIAGNOSTIC TESTS

1. Brain MRI.
2. Ophthalmologic examination for optic atrophy, coloboma, cataracts, retinal abnormalities, lens subluxation, or corneal abnormalities.
3. Echocardiogram.
4. Abdominal ultrasound for polysplenia or asplenia, absent or horseshoe kidney, ureteral or bladder defects, and abdominal situs.
5. Skeletal survey for abnormalities of bone length or structure.

C. GENETIC DIAGNOSTIC TESTS

1. **Karyotype:** Detects abnormal numbers of chromosomes and deletions, duplications, translocations, and inversions large enough to be seen by light microscopy. For indications, see section VI.
2. **Fluorescence in situ hybridization (FISH):** Hybridization of a fluorescently tagged DNA probe to chromosomes allows detection of submicroscopic deletions and duplications. FISH assays are commonly available for the following syndromes: Williams (7q11), Prader-Willi and Angelman (15q11), Miller-Dieker (17p13.3), Smith-Magenis (17p11.2), velocardiofacial and DiGeorge (22q11). Telomere deletions and many other genetic disorders are also testable by FISH. For a complete, updated online list of genetic diagnostic tests, see www.genetests.org.

3. **Deoxyribonucleic acid (DNA) analysis:** Many monogenic disorders now have DNA tests available. Contact your laboratory or www.genetests.org for a list of those available.

V. COMMON SYNDROMES

For more information on common syndromes and other chromosomal abnormalities and syndromes, see Jones.[7]

A. TRISOMY 21 (Incidence: 1:660)

1. **Features:** Presence of 6 of the following 10 cardinal features in the neonate is highly suggestive of the diagnosis of trisomy 21: hypotonia, poor Moro reflex, hyperflexibility, excess skin on back of the neck, flat facies, slanted palpebral fissures, anomalous auricles, pelvic dysplasia, dysplasia of the mid-phalanx of the fifth finger, and a single transverse palmar (simian) crease.
2. **Associated findings:** Mental retardation (100%), hearing loss (75%), eye disease (60%), serous otitis media (50% to 70%), cardiac defects (50%), thyroid disease (15%), gastrointestinal (GI) atresias (12%), atlantoaxial instability (12%), and leukemia (1%).
3. **Testing:** Karyotype for diagnosis, echocardiogram, yearly thyroid function tests, LFTs, complete blood count (CBC), and audiologic evaluation; radiographs of the atlantooccipital junction and ophthalmologic examination by 3 to 5 years of age.[9]
4. **Natural history:** Growth charts for children with trisomy 21 appear in Chapter 20. Approximately 50% of those with congenital heart defects survive to age 30 years; 80% of those without congenital heart defects survive to age 30 years.

B. TRISOMY 18 (Incidence: 1:3000, with 3:1 female predominance)

1. **Features:** Clenched hand, with index finger overlapping third and fifth finger overlapping fourth, intrauterine growth retardation (IUGR), decreased fetal activity, low-arch dermal ridge pattern, inguinal or umbilical hernia, cardiac defects, prominent occiput, low-set ears, micrognathia, rocker bottom feet.
2. **Testing:** Karyotype with FISH analysis allows results within 24 to 48 hours.
3. **Natural history:** Apnea, severe failure to thrive; 50% die by 1 week, 90% by 1 year; profound mental retardation in survivors.

C. TRISOMY 13 (Incidence: 1:5000)

1. **Features:** Holoprosencephaly, polydactyly, scalp skin defects, seizures, deafness, microcephaly, sloping forehead, cleft lip, cleft palate, retinal anomalies, microphthalmia, abnormal ears, single umbilical artery, inguinal hernia, omphalocele, cardiac defects, urinary tract malformations.

2. **Testing:** Karyotype with FISH analysis allows results within 24 to 48 hours.
3. **Natural history:** 44% die within 1 month; >70% die by 1 year; profound mental retardation in survivors.

D. **TURNER SYNDROME—45,X (Incidence: 1:5000)**

1. **Features:** Short female with broad chest, wide-spaced nipples, webbed neck, congenital lymphedema.
2. **Associated findings:** Gonadal dysgenesis (90%), renal anomalies (60%), cardiac defects (20%), most commonly coarctation of the aorta, hearing loss (50%).
3. **Testing:** Karyotype for diagnosis. Baseline echocardiogram, renal ultrasound; blood pressure (BP), hearing, and scoliosis screen with each examination; thyroid function tests and echocardiogram every 1 to 2 years.[10]
4. **Natural history:** Infertility, normal lifespan, mean IQ 90, short stature. Growth charts for girls with Turner syndrome appear in Chapter 20.

E. **FRAGILE X (Incidence: 1:1500 males)**

1. **Features:** Boys—mild to profound mental retardation (6% of boys with mental retardation), cluttered speech, autism (60%), macrocephaly, large ears, prognathism, postpubertal macroorchidism, tall stature. Phenotype most prominent in boys; girls may have only learning disabilities.
2. **Testing:** Fragile X is caused by an expansion of a CGG nucleotide repeat in the *FMR1* gene. The size of the repeat correlates with disease severity. Diagnosis is established by DNA analysis.
3. **Natural history:** Normal lifespan.

F. **MARFAN SYNDROME (Incidence: 2–3:10,000)**

1. **Features:** There are major and minor diagnostic criteria involving the skeletal, ocular, cardiovascular, and pulmonary systems, and skin or integument. Features include but are not limited to tall stature, low upper-to-lower segment ratio, arachnodactyly, joint laxity, scoliosis, pectus excavatum or carinatum, lens subluxation, glaucoma, retinal detachment, dilation with or without dissecting aneurysm of ascending aorta, mitral valve prolapse, lumbosacral dural ectasia by computed tomography (CT) or MRI scans, and inguinal and/or femoral hernias.
2. **Testing:** Slit-lamp examination, echocardiogram, genetic evaluation. Diagnosis is made clinically and requires major criteria in at least two different organ systems and involvement of a third organ system. For a complete list of criteria, see Scriver and associates[3] and De Paepe and colleagues.[11]
3. **Natural history:** Patients with aortic root dilation > 2 standard deviations (SD) above the mean should be treated with atenolol and

followed with a yearly echocardiogram. Significant aortic root dilation requires surgical repair. With corrective surgery, mean age of survival approaches normal life span; this is significantly lower in patients with untreated vascular complications.[12]

G. 22Q11 SYNDROME

1. **Synonyms:** DiGeorge syndrome, velocardiofacial syndrome (VCFS), Shprintzen syndrome, conotruncal anomaly face syndrome (CTAF).
2. **Features:** Congenital heart defects, palatal abnormalities, immune deficiency (defective T-cell function), hypocalcemia (parathyroid involvement), characteristic facial features.
3. **Testing:** FISH analysis for 22q11.2 deletion and routine cytogenetics to evaluate for chromosomal rearrangement (<1% cases). Measure serum calcium, absolute lymphocyte count, B- and T-cell subsets if lymphopenic, renal ultrasound for structural abnormalities, chest x-ray for thoracic vertebral anomalies, baseline cardiac evaluation including echocardiogram.
4. **Natural history:** More than 90% of patients have speech and language delay, learning disabilities, and feeding difficulties. There is an increased risk for mental retardation, and approximately 25% of patients have psychiatric illness. Parents should also be tested because of an up to 28% risk for being carriers of the deletion.

VI. GENETIC CONSULTATION

A. INDICATIONS FOR REFERRAL

1. Known or suspected hereditary disorder.
2. Major physical anomalies, unusual body proportions, short stature, dysmorphic features.
3. Major organ malformation.
4. Developmental delay or mental retardation; learning disabilities in females who have brothers with mental retardation.
5. Complete or partial blindness or hearing loss.
6. Deterioration of motor or speech abilities in a previously thriving child.
7. Maternal exposure to drugs, alcohol, or radiation during pregnancy.
8. Strong family history of cancer.
9. Failure to thrive if routine evaluation is unrevealing.

B. INDICATIONS FOR PRENATAL COUNSELING

1. Genetic disorder or birth defect in one partner.
2. Known carrier of a genetic disorder.
3. Previous child with known or suspected genetic disorder.
4. Maternal age ≥35 years.
5. Family history of known or suspected chromosomal anomaly.
6. Multiple early miscarriages or stillbirths.

7. Member of an ethnic group known to have a high incidence of a specific genetic disorder.

C. INDICATIONS FOR KARYOTYPE

1. Two major *or* one major and two minor malformations (include small for gestational age and mental retardation as major).
2. Features of a specific chromosomal syndrome.
3. At risk for familial chromosomal aberration.
4. Ambiguous genitalia.
5. More than two spontaneous abortions or infertility (karyotype both partners).
6. Girls with short stature.

REFERENCES

1. Epstein CJ (assoc. ed): Genetic disorders and birth defects. In Rudolph AM, Rudolph CD, et al (eds): Rudolph's Pediatrics, 21st ed. Norwalk, CT, Appleton & Lange, 2003.
2. Fernandes J, Sauderbray J-M, Vanden Berghe G: Inborn Metabolic Diseases, 3rd ed. Berlin, Springer-Verlag, 2000.
3. Scriver CR, et al: The Molecular and Metabolic Bases of Inherited Disease, 8th ed. New York, McGraw-Hill, 2001.
4. Seashore M, Wappner R: Genetics in Primary Care and Clinical Medicine. Norwalk, CT, Appleton & Lange, 1996.
5. Seidel HM, Rosenstein BJ, Pathak A: Primary Care of the Newborn, 3rd ed. St. Louis, Mosby, 2001.
6. Hall JG, Froster-Iskenius UG, Allanson JE: Handbook of Normal Physical Measurements. Oxford, UK, Oxford Medical Publications, 1989.
7. Jones K: Smith's Recognizable Patterns of Human Malformation, 5th ed. Philadelphia, WB Saunders, 1997.
8. Gorlin R, Cohen M, Hennekan R: Syndromes of the Head and Neck, 4th ed. New York, Oxford University Press, 2001.
9. American Academy of Pediatrics, Committee on Genetics: Health supervision for children with Down syndrome. Pediatrics 2001;107:442–449.
10. American Academy of Pediatrics, Committee on Genetics: Health supervision for children with Turner syndrome. Pediatrics 2003;111:692–702.
11. De Paepe A, et al: Revised diagnostic criteria for the Marfan syndrome. Am J Med Genet 1996;62:417.
12. American Academy of Pediatrics, Committee on Genetics: Health supervision of children with Marfan syndrome. Pediatrics 1996;98:978–982.

Hematology

Marissa Brunetti, MD and Joanna Cohen, MD

13

I. ANEMIA

A. GENERAL EVALUATION

Anemia is defined by age-specific norms (Fig. 13-1 and Table 13-1). Evaluation includes the following:

1. **Complete history:** Includes melena, hematochezia, blood loss, fatigue, pica, medication exposure, growth and development, nutritional history, ethnic background, and family history of anemia, splenectomy, or cholecystectomy.
2. **Physical examination:** Includes pallor, jaundice (including scleral icterus), glossitis, tachypnea, tachycardia, cardiac murmur, hepatosplenomegaly, and signs of systemic illness.
3. **Initial laboratory tests:** May include a complete blood count (CBC) with red blood cell (RBC) indices, reticulocyte count, blood smear, stool for occult blood, urinalysis, and serum bilirubin.

B. DIAGNOSIS

Anemias may be categorized as macrocytic, microcytic, or normocytic. Table 13-2 gives a differential diagnosis of anemia based on RBC production and cell size. Note that normal ranges for hemoglobin (Hb) and mean corpuscular volume (MCV) are age dependent (see Fig. 13-1 and Table 13-1).

C. EVALUATION OF SPECIFIC CAUSES OF ANEMIA

1. **Iron-deficiency anemia:** Hypochromic/microcytic anemia with a low reticulocyte count and an elevated red cell distribution width (RDW).

a. Serum ferritin reflects total body iron stores after 6 months of age and is the first value to fall in iron deficiency. Ferritin is an acute-phase reactant, and it may be falsely elevated with inflammation or infection. See Chapter 25 for normal ferritin values.

b. Other indicators include low serum iron and/or transferrin levels and an elevated total iron-binding capacity (TIBC). See Chapter 25 for normal iron, transferrin, and TIBC values.

c. Free erythrocyte protoporphyrin (FEP) accumulates when the conversion of protoporphyrin to heme is blocked. FEP is elevated in iron deficiency, plumbism, and erythrocyte protoporphyria. Levels >300 μg/dL are generally found only with lead intoxication.

d. Iron therapy (see Formulary for dosage information) should result in an increased reticulocyte count in 2 to 3 days and an increase in hematocrit (HCT) after 1 to 4 weeks of therapy. Iron stores are generally repleted with 3 months of therapy.

2. **Hemolytic anemia:** Rapid RBC turnover. Etiologies include congenital membranopathies, hemoglobinopathies, enzymopathies, metabolic

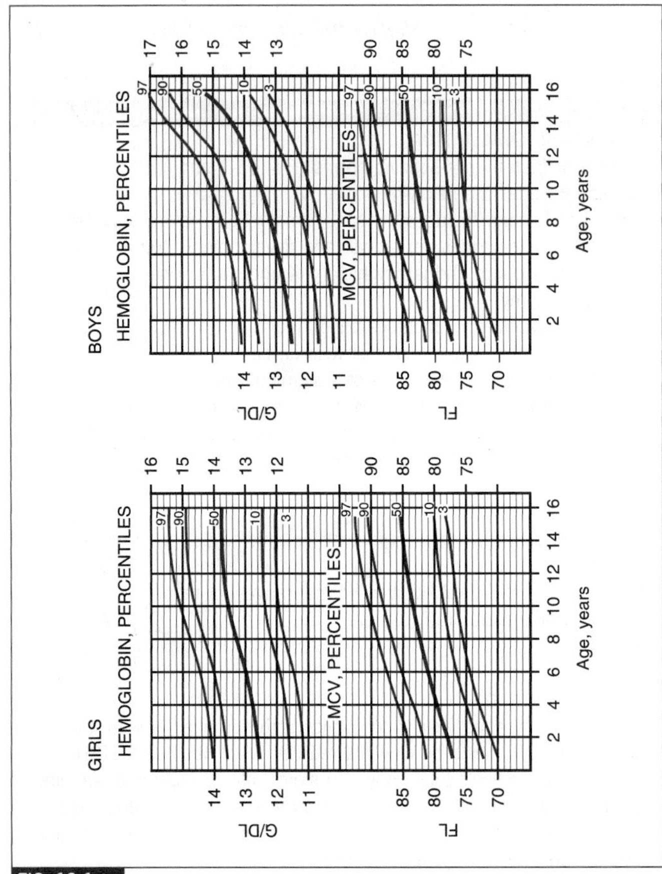

FIG. 13-1

Hemoglobin and mean corpuscular volume by age and gender. *(Data from Dallman PR, Siimes MA: J Pediatr 1979;94:26.)*

defects, and immune-mediated destruction. Useful studies include the following:

a. **Reticulocyte count:** Usually elevated and indicates increased production of RBCs to compensate for increased destruction. Corrected reticulocyte count (CRC): Corrected for differences in HCT, CRC is an indicator of erythropoietic activity. A CRC >1.5 suggests increased RBC production as a result of hemolysis or blood loss.

$$CRC = \%\ \text{reticulocytes} \times \text{patient HCT/normal HCT}$$

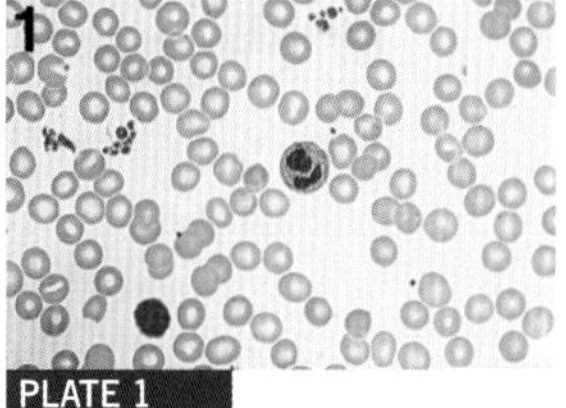

PLATE 1

Normal smear. Round RBCs with central pallor about one third of the cell's diameter, scattered platelets, occasional white blood cells.

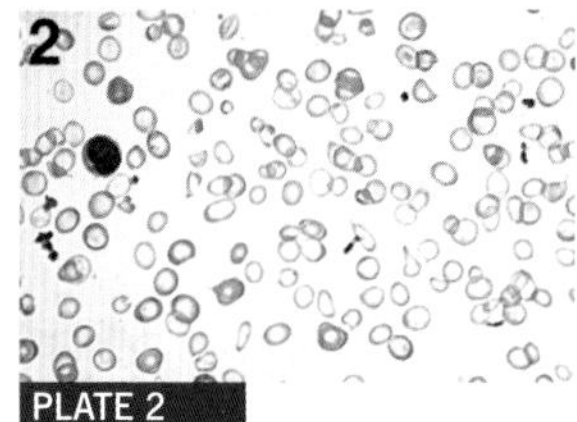

PLATE 2

Iron deficiency. Hypochromic/microcytic RBCs, poikilocytosis, plentiful platelets, occasional ovalocytes, and target cells. Basophilic stippling may also be present, as in lead intoxication and β-thalassemia.

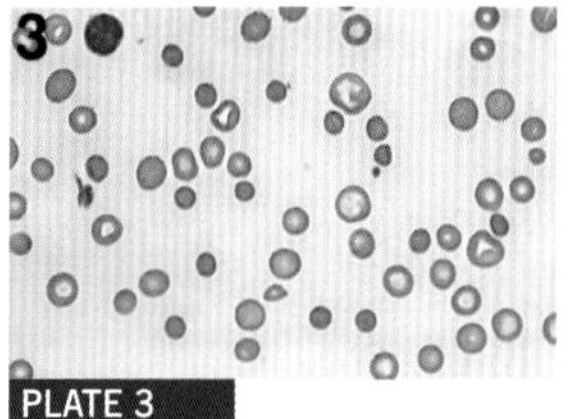

PLATE 3

Spherocytosis. Microspherocytes a hallmark (densely stained RBCs with no central pallor).

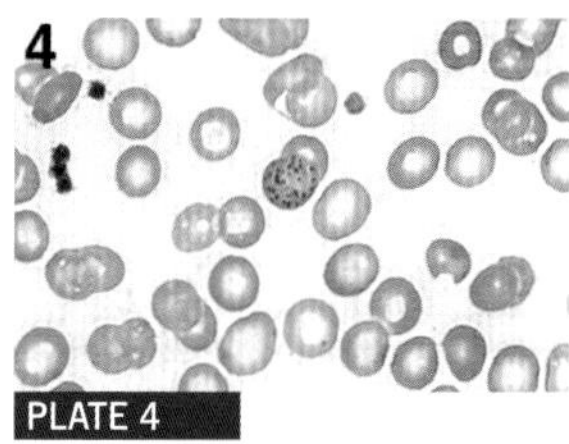

PLATE 4

Basophilic stippling as a result of staining of ribosomal complexes containing RNA throughout the cell; seen with heavy metal intoxication, thalassemia, pyrimidine 5′-nucleotidase deficiency, iron deficiency, and other states associated with ineffective erythropoiesis.

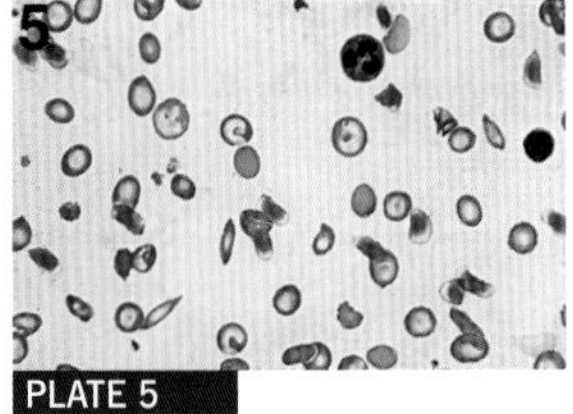

PLATE 5

Hemoglobin SS disease. Sickled cells, target cells, hypochromia, poikilocytosis, Howell-Jolly bodies, nucleated RBCs common (not shown).

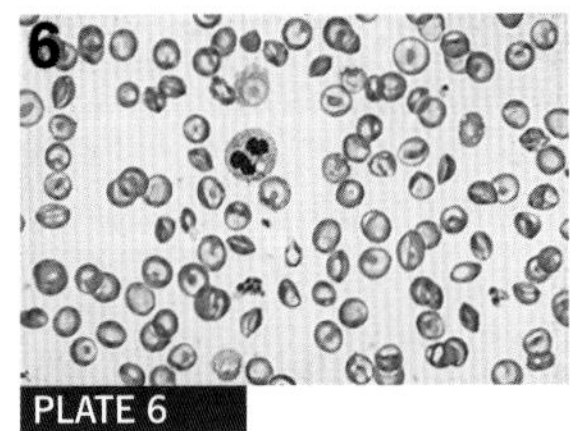

PLATE 6

Hemoglobin SC disease. Target cells, "oat cells," poikilocytosis; sickle forms rarely seen.

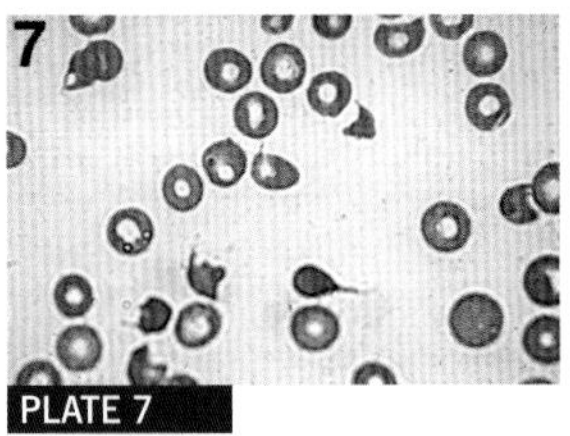

PLATE 7

Microangiopathic hemolytic anemia. RBC fragments, anisocytosis, polychromasia, decreased platelets.

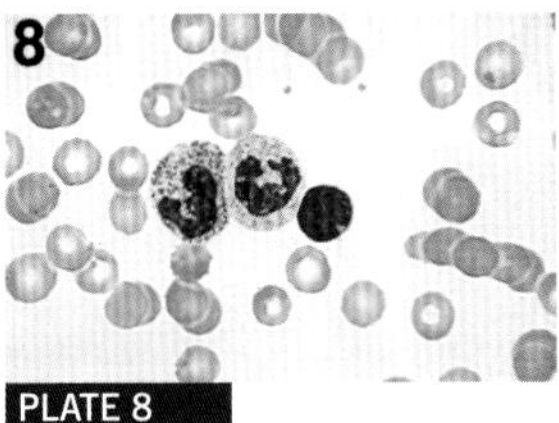

PLATE 8

Toxic granulations. Prominent dark blue primary granules; commonly seen with infection and other toxic states, such as Kawasaki disease.

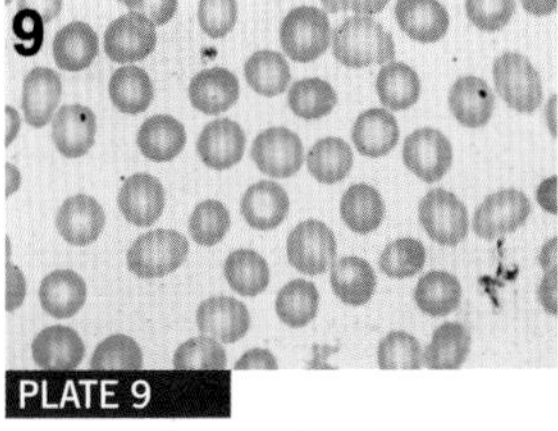

PLATE 9

Howell-Jolly body. Small, dense nuclear remnant in an RBC; suggests splenic dysfunction or asplenia.

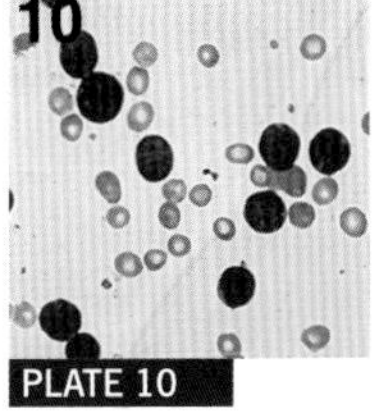

PLATE 10

Leukemic blasts showing large nucleus-to-cytoplasm ratio.

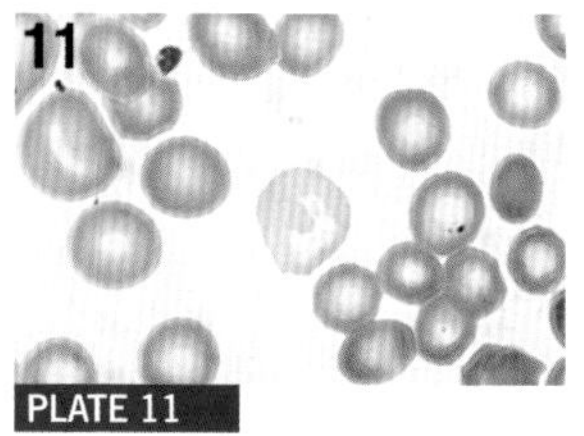

PLATE 11

Polychromatophilia. Diffusely basophilic because of RNA staining; seen with early release of reticulocytes from the marrow.

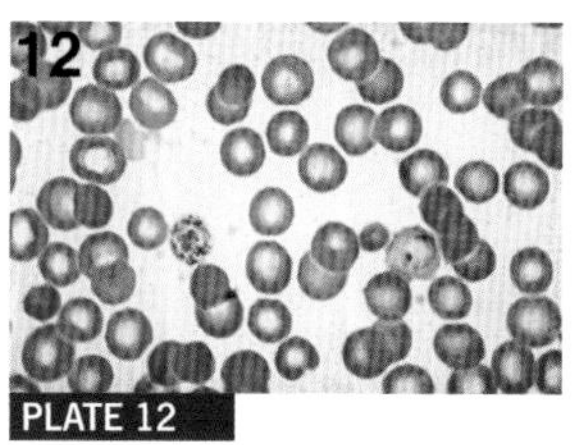

PLATE 12

Intraerythrocytic parasites. Malaria.

TABLE 13–1
AGE-SPECIFIC BLOOD CELL INDICES

Age	Hb (g%)[a]	HCT (%)[a]	MCV (fL)[a]	MCHC (g/% RBC)[a]	Reticulocytes	WBCs ($\times 10^3/mm^3$)[b]	Platelets ($10^3/mm^3$)[b]
26–30 wk gestation[c]	13.4 (11)	41.5 (34.9)	118.2 (106.7)	37.9 (30.6)	—	4.4 (2.7)	254 (180–327)
28 wk	14.5	45	120	31.0	(5–10)	—	275
32 wk	15.0	47	118	32.0	(3–10)	—	290
Term[d] (cord)	16.5 (13.5)	51 (42)	108 (98)	33.0 (30.0)	(3–7)	18.1 (9–30)[e]	290
1–3 day	18.5 (14.5)	56 (45)	108 (95)	33.0 (29.0)	(1.8–4.6)	18.9 (9.4–34)	192
2 wk	16.6 (13.4)	53 (41)	105 (88)	31.4 (28.1)	—	11.4 (5–20)	252
1 mo	13.9 (10.7)	44 (33)	101 (91)	31.8 (28.1)	(0.1–1.7)	10.8 (4–19.5)	—
2 mo	11.2 (9.4)	35 (28)	95 (84)	31.8 (28.3)	—	—	—
6 mo	12.6 (11.1)	36 (31)	76 (68)	35.0 (32.7)	(0.7–2.3)	11.9 (6–17.5)	—
6 mo–2 yr	12.0 (10.5)	36 (33)	78 (70)	33.0 (30.0)	—	10.6 (6–17)	(150–350)
2–6 yr	12.5 (11.5)	37 (34)	81 (75)	34.0 (31.0)	(0.5–1.0)	8.5 (5–15.5)	(150–350)
6–12 yr	13.5 (11.5)	40 (35)	86 (77)	34.0 (31.0)	(0.5–1.0)	8.1 (4.5–13.5)	(150–350)
12–18 yr							
Male	14.5 (13)	43 (36)	88 (78)	34.0 (31.0)	(0.5–1.0)	7.8 (4.5–13.5)	(150–350)
Female	14.0 (12)	41 (37)	90 (78)	34.0 (31.0)	(0.5–1.0)	7.8 (4.5–13.5)	(150–350)
Adult							
Male	15.5 (13.5)	47 (41)	90 (80)	34.0 (31.0)	(0.8–2.5)	7.4 (4.5–11)	(150–350)
Female	14.0 (12)	41 (36)	90 (80)	34.0 (31.0)	(0.8–4.1)	7.4 (4.5–11)	(150–350)

[a]Data are mean (–2 SD).
[b]Data are mean (±2 SD).
[c]Values are from fetal samplings.
[d]<1 mo, capillary hemoglobin exceeds venous: 1 hr: 3.6 g difference; 5 dy: 2.2 g difference; 3 wk: 1.1 g difference.
[e]Mean (95% confidence limits).
Hb, hemoglobin.
Data from Forestier F, et al: Pediatr Res 1986;20:342; Oski FA, Naiman JL: Hematological Problems in the Newborn Infant. Philadelphia, WB Saunders, 1982; Nathan D, Oski FA: Hematology of Infancy and Childhood. Philadelphia; WB Saunders, 1998; Matoth Y, Zaizov R, Varsano I: Acta Paediatr Scand 1971;60:317; and Wintrobe MM: Clinical hematology. Baltimore, Williams & Wilkins, 1999.

TABLE 13-2

CLASSIFICATION OF ANEMIA

Reticulocyte Count	Microcytic Anemia	Normocytic Anemia	Macrocytic Anemia
Low	Iron deficiency Lead poisoning Chronic disease Aluminum toxicity Copper deficiency Protein malnutrition	Chronic disease RBC aplasia (TEC, infection, drug induced) Malignancy Juvenile rheumatoid arthritis Endocrinopathies Renal failure	Folate deficiency Vitamin B_{12} deficiency Aplastic anemia Congenital bone marrow dysfunction (Diamond-Blackfan or Fanconi syndromes) Drug induced Trisomy 21 Hypothyroidism
Normal	Thalassemia trait Sideroblastic anemia	Acute bleeding Hypersplenism Dyserythropoietic anemia II	—
High	Thalassemia syndromes Hemoglobin C disorders	Antibody-mediated hemolysis Hypersplenism Microangiopathy (HUS, TTP, DIC, Kasabach-Merritt) Membranopathies (spherocytosis, elliptocytosis) Enzyme disorders (G6PD, pyruvate kinase) Hemoglobinopathies	Dyserythropoietic anemia I, III Active hemolysis

DIC, disseminated intravascular coagulation; G6PD, glucose-6–phosphate dehydrogenase; HUS, hemolytic-uremic syndrome; TEC, transient erythroblastopenia of childhood; TTP, thrombotic thrombocytopenic purpura.

Data from Nathan D, Oski FA. Hematology of Infancy and Childhood. Philadelphia, WB Saunders, 1988.

b. **Increased plasma aspartate aminotransferase (AST) and lactate dehydrogenase (LDH)** from release of intracellular enzymes.
c. **Haptoglobin:** Binds free Hb; decreased with intravascular and extravascular hemolysis.
d. **Direct Coombs test (DCT):** Tests for the presence of antibody on patient RBCs. Can be falsely negative if affected cells have already been destroyed or antibody titer is low.
e. **Indirect Coombs test (ICT):** Tests for free autoantibody in the patient's serum after RBC antibody binding sites are saturated. Not very sensitive because relies on agglutination and thus will not detect immune hemolytic anemias with only a small amount of immunoglobulin G (IgG) on RBC.
f. **Glucose-6-phosphate dehydrogenase (G6PD) assay:** Used to diagnose G6PD deficiency, an X-linked disorder. May be normal immediately after a hemolytic episode because older, more enzyme-deficient cells have been lysed. See Chapter 29 for a list of oxidizing drugs.
g. **Osmotic fragility test:** Useful in diagnosis of hereditary spherocytosis.
h. **Heinz body preparation:** detects precipitated Hb within RBCs; present in unstable hemoglobinopathies and during oxidative stress (e.g., G6PD deficiency). Requires supravital stain.

3. **Red cell aplasia:** Normocytic, macrocytic, or slightly microcytic, low reticulocyte count, variable platelet and white blood cell (WBC) counts. Bone marrow aspiration evaluates RBC precursors in the marrow to look for bone marrow dysfunction, neoplasm, or specific signs of infection. May not be necessary for the diagnosis of transient erythroblastopenia of childhood (TEC) or aplastic crisis.

a. **Acquired aplasias:**
   (1) **Infectious causes,** including parvovirus in children with rapid RBC turnover (infects RBC precursors), Epstein-Barr virus (EBV), cytomegalovirus (CMV), human herpesvirus type 6 (HHV-6), or human immunodeficiency virus (HIV).
   (2) **TEC:** Occurs from age 6 months to 4 years, with >80% of cases presenting after 1 year of age with a normal or slightly low MCV and low reticulocyte count. There is usually spontaneous recovery within 4 to 8 weeks.
   (3) **Exposures** (drugs, radiation, chemicals).
b. **Congenital aplasias** (macrocytic), including the following:
   (1) **Fanconi anemia:** An autosomal recessive disorder, Fanconi anemia usually presents before 10 years of age and may present with pancytopenia. Patients may have absent thumbs, renal anomalies, microcephaly, or short stature. Chromosomal fragility studies may be diagnostic.
   (2) **Diamond-Blackfan-Oski syndrome:** An autosomal recessive pure RBC aplasia, this syndrome presents in the first year of life. It is associated with congenital anomalies in one third of cases, including triphalangeal thumb, short stature, and cleft lip.
c. **Aplastic anemia** (usually macrocytic).

II. HEMOGLOBINOPATHIES

A. HEMOGLOBIN ELECTROPHORESIS

Hemoglobin electrophoresis involves separation of Hb variants based on molecular charge and size. All positive sickle preparations and solubility tests for sickle Hb (e.g., Sickledex) should be confirmed with electrophoresis or isoelectric focusing (a component of the mandatory newborn screen in many states). See Table 13-3 for interpretation of neonatal Hb electrophoresis patterns.

B. SICKLE CELL ANEMIA

Sickle cell anemia is caused by a genetic defect in β-globin present in 1 in 500 African Americans; 8% of African Americans are carriers.

1. **Diagnosis:** Often made on newborn screen with Hb electrophoresis. The sickle preparation and Sickledex are both rapid tests that are positive in all sickle hemoglobinopathies (e.g., sickle trait [AS], sickle cell anemia [SS], sickle-C [SC], sickle β-thalassemia [Sβ-thal]).

TABLE 13-3

NEONATAL HEMOGLOBIN (Hb) ELECTROPHORESIS PATTERNS*

FA	Fetal Hb and adult normal Hb; the normal newborn pattern.
FAV	Indicates the presence of both HbF and HbA. However, an anomalous band (V) is present, which does not appear to be any of the common Hb variants.
FAS	Indicates fetal Hb, adult normal HbA and HbS, consistent with benign sickle cell trait.
FS	Fetal and sickle HbS without detectable adult normal HbA. Consistent with homozygous sickle Hb genotype (S/S) or sickle β-thalassemia, with manifestations of sickle cell anemia during childhood.
FC†	Designates the presence of HbC without adult normal HbA. Consistent with clinically significant homozygous HbC genotype (C/C), resulting in a mild hematologic disorder presenting during childhood.
FSC	HbS and HbC present. This heterozygous condition could lead to the manifestations of sickle cell disease during childhood.
FAC	HbC and adult normal HbA present, consistent with benign HbC trait.
$FSAA_2$	Heterozygous HbS/β-thalassemia, a clinically significant sickling disorder.
FAA_2	Heterozygous HbA/β-thalassemia, a clinically benign hematologic condition.
F†	Fetal HbF is present without adult normal HbA. Although this may indicate a delayed appearance of HbA, it is also consistent with homozygous β-thalassemia major, or homozygous hereditary persistence of fetal HbF.
FV†	Fetal HbF and an anomalous Hb variant (V) are present.
AF	May indicate prior blood transfusion. Submit another filter paper blood specimen when the infant is 4 mo of age, at which time the transfused blood cells should have been cleared.

*Hemoglobin variants are reported in order of decreasing abundance; for example, FA indicates more fetal than adult hemoglobin.

†Repeat blood specimen should be submitted to confirm the original interpretation.

False-negative test results may be seen in neonates and other patients with a high percentage of fetal Hb.

2. **Complications:** See Table 13-4. A hematologist should generally be consulted.
3. **Health maintenance**[2]**:** Ongoing consultation and clinical involvement with a pediatric hematologist and/or sickle cell program are essential.

a. Pneumococcal vaccine: Heptavalent protein-conjugate vaccine should be provided according to routine childhood schedule. A 23-valent polysaccharide vaccine should be provided after 2 years of age, with a booster after 3 to 5 years of age (see Chapter 15).

b. Influenza vaccine yearly for those 6 months of age and older.

c. Begin prophylaxis with penicillin as soon as diagnosis is made; prophylaxis may be discontinued by age 5 years if patient has had no prior severe pneumococcal infections nor splenectomy and has documented pneumococcal vaccinations, including second 23 valent vaccination. Practice patterns vary. Some continue penicillin indefinitely.

d. Consider supplementation with folic acid.

e. Consider hydroxyurea for severe disease. It increases levels of fetal Hb and decreases HbS content in cells. Has been shown to significantly decrease episodes of vasoocclusive crises, hemolytic crises, acute chest syndrome, number of transfusions, and days spent in the hospital.[3] May decrease mortality in adults.

f. An annual ophthalmologic examination should be performed after 10 years of age.

g. An annual transcranial Doppler examination should be performed between ages 2 and 16 years in patients with SS disease to screen for cerebrovascular accident (CVA).

h. Closely follow growth, development, and school performance.

C. THALASSEMIAS

Thalassemias are defects in α- or β-globin production. Imbalance in production of globin chains leads to precipitation of excess chains, causing ineffective erythropoiesis and shortened survival of mature RBCs.

1. **α-Thalassemias:** Hydrops fetalis (--/--) with Hb Barts (γ4), which cannot deliver oxygen, is usually fatal. HbH disease (β4) (α-/--) causes moderately severe anemia. Both are seen in Southeast Asia. α-Thalassemia trait (α–/α–) or (αα/--) occurs in 1.5% of African Americans and causes mild microcytic anemia. α–/αα are silent carriers.
2. **β-Thalassemia:** Found throughout the Mediterranean, Middle East, India, and Southeast Asia. Ineffective erythropoiesis is more severe in β-thalassemia than α-thalassemia because excess α chains are more unstable than β chains. **Thalassemia major/Cooley's anemia** (β0/β0): Presence of anemia within the first 6 months of life with hepatosplenomegaly and progressive bone marrow expansion, which may lead to "thalassemic face" and other skeletal deformities. Regular

TABLE 13-4

SICKLE CELL DISEASE COMPLICATIONS

Complication	Evaluation	Treatment
Fever (T > 38.5°C)	History and physical CBC with differential Reticulocyte count Blood cultures Chest x-ray, other cultures as indicated	IV antibiotics (third-generation cephalosporin, other antibiotics as indicated) Admit if ill appearing, <3 yr of age, concerning lab results, or complications Some centers use antibiotics with a long half-life and re-evaluate in 24 hours as an outpatient
Vasoocclusive crisis Children <2 yr, dactylitis Children >2 yr, unifocal or multifocal pain	History and physical CBC with differential Reticulocyte count Type and screen	Oral analgesics as an outpatient, as tolerated IV analgesics and IV fluids if outpatient therapy fails (parenteral narcotics in form of PCA and parenteral NSAIDs usually used in combination) Aggressive early treatment of pain is essential
Acute chest syndrome New pulmonary infiltrate with fever, cough, chest pain, tachypnea, dyspnea, or hypoxia	History and physical CBC with differential Reticulocyte count Blood cultures Chest x-ray Type and screen	Admit O_2, incentive spirometry, bronchodilators IV antibiotics (third-generation cephalosporin and macrolide) Analgesia, IV fluids Simple transfusion for moderately severe illness, exchange transfusion for severe or rapidly progressing illness High-dose dexamethasone controversial[1]

Splenic sequestration Acutely enlarged spleen and Hb level 2 g/dL or more below patient's baseline	History and physical CBC Reticulocyte count Type and hold	Serial abdominal exams IV fluids and fluid resuscitation as necessary RBC transfusion or, in severe cases, exchange transfusion for cardiovascular compromise and Hb < 4.5 g/dL. (Autotransfusion may occur with recovery, leading to increased Hb and CHF. Transfuse cautiously)
Aplastic crisis Acute illness with Hb below patient's baseline and low reticulocyte count. May follow viral illnesses, especially parvovirus B19	History and physical CBC with differential Reticulocyte count Type and screen Parvovirus serology and polymerase chain reaction	Admit IV fluids PRBCs for symptomatic anemia Isolation to protect susceptible individuals and women of childbearing age until parvovirus excluded
Other complications Priapism, CVA, TIA, gallbladder disease, avascular necrosis		

Note: CVA requires emergency transfusion guided by a hematologist and a neurologist experienced with sickle cell disease.

transfusions are required to avoid anemia. **Thalassemia intermedia (β+/β+):** Presents at about 2 years of age with moderate, compensated anemia which may become symptomatic, leading to heart failure, pulmonary hypertension, splenomegaly, and bony expansion, usually in the second or third decade of life. **Thalassemia trait/thalassemia minor (β/β+) or (β/β0):** Usually asymptomatic with microcytosis out of proportion to anemia, sometimes with erythrocytosis.

3. **Mentzer index (MCV/RBC)** >13.5 suggests iron deficiency; Mentzer index <11.5 is suggestive of thalassemia minor.

III. NEUTROPENIA

A. DEFINITION

Neutropenia is an absolute neutrophil count (ANC) <1500/mm3, although neutrophil counts vary with age (Table 13-5). Severe neutropenia is defined as an absolute neutrophil count <500/mm3. See Box 13-1 for a differential diagnosis of neutropenia. Children with significant neutropenia are at risk for bacterial and fungal infections. Granulocyte colony-stimulating factor (G-CSF) may be indicated. See Formulary for dosage information. Transient neutropenia secondary to viral illness rarely causes significant morbidity. For management of fever and neutropenia in oncology patients, see Chapter 21.

IV. THROMBOCYTOPENIA

A. DEFINITION

Thrombocytopenia is a platelet count <150,000/mm^3 (see Table 13-1). Clinically significant bleeding is unlikely with platelet counts >20,000/mm^3 in the absence of other complicating factors.

BOX 13-1

DIFFERENTIAL DIAGNOSIS OF CHILDHOOD NEUTROPENIA

Acquired	Congenital
Infection	Cyclic neutropenia
Immune	Severe congenital neutropenia (Kostmann syndrome)
Hypersplenism	Chronic benign neutropenia of childhood
Vitamin B_{12}, folate, copper deficiency	Schwachman syndrome
Drugs or toxic substances	Fanconi syndrome
Aplastic anemia	Metabolic disorders (amino acidopathies, glycogenolysis)
Malignancies or preleukemic disorders	Osteopetrosis
Ionizing radiation	

TABLE 13-5

AGE-SPECIFIC LEUKOCYTE DIFFERENTIAL

	Total Leukocytes*	Neutrophils†		Lymphocytes		Monocytes		Eosinophils	
Age	Mean (range)	Mean (range)	%	Mean (range)	%	Mean	%	Mean	%
Birth	18.1 (9–30)	11 (6–26)	61	5.5 (2–11)	31	1.1	6	0.4	2
12 hr	22.8 (13–38)	15.5 (6–28)	68	5.5 (2–11)	24	1.2	5	0.5	2
24 hr	18.9 (9.4–34)	11.5 (5–21)	61	5.8 (2–11.5)	31	1.1	6	0.5	2
1 wk	12.2 (5–21)	5.5 (1.5–10)	45	5.0 (2–17)	41	1.1	9	0.5	4
2 wk	11.4 (5–20)	4.5 (1–9.5)	40	5.5 (2–17)	48	1.0	9	0.4	3
1 mo	10.8 (5–19.5)	3.8 (1–8.5)	35	6.0 (2.5–16.5)	56	0.7	7	0.3	3
6 mo	11.9 (6–17.5)	3.8 (1–8.5)	32	7.3 (4–13.5)	61	0.6	5	0.3	3
1 yr	11.4 (6–17.5)	3.5 (1.5–8.5)	31	7.0 (4–10.5)	61	0.6	5	0.3	3
2 yr	10.6 (6–17)	3.5 (1.5–8.5)	33	6.3 (3–9.5)	59	0.5	5	0.3	3
4 yr	9.1 (5.5–15.5)	3.8 (1.5–8.5)	42	4.5 (2–8)	50	0.5	5	0.3	3
6 yr	8.5 (5–14.5)	4.3 (1.5–8)	51	3.5 (1.5–7)	42	0.4	5	0.2	3
8 yr	8.3 (4.5–13.5)	4.4 (1.5–8)	53	3.3 (1.5–6.8)	39	0.4	4	0.2	2
10 yr	8.1 (4.5–13.5)	4.4 (1.5–8.5)	54	3.1 (1.5–6.5)	38	0.4	4	0.2	2
16 yr	7.8 (4.5–13.0)	4.4 (1.8–8)	57	2.8 (1.2–5.2)	35	0.4	5	0.2	3
21 yr	7.4 (4.5–11.0)	4.4 (1.8–7.7)	59	2.5 (1–4.8)	34	0.3	4	0.2	3

*Numbers of leukocytes are × $10^3/mm^3$; ranges are estimates of 95% confidence limits; percents refer to differential counts.

†Neutrophils include band cells at all ages and a small number of metamyelocytes and myelocytes in the first few days of life.

From Dallman PR. In Rudolph AM (eds): Pediatrics, 20th ed. New York: Appleton-Century-Crofts; 1996.

B. CAUSES OF THROMBOCYTOPENIA

1. **Idiopathic thrombocytopenic purpura (ITP):** ITP is a diagnosis of exclusion; it can be acute or chronic. WBC count and Hb levels are normal. Hemorrhagic complications are rare with platelet counts >20,000/mm^3. Many patients require no therapy. Treatment options include Rh (D) immune globulin (WinRho; useful only in Rh-positive patients), intravenous immune globulin (see Formulary for IVIG dosing), or corticosteroids (i.e., prednisone 2 mg/kg/day or up to 30 mg/kg methylprednisolone for up to 3 days). Splenectomy or chemotherapy may be considered in chronic cases. Platelet transfusions are not generally helpful but are necessary in life-threatening bleeding.
2. **Neonatal thrombocytopenia:** This may be caused by decreased production, increased consumption, or immune-mediated disease.
   a. Decreased production: Results from aplastic disorders, congenital malignancy such as leukemia, and viral infections.
   b. Increased consumption: Usually result of disseminated intravascular coagulation (DIC) from infection or asphyxia.
   c. Immune mediated: IgG or complement attach to platelets and cause destruction. Specific causes include pre-eclampsia, sepsis, maternal ITP, and platelet alloimmunization.
3. **Platelet alloimmunization:** A common cause of thrombocytopenia in newborns. Transplacental maternal antibodies (usually against PLA-1 antigen/HPA-1a) cause fetal platelet destruction and in utero bleeding. If severe, a transfusion of maternal platelets will be more effective in raising the platelet count than random donor platelets. Diagnosis may be confirmed as follows:
   a. A mixing study of maternal or neonatal plasma and paternal platelets.
   b. Absence of maternal PLA-1 antigen/HPA-1a.
   c. A mixing study with patient plasma and a panel of known minor platelet antigens.
4. **Other causes** of thrombocytopenia include microangiopathic hemolytic anemias, such as DIC and hemolytic-uremic syndrome (HUS), infection causing marrow suppression, malignancy, HIV, drug-induced thrombocytopenia, marrow infiltration, cavernous hemangiomas (Kasabach-Merritt syndrome), thrombocytopenia with absent radii syndrome (TAR), thrombosis, hypersplenism, and other rare inherited disorders (e.g., Wiskott-Aldrich syndrome, Noonan syndrome, chromosomal abnormalities).

V. COAGULATION (Figs. 13-2 and 13-3)

A. TESTS OF COAGULATION

An incorrect anticoagulant-to-blood ratio will give inaccurate results. See Table 13-6 for normal hematologic values.

1. **Activated partial thromboplastin time (aPTT):** Measures intrinsic system; requires factors V, VIII, IX, X, XI, XII, fibrinogen, and

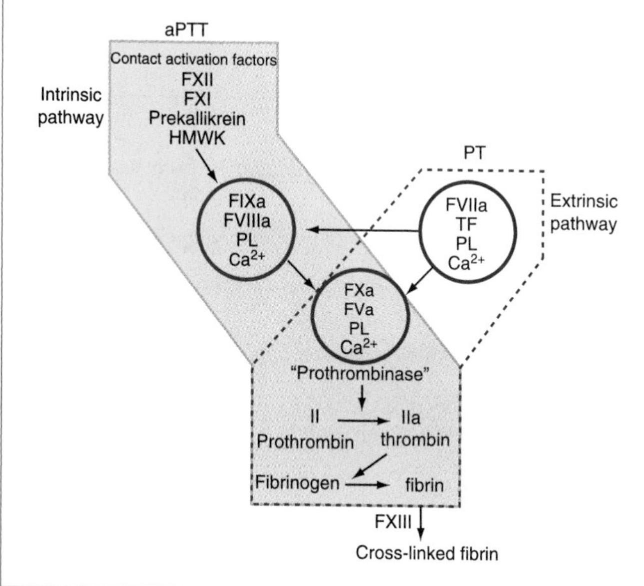

FIG. 13-2

Coagulation cascade. *(Adaptation courtesy of James Casella and Clifford Takemoto.)* Key: F: factor, PL: phospholipid, TF: tissue factor, HMWK: high molecular weight kininogen.

prothrombin. May be prolonged in heparin administration, hemophilia, von Willebrand disease (vWD), DIC, and the presence of circulating inhibitors (e.g., lupus anticoagulants or other antiphospholipid antibodies).

2. **Prothrombin time (PT):** Measures extrinsic pathway; requires fibrinogen, prothrombin, and factors V, VII, and X. May be prolonged in deficiencies of vitamin K–associated factors, malabsorption, liver disease, DIC, warfarin administration, and circulating inhibitors.
3. **Bleeding time (BT):** Evaluates clot formation, including platelet number and function, and von Willebrand factor (vWF). Performed at patient bedside. Always assess the platelet number and check for a history of ingestion of platelet inhibitors, such as nonsteroidal anti-inflammatory drugs (NSAIDs), before a BT test.

B. HYPERCOAGULABLE STATES

Hypercoagulable states present clinically as venous or arterial thrombosis (Table 13-7).

1. **Laboratory evaluation[4]:**

TABLE 13-6
AGE-SPECIFIC COAGULATION VALUES

Coagulation Tests	Preterm Infant 30–36 wk, Day of Life #1	Term Infant, Day of Life #1	1–5 yr	6–10 yr	11–16 yr	Adult
PT (sec)	15.4 (14.6–16.9)	13.0 (10.1–15.9)	11 (10.6–11.4)	11.1 (10.1–12.1)	11.2 (10.2–12.0)	12 (11.0–14.0)
INR	—	—	1.0 (0.96–1.04)	1.0 (0.91–1.11)	1.02 (0.93–1.10)	1.10 (1.0–1.3)
aPTT (sec)	108 (80–168)	42.9 (31.3–54.3)	30 (24–36)	31 (26–36)	32 (26–37)	33 (27–40)
Fibrinogen (g/L)	2.43 (1.50–3.73)	2.83 (1.67–3.09)	2.76 (1.70–4.05)	2.79 (1.57–4.0)	3.0 (1.54–4.48)	2.78 (1.56–4.0)
Bleeding time (min)	—	—	6 (2.5–10)	7 (2.5–13)	5 (3–8)	4 (1–7)
Thrombin time (sec)	14 (11–17)	12 (10–16)	—	—	—	10
II (U/mL)	0.45 (0.20–0.77)	0.48 (0.26–0.70)	0.94 (0.71–1.16)	0.88 (0.67–1.07)	0.83 (0.61–1.04)	1.08 (0.70–1.46)
V (U/mL)	0.88 (0.41–1.44)	0.72 (0.43–1.08)	1.03 (0.79–1.27)	0.90 (0.63–1.16)	0.77 (0.55–0.99)	1.06 (0.62–1.50)
VII (U/mL)	0.67 (0.21–1.13)	0.66 (0.28–1.04)	0.82 (0.55–1.16)	0.85 (0.52–1.20)	0.83 (0.58–1.15)	1.05 (0.67–1.43)
VIII (U/mL)	1.11 (0.50–2.13)	1.00 (0.50–1.78)	0.90 (0.59–1.42)	0.95 (0.58–1.32)	0.92 (0.53–1.31)	0.99 (0.50–1.49)
vWF (U/mL)	1.36 (0.78–2.10)	1.53 (0.50–2.87)	0.82 (0.47–1.04)	0.95 (0.44–1.44)	1.00 (0.46–1.53)	0.92 (0.50–1.58)
IX (U/mL)	0.35 (0.19–0.65)	0.53 (0.15–0.91)	0.73 (0.47–1.04)	0.75 (0.63–0.89)	0.87 (0.59–1.22)	1.09 (0.55–1.63)
X (U/mL)	0.41 (0.11–0.71)	0.40 (0.12–0.68)	0.88 (0.58–1.16)	0.75 (0.55–1.01)	0.79 (0.50–1.17)	1.06 (0.70–1.52)
XI (U/mL)	0.30 (0.08–0.52)	0.38 (0.10–0.66)	0.97 (0.56–1.50)	0.86 (0.52–1.20)	0.74 (0.50–0.97)	0.97 (0.67–1.27)
XII (U/mL)	0.38 (0.10–0.66)	0.53 (0.13–0.93)	0.93 (0.64–1.29)	0.92 (0.60–1.40)	0.81 (0.34–1.37)	1.08 (0.52–1.64)
PK (U/mL)	0.33 (0.09–0.57)	0.37 (0.18–0.69)	0.95 (0.65–1.30)	0.99 (0.66–1.31)	0.99 (0.53–1.45)	1.12 (0.62–1.62)
HMWK (U/mL)	0.49 (0.09–0.89)	0.54 (0.06–1.02)	0.98 (0.64–1.32)	0.93 (0.60–1.30)	0.91 (0.63–1.19)	0.92 (0.50–1.36)
XIIIa (U/mL)	0.70 (0.32–1.08)	0.79 (0.27–1.31)	1.08 (0.72–1.43)	1.09 (0.65–1.51)	0.99 (0.57–1.40)	1.05 (0.55–1.55)

XIIIs (U/mL)	0.81 (0.35–1.27)	0.76 (0.30–1.22)	1.13 (0.69–1.56)	1.16 (0.77–1.54)	1.02 (0.60–1.43)	0.97 (0.57–1.37)
D-Dimer	—	—	—	—	—	Positive titer ≥ 1 : 8
FDPs	—	—	—	—	—	Borderline titer = 1 : 25–1 : 50 Positive titer > 1 : 50
COAGULATION INHIBITORS						
ATIII (U/mL)	0.38 (0.14–0.62)	0.63 (0.39–0.97)	1.11 (0.82–1.39)	1.11 (0.90–1.31)	1.05 (0.77–1.32)	1.0 (0.74–1.26)
α2–M (U/mL)	1.10 (0.56–1.82)	1.39 (0.95–1.83)	1.69 (1.14–2.23)	1.69 (1.28–2.09)	1.56 (0.98–2.12)	0.86 (0.52–1.20)
C1–Inh (U/mL)	0.65 (0.31–0.99)	0.72 (0.36–1.08)	1.35 (0.85–1.83)	1.14 (0.88–1.54)	1.03 (0.68–1.50)	1.0 (0.71–1.31)
α2–AT (U/mL)	0.90 (0.36–1.44)	0.93 (0.49–1.37)	0.93 (0.39–1.47)	1.00 (0.69–1.30)	1.01 (0.65–1.37)	0.93 (0.55–1.30)
Protein C (U/mL)	0.28 (0.12–0.44)	0.35 (0.17–0.53)	0.66 (0.40–0.92)	0.69 (0.45–0.93)	0.83 (0.55–1.11)	0.96 (0.64–1.28)
Protein S (U/mL)	0.26 (0.14–0.38)	0.36 (0.12–0.60)	0.86 (0.54–1.18)	0.78 (0.41–1.14)	0.72 (0.52–0.92)	0.81 (0.60–1.13)
FIBRINOLYTIC SYSTEM						
Plasminogen (U/mL)	1.70 (1.12–2.48)	1.95 (1.60–2.30)	0.98 (0.78–1.18)	0.92 (0.75–1.08)	0.86 (0.68–1.03)	0.99 (0.7–1.22)
TPA (ng/mL)	—	—	2.15 (1.0–4.5)	2.42 (1.0–5.0)	2.16 (1.0–4.0)	4.90 (1.40–8.40)
α2–AP (U/mL)	0.78 (0.4–1.16)	0.85 (0.70–1.0)	1.05 (0.93–1.17)	0.99 (0.89–1.10)	0.98 (0.78–1.18)	1.02 (0.68–1.36)
PAI (U/mL)	—	—	5.42 (1.0–10.0)	6.79 (2.0–12.0)	6.07 (2.0–10.0)	3.60 (0–11.0)

α2–AP, α2–antiplasmin; α2–AT, α2–antitrypsin; α2–M, α2–macroglobulin; ATIII, antithrombin III; HMWK, high-molecular-weight kininogen; PAI, plasminogen activator inhibitor; PK, prekalikrein; TPA, tissue plasminogen activator; VIII, factor VIII procoagulant.

Data from Andrew M, et al: *Blood* 1987;70:165–172; Andrew M, et al: *Blood* 1988;72:1651–1657; and Andrew M, et al: *Blood* 1992;8:1998–2005.

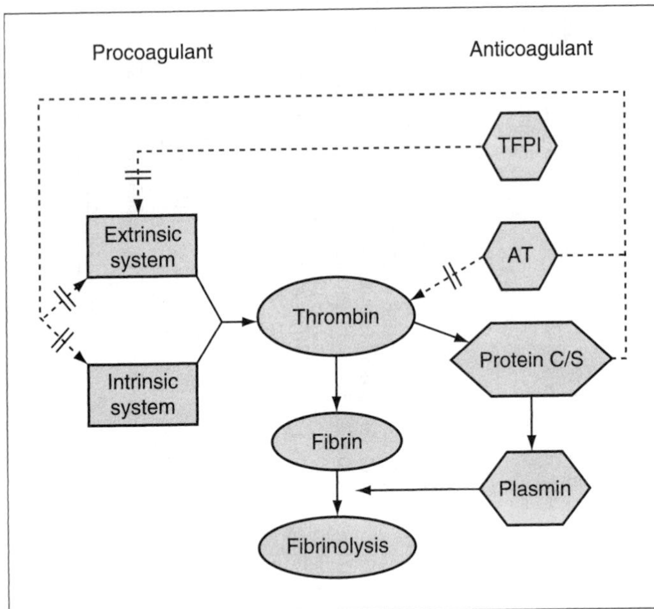

FIG. 13-3

Coagulation cascade. *(Adaptation courtesy of James Casella and Clifford Takemoto.)* Key: AT, antithrombin; TFPI, tissue factor pathway inhibitor.

a. Exclude common acquired causes. Initial laboratory screening includes PT, high-sensitivity aPTT, circulating anticoagulants, mixing study. If aPTT is prolonged, send mixing studies.
b. Extended workup for hypercoagulable states: see Table 13-8. A hematologist should be consulted.
c. The identification of one risk factor, such as an indwelling vascular catheter, does not preclude the search for others, especially when accompanied by a family history of thrombosis.

2. Treatment of thromboses:

a. **Heparin therapy:** For deep venous thrombus or pulmonary embolus.
   (1) Loading dose: 50 to 75 U/kg IV over 30 minutes to 1 hour, followed by maintenance continuous infusion of heparin at 28 U/kg/hr if patient is <1 year old, or 20 U/kg/hr if ≥ 1 year old.
   (2) Obtain aPTT level 6 hours after loading dose and adjust per Table 13-9. Goal is aPTT at 1.5 to 2.5 times baseline aPTT.

TABLE 13-7

HYPERCOAGULABLE CONDITIONS

Congenital	Acquired
Protein C and S deficiency: hereditary, autosomal dominant disorder in which heterozygotes have threefold to sixfold increased risk for venous thrombosis	**Endothelial damage:** causes include vascular catheters, smoking, diabetes, hypertension, surgery, hyperlipidemia
Antithrombin III deficiency: hereditary, autosomal dominant disorder. Homozygotes die in infancy	**Hyperviscosity:** macroglobulinemia, polycythemia, sickle cell disase
Factor V Leiden (activated protein C resistance): 2%–5% of whites are heterozygotes with fivefold to tenfold increased risk for venous thrombosis. 1 in 1000 are homozygotes, with eighty-fold to one hundred-fold increased risk for venous thrombosis	**Platelet activiation:** caused by essential thrombocytosis, oral contraceptives
Homocystinemia: increased levels of homocystine associated with arterial and venous thromboses, often due to MTHFR abnormalities	**Antiphospholipid syndromes:** common in patients with systemic lupus erythematosus or malignancy. May occur during pregnancy or after a viral infection. Associated with venous and arterial thromboses and spontaneous abortions
Others: prothrombin mutation (G20210A), plasminogen abnormalities, fibrinogen abnormalities	**Others:** drugs, malignancy, liver disease, inflammatory disease such as inflammatory bowel disease, paroxysmal nocturnal hemoglobinuria, lipoprotein A, heparin-induced thrombocytopenia

MTHFR = Methyltetrahydrofolate reductase.

TABLE 13-8

EXTENDED WORKUP FOR HYPERCOAGULABLE STATES*

Factors VIII, IX, XI
Activated protein C resistance assay (screening test for factor V Leiden)
Factor V Leiden (DNA-based assay for factor V Leiden)
Factor II 20210A (prothrombin mutation)
Homocystine
Methlytetrahydrofolate reductase genetic testing if homocystine elevated
Dilute Russel viper venom test (antiphospholipid antibody syndrome)
Platelet neutralization procedure (lupus anticoagulant)
Anticardiolipin screening ELISA assay (anticardiolipin antibodies)
Protein C activity and antigen (protein C deficiency and dysfunction)
Protein S activity and antigen (protein S deficiency and dysfunction)
Antithrombin III activity and antigen (antithrombin III deficiency and dysfunction)
Plasminogen activity
Tissue plasminogen activator (TPA) antigen
Plasminogen activator inhibitor activity (measures activity of this TPA inhibitor)
α2–Antiplasmin activity (measures activity of this plasmin inhibitor)

*Where necessary, abnormality tested for is listed in parenthesis.
ELISA, enzyme-linked immunosorbent assay.

TABLE 13-9

ADJUSTMENT AND MONITORING OF HEPARIN THERAPY

aPTT Control Ratio	Rebolus/Dose Interruption	Heparin Infusion Adjustment
<1.2 ×	Repeat original load	Increase by 5 U/kg/hr
1.2–1.4 ×	Repeat half original load	Increase by 3 U/kg/hr
1.5–2.5 ×	None	No change
2.6–3.2 ×	None	Decrease by 3 U/kg/hr
3.3–4.0 ×*	Stop infusion, recheck aPTT in 1 hr Restart infusion when aPTT is in or is projected to be in therapeutic range	Decrease by 5 U/kg/hr
4.0–5.0 ×*	Stop infusion, recheck aPTT in 2 hr Restart infusion when aPTT is in or is projected to be in therapeutic range	Decrease by 7 U/kg/hr
>5.0 ×*	Stop infusion; call hematologist immediately	

*Make sure sample not drawn from heparinized line.
From The Johns Hopkins Hospital laboratory guidelines, 10/98.
Note Draw aPTT 6 hr after bolus dose, and repeat 6–8 hr after every dose adjustment. Repeat daily during stable dosing period. Check platelet count every third day until heparin is discontinued.

(3) Heparin may be reversed with protamine (see Formulary for dosage information).

b. **Low-molecular-weight heparin (LMWH)[5]:** LMWH (or enoxaparin) may be useful in children, although it is less studied and more costly than heparin. LMWH has more specific anti-Xa activity, a longer half-life, and a more predictable dose-to-efficacy ratio.

(1) Dose depends on preparation. See Formulary for enoxaparin dosage information.
(2) Monitor LMWH therapy by following anti-Xa activity. Therapeutic range is 0.5 to 1.0 U/mL for full anticoagulation and 0.2 to 0.4 U/mL for prophylactic dosing.

c. **Warfarin** may be used for long-term anticoagulation, although it carries significant risk for morbidity and mortality. Patient must receive heparin while initiating warfarin therapy secondary to hypercoagulability from decreased protein C and S levels.
(1) Warfarin is usually administered orally at a loading dose for 2 to 3 days, followed by a daily dose sufficient to maintain the PT INR (international normalized ratio) in the desired range, usually 2 to 3 times baseline. See Formulary for warfarin dosing. Infants often require higher daily doses of warfarin. In all patients, levels should be measured every 1 to 2 weeks (Table 13-10).
(2) Warfarin efficacy is greatly affected by dietary intake of vitamin K.
(3) Warfarin is protein bound, and many drugs alter the therapeutic level. Concomitant medicines should be carefully reviewed.
(4) Warfarin effect can be reversed with the administration of vitamin K or fresh-frozen plasma (FFP). Vitamin K dosing for elevated INR is still controversial. Actual dosage recommendations are only present in the adult literature.[6]
(a) INR above desired range and <5: Hold the next warfarin dose and readjust subsequent dosages.

TABLE 13-10

ADJUSTMENT AND MONITORING OF WARFARIN TO MAINTAIN AN INR BETWEEN 2 AND 3*

I. Day 1:	If the baseline INR is 1.0–1.3:
	Dose = 0.2 mg/kg orally
II. Loading Days 2 to 4: If the INR is:	
INR	**Action**
1.1–1.3	Repeat initial loading dose
1.4–1.9	50% of initial loading dose
2.0–3.0	50% of initial loading dose
3.1–3.5	25% of initial loading dose
>3.5	Hold until INR <3.5, then restart at 50% less than previous dose
III. Maintenance Oral Anticoagulation Dose Guidelines	
INR	**Action**
1.1–1.4	Increase by 20% of dose
1.5–1.9	Increase by 10% of dose
2.0–3.0	No change
3.1–3.5	Decrease by 10% of dose
>3.5	Hold until INR <3.5, then restart at 20% less than the previous dose

*Onset of action of warfarin is 36–72 hr, peak effects in 5–7 days. Because of this long half-life, avoid making dose adjustments with excessive frequency.

(b) INR 5–9: Evaluate for risk for bleeding. If low risk, hold the next one to two doses. If high risk, consider also giving a low dose of vitamin K orally (1–2.5 mg for adults).

(c) INR >9: Vitamin K is generally recommended. If there is low risk for bleeding, give vitamin K orally (3–5 mg for adults). If there is high risk for bleeding, give vitamin K orally or intravenously and FFP.

(d) INR ≥20, or life-threatening bleeding: Give vitamin K IV (10 mg for adults) and FFP. Repeat every 12 hours as needed.

d. Anticoagulant therapy alters many coagulation tests.

(1) Heparin alters aPTT, thrombin time, heparin level (anti Xa), mixing studies, and fibrinogen.

(2) Warfarin alters PT, aPTT, dilute Russell Viper Venom test (dRVVT), vitamin K–dependent factors (II, VII, IX, X, protein C and S).

e. Consult a hematologist for thrombolytic therapy.

Note *Children receiving anticoagulation therapy should be protected from trauma. Intramuscular injections are contraindicated. The use of antiplatelet agents and arterial punctures should be avoided.*

C. BLEEDING DISORDERS (Table 13-11 and Fig. 13-4)

1. **Factor VIII deficiency (Hemophilia A):** X-linked disorder characterized by prolonged aPTT and reduced factor VIII activity. PT and BT are normal. Treat with factor VIII concentrate. Recombinant factor VIII is preferred to reduce risk for infection. The factor level is usually raised by 2% per 1 unit of factor VIII per kilogram of body weight (Table 13-12 shows desired level). Factor may need to be redosed based on the clinical scenario. The first dose has a shorter half-life, and a second dose, if needed, is given after 4 to 8 hours. Thereafter, the half-life is approximately 8 to 12 hours, and subsequent doses are usually given every 12 hours. Continuous infusion is often required for surgical patients, usually with a 50-U/kg loading dose, followed by 3 to 4 U/kg/hr. For suspected intracranial bleeding, replace to 100% before diagnostic procedures, such as CT scan.

   Units of factor VIII = weight (kg) × desired % replacement × 0.5

2. **Factor IX deficiency (Hemophilia B or Christmas disease):** X-linked disorder characterized by prolonged aPTT and low factor IX activity. Treat with factor IX concentrate. The factor level is usually raised by 1% for each unit of factor IX concentrate per kilogram of body weight; it has a half-life of 18 to 24 hours. As with factor VIII, a second dose, if needed, should be given at a shorter interval. Recombinant factor IX has a shorter half-life; consider evaluation of in vivo factor survival in each patient.

TABLE 13-11
BLEEDING DISORDERS

Congenital	Acquired
Disorder of platelet number or function Thrombocytopenia: secondary to bone marrow disease or defective megakaryocyte maturation Disorders of platelet function: Bernard-Soulier syndrome, Glanzmann thrombasthenia, storage pool diseases	**Disseminated intravascular coagulation:** characterized by prolonged PT and aPTT, decreased fibrinogen and platelets, increased fibrin degradation products, and D-dimers. Treatment includes identifying and treating underlying disorder. Replacement of depleted coagulation factors with fresh-frozen plasma (FFP) may be necessary in severe cases, especially when bleeding is present—10–15 mL/kg will raise clotting factors 20% . Fibrinogen, if depleted, can be given as cryoprecipitate. Platelet transfusions may also be necessary.
Factor VIII deficiency: see text	**Liver disease:** the liver is the major site of synthesis of factors V, VII, IX, X, XI, XII, XIII, prothrombin, plasminogen, fibrinogen, protein C and S, and ATIII. Treatment with FFP and platelets may be needed, but this will increase hepatic protein load. Vitamin K should be given to patients with liver disease and clotting abnormalities.
Factor IX deficiency: see text	**Vitamin K deficiency:** factors II, VII, IX, X, protein C, and protein S are vitamin K dependent. Early vitamin K deficiency may present with isolated prolonged PT because factor VII has the shortest half-life. Fibrinogen should be normal.
Von Willebrand disease: see text	**Hemolytic-uremic syndrome/thrombotic thrombocytopenic purpura (HUS/TTP):** Characterized by the triad of microangiopathic hemolytic anemia, uremia, and thrombocytopenia. HUS/TTP is often triggered by bacterial enteritis, especially caused by *Escherichia coli* O157:H7, although there are a variety of causes. HUS does not typically include coagulation abnormalities, such as those seen in DIC. Avoid blood products in patients with HUS thought to be secondary to pneumococcal infection. TTP includes the triad of HUS in addition to fever and CNS changes and is more common in older adolescents and adults.

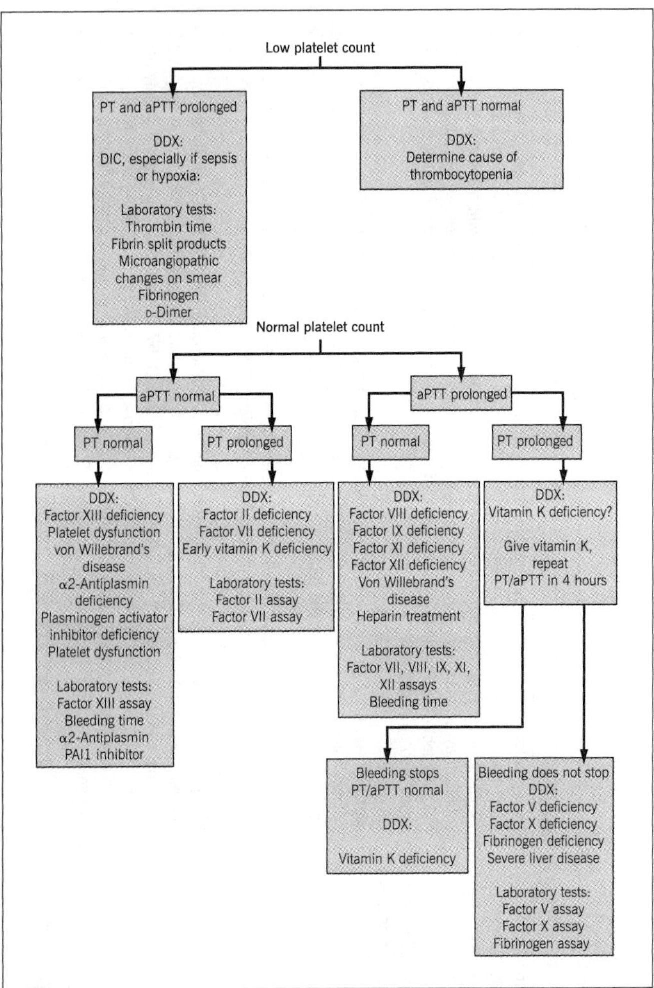

FIG. 13-4

Differential diagnosis of bleeding disorders.

TABLE 13-12

DESIRED FACTOR REPLACEMENT IN HEMOPHILIA

Bleeding Site	Desired Level (%)
Joint or simple hematoma	20–40
Simple dental extraction	50
Major soft tissue bleed	80–100
Serious oral bleeding	80–100
Head injury	100+
Major surgery (dental, orthopedic, other)	100+

Note *All patients with hemophilia should be vaccinated with hepatitis A and hepatitis B vaccines.*

3. **Von Willebrand disease:** The vWF binds platelets to subendothelial surfaces and carries factor VIII. Typical vWD type I is characterized by a prolonged BT and normal platelet count. The aPTT is often mildly or moderately prolonged, and there is decreased ristocetin cofactor activity. Factor VIII and vWF levels are decreased in type 1 disease but may be normal in variants with dysfunctional vWF.

a. In patients with a proven response to desmopressin acetate (DDAVP), bleeding or minor surgical procedures may be treated with DDAVP, intravenously over 20 to 30 minutes, or intranasally (see Formulary for dosage information).

Note *DDAVP may be contraindicated in vWD type 2b because it may exacerbate thrombocytopenia.*

b. For more severe disease or patients with dysfunctional vWF (type 2), the treatment of choice is Humate P (heat-inactivated vWF-enriched concentrate: 40 IU/kg), a similar product containing active vWF, or cryoprecipitate; note the associated infectious risks of these pooled blood products. Concentrates are preferred because they are virally inactivated.

c. Aminocaproic acid, 100 mg/kg IV or by mouth (PO) every 4 to 6 hours (up to 24 g/day); may be useful for treatment of oral bleeding and as prophylaxis for dental extractions.

VI. BLOOD COMPONENT REPLACEMENT

A. BLOOD VOLUME

Blood volume requirements are age specific (Table 13-13).

B. BLOOD PRODUCT COMPONENTS

1. **RBCs:** The decision to transfuse RBCs should be made with consideration of clinical symptoms and signs, the degree of cardiorespiratory or CNS disease, the cause and course of anemia, and

TABLE 13-13
APPROXIMATE BLOOD VOLUME

Age	Total Blood Volume (mL/kg)	Age	Total Blood Volume (mL/kg)
Preterm infants	90–105	4–6 yr	80–86
Term newborns	78–86	7–18 yr	83–90
1–12 mo	73–78	Adults	68–88
1–3 yr	74–82		

Data from Nathan D, Oski FA: Hematology of Infancy and Childhood. Philadelphia, WB Saunders, 1998.

options for alternative therapy, noting the risks for transfusion-associated infections and reactions.

a. **Packed RBC (PRBC) transfusion:** Concentrated RBCs, with HCT of 55% to 70%. A typed and cross-matched blood product is preferred when possible; O-negative (or O-positive) blood may be used if transfusion cannot be delayed. O-negative is preferred for females of child-bearing age to reduce risk for Rh sensitization.
   (1) Unless rapid replacement is required for acute blood loss or shock, infuse no faster than 2 to 3 mL/kg/hr (generally, 10 mL/kg aliquots over 4 hours) to avoid congestive heart failure. A rule of thumb in severe compensated anemia is to give an "X" mL/kg aliquot, where X = patient Hb (mg/dL); that is, if Hb = 5, transfuse 5 mL/kg over 4 hours.

Volume of PRBCs (mL) = EBV (mL) × (desired HCT − actual HCT)/HCT of PRBCs

where EBV is the estimated blood volume and HCT of PRBCs is usually 55% to 70%.

Cross-check: assume 200 mL PRBC per 500-mL unit (40% HCT of donor)/EBV = amount of increase in HCT.

b. **Leukocyte-poor PRBCs**
   (1) **Filtered RBCs:** 99.9% of WBCs removed from product; used for CMV-negative patients to reduce risk for CMV transmission. Also reduces likelihood of a nonhemolytic febrile transfusion reaction.
   (2) **Washed RBCs:** 92% to 95% of white cells removed from product. Similar advantages to leukocyte-poor filtered RBCs. Although filtered leukocyte-poor blood is now more commonly used, washing may be helpful if a patient has pre-existing antibodies to blood products (e.g., patients who have complete IgA deficiency or a history of urticarial transfusion reactions).
c. **Irradiated blood products:**
   (1) Many blood products (PRBCs, platelet preparations, leukocytes, FFP, and others) contain viable lymphocytes capable of proliferation and engraftment in the recipient, causing graft-versus-host disease (GVHD). Irradiation with 1500 cGy before transfusion may prevent

GVHD but does not prevent antibody formation against donor white cells. Engraftment is most likely in young infants, immunocompromised patients, and patients receiving blood from first-degree relatives.

(2) Indications: Intensive chemotherapy, leukemia, lymphoma, bone marrow transplantation, solid organ transplantation, known or suspected immune deficiencies, intrauterine transfusions, and transfusions in neonates.

d. **CMV-negative blood:** Obtained from donors who test negative for CMV. May be given to neonates or other immunocompromised patients, including those awaiting organ or marrow transplant who are CMV negative.

2. Platelets: Indicated to treat severe or symptomatic thrombocytopenia.

a. Single-donor product: Preferred over pooled concentrate for patients with antiplatelet antibodies.

b. Leukocyte-poor: Use if there is a history of significant acute, febrile platelet transfusion reactions.

c. Usually give 4 U/m^2, or approximately 10 mL/kg of normally concentrated platelet product. The platelet count is raised by 10,000 to 15,000/mm^3 by giving 1 U/m^2. For infants and children, 10 mL/kg will increase the platelet count by approximately 50,000/mm^3. Hemorrhagic complications are rare with platelet counts >20,000/mm^3. A transfusion "trigger" of 10,000/mm^3 is recommended by many in the absence of serious bleeding complications. A platelet count >50,000/mm^3 is advisable for minor procedures such as lumbar puncture; >100,000/mm^3 is advisable for major surgery or intracranial operation. Peak post-transfusion concentration is reached 45 to 60 minutes after transfusion. Platelet products should not be refrigerated because this promotes premature platelet activation and clumping.

3. FFP: Contains all clotting factors except platelets. Used in severe clotting factor deficiencies with active bleeding or to reverse the effects of warfarin. Also may replace anticoagulant factors (antithrombin III, protein C, protein S). Used in treatment of DIC, vitamin K deficiency with active bleeding, or thrombotic thrombocytopenic purpura (TTP). The usual amount is 10 to 15 mL/kg; repeat doses as needed. In acquired TTP, plasma exchange is the treatment of choice.

4. Cryoprecipitate: Enriched for factor VIII (5–10 U/mL), vWF, and fibrinogen. Historically useful for children with factor VIII or vWF deficiency in the context of active bleeding, but concentrates are now preferred because of lower risk for viral transmission.

5. Monoclonal factor VIII: Highly purified factor, derived from pooled human blood.

6. Recombinant factor VIII or IX: Highly purified, with less theoretical infectious risk than pooled human products. There is a risk for inhibitor formation, as with other products.

C. PARTIAL PRBC EXCHANGE TRANSFUSION

A partial PRBC exchange transfusion may be indicated for sickle cell patients with acute chest syndrome, stroke, intractable pain crisis, or refractory priapism. Replace with Sickledex-negative cells. Goal is to reduce percentage of HbS to <40%. Follow HCT carefully during transfusion to avoid hyperviscosity, maintaining HCT <35%.

D. COMPLICATIONS OF TRANSFUSIONS

1. **Acute transfusion reactions:**
   a. **Acute hemolytic reaction:** Most often the result of blood group incompatibility. Signs and symptoms include fever, chills, tachycardia, hypotension, and shock. Treatment includes immediate cessation of blood transfusion and institution of supportive measures. Laboratory findings include DIC, hemoglobinuria, and positive Coombs test.
   b. **Febrile nonhemolytic reaction:** Usually the result of host antibody response to donor leukocyte antigens, common in previously transfused patients. Symptoms include fever, chills, and diaphoresis. Stop transfusion and evaluate as described below. Prevention includes premedication with antipyretics, antihistamines, and corticosteroids; and, if necessary, use of leukocyte-poor PRBCs.
   c. **Urticarial reaction:** Reaction to donor plasma proteins. Stop transfusion immediately; treat with antihistamines, and epinephrine and steroids if there is respiratory compromise (see also treatment of anaphylaxis, Chapter 1). Use washed or filtered RBCs with the next transfusion.
   d. **Evaluation of acute transfusion reaction:**
      (1) Patient's urine: Test for hemoglobin.
      (2) Patient's blood: Confirm blood type, screen for antibodies, and repeat DCT on pretransfusion and post-transfusion sera.
      (3) Donor blood: Culture for bacteria.
2. **Delayed transfusion reaction:** Usually due to minor blood group antigen incompatibility with low or absent titer of antibodies at time of transfusion. Occurs 3 to 10 days after transfusion. Symptoms include fatigue, jaundice, and dark urine. Laboratory findings include anemia, a positive Coombs test, new RBC antibodies, and hemoglobinuria.
3. **Transmission of infectious diseases**[7]: Blood supply is tested for HIV types 1 and 2, HTLV types I and II, hepatitis B, and hepatitis C. Data from 2003 estimate the risk for transmitting infection as follows: HIV, 1 in 725,000–835,000; HTLV, 1 in 641,000; hepatitis B, 1 in 63,000–500,000; hepatitis C, 1 in 250,000–500,000; parvovirus, 1 in 10,000. CMV, parvovirus, and hepatitis A may also be transmitted by blood products.
4. **Sepsis:** Sepsis occurs with products that are contaminated with bacteria, particularly platelets, because they are stored at room temperature.

REFERENCES

1. Bernini JC, et al: Beneficial effect of intravenous dexamethasone in children with mild to moderately severe acute chest syndrome complicating sickle cell disease. Blood 1998;92(9):3082–3089.
2. American Academy of Pediatrics, Section on Hematology/Oncology Committee on Genetics: Health supervision in children with sickle cell disease. Pediatrics 2002;109:526–535.
3. Koren A, et al: Effect of hydroxyurea in sickle cell anemia: A clinical trial in children and teenagers with severe sickle cell anemia and sickle beta-thalassemia. Pediatr Hematol Oncol 1999;16(3):221–232.
4. Streiff MB, Bray PF, Kickler TS: Johns Hopkins Hospital Coagulation Laboratory Guide. July 2002.
5. Massicotte P, et al: Low-molecular-weight heparin in pediatric patients with thrombotic disease: A dose finding study. J Pediatr 1996;128:313–318.
6. Hirsh J, et al: Fifth ACCP Consensus Conference on antithrombotic therapy. Chest 1998;114(5):439S–769S.
7. American Academy of Pediatrics: 2003 Red book: Report of the committee on infectious diseases, 26th ed. Elk Grove Village, IL, American Academy of Pediatrics, 2003.

Immunology and Allergy

W. Adam Gower, MD

14

I. ALLERGIC RHINITIS

A. EPIDEMIOLOGY

1. **Most common chronic condition.**
2. **Significant impact on quality of life demonstrated in multiple studies.**
3. **Increases risk for recurrent otitis media, acute and chronic sinusitis.**

B. DIAGNOSIS

1. **History:**
   a. Symptoms:
      (1) Nasal: Congestion, rhinorrhea, pruritus.
      (2) Ocular: Pruritus, tearing.
      (3) Postnasal drip: Sore throat, cough.
   b. Patterns:
      (1) Seasonal: Depends on local allergens.
      (2) Perennial.
   c. Often have other coexisting atopic diseases (eczema, asthma, food allergy).
2. **Physical examination:**
   a. "Allergic facies" with shiners, mouth breathing, transverse nasal crease caused by "allergic salute."
   b. Nasal mucosa may be normal to pink to pale gray.
   c. Injected sclera with or without clear discharge.
3. **Laboratory studies:**
   a. Nasal smear for eosinophils: Quick, easy screen with good positive predictive value.
   b. Total immunoglobulin E (IgE): Too nonspecific.
   c. Peripheral blood eosinophil count: Too nonspecific.
   d. Skin testing: Gold standard.
   e. Radio allergosorbent testing (RAST): Identifies presence of serum IgE to selected antigens.
   f. Imaging studies: Not useful.

C. DIFFERENTIAL DIAGNOSIS

1. **Vasomotor rhinitis:** Symptoms made worse by scents, alcohol, or changes in temperature or humidity.
2. **Rhinitis medicamentosa:** Rebound rhinitis from prolonged use of nasal vasoconstrictors.
3. **Sinusitis:** Acute or chronic.
4. **Nonallergic rhinitis with eosinophilia syndrome (NARES).**
5. **Nasal polyps.**

D. TREATMENT

1. Allergen avoidance:
a. Relies on identification of triggers.
b. May not always be possible.

2. Topical corticosteroids (beclomethasone, fluticasone):
a. Most effective maintenance therapy for nasal congestion.
b. No benefit for ocular symptoms.
c. Adverse effects: No proven effect on long-term growth.

3. Oral antihistamines (diphenhydramine, cetirizine):
a. Newer less sedating preparations preferable (cetirizine).
b. Adverse effects: Sedation with older agents (diphenhydramine), risk for development of tolerance.

4. Leukotriene inhibitors (montelukast).

5. Mast cell stabilizers (cromolyn):
a. Inexpensive and easily available.
b. Most effective as prophylaxis.
c. Few adverse effects.

6. Intranasal antihistamines (azelastine):
a. Effective for acute symptoms.
b. Adverse effects: Bitter taste, systemic absorption with sedation.

7. Decongestants (pseudoephedrine):
a. May be effective in the short term.
b. Adverse effects: Anxiety, insomnia, rebound symptoms.

8. Anticholinergics (ipratropium):
a. Useful for rhinorrhea only.
b. Adverse effects: Drying of nasal mucosa.

9. Immunotherapy:
a. Success rate is high when patients are chosen carefully and when performed by an allergy specialist.
b. Consider when drug side effects are limiting or triggering allergens are difficult to avoid.
c. Not recommended in poorly compliant patients.

II. FOOD ALLERGY

A. EPIDEMIOLOGY

1. Only 5%–8% in pediatric population.

2. Most common allergens in children: Milk, eggs, peanuts, tree nuts, soy, wheat.

B. DIFFERENTIAL DIAGNOSIS OF ADVERSE FOOD REACTION

1. Food intolerance:
a. Nonimmunologic.
b. Based on toxins or other properties of foods.

2. Malabsorption syndromes.

C. MANIFESTATIONS OF FOOD ALLERGY

Often a combination of several syndromes.

1. Anaphylaxis:

a. Uniphasic, biphasic, or protracted patterns.

b. Risk factors for fatal outcome:

(1) History of asthma.

(2) Nut allergy.

(3) Delayed administration of epinephrine.

c. May be associated with exercise.

2. Skin syndromes:

a. Urticaria/angioedema:

(1) Chronic urticaria rarely related to food allergy.

(2) Acute urticaria predicts risk for future anaphylaxis.

b. Atopic dermatitis/eczema:

(1) Food allergy more common in patients with atopic dermatitis.

(2) Treat with allergen avoidance and symptomatic therapy.

3. Gastrointestinal syndromes:

a. Oral allergy syndrome:

(1) Edema of oral mucosa after ingestion of certain fresh fruits and vegetables in patients with pollen allergies.

(2) Inciting antigens destroyed by cooking.

(3) Caused by cross-reactivity of antibodies to pollens.

(4) Rarely progresses beyond the mouth.

b. Allergic eosinophilic gastroenteritis:

(1) Reflux, abdominal pain, diarrhea, early satiety.

(2) Characterized by eosinophilic infiltration of digestive tract.

c. Food-induced enterocolitis:

(1) Presents in infancy.

(2) Vomiting and diarrhea (may contain blood): When severe may lead to lethargy, dehydration, hypotension, acidosis.

(3) Most commonly associated with milk, soy.

d. Infantile proctocolitis:

(1) Confined to distal colon and presents with only diarrhea.

(2) Symptoms of short duration and rarely lead to anemia.

4. Respiratory syndromes:

a. Rhinitis.

b. Asthma.

c. Heiner syndrome:

(1) Precipitating IgG antibody to cow's milk.

(2) Results in pulmonary infiltrates, hemosiderosis, anemia, recurrent pneumonia, and failure to thrive.

D. EVALUATION AND MANAGEMENT OF FOOD ALLERGY (Fig. 14-1)

1. History:

a. Identify specific foods.

b. Establish timing and nature of reactions.

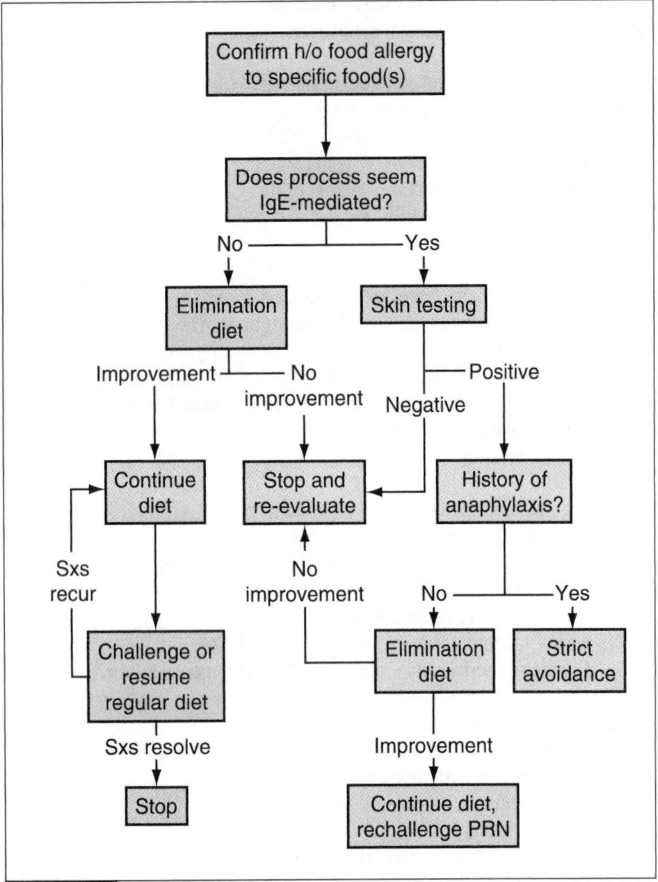

FIG. 14-1

Evaluation and management of food allergy. *(Data from Wood RA: Pediatrics 2003;111(6)1631–1637; and American Gastroenterological Association: Up To Date 2004.)*

2. Physical examination.

3. Skin testing:

a. Skin prick test has poor positive predictive value, but negative test virtually rules out IgE-mediated allergy.

b. Must be done off antihistamines.

c. Intradermal tests have high false-positive rates.

4. RAST:
a. Like skin tests, RAST tests have poor positive predictive value, excellent negative predictive value.
b. IgG testing not useful.
5. Oral food challenges:
a. Must be done under medical supervision with intravenous (IV) access for giving emergency medications if needed.
b. Must be off antihistamines.
c. Most effective when double-blinded using graded doses of disguised food extract.
6. Anti-IgE therapy: Still experimental.

E. NATURAL HISTORY

1. About one third of allergies are lost in 1- to 2-year period (peanut, tree nut, and shell fish allergies rarely outgrown).
2. Most likely to be outgrown with complete avoidance.
3. Skin and RAST tests may remain positive even though symptoms resolve.

III. PENICILLIN ALLERGY

See Figure 14-2.

IV. IMMUNOGLOBULIN THERAPY

A. INTRAVENOUS IMMUNE GLOBULIN (IVIG)

1. Indications:
a. Replacement therapy for antibody-deficient disorders:
   (1) 400–600 mg/kg IV every month to start.
   (2) Adjust dosing to maintain trough IgG level of at least 500 mg/dL.
b. Idiopathic Thrombocytopenic Purpura (ITP):
   (1) 400–1000 mg/kg IV as a single daily dose for 2 to 5 consecutive days, then repeat dose every 3 to 6 weeks based on clinical response and platelet count.
   (2) May also use Rh (D) immunoglobulin in Rh-positive patients.
c. Kawasaki disease:
   (1) 2 g/kg x 1 dose over 10 to 12 hours.
   (2) Must be started within first 10 days of symptoms.
d. Pediatric human immunodeficiency virus (HIV) infection:
   (1) 400 mg/kg every 28 days for hypogammaglobulinemia, recurrent serious bacterial infections, failure to form antibodies to common antigens, or measles prophylaxis.
   (2) 500–1000 mg/kg/day x 3 to 5 days for HIV-associated thrombocytopenia.

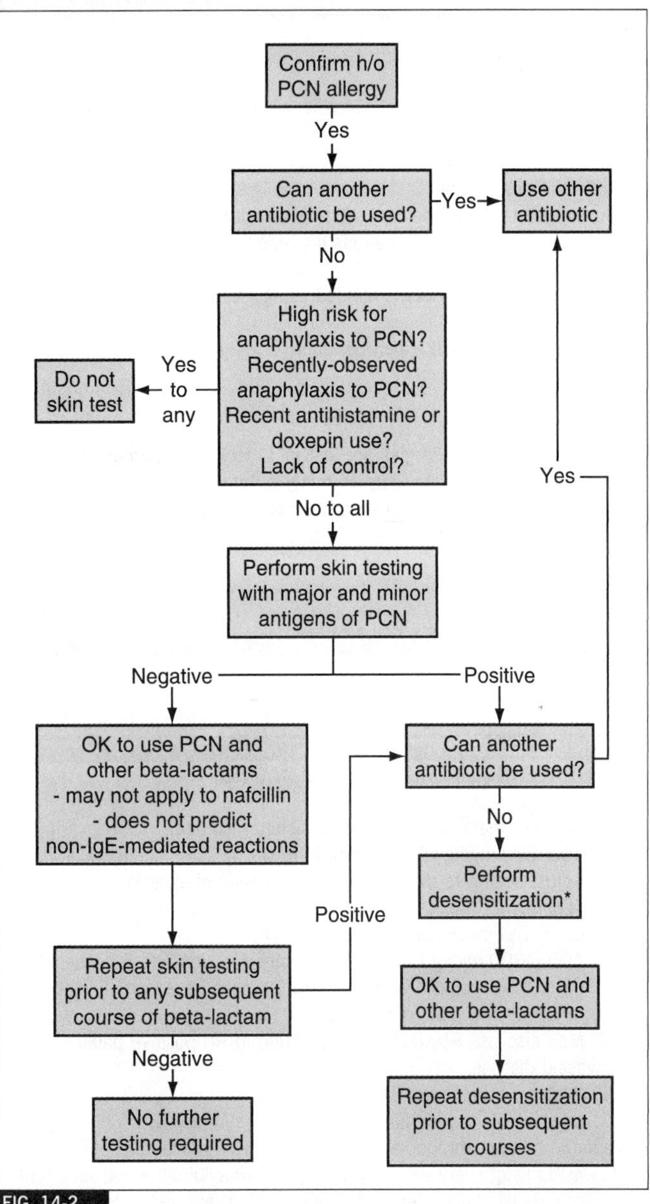

FIG. 14-2

Evaluation and management of penicillin allergy. *May be performed orally (preferred) or parenterally, and multiple protocols are available. Should be done in an ICU setting where adverse reactions can be managed. *(Adapted from O'Dowd LC, Atkins P: Up To Date 2004.)*

e. Bone marrow transplantation:
 (1) 400–500 mg/kg every week for 3 months, then every month.
 (2) May decrease incidence of infection and death but not acute graft-versus-host disease.

f. Other potential uses:
 (1) Guillain-Barré syndrome.
 (2) Toxic shock syndrome.
 (3) Adjuvant in severe cytomegalovirus (CMV) infection.
 (4) Refractory dermatomyositis and polymyositis.
 (5) Low-birth-weight infants.
 (6) Chronic inflammatory demyelinating polyneuropathy.
 (7) Severe systemic viral and bacterial infections.

2. Precautions and adverse reactions:

a. Severe systemic symptoms (hemodynamic changes, anaphylaxis).
b. Less severe reactions (headache, myalgia, fever, chills, nausea, vomiting) may be alleviated by decreasing infusion rate or premedication with antihistamines, antipyretics, and/or IV steroids.
c. Aseptic meningitis.
d. Acute renal failure.
e. Relatively contraindicated in patients with complete IgA deficiency due to trace amounts of IgA in IVIG, although routine screening for IgA deficiency not recommended in potential recipients.

B. INTRAMUSCULAR IMMUNE GLOBULIN (IMIG)

1. Indications:

a. Hepatitis A prophylaxis.
b. Measles prophylaxis.

2. Precautions and adverse reactions:

a. Severe systemic symptoms (hemodynamic changes, anaphylaxis).
b. Local symptoms at the site of injection increase with repeated use.
c. High risk for anaphylactoid reactions if given intravenously.
d. Relatively contraindicated in patients with complete IgA deficiency due to trace amounts of IgA in IMIG.

3. Administration:

a. No more than 5 mL should be given at one site in an adult or large child.
b. Smaller amounts per site (1–3 mL) for smaller children and infants.
c. Administration of more than 15 mL at one time is essentially never warranted.
d. Peak serum levels achieved in 48 to 72 hours, and half-life is 3 to 4 weeks
e. Intravenous or intradermal use of IMIG is absolutely contraindicated.

C. SPECIFIC IMMUNE GLOBULINS

1. Hyperimmune globulins:

a. Prepared from donors with high titers of specific antibodies.
b. Includes HBIG, VZIG, CMV-IG, Rho(D)IG, and others.

2. Monoclonal antibody preparations: palivizumab and others.

TABLE 14-1

SERUM IgG, IgM, IgA, AND IgE LEVELS*

Age	IgG (mg/dL)	IgM (mg/dL)	IgA (mg/dL)	IgE (IU/ml)
Cord blood (term)	1121 (636–1606)	13 (6.3–25)	2.3 (1.4–3.6)	0.22 (0.04–1.28)
1 mo	503 (251–906)	45 (20–87)	13 (1.3–53)	
6 wk				0.69 (0.08–6.12)
2 mo	365 (206–601)	46 (17–105)	15 (2.8–47)	
3 mo	334 (176–581)	49 (24–89)	17 (4.6–46)	0.82 (0.18–3.76)
4 mo	343 (196–558)	55 (27–101)	23 (4.4–73)	
5 mo	403 (172–814)	62 (33–108)	31 (8.1–84)	
6 mo	407 (215–704)	62 (35–102)	25 (8.1–68)	2.68 (0.44–16.3)
7–9 mo	475 (217–904)	80 (34–126)	36 (11–90)	2.36 (0.76–7.31)
10–12 mo	594 (294–1069)	82 (41–149)	40 (16–84)	
1 yr	679 (345–1213)	93 (43–173)	44 (14–106)	3.49 (0.80–15.2)
2 yr	685 (424–1051)	95 (48–168)	47 (14–123)	3.03 (0.31–29.5)
3 yr	728 (441–1135)	104 (47–200)	66 (22–159)	1.80 (0.19–16.9)
4–5 yr	780 (463–1236)	99 (43–196)	68 (25–154)	8.58 (1.07–68.9)†
6–8 yr	915 (633–1280)	107 (48–207)	90 (33–202)	12.89 (1.03–161.3)‡
9–10 yr	1007 (608–1572)	121 (52–242)	113 (45–236)	23.6 (0.98–570.6)§
14 yr				20.07 (2.06–195.2)
Adult	994 (639–1349)	156 (56–352)	171 (70–312)	13.2 (1.53–114)

*Numbers in parentheses are the 95% confidence intervals (CIs).

†IgE data for 4 yr.

‡IgE data for 7 yr.

§IgE data for 10 yr.

From Kjellman NM, Johansson SG, Roth A: Clin Allergy 1976;6:51–59, Jolliff CR, et al: Clin Chem 1982;28:126–128; and Zetterström O, Johansson SG: Allergy 1981;36(8)537–547.

TABLE 14-2

NUMBERS OF T CELLS AND B CELLS*

Age	CD3 (total T cells) (%)†	CD4 (T-helper) (%)†	CD8 (T-suppressor/cytotoxic) (%)†	CD4/CD8 Ratio†	CD19 (B cells) (%)‡
Neonatal	0.6–5.0 (28–76)	0.4–3.5 (17–52)	0.2–1.9 (10–41)	1.0–2.6	0.04–1.1 (5–22)
1 wk–2 mo	2.3–7.0 (60–85)	1.7–5.3 (41–68)	0.4–1.7 (9–23)	1.3–6.3	0.6–1.9 (4–26)
2–5 mo	2.3–6.5 (48–75)	1.5–5.0 (33–58)	0.5–1.6 (11–25)	1.7–3.9	0.6–3.0 (14–39)
5–9 mo	2.4–6.9 (50–77)	1.4–5.1 (33–58)	0.6–2.2 (13–26)	1.6–3.8	0.7–2.5 (13–35)
9–15 mo	1.6–6.7 (54–76)	1.0–4.6 (31–54)	0.4–2.1 (12–28)	1.3–3.9	0.6–2.7 (15–39)
15–24 mo	1.4–8.0 (39–73)	0.9–5.5 (25–50)	0.4–2.3 (11–32)	0.9–3.7	0.6–3.1 (17–41)
2–5 yr	0.9–4.5 (43–76)	0.5–2.4 (23–48)	0.3–1.6 (14–33)	0.9–2.9	0.2–2.1 (14–44)
5–10 yr	0.7–4.2 (55–78)	0.3–2.0 (27–53)	0.3–1.8 (19–34)	0.9–2.6	0.2–1.6 (10–31)
10–16 yr	0.8–3.5 (52–78)	0.4–2.1 (25–48)	0.2–1.2 (9–35)	0.9–3.4	0.2–0.6 (8–24)
Adult	0.7–2.1 (55–83)	0.3–1.4 (28–57)	0.2–0.9 (10–39)	1.0–3.6	0.1–0.5 (6–19)

*Absolute counts ($\times 10^9$/L).

†Normal values (5th to 95th percentile).

‡Normal values (25th to 75th percentile). Values in parentheses 5th to 95th percentile for adult data.

From Comans-Bitter WM et al: J Pediatr 1996;130(3):388–393.

D. IMMUNOLOGIC REFERENCE VALUES

1. Serum IgG, IgM, IgA, and IgE levels (Table 14-1).
2. Lymphocyte enumeration (Table 14-2).
3. Serum IgG subclass levels (Table 14-3).
4. Serum complement levels (Table 14-4).

V. EVALUATION OF A SUSPECTED IMMUNODEFICIENCY

See Table 14-5.

TABLE 14-3

SERUM IgG SUBCLASS LEVELS*

Age (yr)	IgG1 (mg/dL)	IgG2 (mg/dL)	IgG3 (mg/dL)	IgG4 (mg/dL)†
0–1	340 (190–620)	59 (30–140)	39 (9–62)	19 (6–63)
1–2	410 (230–710)	68 (30–170)	34 (11–98)	13 (4–43)
2–3	480 (280–830)	98 (40–240)	28 (6–130)	18 (3–120)
3–4	530 (350–790)	120 (50–260)	30 (9–98)	32 (5–180)
4–6	540 (360–810)	140 (60–310)	39 (9–160)	39 (9–160)
6–8	560 (280–1120)	150 (30–630)	48 (40–250)	81 (11–620)
8–10	690 (280–1740)	210 (80–550)	85 (22–320)	42 (10–170)
10–13	590 (270–1290)	240 (110–550)	58 (13–250)	60 (7–530)
13–adult	540 (280–1020)	210 (60–790)	58 (14–240)	60 (11–330)

*Numbers in parentheses are the 95% confidence intervals (CIs).

†10% of individuals appear to have absent IgG4 levels.

From Schur PH: Ann Allergy 1987;58:89–96, 99.

TABLE 14-4

SERUM COMPLEMENT LEVELS*

Age	C3 (mg/dL)	C4 (mg/dL)
Cord blood (term)	83 (57–116)	13 (6.6–23)
1 mo	83 (53–124)	14 (7.0–25)
2 mo	96 (59–149)	15 (7.4–28)
3 mo	94 (64–131)	16 (8.7–27)
4 mo	107 (62–175)	19 (8.3–38)
5 mo	107 (64–167)	18 (7.1–36)
6 mo	115 (74–171)	21 (8.6–42)
7–9 mo	113 (75–166)	20 (9.5–37)
10–12 mo	126 (73–180)	22 (12–39)
1 yr	129 (84–174)	23 (12–40)
2 yr	120 (81–170)	19 (9.2–34)
3 yr	117 (77–171)	20 (9.7–36)
4–5 yr	121 (86–166)	21 (13–32)
6–8 yr	118 (88–155)	20 (12–32)
9–10 yr	134 (89–195)	22 (10–40)
Adult	125 (83–177)	28 (15–45)

*Numbers in parentheses are the 95% confidence intervals (CIs).

Modified from Jolliff CR, et al: Clin Chem 1982;28:126–128.

TABLE 14-5

EVALUATION OF A SUSPECTED IMMUNODEFICIENCY

Suspected Abnormality	Clinical Findings	Initial Tests	More Advanced Tests
Antibody (e.g., X-linked agammaglobulinemia, IgA deficiency)	Sinopulmonary and systemic infections (pyogenic bacteria) Enteric infections (enterovirus, other viruses, *Giardia* sp.) Autoimmune disease (ITP, hemolytic anemia, IBD)	Immunoglobulin levels (IgG, IgM, IgA) Antibody titers to protein antigens (diphtheria, tetanus) Antibody titers to polysaccharide antigens (≥2-yr-old child) before and after immunization (pneumococcal polysaccharide vaccine)	B-cell enumeration Immunofixation IgG subclass levels
Cell-mediated immunity (e.g., DiGeorge syndrome)	Pneumonia (pyogenic bacteria, fungi, *Pneumocystis carinii*, viruses) Gastroenteritis (viruses, *Giardia* sp. *Cryptosporidium* sp.) Dermatitis/mucositis (fungi)	Total lymphocyte counts HIV ELISA/Western blot Delayed-type hypersensitivity skin test (*Candida* sp., tetanus toxoid, mumps, *Trichophyton* sp.)	T-cell enumeration and subsets (CD3, CD4, CD8) In vitro T-cell proliferation to mitogens, antigens, or allogeneic cells Chest radiograph for thymic hypoplasia FISH 22 for DiGeorge syndrome
Antibody and cell-mediated immunity (e.g., severe combined immunodeficiency, ataxia telangiectasia, Wiskott-Aldrich syndrome, common variable immunodeficiency, hyper-IgM syndrome)	See above	See above	See above ADA assay Alpha-fetoprotein Platelet count/size

continued

TABLE 14-5

EVALUATION OF A SUSPECTED IMMUNODEFICIENCY—cont'd

Suspected Abnormality	Clinical Findings	Initial Tests	More Advanced Tests
Phagocytosis (chronic granulomatous disease, leukocyte adhesion deficiency, Chediak-Higashi syndrome)	Cutaneous infections, abscesses, lymphadenitis (staphylococci, enteric bacteria, fungi, mycobacteria), poor wound healing	WBC/neutrophil count and morphology	Nitroblue tetrazolium (NBT) test Chemotactic assay Phagocytic and bacterial assay
Spleen	Bacteremia/hematogenous infection (pneumococcus, other streptococci, *Neisseria* sp.)	Peripheral blood smear for Howell-Jolly bodies Hemoglobin electrophoresis (HbSS)	Technetium-99 spleen scan
Complement	Bacteria sepsis, autoimmune disease (lupus, glomerulonephritis), angioedema, pyogenic infection, encapsulated bacterial infections (i.e., *Neisseria* sp.)	CH50 (total hemolytic complement)	Alternative pathway assays Individual component assays

From Rosen FS, Cooper MD, Wedgewood R. N Engl J Med 1995; 333(7):431–440 and Shyur SD, Hill HR. J Pediatr 1996; 129(1):8–24.

ADA, Adenosine deaminase; *ELISA*, enzyme-linked immunosorbent assay; *FISH*, fluorescent in situ hybridization; *HIV* human immunodeficiency virus; *IBD*, inflammatory bowel disease; *ITP*, idiopathic thrombocytopenic purpura; *WBC*, white blood cell.

REFERENCES

1. Sampson HA, Sicherer SH, Birnbaum AK: American Gastroenterology Association technical review on the evaluation of food allergy in gastrointestinal disorders. Gastroenterology 2001;120(4):1023–1025.
2. Barrett DJ: Approach to the child with recurrent infections. Up to Date 2004.
3. DeShazo RD, Kemp SF: Clinical manifestations and evaluation of allergic rhinitis (rhinosinusitis). Up To Date 2004. Website: www.uptodate.com
4. Fireman P: Therapeutic approaches to allergic rhinitis: Treating the child. Journal of Allergy and Clinical Immunology 2000;105(6 Pt 2):S616–621.
5. Intravenous immune globulin: Pediatric drug information. Up To Date 2004.
6. Lederman H (ed): The Clinical Presentation of Primary Immunodeficiency Diseases. Towson, MD, Immune Deficiency Foundation, 2002.
7. Lifschitz CH: Dietary protein-induced proctitis/colitis, enteropathy, and enterocolitis of infancy. Up To Date 2004. Website: www.uptodate.com
8. O'Dowd LC, Atkins P: Penicillin and other antibiotic allergy, skin testing, and desensitization. Up To Date 2004. Website: www.uptodate.com
9. Passali D, Mosges R, et al: Consensus conference of allergic rhinitis in childhood. Allergy 1999;54:4–34.
10. Pickering LK (ed): Red book: 2003 Report of the Committee on Infectious Diseases, 26th ed. Elk Grove Village, IL, American Academy of Pediatrics, 2003, pp 55–60, 394.
11. Ressel GW: AHRQ releases review of treatments for allergic and nonallergic rhinitis. American Family Physician 2002;66(11):2164–2167.
12. Sicherer SH: Manifestations of food allergy: Evaluation and management. American Family Physician 1999;59(2):415–424, 429–430.
13. Stone KD: Atopic diseases of childhood. Current Opinion in Pediatrics 2002;14:634–646.
14. Wood RA: The natural history of food allergy. Pediatrics 2003;111(6):1631–1637.

Immunoprophylaxis

Megan E. Partridge, MD

15

I. SOURCES OF INFORMATION

A. PRINTED SOURCES

American Academy of Pediatrics. *Red Book: 2003 Report of the Committee on Infectious Diseases,* 26th ed. Elk Grove Village, IL: American Academy of Pediatrics, 2003.

Updated Recommended Childhood Vaccination Schedule is published each January in *Pediatrics and Morbidity and Mortality Weekly Report*.

Current issues of *Morbidity and Mortality Weekly Report*.

Vaccine package inserts.

B. ELECTRONIC AND TELEPHONE SOURCES

State health departments.

The Centers for Disease Control and Prevention (CDC) can provide telephone consultation and send printed material on vaccines. Call 1-800-232-SHOT.

The American Academy of Pediatrics (AAP) website: www.aap.org.

The Vaccine Adverse Event Reporting System (VAERS) website: www.vaers.org. To submit a report about an adverse event or for questions, call 1-800-822-7967.

National Network for Immunization Information (www.immunizationinfo.org) and Immunization Action Coalition (www.immunize.org).

II. IMMUNIZATION SCHEDULES

A. RECOMMENDED CHILDHOOD IMMUNIZATION SCHEDULE (Fig. 15-1)

B. CATCH-UP IMMUNIZATION SCHEDULES

1. **Lapsed immunizations:** Resume immunization schedule as if the usual interval had elapsed. Repeating doses is not indicated.
2. **Catch-up immunization schedules:**

See Tables 15-1 and 15-2.

a. *Haemophilus influenzae* type b (Hib): See section V.C.

b. *Pneumococcus* conjugate vaccine (PCV7): See Table 15-3.

C. MINIMUM AGE FOR INITIAL VACCINATION AND MINIMUM INTERVALS BETWEEN DOSES OF VARIOUS VACCINES (Table 15-4)

D. GUIDELINES FOR SPACING LIVE AND INACTIVATED ANTIGENS (Table 15-5)

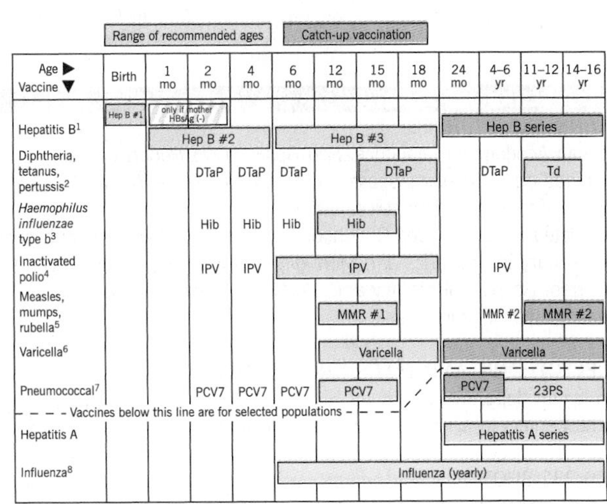

Range of recommended ages
Catch-up vaccination
Age ▶
Vaccine ▼
Birth
1 mo
2 mo
4 mo
6 mo
12 mo
15 mo
18 mo
24 mo
4–6 yr
11–12 yr
14–16 yr
Hepatitis B1
Hep B #1
only if mother HBsAg (-)
Hep B #2
Hep B #3
Hep B series
Diphtheria, tetanus, pertussis2
DTaP
DTaP
DTaP
DTaP
DTaP
Td
Haemophilus influenzae type b3
Hib
Hib
Hib
Hib
Inactivated polio4
IPV
IPV
IPV
IPV
Measles, mumps, rubella5
MMR #1
MMR #2
MMR #2
Varicella6
Varicella
Varicella
Pneumococcal7
PCV7
PCV7
PCV7
PCV7
PCV7
23PS
Vaccines below this line are for selected populations
Hepatitis A
Hepatitis A series
Influenza8
Influenza (yearly)

[1]All infants should receive the first dose of hepatitis B vaccine soon after birth and before hospital discharge; the first dose may also be given by age 2 months if the infant's mother is HBsAg-negative. Only monovalent hepatitis B vaccine can be used for the birth dose.

[2]The fourth dose of DTaP may be administered as early as 12 mo of age if 6 mo have elapsed since the third dose and if the child is unlikely to return at age 15–18 mo. Td is recommended at 11–12 yr of age if at least 5 yr have elapsed since the last dose of DTaP. Subsequent routine Td boosters are recommended every 10 yr.

[3]If PRP-OMP is administered at 2 and 4 mo of age, a dose at 6 mo is not required. DTaP/Hib combination products ***should not*** be used for primary immunization in infants at 2, 4, or 6 mo of age until FDA approved for these ages.

[4]An all-IPV schedule is recommended for routine childhood polio vaccination in the United States. All children should receive four doses of IPV at ages 2 mo, 4 mo, 6–18 months, and 4–6 yr. OPV is acceptable in special circumstances: children of parents who do not accept the number of injections, late initiation of immunization that would require an unacceptable number of injections, and imminent travel to polio-endemic areas. OPV remains the vaccine of choice for mass immunization campaigns to control outbreaks caused by wild poliovirus.

[5]The second dose of MMR is recommended routinely at 4–6 yr of age but may be administered during any visit, provided at least 4 weeks have elapsed since the first dose. Those who have not previously received the second dose should complete the schedule by the 11–12 yr visit.

[6]Varicella vaccine is recommended at any visit for susceptible children ≥1 yr of age. Susceptible persons ≥13 yr of age should receive two doses given at least 4 weeks apart.

[7]The heptavalent pneumococcal conjugate vaccine (PCV7) is recommended for all children ages 2–23 mo. It is also recommended for certain children ages 24–59 mo. Pneumococcal polysaccharide vaccine (23PS) is recommended in addition to PCV7 for certain high-risk groups (see p. 335 for further information).

[8]Influenza vaccine is recommended annually for certain high-risk children ≥6 mo (see pp. 327, 329-330) and can be administered to all others wishing to obtain immunity.

FIG. 15-1

Recommended childhood immunization schedule, United States, 2003. *Dark bars* indicate vaccines to be given if previous recommended doses were missed or given earlier than the recommended minimum age. Combination vaccines may be used when vaccine components are indicated, as long as other components are not contraindicated. Note that DTaP-IPV-HepB (Pediarix) given according to the vaccination schedule will result in the administration of an extra dose of HepB, which is acceptable according to the American Academy of Pediatrics (AAP). Most recent recommendations can be found on the Centers for Disease Control and Prevention (CDC) or AAP websites. *(Modified from the CDC Advisory committee on Immunization Practices [Online]. Available: www.cdc.gov/nip/acip.)*

TABLE 15-1

RECOMMENDED IMMUNIZATION SCHEDULES FOR CHILDREN (AGE 4 MO–6 YR) WHO ARE LATE OR ARE >1 MO BEHIND

	Dose 1–2	Dose 2–3	Dose 3–4
DTaP[a]	4 wk	4 wk	6 mo
IPV	4 wk	4 wk	4 wk
HepB	4 wk	3 wk (at 16 wk after dose 1)	
MMR	4 wk		
Hib	4 wk (if dose 1 given at <1 yr)	4 wk (if current age ≤1 yr)	8 wk (final dose; give only in children 1–5 yr who got 3 doses before age 1 yr)
	8 wk (final dose; if dose 1 given at 12–14 mo age)	If current age ≥1 yr and dose 1 given at <15 mo	
	No further doses if dose 1 given at ≥15 mo	No further doses if previous dose given at ≥15 mo	
PCV7	4 wk (if dose 1 at <1 yr and current age <2 yr	4 wk (if current age <1 yr)	8 wk (final dose; give only in children 1–5 yr who got 3 doses before age 1 yr)
	8 wk (final dose, if dose 1 given at ≥12 mo or currently 24–59 mo)	8 wk (final dose if current age ≥12 mo)	
	No further doses in healthy children if dose 1 given at ≥24 mo	No further doses in healthy children if dose given 1 at ≥24 mo	

[a]Allow 6 mo between doses 4 and 5. Dose 5 is not needed if dose 4 is given after 4 yr of age.

Data from American Academy of Pediatrics: Red Book: 2003 Report of the Committee on Infectious Diseases, 26th ed. Elk Grove Village, IL, American Academy of Pediatrics, 2003.

TABLE 15-2

RECOMMENDED IMMUNIZATION SCHEDULES FOR ADOLESCENTS (AGE 7–18 YR) WHO ARE LATE OR ARE >1 MO BEHIND

Dose 1–2	Dose 2–3	Dose 3–Booster
Td: 4 wk	6 mo	6 mo: if dose 1 given <12 mo and current age <11 yr 5 yr: if dose 1 given at >12 mo and dose 3 given at <7 yr and current age ≥11 yr 10 yr: if dose 3 given at ≥7 yr
IPV: 4 wk	4 wk	
HepB: 4 wk	8 wk (and 16 wk after dose 1)	
MMR: 4 wk		
Varicella: 4 wk		

Data from American Academy of Pediatrics: Red Book: 2003 Report of the Committee on Infections Diseases, 26th ed. Elk Grove Village, IL, American Academy of Pediatrics, 2003.

TABLE 15-3

CATCH-UP IMMUNIZATION SCHEDULE FOR PCV7 IN PREVIOUSLY UNVACCINATED CHILDREN

Age at First Dose	Primary Series	Booster Dose[a]
2–6 mo	3 doses, 6–8 wk apart	1 dose at 12–15 mo of age
7–11 mo	2 doses, 6–8 wk apart	1 dose at 12–15 mo of age
12–23 mo	2 doses, 6–8 wk apart	
≥24 mo	1 dose	

[a]Booster doses to be given at least 6 to 8 weeks after the final dose of the primary series.

Data from American Academy of Pediatrics Committee on Infectious Diseases: Red Book: 2003 Report of the Committee on Infectious Diseases, 26th ed. Elk Grove Village, IL, American Academy of Pediatrics, 2003.

TABLE 15-4

MINIMUM AGE FOR INITIAL VACCINATION AND MINIMUM INTERVAL BETWEEN VACCINE DOSES, BY TYPE OF VACCINE

		Minimum Interval from Dose to Dose		
Vaccine	Minimum Age for First Dose[a]	1 to 2[a]	2 to 3[a]	3 to 4
DTaP[b,c]	6 wk	1 mo	1 mo	6 mo
Hib (PRP-OMP)[c]	6 wk	1 mo	2 mo[d]	—
PCV7	6 wk	1 mo[e]	1 mo[e]	2 mo[e]
IPV	6 wk	1 mo	1 mo	1 mo[f]
MMR	12 mo[g]	1 mo	—	—
HBV[c]	Birth	1 mo	2 mo[h]	—
Varicella	12 mo	1 mo[i]	—	—
HAV	2 yr	6 mo	—	—
Influenza[j]	6 mo	1 mo	—	—

[a]These minimum acceptable ages and intervals may not correspond with the optimal recommended ages and intervals for vaccination. See Fig. 15–1.

[b]The total number of doses of diphtheria and tetanus toxoids should not exceed six each before the seventh birthday. If the fourth dose is given after the fourth birthday, the fifth (booster) dose is not needed.

[c]The combination vaccines Pediarix (DTaP/IPV/HepB) and Comvax (HepB-Hib) should not be given to infants younger than 6 weeks of age.

[d]The booster dose of Hib vaccine recommended after the primary vaccination series should be administered no earlier than 12 mo of age.

[e]See Table 15–3 for recommendations of number of doses at different ages.

[f]If the third dose is given after the fourth birthday, the fourth (booster) dose is not needed.

[g]Although the age for measles vaccination may be as young as 6 mo in outbreak areas where cases are occurring in children <1 yr of age, children initially vaccinated before the first birthday should be revaccinated at 12–15 mo of age, and an additional dose of vaccine should be administered at the time of school entry or according to local policy. Doses of MMR or other measles-containing vaccine should be separated by at least 1 mo.

[h]This final dose is recommended at least 4 mo after the first dose, at least 2 mo after the second dose, and no earlier than 6 mo of age.

[i]A second dose of varicella is indicated only in children ≥13 yr.

[j]Two doses of influenza are commended for children 6 mo–9 yr of age who have never received the vaccine. Only one dose is required for children 9 yr or older, as well as children 6 mo–9 yr who have received the vaccine in the past.

Data from American Academy of Pediatrics: Red Book: 2003 Report of the Committee on Infectious Diseases, 26th ed. Elk Grove Village, IL, American Academy of Pediatrics, 2003.

TABLE 15-5

GUIDELINES FOR SPACING LIVE AND INACTIVATED VACCINES

Antigen Combination	Minimum Interval Between Doses
≥2 inactivated or inactivated and live	None, can give simultaneously
≥2 live parenteral	28–day minimum interval, if not given at same time

Data from American Academy of Pediatrics: Red Book: 2003 Report of the Committee on Infectious Diseases, 26th ed. Elk Grove, IL, American Academy of Pediatrics, 2003, Table 1.5, p 23.

III. IMMUNIZATION GUIDELINES

A. VACCINE INFORMED CONSENT

Vaccine information statements (VISes) can be obtained from local health departments, the CDC, the AAP, and vaccine manufacturers. For vaccines that do not currently have VISes, the CDC produces "important information" statements. The most recent VIS must be provided to the patient (nonminor) or parent/guardian with documentation of version date and date vaccine administered.

B. VACCINE ADMINISTRATION

1. **Volume/dose:** Unless otherwise specified, all pediatric immunization doses are 0.5 mL.
2. **Preferred sites of administration of intramuscular (IM) and subcutaneous (SC) vaccines follow:**

a. Less than 18 months old: Anterolateral thigh.

b. Toddlers: Anterolateral thigh or deltoid (deltoid preferred if large enough).

c. Adolescents and young adults: Deltoid.

3. **Route:**

a. IM: Deep into muscle to avoid tissue damage from adjuvants, usually with a 22- to 25-gauge needle, $^{7}/_{8}$- to 1-inch long in infants and toddlers and 1 to 2 inches long in adolescents and young adults.

b. SC: Into pinched skinfold with a 23- to 25-gauge needle $^{5}/_{8}$- to $^{3}/_{4}$-inch long.

4. **Simultaneous administration:** Routine childhood vaccines, including live viral vaccines, are safe and effective when administered simultaneously at different sites, generally 1 to 2 inches apart. If given at separate times, the interval between administration of live viral vaccines should be >1 month.

C. MISCONCEPTIONS REGARDING VACCINE ADMINISTRATION

Vaccines may be given despite the presence of the following:

1. **Mild acute illness, regardless of fever.**
2. **Convalescent phase of illness.**
3. **Recent exposure to infectious disease.**

4. Mild to moderate local reaction to previous dose of vaccine (soreness, redness, swelling).
5. Current antimicrobial therapy.
6. Prematurity (see also section IV.D).
7. Malnutrition.
8. Allergy to penicillin or other antibiotics, except anaphylactic reaction to neomycin or streptomycin.
9. Pregnancy of mother or another household contact (except varicella vaccine may be deferred if there is a pregnant, varicella-susceptible household contact).
10. Breast-feeding.
11. Unimmunized household contact.
12. Family history of adverse event to immunization.

D. EGG ALLERGIES

1. Skin testing is *not* needed in children with egg allergies before the administration of the measles-mumps-rubella (MMR) vaccine (refer to section V.H for details).
2. Skin testing with yellow fever vaccine is recommended before administration in children with a history of immediate hypersensitivity reaction (e.g., anaphylaxis or generalized urticaria) to eggs.
3. Immediate hypersensitivity reaction to eggs is a contraindication to both the parenteral and intranasal influenza vaccines.

Less severe or local manifestations of allergy to egg are not contraindications to influenza vaccine.

IV. IMMUNOPROPHYLAXIS GUIDELINES FOR SPECIAL HOSTS

A. IMMUNOCOMPROMISED HOSTS

1. Congenital immunodeficiency disorders:

a. Live bacterial and live viral vaccines are generally contraindicated. See the AAP Red Book[1] for details regarding individual immunodeficiencies.
b. Inactivated vaccines should be given according to the routine schedule. Immune response may vary and may be inadequate.
c. Immunoglobulin (Ig) therapy may be indicated.
d. Household contacts: Immunize according to the routine childhood immunization schedule. A yearly influenza vaccine is recommended.

2. Known or suspected human immunodeficiency virus (HIV) disease:

a. Inactivated vaccines should be given according to the routine immunization schedule (see Fig. 15-1).
b. See Table 15-6, (see Table 3.17 in AAP Red Book).[1]
c. MMR vaccine should be given to asymptomatic or mildly symptomatic patients with $CD4^+$ T-lymphocyte counts ≥15%. Immunize at 12 months of age; the second dose should be administered 1 month after the first dose to ensure optimal seroconversion.

TABLE 15-6
RECOMMENDATIONS FOR ROUTINE IMMUNIZATION OF HIV-INFECTED CHILDREN

	Administer	Consider	Do Not Administer
Known Asymptomatic HIV infection	HepB, DtaP, IPV, MMR, Hib, PCV, influenza	Varicella	BCG
Symptomatic HIV infection	HepB, DtaP, IPV, MMR, Hib, PCV, influenza	Varicella	BCG

Data from American Academy of Pediatrics: Red Book: 2003 Report of the committee on Infectious Diseases, 26th ed. Elk Grove, IL, American Academy of Pediatrics, 2003, Table 3.27.

d. Varicella vaccine should be considered in asymptomatic or mildly symptomatic patients with $CD4^+$ T-lymphocyte counts ≥25%. Give two doses 3 months apart.
e. A booster dose of the 23-valent pneumococcal polysaccharide vaccine (23PS) is recommended at 2 and 5 years of age, in addition to the routine PCV7 vaccines.
f. Influenza: Immunize all patients at the start of the influenza season as early as 6 months of age and yearly thereafter.
g. Passive immunoprophylaxis or chemoprophylaxis should be considered in all HIV-infected children after exposure to any vaccine-preventable disease.

3. Oncology patients: See Table 15-7.

4. Functional or anatomic asplenia (including sickle cell disease):

a. Penicillin prophylaxis: See Chapter 21.
b. Pneumococcal vaccine:
   (1) Children ≤5 years at diagnosis: See Table 15-8.
   (2) Children >5 years at diagnosis: Immunization with a single dose of either PCV7 or 23PS is acceptable. If both vaccines are given, their administration should be separated by 6 to 8 weeks. A second dose of 23PS may be given in 5 years. Data are insufficient for the most effective combination of the pneumococcal vaccines in older children.
c. Meningococcal vaccine at 2 years of age or at diagnosis if ≥2 years old.
d. Ensure that Hib series is completed; children ≥5 years who never received Hib immunization should receive one dose.
e. Children ≥2 years of age undergoing elective splenectomy should receive one or both of the pneumococcal vaccines and the meningococcal vaccine at least 2 weeks before surgery to ensure optimal immune response. Children <2 years of age should receive PCV7 before surgery.

TABLE 15-7

IMMUNIZATION FOR ONCOLOGY PATIENTS[a]

Vaccine: Indications and comments

DtaP: Indicated for incompletely immunized children <7 yr, even during active chemotherapy

Td: Indicated 1 yr after completion of therapy in children ≥7 yr

Hib: Indicated for incompletely immunized children if <7 yr

HBV: Indicated for incompletely immunized children

23Ps: Indicated for asplenic patients

PCV7: Indicated for incompletely immunized children <5 yr

Meningococcus: Consider in asplenic patients

IPV: Indicated for incompletely immunized children; IPV also recommended for all household contacts requring immunization to reduce the risk for vaccine-associated polio

MMR: Contraindicated until child is in remission and finished with all chemotherapy for 3–6 mo; may need to reimmunize after chemotherapy if titers have fallen below protective levels

Influenza: Defer in active chemotherapy; may give as early as 3–4 wk after remission and off chemotherapy if during influenza season; peripheral granulocyte and lymphocyte counts should be >1000/mm^3; should also be given to household contacts of children with cancer

Varicella: Consider immunizing children who have remained in remission and have finished chemotherapy for >1 yr; with absolute lymphocyte count of >700/mm^3 and platelet count of >100,000/mm^3 within 24 hr of immunization; check titers of previously immunized children to verify protective levels of antibodies

[a]Immune reconstitution is slower for oncology patients who have received bone marrow transplants. See Centers for Disease Control and Prevention: MMWR 2000;49(No. RR-10):1–147 for vaccine schedule.

B. CORTICOSTEROID ADMINISTRATION

Only live viral and live bacterial vaccines are potentially contraindicated (see Table 15-9 for details).

C. PATIENTS TREATED WITH IMMUNOGLOBULIN OR OTHER BLOOD PRODUCTS

See the AAP Red Book[1] for suggested intervals between immunoglobulin or blood product administration and MMR or varicella immunization.

D. PRETERM AND LOW-BIRTH-WEIGHT INFANTS (<2500 g)

Immunize according to chronologic age using regular vaccine dosage.

1. **Hepatitis B virus (HBV):** Initiation of HBV vaccine may be delayed for infants of hepatitis B surface antigen (HBsAg)-negative mothers until the child is >2 kg or 2 months of age, whichever is earlier.
2. **Influenza:** Give 2 doses 1 month apart each fall to all preterm infants >6 months of age. Household contacts should also receive influenza vaccine.

TABLE 15-8

RECOMMENDATIONS FOR PNEUMOCOCCAL IMMUNIZATION WITH PCV7 OR 23PS VACCINE FOR CHILDREN AT HIGH RISK OF PNEUMOCOCCAL DISEASE

Age	Previous Doses	Recommendations
≤23 mo	None	PCV7 as in Table 15–3
24–59 mo	1–3 doses of PCV7	1 dose of PCV7 First dose of 23PS vaccine at 24 mo, at least 6–8 wk after last dose of PCV7 Second dose of 23PS vaccine, 3–5 yr after first dose of 23PS vaccine
24–59 mo	4 doses of PCV7	First dose of 23PS vaccine at 24 mo, at least 6–8 wk after last dose of PCV7 Second dose of 23PS vaccine, 3–5 yr after first dose of 23PS vaccine
24–59 mo	None	Two doses of PCV6–8 wk apart First dose of 23PS vaccine, 6–8 wk after last dose of PCV7 Second dose of 23PS vaccine, 3–5 yr after first dose of 23PS vaccine
24–59 mo	1 dose of 23PS	Two doses of PCV 7, 6–8 wk apart, beginning at least 6–8 wk after last dose of 23PS vaccine One dose of 23PS vaccine, 3–5 yr after first dose of 23PS vaccine

Data from American Academy of Pediatrics: Red Book: 2003 Report of the Committee on Infectious Diseases, 26th ed. Elk Grove Village, IL, American Academy of Pediatrics, 2003.

TABLE 15-9

LIVE VIRUS IMMUNIZATION FOR PATIENTS RECEIVING CORTICOSTEROID THERAPY

Steroid Dose	Recommended Guidelines
Topical or inhaled therapy or local injection of steroids	Live virus vaccines may be given unless there is clinical evidence of immunosuppression; if suppressed, wait 1 mo after cessation of therapy to give live vaccines
Physiologic maintenance doses of steroids	Live virus vaccines may be given
Low-dose steroids (<2 mg/kg/day prednisone or equivalent, or <20 mg/day if >10 kg)	Live virus vaccines may be given
High-dose steroids (≥2 mg/dg/day prednisone or equivalent, or 20 mg/day if >10 kg)	
Duration of therapy <14 days	May give live virus vaccines immediately after cessation of therapy
Duration of therapy ≥14 days	Do not give live virus vaccines until therapy has been discontinued for 1 mo
Children with immunosuppressive disorders receiving steroid therapy	Live virus vaccines are contraindicated, except in special circumstances

From American Academy of Pediatrics: Red Book: 2003 Report of the Committee on Infectious Diseases, 26th ed. Elk Grove Village, IL, American Academy of Pediatrics, 2003.

E. PREGNANCY

Live virus vaccines are generally contraindicated during pregnancy, with the exception of the parenteral form of the influenza vaccine. The parenteral influenza vaccine should be given to all women who will be >14 weeks' gestation during the influenza season and is considered safe at any stage of pregnancy. The intranasal form is contraindicated during pregnancy. Pregnant women not immunized or incompletely immunized against tetanus should receive Td to prevent neonatal tetanus. Pregnant women not immunized or incompletely immunized against polio should receive the inactivated poliomyelitis vaccine (IPV). When indicated, hepatitis A virus (HAV) and HBV vaccines may be given to pregnant women. Pneumococcal vaccines should be deferred during pregnancy, although 23PS has been administered safely.

F. ADOLESCENT AND COLLEGE POPULATION

Refer to the CDC website (www.cdc.gov) for immunization recommendations. Information on immunizations required for foreign travel is also available at this website.

V. IMMUNOPROPHYLAXIS GUIDELINES FOR SPECIFIC DISEASES

A. GUIDE TO CONTRAINDICATIONS AND PRECAUTIONS TO IMMUNIZATIONS (Table 15-10)

B. DIPHTHERIA/TETANUS/PERTUSSIS VACCINES AND TETANUS IMMUNOPROPHYLAXIS

1. Description:

a. DTaP: Diphtheria and tetanus toxoids combined with acellular pertussis vaccine; preferred formulation for children <7 years.
b. DT: Diphtheria and tetanus toxoids without pertussis vaccine; use in children <7 years in whom pertussis vaccine is contraindicated.
c. Td: Tetanus toxoid with one third to one sixth the dose of diphtheria toxoid of other preparations; use in individuals ≥7 years.
d. DTP: Diphtheria and tetanus toxoids combined with whole-cell pertussis vaccine; no longer marketed in the United States.

2. Indications:

a. Routine: See Figure 15-1.
b. Tetanus prophylaxis in wound management: See Table 15-11.
c. Unimmunized pregnant women: Two doses of Td 4 weeks apart; the second dose should be ≥2 weeks before delivery.
d. Pregnant women who have not completed a primary series: Give Td as soon as possible.

3. Precautions/contraindications: See Table 15-10.

4. Children with neurologic disorders:

a. Seizures
   (1) Poorly controlled or new-onset seizures: Defer pertussis immunization until seizure disorder is well controlled and

Text continues on p. 392

TABLE 15-10

GUIDE TO CONTRAINDICATIONS AND PRECAUTIONS TO IMMUNIZATIONS, 2003*

Vaccine	Contraindications	Precautions[1]	Not Contraindications (Vaccines May Be Given)
General for all vaccines (DTaP, IPV, MMR, Hib, pneumococcal, hepatitis B, varicella, hepatitis A, influenza)	Anaphylactic reaction to a vaccine contraindicates further doses of that vaccine Anaphylactic reaction to a vaccine constituent contraindicates the use of vaccines containing that substance	Moderate or severe illnesses with or without a fever Latex allergy[2]	Mild to moderate local reaction (soreness, redness, swelling) after a dose of an injectable antigen Low-grade or moderate fever after a previous vaccine dose Mild acute illness with or without low-grade fever Current antimicrobial therapy Convalescent phase of illnesses Prematurity (same dosage and indications as for healthy, full-term infants)

From American Academy of Pediatrics: Red Book: 2003 Report of the Committee on Infectious Diseases, 26th ed. Elk Grove Village, IL, American Academy of Pediatrics, 2003, Appendix III, p 798.

*This information is based on the recommendations of the Advisory Committee on Immunization Practices (ACIP) and the Committee on Infectious Diseases of the American Academy of Pediatrics (AAP). Sometimes, these recommendations vary from those in the manufacturers' package inserts. For more detailed information, health care professionals should consult the published recommendations of the ACIP, AAP, and the manufacturers' package inserts. These guidelines, originally issued in 1993, have been updated to give current recommendations as of 2003 (based on information available as of February 2003).

DTaP indicates diphtheria and tetanus toxoids and acellular pertussis; DTP, diphtheria and tetanus toxoids and pertussis; IPV, inactivated poliovirus; MMR, measles-mumps-rubella; Hib, *Haemophilus influenzae* type b; GBS, Guillain-Barré syndrome; HIV, human immunodeficiency virus; PPD, purified protein derivative (tuberculin).

[1]The events or conditions listed as precautions, although not contraindications, should be reviewed carefully. The benefits and risks of administering a specific vaccine to a person under the circumstances should be considered. If the risks are believed to outweigh the benefits, the immunization should be withheld; if the benefits are believed to outweigh the risks (for example, during an outbreak or foreign travel), the immunization should be given. Whether and when to administer DTaP to children with proven or suspected underlying neurologic disorders should be decided on an individual basis.

[2]If a person reports a severe (anaphylactic) allergy to latex, vaccines supplied in vials or syringes that contain natural rubber should not be administered unless the benefits of immunization outweigh the risks of an allergic reaction to the vaccine. For latex allergies other than anaphylactic allergies (e.g., a history of contact allergy to latex gloves), vaccines supplied in vials or syringes that contain dry natural rubber or latex can be administered.

TABLE 15-10

GUIDE TO CONTRAINDICATIONS AND PRECAUTIONS TO IMMUNIZATIONS, 2003*—cont'd

Vaccine	Contraindications	Precautions[1]	Not Contraindications (Vaccines May Be Given)
General for all vaccines —cont'd			Recent exposure to an infectious disease History of penicillin or other nonspecific allergies or fact that relatives have such allergies Pregnancy of mother or household contact Unimmunized household contact Immunodeficient household contact Breastfeeding (nursing infant OR lactating mother)
DTaP	Encephalopathy within 7 days of administration of previous dose of DTaP/DTP	Temperature of 40.5°C (104.8°F) within 48 h after immunization with a previous dose of DTaP/DTP Collapse or shock-like state hypotonic-(hyporesponsive episode) within 48 h of receiving a previous dose of DTaP/DTP Seizures within 3 days of receiving a previous dose of DTaP/DTP[3] Persistent inconsolable crying lasting 3 h, within 48 h of receiving a previous dose of DTaP/DTP GBS within 6 wk after a dose[4]	Family history of seizures[3] Family history of sudden infant death syndrome Family history of an adverse event after DTaP/DTP administration

[3]Acetaminophen given before administering DTaP and thereafter every 4 hours for 24 hours should be considered for children with a personal or family (i.e., siblings or parents) history of seizures.

[4]The decision to give additional doses of DTaP should be made on the basis of consideration of the benefit of further immunization versus the risk of recurrence of GBS. For example, completion of the primary series in children is justified.

TABLE 15-10

GUIDE TO CONTRAINDICATIONS AND PRECAUTIONS TO IMMUNIZATIONS, 2003*—cont'd

Vaccine	Contraindications	Precautions[1]	Not Contraindications (Vaccines May Be Given)
IPV	Anaphylactic reactions to neomycin, streptomycin, or polymyxin B	Pregnancy	
MMR[5,6]	Pregnancy Anaphylactic reaction to neomycin or gelatin Known altered immunodeficiency (hematologic and solid tumors, congenital immunodeficiency, severe HIV infection, and long-term immunosuppressive therapy)	Recent (within 3 to 11 mo, depending on product and dose) Immune Globulin administration[7] Thrombocytopenia or history of thrombocytopenic purpura[7] Tuberculosis or positive PPD[8]	Simultaneous tuberculin skin testing[9] Breastfeeding Pregnancy of mother of recipient Immunodeficient family member or household contact Infection with HIV Nonanaphylactic reactions to gelatin or neomycin

[5]A theoretic risk exists that the administration of multiple live-virus vaccines within 30 days (4 weeks) of one another if not given on the same day will result in suboptimal immune response. No data substantiate this risk, however.

[6]An anaphylactic reaction to egg ingestion previously was considered a contraindication unless skin testing and, if indicated, desensitization had been performed. However, skin testing no longer is recommended as of 1997.

[7]The decision to immunize should be made on the basis of consideration of the benefits of immunity to measles, mumps, and rubella versus the risk of recurrence or exacerbation of thrombocytopenia after immunization or from natural infections of measles or rubella. In most instances, the benefits of immunization will be much greater than the potential risks and justify giving MMR, particularly in view of the even greater risk of thrombocytopenia after measles or rubella disease. However, in previous episode of thrombocytopenia occurred in temporal proximity to immunization, not giving a subsequent dose may be prudent.

[8]A theoretic basis exists for concern that measles vaccine might exacerbate tuberculosis. Consequently, before administering MMR to people with untreated active tub culosis, initiating antituberculosis therapy is advisable.

[9]Measles immunization may suppress tuberculin reactivity temporarily. MMR vaccine may be given after, or on the same day as, tuberculin testing. If MMR has been given recently, postpone the tuberculin skin test until 4 to 6 weeks after administration of MMR.

TABLE 15-10

GUIDE TO CONTRAINDICATIONS AND PRECAUTIONS TO IMMUNIZATIONS, 2003*—cont'd

Vaccine	Contraindications	Precautions[1]	Not Contraindications (Vaccines May Be Given)
Hib	None	—	—
Hepatitis B	Anaphylactic reaction to baker's yeast	Prematurity[10]	Pregnancy
Pneumococcal	None	—	—
Varicella[5]	Pregnancy Anaphylactic reaction to neomycin or gelatin Infection with HIV[11]	Recent Immune Globulin administration Family history of immunodeficienty[13]	Pregnancy of mother of recipient Immunodeficiency in a household contact Household contact with HIV

[10]For preterm infants weighing less than 2 kg at birth and born to hepatitis B surface antigen (HBsAg)-negative mothers, initiation of immunization should be delayed until just before hospital discharge if the infant weighs 2 kg or more, or until approximately 2 months of age, when other routine immunizations are given, to improve response. All preterm infants born to HBsAg-positive mothers should receive immunoprophylaxis (Hepatitis B Immune Globulin and vaccine) beginning as soon as possible after birth, followed by appropriate postimmunization testing.

[11]Varicella vaccine should be considered for asymptomatic or mildly symptomatic HIV-infected children, specifically children in Centers for Disease Control and Prevention class N1 or A1, with age-specific T-cell percentages of 25% or higher.

TABLE 15-10

GUIDE TO CONTRAINDICATIONS AND PRECAUTIONS TO IMMUNIZATIONS, 2003*—cont'd

Vaccine	Contraindications	Precautions[1]	Not Contraindications (Vaccines May Be Given)
	Known altered immunodeficiency (hematologic and solid tumors, congenital immunodeficiency, and long-term immunosuppressive therapy)[12]		
Hepatitis A	Anaphylactic reaction to 2-phenoxyethanol or alum	Pregnancy	
Influenza	Anaphylactic reaction to eggs	GBS within 6 wk after a previous influenza immunization	Pregnancy

[12]Varicella vaccine should not be administered to people who have cellular immunodeficiencies, but people with impaired humoral immunity may be immunized.

[13]Varicella vaccine should not be administered to a person who has a family history of congenital or hereditary immunodeficiency in parents or siblings unless that person's immune competence has been substantiated clinically or verified by a laboratory.

TABLE 15-11

INDICATIONS FOR TETANUS PROPHYLAXIS

Prior Tetanus	Clean, Minor Wounds		All Other Wounds	
Toxoid Doses	Tetanus Vaccine[a]	TIG	Tetanus Vaccine[a]	TIG
Unknown or <3	Yes	No	Yes	Yes
≥3, last <5 yr ago	No	No	No	No[b]
≥3, last 5–10 yr ago	No	No	Yes	No[b]
≥3, last >10 yr ago	Yes	No	Yes	No[b]

[a]Vaccine choice for child <7 yr old is DTaP (DT if pertussis is contraindicated). For child ≥7 yr, Td is the vaccine of choice.

[b]Any child with HIV infection or who is within the first year after bone marrow transplantation should receive TIG for any tetanus-prone wound regardless of vaccination status.

TIG, tetanus immune globulin: 250 U IM.

Data from American Academy of Pediatrics: Red Book: 2003 Report of the Committee on Infectious Diseases, 26th ed. Elk Grove Village, IL, American Academy of Pediatrics, 2003.

progressive neurologic disorder is excluded; then use DTaP and antipyretics for 24 hours after immunization.

(2) Personal or family history of febrile seizures: Use DTaP and antipyretics for 24 hours after immunization.

b. Known or suspected progressive neurologic disorder: Defer pertussis immunization until diagnosis and treatment are established and neurologic condition is stable. Progressive disorders may merit permanent deferral of pertussis immunization. Reconsider pertussis immunization at each visit. Use DT if pertussis vaccine is permanently deferred.

Note *Children <1 year with neurologic disorders necessitating temporary deferment of pertussis vaccine should not receive DT because the risk for diphtheria and tetanus is low in the first year of life. After the first birthday, initiate either DT or DTaP immunization as clinically indicated previously.*

5. **Side effects:**
   a. Minor side effects within 3 days: Erythema (26% to 39%), drowsiness (40% to 47%), swelling (15% to 30%), anorexia (19% to 25%), fussiness (14% to 19%), vomiting (7% to 13%), pain (4% to 11%), body temperature >38.3°C (3% to 5%).
   b. Moderate to severe side effects: Persistent crying >3 hours (1/100), seizures (1/1750), hypotonic-hyporesponsive episode (1/1750), anaphylaxis (1/50,000), body temperature ≥40.5°C (rare).
6. **Administration:** DTaP, DT, and Td are all given in a dose of 0.5 mL IM.
7. **Special considerations:**
   a. Pertussis exposure: Immunize all unimmunized or partially immunized close contacts <7 years.

(1) Give fourth dose of DTaP if third dose was given >6 months prior.
(2) Give booster dose of DTaP if last dose was given >3 years prior and child is <7 years old.

b. Chemoprophylaxis for all household and other close contacts: Treat with erythromycin for 14 days to limit secondary transmission regardless of immunization status because pertussis immunity may wane. Estolate preparation may be better tolerated (see Formulary). Azithromycin, clarithromycin, and trimethoprim-sulfamethoxazole are possible alternatives.

Note *The total number of DT and DTaP immunizations should not exceed six by the 7th birthday.*

C. *HAEMOPHILUS INFLUENZAE* TYPE B IMMUNOPROPHYLAXIS

1. Description:

The three licensed vaccines consist of a capsular polysaccharide antigen (PRP) conjugated to a carrier protein. It is not necessary to use the same formulation for the entire series. Vaccines do not confer protection against the disease associated with the carrier (e.g., PRP-T does not protect against tetanus).

a. PRP-OMP: Conjugated to outer membrane protein of *Neisseria meningitidis;* requires only two doses in primary series (2 and 4 months) plus booster at 12 to 15 months. If PRP-OMP is used only for part of the immunization series, the recommended number of doses to complete the series is based on the other Hib conjugate vaccine used. Children without prior DTaP vaccine may respond better to PRP-OMP than to other formulations.
b. HbOC: Conjugated to mutant diphtheria toxin.
c. PRP-T: Conjugated to tetanus toxoid.
d. PRP-OMP/HepB (Comvax): See section V.O.

2. Indications:

a. Routine: See Figure 15-1.
b. Children not immunized against Hib before 7 months of age: Give all doses 2 months apart (minimum of 1 month apart). If initiating Hib immunization at 7 to 11 months, give three doses; at 12 to 14 months, give two doses; and at 15 to 59 months, give one dose. Immunization is not necessary for immunocompetent children ≥60 months.
c. Unimmunized children >15 months with underlying conditions predisposing to invasive Hib disease (e.g., IgG2 deficiency, HIV) require two doses of vaccine given 2 months apart.
d. Children undergoing splenectomy may benefit from an additional dose 7 to 10 days before procedure, even if series was previously completed.
e. Children with invasive Hib disease at age <24 months: Begin Hib immunization 1 month after acute illness, and continue as if previously

unimmunized. Vaccination is not required if invasive disease develops after 24 months of age.

Note *Consider immunologic workup for children who contract invasive Hib disease after completing the immunization series.*

3. **Precautions/contraindications:** See Table 15-10.
4. **Side effects:** Local pain, redness, and swelling in 25% of recipients (mild, lasting <24 hours)
5. **Administration:** Dose is 0.5 mL IM.
6. **Special considerations:** Consider prophylactic rifampin to selected household and child care contacts of children with invasive Hib disease; see the AAP Red Book[1] for details because this issue is controversial.

D. HEPATITIS A VIRUS IMMUNOPROPHYLAXIS

1. **Description: Hepatitis A (HAV) vaccine is an inactivated adsorbed vaccine; two brands are available, Harvix and Vaqta (preservative free). It is licensed only for children ≥2 years.**
2. **Indications:**
   a. Children living in regions of elevated hepatitis A rates (consult local public health authority). See Figure 15-2 for schedule.
   b. Travelers to or residents of endemic areas.
   c. After exposure to HAV if future exposure is likely.
   d. Military personnel.
   e. Homosexual or bisexual men.
   f. Users of illicit injection drugs.
   g. Patients with clotting factor disorders.
   h. Patients with chronic liver disease, including HBV or hepatitis C (HCV).
   i. Persons at risk for occupational exposure.
   j. Immunocompromised individuals may be immunized, although efficacy is not established in immunocompromised children.
   k. Consider use in staff of institutions with ongoing or recurrent outbreaks.
3. **Precautions/contraindications:** See Table 15-10.
4. **Side effects:** Local reactions are typically mild and include induration, redness, swelling (18%); headache (12%); fever (6%); fatigue, malaise, anorexia, nausea (1% to 10%). No serious adverse events have been reported.
5. **Administration:** See Table 15-12 for dose and schedule; give IM.
6. **Special considerations:**
   a. Pre-exposure immunoprophylaxis for travelers:
      (1) HAV vaccine is preferred for travelers ≥2 years old; a single dose usually provides adequate immunity if time does not allow further doses before travel.

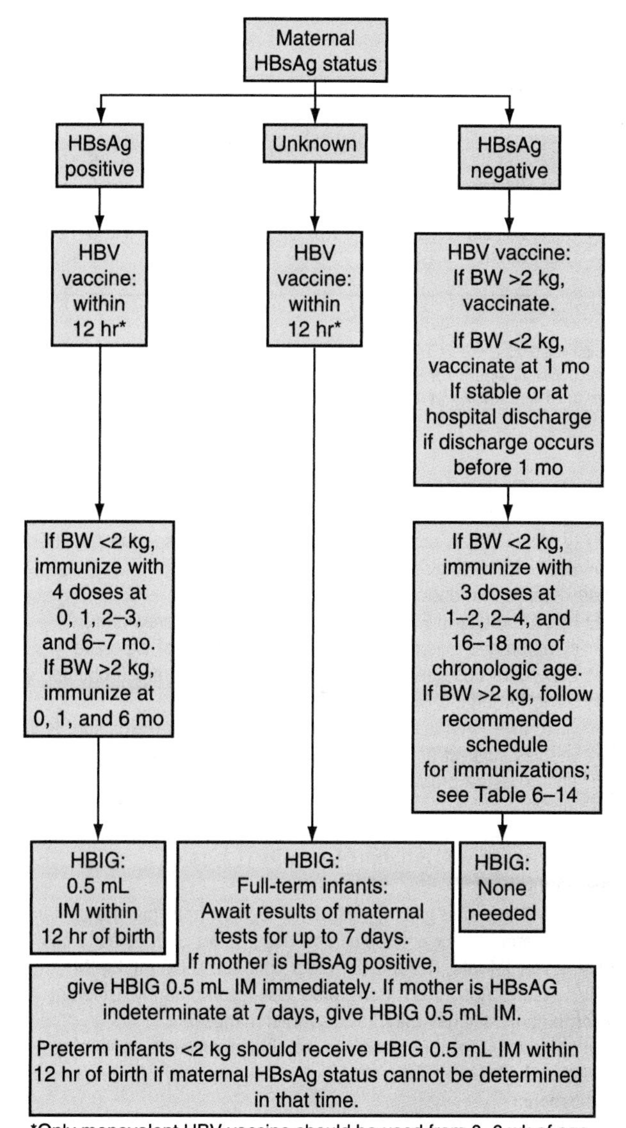

FIG. 15-2

Management of neonates born to mothers with unknown or positive HbsAg status. BW, birth weight. *(Data from American Academy of Pediatrics: Red Book: 2003 Report of the Committee on Infectious Diseases, 26th ed. Elk Grove Village, IL: American Academy of Pediatrics, 2003.)*

TABLE 15-12

RECOMMENDED DOSAGES AND SCHEDULES FOR HAV VACCINES

Age (yr)	Vaccine	Antigen	Volume (mL)	No. of Doses	Schedule
2–18	Havrix (SB)	720 ELU	0.5	2	Initial and 6–12 mo later
	Vaqta (Merck)	25 U	0.5	2	Initial and 6–18 mo later
≥19	Havrix (SB)	1440 ELU	1.0	2	Initial and 6–12 mo later
	Vaqta (Merck)	50 U	1.0	2	Initial and 6–12 mo later
>18	Twinrix* (SB)	720 ELU	1.0	3	Initial and 1 and 6 mo later

*Twinrix is a combination of hepatits B (Energix-B, 20 μg) and hepatitis A (Havrix, 720 ELU) vaccines.

SB, SmithKline Beecham; ELU, enzyme-linked immunoassay units; U, antigen units.

Data from American Academy of Pediatrics: Red Book: 2003 Report of the Committee on Infectious Diseases, 26th ed. Elk Grove Village, IL, American Academy of Pediatrics, 2003.

(2) Ig, given IM, is protective for up to 5 months; see the AAP Red Book[1] for dosing.

b. Postexposure immunoprophylaxis:

(1) Ig 0.02 mL/kg IM is 80% to 90% effective in preventing symptomatic infection if given within 2 weeks of exposure. Maximum dose per site is 3 mL for infants and small children and 5 mL for large children and adults.

(2) Also, give HAV vaccine if ≥2 years old and future exposure is likely. Studies suggest that HAV vaccine alone may be effective for postexposure prophylaxis, but data are insufficient to recommend alone.

E. HEPATITIS B VIRUS IMMUNOPROPHYLAXIS

1. Description:

a. Hepatitis B immune globulin (HBIG): Prepared from plasma containing high-titer anti-HBsAg antibodies and negative for antibodies to HIV and HCV. Dose: Infants, 0.5 mL IM; older children, 0.06 mL/kg IM.

b. HBV vaccine: Adsorbed HBsAg produced recombinantly. Different recombinant vaccines may be used interchangeably.

c. See section V.O for information on combined vaccines containing hepatitis B (Pediarix, Twinrix).

2. Indications:

a. Routine: See Figure 15-1.

b. Infants of mothers who are HBsAg positive or indeterminate: See Figure 15-2.

3. Precautions/contraindications: See Table 15-11.

4. Side effects: Pain at injection site (3%–29%) or fever >37.7°C (1%–6%); immediate hypersensitivity reaction is very rare.

5. Administration:

a. See Table 15-13 for dose; give IM in the anterolateral thigh or deltoid; administration in the buttocks or intradermally is not recommended due to decreased immunogenicity.

b. HBV vaccines are interchangeable between different manufacturers, but interchangeability of Pediarix may be limited by the DTaP component. See section V.O.

6. Special considerations: See Table 15-14 for HBV prophylaxis after percutaneous exposure to blood.

See Figure 15-2 for management of neonates born to mothers with unknown or positive HBsAg status.

F. INFLUENZA VACCINE AND CHEMOPROPHYLAXIS

1. Description:

a. Inactivated influenza vaccines are produced in embryonated eggs.

b. Vaccines contain three viral strains (usually two type A and one type B), based on expected prevalent influenza strains for the upcoming winter.

c. Preparations:

(1) Inactivated whole virus vaccine is no longer available in the United States.

(2) Split-virus vaccines: Subvirion or purified surface antigen vaccines available; licensed for children >6 months of age.

(3) Live, attenuated intranasal vaccine (LAIV) was introduced in 2003. LAIV is not approved for children <60 months of age. Licensed for use in healthy persons 5 to 49 years of age, with no preference given to the inactivated or the intranasal vaccine.[2]

TABLE 15-13

RECOMMENDED DOSE FOR HBV VACCINES[a]

Patient Group	Recombivax Dose (μcg)[b]	Engerix-B Dose (μcg)[c]
Up to 19 yr	5	10
11–15 yr[d]	10[c]	—
≥20 yr	10	20
Patients undergoing dialysis and other immunosuppressed adults	40	40

[a]Vaccines are administered on a three- or four-dose schedule. Four doses are given if HBV is administered at birth, and a combination vaccine is used to complete the series.

[b]Recombivax HB is available from Merck & Co. in pediatric, adult, and dialysis patient formulations.

[c]Engerix-B is available from GlaxoSmithKline Biologicals; it is also available as combination vaccines: (1) Twinrix (Hepatitis B/Hepatitis A); (2) Pediarix (DTap/IPV/Hepatitis B). See section O for details.

[d]May use alternative two-dose regimen 6 months apart.

Data from American Academy of Pediatrics: Red Book: 2003 Report of the Committee on Infectious Diseases, 26th ed. Elk Grove Village, IL, American Academy of Pediatrics, 2003.

TABLE 15-14
HBV PROPHYLAXIS AFTER PERCUTANEOUS EXPOSURE TO BLOOD

	HBsAg Status of Source of Blood		
Exposed Person	Positive	Negative	Unknown
Unimmunized	HBIG Start vaccine series	Start vaccine series	Start vaccine series If source known to be high risk, treat as if HBsAg positive
Immunized			
Known responder	No treatment	No treatment	No treatment
Known nonresponder[a]	HBIG Start vaccine series	Start vaccine series	Start vaccine series If source known to be high risk, treat as if HBsAg positive
Response unknown	Test exposed person for anti-HBs If <10 mIU/mL, give HBIG, reimmunize If ≥10 mIU/mL, no treatment	No treatment	Test exposed person for anti-HBs If <10 mIU/mL, reimmunize If ≥10 mIU/mL, no treatment

[a]If patient has previously failed to respond to second vaccine series, two doses of HBIG (0.06 mL/kg) given 1 mo apart is recommended.
Data from American Academy of Pediatrics: Red Book: 2003 Report of the Committee on Infectious Diseases, 26th ed. Elk Grove Village, IL, American Academy of Pediatrics, 2003.

2. Indications:

a. High-risk children:
   (1) Asthma and other chronic pulmonary diseases.
   (2) Hemodynamically significant cardiac disease.
   (3) Immunosuppressive disorders and therapy.
   (4) HIV infection.
   (5) Sickle cell anemia and other hemoglobinopathies.
   (6) Diseases requiring long-term aspirin therapy.
   (7) Chronic renal disease.
   (8) Chronic metabolic disease, including diabetes mellitus.

b. Close contacts of high-risk children, children younger than 24 months, and adults: including household contacts, health care workers, and day-care providers. Also, consider chemoprophylaxis of these individuals.

c. Consider immunization for other high-risk persons:
   (1) Pregnant women who will be in their second or third trimester during influenza season (only the IM inactivated vaccine is approved).
   (2) International travel to areas with influenza outbreaks.
   (3) Institutional settings, including colleges and other residential facilities.

d. Annual immunization should be encouraged in healthy children 6 to 24 months of age and their close contacts.

3. Precautions/contraindications: See Table 15-10.

4. Side effects:

a. Fever 6 to 24 hours after immunization in children <2 years; rare in children >2 years.

b. Local reactions uncommon in children <13 years; 10% in children ≥13 years.

c. Side effects and immunogenicity are similar for whole and split-virus vaccines in children >12 years of age.

d. Guillain-Barré syndrome (GBS): Influenza immunization has been associated with GBS in about 1 per million persons ≥45 years of age; GBS has not been associated with influenza immunization in children.

e. LAIV: nasal congestion (20%–75%), headache (2%–46%), fever (0%–26%), and abdominal pain (2%).

5. Administration:

a. Administer annually during the fall in preparation for winter influenza season.

b. Dosage and schedule: See Table 15-15; give inactivated vaccine IM.

6. Special considerations:

a. Children receiving chemotherapy have poor seroconversion rates until chemotherapy is discontinued for 3 to 4 weeks and absolute neutrophil and lymphocyte counts are >1000/mm^3.

b. Immunization may be delayed in patients on prolonged high-dose steroids (equivalent to 2 mg/kg/day or >20 mg/day of prednisone) until dose is decreased, only if time allows before the influenza season.

TABLE 15-15

INFLUENZA VACCINE DOSAGE AND SCHEDULE

Age	Volume (mL)	Number of Doses
6–35 mo	0.25	1 or 2[a]
3–8 yr	0.5	1 or 2[a]
≥9 yr	0.5	1

[a]Two doses, at least 1 mo apart, are recommended for children <9 yr receiving influenza vaccine for the first time. Try to give the second dose before December.

Data from American Academy of Pediatrics: Red Book: 2003 Report of the Committee on Infectious Diseases, 26th ed. Elk Grove Village, IL, American Academy of Pediatrics, 2003.

c. Infants <6 months of age with high-risk conditions should not be immunized and should not receive chemoprophylaxis. However, close contacts of these infants should receive both the vaccine and chemoprophylaxis.
d. LAIV should not be administered until >48 hours after completing antiviral therapy for influenza.[2]

7. Chemoprophylaxis for influenza A and B[3]:

a. See Table 15-16.
b. Indications:
   (1) High-risk children immunized after influenza is present in the community or if likely to be exposed to individuals infected with influenza. In children <9 years of age, give for 6 weeks after first dose of vaccine or 2 weeks after second dose, depending on whether child is scheduled for 1 or 2 doses of vaccine.
   (2) Unimmunized individuals in close contact with or providing care to high-risk individuals.
   (3) Immunodeficient individuals unlikely to have protective response to vaccine.
   (4) Individuals at high risk for influenza infection with contraindication to vaccine.
   (5) Immunized high-risk individuals if vaccine strain different from circulating strain.
   (6) Healthy children with severe illness from influenza.
c. Chemoprophylaxis is not a substitute for immunization and does not interfere with the immune response to the inactivated virus vaccine.

TABLE 15-16

ANTIVIRAL DRUGS FOR INFLUENZA[a]

	Amantidine[b]	Rimantadine[b]	Zanamivir[c]	Oseltamivir[c]
Virus	A	A	A and B	A and B
Administration	Oral	Oral	Inhalational	Oral
Licensed ages	≥1 yr of age	≥13 yr of age	≥7 yr of age	≥1 yr of age
Prophylaxis indications	≥1 yr of age	≥1 yr of age	Not licensed	≥13 yr of age
Adverse effects	CNS, anxiety	CNS, anxiety	Bronchospasm	Nausea, vomiting

[a]All drugs, except zanamivir, require dosage adjustment in patients with renal failure.
[b]Antiviral therapy should be started as soon as possible and discontinued 24–48 hours after symptoms resolve. Both drugs, especially amantidine, may increase the risk for seizures in children with epilepsy. Resistance occurs but has not been proved clinically significant.
[c]Neuraminidase inhibitors should be given within 2 days of onset of symptoms and continued for a 5–day course. Resistance is uncommon but clinical significance is not fully known.
Data from American Academy of Pediatrics: Red Book: 2003 Report of the Committee on Infectious Diseases, 26th ed. Elk Grove Village, IL, American Academy of Pediatrics, 2003, Table 3.29, p 385.

d. Do not administer for chemoprophylaxis at least 2 weeks after administration of LAIV.

G. LYME IMMUNOPROPHYLAXIS

Vaccine is no longer available.

H. MEASLES/MUMPS/RUBELLA IMMUNOPROPHYLAXIS

1. Description:

a. MMR: Combined vaccine composed of live, attenuated viruses. Measles and mumps vaccines are grown in chick embryo cell culture; rubella vaccine is prepared in human diploid cell culture.

b. Monovalent measles, rubella, and measles/rubella (MR) formulations are available.

c. Ig: Intramuscular and intravenous immunoglobulin (IVIG) preparations contain similar concentration of measles antibody.

2. Indications:

a. Routine: See Figure 15-1.

b. Screen all women of childbearing age for susceptibility to rubella. People are considered susceptible to rubella unless they have documentation of one dose of rubella-containing vaccine or serologic evidence of immunity. If susceptible, immunize with one dose of MMR unless pregnant.

c. Screen all adolescents and young adults for susceptibility to measles. People are considered susceptible to measles unless they have had two measles-containing vaccines given 1 month apart after 12 months of age, physician-diagnosed disease, or laboratory evidence of immunity.

d. Immunize people traveling to foreign countries with MMR. Young children may need to be immunized at a younger age than recommended for routine immunization. See the AAP Red Book[1] for details.

3. Precautions/contraindications: See Table 15-10.

4. Misconceptions: The following are *not* contraindications to MMR administration:

a. Anaphylactic reaction to eggs: Consider observing patient for 90 minutes after vaccine administration. Skin testing is not predictive of hypersensitivity reaction and therefore is not recommended.

b. Allergy to penicillin.

c. Exposure to measles.

d. History of seizures: There is a slightly increased risk for seizure after immunization. Temperature should be followed and treated with antipyretics.

5. Side effects:

a. Minor side effects 7 to 12 days after immunization: Body temperature to 39.4°C develops 6 to 12 days after MMR vaccine and lasts 1 to 5 days (5%–15%); transient rash (5%).

b. Moderate to severe side effects: Febrile seizures (rare); transient thrombocytopenia (1 in 25,000 to 1 in 2 million) 2 to 3 weeks after immunization; encephalitis and encephalopathy (<1 in 1 million).

6. Administration:

a. Dose is 0.5 mL SC.

b. See AAP Red Book[1] for suggested intervals between Ig administration and MMR vaccination.

c. Purified protein derivative (PPD) testing may be done on the day of immunization; otherwise, postpone PPD 4 to 6 weeks because of suppression of response.

7. Special considerations:

a. Measles postexposure immunoprophylaxis.

(1) Vaccine prevents or modifies disease if given within 72 hours of exposure.

(2) Ig prevents or modifies disease if given within 6 days of exposure. Indicated in susceptible household contacts, pregnant women, children <1 year of age, and immunocompromised individuals. Dosage is as follows:

(a) Standard-dose Ig for children and pregnant women: 0.25 mL/kg (maximum dose, 15 mL) IM.

(b) High-dose Ig for immunocompromised children (including those with HIV infection): 0.5 mL/kg (maximum dose, 15 mL) IM. Not required if IVIG received within 3 weeks before exposure.

b. Rubella postexposure immunoprophylaxis: Ig may modify rubella disease but does not prevent congenital rubella syndrome; therefore, it is not recommended for exposed pregnant women.

I. MENINGOCOCCUS IMMUNOPROPHYLAXIS

1. Description: Quadrivalent serogroup-specific vaccine made from purified capsular polysaccharide antigen from groups A, C, Y, and W-135. Immunogenicity of serogroup antigens varies with age of child. No vaccine is available for group B because of poor immunogenicity.

2. Indications:

a. High-risk children ≥2 years of age include the following:

(1) Functional or anatomic asplenia.

(2) Terminal complement or properdin deficiencies.

b. Possible adjunct to postexposure chemoprophylaxis in an outbreak setting.

c. Consider in college freshmen, particularly those living in dormitories or residence halls.

d. Travelers to endemic or hyperendemic areas.

e. U.S. military recruits.

3. Precautions/contraindications: See Table 15-10.

4. Side effect: Mild: localized erythema lasting 1 to 2 days occurs infrequently.

5. Administration: Dose is 0.5 mL SC.

6. **Postexposure chemoprophylaxis:** Antibiotics should be given to exposed household, child care, and nursery school contacts within 24 hours of primary case diagnosis. Individuals with potential contact with oral secretions of infected patient should also receive chemoprophylaxis.
a. Rifampin is the drug of choice (See Formulary for dosage information).
b. Ciprofloxacin (500 mg single dose) may be given to persons ≥18 years.
c. Ceftriaxone (125 mg single dose in children ≤15 years, 250 mg single dose in children >15 years).

J. PNEUMOCOCCUS IMMUNOPROPHYLAXIS

1. **Description:**
a. PCV7: Pneumococcal conjugate vaccine includes seven purified capsular polysaccharides of *Streptococcus pneumoniae*, each coupled to a variant of diphtheria toxin. Serotypes are 4, 9V, 14, 19F, 23F, 18C, and 6B, which account for 88% of cases of bacteremia, 82% of cases of meningitis, and more than 70% of acute otitis media (AOM) among children <6 years old.
b. 23PS: Purified capsular polysaccharide includes antigen from 23 serotypes of *S. pneumoniae.* 23PS is not approved for use in children <2 years.
2. **Indications:**
a. Routine: See Figure 15-1.
b. See Table 15-3 for catch-up schedule for previously unvaccinated children ages 7 to 24 months.
c. See Table 15-6 for an immunization schedule of high-risk children ages 23 to 59 months, including those with the following conditions:
 (1) Sickle cell disease, functional or anatomic asplenia.
 (2) HIV infection.
 (3) Congenital immune deficiency.
 (4) Chronic renal insufficiency, including nephrotic syndrome.
 (5) Immunosuppression, including malignant neoplasms, leukemias, lymphomas, and Hodgkin disease, and solid organ transplantation.
 (6) Chronic cardiac disease.
 (7) Chronic pulmonary disease (including asthma treated with high-dose oral corticosteroid therapy).
 (8) Cerebrospinal fluid (CSF) leaks.
 (9) Diabetes mellitus.
d. Consider immunization in the following children, who are considered to be at moderate risk for invasive pneumococcal infection:
 (1) All children ages 24 to 35 months.
 (2) Children ages 36 to 59 months attending out-of-home care.
 (3) Children ages 36 to 59 months who are of American Indian, Alaska Native, or African American descent.

3. **Precautions/contraindications:** See Table 15-10.
4. **Side effects:** Pain and erythema at injection site (common); fever within 1 to 2 days after administration (less common); severe systemic reactions such as anaphylaxis (rare).
5. **Administration:**
a. Dose for both PCV7 and 23PS is 0.5 mL given IM.
b. Concurrent administration of PCV7 and 23PS vaccines is not recommended. Either vaccine may be given concurrently with other vaccines in a separate syringe at a separate injection site.
c. Give vaccine 2 weeks or more before elective splenectomy, chemotherapy, radiotherapy, or immunosuppressive therapy; or give 3 months after chemotherapy or radiotherapy.
6. **Special considerations:**
a. Passive immunoprophylaxis with IVIG is recommended for some children with congenital or acquired immune deficiencies.
b. See functional or anatomic asplenia, section IV.
c. PCV7 may provide a modest decrease in recurrent AOM and therefore may be beneficial in children 24 to 59 months of age with either recurrent AOM or with AOM requiring tympanostomy tube placement.

K. POLIOMYELITIS IMMUNOPROPHYLAXIS

1. **Description:**
a. IPV: Trivalent enhanced-potency vaccine of formalin-inactivated poliovirus types 1, 2, and 3 grown in human diploid or Vero cells.
b. OPV: No longer available in the United States. Children who have received the appropriate number of doses of OPV in other countries should be considered adequately immunized.
c. Combined vaccine (DTaP, HepB, Pediarix, IPV): See section V.O.
2. **Indications:**
a. Routine: See Figure 15-1.
b. Unimmunized or partially immunized individuals who are at imminent risk for exposure to poliovirus (dose interval may be 4 weeks).
3. **Precautions/contraindications:** See Table 15-10.
4. **Side effects:** No serious side effects have been associated with use of the IPV vaccine.
5. **Administration:** Dose is 0.5 mL SC.

L. RABIES IMMUNOPROPHYLAXIS (Table 15-17)

1. **Description:**
a. Three rabies vaccines are available for prophylaxis:
   (1) Human diploid cell vaccine (HDCV).
   (2) Rabies vaccine adsorbed (RVA).
   (3) Purified chicken embryo cell (PCEC).
b. Human rabies immune globulin (RIG): Anti-rabies Ig prepared from plasma of donors hyperimmunized with rabies vaccine.

TABLE 15-17

RABIES POSTEXPOSURE PROPHYLAXIS

Animal Type	Evaluation and Disposition of Animal	Postexposure Prophylaxis Recommendations
Dogs, cats, ferrets	Health and available for 10 days' observation	Do not begin prophylaxis unless animal develops symptoms of rabies
	If rabid or suspected rabid, euthanize animal and test brain	Immediate immunization and RIG
	Unknown (escaped)	Consult public health officials
Skunk, raccoon, bat[a], fox, most other carnivores	Regard as rabid unless animal is euthanized and brain is negative for rabies by fluorescein antibody test	Immediate immunization and RIG[b]
Livestock, rodents, rabbit, other mammals	Consider individually	Consult public health officials; these bites rarely require treatment

[a]In the case of direct contact between a human and a bat, consider prophylaxis even if a bite, scratch, or mucous membrane exposure is not apparent.

[b]Treatment may be discontinued if animal fluorescent antibody is negative.

Data from American Academy of Pediatrics: Red Book: 2003 Report of the Committee on Infectious Diseases, 26th ed. Elk Grove Village, IL, American Academy of Pediatrics, 2003.

2. Indications:

a. Preexposure prophylaxis: Indicated for high-risk groups, including veterinarians, animal handlers, laboratory workers, children living in high-risk environments, those traveling to high-risk areas, spelunkers.

(1) Three injections of vaccine on days 0, 7, and 21 or 28.

(2) Rabies serum antibody titers should be followed at 6-month intervals for those at continuous risk and at 2-year intervals for those with risk for frequent exposure; give booster doses only if titers are nonprotective.

b. Postexposure prophylaxis (see Table 15-17).

3. Precautions/contraindications: See Table 15-10.

4. Side effects: Side effects are uncommon in children. Local reactions in 25%; mild systemic reactions, such as headache, abdominal pain, and dizziness in 20%; neurologic illness similar to GBS or focal central nervous system (CNS) disorder (reported with HDCV, but not believed to be causally related); immune complex-like reaction (urticaria, arthralgia, angioedema, vomiting, fever, and malaise) 2 to 21 days after immunization with HDCV, rare in primary series, 6% after booster dose.

5. Administration: Dose is 1 mL IM for HDCV, RVA, and PCEC.

6. Postexposure prophylaxis:

a. General wound management:

(1) Clean immediately with soap and water.

(2) Avoid suturing wound unless indicated for functional reasons.

(3) Consider tetanus prophylaxis and antibiotics if indicated.

b. Indications: Infectious exposures include bites, scratches, or contamination of open wound or mucous membrane with infectious material of a rabid animal or human.

Note *Report all patients suspected of rabies infection to public health authorities.*

c. Administration:

(1) Vaccine and RIG should be given jointly except in previously immunized patients (no RIG required). If the vaccine is not immediately available, give RIG alone and vaccinate later. If RIG is not available, give the vaccine alone. RIG may be given later, if it can be administered within 7 days after initiating immunization.

(2) Vaccine for postexposure prophylaxis:

(a) Do not administer in same part of body or in same syringe as RIG.

(b) Deltoid muscle except infants, in whom anterolateral thigh is appropriate.

(c) Routine serologic testing not indicated.

(d) Unimmunized: 1 mL IM on days 0, 3, 7, 14, and 28.

(e) Previously immunized: 1 mL IM on days 0 and 3. Do not give RIG.

(3) RIG: Recommended dose of 20 IU/kg should not be exceeded. Infiltrate around the wound and give remainder IM.

M. RESPIRATORY SYNCYTIAL VIRUS (RSV) IMMUNOPROPHYLAXIS

1. Description:

a. No vaccine is available.

b. Palivizumab (monoclonal RSV-Ig): Humanized mouse monoclonal IgG to RSV, recombinantly produced for IM administration.

c. Polyclonal RSV-IVIG: Ig pooled from donors with high serum titers of RSV-neutralizing antibody, for IV administration. Provides some protection against other respiratory viruses.

2. Indications:

a. Infants and children <2 years of age with chronic lung disease (CLD) who have required medical therapy (oxygen, bronchodilators, diuretics, or corticosteroids) within the 6 months before the RSV season. Palivizumab is preferred. Data are limited, but these patients may also benefit from prophylaxis during a second RSV season.

b. Infants <32 weeks' estimated gestational age (EGA) at birth who do not have CLD may benefit from prophylaxis with palivizumab.

(1) EGA ≤28 weeks: Consider until 12 months of age.

(2) EGA 29 to 32 weeks: Consider until 6 months of age.

c. Prophylaxis should be considered in infants born between 32 and 35 weeks' gestation with two or more of the following risk factors:

(1) Child-care attendance.

(2) School-aged siblings.

(3) Exposure to environmental air pollutants, such as tobacco smoke.

(4) Congenital abnormalities of airways.

(5) Severe neuromuscular disease.

Note *These risk factors are considered additive.*

d. Children ≤24 months of age with significant cyanotic and acyanotic heart disease should be considered for prophylaxis with palivizumab.

e. Infants <12 months of age with congenital heart disease should be considered for prophylaxis with palivizumab, especially if they:

(1) Are receiving medication to treat congestive heart failure.

(2) Have moderate to severe pulmonary hypertension.

(3) Have a cyanotic heart lesion.

f. Children with severe immunodeficiency may benefit from RSV-IVIG, although its use has not been evaluated in randomized trials.

3. Precautions/contraindications: See Table 15-10.

4. Side effects:

a. Palivizumab: Side effects are comparable to placebo.

b. RSV-IVIG: See Formulary.

(1) Fever in 6% (2% in placebo group).
(2) 8% of children with CLD required extra diuretics around the time of administration.

5. **Administration:** Give RSV-IVIG or palivizumab at onset of RSV season, typically in November, and then monthly during the RSV season, which usually ends in March. In general, five total doses are given. Consult the local health department for the optimal schedule.
a. Palivizumab: Dose is 15 mg/kg IM monthly.
b. Polyclonal RSV-IVIG: Dose is 15 mL/kg (750 mg/kg) IV monthly. Must defer live vaccines (e.g., MMR and varicella) for 9 months after the last dose.

N. VARICELLA IMMUNOPROPHYLAXIS

1. **Description:**
a. Vaccine: Cell-free live attenuated varicella virus vaccine.
b. Varicella-zoster immune globulin (VZIG): Prepared from plasma-containing high-titer antivaricella antibodies.
2. **Indications:**
a. Routine: See Figure 15-1.
b. Aim to immunize before the 13th birthday because two doses are needed after that time.
3. **Precautions/contraindications:** See Table 15-10.
4. **Misconceptions:** Vaccine may be given in the following circumstances:
a. Certain children with acute lymphoblastic leukemia in remission >1 year may be immunized under a research protocol. Approval must be obtained by the appropriate institutional review board.
b. Household contacts of immunocompromised hosts: If a rash develops in the immunized child, avoid direct contact if possible.
c. Household contacts of pregnant women.
5. **Side effects:**
a. Local reaction, 20% to 35%; mild varicelliform rash within 5 to 26 days of vaccine administration, 3% to 5%.
b. Vaccine rash often very mild, but patient may be infectious; reversion to wild-type virus has not been reported. Most varicelliform rashes that occur within 2 weeks of vaccination are due to wild-type VZV infection.
6. **Administration:**
a. Dose is 0.5 mL SC.
b. May give simultaneously with MMR; otherwise, allow at least 1 month between MMR and varicella vaccines.
c. Do not give for 5 months after VZIG; do not give concurrently with VZIG.
d. Avoid salicylates for 6 weeks after vaccine administration if possible.
7. **Postexposure prophylaxis:**
a. Indications: VZIG should be administered within 96 hours of exposure to individuals who are at high risk for severe varicella and who have

had a significant exposure (see below). Repeat VZIG every 3 weeks if exposure is ongoing or repeated.

(1) Individuals at high risk for severe varicella include the following:
   (a) Immunocompromised individuals without a history of varicella.
   (b) Susceptible pregnant women.
   (c) Newborn infant with onset of varicella in mother from 5 days before to 2 days after delivery (even if mother received VZIG during pregnancy).
   (d) Hospitalized preterm infant who was born before 28 weeks' gestation or who weighs <1000 g, regardless of maternal history.
   (e) Hospitalized preterm infant who was born at ≥28 weeks' gestation to a susceptible mother.

(2) Significant exposures include the following:
   (a) Household contact.
   (b) Face-to-face indoor play.
   (c) Onset of varicella in the mother of a newborn from 5 days before to 2 days after delivery.
   (d) Hospital exposures: Roommate, face-to-face contact with infectious individual, visit by contagious individual, or intimate contact with person with active zoster lesions.

Note *For VZIG recipients, incubation period may be up to 28 days instead of 21 days.*

b. VZIG dose is 12.5 U/kg IM (maximum dose, 625 U; minimum dose, 125 U). Do not give intravenously. Local discomfort is common.

c. Varicella vaccine should be administered to susceptible immunocompetent children within 72 hours after varicella exposure. If the child was exposed at the same time as the index case, the vaccine may not protect against the disease. Susceptible immunocompromised children should receive VZIG as soon as possible.

O. COMBINED VACCINES

1. DTaP-HepB-IPV (Pediarix):

a. Description: DTap, IPV, and Hepatitis B (Energix-B, 20 μg).

b. Indications:
   (1) Routine: Use when vaccine components are indicated, so long as other components are not contraindicated. Administered in a three-dose schedule, preferably at 2, 4, and 6 months of age. See Figure 15-1.
   (2) Should not be administered to infants <6 weeks of age or to children >7 years of age.

c. If used as the third dose to complete the hepatitis B series, it should be administered at 6 months of age or older.

d. Pediarix should not be used as a booster dose following the three-dose primary DTaP series because there are insufficient data on safety and efficacy on use as a booster dose.
e. Side effects: Higher rates of fever are reported with combined vaccine than with three vaccines administered separately.
f. Precautions/contraindications: See Table 15-10.

2. Hep A-Hep B (Twinrix):

a. Description: Energix-B (20 μg) and Havrix (720 ELU).
b. Indications: Routine: See Figure 15-1.
c. Licensed for use in patients ≥18 years of age.
d. Administered in a three-dose schedule given at 0, 1 month, and at least 6 months later.

3. PRP-OMP/HepB (Comvax):

a. Description: PRP-OMP and Recombivax (5 μg).
b. Indications: Routine: See Figure 15-1.
c. Licensed for use at 2, 4, and 12 to 15 months of age.

REFERENCES

1. American Academy of Pediatrics. Red Book: 2003 Report of the Committee on Infectious Diseases, 26th ed. Elk Grove Village, IL: American Academy of Pediatrics, 2003.
2. Using live, attenuated influenza vaccine for prevention and control of influenza: Supplemental Recommendations of the Advisory Committee on Immunization Practices (ACIP). MMWR Morb Mortal Wkly Rep 2003;52 [RR13]:1–8.
3. Centers for Disease Control and Prevention: Guidelines for preventing opportunistic infections among hematopoietic stem cell transplant recipients: Recommendations of CDC, the Infectious Disease Society of America, and the American Society of Blood and Marrow Transplantation. MMWR Morb Mortal Wkly Rep 2000;49(No. RR-10):1–147.

Microbiology and Infectious Disease

Kabuiya Kimani, MD

16

I. MICROBIOLOGY

A. COLLECTION OF SPECIMENS FOR BLOOD CULTURE

1. **Preparation:** Proper specimen collection is essential to minimize contamination. Clean venipuncture site with 70% isopropyl ethyl alcohol. Apply tincture of iodine or 10% povidone-iodine and allow to dry for at least 1 minute, or scrub site with 2% chlorhexidine. Clean blood culture bottle injection site with alcohol only.
2. **Collection:** Obtain 1 to 2 mL for a neonate, 2 to 3 mL for an infant, 3 to 5 mL for a child, and 10 to 20 mL for an adolescent. There is a higher culture yield with higher volume blood cultures.

B. RAPID MICROBIOLOGIC IDENTIFICATION OF COMMON AEROBIC BACTERIA (Fig. 16-1)

C. CHOOSING APPROPRIATE ANTIBIOTIC BASED ON SENSITIVITIES

1. **Definitions**[1,2]**:**
   a. **Minimum inhibitory concentration (MIC):** The lowest concentration of an antimicrobial agent that prevents visible growth after an 18- to 24-hour incubation period.
   b. **Minimum bactericidal concentration (MBC):** The lowest concentration of an antimicrobial agent that kills >99.9% of organisms, as measured by subculturing to antibiotic-free media after 18- to 24-hour incubation.
2. **Common pitfalls:** See Table 16-1 for clinically significant, common discrepancies between in vitro (laboratory reported) and in vivo antibiotic sensitivity profiles.

II. INFECTIOUS DISEASE

A. FEVER EVALUATION AND MANAGEMENT GUIDELINES (Figs. 16-2 and 16-3)

B. COMMON PEDIATRIC INFECTIONS: GUIDELINES FOR INITIAL MANAGEMENT (Table 16-2)

C. CONGENITAL INFECTIONS

1. **Intrauterine infections:** TORCH infections (toxoplasmosis; others such as syphilis, varicella-zoster [VZV], and other viruses; rubella; cytomegalovirus [CMV]; and herpes simplex virus [HSV]) often present in the neonate with overlapping findings: intrauterine growth retardation (IUGR), microcephaly, hepatosplenomegaly, rash, central nervous system (CNS) manifestations, early jaundice, and low platelets.[5] Table 16-3 helps differentiate possible infections based on clinical features.

Text continues on p. 423

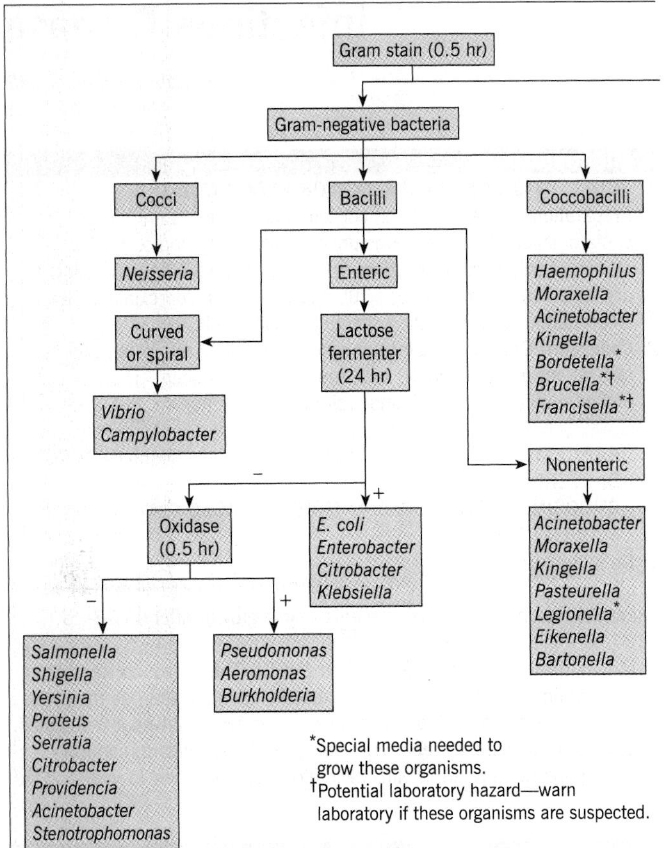

FIG. 16-1

Algorithm demonstrating identification of aerobic bacteria. Numbers in parentheses indicate the time required for the tests.

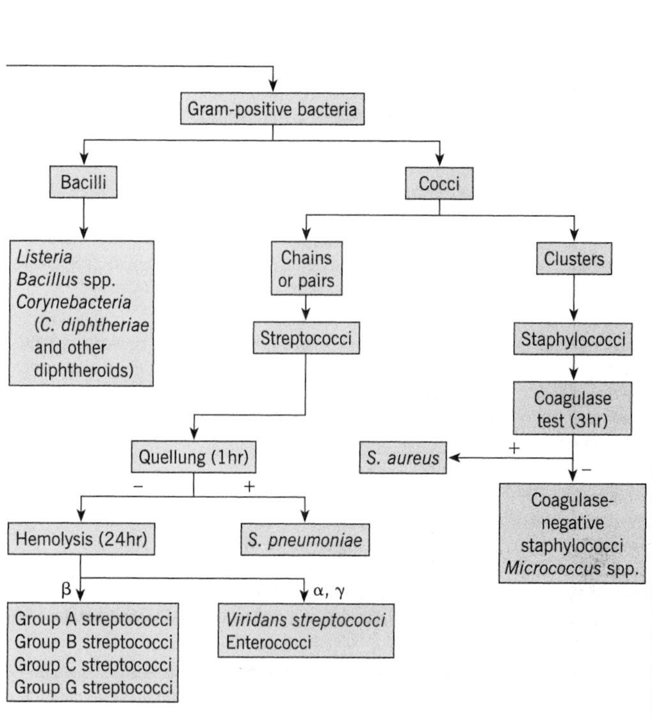
Gram-positive bacteria
Bacilli
Cocci
Listeria
Bacillus spp.
Corynebacteria
(C. diphtheriae
and other
diphtheroids)
Chains
or pairs
Clusters
Streptococci
Staphylococci
Coagulase
test (3hr)
Quellung (1hr)
S. aureus
+
−
Coagulase-
negative
staphylococci
Micrococcus spp.
Hemolysis (24hr)
S. pneumoniae
β
α, γ
Group A streptococci
Group B streptococci
Group C streptococci
Group G streptococci
Viridans streptococci
Enterococci

TABLE 16-1

COMMON PITFALLS BETWEEN IN VITRO AND IN VIVO ANTIBIOTIC SENSITIVITY PROFILES

Bacteria	Pitfall
Staphylococci	If methicillin-resistant Staph Aureus (MRSA) is reported as having susceptibility to clindamycin but resistance to erythromycin, a D test (double disc diffusion assay) is recommended to look for in vitro inducible macrolide-lincosamide-streptogramin B (MLS_B) resistance. If the D test is positive, suspect that MRSA may have inducible resistance to clindamycin and consider using vancomycin.
Salmonella	Despite in vitro susceptibility to aminoglycosides, salmonella are not susceptible in vivo to this class of antibiotics.
Enterobacter spp. *Citrobacter* spp. *Pseudomonas aeruginosa* *Serratia* spp. *Providencia* spp.	All are inducibly resistant to all cephalosporins; therefore, cephalosporins should not be used as sole treatment for invasive or serious infections caused by these organisms. Because β-lactamase inhibitors are potent inducers of cephalosporin resistance, and they do not overcome resistance in these organisms. β-lactamase inhibitors should not be used.[3]
Pseudomonas and related species *P. aeruginosa* *Acinetobacter* spp. *Burkholderia cepacia* *Stenotrophomonas maltophilia*.	*Burkholderia* and *Stenotrophomonas* species are resistant to aminoglycosides and often are only susceptible to TMP-SMX, the drug of choice in most cases for these organisms. *P. aeruginosa* and *Acinetobacter* species, on the other hand are usually susceptible to aminoglycosides, but resistant to TMP-SMX (despite reported in vitro susceptibility).
Enterococci	Intrinsic resistance to most antibiotic classes necessitates double-agent therapy for synergy and bacterial killing in the treatment of invasive infections. Recommended therapy is ampicillin (vancomycin if ampicillin resistant). Add an aminoglycoside (preferably gentamicin; streptomycin also active) for serious invasive infections. Other antiblotics with activity against enterococci include amoxicillin, penicillin, piperacillin, and imipenem. Vancomycin-resistant enterococcus (VRE) is usually *Enterococcus faecium*, though rarely *E. faecalis*. Linezolid is active against most enterococcal isolates, including VRE. Quinupristin/dalfopristin (Synercid) is active against most *E. faecium*, including VRE, but not against *E. faecalis*. The following antibiotics are *not* clinically active against enterococci: all cephalosporins, antistaphylococcal penicillins (e.g., oxacillin), macrolides, clindamycin, and quinolones.

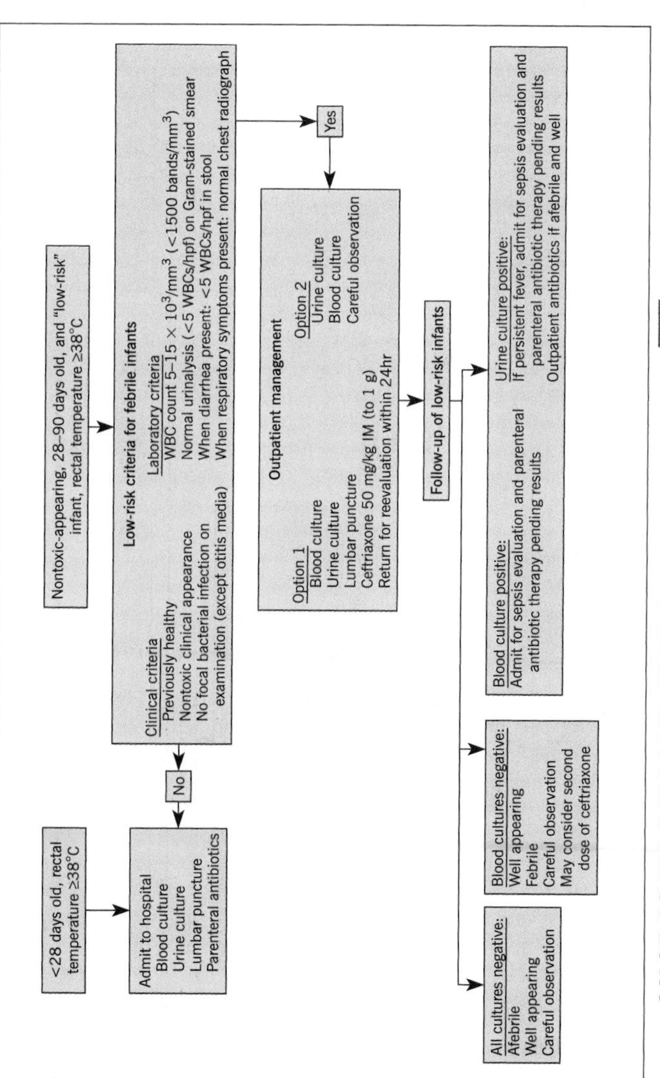

FIG. 16-2

Algorithm for the management of a previously healthy infant <90 days of age with a fever without localizing signs. This algorithm is a suggested, but not exhaustive, approach to management. hpf, high-power field. *(Modified from Baraff LJ, et al: Ann Emerg Med 2000;36[6]:602–614.)*

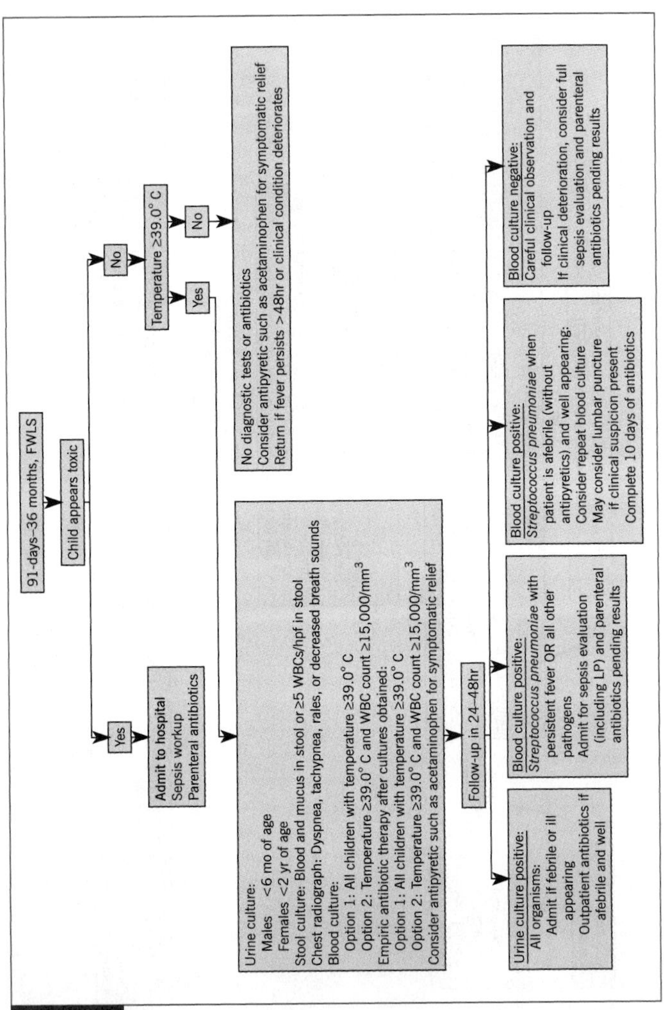

FIG. 16-3

Algorithm for the management of a previously healthy child 91 days to 36 months of age with a fever without localizing signs (FWLS). This algorithm is a suggested, but not exhaustive, approach to management. *(Modified from Baraff LJ, et al: Pediatrics 1993;92:5–9.)*

TABLE 16-2
COMMON PEDIATRIC INFECTIONS: GUIDELINES FOR INITIAL MANAGEMENT

Infectious Syndrome	Usual Etiology	Suggested Empiric Therapy	Suggested Length of Therapy/Comments
Bacteremia (outpatient)	*Streptococcus pneumoniae, GAS, Neisseria meningitidis, Escherichia coli, Salmonella*	Empiric: Ceftriaxone or cefotaxime	7–10 days (longer for some pathogens). Occult bacteremia with susceptible *S. pneumoniae* may be treated with amoxicillin if afebrile, well, and without focal complications.
Bites			
Human	Streptococci, *Staphylococcus aureus, Staphylococcus epidermidis*, oral anaerobes, *Eikenella corrodens*	PO: Amoxicillin/clavulanate or cefotaxime and clindamycin Alt: TMP/SMX + clindamycin IV: Ampicillin/sulbactam	5–7 days. Cleaning, irrigation, and debridement most important. Assess tetanus immunization status, risk of hepatitis B and HIV. Antibiotic prophylaxis routinely used for human bites.
Dog/cat	Human bite pathogens *plus Pasteurella multocida*	Same	7–10 days. Assess tetanus immunization status, risk of rabies. Antibiotic prophylaxis for all cat bites and selected dog bites.
Cellulitis	GAS, *S. aureus* (MSSA or MRSA)	PO: Cephalexin. If penicillin allergic or MRSA common in population, clindamycin IV: Oxacillin Alt: Clindamycin	3 days after acute inflammation resolves (usually 7–10 days).
Conjunctivitis			
Neonatal	*Chlamydia trachomatis* (onset 3–10 days)	PO: Erythromycin, other macrolides	14 days. Topical ineffective in preventing pneumonia.
	Neisseria gonorrhoeae (onset 2–4 days)	IM/IV: Ceftriaxone, cefotaxime	Localized to eye: Single dose. Disseminated: 7 days of parenteral therapy.
Suppurative	*S. pneumoniae, H. influenzae*	Ophthalmic; erythromycin or bacitracin/polymyxin B, or polymyxin B/TMP	5 days. Ointments preferred for infants or young children and eyedrops for older chilren and adolescents.

continued

TABLE 16-2

COMMON PEDIATRIC INFECTIONS: GUIDELINES FOR INITIAL MANAGEMENT—*cont'd*

Infectious Syndrome	Usual Etiology	Suggested Empiric Therapy	Suggested Length of Therapy/Comments
Gastroenteritis			
Community acquired	Viruses, *Escherichia coli*	Antibiotic therapy strongly discouraged because of possible increased risk for hemolytic-uremic syndrome occurring in patients with *E. coli* 0157:H7 treated with antibiotics[4]	Primary treatment: fluid and electrolyte replacement.
	Salmonella	Cefotaxime or ceftriaxone Alt: Azithromycin	10–14 days for infants <6 mo, bacteremia, toxicity or immunocompromised status. Antiblotics generally not indicated otherwise.
	Shigella	TMP/SMX. Alt: Ceftriaxone or oral cefixime	5 days.
	Yersinia	TMP/SMX, aminoglycosides, cefotaxime, tetracycline (>8 yr)	Usually no antibiotic therapy is recommended except with bacteremia, extraintestinal infections, or immunocompromised hosts.
	Campylobacter	Azithromycin or Erythromycin	5–7 days. Shortens duration and fecal excretion.
Nosocomial	*Clostridium difficile*	Metronidazole	7 days. Community organisms unlikely after 72 hr of hospitalization.
Lymphadenitis	Viruses, Group A strep, *Mycobacterium TB, S. aureus,* anaerobes, atypical mycobacteria, actinomyces, *B. henselae* (cat scratch)	PO: Augmentin or cloxacillin Alt: Cephalexin IV: Oxacillin or Nafcillin Alt: Cefazolin	Surgical incision with *M. TB*. Needle aspiration with *B. henselae*.

Mastoiditis (acute)	*S. pneumoniae, Streptococcus pyogenes, S. aureus, H. influenzae*	Oxacillin plus cefotaxime or ceftriaxone Alt: Amoxicillin/clavulanic acid	10 days.
Meningitis			
Neonate. <1 mo	GBS, Enterobacteriaceae, (esp. *E. coli*) *Listeria monocytogenes*	Ampicillin and cefotaxime Alt: Ampicillin and gentamicin	14–21 days for GBS and *Listeria*. 21 days for Enterobacteriaceae (cefotaxime, aminoglycoside).
1–3 mo	GBS, *S. pneumoniae, H. influenzae, N. meningitidis*, Enterobacteriaceae	Ampicillin and cefotaxime	10–14 days for *S. pneumoniae*, 7 days for *N. meningitidis*, 7–10 days for *H. influenzae*.
Infants >3 mo and childen	*S. pneumoniae, N. meningitidis, H. influenzae,* neonatal pathogens	Cefotaxime or ceftriaxone. Vancomycin should be also added empirically for possible penicillin-resistant *S. pneumoniae*, until susceptibility is known.	Dexamethasone use except for *H. Flu* uncertain. Recommended with evidence of increased ICP to be given before or with first antibiotic dose. See *Red Book*[8] *2003* for chemoprophylaxis recommendations for contacts of meningococcal and Hib disease.
Orbital cellulitis	*S. pneumoniae, H. influenzae (nontypeable), Moraxella catarrhalis, S. aureus,* GAS	Cefotaxime or ceftriaxone *plus* clindamycin or oxacillin.	10 days. Monitor for cavernous thrombosis.
Osteomyelitis	*S. aureus,* GAS	Semisynthetic penicillin (oxacillin, nafcillin). Alt: Clindamycin or vancomycin.	4–6 wk.
Foot puncture	Add *Pseudomonas*	Add ceftazidime.	
Sickle cell disease	Add *Salmonella*	Add cefotaxime.	

continued

TABLE 16-2

COMMON PEDIATRIC INFECTIONS: GUIDELINES FOR INITIAL MANAGEMENT—*cont'd*

Infectious Syndrome	Usual Etiology	Suggested Empiric Therapy	Suggested Length of Therapy/Comments
Otitis media (acute)	*S. pneumoniae, H. influenzae* (nontypeable), *M. catarrhalis*, viral	Firstline: Amoxicillin or high-dose amoxicillin (80–100 mg/kg/day). Alt for penicillin allergy: Cefuroxime, cefdinir, cefprozil, azithromycin. Persistent otitis media (after 3 days): Amoxicillin/clavulanic acid, cefuroxime, or ceftriaxone (IM/IV).	5–10 days. For persistent otitis media (at 2–3 days follow-up) despite antibiotic therapy, consider tympanocentesis. Short course 5–7 days for >2 yr old without language or hearing deficil.
Otitis externa (uncomplicated)	*Pseudomonas*, Enterobacteriaceae, *Proteus*	Eardrops: Polymyxin B/neomycin/hydrocortisone. Alt: Ofloxacin drops.	7–10 days.
Periorbital cellulitis (preseptal)	Associated with sinusitis: See sinusitis Associated with skin lesion: See cellulitis Hematogenous (<2 yr): See bacteremia	IV: Oxacillin + cefotaxime. PO: Amoxicillin/clavulanate.	10–14 days.
Pharyngitis	GAS, Group C and G strep, viral, mononucleosis	PO: Penicillin VK. IM: Benzathine penicillin G × 1 dose. Alt: Erythromycin, cephalexin.	10 days. TMP/SMX *not* effective. 10 days.

Pneumonia			
Neonatal	*E. coli*, GBS, *S. aureus*, *Listeria monocytogenes*, *C. trachomatis*	Ampicillin + gentamicin or ampicillin + cefotaxime.	10–21 days. Blood cultures indicated. Effusions should be drained, Gram stain of fluid obtained.
3 wk–4 mo	*Chlamydia trachomatis*, *S. pneumoniae*, viruses	Erythromycin. Alt:	10 days.
Infant/child (6 wk–4 yr)		PO: Azithromycin IV: Cefotaxime (if febrile)	
Lobar	*S. pneumoniae*	PO: Amoxicillin. Alt: Clindamycin. IV: Ceftriaxone, cefotaxime.	7–10 days.
Atypical	*Bordetella pertussis*	Erythromycin (estolate preparation preferred), azithromycin, or clarithromycin.	14 days for erythromycin, 5 days for azithromycin, 7 days for clarithromycin. Chemoprophylaxis indicated for close contacts.
	Respiratory viruses	No antibiotics indicated.	
	Influenza	Zanamivir for flu A and B (>7 yo) Oseltamivir for flu A and B (>1 yo) Amantadine for flu A (>1 yo) Rimantadine for flu A (>13 yo)	Reduces symptoms notably if given within 36 hours after onset of symptoms.
≥4 yr			
Lobar	*S. pneumoniae*	PO: Amoxicillin. Alt: Erythromycin. IV: Ceftriaxone, or cefotaxime PLUS PO/IV macrolide.	7–10 days.
		Clarithromycin.	10 days.
		Azithromycin.	5 days.
Atypical	*Mycoplasma pneumoniae* or *Chlamydia pneumoniae*	Clarithromycin or azithromycin. Alt: Doxycycline or erythromycin.	14–21 days (5 days if using azithromycin).
	Influenza	Zanamivir or oseltamivir.	See comments above.

continued

TABLE 16-2

COMMON PEDIATRIC INFECTIONS: GUIDELINES FOR INITIAL MANAGEMENT—*cont'd*

Infectious Syndrome	Usual Etiology	Suggested Empiric Therapy	Suggested Length of Therapy/Comments
Septic arthritis			
<5 yr	*S. aureus,* GBS, Hib, GNB	See osteomyelitis.	3–4 wk IV. May switch to PO after response. Aspiration of affected joint recommended.
>5 yr	*S. aureus,* GAS		
Adolescent	Add *Neisseria gonorrhoeae*	See Table 16-10	
Sinusitis			
Acute	*S. pneumoniae, H. influenzae, M. catarrhalis*	See otitis media. Seriously ill child: Vancomycin and cefotaxime or ceftriaxone.	10–14 days.
Chronic	Add *S. aureus,* anaerobes	Amoxicillin/clavulanate or cefpodoxime.	21 days and 7 days after resolution of symptoms.
UTI			
Uncomplicated	*E. coli, Proteus, Staph suprophyticus* Enterococci	PO: TMP/SMX, cefixime. IV: Cefotaxime *or* ampicillin and gentamicin.	7–14 days (cystitis vs. pyelonephritis and age dependent).
Abnormal host/ urinary tract	Add *Pseudomonas*	Ampicillin and gentamicin, zosyn, or timentin.	14–21 days. Parenteral until afebrile × 24 hr.
Ventriculoperitoneal shunt, infected	*S. epidermidis, S. aureus,* Enterobacteriaceae	Vancomycin + cefotaxime or ceftriaxone. Add aminoglycoside if culture suggests Enterobacteriaceae. Consider adding rifampin.	10–21 days depending on organism and response. Shunt removal or revision may be necessary.

Alt, alternative; GAS, group A streptococci; GBS, group B streptococci; Hib, *Haemophilus influenzae* type b; TMP/SMX, trimethoprim-sulfamethoxazole.

TABLE 16-3

COMMON ETIOLOGIES OF CONGENITAL INFECTIONS AND THEIR ASSOCIATED CLINICAL FINDINGS

Congenital Infection	Clinical Finding
Rubella	IUGR, cataracts, cardiac anomalies, deafness
Toxoplasma	Retinopathy, cerebral calcifications, hydrocephalus
CMV	Jaundice, hepatosplenomegaly, microcephaly, thrombocytopenia
Syphilis	Hepatosplenomegaly, bone abnormalities, rash
HSV	Rash, retinopathy, meningoencephalitis

Initial evaluation of a neonate depends on level of suspicion and severity of clinical findings.[6] Consider head computed tomography (CT) or head ultrasound (intracerebral calcifications), long-bone films (metaphyseal abnormalities), ophthalmologic examination (keratoconjunctivitis and chorioretinitis), brainstem evoked responses for hearing evaluation, blood, urine, and cerebrospinal fluid (CSF) evaluation (cultures, serology, counts) as part of initial investigation. **See Table 16-4 for specific diagnostic criteria and therapy for the most common intrauterine infections.**

Note *HSV and VZV usually present as perinatal infections and rarely as an intrauterine infection. See Table 16-4 for descriptions.*

2. **Group B streptococcal (GBS) infection:**

a. **Presentation:**

(1) **Early-onset disease (<7 days old):** Respiratory distress, apnea, shock, pneumonia, and less often, meningitis.

(2) **Late-onset disease (1 week to 3 months):** Bacteremia, meningitis, osteomyelitis, septic arthritis, and cellulitis.

b. **Maternal intrapartum antibiotic prophylaxis (IAP):** To prevent early-onset GBS, the chemoprophylaxis regimen is penicillin or ampicillin. For penicillin-allergic patients with low anaphylaxis risk, may use cefazolin; otherwise, use clindamycin or erythromycin. For resistant organisms or if susceptibility is unknown, use vancomycin. IAP is recommended for women with vaginal or anorectal screening cultures positive for GBS at 35 to 37 weeks' gestation *or* one or more of the following risk factors:

(1) Previous infant with invasive disease.

(2) GBS bacteruria during pregnancy.

(3) Delivery at <37 weeks' gestation.

(4) Ruptured membranes for ≥18 hours.

(5) Intrapartum temperature >38°C (100.4°F).

(6) Unknown GBS status.

TABLE 16-4

DIAGNOSTIC CRITERIA AND THERAPY FOR COMMON INTRAUTERINE AND PERINATAL INFECTIONS

Disease	Diagnostic Criteria	Therapy
Cytomegalovirus (CMV)	CMV IgM from serum, CMV culture and early antigen from urine between 2 days and 1 wk of age.	Treatment of symptomatic infants with ganciclovir may decrease hearing loss but efficacy data are limited.
Enterovirus	Cultures from throat, stool, rectal swab; CSF for culture and PCR.	IVIG Pleconaril is an orally active agent that appears to be a safe and effective treatment of severe enteroviral illness in neonates and other age groups.[7] It is currently available on a compassionate care basis from the manufacturer, Viropharma in Exton, PA (610) 458-7300 or www.viropharma.com.
Hepatitis B	Check maternal HepBsAg status. If a HepBsAg-positive mother is also HepBeAg positive, the infant has a 90% chance of acquiring chronic hepatitis B infection if not given appropriate prophylaxis.	See Chapter 15 for initial management. To monitor success of efforts to prevent perinatal transmission of HBV, obtain HepBsAg and anti-HBs 1–3 mo after completion of Hep B series (series should be at birth, 1 mo, 6 mo). If HepBsAg is negative on follow-up, but anti-HBs concentration is <10 mIU/mL, infant should repeat vaccine series (0, 1, and 6 mo) with testing of anti-HBs 1 mo after series.
Hepatitis C	Check maternal HepC antibody status. If possible, check infant's HepC Ab status at 1 yr of age. If symptomatic, however, and earlier diagnosis needed, HCV PCR or HCV RNA can be checked at 1–2 mo of age.	No therapy until HCV status ascertained at 1 yr of life. Treatment with interferon-α and ribavirin is under investigation in children.
Herpes simplex virus (HSV)	HSV culture of blood, urine, CSF, skin vesicles, and surface cultures from conjunctiva, nasopharynx, throat, and rectum. Surface cultures obtained before 24–48 hr of life may indicate colonization from intrapartum exposure, without infection. Positive cultures obtained from any of these sites >48 hr after birth indicate viral replication suggestive of infection rather than colonization.[8]	Parenteral acyclovir 60 mg/kg/day divided Q8 hours for 14 days if only SEM disease; give 60 mg/kg/day for 21 days if CNS or disseminated disease. Infants with ocular involvement should also get topical ophthalmologic drug (1%–2% trifluridine, 1% iododeoxyuridine, or 3% vidarabine).

HIV	See section II.E	
Parvovirus	Parvovirus PCR and IgM antibody from serum.	Intrauterine blood transfusions may be indicated in selected cases. Infant treatment is supportive.
Rubella	Rubella virus can usually be obtained from nasal specimens. Throat swabs, blood, urine, and CSF can also yield virus. Check serum for rubella IgM.[9] Knowledge of maternal rubella immune status at onset of pregnancy is the most helpful piece of information. If checked late in pregnancy, infection early in pregnancy cannot be excluded.	Postexposure prophylaxis with immunoglobulin is not routinely recommended. Mothers with nonimmune status should be vaccinated in the immediate postpartum period, even if breast-feeding.
Syphilis	See section II.C.5.	
Toxoplasmosis	*Prenatal diagnosis*: A definitive diagnosis can be made by detecting either the parasite in fetal blood or amniotic fluid, or documenting *Toxoplasmosis gondii* IgM or IgA antibody in fetal blood. *T gondii* DNA by PCR from amniotic fluid also can be valid. *Postnatal diagnosis*: Attempts should be made to isolate *T. gondii* from placenta, umbilical cord, or assay for *T. gondii* by PCR from peripheral blood, CSF, and amniotic fluid. A positive IgM or IgA within 6 mo of life, or persistently positive IgG titers beyond 1 yr of life can also be diagnostic.	Treatment indicated for chorioretinitis, meningitis, or significant organ damage. Treat with pyrimethamine in combination with sulfasalazine and leucovorin. Add prednisone for congenital toxo and chorioretinitis.
Varicella (VZV)	Direct fluorescent antigen (DFA) from vesicle scraping is rapid and sensitive. VZV PCR from body fluid or tissue is also very sensitive. Virus may be cultured from vesicle base during first 3–4 days of eruption. It can be difficult to distinguish VZV from HSV lesions clinically.	*Maternal*: Acyclovir may be beneficial during pregnancy. VZIG after exposure for susceptible pregnant women is recommended. *Infant*: VZIG immediately if maternal rash develops between 5 days before and 2 days after birth. Acyclovir if neonate develops varicella.

Note *Women with known negative results from vaginal and rectal GBS screening cultures within 5 weeks of delivery do not require IAP even if any of the intrapartum risk factors develop.*

Routine IAP is not recommended for GBS colonized women undergoing planned cesarean section who have not begun labor or had ruptured membranes.

c. **Management of neonates:** Figure 16-4 shows the management of neonates born to mothers for whom intrapartum prophylaxis of GBS is indicated.

d. **Treatment of neonatal GBS disease:** Penicillin G or ampicillin, plus an aminoglycoside (usually gentamicin). Duration of therapy depends on extent of disease. Alternative: cefotaxime.

3. **Perinatal viral infections:**

a. **VZV:** If a mother develops varicella from 5 days before to 2 days after delivery, varicella infection in the infant can be severe and even fatal. Neonates usually look well at birth, then develop vesicles between 3 to 10 days of life. Dissemination can result in pneumonitis, encephalitis, purpura fulminans, widespread bleeding, hypotension, and death. If mother develops varicella more than 5 days before delivery and infant's gestational age is more than 28 weeks, severity of disease tends to be milder secondary to transplacental transfer of antibody.[9] **See Table 16-4 for diagnosis and treatment.**

b. **Herpes simplex virus:** Neonatal HSV infections are often severe, with high mortality and morbidity despite therapy. HSV infection can present as (1) **disseminated disease** with lung and severe liver disease, (2) **localized CNS infection,** or (3) **disease localized to skin, eye, mouth (SEM).** Initial symptoms can occur any time in the first 4 to 5 weeks of life. Disseminated disease often occurs in the first week of life. CNS disease presents latest, often in the second or third week of life.[8] **See Table 16-4 for diagnosis and treatment.**

c. **Enterovirus:** Neonates (usually <2 weeks old) who develop enterovirus infections can develop severe disease with major systemic manifestations (hepatic necrosis, myocarditis, encephalitis, pneumonia, necrotizing enterocolitis [NEC], and disseminated intravascular coagulation [DIC]) mimicking overwhelming bacterial infection. Death is typically caused by hepatic failure or myocarditis.[7] See Table 16-4 for diagnosis and treatment.

4. **Hydrops fetalis:** Infectious causes of hydrops account for 8% of all cases; the most common causes of nonimmune hydrops fetalis are parvovirus B19, CMV, HSV, *Toxoplasma gondii* infection, and *Treponema pallidum* infection. Less common agents include enterovirus, adenovirus, rubella, polio, influenza B, respiratory syncytial virus (RSV), *Listeria* species, *Leptospira* species, *Trypanosoma cruzii, Chlamydia* species, and *Ureaplasma urealyticum*.[10] Specific serology or cultures for the more common etiologic agents are indicated when

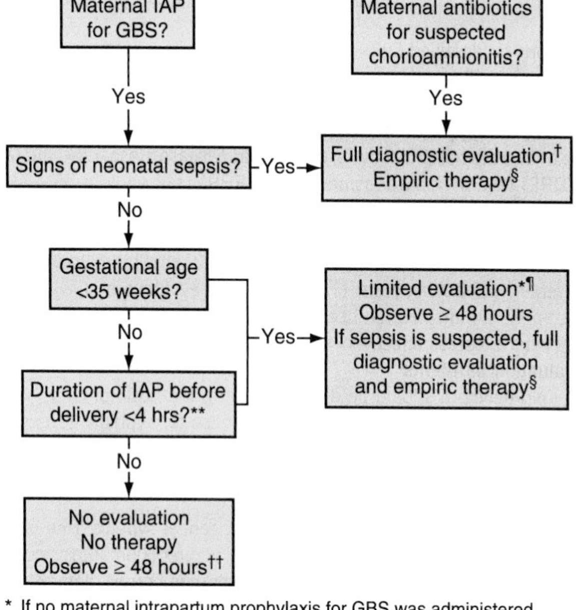

* If no maternal intrapartum prophylaxis for GBS was administered despite an indication being present, data are insufficient on which to recommend a single management strategy.

† Includes complete blood cell count and differential, blood culture, and chest radiograph if respiratory abnormalities are present. When signs of sepsis are present, a lumbar puncture, if feasible, should be performed.

§ Duration of therapy varies depending on results of blood culture, cerebrospinal fluid findings, if obtained, and the clinical course of the infant. If laboratory results and clinical course do not indicate bacterial infection, duration may be as short as 48 hours.

¶ CBC with differential and blood culture.

** Applies only to penicillin, ampicillin, or cefazolin and assumes recommended dosing regimen.

†† A healthy-appearing infant who was ≥38 weeks' gestation at delivery and whose mother received ≥4 hours of intrapartum prophylaxis before delivery may be discharged home after 24 hours if other discharge criteria have been met and a person able to comply fully with instructions for home observation will be present. If any one of these conditions is not met, the infant should be observed in the hospital for at least 48 hours and until criteria for discharge are achieved.

FIG. 16-4

Empiric management of neonate born to a mother who received intrapartum antimicrobial prophylaxis (IAP) to prevent early-onset group B streptococcal disease. This algorithm is a suggested, but not exclusive, approach to management. *(From MMWR Recommendations and Reports. 2002;51[RR-11]:1–22.)*

hydrops is identified by ultrasound. See respective sections for appropriate diagnostic workup.

5. **Congenital syphilis:**

a. **Testing during pregnancy:** All pregnant women should be screened with a nontreponemal antibody test **(Venereal Disease Research Laboratory [VDRL] test or Rapid Plasma Reagin [RPR] test)** early in pregnancy and preferably again at delivery. In areas of high prevalence and in patients considered high risk, a test early in the third trimester is also indicated. Positive screening for RPR or VDRL should be confirmed with a treponemal antibody test (FTA). If there is evidence of infection, treatment is indicated, and serologies (RPR or VDRL titers) should be followed to assess effectiveness of therapy.

b. **Evaluation of infants:**
   (1) No newborn should be discharged from the hospital without determining the mother's serologic status for syphilis. Testing of cord blood or infant serum is not adequate for screening.
   (2) All infants of women diagnosed with syphilis should have a venous nontreponemal antibody test.
   (3) An infant should be evaluated for congenital syphilis if he or she is born to a mother who has a positive nontreponemal test, confirmed by a positive treponemal test, and who has one or more of the following:
      (a) No treatment, inadequate treatment, or undocumented treatment.
      (b) Treatment with nonpenicillin regimen; for example, erythromycin (a pregnant woman with syphilis and a penicillin allergy history should be treated with penicillin after desensitization).
      (c) Treated less than 1 month before delivery.
      (d) Appropriately treated but expected decrease of fourfold or more in RPR or VDRL titers did not occur.
      (e) Had insufficient serologic follow-up to ensure that she responded appropriately to treatment by demonstrating a fourfold or greater decrease in titers in 3 months after course of treatment.
      (f) Maternal titer has increased fourfold, infant titer is at least fourfold greater than mother's, or the infant is symptomatic.
   (4) Further evaluation of infants with the preceding conditions should include the following:
      (a) Physical examination (e.g., rash [vesiculobullous], hepatomegaly, generalized lymphadenopathy, persistent rhinitis).
      (b) Quantitative nontreponemal test on infant's serum (cord blood not adequate).
      (c) Examine CSF for protein, cell count, and VDRL test. CSF VDRL is specific but *not* sensitive. (Do not perform RPR or FTA-ABS test [fluorescent treponemal antibody absorption] on CSF.)
      (d) Radiologic studies: Long-bone films for diaphyseal periostitis, osteochondritis.

(e) If available, antitreponemal immunoglobulin M (IgM) through a testing method recognized by the Centers for Disease Control and Prevention (CDC) either as a standard or provisional method.
(f) Complete blood cell (CBC) count and platelet count.
(g) Other tests as clinically indicated (e.g., chest radiograph, liver function tests [LFTs]).

(5) Guide for interpretation of the syphilis serology of mothers and their infants[8] (Table 16-5).

TABLE 16-5

GUIDE FOR INTERPRETATION OF THE SYPHILIS SEROLOGY OF MOTHERS AND THEIR INFANTS

Nontreponemal Test (e.g., VDRL, RPR, ART)		Treponemal Test (e.g., MHA-TP, FTA-ABS)		
Mother	Infant	Mother	Infant	Interpretation*
–	–	–	–	No syphilis or incubating syphilis in the mother and infant
+	+	–	–	No syphilis in mother (false-positive nontreponemal test with passive transfer to infant)†
+	+ or –	+	+	Maternal syphilis with possible infant infection; or mother treated for syphilis during pregnancy; or mother with latent syphilis and possible infection of infant‡
+	+	+	+	Recent or previous syphilis in the mother; possible infection in infant
–	–	+	+	Mother successfully treated for syphilis before or early in pregnancy with passive transmission of + FTA-ABS; or mother with Lyme disease, yaws, or pinta (i.e., false-positive serology)†

*Table presents a guide and not the definitive interpretation of serologic tests for syphilis in mothers and their newborns. Other factors that should be considered include the timing of maternal infection, the nature and timing of maternal treatment, quantitative maternal and infant titers, and serial determination of nontreponemal test titers in both mother and infant.

†False-positive nontreponemal reagin tests can occur with acute bacterial or viral infections, early HIV infection, vaccination, and a variety of autoimmune diseases. Some illnesses (e.g., systemic lupus erythematosus) can also give false-positive treponemal tests. Other spirochetal illnesses (relapsing fever, yaws, pinta, leptospirosis, rat-bite fever) can also yield both positive nontreponemal and treponemal tests. Lyme disease gives a false-positive FTA-ABS, but a negative nontreponemal test.[2]

‡Mothers with latent syphilis may have nonreactive nontreponemal tests.

ART, automated reagin test; *MHA-TP*, microhemagglutination test for *T. pallidum*.

Modified from Pickering LK (ed): 2003 Red Book: Report of the Committee on Infectious Diseases, 26th ed. Elk Grove Village, IL, American Academy of Pediatrics, 2003.

(6) Treatment of neonates with proven or possible congenital syphilis (Table 16-6): Follow nontreponemal serologic tests at 3, 6, and 12 months after treatment. See Table 16-7 for guidance in interpreting follow-up serology.
(7) Treatment of syphilis (postneonatal) (Table 16-8).

D. SELECTED SEXUALLY TRANSMITTED DISEASES

1. Pelvic inflammatory disease (PID) (Table 16-9).

2. Therapy for chlamydia, gonorrhea, and PID (Table 16-10).

TABLE 16-6

TREATMENT OF NEONATES WITH PROVEN OR POSSIBLE CONGENITAL SYPHILIS

Clinical Status	Antimicrobial Therapy[a]
Proven or highly probable disease[b]	Aqueous crystalline penicillin G 50,000 U/kg/dose IV Q12 hr for the first week, then Q8hr for a total course of 10 days[c,d]
Asymptomatic, normal CSF and radiologic examination—maternal treatment history as follows:	
• None, inadequate penicillin treatment,[e] undocumented, failed, or reinfected	Aqueous crystalline penicillin G IV for 10–14 days[c,d] (see dosing above) ***or*** Clinical, serologic follow-up and benzathine penicillin G 50,000 U/kg IM, single dose[f]
• Adequate therapy given >1 mo before delivery, mother's response to treatment demonstrated by a fourfold decrease in titer of a nontreponemal serologic test, no evidence of reinfection or relapse	Clinical, serologic follow-up and benzathine penicillin G 50,000 U/kg IM, single dose[f]

[a]See Formulary for further drug information.
[b]Proven or probable disease if:
1) Physical or radiologic evidence of active disease.
2) Infant's nontreponemal titer is at least four times higher than the mother's titer.
3) CSF VDRL is reactive or CSF cell count and/or protein is abnormal.
4) Positive antitreponemal IgM test.
5) Placenta or umbilical cord is positive for treponemes organisms using specific fluorescent antibody staining.
[c]If more than 1 day of therapy is missed, the entire course should be restarted.
[d]Alternatively, some experts recommend procaine penicillin G 50,000 U/kg IM daily for 10–14 days, but CSF levels may be inadequate.
[e]Mother's penicillin dose unknown, undocumented, inadequate, *or* lack of fourfold or greater decrease in nontreponemal antibody titer in mother.
[f]Some experts recommend aqueous crystalline penicillin G as for proven or highly probable disease (see text). Other experts would follow the infant without giving antibiotic therapy if both clinical and serologic follow-up can be ensured.
Modified from Pickering LK (ed): 2003 Red Book: Report of the Committee on Infectious Diseases, 26th ed. Elk Grove Village, IL, American Academy of Pediatrics, 2003.

TABLE 16-7

INTERPRETATION OF SYPHILIS SEROLOGY AFTER TREATMENT OF SUSPECTED CONGENITAL SYPHILIS

Actual Congenital Syphilis Infection Status	Rapid Plasma Reagin (RPR)	Fluorescent Treponemal Antibody (FTA)	Comments
Not congenitally infected	Titers decrease fourfold by 3 mo; negative by 6 mo	Negative by 12–18 mo	Both RPR and FTA are waning passive maternal antibodies
Congenitally infected and successfully treated	Same as above	Long-lasting positive (may be lifelong)	—
Congenitally infected but *not* successfully treated	Increase or less than fourfold decrease by 3 mo	Long-lasting positive (may be lifelong)	Needs complete reevaluation and treatment for syphilis

E. HUMAN IMMUNODEFICIENCY VIRUS (HIV) AND ACQUIRED IMMUNODEFICIENCY SYNDROME (AIDS)

For the most recent information on the diagnosis and management of children with HIV infection, check the recommendations at **www.aidsinfo.nih.gov.**

1. **Counseling and testing:** Legal requirements vary by state. Counseling includes informed consent for testing, implications of positive test results, and prevention of transmission. All pregnant women should be offered counseling and testing, regardless of risk factors, so that they can make an informed decision regarding therapy aimed at reducing transmission to their infants. When maternal HIV status has not been determined before delivery, mother and/or newborn should undergo HIV antibody testing after counseling and consent of the mother (unless state law allows newborn testing without consent).
2. **Diagnosis of HIV in children:**

a. **Infected child:**

(1) Child <18 months of age is considered HIV infected if he or she has positive results on two separate blood samples (excluding cord blood) from one or more of the following HIV detection tests:

(a) HIV culture.

(b) HIV polymerase chain reaction (DNA PCR preferred but RNA PCR also used).

(2) Child >18 months of age is considered HIV infected if he or she:

(a) Is HIV antibody positive by repeated reactive enzyme immunoassay (EIA) and confirmatory test (e.g., Western blot or immunofluorescence assay [IFA]), *or*

(b) Meets the criteria for a child <18 months of age.

TABLE 16-8

TREATMENT FOR SYPHILIS (POSTNEONATAL)

Type or Stage	Firstline Drug and Dosage	Alternatives
Congenital syphilis (diagnosed >4 wk of age)	Aqueous crystalline penicillin 200,000–300,000 U/kg/24 hr IV Q6hr × 10–14 days	—
Early acquired syphilis of <1 yr duration	Benzathine benzylpenicillin 50,000 U/kg (maximum 2.4 × 10^6 U) IM × 1 dose (*Note*: Must examine CSF to exclude asymptomatic neurosyphilis in children)	Tetracycline 500 mg PO Q6hr × 14 days (for <8 yr) *or* Doxycycline 4 mg/kg/24 hr (maximum 200 mg) PO Q12hr × 14 days (for >8 yr).
Syphilis of >1 yr duration (late syphilis)	Benzathine benzylpenicillin 50,000 U/kg/dose (maximum 2.4 × 10^6 U) IM every wk × 3 successive weeks	Tetracycline 500 mg PO Q6hr × 28 days (for >8 yr) *or* Doxycycline 4 mg/kg/24 hr (maximum 200 mg) PO Q12hr × 28 days (for >8 yr).
Neurosyphilis	Aqueous crystalline benzylpenicillin 200,000–300,000 U/kg/day IV Q4–6hr (maximum 4 × 10^6 U IV Q4hr) × 10–14 days; may be followed by benzathine penicillin 50,000 U/kg/dose (maximum 2.4 × 10^6 U) IM every week ×3 wk	Aqueous procaine benzylpenicillin 2.4 × 10^6 U IM Q24hr × 10–14 days + probenecid 500 mg PO Q6hr × 10–14 days; may be followed by benzathine penicillin 50,000 U/kg/dose (maximum 2.4 × 10^6 U) IM every week ×3 wk. (If penicillin allergic, especially if <9 yr, consider penicillin desensitization and administration in an appropriate setting. Also, patient should be managed in consultation with a specialist.)

Modified from Pickering LK (ed): 2003 Red Book: Report of the Committee on Infectious Diseases, 26th ed. Elk Grove Village, IL, American Academy of Pediatrics, 2003.

b. **Perinatally exposed child:** A child is considered exposed when he or she does not meet the aforementioned criteria, *and*
   (1) Is HIV seropositive by EIA and confirmatory test (e.g., Western blot or IFA) and is <18 months old at the time of the test, *or*
   (2) Has unknown antibody status but was born to a mother known to be infected with HIV.

Text continues on p. 437

TABLE 16-9

DIAGNOSIS OF PELVIC INFLAMMATORY DISEASE

Etiology	Diagnostic Criteria	Diagnostic Techniques	Admission Criteria
1. *Neisseria gonorrhoeae* 2. *Chlamydia trachomatis* 3. Lower genital tract flora (*Haemophilus influenzae*, gram-negative rods, anaerobes, *Streptococcus agalactiae*)	Minimal criteria (all of the following): 1. Lower abdominal tenderness 2. Adnexal tenderness 3. Cervical motion tenderness 4. Absence of other etiology Additional criteria (one or more of the following): 1. Temperature ≥38.3°C 2. Abnormal cervical or vaginal discharge 3. Elevated erythrocyte sedimentation rate (ESR) 4. Elevated C-reactive protein (CRP) 5. Laboratory confirmation of infection with *N. gonorrhoeae* or *C. trachomatis* Other: 1. Endometriosis 2. Tubo-ovarian abscess (TOA)	*Chlamydia trachomatis* 1. *Definitive*: Tissue culture (only acceptable method for evaluation of child abuse). 2. *Presumptive*: Antigen detection through fluorescent staining with DNA probe, enzyme immunoassay (EIA), or monoclonal antibody (DFA); nucleic acid amplification test (NAAT) may be used on urine or cervical samples; DNA probe not reliable on bloody specimens; serologies not available. *Neisseria gonorrhoeae* 1. *Definitive*: Tissue culture (selective media with carbon dioxide incubation for transport). 2. *Presumptive*: Gram-negative intracellular diplococci on smear, or EIA or DNA probe of specimen; PCR or LCR may be used on urine or cervical sample.	1. Cannot exclude diagnosis of surgical abdomen (such as appendicitis) 2. Presence of tubo-ovarian abscess 3. Pregnancy 4. Immunodeficiency 5. Inability to tolerate or follow outpatient oral regimen 6. Failure to respond to oral antibiotic therapy 7. Clinical follow-up cannot be arranged (especially in adolescents)

TABLE 16-10

THERAPY FOR CHLAMYDIA, GONORRHEA, AND PELVIC INFLAMMATORY DISEASE

Type or Stage	Firstline Drug and Dosage	Alternatives
CHLAMYDIA TRACHOMATIS		
Urethritis, cervicitis, or proctitis	Doxycycline 100 mg PO bid × 7 days (if >9 yr) *or* Azithromycin 1 g PO × 1 dose	Erythromycin base 500 mg PO qid × 7 days *or* Erythromycin ethylsuccinate 800 mg PO qid × 7 days *or* Ofloxacin 300 mg PO bid × 7 days (if >18 yr)
Infection in pregnancy	Erythromycin base 500 mg PO qid × 7 days *or* 250 mg PO qid × 14 days	Erythromycin ethylsuccinate 400 mg PO qid × 14 days *or* Azithromycin 1 g PO × 1 dose *or* amoxicillin 500 mg PO TID × 7 days (alternative but less effective regimen).
Neonatal ophthalmia	Erythromycin base 50 mg/kg/24 hr PO or IV ÷ qid × 14 days	Topical treatment is ineffective.
Neonatal pneumonia	Erythromycin base 50 mg/kg/24 hr PO or IV ÷ qid × 14 days	*Note*: Association between PO erythromycin and pyloric stenosis has been reported.
GONORRHEA*		
Newborns		
Sepsis, arthritis, meningitis, scalp abscess	Ceftriaxone 25–50 mg/kg/24 hr IV/IM Q24 hr × 7 days (10–14 days if meningitis) *or*	—
Neonatal ophthalmia	Ceftriaxone 25–50 mg/kg (maximum 125 mg) IV/IM × 1 dose plus saline irrigation *or* Cefotaxime 100 mg/kg per dose IM/IV × 1 dose	All infants should receive silver nitrate, tetracycline, or erythromycin ointment instilled into each eye within 1 hr of birth. *Note*: All infants with GC conjunctivitis should be evaluated for possible sepsis/disseminated disease and the need to be treated for a longer time.

Prepubertal children who weigh <100 lb (45 kg)		
Uncomplicated urethritis, vulvovaginitis, proctitis, or pharyngitis	Ceftriaxone 125 mg IM × 1 dose	Spectinomycin 40 mg/kg (maximum 2 g) IM × 1 dose and erythromycin 50 mg/kg/day in 4 divided doses × 7 days *or* azithromycin 20 mg/kg (max 1 g) × 1 dose.
Bacteremia, peritonitis, or arthritis	Ceftriaxone 50 mg/kg/24 hr (maximum 1 g) IM/IV Q24 hr × 7–10 days and erythromycin, doxycycline, or azithromycin	—
Children who weigh ≥100 lb (45 kg) and are ≥9 yr		
Uncomplicated endocervicitis or urethritis	Ceftriaxone 125 mg IM × 1 dose *or* Cefixime 400 mg PO × 1 dose *or* Ciprofloxacin 500 mg PO × 1 dose (if >18 yr) *or* Ofloxacin 400 mg PO × 1 dose (if >18 yr) *plus* Azithromycin 1 g PO × 1 dose *or* Doxycycline 100 mg PO bid × 7 days	
Pharyngitis	Same as uncomplicated endocervicitis or urethritis therapy	—
Disseminated gonococcal infections	Ceftriaxone 1 g/24 hr IV/IM Q24 hr × 7 days	Cefotaxime or ceftizoxime 1 g IV Q8 hr × 7 days. For persons allergic to β-lactam drugs: Spectinomycin 2 g IM Q12 hr × 7 days *or* Ciprofloxacin 500 mg IV Q12 hr *or* Ofloxacin 400 mg IV Q12 hr.

continued

TABLE 16-10
THERAPY FOR CHLAMYDIA, GONORRHEA, AND PELVIC INFLAMMATORY DISEASE—*cont'd*

Type or Stage	Firstline Drug and Dosage	Alternatives
Bacteremia or arthritis	Ceftriaxone 50 mg/kg/day (maximum dose 1 g) IM or IV Q24 hr × 10–14 days	—
Pelvic Inflammatory Disease (PID)		
Inpatient	Cefoxitin 2 g IV Q6 hr *or*	Clindamycin 900 mg IV Q8 hr ***plus***
	Cefotetan 2 g IV Q12 hr ***plus***	Gentamicin 2 mg/kg loading dose ***plus***
	Doxycycline 100 mg IV/PO Q12 hr	Gentamicin 1.5 mg/kg IV Q8 hr
	If clinical improvement after 24 hrs follow with: Doxycycline 100 mg PO Q12 hr *or* Clindamycin 600 mg PO TID (for total of 14 days)	Same
Outpatient	Doxycycline 100 mg PO bid × 14 days ***plus***	(>18 years)
	Cefoxitin 2 g IM × 1 dose and probenicid 1 g PO × 1 dose *or*	Ofloxacin 400 mg PO bid × 14 days *or*
	Ceftriaxone 250 mg IM × 1 dose	Levofloxacin 500 mg PO daily × 14 days

*Therapy should include treatment for presumed concomitant chlamydial infection.

From Centers for Disease Control and Prevention: Guidelines for treatment of sexually transmitted diseases MMWR 2002;51(RR-6).

c. **Exclusion of HIV infection in a perinatally exposed child:** HIV can be reasonably excluded in an exposed asymptomatic infant with two negative HIV DNA PCR studies, one obtained at age 1 month or older and the other at age 4 months or older.

HIV is definitively excluded if HIV antibody testing is negative at 18 months in an asymptomatic non-breast-feeding child with negative HIV DNA PCR studies (as above).

3. **Pediatric HIV immunologic categories (Table 16-11).**
4. **Guidelines for prophylaxis against first episode of opportunistic infections (Table 16-12).**
5. **Management of perinatal HIV exposure:** Recommendations provided are current at the time of publication; check the recent recommendations for most current therapy at **www.aidsinfo.nih.gov.**

a. **Prevention of vertical transmission:** Use of antiretroviral therapy during pregnancy, during delivery, and in the newborn dramatically reduces HIV transmission. Bottle-feeding of formula is also recommended to reduce transmission through breast milk.

(1) **Pregnancy:** All HIV-infected women should be offered antiretroviral therapy for their own health, consistent with the standards of nonpregnant adults. Zidovudine (ZDV) should generally be included in the pregnant woman's regimen because ZDV given during pregnancy (initiated at 14–34 weeks' gestation) and then given to the infant at delivery and for 6 weeks postnatally significantly reduces vertical transmission of HIV. For prevention of vertical transmission ZDV with or without other antiretrovirals is commonly given to women without an indication for antiretrovirals for their own health. Higher viral loads have been associated with increased risk for transmission. Elective cesarean section (before onset of labor or membrane rupture) has been shown to decrease transmission in women not receiving antiretroviral therapy and in those with high viral loads.

16

MICROBIOLOGY AND INFECTIOUS DISEASE

TABLE 16-11

1994 REVISED PEDIATRIC HIV CLASSIFICATION SYSTEM: IMMUNOLOGIC CATEGORIES BASED ON AGE-SPECIFIC CD4+ LYMPHOCYTE COUNT AND PERCENT

	Age of Child		
Immunologic Category	<12 mo cells/μL (%)	1–5 yr cells/μL (%)	6–12 yr cells/μL (%)
1: No suppression	≥1500 (≥25)	≥1000(≥25)	≥500(≥25)
2: Moderate suppression	750–1499 (15–24)	500–999 (15–24)	200–499 (15–24)
3: Severe suppression	<750 (<15)	<500 (<15)	<200 (<15)

From Centers for Disease Control and Prevention: MMWR 1994;43(RR–12).

TABLE 16-12

PROPHYLAXIS FOR FIRST EPISODE OF OPPORTUNISTIC DISEASE IN HIV-INFECTED INFANTS AND CHILDREN

		Preventive Regimens	
Pathogen	Indication	First Choice	Alternatives
STRONGLY RECOMMENDED AS STANDARD OF CARE			
Pneumocystis carinii	HIV-infected or HIV-indeterminate infants 4–6 wk → 12 mo of age; HIV-children 1–5 yr with CD4+ count <500 µL or CD4+ percent <15%; HIV-infected children 6–12 yr with CD4+ count <200 µL or CD4+ percent <15%	TMP/SMX 150/750 mg/m²/day in two divided doses PO 3×/week on consecutive days. Acceptable altemative dosage schedules: Single dose PO 3×/week on consecutive days. Two divided doses PO every day. Two divided doses PO 3×/week on alternate days.	Aerosolized pentamidine (children ≥5 yr) 300 mg via Respirgard II inhaler monthy; dapsone (children ≥1 mo) 2 mg/kg (maximum 100 mg) PO every day or 4 mg/kg (maximum 200 mg) PO every week; atovaquone daily.
Mycobacterium tuberculosis			
Isoniazid sensitive	Tuberculin skin test reaction ≥5 mm *or* prior positive TST result without treatment *or* contact with case of active tuberculosis	Isoniazid 10–15 mg/kg (maximum 300 mg) PO every day × 9 mo *or* 20–30 mg/kg (maximum 900 mg) PO biweekly × 9 mo.	Rifampin 10–20 mg/kg (maximum 600 mg) PO or IV every day × 4–6 mo.
Isoniazid resistant	Same as above; high probability of exposure to isoniazid-resistant tuberculosis	Rifampin 10–20 mg/kg (maximum 600 mg) PO every day × 4–6 mo.	Uncertain.
Multidrug (isoniazid and rifampin) resistant	Same as above; high probability of exposure to multidrug-resistant tuberculosis	Choice of drug requires consultation with public health authorities.	None.
Mycobacterium avium complex	For children <1 yr, CD4+ count <750/µL 1–2 yr, CD4+ count <500/µL 2–6 yr, CD4+ count <75/µL ≥6 yr, CD4+ count <50/µL	Clarithromycin 7.5 mg/kg (maximum 500 mg) PO bid *or* azithromycin 20 mg/kg (maximum 1200 mg) PO once weekly.	Azithromycin 5 mg/kg (max 250 mg) PO q day; Children ≥6 yr: Rifabutin 300 mg PO q day.

Varicella zoster virus	Significant exposure to varicella with no history of chickenpox or shingles	VZIG 1 vial (1.25)/10 kg (maximum 5 vials) IM, administered ≤96 hr after exposure, ideally within 48 hr.	None.
GENERALLY RECOMMENDED			
*Toxoplasma gondii**	IgG antibody to *Toxoplasma* and severe immunosuppression	TMP/SMX 150/750 mg/m^2/day in 2 divided doses PO every day.	*Dapsone (children ≥1 mo):* 2 mg/kg or 15 mg/m^2 (maximum 25 mg) PO every day *plus* pyrimethamine 1 mg/kg PO every day *plus* leucovorin 5 mg PO daily every 3 days. Atovaquone can also be used.
Varicella zoster virus	HIV infected children who are asymptomatic and not immunosuppressed	Varicella zoster vaccine	None.
Influenza virus	All patients (annually before flu season)	Inactivated split trivalent influenza virus	Oseltamivir for children >13 yr (during flu A or B outbreak); Rimantidine or amantadine for ages >1 yr (during flu A outbreak).
NOT RECOMMENDED FOR MOST PATIENTS; INDICATED FOR USE ONLY IN UNUSUAL CIRCUMSTANCES			
Cryptococcus neoformans	Severe immunosuppression	Fluconazole 3–6 mg/kg PO every day.	Itraconazole 2–5 mg/kg PO Q12–24 hr.
Histoplasma capsulatum	Severe immunosuppression, endemic geographic area	Itraconazole 2–5 mg/kg PO Q12–24 hr.	None.
Cytomegalovirus (CMV)†	CMV antibody positivity and severe Immunosuppression	Oral ganciclovir 30 mg/kg PO TID	None.

*Protection against *Toxoplasma* is provided by the preferred anti-*Pneumocystis* regimens. Pyrimethanine alone probably provides little, if any, protection.

†Oral ganciclovir and perhaps valganciclovir result in reduced CMV shedding in CMV-infected children. Acyclovir is not protective against CMV.

BIW, Twice a week; *TMP/SMX*, trimethoprim-sulfamethoxazole.

From 2002 USPHS/IDSA Guidelines for prevention of opportunistic infections in persons infected with HIV. MMWR 2002;51(RR–08).

(2) **Labor:** During labor, intravenous (IV) ZDV in a loading dose of 2 mg/kg over 1 hour, followed by continuous infusion of 1 mg/kg/hour until delivery. Invasive procedures such as fetal scalp electrode monitoring are generally avoided. Consider adding nevirapine (NVP) for high-risk situations such as high viral load in mother, no prenatal care, or break in infant's skin.

(3) **Newborn:** To reduce the risk for HIV infection, the newborn is given ZDV, 2 mg/kg/dose PO every 6 hours (or 1.5 mg/kg/dose IV every 6 hours until tolerating PO) for first 6 weeks of life. Initiate preferably within 12 hours of birth. For premature infants (<35 weeks' gestation), use 1.5 mg/kg/dose PO (1.5 mg/kg/dose IV) every 12 hours initially, then increase to 1.5 mg/kg/dose PO every 8 hours at 2 weeks if gestational age >30 weeks, or at 4 weeks if gestational age <30 weeks. In high-risk situations in which the mother received intrapartum NVP >1 hour before delivery, give a single dose of 2 mg/kg PO to the neonate at 48 to 72 hours of life. In high-risk situations in which the mother did not receive intrapartum NVP or received it <1 hour before delivery, some experts give one dose of 2 mg/kg/dose PO immediately after birth, and a second dose at 48 to 72 hours of life. Monitor ZDV toxicity with periodic CBCs with differential count. The main toxicities are anemia and neutropenia.

b. **Ongoing management of indeterminate infants:**

(1) ***Pneumocystis carinii*** **pneumonia (PCP) prophylaxis** with trimethoprim-sulfamethoxazole (TMP/SMX) should be initiated for all HIV-exposed infants at 4 to 6 weeks of life. PCP prophylaxis should be continued until HIV infection is reasonably excluded. Dose is 75 mg/m^2/dose TMP PO twice daily for 3 consecutive days per week. Alternatives: dapsone, atovaquone. **See Table 16-12** for PCP prophylaxis medications and dosing.

(2) **HIV diagnostic tests (DNA PCR)** should be obtained on the infant between birth and 2 weeks of life (cord blood should not be used), at 1 to 2 months, and again at 4 to 6 months to determine infection status. A positive test should be immediately repeated for confirmation of infection. If all tests are negative, the infant should be tested for HIV antibody at 12 and 18 months of age to document disappearance of the antibody.

(3) **Clinical monitoring:** Infants should be evaluated at routine well-child visits for signs and symptoms of HIV infection. In addition to HIV diagnostic tests, T-cell subsets and quantitative HIV RNA are obtained for HIV monitoring, and CBC with differential and chemistries are obtained for toxicity monitoring. Any suspicious clinical or laboratory findings merit careful and close follow-up. Avoid breast-feeding.

6. **Management of HIV-infected infants and children:**

Note *Primary care physicians are encouraged to participate in the care and management of HIV-infected children in consultation with specialists who have expertise in the care of such children. Knowledge about antiretroviral therapy is changing, and in areas where enrollment into clinical trials is possible, it should be encouraged.*

a. **Criteria for initiation of antiretroviral therapy:**
   (1) Initiation of antiretroviral therapy depends on virologic, immunologic, and clinical status.
   (2) All HIV-infected infants (<12 months of age) regardless of immunologic, virologic, or clinical status, should usually be started on antiretroviral therapy.
   (3) Antiretroviral therapy should be initiated in children with evidence of immune suppression as indicated by CD4 lymphocyte absolute number or percentage in Immunologic Category 2 or 3 (see Table 16-11).
   (4) Therapy should be initiated in any child with clinical symptoms related to HIV infection.
   (5) For asymptomatic HIV-infected children >1 year of age with normal immune status, consideration should be given to initiating therapy.

b. **Antiretroviral regimen:** For the most recent recommendations, refer to **www.aidsinfo.nih.gov.** Data support the use of combination therapy for initial and ongoing therapy (except ZDV monotherapy for chemoprophylaxis in an exposed infant as previously listed). If an infant is identified as HIV infected while receiving ZDV prophylaxis, therapy should be changed to combination therapy.

c. **Clinical and laboratory monitoring in HIV-infected children:** Immune status, viral load, and evidence of HIV progression and drug toxicity should be monitored on a regular basis (about every 3 months). Careful attention to routine aspects of pediatric care, such as growth, development, and vaccines, is essential.

7. **Immunizations in HIV-infected or HIV-exposed infants and children:** Perinatally exposed infants should receive all scheduled U.S. infant immunizations. Measles-mumps-rubella (MMR) and varicella vaccine can be given to selected HIV-infected children (see Chapter 15). HIV-infected children should receive PPS23 at 2 and 5 years of age. Influenza vaccine should be given annually in the fall to all infected children ≥ 6 months of age as well as children ≥6 months of age who have HIV-infected household contacts.

F. TUBERCULOSIS

1. **Recommended tuberculosis testing:**

a. Tuberculin skin test (TST) recommendations (from American Academy of Pediatrics: 2003 Red Book. Chicago, The Academy, 2003): Bacille

Calmette-Guérin (BCG) immunization is not a contraindication to tuberculin skin testing.

(1) Immediate testing:
   (a) Contacts of people with confirmed or suspected infectious tuberculosis (contact investigation).
   (b) Children with clinical or radiographic findings of tuberculosis.
   (c) Children emigrating from or with history of travel to TB endemic areas (e.g., Asia, the Middle East, Africa, Latin America); children with close contacts from TB endemic areas.

(2) Annual testing (initial TST is at the time of diagnosis or circumstance, beginning as early as age 3 months):
   (a) HIV-infected children.
   (b) Incarcerated adolescents.

(3) Testing every 2 to 3 years: Children with ongoing exposure to the homeless, HIV-infected people, nursing home residents, institutionalized or incarcerated adolescents or adults, illicit drug users, and migrant farm workers.

(4) Testing at 4 to 6 and 11 to 16 years of age:
   (a) Children of immigrants (with unknown TST status) from endemic countries (continued personal exposure by travel to endemic areas and contact with people from the endemic areas are indications for repeat TST).
   (b) Children without specific risk factors residing in high-prevalence areas (may vary within each region of country).

(5) Children at increased risk for progression of infection to disease: Medical conditions such as diabetes mellitus, chronic renal failure, malnutrition, and congenital or acquired immunodeficiencies. Immunodeficiency itself may increase risk for progression to severe disease; therefore, if exposure is likely, immediate and periodic TST should be considered; TST should always be performed before initiation of immunosuppressive therapy.

b. Standard TST is the Mantoux test. The tine test (multipuncture test) is no longer recommended.

(1) Inject 5 tuberculin units (5TU) of purified protein derivative (0.1 mL) intradermally on the volar aspect of the forearm to form a 6- to 10-mm weal. Results of skin testing (in millimeters of induration) should be read 48 to 72 hours later by qualified medical personnel.

(2) Definition of positive Mantoux test (regardless of whether BCG has been previously administered). See Table 16-13.

2. Drug therapy:

a. Treatment of latent tuberculosis infection (formerly "prophylaxis"):

(1) Indications:
   (a) Children with positive tuberculin tests but no evidence of clinical disease.
   (b) Recent contacts, especially HIV-infected children, of people with

TABLE 16-13

DEFINITIONS OF POSITIVE TUBERCULIN SKIN TESTING[8]

Induration ≥5 mm
Children in close contact with known or suspected contagious cases of tuberculosis
Children suspected to have tuberculosis based on clinical or radiographic findings
Children on immunosuppressive therapy or with immunosuppressive conditions (including HIV infection)
Induration ≥10 mm
Children at increased risk for dissemination based on young age (<4 yr) or with other medical conditions (cancer, diabetes mellitus, chronic renal failure, or malnutrition)
Children with increased exposure: those born in or whose parents were born in endemic countries; those with travel to endemic countries; those exposed to HIV-infected adults, homeless, illicit drug user, nursing home residents, incarcerated or institutionalized persons, migrant farm workers
Induration ≥15 mm
Children 4 yr or older without any risk factors

infectious tuberculosis, even if tuberculin test and clinical evidence are not indicative of disease.

(2) Recommendations (see Formulary for specific doses) see Table 16-14

b. Treatment for active tuberculosis disease (for details, see Pickering LH [ed]: 2003 Red Book. Chicago, American Academy of Pediatrics, 2003) (see Table 16-14).

G. SELECTED TICK-BORNE ILLNESSES

1. **Lyme disease:**

a. **Presentation:**

(1) **Early localized disease:** Clinical manifestations appear between 3 and 32 days after tick bite and include erythema migrans (annular rash at site of bite, target lesion with clear or necrotic center), fever, headache, myalgia, malaise.

(2) **Early disseminated disease:** Appears some 3 to 10 weeks after the tick bite and includes secondary erythema migrans with multiple, smaller target lesions, cranioneuropathy (especially facial nerve palsy), systemic symptoms as previously listed, and lymphadenopathy; 1% may develop carditis with heart block or aseptic meningitis.

(3) **Late disease:** Intermittent, recurrent symptoms occur 2 to 12 months from initial tick bite and include pauciarticular arthritis affecting large joints (7% of those untreated), peripheral neuropathy, encephalopathy.

b. **Transmission:** Disease is caused by spirochete *Borrelia burgdorferi.* Inoculation occurs by a deer tick, *Ixodes scapularis* or *Ixodes pacificus*. After a bite from an infected deer tick, the spirochete disseminates

TABLE 16-14

RECOMMENDED TREATMENT REGIMENS FOR DRUG-SUSCEPTIBLE TUBERCULOSIS IN INFANTS, CHILDREN, AND ADOLESCENTS

Infection or Disease Category	Regimen*	Remarks
Asymptomatic infection (positive skin test, no disease)	Prophylaxis	If daily therapy is not possible, therapy twice a week may be used for 9 mo. HIV-infected children should be treated for 12 mo. Also indicated for contacts of people with infectious tuberculosis, even if tuberculin test is negative, including all children <4 yr with household TB contacts.
Isoniazid susceptible	9 mo of isoniazid Q24 hr	Repeat TST 12 wk after contact with TB is broken; if negative (in normal host), may discontinue prophylaxis; if positive (and no evidence of TB disease), complete prophylactic regimen.
Isoniazid resistant	6 mo of rifampin Q24 hr	For management of neonates born to mothers with evidence of TB infection, see *2003 Red Book*.[8]
Isoniazid/rifampin resistant*	Consultation with a tuberculosis specialist	
Pulmonary	**6-mo regimens**	
	2 mo of isoniazid, rifampin, and pyrazinamide Q24 hr, followed by 4 mo of isoniazid and rifampin daily *or*	If possible drug resistance is a concern, another drug (ethambutol or an aminoglycoside) is added to the initial three-drug therapy until drug susceptibilities are determined.
	2 mo of isoniazid, rifampin, and pyrazinamide daily, followed by 4 mo of isoniazid and rifampin twice a week	Drugs can be given 2 or 3 times/wk under direct observation in the initial phase if nonadherence is likely.

	6-mo alternative regimens (for hilar adenopathy only): 6 mo of isoniazid and rifampin	
Extrapulmonary: meningitis, disseminated (miliary), bone/joint disease	2 mo of isoniazid, rifampin, pyrazinamide, and an aminoglycoside or ethionamide once a day, followed by 10 mo of isoniazid and rifampin Q24 hr (12 mo total) *or*	An aminoglycoside is given with initial therapy until drug susceptibility is known.
	2 mo of isoniazid, rifampin, pyrazinamide, and streptomycin Q24 hr, followed by 10 mo of isoniazid and rifampin twice a week (12 mo total)	For patients who may have acquired tuberculosis in geographic areas where resistance to streptomycin is common: capreomycin (15–30 mg/kg/day) or kanamycin (15–30 mg/kg/day) may be used instead of streptomycin.
Other (e.g., cervical lymphadenopathy)		See Pulmonary.

*Duration of therapy is longer in HIV-infected persons, and additional drugs may be indicated.

Modified from Pickering LK (ed): 2003 Red Book: Report of the Committee on Infectious Diseases, 26th ed. Elk Grove Village, IL, American Academy of Pediatrics, 2003.

systemically through the blood and lymphatics. Of note, transmission of *B. burgdorferi* from infected ticks requires a prolonged time (24–48 hours) of tick attachment. Lyme disease occurs commonly in New England and the Middle Atlantic, Upper Midwest, and Pacific Northwest. April to October is the peak season.

c. **Diagnosis:** Most cases of early Lyme disease can be diagnosed clinically by the characteristic erythema migrans rash or illness compatible with early or late disease (e.g., meningitis, facial palsy, arthritis). Serologic confirmation of diagnosis is with immunoassays for *B. burgdorferi*–specific immunoglobulin M (IgM), which begins at 3 to 4 weeks and peaks at 6 to 8 weeks after disease onset, and with *B. burgdorferi*–specific IgG, which rises weeks to months after symptoms appear and persists. False-positive results of these assays occur as a result of cross-reactivity with viral infections, other spirochetal infections, and autoimmune diseases. Western blot assays should be used to confirm positive enzyme-linked immunosorbent assay (ELISA). Lyme disease–specific antibodies can be isolated from CSF in patients with CNS involvement.

d. **Treatment:** Therapy depends on the stage of disease. Antibiotic prophylaxis is not routinely recommended for ticks attached <24 to 48 hours. For early localized disease, doxycycline for 14 to 21 days is the treatment of choice for patients ≥8 years of age. Amoxicillin is recommended for younger children. The following early disseminated and late-onset disease manifestations are treated by the same oral regimen as early disease, with treatment extended as indicated: multiple erythema migrans therapy for 21 days, isolated facial palsy treatment for 21 to 28 days, and arthritis treatment for 28 days. Persistent or recurrent arthritis (>2 months) and carditis may be treated with 14 to 21 days of ceftriaxone or 14 to 28 days of parenteral penicillin. Meningitis or encephalitis should be treated with ceftriaxone or parenteral penicillin for 30 to 60 days.

2. **Rocky Mountain spotted fever:**

a. **Presentation:** The incubation period ranges from 2 to 14 days. Clinical manifestations include fever, headache, and a characteristic rash that usually occurs by day 6 of illness and is initially erythematous and macular and progresses to maculopapular and petechial. The rash usually appears on the wrists and ankles and spreads proximally. Palms and soles are often involved. Other symptoms include myalgia, nausea, anorexia, abdominal pain, and diarrhea. Thrombocytopenia, hyponatremia, and anemia may develop. White blood count is usually normal. Severe disease may manifest in CNS, cardiac, pulmonary, gastrointestinal tract and renal involvement, disseminated intravascular involvement, and shock leading to death.

b. **Transmission:** Disease is caused by *Rickettsia rickettsii*, an obligate intracellular pathogen transmitted to humans by a tick bite. Incidence is highest between April and September. Most cases are reported in the south Atlantic, southeastern, and south central states, although the disease is widespread in the United States and also occurs in Canada, Mexico, and Central and South America.

c. **Diagnosis:** Diagnosis is by rickettsial group-specific serologic tests. However, they may be negative early in the illness. A fourfold or greater change between acute- and convalescent-phase serum specimens is diagnostic when determined by indirect immunofluorescence antibody (IFA) assay, enzyme immunoassay, or complement fixation, latex agglutination, indirect hemagglutination, or microagglutination tests. A probable diagnosis can be established by a single serum titer of 1:64 or greater by IFA assay. Culture of *R. rickettsii* is generally not attempted because of the danger of transmission to laboratory personnel. *R. rickettsii* can be obtained by immunohistochemical staining of tissue specimens obtained before initiation of antimicrobial therapy. This method is highly specific but not sensitive.

d. **Treatment:** Doxycycline is the recommended drug for children of any age. Chloramphenicol is an alternative, although it is less favored because of serious side effects, the need to monitor levels, and lack of an oral preparation in the United States. Treatment is initiated on the basis of clinical features and epidemiologic considerations. Treatment usually lasts 7 to 10 days and is continued until the patient is afebrile for at least 3 days and has demonstrated clinical improvement.

3. **Ehrlichiosis:**

a. **Presentation:** Ehrlichiosis is caused by three distinct tick-borne pathogens, namely *Ehrlichia chaffeensis* (human monocytic ehrlichiosis or HME), *Anaplasma phagocytophilia* agent (human granulocytic ehrlichiosis or HGE), and *Ehrlichia ewingii*. Infection is characterized by an acute systemic febrile illness usually accompanied by one or more systemic manifestations including headache, chills, malaise, myalgia, arthralgia, nausea, vomiting, anorexia, and acute weight loss. Leukopenia, anemia, and hepatitis are common. Rash is variable in location and appearance and is more common in HME than HGE. More severe manifestations include pulmonary infiltrates, bone marrow hypoplasia, respiratory failure, encephalopathy, meningitis, disseminated intravascular coagulation, spontaneous hemorrhage, and renal failure.

b. **Transmission:** *Ehrlichia* infections caused by *E. chaffeensis* and *E. ewingii* are associated with the bite of a lone star tick (*Amblyomma americanum*), although other tick species may be vectors. HGE is transmitted by the deer tick (*Ixodes scapularis*). Mammalian reservoirs for agents of human ehrlichiosis include white-tailed deer and white-footed mice. Most HME infections occur in the southeastern and south central United States. Most cases of HGE are reported from north central and northeastern United States. Most human infections occur between April and September, with peak occurrence from May through July.

c. **Diagnosis:** Diagnosis is confirmed by isolation of *Ehrlichia* organisms from blood or CSF, a fourfold or greater change in antibody titer by IFA assay between acute and convalescent serum specimens, PCR assay amplification of ehrlichial DNA from a clinical specimen or detection of an intraleukocytoplasmic cluster of bacteria in conjunction with a single IFA titer of ≥64. PCR from acute-phase peripheral blood of patients with ehrlichiosis seems sensitive, specific, and promising for early diagnosis.

d. **Treatment:** Doxycycline is the drug of choice. The recommended dosage is 4.4 mg/kg per day given every 12 hours IV or PO (maximum, 100 mg/dose). Ehrlichiosis may be severe or fatal in untreated patients, and treatment should therefore be initiated early. Failure to respond within the first 3 days should suggest infection with an agent other than *Ehrlichia* species. Treatment should be continued for at least 3 days after defervescence for a minimum total course of 5 to 10 days.

H. FUNGAL AND YEAST INFECTIONS

1. Place specimen (nail or skin scrapings, biopsy specimens, fluids from tissues or lesions) in 10% KOH on glass slide to look for hyphae, pseudohyphae.
2. Germ tube screen of yeast (3 hours) for *Candida albicans*: all germ tube–positive yeast are *C. albicans*, but not all *C. albicans* are germ tube–positive.
3. Common community-acquired fungal infections, etiology, and treatment are listed in Table 16-15.

I. EXPOSURES TO BLOOD-BORNE PATHOGENS AND POSTEXPOSURE PROPHYLAXIS (PEP)

1. HIV[12]:

a. **Occupational exposure:** Risk for occupational transmission of HIV:
   (1) **Needle sticks:** Three infections for every 1000 exposures (0.3%). Risk is greater when the exposure involves a larger volume of blood and/or higher titer of HIV, as in a deep injury, visible blood on the device causing the injury, a device previously used in the source patient's vein or artery, or a source patient in the late stages of HIV infection.
   (2) **Mucous membrane exposure:** One infection for every 1000 exposures (0.1%). The risk may be higher when the exposure involves a larger volume of blood and a higher titer of HIV, prolonged skin contact, extensive surface area of exposure, or skin integrity that is visibly compromised.

b. **Nonoccupational HIV exposure in children and adolescents:**
   (1) **Injury from needles of discarded syringes:** There are no confirmed reports of HIV acquisition from percutaneous injury by a needle found in the community. The risk for transmission from a "found needle" (i.e., a needle discarded in a public place) is low. However, if the needle or syringe is found to have visible blood and

TABLE 16-15

COMMON COMMUNITY-ACQUIRED FUNGAL INFECTIONS

Disease	Usual Etiology	Suggested Therapy	Suggested Length of Therapy
Tinea capitis (ringworm of scalp)	*Trichophyton tonsurans*, *Microsporum canis*	Oral griseofulvin: Give with fatty foods. Fungal shedding decreased with 1%–2.5% selenium sulfide shampoo. Alt: Terbinafine itraconozole or fluconazole	4–6 wk or 2 wk after clinical resolution
Tinea corporis/ pedis (ringworm of body/feet)	*Trichophyton rubrum*, *Trichophyton mentagrophytes*, *Microsporum canis*	Topical antifungal (miconazole, clotrimazole)	4 wk
		Terbinafine	2 wk
Oral candidiasis (thrush)	*Candida albicans*, *Candida tropicalis*	Nystatin suspension or clotrimazole troches.	3 days after clinical resolution
Candidal skin infections (intertriginous)	*Candida albicans*	Topical nystatin, miconazole, clotrimazole	3 days after clinical resolution
Tinea unguium (ringworm of nails)		Oral terbinafine	6 wk
		or itraconazole	3 mo
		or fluconazole	3–6 mo

the source is known to be HIV infected, PEP should be considered. Testing the syringe for HIV is not practical or reliable.

(2) **Repeated sexual encounters or a single episode of sexual abuse:** Risk is highest with unprotected receptive anal intercourse (0.5%–3.2%), intermediate with receptive vaginal intercourse (0.05%–0.15%), and lowest with insertive vaginal intercourse (0.03%–0.09%). If the exposure source has genital ulcer disease or another sexually transmitted infection or if there was tissue damage, the risk for HIV transmission is higher, increasing the benefit of PEP relative to the burden and risk for drug toxicity.

(3) **Human milk:** In the United States, women who are HIV infected should be counseled not to breast-feed. An infant who has a single exposure to human milk from a woman with HIV infection is estimated to have 100 times lower risk than that of other mucous membrane exposures, and PEP is likely not warranted.

(4) **Human bites:** Transmission is extremely rare even when saliva is contaminated with blood for reasons that include saliva inhibits HIV infectivity, HIV is rarely isolated from saliva, and concentrations of HIV in saliva of HIV-infected persons is low even in the presence of periodontal disease.

c. **Prophylaxis:**

(1) Optimally, PEP should be initiated as soon as possible but certainly within 72 hours.

(2) A clinician with experience in the treatment of individuals with HIV infection should be consulted before initiating therapy. Many clinicians would use the three-drug combination of zidovudine [ZDV], lamivudine [3TC], and nelfinavir [NFV]. However, a 28-day course of a two-drug regimen is easier and may have fewer side effects, for which reason some clinicians may choose to use ZDV and 3TC. This two-drug regimen is available as a single tablet, Combivir, enhancing ease of use for older children.

(3) Use of ZDV alone as PEP is no longer recommended.

For most recent recommendations, refer to CDC guidelines. The CDC's postexposure prophylaxis hotline (open 24 hr/day) is 888-448-4911.

2. **Hepatitis B:** Recommendations for hepatitis B prophylaxis after percutaneous exposure to blood that contains (or might contain) HBsAg include hepatitis B immune globulin (HBIG) and initiation of hepatitis B vaccine series. For details, see Chapter 15.

J. INFECTIOUS DISEASES IN INTERNATIONALLY ADOPTED CHILDREN

For more information, see www.cdc.gov/travel/other/adoption.htm.

REFERENCES

1. Gilbert ON, Moellering RC, Sande MA: The Sanford Guide to Antimicrobial Therapy, 33rd ed. VT, Antimicrobial Therapy, 2003.
2. Mandell GL, Bennett JE, Dolin R: Principles and Practice of Infectious Disease. New York, Churchill Livingstone, 1995.
3. Livermore DM. β-Lactamases in laboratory and clinical resistance. Clin Microbiol Rev 1995;8:557.
4. Wong CS, et al: The risk of hemolytic-uremic syndrome after antibiotic treatment of Escherichia coli o157:H7 infections. N Engl J Med 2000;342:1930.
5. Gomella TA: Neonatology: Management, procedures, on-call problems, diseases and drugs. Norwalk, CT, Appleton & Lange, 1999.
6. McMillan JA, et al. (eds): Oski's Pediatrics: Principles and Practice, 3rd ed. Philadelphia, Lippincott Williams and Wilkins, 1999.
7. Robart HA, et al: Treatment of potentially life-threatening enterovirus infections with pleconaril. Clin Infect Dis 2000;32:228.
8. Pickering LK (ed): 2003 Red Book: Report of the Committee on Infectious Diseases, 26th ed. Elk Grove Village, IL, American Academy of Pediatrics, 2003.
9. Long S, Pickering LK, Prober CG (eds): Principles and Practice of Pediatric Infectious Diseases. Edinburgh, Churchill Livingstone, 2003.

10. Barron SD, Pass RF: Infectious causes of hydrops fetalis. Semin Perinatol 1995;19:493.
11. Council of State and Territorial Epidemiologists; AIDS Program, Center for Infectious Diseases: Revision of the CDC surveillance case definition for acquired immunodeficiency syndrome. MMWR Morb Mortal Wkly Rep 1987;36(Suppl 1):1S–5.
12. Centers for Disease Control and Prevention: Updated U.S. Public Health Service guidelines for the management of occupational exposures to HBV, HCV, and HIV and recommendations for postexposure prophylaxis. MMWR Morb Mortal Wkly Rep 2001;50(RR-11).
13. MMWR Recommendations and Reports. MMWR Morb Mortal Wkly Rep 2002;51(RR-11):1–22.
14. Siberry G, Parsons G, Hutton N: Management of infants born to HIV infected mothers. Hopkins HIV Rep 2003;15(6):7–9, 12.
15. Havens P, et al: Postexposure prophylaxis in children and adolescents for nonoccupational exposure to human immunodeficiency virus. Pediatrics 2003;111(6):1475–1489.

[illegible] infectious [illegible]

[illegible]

[illegible] Centers for Disease Control and Prevention [illegible]

[illegible] guidelines for the management of occupational exposures to HBV, HCV, and HIV and recommendations for postexposure prophylaxis. [illegible]

[illegible]

[illegible]

Neonatology

Theodora A. Stavroudis, MD

17

I. FETAL ASSESSMENT

A. FETAL ANOMALY SCREENING

1. **Routine ultrasound: performed at 18 to 20 weeks gestation.**
2. **Maternal α-fetoprotein (AFP)** (Table 17-1).
3. **Amniotic fluid volume (AFV) estimation** (Table 17-2).
4. **Fetal karyotyping:**

a. Amniocentesis: 20 to 30 mL of amniotic fluid is withdrawn under ultrasound guidance after 16 to 18 weeks gestation. Detects chromosomal abnormalities, metabolic disorders, and neural tube defects. Complications include pregnancy loss (<5/1000), chorioamnionitis (<1/1000), leakage of amniotic fluid (1/300), fetal scarring or dimpling of the skin.

b. Chorionic villus sampling: Segment of placenta obtained either transcervically or transabdominally at 8 to 11 weeks gestation. Detects chromosomal abnormalities and metabolic disorders but cannot detect neural tube defects or measure AFP. Complications include pregnancy loss (0.5%–2%), maternal infection, increased risk for fetomaternal hemorrhage, and fetal limb and jaw malformation.

B. ESTIMATION OF GESTATIONAL AGE

1. **Last menstrual period (LMP):** Nägele's rule, most accurate determination of gestational age. EDC = 280 days + 7 days from LMP.
2. **Ultrasound:** Crown–rump length obtained between 6 and 12 weeks gestation predicts gestational age ±3 to 4 days. After 12 weeks, the biparietal diameter is accurate within 10 days, and beyond 26 weeks, accuracy diminishes to ±3 weeks.

C. EXPECTED BIRTH WEIGHT

1. **By gestational age** (Table 17-3).

D. INTRAPARTUM FETAL HEART RATE (FHR) MONITORING

1. **Normal baseline FHR is 120 to 160 bpm. Mild bradycardia is 100 to 120 bpm. Severe bradycardia is <90 bpm.**
2. **Normal beat-to-beat variability:** Deviation from baseline of >6 bpm. Absence of variability is <2 bpm from baseline and is a sign of potential fetal distress, particularly when combined with variable or late decelerations.
3. **Accelerations:** Associated with fetal movement, are benign, and indicate fetal well-being.

TABLE 17-1
MATERNAL α-FETOPROTEIN ASSOCIATIONS

Elevated (>2.5 multiples of the median)	Low (<0.75 multiples of the median)
Incorrect gestational dating	Underestimation of gestational age
Neural tube defects	Intrauterine growth retardation
Anencephaly	Trisomy 13
Multiple pregnancy	Trisomy 18
Turner syndrome	Down syndrome
Omphalocele	
Cystic hygroma	
Epidermolysis bullosa	
Renal agenesis	

TABLE 17-2
AMNIOTIC FLUID VOLUME ESTIMATION

Oligohydramnios (<500 mL)	Polyhydramnios (>2 L)
Renal and urologic anomalies:	GI anomalies: gastroschisis, duodenal
Potter syndrome	atresia, tracheoesophageal fistula,
Lung hypoplasia	diaphragmatic hernia
	CNS anomalies: anencephaly, Werdnig-
Limb deformities	Hoffman syndrome
Premature rupture of membranes	Chromosomal trisomies
Placental insufficiency	Maternal diabetes
	Cystic adenomatoid malformation of the lung

TABLE 17-3
PREDICTED ENDOTRACHEAL TUBE SIZE AND EXPECTED BIRTH WEIGHT BY GESTATIONAL AGE*

Gestational Age (wk)	Weight (g)	ETT Size (mm)	ETT Depth of Insertion (cm from upper lip)
24	700	2.5	7
26	900	2.5	7
28	1100	2.5–3.0	7
30	1350	3.0	7
32	1650	3.0	7
34	2100	3.5	8
36	2600	3.5	8
38	3000	3.5–4.0	9

*Weight is the 50th percentile for age.

ETT, endotracheal tube.

Data from Usher R, McLean F: J Pediatr 1969;74:901 and Welty SE: Pediatrics 2000;106(3): e29.

4. **Deceleratons:**

a. Early decelerations: Begin with the onset of contractions. The heart rate reaches the nadir at the peak of the contraction and returns to baseline as the contraction ends. Occur secondary to changes in vagal tone after brief hypoxic episodes or head compression and are benign.

b. Variable decelerations: Represent umbilical cord compression and have no uniform temporal relationship to the onset of the contraction. They are considered severe when the heart rate drops to <60 bpm for about 60 seconds with slow recovery to baseline.

c. Late decelerations: Occur after the peak of contraction, persist after the contraction stops, and show a slow return to baseline. Result from uteroplacental insufficiency and indicate fetal distress.

II. NEWBORN RESUSCITATION

A. NALS ALGORITHM FOR NEONATAL RESUSCITATION (Fig. 17-1)

For infants with meconium in the amniotic fluid, the mouth, pharynx, and nose should be suctioned before delivery of the thorax and before drying and stimulating the infant. For indications for intubation with meconium staining, refer to Figure 17-1.[1]

B. ENDOTRACHEAL TUBE SIZE AND DEPTH OF INSERTION

C. VENTILATORY SUPPORT (see Chapter 4)

D. VASCULAR ACCESS (see Chapter 3 for umbilical venous catheter and umbilical artery catheter placement)

III. NEWBORN ASSESSMENT

A. VITAL SIGNS

Average heart rate and respiratory rate are 120 to 160 bpm and 40 to 60 breaths/min, respectively. Arterial blood pressure is related to birth weight and gestational age (see Chapter 6). Normal core temperature in the neonate is 36.5° to 37.5°C rectally. (See Chapter 20 for height, weight, and head circumference growth charts in the premature infant.)

B. APGAR SCORES (Table 17-4)

APGAR scores are assessed at 1 and 5 minutes and may be repeated at 5-minute intervals for infants with 5-minute scores <7.[2]

C. NEW BALLARD GESTATIONAL AGE ESTIMATION

The Ballard score is most accurate when performed between 12 and 20 hours of age.[3] The approximate gestational age is calculated based on the sum of the neuromuscular and physical maturity ratings (Fig. 17-2).

1. **Neuromuscular maturity:**

a. Posture: Observe infant quiet and supine. Score 0 for arms, legs extended; 1 for starting to flex hips and knees, arms extended; 2 for

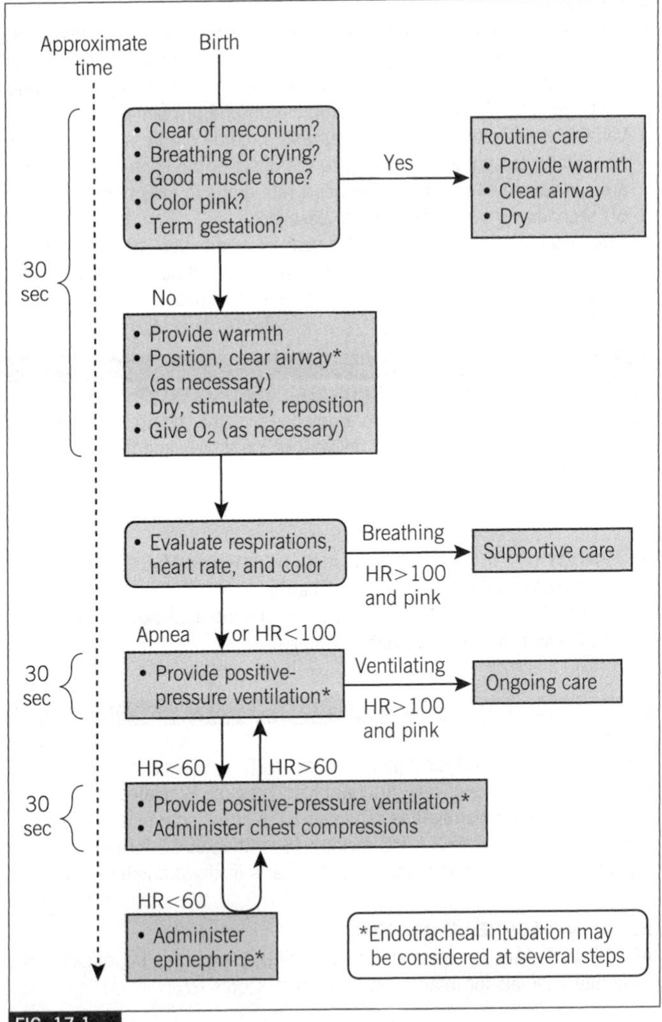

FIG. 17-1

Overview of resuscitation in the delivery room. *(From Welty SE: Is oxidant stress in the causal pathway to BPD? Pediatrics 2000;106[3]:e29.)*

TABLE 17-4

APGAR SCORES

Score	0	1	2
Heart rate	Absent	<100 bpm	>100 bpm
Respiratory effort	Absent, irregular	Slow, crying	Good
Muscle tone	Limp	Some flexion of extremities	Active motion
Reflex irritability (nose suction)	No response	Grimace	Cough or sneeze
Color	Blue, pale	Acrocyanosis	Completely pink

Data from Apgar V: Anesth Analg 1953;32:260.

stronger flexion of legs, arms extended; 3 for arms slightly flexed, legs flexed and abducted; and 4 for full flexion of arms, legs.

b. Square window: Flex hand on forearm enough to obtain fullest possible flexion without wrist rotation. Measure angle between the hypothenar eminence and the ventral aspect of the forearm.

c. Arm recoil: With infant supine, flex forearms for 5 seconds, fully extend by pulling on hands, then release. Measure the angle of elbow flexion to which the arms recoil.

d. Popliteal angle: Hold infant supine with pelvis flat, thigh held in the knee-chest position. Extend leg by gentle pressure and measure the popliteal angle.

e. Scarf sign: With baby supine, pull infant's hand across the neck toward the opposite shoulder. Determine how far the elbow will go across. Score 0 if elbow reaches opposite axillary line; 1 if past midaxillary line; 2 if past midline; and 3 if elbow unable to reach midline.

f. Heel-to-ear maneuver: With baby supine, draw foot as near to the head as possible without forcing it. Observe distance between foot and head and degree of extension at the knee.

2. **Physical maturity: Based on the developmental stage of eyes, ears, breasts, genitalia, skin, lanugo, and plantar creases.**

D. SELECTED ANOMALIES, SYNDROMES, AND MALFORMATIONS

1. **Extradural fluid collections (Fig. 17-3): caput succedaneum, cephalohematoma, and subgaleal hemorrhage.**
2. **Miscellaneous syndromes and teratogenic malformations (see Chapter 12 for more common syndromes and genetic disorders):**

a. **VATER association: V**ertebral anomalies, **A**nal anomalies and anal atresia, **T**racheoesophageal fistula, **E**sophageal atresia, and **R**adial defects. May also include vascular (cardiac) defects and renal defects.

b. **CHARGE association: C**oloboma, **H**eart disease, choanal **A**tresia, **R**etarded growth and development (may include central nervous system [CNS] anomalies), **G**enital anomalies (may include hypogonadism), **E**ar abnormalities or deafness.

Neuromuscular maturity

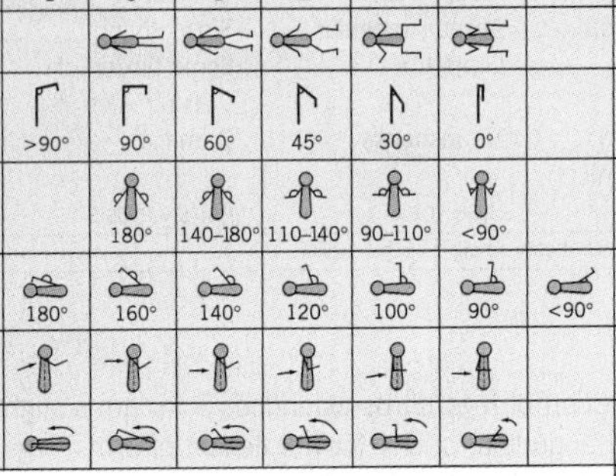

Neuromuscular maturity sign	Score −1	0	1	2	3	4	5	Record score here
Posture								
Square window (wrist)	>90°	90°	60°	45°	30°	0°		
Arm recoil		180°	140–180°	110–140°	90–110°	<90°		
Popliteal angle	180°	160°	140°	120°	100°	90°	<90°	
Scarf sign								
Heel to ear								

TOTAL NEUROMUSCULAR MATURITY SCORE

Physical maturity

Physical maturity sign	Score −1	0	1	2	3	4	5	Record score here
Skin	Sticky, friable, transparent	Gelatinous, red, translucent	Smooth, pink, visible veins	Superficial peeling and/or rash, few veins	Cracking, pale areas, rare veins	Parchment, deep cracking, no vessels	Leathery, cracked, wrinkled	
Lanugo	None	Sparse	Abundant	Thinning	Bald areas	Mostly bald		
Plantar surface	Heel–toe: 40–50mm: −1 <40mm: −2	>50mm, no crease	Faint red marks	Anterior transverse crease only	Creases anterior two thirds	Creases over entire sole		
Breast	Imperceptible	Barely perceptible	Flat areola, no bud	Stippled areola, 1–2mm bud	Raised areola, 3–4mm bud	Full areola, 5–10mm bud		
Eye/ear	Lids fused: loosely: −1 tightly: −2	Lids open, pinna flat, stays folded	Sl. curved pinna, soft, slow recoil	Well-curved pinna, soft but ready recoil	Formed and firm, instant recoil	Thick cartilage, ear stiff		
Genitals (male)	Scrotum flat, smooth	Scrotum empty, faint rugae	Testes in upper canal, rare rugae	Testes descending, few rugae	Testes down, good rugae	Testes pendulous, deep rugae		
Genitals (female)	Clitoris prominent and labia flat	Prominent clitoris and small labia minora	Prominent clitoris and enlarging minora	Majora and minora equally prominent	Majora large, minora small	Majora cover clitoris and minora		

TOTAL PHYSICAL MATURITY SCORE

Score

Neuromuscular____
Physical____
Total____

Maturity rating

Score	−10	−5	0	5	10	15	20	25	30	35	40	45	50
Weeks	20	22	24	26	28	30	32	34	36	38	40	42	44

Gestational age (weeks)

By dates____
By ultrasound____
By exam____

FIG. 17-2

Neuromuscular and physical maturity (New Ballard Score). *(Modified from Ballard JL, et al: J Pediatr 1991;119:417–423.)*

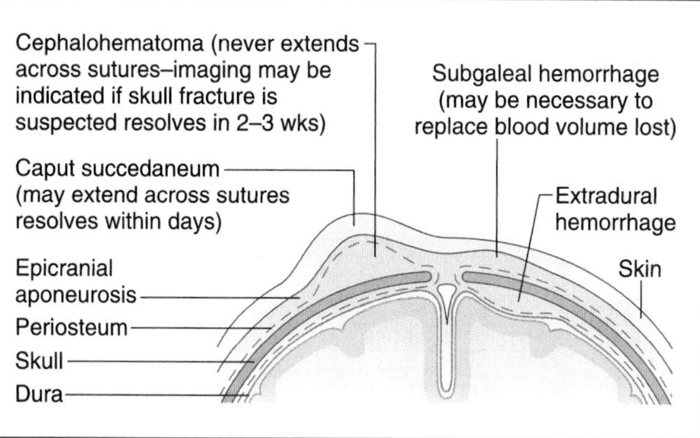

FIG. 17-3
Types of extradural fluid collections seen in newborn infants.

c. **Infant of a diabetic mother:** Sacral agenesis, femoral hypoplasia, heart defects, and cleft palate. May also include preaxial radial defects, microtia, cleft lip, microphthalmos, holoprosencephaly, microcephaly, anencephaly, spina bifida, hemivertebra, urinary tract defects, and polydactyly.
d. **Fetal alcohol syndrome:** Short palpebral fissures, epicanthal folds, flat nasal bridge, long philtrum, thin upper lip, small hypoplastic nails, and small for gestational age. May be associated with cardiac defects.
e. **Fetal hydantoin syndrome:** Broad, low nasal bridge, hypertelorism, epicanthal folds, ptosis, prominent malformed ears, hypoplasia of fifth nail of toe or finger.
f. **Fetal valproate syndrome:** Neural tube defects, fused metopic suture, trigonocephaly, epicanthal folds, midface hypoplasia, anteverted nostrils, oral cleft, heart defects, hypospadias, clubfeet, and psychomotor retardation.

IV. FLUIDS, ELECTROLYTES, AND NUTRITION

A. FLUIDS

1. **Insensible water loss in preterm infants** (Table 17-5).
2. **Water requirements of newborns** (Table 17-6).

B. GLUCOSE

1. **Requirements: Preterm neonates require about 5 to 6 mg/kg/min of glucose to maintain euglycemia (40 to 100 mg/dL).[4] Term neonates require about 3 to 5 mg/kg/min of glucose to maintain euglycemia. The formula to calculate rate of glucose infusion follows:**

TABLE 17-5
INSENSIBLE WATER LOSS IN PRETERM INFANTS*

Body Weight (g)	Insensible Water Loss (mL/kg/day)
<1000	60–70
1000–1250	60–65
1251–1500	30–45
1501–1750	15–30
1751–2000	15–20

*Estimates of insensible water loss at different body weights during the first few days of life.
Data from Veille JC: Clin Perinatol 1988;15:863.

TABLE 17-6
WATER REQUIREMENTS OF NEWBORNS

	Water Requirements (mL/kg/24 hr) by Age		
Birth Weight (g)	1–2 days	3–7 days	7–30 days
<750	100–250	150–300	120–180
750–1000	80–150	100–150	120–180
1000–1500	60–100	80–150	120–180
<1500	60–80	100–150	120–180

Data from Taeusch HW, Ballard RA (eds): Schaffer and Avery's Diseases of the Newborn, 7th ed. Philadelphia, WB Saunders, 1998.

glucose (mg/kg/min) = (% glucose in solution × 10) × (rate of infusion per hour)/60 × weight (kg)

2. **Management of hyperglycemia and hypoglycemia** (Tables 17-7 and 17-8).

C. ELECTROLYTES, MINERALS, AND VITAMINS

1. **Electrolyte requirements** (Table 17-9).
2. **Mineral and vitamin requirements:**

a. Infants born at <34 weeks' gestation have higher calcium, phosphorus, sodium, iron, and vitamin D requirements and require breast-milk fortifier or special preterm formulas with iron. Fortifier should be added to breast milk only after the second week of life.

b. Iron: Enterally fed preterm infants require elemental iron supplementation of 2 mg/kg/day after 4 to 8 weeks of age.

D. NUTRITION

1. **Growth and caloric requirements** (Table 17-10).
2. **Total parenteral nutrition (see Chapter 20).**

V. CYANOSIS IN THE NEWBORN

A. DIFFERENTIAL DIAGNOSIS (FIG. 17-4)

B. EVALUATION

1. **Physical examination:** Note central versus peripheral and persistent versus intermittent cyanosis, degree of respiratory effort, single versus

TABLE 17-7

MANAGEMENT OF HYPERGLYCEMIA AND HYPOGLYCEMIA

	Hypoglycemia	Hyperglycemia
Definition	Serum glucose <40 in term and preterm infants	Serum glucose >125 mg/dL in term infants, >150 mg/dL in preterm infants
Differential diagnosis	Insufficient glucose delivery Decreased glycogen stores Increased circulating insulin (infant of a diabetic mother, maternal drugs, Beckwith-Wiedemann syndrome, tumors) Endocrine and metabolic disorders Sepsis Hypothermia Polycythemia Asphyxia Shock	Excess glucose administration Sepsis Hypoxia Hyperosmolar formula Transient neonatal diabetes mellitus Medications
Evaluation	Ensure venous sample confirms bedside testing Assess for symptoms Calculate glucose delivery to infant Serum glucose CBC with differential Blood cultures Urine analysis Urine cultures Electrolytes Lumbar puncture if warranted Insulin and C-peptide levels if warranted	
Management	Change dextrose infusion rates gradually. Generally, it should not exceed 2 mg/kg/min in a 2-hour interval. (See Table 17–9 for further guidelines). Monitor glucose levels every 30–60 min until normal values have been established.	Gradually decrease glucose infusion rate if receiving >5 mg/kg/min. Monitor glucosuria. Consider insulin infusion for persistent hyperglycemia. Consider consulting an endocrinologist.

split S2, and presence or absence of a heart murmur. Acrocyanosis is often a normal finding in newborns.

2. **Clinical tests:** Oxygen challenge test (see Chapter 6), preductal and postductal arterial blood gas (ABG) levels, or pulse oximetry to assess for right-to-left shunt, transillumination of chest for possible pneumothorax.
3. **Other data:** Complete blood count (CBC) with differential, serum glucose, chest radiograph, electrocardiogram, echocardiography.

TABLE 17-8
GUIDELINES FOR TREATMENT OF NEONATAL HYPOGLYCEMIA

Plasma Glucose (mg/dL)—Venous Sample	Asymptomatic or Mildly Symptomatic	Symptomatic
35–45	Breast-feed or give formula or D_5W by nipple/gavage	IV glucose ($D_{5-12.5}W$) at 4–6 mg/kg/min*
25–34	IV glucose ($D_{5-12.5}W$) at 6–8 mg/kg/min*	IV glucose ($D_{5-12.5}W$) at 6–8 mg/kg/min*
<25	Minibolus of 2 mL/kg ($D_{10}W$) and continue at a rate to provide 6–8 mg/kg/min†	

*Changes in infusion rates should not exceed 2 mg/kg/min per change.

†If blood glucose <25 mg/dL and IV access is not available, give glucagon, 0.1 mg/kg per dose (maximum, 1 mg/dose) IM or SC every 30 minutes. Not as effective in small-for-gestational-age (SGA) or extremely premature infants.

Modified from Cornblath M: In Donn SM, Fisher CW (eds): Risk Management Techniques in Perinatal and Neonatal Practice. Armonk, NY, Futura, 1996.

TABLE 17-9
ELECTROLYTE REQUIREMENTS

	Before 48 Hours of Life	After 48–72 Hours of Life
Sodium	None, unless serum sodium <135 mEq/L without evidence of volume overload	Term infants: 2–3 mEq/kg/day Preterm infants: 3–5 mEq/kg/day
Potassium	None	1–2.5 mEq/kg/day if adequate urine output is established and serum level <4.5 mEq/L

TABLE 17-10
INFANT GROWTH AND CALORIC REQUIREMENTS

		Preterm Infants	Term Infants
Growth* (after 10 days of life)		15–20 g/kg/day	10 g/kg/day
Caloric Requirments*	Maintaining weight	50–75 kcal/kg/day	
	Adequate growth	115–130 kcal/kg/day (may be up to 150 kcal/kg/day for VLBW infants)	100–120 kcal/kg/day

*Rates and requirements presume healthy infants in thermoneutral environments.

VLBW, very-low-birth-weight.

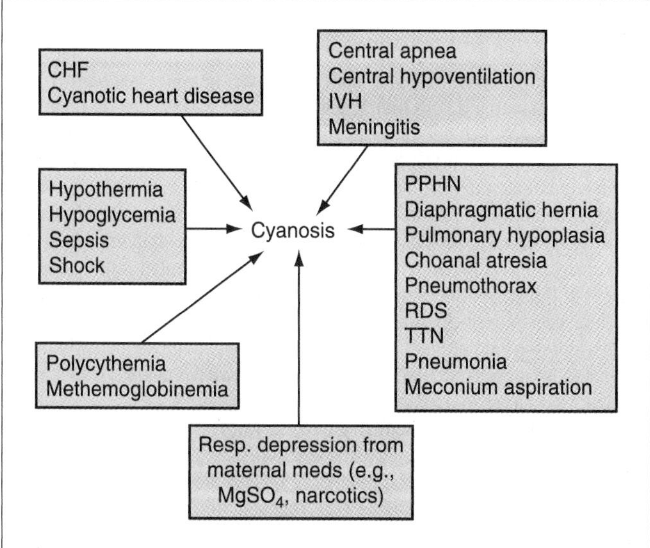

FIG. 17-4
Causes of cyanosis in the newborn.

Consider blood, urine, and cerebrospinal fluid (CSF) cultures if sepsis is suspected, and methemoglobin level if cyanosis does not match degree of hypoxemia.

VI. RESPIRATORY DISEASES

A. GENERAL RESPIRATORY CONSIDERATIONS

1. Exogenous surfactant therapy:

a. Indications: Respiratory distress syndrome in preterm infants, meconium aspiration, pneumonia, persistent pulmonary hypertension.

b. Administration: Each preparation has specific dosing instructions. If the infant is ″ 26 weeks gestation, the first dose is typically given in the delivery room when stabilized, repeat dosing may follow at 6-hour intervals.

c. Complications: Pneumothorax, pulmonary hemorrhage.

2. Supplemental O_2: Adjust inspired oxygen to maintain O_2 saturation between 88% and 92% until the retina is fully vascularized, 94% to 98% if the retinas are mature, and >97% in cases of pulmonary hypertension. Consider oxygen hoods, nasal cannula modalities.

B. RESPIRATORY DISTRESS SYNDROME (RDS)

1. **Definition:** A deficiency of pulmonary surfactant, a phospholipid protein mixture that decreases surface tension and prevents alveolar collapse. It is produced by type II alveolar cells in increasing quantities from 32 weeks' gestation. Factors that accelerate lung maturity include maternal hypertension, sickle cell disease, narcotic addiction, intrauterine growth retardation (IUGR), prolonged rupture of membranes, fetal stress, and exogenous antenatal steroids.
2. **Incidence:** 60% in infants <30 weeks' gestation without steroids, but decreases to 35% for those who have received antenatal steroids. Between 30 and 34 weeks' gestation, 25% in untreated infants and 10% in those who have received antenatal steroids. For infants >34 weeks' gestation, incidence is 5%.
3. **Risk factors:** Prematurity, maternal diabetes, cesarean section without antecedent labor, perinatal asphyxia, second twin, previous infant with RDS.
4. **Clinical presentation:** Respiratory distress worsens during the first few hours of life, progresses over 48 to 72 hours, and subsequently improves. Recovery is accompanied by brisk diuresis. Classically, on chest radiograph, lung fields have a "reticulogranular" pattern that may obscure the heart border.
5. **Management:**
   a. Support ventilation and oxygenation.
   b. Surfactant therapy.
6. **Intrauterine acceleration of fetal lung maturation:** Maternal administration of steroids antenatally has been shown to decrease neonatal morbidity and mortality. In particular, the risk for RDS is decreased in babies born >24 hours and <7 days after maternal steroid administration.

C. PERSISTENT PULMONARY HYPERTENSION OF THE NEWBORN (PPHN)

1. **Etiology:** Idiopathic or secondary to conditions leading to increased pulmonary vascular resistance. Most commonly seen in term or post-term infants, infants born by cesarean section, and infants with a history of fetal distress and low Apgar scores. Usually presents within 12 to 24 hours of birth. Accounts for up to 2% of all neonatal admissions to the intensive care unit (ICU).
   a. Vasoconstriction secondary to hypoxemia and acidosis (neonatal sepsis).
   b. Interstitial pulmonary disease (meconium aspiration syndrome, pneumonia).
   c. Hyperviscosity syndrome (polycythemia).
   d. Pulmonary hypoplasia, either primary or secondary to congenital diaphragmatic hernia or renal agenesis.
2. **Diagnostic features:**

a. Severe hypoxemia (Pao_2 <35 to 45 mmHg in 100% O_2) disproportionate to radiologic changes.
b. Structurally normal heart with right-to-left shunt at foramen ovale or ductus arteriosus; decreased postductal oxygen saturations compared with preductal values. (Difference of at least 7 to 15 mmHg between preductal and postductal Pao_2 is significant.)
c. Must distinguish from cyanotic heart disease. Infants with heart disease will have an abnormal cardiac examination and show little to no improvement in oxygenation with increased Fio_2 and hyperventilation. See Chapter 6 for interpretation of oxygen challenge test.

3. Principles of therapy:

a. Consider transfer to a tertiary care center.
b. Minimal handling and limited invasive procedures. Sedation and occasionally paralysis of intubated babies may be necessary.
c. Maintenance of systemic blood pressure with reversal of right-to-left shunt through volume expanders and/or inotropes.
d. Optimize oxygen-carrying capacity with blood transfusions as needed.
e. Administer broad-spectrum antibiotics.
f. Mild hyperventilation to induce respiratory alkalosis (Pco_2 in low 30s) or bicarbonate infusion to induce metabolic alkalosis with pH 7.55 to 7.60. Both may improve oxygenation. Avoid severe hypocarbia (Pco_2 <25), which can be associated with myocardial ischemia and decreased cerebral blood flow. Hyperventilation may result in barotrauma, which predisposes to chronic lung disease. Consider high-frequency ventilation.
g. Nitric oxide, a selective pulmonary vasodilator, may be beneficial. Blended with ventilatory gases and titrated to effect, 2 to 80 ppm. Unlikely to be efficacious >40 ppm. Complications include methemoglobinemia (reduce NO dose for methemoglobin >4%), NO_2 poisoning (reduce NO dose for NO_2 concentration >1–2 ppm).
h. Consider extracorporeal membrane oxygenation (ECMO) if infant has severe cardiovascular instability, if oxygenation index (OI) is >40 for more than 3 hours, or if alveolar-arterial gradient (Aao_2) is ≥610 for 8 hours (see Chapter 4 for the calculation of OI and Aao_2. Pao_2 should be measured at a postductal site). Patients typically need to be >2000 g and >34 weeks' gestation. Infants need a head ultrasound and an echocardiogram before going on ECMO.
i. Mortality: Depends on the etiology, but overall mortality rates in North American centers approximate 30% to 40%.

VII. APNEA AND BRADYCARDIA

A. APNEA[5]

1. **Definition:** Respiratory pause >20 seconds, or a shorter pause associated with cyanosis, pallor, hypotonia, or bradycardia <100 bpm. In preterm infants, apneic episodes may be central (no

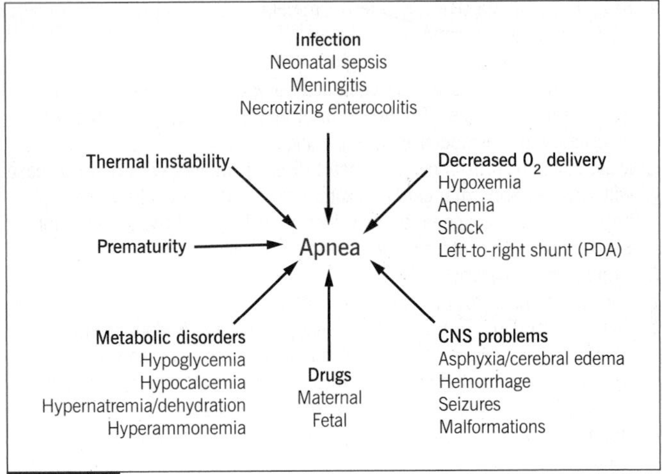

FIG. 17-5
Causes of apnea in the newborn. *(From Klaus MH, Fanaroff AA: Care of the High-Risk Neonate, 4th ed. Philadelphia, WB Saunders, 1993.)*

diaphragmatic activity), obstructive (upper airway obstruction), or mixed central and obstructive. Common causes of apnea in the newborn are listed in Figure 17-5.

2. **Incidence:** Apnea* occurs in most infants born at <28 weeks gestation, about 50% of infants born at 30 to 32 weeks gestation, and <7% of infants born at 34 to 35 weeks gestation. It usually resolves by 34 to 36 weeks postconceptual *age, but may persist after term in infants born* at >25 weeks gestation.
3. **Management:**
a. Consider pathologic causes for apnea.
b. Pharmacotherapy with theophylline, aminophylline, caffeine, or doxapram (see Formulary for dosage information).
c. Continuous positive-airway pressure or mechanical ventilation (see Chapter 24 for details).

B. BRADYCARDIA WITHOUT CENTRAL APNEA

Obstructive apnea, mechanical airway obstruction, gastroesophageal reflux (GER), increased intracranial pressure (ICP), increased vagal tone (defecation, yawning, rectal stimulation, placement of nasogastric tube), electrolyte abnormalities, heart block.

* of prematurity

VIII. CARDIAC DISEASES

A. PATENT DUCTUS ARTERIOSUS (PDA)

1. **Summary:** Failure of the ductus arteriosus to close in the first few days of life or reopening after functional closure. Typically results in left-to-right shunting of blood once pulmonary vascular resistance (PVR) has decreased. If the PVR remains high, blood may be shunted right to left, resulting in hypoxemia (see Persistent Pulmonary Hypertension, section VI.C).
2. **Incidence:** Up to 60% in preterm infants weighing <1500 g, higher in those <1000 g. Female-to-male ratio is 2 : 1. Obligatory PDA is found in 10% of infants with congenital heart disease.
3. **Risk factors:** Most often related to hypoxia and immaturity. Term infants with PDA usually have structural defects in the walls of the ductal vessel.
4. **Diagnosis:**

a. Examination: A systolic murmur that may be continuous and is best heard at the left upper sternal border (LUSB) or left infraclavicular area. May have apical diastolic rumble because of increased blood flow across the mitral valve in diastole. Bounding peripheral pulses with widened pulse pressure if large shunt. Hyperactive precordium and palmar pulses may also be present.

b. Electrocardiogram (ECG): Normal or left ventricular hypertrophy in small to moderate PDA. Bilateral ventricular hypertrophy in large PDA.

c. Chest radiograph: May have cardiomegaly and increased pulmonary vascular markings depending on size of the shunt.

d. Echocardiogram.

5. **Management:**

a. Indomethacin: A prostaglandin synthetase inhibitor; 80% closure rate in preterm infants.

   (1) For dosage information and contraindications, see Formulary.

   (2) Complications: Transient decrease in glomerular filtration rate (GFR) and subsequent decreased urine output; transient gastrointestinal (GI) bleeding (not associated with an increased incidence of necrotizing enterocolitis [NEC]); and prolonged bleeding time and disturbed platelet function for 7 to 9 days independent of platelet number (not associated with increased incidence of intracranial hemorrhage).

b. Surgical ligation of the duct.

B. CYANOTIC HEART DISEASE

See Chapter 6.

IX. HEMATOLOGIC DISEASES

A. UNCONJUGATED HYPERBILIRUBINEMIA IN THE NEWBORN[6]

1. **Summary:** During the first 3 to 4 days of life, infants' serum bilirubin increases from cord bilirubin levels of 1.5 mg/dL to 6.5 ± 2.5 mg/dL.

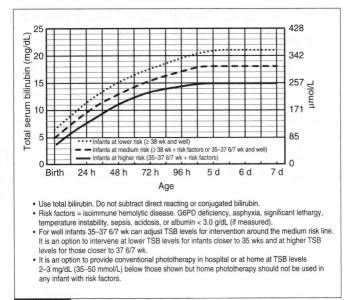

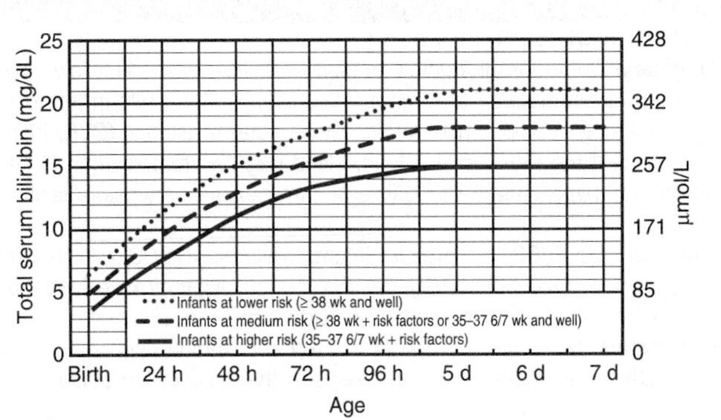

- Use total bilirubin. Do not subtract direct reacting or conjugated bilirubin.
- Risk factors = isoimmune hemolytic disease. G6PD deficiency, asphyxia, significant lethargy, temperature instability, sepsis, acidosis, or albumin < 3.0 g/dL (if measured).
- For well infants 35–37 6/7 wk can adjust TSB levels for intervention around the medium risk line. It is an option to intervene at lower TSB levels for infants closer to 35 wks and at higher TSB levels for those closer to 37 6/7 wk.
- It is an option to provide conventional phototherapy in hospital or at home at TSB levels 2–3 mg/dL (35–50 mmol/L) below those shown but home phototherapy should not be used in any infant with risk factors.

FIG. 17-6

Guidelines for phototherapy in infants 35 weeks gestation or more.

The maximum rate of increase in bilirubin for otherwise normal infants with nonhemolytic hyperbilirubinemia is 5 mg/dL/24 hr or 0.2 mg/dL/hr. Visible jaundice or a total bilirubin concentration >5 mg/dL on the first day of life is outside the normal range and suggests a potentially pathologic cause. Infants <37 weeks gestation tend to have maximum serum indirect bilirubin levels 30% to 50% higher compared with term infants. Treatment guidelines for preterm infants (Table 17-11) differ from those for term infants (Figs. 17-6 and 17-7).

2. **Evaluation:**

a. Maternal prenatal testing: ABO and Rh (D) typing and serum screen for isoimmune antibodies.

b. Infant or cord blood: Evaluation of blood smear, direct Coombs test, blood type, and Rh typing if mother has not had prenatal blood typing or she is blood type O or Rh negative.

3. **Management:**

a. Phototherapy:

(1) Preterm newborn (see Table 17-11): Bilirubin levels may significantly increase in the infant who is <36 weeks' gestation, weighs <2500 g, and is breast-feeding. These infants may require phototherapy at lower bilirubin levels.

(2) Term newborn (see Fig. 17-6): Intensive phototherapy should produce a decline of the total serum bilirubin (TSB) level of 1 to

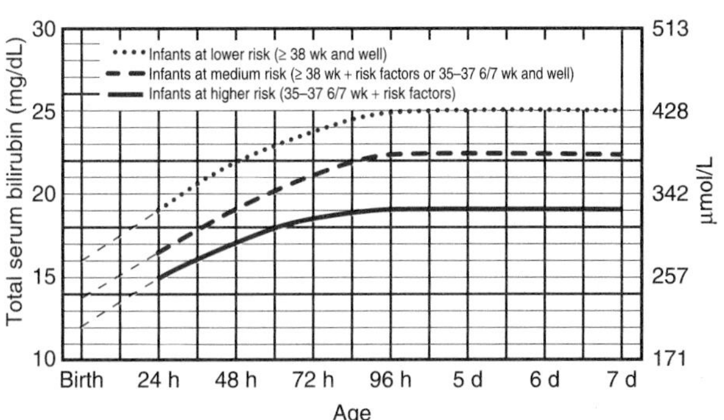

- The dashed lines for the first 24 hours indicate uncertainty due to a wide range of clinical circumstances and a range of responses to phototherapy.
- Immediate exchange transfusion is recommended if infant shows signs of acute bilirubin encephalopathy (hypertonia, arching, retrocollis, opisthotonos, fever, high pitched cry) or if TBS is ≥ 5 mg/dL (85 μmol/L) above these lines.
- Risk factors: isoimmune hemolytic disease, G6PD deficiency, asphyxia, significant lethargy, temperature instability, sepsis, acidosis.
- Measure serum albumin and calculate B/A ratio (see legend)
- Use total bilirubin. Do not subtract direct reacting or conjugated bilirubin.
- If infant is well and 35–37 6/7 wk (median risk) can individualize TSB levels for exchange based on actual gestational age.

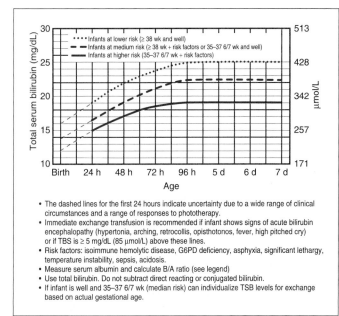

FIG. 17-7

Guidelines for exchange transfusion in infants 35 or more weeks gestation.

2 mg/dL within 4 to 6 hours. The TSB level should continue to fall and remain below the threshold level for exchange transfusion. If this does not occur, it is considered a failure of phototherapy.

b. Neonatal exchange transfusion (see Table 17-11 and Fig. 17-7): To complete double-volume exchange, transfuse 160 mL/kg for full-term infant and 160 to 200 mL/kg for preterm infant. During the exchange, blood is removed through the umbilical artery catheter, and an equal volume is infused through the venous catheter. If unable to pass an arterial catheter, use a single venous catheter. Exchange in 15-mL increments in vigorous full-term infants, smaller volumes for smaller,

TABLE 17-11

GUIDELINES FOR USE OF PHOTOTHERAPY IN PRETERM INFANTS <1 WEEK OF AGE

Weight (g)	Phototherapy (mg/dL)	Consider Exchange Transfusion (mg/dL)
500–1000	5–7	12–15
1000–1500	7–10	15–18
1500–2500	10–15	18–20
>2500	>15	>20

NEONATOLOGY 17

less stable infants. Withdraw and infuse blood 2 to 3 mL/kg/min to avoid mechanical trauma to patient and donor cells. Complications include emboli, thromboses, hemodynamic instability, electrolyte disturbances, coagulopathy, infection, and death.

Note *CBC, reticulocyte count, peripheral smear, bilirubin, Ca^{2+}, glucose, total protein, infant blood type, Coombs test, and newborn screen should be performed on a pre-exchange sample of blood because they are of no diagnostic value on postexchange blood. If indicated, save pre-exchange blood for serologic or chromosome studies.*

B. CONJUGATED HYPERBILIRUBINEMIA

1. **Definition:** Direct bilirubin is >2.0 mg/dL and is >10% of the total serum bilirubin.
2. **Etiology:** biliary obstruction/atresia, choledochal cyst, hyperalimentation, α_1-antitrypsin deficiency, hepatitis, sepsis, infections (especially urinary tract infections), hypothyroidism, inborn errors of metabolism, cystic fibrosis, red blood cell abnormalities.
3. **Management:** Phenobarbital for infants not on full feeds. Actigall for infants on full feeds.

C. POLYCYTHEMIA

1. **Definition:** Venous hematocrit >65% confirmed on two consecutive samples. May be falsely elevated when sample obtained by heel stick.
2. **Etiology:** Delayed cord clamping; twin–twin transfusion; maternal–fetal transfusion; intrauterine hypoxia; trisomy 13, 18, or 21; Beckwith-Wiedemann syndrome; maternal gestational diabetes; neonatal thyrotoxicosis; and congenital adrenal hyperplasia.
3. **Clinical findings:** Plethora, respiratory distress, cardiac failure, tachypnea, hypoglycemia, irritability, lethargy, seizures, apnea, jitteriness, poor feeding, thrombocytopenia, hyperbilirubinemia.
4. **Complications:** Hyperviscosity predisposes to venous thrombosis and CNS injury. Hypoglycemia may result from increased erythrocyte utilization of glucose.
5. **Management:** Partial exchange transfusion for symptomatic infants with isovolemic replacement of blood with isotonic fluid. Blood is exchanged in 10- to 20-mL increments to reduce hematocrit (HCT) to <55. (See Chapter 9 to calculate the amount of blood to be exchanged. Use birth weight (kg) × 90 for estimated blood volume [EBV].)

X. GASTROINTESTINAL DISEASES

A. NECROTIZING ENTEROCOLITIS (NEC)

1. **Definition:** NEC is serious intestinal inflammation and injury thought to be secondary to bowel ischemia, immaturity, and infection.
2. **Incidence:** NEC is more common in preterm infants (3%–4% of infants <2000 g) and African-American infants. There is no gender predominance.

TABLE 17-12
CONSIDERATIONS IN BILIOUS EMESIS

	Bilious Emesis	
Pathophysiology	Proximal Intestinal Obstruction	Distal Intestinal Obstruction
Differential Diagnosis	Duodenal atresia Annular pancreas Malrotation with or without volvulus Jejunal obstruction/atresia	Ileal atresia Meconium ileus Colonic atresia Meconium plug—hypoplastic left colon syndrome Hirschsprung disease
Physical examination	Abdominal distention not prominent	Abdominal distention
Diagnosis	Abdominal x-ray: "double bubble" Upper GI	Abdominal x-ray: dilated loops of bowel Contrast enema Sweat test Mucosal rectal biopsy

3. **Risk factors:** Prematurity, asphyxia, hypotension, polycythemia-hyperviscosity syndrome, umbilical vessel catheterization, exchange transfusion, bacterial and viral pathogens, enteral feeds, PDA, congestive heart failure, cyanotic heart disease, RDS, in utero cocaine exposure.
4. **Clinical findings:**
a. Systemic: Temperature instability, apnea, bradycardia, metabolic acidosis, hypotension, disseminated intravascular coagulation (DIC).
b. Intestinal: Elevated pregavage residuals with abdominal distention, blood in stool, absent bowel sounds, and/or abdominal tenderness or mass. Elevated pregavage residuals in the absence of other clinical symptoms rarely raise suspicion of NEC.
c. Radiologic: Ileus, intestinal pneumatosis, portal vein gas, ascites, pneumoperitoneum.
5. **Management:** No food or water by mouth (NPO), nasogastric (NG) tube decompression, maintain adequate hydration and perfusion, antibiotics for 7 to 14 days, surgical consultation. Surgery is performed for signs of perforation or necrotic bowel.

B. BILIOUS EMESIS (Table 17-12)
Must eliminate malrotation as an etiology because its complication is a surgical emergency.

C. ABDOMINAL WALL DEFECTS
Omphalocele and gastroschisis (Table 17-13).

XI. NEUROLOGIC DISEASES
A. INTRAVENTRICULAR HEMORRHAGE (IVH)
1. **Definition:** Intracranial hemorrhage usually arising in the germinal matrix and periventricular regions of the brain.

TABLE 17-13

DIFFERENCES BETWEEN OMPHALOCELE AND GASTROSCHISIS

	Omphalocele	Gastroschisis
Position	Central abdominal	Right paraumbilical
Hernia sac	Present	Absent
Umbilical ring	Absent	Present
Umbilical cord insertion	At the vertex of the sac	Normal
Herniation of other viscera	Common	Rare
Extraintestinal anomalies	Frequent	Rare
Intestinal infarction, atresia	Less frequent	More frequent

2. **Incidence:** About 30% to 40% of infants weighing <1500 g; 50% to 60% of infants weighing <1000 g. Highest incidence in first 72 hours of life, 60% within 24 hours, 85% within 72 hours, <5% after 1 week postnatal age.
3. **Diagnosis and classification:** Ultrasonography is used in the diagnosis and classification of IVH. Routine screening is indicated in infants <32 weeks' gestational age within the first week of life and should be repeated in the second week. The grade is based on the maximum amount of hemorrhage seen by 2 weeks of age.
   a. Grade I: Hemorrhage in germinal matrix only.
   b. Grade II: IVH without ventricular dilatation.
   c. Grade III: IVH with ventricular dilatation (30%–45% incidence of motor and cognitive impairment).
   d. Grade IV: IVH with periventricular hemorrhagic infarct (60%–80% incidence of motor and cognitive impairment).
4. **Prophylaxis:** Maintain acid-base balance and avoid fluctuations in blood pressure. Indomethacin is considered for IVH prophylaxis in some newborns (<28 weeks' gestation, birth weight <1250 g) and is most efficacious if given in the first 6 hours of life (see Formulary for dosage information).
5. **Outcome:** Infants with grade III and IV hemorrhages have a higher incidence of neurodevelopmental handicap and an increased risk for posthemorrhagic hydrocephalus.

B. PERIVENTRICULAR LEUKOMALACIA (PVL)

1. **Definition and ultrasound findings:** Ischemic necrosis of periventricular white matter characterized by CNS depression within first week and ultrasound findings of cysts with or without ventricular enlargement caused by cerebral atrophy.
2. **Incidence:** More common in preterm infants but also occurs in term infants; 3.2% in infants <1500 g.
3. **Etiology:** Primarily ischemia-reperfusion injury, hypoxia, acidosis, hypoglycemia, acute hypotension, low cerebral blood flow.
4. **Outcome:** Commonly associated with cerebral palsy with or without sensory and cognitive deficit.

TABLE 17-14

OPIATE WITHDRAWAL

	Signs and Symptoms of Opiate Withdrawal
W	Wakefulness
I	Irritability, insomnia
T	Tremors, temperature variation, tachypnea, twitching (jitteriness)
H	Hyperactivity, high-pitched cry, hiccoughs, hyperreflexia, hypertonia
D	Diarrhea (explosive), diaphoresis, disorganized suck
R	Rubmarks, respiratory distress, rhinorrhea, regurgitation
A	Apnea, autonomic dysfunction
W	Weight loss
A	Alkalosis (respiratory)
L	Lacrimation (photophobia), lethargy
S	Seizures, sneezing, stuffy nose, sweating, sucking (nonproductive)

C. NEONATAL SEIZURES (see Chapter 19)

D. NEONATAL ABSTINENCE SYNDROME

Onset of symptoms usually occurs within the first 24 to 72 hours of life (methadone may delay symptoms until 96 hours or later). The duration of symptoms may last 8 weeks and persist for 4 months. Table 17-14 shows signs and symptoms of opiate withdrawal.

E. PERIPHERAL NERVE INJURIES (Table 17-15)

1. **Etiology:** Result from lateral traction on the shoulder (vertex deliveries) or the head (breech deliveries).
2. **Clinical features (See** Table 17-15**).**
3. **Management:** Evaluate for associated trauma (clavicular and humeral fractures, shoulder dislocation, facial nerve injury and cord injuries). Treatment includes immobilization for 7 to 10 days. Full recovery is seen in 85%–95% of cases in the first year of life.

TABLE 17-15

PLEXUS INJURIES

Plexus Injury	Spinal Level Involved	Clinical Features
Erb-Duchenne palsy (90% of cases)	C5 to C6 Occasionally involves C4	Adduction and internal rotation of the arm. Forearm is pronated. Wrist is flexed. Diaphragm paralysis may occur if C4 is involved.
Total palsy (8%–9% of cases)	C5 to T1 Occasionally involves C4	Upper arm, lower arm, and hand are involved. Horner syndrome (ptosis, anhydrosis, and miosis) exists if T1 is involved.
Klumpke paralysis (<2% of cases)	C7 to T1	Hand flaccid with little control Horner syndrome if T1 is involved

XII. RETINOPATHY OF PREMATURITY (ROP)[7]

A. DEFINITION

ROP is the interruption of the normal progression of retinal vascularization.

B. ETIOLOGY

Exposure of the immature retina to high oxygen concentrations can result in vasoconstriction and obliteration of the retinal capillary network, followed by vasoproliferation. Risk is greatest in the most immature infant.

C. DIAGNOSIS

All infants born <28 weeks gestation, and any infant born weighing 1500 to 2000 g or at <35 weeks gestation who requires oxygen should have a dilated funduscopic examination either 4 to 6 weeks after birth or 31 to 33 weeks gestation to screen for ROP.

D. CLASSIFICATION

ROP is described by the stage of disease, the highest zone of the retina involved (Fig. 17-8), the number of clock hours or 30-degree sectors involved, and the presence or absence of plus disease.

1. **Stage 1: Demarcation line separates avascular from vascularized retina.**
2. **Stage 2: Ridge forms along demarcation line.**
3. **Stage 3: Extraretinal fibrovascular proliferation tissue forms on ridge.**
4. **Stage 4: Retinal detachment.**
5. **Plus disease: Tortuosity and engorgement of blood vessels near the optic disc; may be present at any stage.**

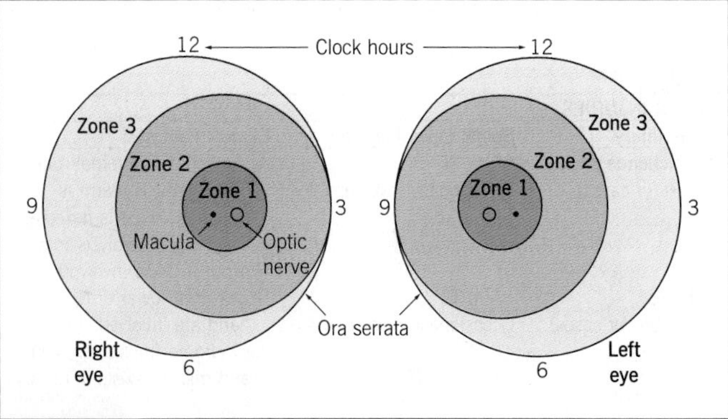

FIG. 17-8

Zones of the retina. *(From American Academy of Pediatrics: Pediatrics 1994;94[4 Pt 1]:558–565.)*

E. MANAGEMENT

Laser treatment is recommended when there are five contiguous or eight total 30-degree sectors of stage 3 in zone 1 or in zone 2 if accompanied by plus disease; the risk for blindness if untreated is 50%. An infant with stage 3 ROP in zone 2, stage 2 ROP with plus disease in zone 2, or any stage disease in zone 1 should have ophthalmologic examinations weekly to monitor progression of the ROP. All other infants should have ophthalmologic examinations every 2 weeks until the retina is fully vascularized.

XIII. CONGENITAL INFECTIONS

See Chapter 16.

REFERENCES

1. Wiswell TE, et al: Delivery room management of the apparently vigorous meconium-stained neonate: Results of the multicenter, international collaborative trial. Pediatrics 2000;105:1.
2. Apgar V: A proposal for new method of evaluation of the newborn infant. Anesth Analg 1953;32:260.
3. Ballard JL, et al: New Ballard Score, expanded to include extremely premature infants. J Pediatr 1991;119:417–423.
4. Cornblath M: Neonatal hypoglycemia. In Donn SM, Fisher CW (eds): Risk Management Techniques in Perinatal and Neonatal Practice. Armonk, NY, Futura, 1996.
5. Klaus MH, Fanaroff AA: Care of the High-Risk Neonate, 4th ed. Philadelphia, WB Saunders, 1993.
6. American Academy of Pediatrics Subcommittee on Hyperbilirubinemia: Management of hyperbilirubinemia in the newborn infant 35 or more weeks of gestation. Pediatrics 2004;114(1):297–316. Erratum in Pediatrics 2004;114(4): 1138.
7. Ben-Sira I, et al: An international classification of retinopathy of prematurity. Pediatrics 1984;74:127.
8. American Academy of Pediatrics: Clinical Practice Guideline. Pediatrics 2001;108:809–811.
9. American Academy of Pediatrics: Clinical Practice Guideline. Pediatrics 2004;114:297–316.
10. Annual Summary of Vital Statistics. Pediatrics 2003;112:1215–1230.

Nephrology

Stephanie O. Omokaro, MD

18

I. EPIDEMIOLOGY[1]

According to the 2002 U.S. Renal Data System (USRDS) Annual Data Report, the incidence of end-stage renal disease in patients aged 0 to 19 years in the United States is 15 per 1 million population. Although primary etiologies vary with age, structural anomalies predominate. Growth impairment is by far the best-documented complication of chronic renal disease. Hypertension in children with chronic renal insufficiency (CRI) is reported to be 38% to 78%. Although infrequent in congenital renal disease, it is almost universal in primary glomerular disease as well as in renal injury secondary to systemic disease.

II. CLINICAL MANIFESTATIONS OF RENAL DISEASE

A. HEMATURIA[2–9]

1. **Gross hematuria:** Bright red blood, clots in urine, or tea-colored urine.
2. **Microscopic hematuria:** >5 red blood cells (RBCs) per high-power field (hpf) on more than two occasions. Significant or persistent hematuria can be defined as three positive urinalyses, based on dipstick and microscopic examination over a 2- to 3-week period.
3. **Etiology:** Gross hematuria occurs with kidney stones, trauma, and arteriovenous malformations. It can also occur with acute tubular necrosis and renal vein thrombosis. Asymptomatic hematuria alone, without proteinuria, is often not indicative of significant kidney disease. However, a number of glomerular diseases, including immunoglobulin A (IgA) nephropathy and Alport nephritis, can present with recurrent gross hematuria.
4. **Suggested evaluation of persistent hematuria** (Fig. 18-1):

a. Examination of urine sediment, urine dipstick for protein, urine culture, sickle cell screen, urine calcium–to–creatinine (Ca/Cr) ratio, family history, medication history, and audiology screen if indicated.
b. Serum electrolytes, blood urea nitrogen (BUN), serum creatinine (Cr), serum total protein and albumin, complete blood count (CBC) with smear, immunoglobulins, and hepatitis serologies; consider testing for human immunodeficiency virus (HIV).
c. ASO titers, C3, C4, and antinuclear antibodies (ANAs).
d. Renal ultrasonography and other indicated radiologic studies.

5. **Management algorithm** (Fig. 18-2).

B. PROTEINURIA[8,9]

1. **More likely than hematuria to indicate significant renal disease.** Protein can be found in the urine of healthy children, with a reasonable upper limit being 150 mg/24 hr (4 mg/m2/hr). It is commonly detected

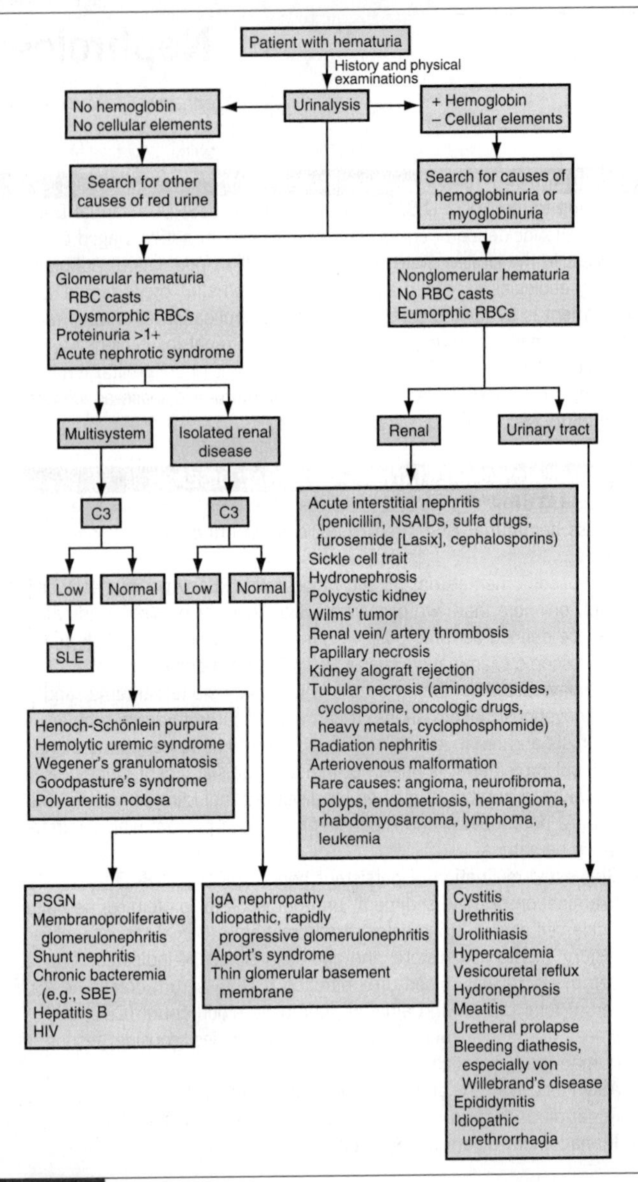

FIG. 18-1

A diagnostic strategy for hematuria. HIV, human immunodeficiency virus; NSAIDs, nonsteroidal anti-inflammatory drugs; PSGN, poststreptococcal glomerulonephritis; RBC, red blood cell; SBE, subacute bacterial endocarditis; SLE, systemic lupus erythematosus.

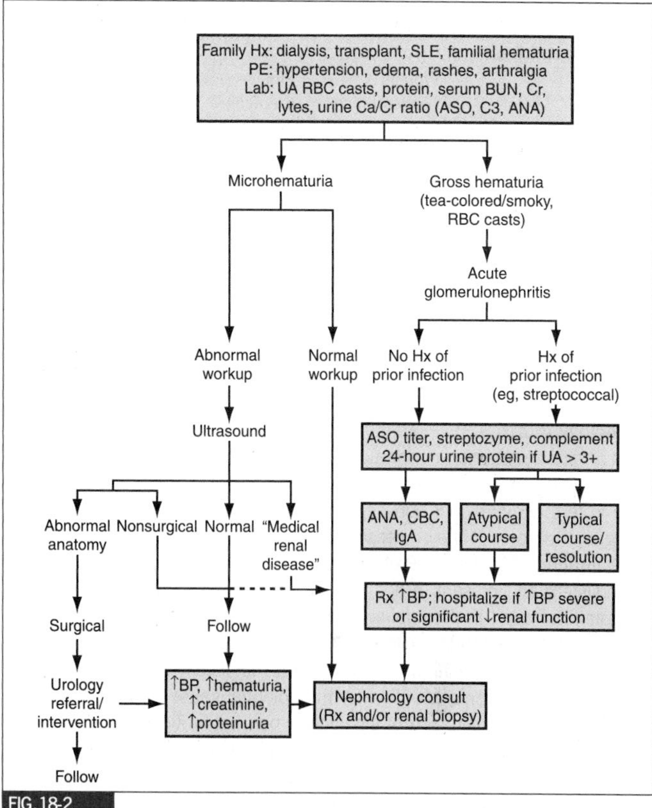

FIG. 18-2

Management algorithm for hematuria. *(Data from Hay WW, et al: Current Pediatric Diagnosis and Treatment, 14th ed. Stamford, CT, Appleton & Lange, 1999.)*

by dipstick with results of negative, trace, 1+ (~30 mg/dL), 2+ (~100 mg/dL), 3+ (~300 mg/dL), and 4+ (>2000 mg/dl). Dipstick is useful primarily for albuminuria and is not an accurate measure of protein excretion. Persistent proteinuria should be precisely quantified by a timed 24-hr urine collection (**Table 18-1**). If unable to obtain, a timed urine excretion can be estimated by the ratio of urine protein to creatine concentrations in a first morning voided specimen (or spot urine). Ratios (mg/mg) <0.5 in children who are <2 years old and <0.2 in older children are normal. A ratio >2 suggests nephrotic range proteinuria.

TABLE 18-1
24-HOUR URINE PROTEIN EXCRETION IN CHILDREN OF DIFFERENT AGES (NORMAL RANGES)

Age	Protein Concentration (mg/L)	Protein Excretion (mg/24 hr)	Protein Excretion (mg/24 hr/m^2 BSA)
Premature (5–30 days)	88–845	29 (14–60)	182 (88–377)
Full-term	94–455	32 (15–68)	145 (68–309)
2–12 mo	70–315	38 (17–85)	109 (48–244)
2–4 yr	45–217	49 (20–121)	91 (37–223)
4–10 yr	50–223	71 (26–194)	85 (31–234)
10–16 yr	45–391	83 (29–238)	63 (22–181)

From Cruz C, Spitzer A: Contemp Pediatr 1998;15(9):89.

2. **Etiology** (Fig. 18-3)**:** Proteinuria can be usefully differentiated into nephrotic versus non-nephrotic. Non-nephrotic proteinuria, generally <40 mg/m^2/hr in adults, is rarely associated with edema. It is important to note that significant non-nephrotic proteinuria is one of the earliest signs of chronic kidney disease.
3. **Evaluation** (Fig. 18-4)**:** Proteinuria is not significant unless it is persistent and present in both supine and standing positions. When no protein is found in the supine position, the patient likely has benign orthostatic proteinuria.
4. **Management:** If proteinuria is significant (persistent and nonorthostatic), an evaluation for the potential cause of proteinuria is indicated. The evaluation of significant, non-nephrotic proteinuria includes a comprehensive metabolic panel, serum creatinine, albumin, evaluation of hepatitis B, C, C3, and C4 and ANA, and renal sonogram to evaluate for structural causes. A 24-hr urine protein and creatinine should be obtained. If the protein level is persistently >4 mg/m^2/hr or if this subgroup has worsening proteinuria, a renal biopsy is recommended.

C. EDEMA[3]

Secondary to excessive accumulation of both Na^+ and water. Causes of generalized edema include:

1. **Inability to excrete Na^+ with or without water (e.g., glomerular diseases resulting in decreased glomerular filtration rate [GFR], excess salt intake).**
2. **Decreased oncotic pressure (e.g., nephrotic syndrome, protein-losing enteropathy, congestive heart failure [CHF]).**
3. **Reduced cardiac output (e.g., CHF, pericardial disease, hepatic failure).**
4. **Mineralocorticoid excess (e.g., hyperreninemia, hyperaldosteronism).**

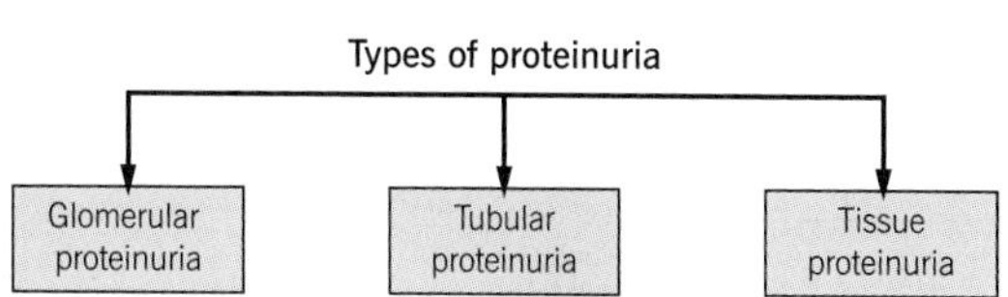

A. GLOMERULAR

1. Transient proteinuria: Most common in children. Associated with exercise, stress, dehydration, postural changes, cold exposure, fever, seizures, congestive heart failure, and vasoactive drugs. Serial urine tests should be negative for protein.

2. Orthostatic proteinuria: Common, not associated with renal pathology. Repeat measure of excreted urinary protein in recumbent position should be negative. Rarely exceeds 1 g/dy (see Table 18-2).

3. Proteinuria secondary to glomerulopathies

a. Primary glomerular disease: Minimal change disease, focal segmental glomerulonephritis, membranous glomerulonephritis, IgM nephropathy, IgA nephropathy.

b. Secondary glomerular disease: medications (e.g., NSAIDs, captopril, lithium), postinfectious (poststreptococcal, hepatitis B, chronic shunt infections, subacute bacterial endocarditis), infectious (bacterial, fungal, viral), neoplastic (solid tumors, leukemia), multisystem (systemic lupus erythematosus, Henoch-Schönlein purpura, sickle cell disease), reflux nephropathy, congenital nephrotic syndrome.

B. TUBULAR

1. Overload proteinuria: Occurs when excessive amount of low-molecular-weight proteins overwhelms the tubular reabsorption capacity (e.g., light chains: multiple myeloma; lysozyme: monocytic and myelocytic leukemias; myoglobin: rhabdomyolysis; hemoglobin: hemolysis).

2. Tubular dysfunction or disorders: Occurs when normal amounts of low-molecular-weight proteins (e.g., amino acids) are not adequately reabsorbed because of damaged or dysfunctional tubular cells (Fanconi's syndrome, Lowe's syndrome, reflux nephropathy, cystinosis, drugs/heavy metals [mercury, lead, cadmium, outdated tetracyclines]), ischemic tubular injury, and renal hypoplasia/dysplasia.

C. TISSUE

1. **Acute inflammation of urinary tract**
2. **Uroepithelial tumors**

FIG. 18-3

Types of proteinuria. NSAIDs, nonsteroidal anti-inflammatory drugs.

D. OLIGURIA[10]

Urine output <300 mL/m^2/24 hr, or <0.5 mL/kg/hr in children and <1.0 mL/kg/hr in infants. May be a normal physiologic response to water with or without salt depletion (prerenal state) or a reflection of renal failure that is associated with azotemia.

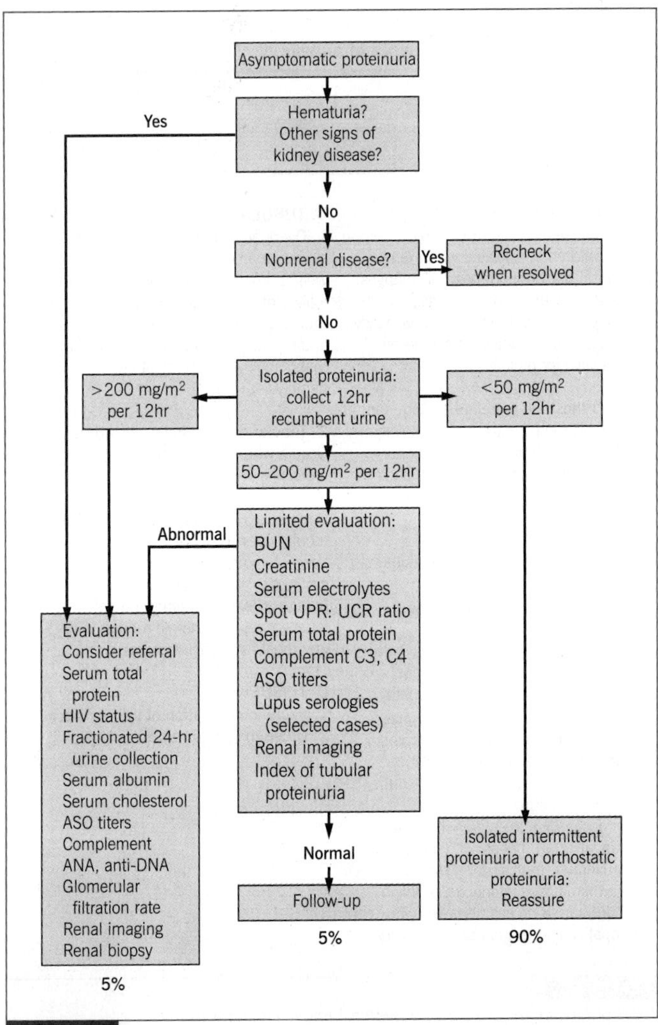

FIG. 18-4

Suggested evaluation of proteinuria in asymptomatic patients. *(From Cruz C, Spitzer A: Contemp Pediatr 1998;15[9]:89.)*

TABLE 18-2

LABORATORY DIFFERENTIATION OF OLIGURIA

Test	Prerenal	Renal
FENa	<1%	>3%
BUN/Cr ratio	>20:1	<10:1
Urine specific gravity	>1.015	<1.010

BUN, blood urea nitrogen; Cr, creatinine; FENa, fractional excretion of sodium.

1. **BUN/Cr ratio (both in mg/dL)[11]:**
a. Normal ratio: 10–20; suggests intrinsic renal disease in the setting of oliguria.
b. >20: Suggests dehydration, prerenal azotemia, or gastrointestinal (GI) bleeding.
c. <5: Suggests liver disease, starvation, inborn error of metabolism.
2. **Laboratory differentiation of oliguria (Table 18-2).**

E. POLYURIA[10]

Water conservation is dependent on antidiuretic hormone (ADH) and its effects on the distal renal tubules. Etiologies include:

1. **Central diabetes insipidus:** ADH deficiency may be idiopathic or acquired (through infection or pituitary trauma).
2. **Nephrogenic diabetes insipidus (DI):** Unresponsive receptors may be hereditary or acquired (through interstitial nephritis, sickle cell disease, or chronic renal insufficiency).
3. **Psychogenic polydipsia.**

III. GLOMERULAR DISEASES[9,10]

Injury to glomeruli results in either inflammatory or noninflammatory lesions. Many glomerular disorders involve both lesions.

A. INFLAMMATORY LESIONS (NEPHRITIC)

Consist of necrotic areas that result in loss of large particles such as RBCs as well as edematous areas resulting in decreased filtration. Nephritic disorders clinically present with fluid retention, hypertension, oliguria, and hematuria. The classic example is poststreptococcal glomerulonephritis.

B. NONINFLAMMATORY (NEPHROTIC) LESIONS

Result in leakage through the injured glomerular basement membrane. Nephrotic disorders, when uncomplicated, do not compromise filtration. The classic example is minimal change disease.

C. NEPHROTIC SYNDROME

The most severe form of proteinuria.[9,12] It is classically characterized by proteinuria (>40 mg/m^2/hr), hypercholesterolemia (>200 mg/dL), hypoproteinemia (<2 g/dL), and edema. Clinically, hypoalbuminemia with concomitant decrease in oncotic pressure results in generalized edema. The initial swelling occurs on the face (especially periorbital) as well as in the pretibial area. Prominent swelling of the scrotum and labia can also be seen. Decreased oncotic pressure also results in compromised splanchnic flow leading to abdominal pain.

1. **Etiology:** Nephrotic syndrome is exclusively a glomerular disorder that can be primary in the kidney or secondary to other systemic disorder resulting in injury. The three most common histologic causes, accounting for >90% of the cases, are minimal-change disease, focal segmental glomerulosclerosis, and membranoproliferative glomerulonephritis.[9,12]
2. **Management:** Is aimed at restoring intravascular volume and encouraging diuresis in order to avoid fluid overload. Steroids and optimal nutrition (high-quality proteins) are also recommended. Most patients with minimal-change disease are steroid responsive with full clearing of proteinuria, but relapse is the rule rather than the exception.

IV. TUBULAR DISORDERS[8–10,13–15]

A. RENAL TUBULAR ACIDOSIS (RTA)

Refers to a group of transport defects in the reabsorption of bicarbonate (HCO_3^-), the excretion of hydrogen ions (H^+), or both, which results in abnormal urine acidification. The defect results in a persistent nonanion gap metabolic acidosis accompanied by hyperchloremia. The RTA syndromes often do not progress to renal failure but are instead characterized by a normal GFR. Clinical presentation is characterized by failure to thrive, polyuria, constipation, vomiting, and dehydration (Table 18-3).

B. TYPE 1 (DISTAL) RTA

May be hereditary or secondary to a systemic disorder (e.g., obstructive uropathy, sickle cell nephropathy, toxins). The defect is in hydrogen ion secretion in the distal renal tubules resulting in 15% of the filtered sodium bicarbonate being lost in the urine. Laboratory findings include hyperchloremic metabolic acidosis, mild hypokalemia, and alkaline urine. It is characteristically complicated by hypercalciuria progressing to nephrocalcinosis and nephrolithiasis (urine Ca^{2+}/Cr >0.21 mg/mg). Treatment is easily achieved with 1–3 mEq/kg/day $NaHCO_3$ (Bicitra or Polycitra), a characteristic which distinguishes it from type II RTA.

C. TYPE II (PROXIMAL) RTA

May be hereditary (part of Fanconi syndrome) or a secondary process (tubular immaturity in premature infants). The defect is in the proximal tubule caused by a lowering of the renal threshold for bicarbonate

TABLE 18-3

BIOCHEMICAL AND CLINICAL CHARACTERISTICS OF THE VARIOUS TYPES OF RENAL TUBULAR ACIDOSIS

	Distal Type I	Type 1 With HCO_3^- Wasting	Proximal Type II	Hyperkalemic Type IV
AT SUBNORMAL (HCO_3^-)*				
Minimal urine pH	>5.5	>5.5	<5.5	<5.5
Urinary citrate excretion	↓	↓	↑	?
Plasma K^+ concentration	nl or ↓	nl or ↓	Usually ↓	↑
Urine anion gap†	Positive	Positive	Positive or ? negative	Positive
AT NORMAL (HCO_3^-)				
Plasma K^+ concentration	nl	nl	nl or ↓	nl or ↑
Therapeutic alkali requirement (mEq/kg/day)	1–3	5–10	5–20	1–5
Nephrocalcinosis/nephrolithiasis	Common	Common	Rare	Absent

*Plasma bicarbonate concentration.

†Urine anion gap = $[Na^+] + [K^+] - [Cl^-]$ (based on urine electrolytes).

nl, normal; TA, titratable acid.

From Holliday MA, et al: Pediatric Nephrology. Baltimore, Williams & Wilkins, 1994.

reabsorption (it requires a lower serum pH to trigger bicarbonate reabsorption from the urine). Laboratory findings include hyperchloremic metabolic acidosis and hypokalemia.

D. TYPE III (COMBINED PROXIMAL AND DISTAL) RTA

Infants with mild type I and mild type II defects were previously classified as type III RTA. Studies have shown that this is not a genetic entity itself. This has resulted in reclassification as a subtype of type I RTA that occurs primarily in premature infants.

E. TYPE IV RTA (MINERALOCORTICOID DEFICIENCY, ALDOSTERONE DEPENDENT)

This disorder is due to mineralocorticoid deficiency (e.g., adrenal failure, congenital adrenal hyperplasia [CAH], diabetes mellitus, pseudohypoaldosteronism, interstitial nephritis). Laboratory findings include hyperchloremic acidosis and distinguishing hyperkalemia. Nephrocalcinosis is rare. Patients are treated with 1–4 mEq/kg/day of Bicitra or Polycitra, potassium-sparing drugs are discontinued, and addition of fludrocortisone (0.05–0.15 mg/m^2/day) as well as potassium binders may be required.

F. FANCONI SYNDROME

A generalized dysfunction of the proximal tubule resulting not only in bicarbonate loss but also in variable wasting of phosphate, glucose, and amino acids. It may be hereditary, as in cystinosis and galactosemia, or acquired through toxin injury and other immunologic factors. It is clinically characterized by rickets and impaired growth.

V. URINALYSIS, URINE DIPSTICK

It is best if the urine specimen is evaluated within 1 hour after voiding, and ideally after the first morning void.

A. TURBIDITY

Cloudy urine can be normal and is most often the result of crystal formation at room temperature. Uric acid crystals form in acidic urine, and phosphate crystals form in alkaline urine. Cellular material and bacteria can also cause turbidity.

B. SPECIFIC GRAVITY

Specific gravity is measured in a refractometer, which requires one drop of urine, and is based on the principle that the refractive index (RI) of a solution is related to the content of dissolved solids present. The RI varies with, but is not identical to, specific gravity. The refractometer measures RI but is calibrated for specific gravity. Glucose, abundant protein, and iodine-containing contrast materials can give falsely high readings. Normal specific gravity is between 1.003 and 1.030.

C. PH

pH levels are estimated using indicator paper or dipstick. To improve accuracy, use a freshly voided specimen and pH meter. Levels can be inappropriately high with hypokalemia, and they can also be used to assess various types of renal tubular acidosis (see Table 18-3).

D. PROTEIN

See Section IIB and related figures.

Normal: <4 mg of protein/m²/hr; significant: 4–40 mg/m²/hr; nephrotic range: >40 mg/m²/hr.[3]

E. SUGARS

Normally, urine does not contain sugars. Glucosuria is suggestive but not diagnostic of diabetes mellitus or proximal renal tubular disease (see section VIII). The presence of other reducing sugars can be confirmed by chromatography.

1. **Dipstick:** Easiest method but only detects glucose. False-negative results occur with high levels of ascorbic acid (used as preservative in antibiotics) in urine.
2. **Clinitest tablet (Ames Co.):** Nonspecific test; changes color if urine is positive for reducing substances, including reducing sugars (glucose, fructose, galactose, pentoses, lactose), amino acids, ascorbic acid, chloral hydrate, chloramphenicol, creatinine, cysteine, glucuronates, hippurate, homogentisic acid, isoniazid, acetoacetic acid, acetone, nitrofurantoin, oxalate, total parenteral nutrition (TPN), penicillin, salicylates, streptomycin, sulfonamides, tetracycline, and uric acid. Because sucrose is not a reducing sugar, it is not detected by Clinitest.

F. KETONES

Except for trace amounts, ketonuria suggests ketoacidosis, usually from either diabetes mellitus or catabolism induced by inadequate intake. Neonatal ketoacidosis may occur with a metabolic defect, such as propionic acidemia, methylmalonic aciduria, or a glycogen storage disease.

1. **Dipstick:** Detects acetoacetic acid best, acetone less well; does not detect β-hydroxybutyrate. False-positive results may occur after phthalein administration or with phenylketonuria.
2. **Acetest tablet (Ames Co.):** Detects only acetoacetic acid and acetone.

G. HEMOGLOBIN, MYOGLOBIN

Dipstick reads positive with intact RBCs, hemoglobin, and myoglobin and can detect as few as 3 to 4 RBCs/hpf. False-positive results can occur with the presence of bacterial peroxidases, high ascorbic acid concentrations, and povidone-iodine (Betadine) (i.e., from fingers of medical staff).

TABLE 18-4

URINALYSIS FOR BILIRUBIN/UROBILINOGEN

	Normal	Hemolytic Disease	Hepatic Disease	Biliary Obstruction
Urine urobilinogen	Normal	Increased	Increased	Decreased
Urine bilirubin	Negative	Negative	+/–	Positive

H. BILIRUBIN, UROBILINOGEN

Dipstick measures each individually. Urine bilirubin will be positive with conjugated hyperbilirubinemia; in this form, bilirubin is water soluble and excreted by the kidney. Urobilinogen will be increased in cases of hyperbilirubinemia in which there is no obstruction to enterohepatic circulation (Table 18-4).

VI. URINALYSIS, MICROSCOPY

A. RBCS

Centrifuged urine usually contains fewer than 5 RBCs/hpf. Significant hematuria is 5 to 10 RBCs/hpf and corresponds to a Chemstrip reading of 50 RBCs/hpf or Labstix reading "trace hemolyzed" or "small." Microscopy is used to differentiate hemoglobinuria or myoglobinuria from hematuria (intact RBCs). In addition, examination of RBC morphology by phase-contrast microscopy may help to localize the source of bleeding. Dysmorphic, small RBCs suggest a glomerular origin, whereas normal RBCs suggest lower tract bleeding.

1. **Differentiation between hemoglobinuria and myoglobinuria:**
   a. History: Hemoglobinuria is seen with intravascular hemolysis or in hematuric urine that has been standing for an extended period. Myoglobinuria is seen in crush injuries, vigorous exercise, major motor seizures, fever and malignant hyperthermia, electrocution, snake bites, ischemia, some muscle and metabolic disorders, and some infections such as influenza.
   b. Laboratory studies: Clinical laboratories may use many techniques to measure hemoglobin or myoglobin directly. Other laboratory data may also be used to identify the source of urinary pigment indirectly. For example, in nephropathy from myoglobinuria, the BUN/Cr ratio is low (creatinine is released from damaged muscles), and the creatine phosphokinase (CPK) level is high.
2. **Suggested evaluation of persistent hematuria: See section IIA and related figures.**

B. SEDIMENT

Using light microscopy, unstained, centrifuged urine can be examined for formed elements, including casts, cells, and crystals.

C. EPITHELIAL CELLS

Squamous epithelial cells (>10 per low-power field) are useful as an index of possible contamination by vaginal secretions in females or by foreskin in uncircumcised males.

D. WHITE BLOOD CELLS (WBCs)

Greater than 5 WBCs/hpf of properly spun urine specimen is suggestive of a urinary tract infection (UTI). Sterile pyuria is rare in the pediatric population. If present, it is usually transient and accompanies systemic infection, for example, with Kawasaki disease. May also be a sign of urolithiasis.

E. BACTERIA, URINE GRAM STAIN

Gram stain is used to screen for UTIs. One organism per high-power field in uncentrifuged urine represents at least 10^5 colonies/mL.

VII. EVALUATION AND MANAGEMENT OF UTIs[16,17]

Note *These recommendations are suggestions and vary from institution to institution and physician to physician. Use them together with the routinely practiced guidelines of your institution.*

A. EPIDEMIOLOGY

Among children 2 months to 2 years of age who present with fever, 5% to 10% are diagnosed with a UTI. Prevalence is dependent on sex and age. Regardless of age, girls are more prone to UTIs than boys. In children younger than 1 year with fever, 6.5% of girls have a UTI, compared with 3.3% of boys. In older children, the prevalence is 8.1% of girls versus 1.9% of boys. Of the children who develop a UTI, 32% to 40% have recurrent UTI, 20% to 35% demonstrate vesicoureteral reflux, and 10% to 20% develop renal scarring; of these, 10% to 30% develop hypertension.[17]

B. CLINICAL CHARACTERISTICS

1. **May indicate a significant urogenital anomaly (obstructive uropathy or vesicoureteral reflux), which often progress to renal scarring, hypertension, and chronic renal failure.**
2. **Accurate diagnosis requires a urine culture using invasive collection methods.**
3. **Young children usually present with nonspecific symptoms, therefore requiring a higher index of suspicion.**
4. **Children younger than 5 years have an increased risk for renal scarring after a single UTI.**

C. HISTORY

Voiding history (stool, urine) with stream characteristics in toilet-trained children, sexual intercourse, sexual abuse, circumcision, masturbation, pinworms, prolonged baths, bubble baths, evaluation of growth curve, recent antibiotic use, and family history or vesicoureteral reflux, recurrent UTIs, or chronic kidney disease.

D. PHYSICAL EXAMINATION

Vital signs, especially blood pressure (BP); abdominal examination for flank masses, bowel distention, evidence of impaction; meatal stenosis or circumcision in males; vulvovaginitis or labial adhesions in females; neurologic examination of lower extremities; perineal sensation and reflexes; rectal and sacral examination (for anteriorly placed anus).

E. LABORATORY STUDIES

Urinalysis with microscopic examination and urine culture (Table 18-5).

Note *All tests must be confirmed with a urine culture. Also helpful if available are the following studies:*

1. **Nitrite test:** Detects nitrites produced by the reduction of dietary nitrates by urinary gram-negative bacteria (especially *Escherichia coli* and *Klebsiella* and *Proteus* species). A positive test is virtually diagnostic of UTI. False-negative results can occur with inadequate dietary nitrates, insufficient time for bacterial proliferation, inability of bacteria to reduce nitrates to nitrites (many gram-positive organisms such as *Enterococcus* and *Mycobacterium* species and fungi), and large volumes of dilute urine.

TABLE 18-5

URINALYSIS WITH MICROSCOPIC EXAMINATION AND URINE CULTURE

Method of Collection	Colony Count (Pure Culture)	Probability of Infection (%)
Suprapubic aspiration	Gram-negative bacilli: any number	>99
	Gram-positive cocci: more than a few thousand	
Transurethral catheterization	>100,000	95
	10,000–100,000	Infection likely
	1000–10,000	Suspicious; repeat
	<1000	Infection unlikely
Clean-voided (boy)	>10,000	Infection likely
Clean-voided (girl)	3 specimens >100,000	95
	2 specimens >100,000	90
	1 specimen >100,000	80
	50,000–100,000	Suspicious; repeat
	10,000–50,000	Symptomatic, suspicious; repeat
	10,000–50,000	Asymptomatic, infection unlikely
	<10,000	Infection unlikely

2. **Leukocyte esterase test:** Detects esterases released from broken-down leukocytes, an indirect test for WBCs that may or may not be present with a UTI.
3. **BUN/Cr ratio.**

F. CULTURE-POSITIVE UTI

Treatment should be based on urine culture and sensitivities if possible; for empiric therapy, see Chapter 16.

1. **Upper versus lower UTI: Differentiating pyelonephritis (upper UTI) from cystitis (lower UTI) is essentially a clinical diagnosis that is suggested by the presence of fever, systemic symptoms and costovertebral angle tenderness. A fever that persists for greater than 48 hours after initiating appropriate antibiotics is also suggestive of pyelonephritis. Although ^{99m}Tc-dimercaptosuccinic acid (DMSA) is the "gold standard" to diagnose pyelonephritis, infants with a febrile UTI are assumed to have pyelonephritis without diagnosis and are treated as such.**

a. Organisms: 75% to 90% of all pediatric UTIs are caused by *E. coli*. Other common pathogens include *Klebsiella* and *Proteus* species, *Staphylococcus saprophyticus*, and *Staphylococcus aureus*. Group B strep (GBS) and other blood-borne pathogens are important in neonatal UTIs, whereas enterococcus and pseudomonal species are more prevalent in abnormal hosts (i.e., recurrent UTI, abnormal anatomy, neurogenic bladder, hospitalized patients, or those with frequent catheterizations).

b. Treatment considerations: All febrile children younger than 4 weeks should be hospitalized and treated with IV antibiotics given the risk for bacteremia and meningitis. Studies show that oral treatment is equally efficacious to 3 days of parenteral antibiotics followed by 11 days of oral antibiotics. The American Academy of Pediatrics (AAP) recommends parenteral antibiotics for children who are toxic, dehydrated, and unable to tolerate oral medication due to vomiting or noncompliance. AAP also recommends 7–14 days of treatment for all UTIs.

Studies comparing duration are inconclusive, but experts recommend 7–10 days for uncomplicated cases and 14 days for toxic children and those with pyelonephritis (any febrile UTI).

c. Inadequate response to therapy: Repeat urine culture in children with the expected response is controversial and thought to be unnecessary by the AAP. A repeat culture, as well as renal ultrasound, to rule out abscess or obstruction is indicated in children with poor response to therapy. Repeat cultures should also be considered in patients with recurrent UTIs to rule out persistent bacteruria.

d. Antibiotic prophylaxis (Table 18-6): Low-dose antibiotic prophylaxis is recommended in all children with diagnosed vesicoureteral reflux and obstructive disease as well as in children pending evaluation with renal

TABLE 18-6

ANTIBIOTIC PROPHYLAXIS

Grade	Age (yr)	Scarring	Initial Treatment	Follow-Up
I–II	Any	Yes/no	Antibiotic prophylaxis	No consensus
III–IV	0–5	Yes/no	Antibiotic prophylaxis	Surgery
III–IV	6–10	Yes/no	Unilateral: antibiotic prophylaxis Bilateral: surgery	Surgery
V	<1	Yes/no	Antibiotic prophylaxis	Surgery
V	1–5	No	Unilateral: antibiotic prophylaxis	Surgery
V	1–5	No	Bilateral: surgery	
V	1–5	Yes	Surgery	
V	6–10	Yes/no	Surgery	

ultrasound and voiding cystourethrogram (VCUG). Prophylaxis in children with recurrent infections but normal anatomy is controversial and is based on individualized decisions.

2. **Imaging studies[18,19] (Fig. 18-5): A renal ultrasound and VCUG to rule out obstructive disease or vesicoureteral reflux should be done in all male patients with their first UTI, all female patients younger than 5 years, and all children with recurrent UTI.**

a. Abdominal radiograph: If indicated to check stool pattern and to rule out spinal dysraphism.

b. Renal sonography: A noninvasive, nonionizing evaluation for gross structural defects, lesions that are obstructive, positional abnormalities, and renal size and growth. Indications regarding appropriate use remain controversial.

c. VCUG: Performed when the patient is asymptomatic and cleared of bacteriuria. May be substituted with radionucleotide cystography (RNC), which has 1/100 the radiation exposure of a VCUG and increased sensitivity for transient reflux. RNC does not visualize urethral anatomy, is not sensitive for low-grade reflux, and cannot grade reflux.

d. DMSA: ^{99m}Tc DMSA scan can detect areas of decreased uptake that may represent acute pyelonephritis or renal scarring but does not differentiate between the two. Routine use is not recommended but may be indicated in patients with an abnormal VCUG or renal sonography, in patients with history of asymptomatic bacteriuria and fever or prenatally diagnosed vesicoureteral reflux (VUR), and in neonates and infants secondary to high incidence of hematologic spread and difficult examination. Repeat in 3–6 months if initial study is positive to evaluate for persistent infection and renal scarring.

e. DTPA/MAG-3: May also be used for indications given above for DMSA use. Provides quantitative assessment of renal function and drainage of dilated collecting system, as in cases of hydronephrosis in the absence of VUR or ureteropelvic junction (UPJ) obstruction.

3. **Asymptomatic bacteriuria: Defined as bacteria in urine on microscopy and Gram stain in an afebrile, asymptomatic patient without pyuria.**

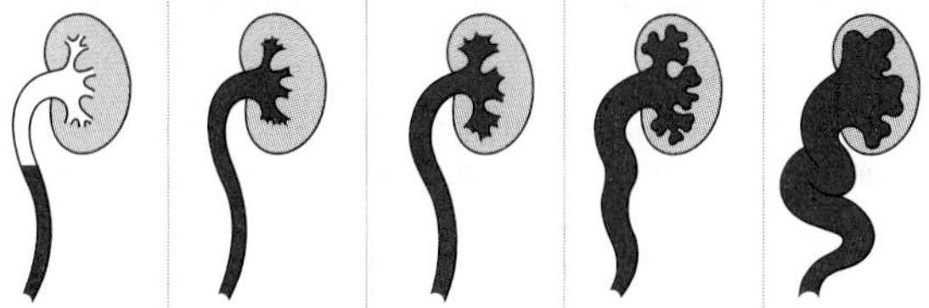

Grade I	Grade II	Grade III	Grade IV	Grade V
Ureter only	Ureter, pelvis, calyces; no dilatation, normal calyceal fornices	Mild or moderate dilatation and/or tortuosity of ureter; mild or moderate dilatation of the pelvis, but no or slight blunting of the fornices	Moderate dilatation and/or tortuosity of the ureter; mild dilatation of renal pelvis and calyces; complete obliteration of sharp angle of fornices, but maintenance of papillary impressions in majority of calyces	Gross dilatation and tortuosity of ureter; gross dilatation of renal pelvis and calyces; papillary impressions are no longer visible in majority of calyces

FIG. 18-5

International classification of vesicoureteral reflux. *(Modified from Rushton H: Pediatr Clin North Am 1997:44:5; and International Reflux Committee: Pediatrics 1981;67:392.)*

Antibiotics are not necessary if voiding habits and urinary tract are normal. Prophylaxis may be necessary in patients with bacteriuria and voiding dysfunction. DMSA may be helpful in differentiating pyelonephritis from fever and coincidental bacteriuria.

4. Nonsurgical management of VUR[18,19]: Amoxicillin recommended in first 2 months of life, otherwise trimethoprim-sulfamethoxazole (TMP/SMX) or nitrofurantoin (Macrodantin) with urine cultures every 4 months and when febrile. There is no need to discontinue antibiotics before screening urine culture. Change antibiotic therapy if patient has breakthrough UTIs while on prophylactic regimen. Repeat VCUG in 12 to 18 months to determine whether VUR has resolved. Surgical correction is indicated in children >2 years old with high-grade reflux (grades IV or V) and children with breakthrough pyelonephritis (especially with DMSA changes) while on prophylaxis.

5. Referral to pediatric urology: Consider referral in children with abnormal voiding function on imaging, neurogenic bladder, abnormal anatomy (grade 3 VUR or higher), recurrent UTI, or poor response to appropriate antibiotics.

VIII. RENAL FUNCTION TESTS

A. TESTS OF GLOMERULAR FUNCTION

1. Creatinine clearance (Ccr):

a. Timed urine specimen: Standard measure of GFR; closely approximates inulin clearance in the normal range of GFR. When GFR is low, Ccr is greater than inulin clearance. Ccr is usually inaccurate in children with obstructive uropathy or problems with bladder emptying.

$$\text{Ccr (mL/min/1.73m}^2) = (U \times [V/P]) \times 1.73/\text{BSA}$$

where U (mg/dL) is urinary creatinine concentration, V (mL/min) is total urine volume (mL) divided by the duration of the collection (min) (24 hours = 1440 minutes); P (mg/dL) is serum creatinine concentration (may average two levels), and BSA (m^2) is body surface area.

b. Estimated GFR from plasma creatinine: Useful when a timed specimen cannot be collected; reasonable estimate of GFR for children with relatively normal renal function and body habitus. If habitus is markedly abnormal or a precise measurement of GFR is needed, more standard methods of measuring GFR must be used.

$$\text{Estimated GFR (mL/min/1.73m}^2) = kL/\text{Pcr}$$

where k is proportionality constant, L is height (cm), and Pcr is plasma creatinine (mg/dL) (Table 18-7).

2. Glomerular function as determined by nuclear medicine scans. Normal values of GFR (measured by inulin clearance) are shown in Table 18-8.

B. TESTS OF TUBULAR FUNCTION

1. Proximal tubule:

a. Proximal tubule reabsorption: The proximal tubule is responsible for the reabsorption of electrolytes, glucose, and amino acids. Studies to determine proximal tubular function compare urine and blood levels of

TABLE 18-7

PROPORTIONALITY CONSTANT FOR CALCULATING GFR

	k Values
Low birth weight during first year of life	0.33
Term AGA during first year of life	0.45
Children and adolescent girls	0.55
Adolescent boys	0.70

AGA, appropriate for gestational age.

From Schwartz GJ, Brion LP, Spitzer A: Pediatr Clin North Am 1987;34:571.

TABLE 18-8
NORMAL VALUES OF GFR

Age	GFR (Mean) (mL/min/1.73 m²)	Range (mL/min/1.73 m²)
Neonates <34 wk gestational age		
2–8 days	11	11–15
4–28 days	20	15–28
30–90 days	50	40–65
Neonates >34 wk gestational age		
2–8 days	39	17–60
4–28 days	47	26–68
30–90 days	58	30–86
1–6 mo	77	39–114
6–12 mo	103	49–157
12–19 mo	127	62–191
2 yr–adult	127	89–165

From Holliday MA et al: Pediatric Nephrology. Baltimore, Williams & Wilkins, 1994.

specific compounds arriving at a percentage of tubular reabsorption (Tx):

$$Tx = 1 - [(Ux/Px)/(Ucr/Pcr)] \times 100\%$$

where Ux = concentration of compound in urine; Px = concentration of compound in plasma; Ucr = concentration of creatinine in urine; Pcr = concentration of creatinine in plasma. This formula can be used for amino acids, electrolytes, calcium, and phosphorus.

b. Glucose reabsorption: The glucose threshold is the plasma glucose concentration at which significant amounts of glucose appear in the urine. The presence of glucosuria must be interpreted in relation to simultaneously determined plasma glucose concentration. If the plasma glucose concentration is <120 mg/dL, and glucose is present in the urine, this implies incompetent tubular reabsorption of glucose and proximal renal tubular disease.

c. Bicarbonate reabsorption: The majority of bicarbonate reabsorption occurs in the proximal tubule. Abnormalities in reabsorption lead to type II RTA (see Table 18-3).

2. Distal tubule:

a. Urine acidification: A urine acidification defect (distal renal tubular acidosis) should be suspected when random urine pH values are >6 in the presence of moderate systemic metabolic acidosis. Acidification defects should be confirmed by simultaneous venous or arterial pH, plasma bicarbonate concentration, and pH meter (not dipstick) determination of the pH of fresh urine.

b. Urine concentration occurs in the distal tubule[20]: A random urine specific gravity of 1.023 or more indicates intact concentrating ability within the limits of clinical testing; no further tests are indicated. A first-

TABLE 18-9

AGE-ADJUSTED CALCIUM/CREATININE RATIOS

Age	Ca^{2+}/Cr Ratio (mg/mg Ratio) (95th Percentile for Age)
<7 mo	0.86
7–18 mo	0.60
19 mo–6 yr	0.42
Adults	0.22

From Sargent JD, et al: J Pediatr 1993;123:393.

voided specimen after an overnight fast is adequate to test concentrating ability. (For more formal testing, see the water deprivation test in Chapter 9.)

c. Urine calcium: Hypercalciuria is seen usually with distal renal tubular acidosis, vitamin D intoxication, hyperparathyroidism, steroids, immobilization, excessive calcium intake, and loop diuretics. It may be idiopathic (associated with hematuria and renal calculi). Diagnosis is as follows:
   (1) 24-hour urine: Calcium >4 mg/kg/24 hr.
   (2) Spot urine: Determine Ca/Cr ratio. It is recommended that an abnormally elevated spot urine Ca/Cr ratio be followed up with a 24-hr urine calcium determination (Table 18-9).

IX. ACUTE RENAL FAILURE

Sudden decline in renal function with increasing BUN/Cr ratio; with or without changes in urine output. Causative factors include impaired renal perfusion, acute renal disease, renal ischemia, or obstructive uropathy.

A. ETIOLOGY

Causes are generally subdivided into three categories:

1. **Prerenal: Most common etiology in children; usually a result of dehydration, although other forms of impaired perfusion can be a cause.**
2. **Renal:**
a. Parenchymal disease through arterial or glomerular lesions.
b. Acute tubular necrosis (ATN): Diagnosis of exclusion; when no evidence of renal parenchymal disease is present and prerenal and postrenal causes have been eliminated if possible.
3. **Postrenal: Obstruction of the urinary tract found often in neonates with anatomic abnormalities.**

B. CLINICAL PRESENTATION

Presenting symptoms include pallor, decreased urine output, edema, hypertension, vomiting, and lethargy. The hallmark of early renal failure is oliguria.

C. ACUTE TUBULAR NECROSIS

ATN is clinically defined by three phases:

1. **Oliguric phase:** A period of severe oliguria that lasts about 10 days. If period of oliguria or anuria persists for longer than 3–6 weeks, then renal recovery from ATN is highly unlikely.
2. **Diuretic phase:** Begins with an increase in urine output to passage of large volumes of isosthenuric urine containing sodium levels of 80–150 mEq/L.
3. **Recovery phase:** Signs and symptoms usually resolve rapidly, but polyuria may persist for days to weeks.

D. TREATMENT CONSIDERATIONS

1. Placement of indwelling catheter to monitor urine output.
2. Prerenal and postrenal factors should be excluded, and the intravascular volume maintained with appropriate fluids in consultation with a pediatric nephrologist.

E. COMPLICATIONS

Often dependent on clinical severity but usually includes fluid overload (hypertension, CHF, pulmonary edema), electrolyte disturbances (hyperkalemia), metabolic acidosis, hyperphosphatemia, and uremia.

X. ACUTE DIALYSIS

A. INDICATIONS

1. **Acute dialysis is indicated when metabolic or fluid derangements are not controlled by aggressive medical management alone. Generally accepted criteria include the following, although a nephrologist should always be consulted:**

a. Volume overload with evidence of pulmonary edema or hypertension that is refractory to therapy.
b. Hyperkalemia >6.0 mEq/L if hypercatabolic or >6.5 mEq/L despite conservative measures.
c. Metabolic acidosis with pH <7.2 or HCO_3^- <10.
d. BUN >150; lower if rising rapidly.
e. Neurologic symptoms secondary to uremia or electrolyte imbalance.
f. Calcium and phosphorus imbalance (e.g., hypocalcemia with tetany or seizures in the presence of a very high serum phosphate level).

2. **Dialyzable toxin or poison (e.g., lactate, ammonia, alcohol, barbiturates, ethylene glycol, isopropanol, methanol, salicylates, theophylline).**

B. TECHNIQUES[21]

1. **Peritoneal dialysis (PD):** Requires catheter to access the peritoneal cavity. May be used acutely or chronically, as in continuous ambulatory or continuous cycling peritoneal dialysis.

2. **Hemodialysis (HD):** Requires placement of special vascular access devices. May be the method of choice for certain toxins (e.g., ammonia, uric acid, poisons) or when there are contraindications to peritoneal dialysis.
3. **Continuous arteriovenous hemofiltration/hemodialysis (CAVH/D) and continuous venovenous hemofiltration/hemodialysis (CVVH/D):** CAVH and CVVH are therapies with the primary goal of continuous generation of a plasma ultrafiltrate. Indications include fluid management, renal failure with profound hemodynamic instability, electrolyte disturbances, and intoxication with substances that are freely filtered across the particular ultrafiltration membrane used. CAVH and CVVH can be helpful in the management of oliguric patients who are in need of better nutritional support, postoperative cardiac patients, and patients with septicemia. These therapies also require special vascular access devices.

C. PD, HD, AND CAVH/CVVH (Table 18-10)

XI. CHRONIC RENAL FAILURE

Kidney damage for >3 months, as defined by structural or functional abnormalities, with or without decreased GFR, or a GFR <60 mL/min/1.73m^2 for >3 months with or without kidney damage.

A. ETIOLOGY

Close association with age at which renal failure is first detected. Chronic renal failure (CRF) in children younger than 5 years is most commonly a result of anatomic abnormalities (hypoplasia, dysplasia, malformations), whereas older children predominantly have acquired glomerular diseases (glomerulonephritis, hemolytic-uremic syndrome) or hereditary disorders (Alport syndrome, cystic disease).

B. CLINICAL PRESENTATION

Usually nonspecific, including headache, fatigue, lethargy, anorexia, vomiting, polydipsia, polyuria, rickets, and growth failure.

C. TREATMENT CONSIDERATIONS

Management involves close monitoring of clinical and laboratory status. Routine lab studies include hemoglobin, electrolytes (hyponatremia, hyperkalemia, acidosis), BUN/Cr ratio, calcium and phosphorus levels, and alkaline phosphatase activity (osteodystrophy). Periodic monitoring of intact parathyroid hormone (PTH), bone imaging, echocardiogram, and nutrition labs may also be useful.

D. COMPLICATIONS (Table 18-11)

TABLE 18-10

PD VERSUS HD VERSUS CAVH/CVVH

Advantages	Disadvantages
PD	
Rapid training	Catheter malfunction
Technical simplicity	Infection
Greater mobility	Poor appetite
Minimal dietary restriction	Poor body image
Feel better than HD patients	Parental "burnout" (emotional exhaustion)
Steady State chemistries	Elevated serum lipid levels
Can live far from medical center	
Cheaper than hemodialysis	
Improved growth rate	
Fewer blood transfusions	
HD	
Rapid fluid removal	Risk of hemodynamic instability
Rapid removal of dialyzable toxins, hyperkalemia, hyperammonianemia	Associated with rapid osmolar changes and decreased systemic vascular resistance
Intermittent	Large volume shifts in between treatments
	Required vascular access
	Risk of infection
HEMOFILTRATION	
Hemodynamic stability	Today body heparinization (bleeding)
Continuous therapy/around the clock	Clotting of filter
Avoids rapid osmolar and diminished systemic vascular resistance of HD	Inadequate removal of fluid or solutes in certain patients
Stabilizes volume and composition of body fluids	Infection of access catheter or substitution fluid
Avoids rapid shifts in electrolyte levels	Leaking from blood lines
Controlled fluid and solute removal	
Slow correction of fluid and electrolyte abnormalities	
Can replace ultrafiltrate with large amounts of hyperalimentation fluid	

Adapted from Rogers MC: Textbook of Pediatric Intensive Care. Baltimore, Williams & Wilkins, 1992.

XII. CHRONIC HYPERTENSION

Note *For management of acute hypertension, see Chapter 4.*

A. DEFINITION

For the definition of chronic hypertension, see Chapter 6.

1. **Normal BP:** Systolic and diastolic BP <90th percentile for age, gender, height, and weight.
2. **High-normal BP:** Average systolic and/or diastolic BP between the 90th and 95th percentiles for age, gender, height, and weight.
3. **Significant hypertension:** The average of three separate systolic and/or diastolic blood pressures >95th percentile for age, gender, height, and weight.
4. **Severe hypertension:** The average of three systolic and/or diastolic blood pressures >99th percentile for age, gender, height, and weight.

TABLE 18-11

CLINICAL MANIFESTATIONS OF CHRONIC RENAL FAILURE

Manifestation	Mechanisms
Accumulation of nitrogenous waste products (azotemia)	Decline in glomerular filtration rate
Acidosis	Urinary bicarbonate wasting Decreased ammonia excretion Decreased acid excretion
Sodium wasting	Solute diuresis Tubular damage Function tubular adaptation for sodium excretion
Sodium retention	Nephrotic syndrome Congestive heart failure Anuria Excessive salt intake
Urinary concentrating defect	Nephron loss Solute diuresis Increased medullary blood flow
Hyperkalemia	Decline in glomerular filtration rate Acidosis Excessive potassium intake Hypoaldosteronism
Renal osteodystrophy	Decreased intestinal calcium absorption Impaired production of 1,25-dihydroxy vitamin D by the kidneys Hypocalcemia and hyperphosphatemia Secondary hyperparathyroidism
Growth retardation	Protein-calorie deficiency Renal osteodystrophy Acidosis Anemia Inhibitors of insulin-like growth factors Unknown factors
Anemia	Decreased erythropoietin production Low-grade hemolysis Bleeding Decreased erythrocyte survival Inadequate iron intake Inadequate folic acid intake Inhibitors of erythropoiesis
Bleeding tendency	Thrombocytopenia Defective platelet function
Infection	Defective granulocyte function
Neurologia (fatigue, poor concentration, headache, drowsiness, loss of memory, slurred speech, muscle weakness and cramps, seizures, coma, peripheral neuropathy, asterixis)	Uremic factors Aluminum toxicity

TABLE 18-11

CLINICAL MANIFESTATIONS OF CHRONIC RENAL FAILURE—cont'd

Manifestation	Mechanisms
Gastrointestinal ulceration	Gastric acid hypersecretion—gastritis Reflux Decreased motility
Hypertension	Sodium and water overload Excessive renin production
Hypertriglyceridemia	Diminished plasma lipoprotein lipase activity
Pericarditis and cardiomyopathy	Unknown
Glucose intolerance	Tissue insulin resistance

Data from Brenner BM: Brenner & Rector's The Kidney, 6th ed. Philadelphia, WB Saunders, 2000.

B. CAUSES OF HYPERTENSION IN NEONATES, INFANTS, AND CHILDREN (Table 18-12)

C. EVALUATION OF CHRONIC HYPERTENSION[22–24]

1. Rule out causes: Rule out "factitious" causes of hypertension (improper cuff size—proper cuff size is two thirds of upper arm length—or measurement technique [i.e., manual versus Dyna map]), "nonpathologic" causes of hypertension (fever, pain, anxiety, muscle spasm), and iatrogenic mechanisms (medications and excessive fluid administration).

TABLE 18-12

CAUSES OF HYPERTENSION BY AGE GROUP

	Cause	
Age	Most Common	Less Common
Neonates/infants	Renal artery thrombosis after umbilical artery catheterization Coarctation of the aorta Renal artery stenosis	Bronchopulmonary dysplasia Medications Patent ductus arteriosus Intraventricular hemorrhage
1–10 yr	Renal parenchymal disease Coarctation of aorta	Renal artery stenosis Hypercalcemia Neurofibromatosis Neurogenic tumors Pheochromocytoma Mineralocorticoid ↑ Hyperthyroidism Transient hypertension Hypertension induced by immobilization Sleep apnea Essential hypertension Medications
11 yr to adolescence	Renal parenchymal disease Essential hypertension	All diagnoses listed above

Modified from Sinaiko A: N Engl J Med 1996;335:26.

2. History and physical examination: Headache, blurred vision, history of UTIs, family history of renal dysfunction or hypertension, pitting edema, dyspnea on exertion, jugular venous distention; or displaced point of maximal impulse (PMI).
3. Laboratory studies: Urinalysis with microscopic evaluation, urine culture, serum electrolytes, CBC, creatinine, BUN, calcium, uric acid, cholesterol, and plasma renin level.
4. Imaging: Renal ultrasonography, including renal artery Doppler and other imaging studies as indicated (echocardiography, renal arteriography).
5. Consider toxicology screen, human chorionic gonadotropin (hCG), thyroid function tests, urine catecholamines, plasma and urinary steroids.
6. Refer any patient with significant hypertension to a pediatric nephrologist.

D. TREATMENT OF HYPERTENSION

1. **Nonpharmacologic:** Aerobic exercise, salt restriction, smoking cessation, and weight loss, indicated in patients with systolic BP and/or diastolic BP >90th percentile.
2. **Pharmacologic:** Indicated in patients with significant hypertension (especially diastolic hypertension).
3. **Parenteral:** Acute hypertensive crisis.

E. ANTIHYPERTENSIVE MEDICATIONS FOR CHRONIC HYPERTENSIVE THERAPY (Box 18-1)

BOX 18-1

ANTIHYPERTENSIVE MEDICATIONS

CALCIUM CHANNEL BLOCKERS: ACT ON VASCULAR SMOOTH MUSCLES

Benefits

Renal perfusion/function minimally affected; ideal for post-renal-transplant hypertension, especially in association with cyclosporine use; ideal in low renin/volume-dependent hypertension

Nifedipine

No effect on cardiac conduction; available in short- and long-acting form; variable GI absorption and sublingual route may cause precipitous drop in BP

Verapamil

Depresses cardiac pacemaker, inhibits cyclosporine metabolism

Amlodipine

Once-daily dose, tasteless, odorless, easily made into suspension with 90% GI absorption

ACE INHIBITORS (CAPTOPRIL, ENALAPRIL): BLOCK ANGIOTENSIN I → ANGIOTENSIN II

Benefits

Decreases proteinuria while preserving renal function; ↑ potency and duration in neonatal and infantile hypertension; ↓ pulmonary vascular resistance and mean arterial pressure with little ↓ in heart rate

continued

Side Effects

Elimination dependent on creatinine clearance; may cause hyperkalemia; contraindicated in compromised renal perfusion and in pregnancy; associated with rash, cough, angioedema, and marrow depression

---

DIURETICS

Thiazides

Effective in primary hypertension; not effective when GFR <50% of normal; side effects: hypokalemia, hypercalcemia, hyperuricemia, hyperlipidemia

Furosemide/Bumetanide

Useful in renal failure; bumetanide has 40 times more diuretic activity than furosemide, but varies with patient/route; side effects: hypokalemia, hyponatremia, ototoxicity (high-dose intravenous [IV] administration)

K^+ Sparing

Spironolactone, triamterene, amiloride; modest antihypertensive medication; anti-androgenic effects

---

β-BLOCKERS

Benefits

↓ Heart rate, ↓ cardiac output, ↓ renin release

Side Effects

May exacerbate underlying collagen vascular disease or Raynaud disease; may cause exaggerated hypoglycemic response in diabetes mellitus and suppress hypoglycemic symptomatology; may cause nightmares, confusion, agitation, depression, contraindicated in persons with congestive heart failure, reactive airways disease, or pulmonary insufficiency

Selective β_1 blockers: Metoprolol, atenolol

Nonselective β-blockers: Propranolol, nadolol (once-daily dosing)

α_1 BLOCKERS (PRAZOSIN): BLOCK VASOCONSTRICTION

Benefits

Effective in patients with renal failure, distorted lipid profile, Raynaud disease/collagen vascular disease

Side Effects

Nausea, palpitations, worsening of narcolepsy, dizziness/syncope

---

COMBINED α- AND β-BLOCKER

Labetalol (↓ peripheral resistance, ↓ heart rate) extremely potent; postural hypotension; can be used in hypertensive crisis

---

CENTRALLY ACTING α STIMULATORS (CLONIDINE, α-METHYLDOPA)

Stimulates brainstem α_2 receptors → peripheral adrenergic drive

Benefits

↓ Intraocular pressure, ↓ opiate withdrawal, effective in renal failure, less hyponatremia and orthostatic symptomatology

Side Effects

Dry mouth, sedation/agitation, constipation, sudden withdrawal → rebound hypertension

---

VASODILATORS (HYDRALAZINE, NITROPRUSSIDE, MINOXIDIL)

Direct action on vascular smooth muscle. Very potent, used in hypertensive crisis, reflex ↑ heart rate, Na^+ and H_2O retention, therefore combine with diuretics/ β-blockers

---

Modified from Hospital for Sick Children: The HSC Handbook of Pediatrics, 9th ed. St Louis, Mosby, 1997; Sinaiko A: Pediatr Nephrol 1994;8:603; and Khattak S, et al: Clin Pediatr 1998;37:31.

REFERENCES

1. NIH Guide: Prospective Study of Chronic Kidney Disease in Children [Online]. Available: www.grants.nih.gov.
2. Roy S III: Hematuria. Pediatr Ann 1996;2(5):284.
3. Norman ME: An office approach to hematuria and proteinuria. Pediatr Clin North Am 1987;34:545.
4. Feld L, et al: Hematuria: An integrated medical and surgical approach. Pediatr Clin North Am 1997;44:1191.
5. Cilento B, Stock J, Kaplan G: Hematuria in children: A practical approach. Urol Clin North Am 1995;22:43.
6. Fitzwater D, Wyatt R: Hematuria. Pediatr Rev 1994;15:102.
7. Belman A: Vesicoureteral reflex. Pediatr Clin North Am 1997;44:5.
8. Behrman RE: Nelson Textbook of Pediatrics, 16th ed. Philadelphia, WB Saunders, 2000.
9. Sabella C, et al: The Cleveland Clinic Intensive Review of Pediatrics. Philadelphia, Lippincott Williams & Wilkins, 2003.
10. Haynes TS: BIOTEST Study Aids. Ventura, CA, Biotest Publishing, 2002.
11. Greenhill A, Gruskin AB: Laboratory evaluation of renal function. Pediatr Clin North Am 1976;23:661.
12. Roth K S, et al: Nephrotic syndrome: Pathogenesis and management. Pediatr Rev 2002;23:7.
13. Brenner BM: Brenner and Rector's The Kidney, 6th ed. Philadelphia, WB Saunders, 2000.
14. Rodriguez Soriano J: Frontiers in nephrology: Renal tubular acidosis. J Am Soc Nephrol 2002;13:8.
15. Hay WW, et al: Current Pediatric Diagnosis and Treatment, 14th ed. Stamford, CT, Appleton & Lange, 1999.
16. Chon CH, et al: Pediatric urinary tract infections. Pediatr Clin North Am 2001;48:8.
17. Layton KL: Diagnosis and management of pediatric urinary tract infections. Clin Fam Pract 2003;5:2.
18. American Academy of Pediatrics, Committee on Quality Improvement, Subcommittee on Urinary Tract Infection: Practice parameter: The diagnosis, treatment, and evaluation of the initial urinary tract infection in febrile infants and young children. Pediatrics 1999;103(4):843–852.
19. Hoberman A, et al: Oral versus initial intravenous therapy for urinary tract infections in young febrile children. Pediatrics 1999;104.
20. Edelmann CM Jr, et al: A standardized test of renal concentrating capacity in children. Am J Dis Child 1967;114:639.
21. Rogers MC: Textbook of Pediatric Intensive Care. Baltimore, Williams & Wilkins, 1992.
22. Sinaiko A: Hypertension in children. N Engl J Med 1996;335:26.
23. Rocella E, et al: Update on the 1987 task force report on high blood pressure in children and adolescents: A working group report from the National High Blood Pressure Education program. Pediatrics 1996;98(4):649–658.
24. Sadowski R, Falkner B: Hypertension in pediatric patients. Am J Kidney Dis 1996;27:3.
25. Cruz C, Spitzer A: When you find protein or blood in urine. Contemp Pediatr 1998;15(9):89.

26. Hellerstein S: Urinary tract infections: Old and new concepts. Pediatr Clin North Am 1995;42:6.
27. Liao J, Churchill B: Pediatric urine testing. Pediatr Clin North Am 2001;48:6.
28. Feld G, et al: Hematuria. Pediatr Clin North Am 1997;44:5.

Neurology

Jennifer Huffman, MD, and Ai Sakonju, MD

19

I. NEUROLOGIC EXAMINATION[1]

A complete neurologic examination is rarely productive in the absence of specific concerns raised by the history and must be evaluated relative to developmental norms.

A. MENTAL STATUS

Patient should be alert and oriented to time, person, place, and current situation. Assess attentiveness and behavior in infants.

B. CRANIAL NERVES (Table 19-1)

C. MOTOR

1. **Muscle bulk.**
2. **Tone:** High, low.
   a. Passive: Resting resistance to examiner's movement.
   b. Active: Regulation of power with defined movements (e.g., posture, gait, pull to stand).
   c. Note anatomic distribution of abnormalities. Regional increase in tone (e.g., adducted thumbs, limited hand supination, equinus of feet) suggests CNS dysfunction. Note quality (e.g., rigid, spastic).
3. **Power, Strength:** Observe and describe activity (e.g., rising from the floor). Quantify (e.g., distance of standing broad jump, time to run 30 feet, time to climb stairs).

Strength Rating Scale

0/5: No movement, i.e., no palpable tension at the tendon
1/5: Flicker of movement or less than full range of movement in a gravity-neutral plane
2/5: Full range of movement in a gravity-neutral plane
3/5: Full range of movement against gravity but not resistance
4/5: Subnormal strength against resistance
5/5: Normal strength against resistance

D. SENSORY (Fig. 19-1)

Primary disorders of sensation are rare in children. Evaluation of the following spinal cord pathways and tests may be useful in anatomic localization.

1. **Anterior cord:** Pin and temperature sensation.
2. **Posterior cord:** Vibratory and joint position sense; Romberg test (test of proprioceptive function).
3. **Spinal level:** Best assessed by pinprick and temperature. If concerned about spinal cord injury, ask about bowel and bladder function.

TABLE 19-1

CRANIAL NERVES

Function/Region	Cranial Nerve	Test/Observation
Olfactory	I	Smell (e.g., coffee, vanilla, peppermint)
Vision	II	Acuity, fields, fundus
Pupils	II, III	Sympathetics, size, reaction to light, accommodation
Eye movements and eyelids	III, IV, VI	Range and quality of eye movements, saccades, pursuits, nystagmus, ptosis
Sensation	V	Corneal reflexes, facial sensation
Muscles of mastication	V	Clench teeth
Facial strength	VII	Observe degree of expression of emotions, eye closure strength, smile, puff out cheeks
Hearing	VIII	Localize sound, attend to finger rub
Mouth, pharynx	VII, IX, X, XII	Swallowing, speech quality (labial, lingual, or palatal articulation deficits), symmetric palatal elevation, tongue protrusion
Head control	XI	Lateral head movement, shoulder shrug

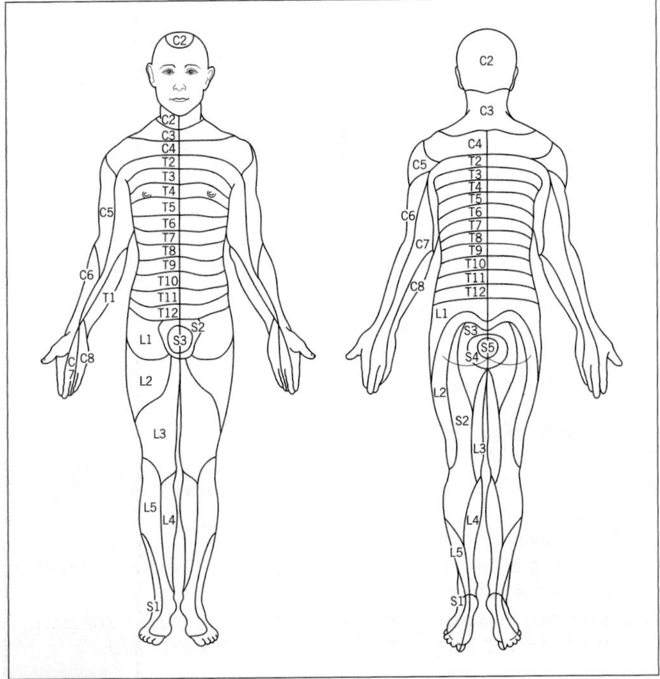

FIG. 19-1

Dermatomes. *(From Athreya BH, Silverman BK: Pediatric physical diagnosis. Norwalk, CT, Appleton-Century-Crofts, 1985.)*

TABLE 19-2

UPPER AND LOWER MOTOR NEURON FINDINGS

	Upper	Lower
Power	Decreased	Decreased
Reflexes	Increased	Decreased
Tone	Increased	Normal or decreased
Babinski	Present	Absent

TABLE 19-3

MUSCLE STRETCH REFLEXES

Reflex	Site
Biceps	C5, C6
Brachioradialis	C5, C6
Triceps	C7, C8
Knee	L(2,3)4
Ankle	L5–S2

E. TENDON REFLEXES

Assessment of tendon reflexes is most helpful in localizing other abnormalities, especially in the presence of weakness or asymmetry. Isolated abnormality of reflexes, in the setting of normal strength and coordination, has little significance. Combined with weakness, brisk reflexes indicate upper motor neuron disorder; absent reflexes suggest motor neuron, nerve, or muscle causes (Table 19-2). In muscle disease, reflexes are usually diminished commensurate with power. Selective reflex dropout can help localize a spinal cord, root, or nerve lesion (Table 19-3).

Reflex rating scale:

- 0: None
- 1+: Diminished
- 2+: Normal
- 3+: Increased (reflexes cross neighboring joint or cross to other side)
- 4+: Hyperactive with clonus

F. COORDINATION AND MOVEMENT

Evaluate general coordination while watching activities (e.g., throwing a ball, dressing, writing, or drawing). Tests for cerebellar function include rapid alternating and repetitive movements, finger to nose, heel to shin, orbiting, walking, and running. Note involuntary movements (e.g., tremor, dystonia, chorea, athetosis, tics, myoclonus) and conditions under which they are enhanced or suppressed. Note abnormal gait (e.g., waddling, wide based, tiptoed).

II. HEADACHES[2]

A. EVALUATION OF HEADACHES

1. **History and physical examination:** Differentiate between acute, acute recurrent, chronic nonprogressive, and chronic progressive (Boxes

19-1 and 19-2). Careful general, neurologic, and funduscopic examinations should be performed (Tables 19-4 and 19-5).

2. **Studies:**

a. Computed tomography (CT) without contrast or magnetic resonance imaging (MRI): Obtain for focal neurologic findings, suspected increased intracranial pressure (ICP), atypical or progressive pattern, seizures, abrupt-onset severe headache (see Chapter 23 for advantages of each modality). Note that CT provides poor imaging of the posterior fossa.

b. Lumbar puncture (LP): Fever, infection, papilledema, sudden severe headache (evaluate opening pressure if concern for pseudotumor). Contraindicated in increased ICP or mass effect secondary to risk for herniation.

3. **Warning signs:** Pain that awakens child from sleep, increases in morning with rising or with Valsalva maneuver; headache associated

BOX 19-1

DIFFERENTIAL DIAGNOSIS OF ACUTE HEADACHE

Evaluation of the first acute headache should exclude pathologic causes listed below before consideration of more common etiologies.

1. Increased intracranial pressure (ICP): Trauma, hemorrhage, tumor, hydrocephalus, pseudotumor cerebri, abscess, arachnoid cyst, cerebral edema
2. Decreased ICP: After ventriculoperitoneal (VP) shunt, lumbar puncture (LP), cerebrospinal fluid (CSF) leak from basilar skull fracture
3. Meningeal inflammation: Meningitis, leukemia, subarachnoid or subdural hemorrhage
4. Vascular: Vasculitis, arteriovenous malformation (AVM), hypertension, cerebrovascular accident (CVA)
5. Bone, soft tissue: Referred pain from scalp, eyes, ears, sinuses, nose, teeth, pharynx, cervical spine, temporomandibular joint
6. Infection: Systemic infection, encephalitis, sinusitis, etc.

BOX 19-2

DIFFERENTIAL DIAGNOSIS OF RECURRENT OR CHRONIC HEADACHES

1. Migraine (with or without aura)
2. Tension
3. Analgesic rebound
4. Caffeine withdrawal
5. Sleep deprivation (e.g., in overweight children with sleep apnea) or chronic hypoxia
6. Tumor
7. Psychogenic: conversion disorder, malingering

TABLE 19-4

EVALUATION OF HEADACHE BY HISTORY

Questions	Comments
How many different kinds of headache do you have?	• A mixed picture implies multifactorial etiology.
What has been the course of the headache?	• Try to characterize as acute, acute recurrent, chronic nonprogressive, or chronic progressive.
Can you describe a typical episode?	• Is there a warning before the episode (e.g., visual aura)? • Where does it hurt? • What is the pain like? • How long do the headaches last? • How often do they occur? • How severe are they? Do they interfere with activities? • Is there abdominal pain, nausea, and/or vomiting?
Are there focal neurologic signs or symptoms?	• *Examples:* visual disturbance, paresthesia, or weakness occurring before, during, or after the headache
Does the child look sick?	• Children who have migraines look unwell during an attack.
What makes the headaches worse?	• Activities that raise intracranial pressure (e.g., coughing, bending over) • Bright light or noise
What helps the headaches?	• Sleep often helps a migraine headache. • Dark, quiet room? Cold cloth over forehead?
What time of day do the headaches occur?	• Headaches that waken the child may be due to increased intracranial pressure. • Headaches in the late afternoon may be due to low blood glucose levels precipitating migraine.
Can you identify precipitating factors?	• Are they related to the school week or term? • Certain foods, lack of sleep, stress, excitement, exercise, menstrual cycle, exertion, illness
What medications and dosages have you used?	• Was the medicine appropriate? Was the dose correct? Was the medicine used correctly?
Is there a family history of headaches?	• Many parents who have migraines attribute their headaches to other causes (e.g., sinus headaches). Ask parents to describe their headaches. Did they have headaches when they were younger?

From Forsyth R, Farrell K: Pediatr Rev 1999;20(2):39–45.

TABLE 19-5
PHYSICAL AND NEUROLOGIC EXAMINATION OF THE CHILD WHO HAS HEADACHES

Feature	Significance
Growth parameters	Chronic illness may affect linear growth Hypothalamopituitary dysfunction may disturb growth
Head circumference	Increased intracranial pressure before fusion of the sutures may accelerate head growth
Skin	Evidence of trauma or a neurocutaneous disorder
Blood pressure	Hypertension
Neurologic examination	Signs of increased intracranial pressure Focal abnormality
Cranial bruits	May reflect an intracranial arteriovenous malformation

From Forsyth R, Farrell K: Pediatr Rev 1999;20(2):39–45.

with emesis, neurologic signs, changes in chronic pattern, and altered mental status (e.g., change in mood, personality, and school performance). *Note:* The classic headache secondary to subarachnoid hemorrhage (SAH) is acute, severe, continuous, and generalized—the "worst headache of my life" or "thunder clap" headache. It may be associated with nausea, emesis, meningismus, focal neurologic symptoms, and loss of consciousness. If SAH is suspected, CT without contrast is the preferred method of evaluation, then LP (if CT is negative) to rule out xanthochromia (develops about 12 hours after event). Send tubes 1 and 4 of cerebrospinal fluid (CSF) sample for cell counts and xanthochromia. There is a persistently high red blood cell (RBC) count and xanthochromia if SAH exists. Significant decline of the RBC count between tubes 1 and 4 in the absence of xanthochromia suggests microtrauma from the LP. **To correct the WBC in traumatic taps, allow 1 WBC for every 700 (500–1500) RBCs.**
Or, true CSF WBC = (CSF WBC − serum WBC) × (CSF RBC/serum RBC).[3]

B. MIGRAINE HEADACHE

1. **Characteristics:** Chronic recurrent; throbbing, pulsatile, or pressure-like in children; usually bifrontal in children, unilateral in adolescents and adults; relieved by sleep; many potential triggers (e.g., stress, caffeine, diet, menses, sleep disruption); hereditary predisposition. Associated symptoms include nausea, vomiting, abdominal pain, photophobia, phonophobia, paresthesia, tinnitus, vertigo; rare associated symptoms include focal weakness, aphasia, ataxia, confusion.
2. **Classification:**
a. With aura: "Classic," often frontotemporal, usually unilateral, may have associated neurologic complications. Aura is any preceding neurologic

abnormality (e.g., visual aberrations, associated symptoms listed above).

b. Without aura: "Common," often bifrontal.

3. **Associated neurologic deficits (rare):** Paresthesia, visual-field cuts, aphasia, hemiplegia, ophthalmoplegia, vertigo, ataxia, confusion.

4. **Treatment:** Includes reassurance and education.

a. Acute symptomatic: Dark and quiet room, sleep, nonsteroidal anti-inflammatory drugs (NSAIDs) (i.e., naproxen, ketorolac), antiemetics (metoclopramide), triptans (sumatriptan), isometheptene, ergotamine, sedative-analgesic combinations (see Formulary for dosage information).

b. Chronic treatment (if frequency more than three or four per month or if migraines interfere with daily functioning or school):

(1) Avoid triggers and stress, improve general health with balanced diet restrictive of certain "migraine-causing" foods (see www.musc.edu/pedres/neurology/migraine_diet.html or www.uth.tmc.edu/pain/pl-migr.html), aerobic exercise, regular sleep.

(2) Explore issues of secondary gain and role of pain in family's relationships. Offer counseling when appropriate; also consider biofeedback.

(3) Consider medications, such as β-blockers (propranolol), calcium-channel blockers (verapamil), tricyclics (amitriptyline, nortriptyline), anticonvulsants (valproic acid, gabapentin, topiramate), and cyproheptadine.

(4) The natural history of chronic headache includes spontaneous improvement. Delayed treatment may be indicated. No child should be on chronic therapy without re-evaluation. Avoid medication overuse (>2–3 doses/wk), which can lead to rebound headache. Refer any child with focal deficits to a child neurologist.

III. PAROXYSMAL EVENTS

A. DIFFERENTIAL DIAGNOSIS OF RECURRENT EVENTS THAT MIMIC EPILEPSY IN CHILDHOOD (Table 19-6)

B. SEIZURE DISORDERS[4,5]

1. **Seizure:** Paroxysmal synchronized discharge of cortical neurons resulting in alteration of function (motor, sensory, cognitive).
2. **Epilepsy:** Two or more seizures not precipitated by a known cause (e.g., infection, tumor).
3. **Status epilepticus:** Prolonged or recurrent seizures lasting at least 30 minutes without the patient regaining consciousness. See Chapter 1 for treatment.
4. **Seizure etiology:** Fever, acquired cortical defect (stroke, neoplasm, infection, trauma), inborn error of metabolism, congenital brain malformation, neurocutaneous syndrome, neurodegenerative disease, toxins/drugs, electrolyte disturbances, idiopathic (epilepsy).

TABLE 19-6

DIFFERENTIAL DIAGNOSIS OF RECURRENT EVENTS THAT MIMIC EPILEPSY IN CHILDHOOD

Event	Differentiation From Epilepsy
Pseudoseizure (psychogenic seizure)	No EEG changes except movement artifact during event; movements thrashing rather than clonic; brief/absent postictal period; most likely to occur in patient with epilepsy
Paroxysmal vertigo (toddler)	Patient frightened and crying; no loss of awareness; staggers and falls, vomiting, dysarthria
GER in infancy, childhood	Paroxysmal dystonic posturing associated with meals (Sandifer syndrome)
Breath-holding spells (18 mo–3 yr)	Loss of consciousness and generalized convulsion always provoked by an event that makes child cry
Syncope	Loss of consciousness with onset of dizziness and clouded or tunnel vision; slow collapse to floor; triggered by postural change, heat, emotion, etc.
Cardiogenic syncope	Abnormal ECG/Holter monitor finding (e.g., prolonged QT, atrioventricular block, other arrhythmias); exercise a possible trigger; episodic loss of consciousness without consistent convulsive movement
Cough syncope	Prolonged cough spasm during sleep in asthmatic, leading to loss of consciousness, often with urinary incontinence
Paroxysmal dyskinesias	May be precipitated by sudden movement or startle; not accompanied by change in alertness
Shuddering attacks	Brief shivering spells with continued awareness
Night terrors (4–6 yr)	Brief nocturnal episodes of terror without typical convulsive movements
Rages (6–12 yr)	Provoked and goal-directed anger
Tics/habit spasms	Involuntary, nonrhythmic, repetitive movements not associated with impaired consciousness; suppressible
Narcolepsy	Sudden loss of tone secondary to cataplexy; emotional trigger; no postictal state or loss of consciousness; EEG with recurrent REM sleep attacks
Migraine (confusional)	Headache or visual changes that may precede attack; family history of migraine; autonomic or sensory changes that can mimic focal seizure; EEG with regional area of slowing during attack

ECG, electrocardiography; EEG, electroencephalography; GER, gastroesophageal reflux; REM, rapid eye movement.

From Murphy JV, Dehkharghani F: Epilepsia 1994;35(Suppl 2):S7–S17.

5. **Diagnosis:** Establish etiology and seizure type (e.g., primary generalized or primary partial [Box 19-3]), which generally determines treatment.
6. **Studies:**
a. Depend on clinical scenario. Consider assessment of glucose, sodium, potassium, calcium, magnesium, phosphate, blood urea nitrogen

BOX 19-3
INTERNATIONAL CLASSIFICATION OF EPILEPTIC SEIZURES

I. Partial seizures (seizures with focal onset)
  A. Simple partial seizures (consciousness unimpaired)
    1. With motor signs
    2. With somatosensory or special sensory symptoms
    3. With autonomic symptoms or signs
    4. With psychic symptoms (higher cerebral functions)
  B. Complex partial seizures (consciousness impaired)
    1. Starting as simple partial seizures
      (a) Without automatisms
      (b) With automatisms
    2. With impairment of consciousness at onset
      (a) Without automatisms
      (b) With automatisms
  C. Partial seizures evolving into secondarily generalized seizures
II. Generalized seizures
  A. Absence seizures: brief lapse in awareness without postictal impairment (atypical absence seizures may have the following: mild clonic, atonic, tonic, automatism, or autonomic components)
  B. Myoclonic seizures: brief, repetitive, symmetric muscle contractions (loss of tone)
  C. Clonic seizures: rhythmic jerking; flexor spasm of extremities
  D. Tonic seizures: sustained muscle contraction
  E. Tonic-clonic seizures
  F. Atonic seizures: abrupt loss of muscle tone
III. Unclassified epileptic seizures

From Committee on Classification and Terminology of the International League Against Epilepsy: Epilepsia 1996;38(11):1051–1059.

(BUN), creatinine, complete blood count (CBC), toxicology screen, blood pressure (supine and upright), electroencephalography (EEG) with video monitoring, electrocardiography, head CT and/or MRI, LP, tilt table, and sleep study. If febrile, consider age-appropriate sepsis evaluation.

b. Although imaging is typically not indicated in epilepsy, head CT without contrast can detect mass lesions, acute hemorrhage, hydrocephalus, and calcifications secondary to congenital disease such as cytomegalovirus (CMV) infection (head ultrasound may be used in early infancy and requires open fontanelles).
c. Brain MRI with contrast should be obtained in infants with epilepsy, children with recurrent partial seizures, focal neurologic deficits, or developmental delay. Otherwise, MRI is not routinely indicated in the evaluation of a first-time seizure.
d. EEG is recommended in all children with nonfebrile seizures to classify

the seizure type and epilepsy syndrome.[6] However, this is controversial, and routine interictal EEGs are frequently normal; repeat EEGs, prolonged EEG monitoring with video, or studies done with sleep deprivation or photic stimulation may be more informative.

7. **Treatment:**

a. Educate parents and patient regarding how to live with epilepsy.[7] Review seizure first aid and cardiopulmonary resuscitation (CPR). Recommend that the child participate in activities but have supervision during bathing or swimming. Individualize other restrictions. Know driver's license laws in the state. Advocate teacher and school awareness.

b. Pharmacotherapy (Table 19-7): Weigh the risk for more seizures without therapy against the risk for treatment side effects plus residual seizures despite therapy. Treatment of single, first, afebrile seizure is not indicated routinely. Reserve pharmacotherapy for recurrent afebrile seizures. Monotherapy may reduce complications; polytherapy increases risk of complications and side effects more than efficacy. See Table 19-7 for information regarding commonly used medications.

c. The ketogenic diet is a high-fat, low-carbohydrate therapy used for intractable seizures. Urine ketones can be monitored, and side effects (e.g., acidosis with bicarbonate value as low as 10–15, kidney stones [6%], constipation), can occur.

d. Vagus nerve stimulation (VNS) employs a subcutaneous, 5-cm, programmable device to periodically stimulate the vagus nerve.

C. SPECIAL SEIZURE SYNDROMES

1. **Simple febrile seizure[8–10]:** Brief, generalized, tonic-clonic seizure associated with a febrile illness, but without any central nervous system (CNS) infection or other known neurologic cause. Genetic predisposition has been noted.

a. **Incidence:** 2% to 5% of children 6 months to 5 years of age.

b. **Evaluation for "atypical" features (Fig. 19-2):** Onset more than 24 hours after onset of fever, duration >15 minutes, focality of seizure, more than one discrete seizure during illness, abnormal neurologic examination. Consider further evaluation if any one of these is present. Also include evaluation for source of fever.

c. **Treatment:** Prophylactic antiepileptic drugs and antipyretics are not indicated for typical febrile seizures. Educate parents about benign nature of events and basic first aid for seizures. Rarely, rectal diazepam as needed (PRN) for seizures may be used for patients with significant parental anxiety or frequent and prolonged febrile seizures, although side effects of lethargy, drowsiness, and ataxia may mask the evolving signs of a CNS infection.

d. **Outcome:**

(1) Risk for recurrence is 30% after first febrile seizure, 50% after second episode, declines to near 0% by age 5 years. Recurrence

TABLE 19-7
COMMONLY USED ANTICONVULSANTS, IN ALPHABETICAL ORDER

Anticonvulsant (Trade Name)	Typical Target Dosage (mg/kg/day)	Standard Therapeutic Levels (mg/dL)	Efficacy (Generalized/Partial)	Side Effects
Carbamazepine (Tegretol, Carbatrol)	10–20	8–12	P	Sedation, ataxia, diplopia, Stevens-Johnson, blood dyscrasias, hepatoxicity
Clonazepam (Klonopin)	0.05–0.2	N/A	G/P	Sedation, drooling, dependence
Ethosuximide (Zarontin)	10–20	40–100	G	Gastrointestinal upset
Felbamate (Felbatol)	15–45	40–100	G/P	Weight loss, hepatotoxicity, sleep disturbances, aplastic anemia (1:7900)
Gabapentin (Neurontin)	20–40	3–18	P	Weight gain, leg edema
Lamotrigine (Lamictal)	5–15	3–18	G/P	Rash (increased risk with combination valproate)
Levetiracetam (Keppra)	10–40	30–60	P	Behavioral changes, irritability, rare psychosis
Oxcarbazepine (Trileptal)	10–30 (3:2 ratio compared with carbamazepine)	MHD level (5–40)	P	Hyponatremia
Phenobarbital (Luminal)	5–10	15–40	P	Cognition, sedation
Phenytoin (Dilantin)	5–10	10–20	P	Hirsutism, gingival hyperplasia, teratogenicity, rash, purple-glove syndrome with infusion
Tiagabine (Gabitril)	1–2	N/A	P	Can worsen generalized seizures
Topiramate (Topamax)	1–9	2–20	G/P	Cognitive side effects, weight loss, renal stones, acidosis, glaucoma
Valproic acid (Depakote, Depakene)	10–20	50–100	G/P	Weight gain, alopecia, hepatotoxicity, pancreatitis, polycystic ovarian disease
Zonisamide (Zonegran)	5–10	20–40	G/P	Renal stones, weight loss, hyphidrosis

MHD, 10-Monohydroxy metabolite.
*Personal communication with Eric Kossoff, MD.

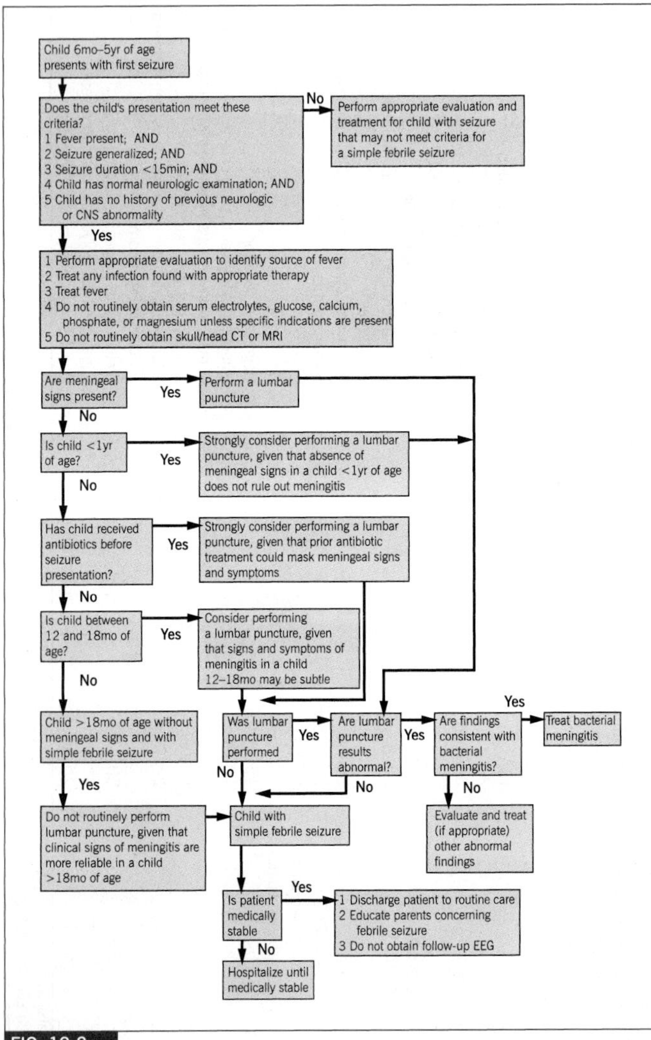

FIG. 19-2

Guidelines for febrile seizure evaluation. *(From American Academy of Pediatrics: Pediatrics 1996;97[5]:769–772.)*

risk greater with younger age (<18 months), family history, temperature <40°C, and fever <1 hour.

(2) Risk for epilepsy: 2% versus 1% in the general population. Increased further in children with two or more of the following: atypical febrile seizures, previously abnormal development or neurologic disorder, family history of afebrile seizures.

2. **Neonatal seizure**[11]**:** Various paroxysmal behaviors or electrical events. May be tonic, myoclonic, clonic, or subtle (blinking, chewing, bicycling, apnea) because of immature CNS.

a. **Etiologies of neonatal seizure:** Almost always a symptom of acute brain disorder. Hypoxic-ischemic encephalopathy (35%–42%); intracranial hemorrhage or infarction (15%–20%); CNS infection (12%–17%); CNS malformation (5%); metabolic (e.g., hypoglycemia, hypocalcemia, pyridoxine deficiency, toxins) (3%–5%); others, including inborn errors of metabolism (5%–20%).

b. **Evaluation:** Search for acute cause. Basic laboratory screens (including glucose, calcium, sodium, magnesium, and toxicology screen), sepsis workup including LP, head CT, and EEG. If basic laboratory screen is unremarkable and patient has recurrent seizures, is encephalopathic, or has signs of inborn error of metabolism, then evaluate for these disorders: plasma amino acids, urine organic acids, ammonia, lactate, pH; consider CSF amino acids, pyruvate, urine sulfites, very long chain fatty acids, and neurotransmitters. Prolonged or repeated EEG examinations are often needed because clinical-electrical dissociation is common.

c. **Treatment:** Treat underlying disorder. Prevent secondary hypoxic-ischemic or metabolic complications. Treat acute symptomatic recurring seizures quickly using combined clinical and EEG end points. Consider trial of pyridoxine IV while EEG is recording. Maintain anticonvulsants for sufficient period of time for acute cause to subside (days to weeks); for most acute symptomatic seizures, drugs can be safely stopped before discharge from nursery (Box 19-4).

3. **Infantile spasms:** Head nodding with flexion or extension of the trunk and extremities, often in clusters during drowsiness or awakening. May be triggered by unexpected stimuli. EEG may show hypsarrhythmia. Usual onset after 2 months, peak onset 4 to 6 months. MRI examination is indicated.

a. **Etiologies:**

(1) Symptomatic (67%): CNS malformation, any acquired infantile brain injury, tuberous sclerosis, inborn errors of metabolism.

(2) Cryptogenic (33%): Associated with better outcome, less mental retardation.

b. **Treatment:** Should be initiated as soon as possible to improve outcome. Adrenocorticotropic hormone (ACTH) (see corticotropin in Formulary for dosage information). Alternatives include valproic acid, benzodiazepine

BOX 19-4

TREATMENT OF NEONATAL SEIZURES

1. Establish airway, ensure oxygenation and circulation.
2. Treat metabolic abnormalities (see Formulary for dosage information and see Chapter 12 for workup of metabolic disorder)
   Hypoglycemia
   Hypocalcemia
   Evaluate for hypomagnesemia if persistent hypocalcemia
3. Treat with medications (see Formulary for dosage information)
   Phenobarbital
   If this fails, add fosphenytoin and/or a benzodiazepine (e.g., lorazepam, diazepam)
   Consider pyridoxine with concurrent EEG monitoring during ictal episode for intractable seizures.

Modified from Scher MS: Clin Perinatol 1997;24(4):735–772.

(clonazepam), and ketogenic diet. New therapies include vigabatrin, topiramate, zonisamide, and surgery.

c. Outcome: Often poor, correlates best with underlying brain pathology. Of cryptogenic cases, 30% to 70% may have good outcome with treatment.

IV. HYDROCEPHALUS

A. DIAGNOSIS

Assess increasing head circumference, misshapen skull, frontal bossing, bulging large anterior fontanelle, increased ICP (sunset sign, increased tone/reflexes, vomiting, irritability, papilledema), and developmental delay. Obtain head CT if increase in head circumference crosses more than 2 percentile lines or if patient is symptomatic. Differentiate hydrocephalus from megalencephaly or hydrocephalus ex vacuo.

B. TREATMENT[12]

1. Medical:

a. Emergently manage acute increase of ICP (see Chapter 4).
b. Slowly progressive hydrocephalus: Acetazolamide may be effective in children 2 weeks to 10 months of age with slowly progressive communicating hydrocephalus (see Formulary for dosing).

2. Surgical: CSF shunting.

a. Shunt types: Ventriculoperitoneal (VP) shunts are used most commonly. Ventriculoatrial and pleural shunts are associated with cardiac arrhythmias, pleural effusions, and higher rates of infection.
b. Shunt complications: Shunt dysfunction may be caused by infection, obstruction (clogging or kinking), disconnection, and migration of proximal and distal tips. Patient will develop signs of increased ICP with shunt malfunction.

C. EVALUATION OF SHUNT INTEGRITY

Obtain shunt series (skull, neck, chest, and abdominal radiographs) to look for kinking or disconnection. Obtain head CT to evaluate shunt position, ventricular size, and evidence of increased ICP. Referral to a neurosurgeon is then warranted to test shunt function and for possible percutaneous shunt drainage.

V. ATAXIA[13]

A. DIFFERENTIAL DIAGNOSIS OF ACUTE OR RECURRENT ATAXIA (Box 19-5)

B. DIFFERENTIAL DIAGNOSIS OF CHRONIC OR PROGRESSIVE ATAXIA (Box 19-6)

C. EVALUATION

Depends on clinical scenario; consider CBC, electrolytes, blood and urine toxicology screens, brain imaging, LP, EEG, urine for vanillylmandelic acid (VMA) and homovanillic acid (HVA), and imaging of the chest and abdomen if neuroblastoma is suspected.

VI. STROKE[14]

A. ETIOLOGY

Risk factors for childhood stroke include, but are not limited to, congenital heart disease (most common), arteriovenous ischemia secondary to infections (e.g., meningitis), coagulation disorders or hematologic disorders (most commonly sickle cell disease), head or neck trauma, and drugs.

B. DIFFERENTIAL DIAGNOSIS (Box 19-7)

Stroke should be considered in the differential diagnosis for any child who presents with acute-onset focal neurologic deficit, focal seizures with prolonged postictal paralysis, new-onset refractory focal status epilepticus, altered mental status, or unexplained encephalopathy.

C. INITIAL WORKUP

Acute diagnostic evaluation entails an urgent noncontrast head CT (to exclude hemorrhage) and initial laboratory studies, including CBC, comprehensive metabolic panel, prothrombin time (PT), partial thromboplastin time (PTT), international normalization ratio (INR), and a urine toxicology screen. MRI with diffusion-weighted imaging and magnetic resonance angiography should be performed, but the urgency of the study may vary from acute to within 24 to 48 hours on a case-by-case basis. Less acute studies include echocardiogram, erythrocyte sedimentation rate (ESR), lipid panel, human immunodeficiency virus (HIV) testing, and further evaluation for coagulation disorders, systemic lupus erythematosus (SLE), and other metabolic and rheumatologic diseases.

BOX 19-5

DIFFERENTIAL DIAGNOSIS OF ACUTE OR RECURRENT ATAXIA

1. Drug ingestion (e.g., phenytoin, carbamazepine, sedatives, hypnotics, and phencyclidine) or intoxication (e.g., alcohol, ethylene glycol, hydrocarbon fumes, lead, mercury, or thallium)
2. Postinfectious (cerebellitis [e.g., varicella], acute disseminated encephalomyelitis [ADEM])
3. Head trauma
4. Basilar migraine
5. Benign paroxysmal vertigo (migraine equivalent)
6. Brain tumor or neuroblastoma (if accompanied by opsoclonus or myoclonus [i.e., "dancing eyes, dancing feet"])
7. Hydrocephalus
8. Infection (e.g., labyrinthitis, abscess)
9. Seizure
10. Vascular events (e.g., cerebellar hemorrhage or stroke)
11. Miller-Fisher variant of Guillain-Barré syndrome (ataxia, ophthalmoplegia, and areflexia)
12. Inherited ataxias
13. Inborn errors of metabolism (e.g., mitochondrial disorders, amino acidopathies, urea cycle defects)
14. Conversion reaction
15. Multiple sclerosis

BOX 19-6

DIFFERENTIAL DIAGNOSIS OF CHRONIC OR PROGRESSSIVE ATAXIA

1. Hydrocephalus
2. Hypothyroidism
3. Tumor or paraneoplastic syndrome
4. Low vitamin E levels (e.g., cystic fibrosis)
5. Wilson disease
6. Inborn errors of metabolism
7. Inherited ataxias (e.g., ataxia telangiectasia, Friedreich ataxia)

BOX 19-7

DIFFERENTIAL DIAGNOSIS OF CHILDHOOD STROKE*

1. Hemiplegic migraine
2. Focal seizure with postictal (Todd's) paralysis
3. Cervical spinal cord injury (deficits spare the face)
4. Ischemic stroke
5. Hemorrhagic stroke

*Personal communication, Lori Jordan, MD.

D. MANAGEMENT

There are no evidence-based guidelines for evaluation or management of stroke in children. However, supportive care is critical and should proceed rapidly and parallel with initial workup. Ensure airway patency, and provide supplemental oxygen to maintain Sao_2 >94%. Optimize cerebral perfusion pressure with adequate fluid volume and maintenance of median blood pressure for age. Treatment of hypertension is controversial. Unless blood pressure is extremely elevated, do not use acute antihypertensive therapy because hypertension may be a compensatory reaction to maintain cerebral perfusion. Monitor neurologic status frequently. Aim for normoglycemia (blood glucose, 60–120 mg/dL). Treat hyperthermia with goal temperature <37°C. Treat seizures aggressively. The role of antiplatelet and anticoagulation therapy is controversial and should be considered on a case-by-case basis. Urgent consultation with a neurologist is indicated, along with transfer to a tertiary care center with expertise in childhood stroke.

REFERENCES

1. Athreya BH, Silverman BK: Pediatric Physical Diagnosis. Norwalk, CT, Appleton-Century-Crofts, 1985.
2. Forsyth R, Farrell K: Headache in childhood. Pediatr Rev 1999;20(2):39–45.
3. Fishman, Robert A: Cerebral Spinal Fluid in Diseases of the Nervous System. Philadelphia, WB Saunders, 1992, p 190.
4. Murphy JV, Dehkharghani F: Diagnosis of childhood seizure disorder. Epilepsia 1994;35(Suppl. 2):S7–17.
5. Committee on Classification and Terminology of the International League Against Epilepsy: Classification of epilepsia: Its applicability and practical value of different diagnostic categories. Epilepsia 1996;38(11):1051–1059.
6. Hirtz D, et al: Practice parameter: Evaluating a first nonfebrile seizure in children. Neurology 2000;55(5):616–623.
7. Freeman J, et al: Seizures and Epilepsy in Childhood: A Guide to Parents, 3rd ed. Baltimore, Johns Hopkins University Press, 2000.
8. American Academy of Pediatrics Subcommittee: Practice parameter: The neurodiagnostic evaluation of the child with a first simple febrile seizure. Pediatrics 1996;97(5):769–772.
9. American Academy of Pediatrics Subcommittee: Practice parameter: Long-term treatment of the child with simple febrile seizures. Pediatrics 1999;103(6):1307–1309.
10. Baumann RJ, Duffner PK: Treatment of children with simple febrile seizures: The AAP practice parameter. Pediatr Neurol 2000;23(1):11–17.
11. Scher MS: Seizures in the newborn infant: Diagnosis, treatment and outcomes. Clin Perinatol 1997;24(4):735–772.
12. Rogers M (ed): Textbook of Pediatric Intensive Care, 3rd ed. Baltimore, Williams & Wilkins, 1996.
13. Dinolfo EA: Evaluation of ataxia. Pediatr Rev 2001;22(5):177–178.
14. Ichord, R: Treatment of pediatric neurologic disorders. In Singer H, Kossoff E, Crawford T, Hartman A (eds): Treatment of Pediatric Neurologic Disorders, in press.

Nutrition and Growth

Kristin N. Fiorino, MD, and Jeanne M. Cox, MS, RD, CSP

20

I. WEBSITES

A. PROFESSIONAL AND GOVERNMENTAL ORGANIZATIONS

www.cdc.gov (The Centers for Disease Control and Prevention website has growth charts and nutrition information.)
www.eatright.org (The American Dietetic Association)
www.clinnutr.org (American Society for Parenteral and Enteral Nutrition)

B. FORMULA COMPANY WEBSITES FOR COMPLETE AND UP-TO-DATE PRODUCT INFORMATION

www.meadjohnson.com
www.nestle.com
www.rosspediatrics.com
www.Pbmproducts.com
www.hormelhealthlab.com
www.novartisnutrition.com

II. ASSESSMENT OF NUTRITIONAL STATUS

A. ELEMENTS OF NUTRITIONAL ASSESSMENT

1. Anthropometric measurements (weight, length/height, head circumference, body mass index [BMI], skin folds); data are plotted on growth charts according to age and compared with a reference population.
2. Clinical assessment (general appearance, including hair, skin, oral mucosa, and gastrointestinal symptoms of nutritional deficiencies).
3. Dietary evaluation (feeding history, current intake).
4. Physical activity and exercise.
5. Laboratory findings (comparison to age-based norms).

B. INDICATORS OF NUTRITIONAL STATUS[1]

1. Ideally, growth should be evaluated over time, but one measurement can be used for screening. Height and weight should be plotted on a growth chart. BMI should be determined and plotted for children >3 years of age. See growth charts.
2. BMI is defined as an index of healthy weight and as a predictor of morbidity and mortality risk. It is used to classify underweight and overweight individuals.[2] Use formula below to calculate BMI or, alternatively, see Figure 20-11 *A* and *B*.[3]

$$\text{BMI} = \text{wt (kg)}/[\text{height (m)}]^2$$

Interpretation of growth charts:[3]

a. Stunting, shortness: Length or height for age <5th percentile.

b. Underweight:
   Children <3 years, weight for length <5th percentile.
   Children >3 years, BMI for age <5th percentile.
c. Risk for overweight:
   Children >3 years, BMI for age 85th to 95th percentile.
d. Overweight:
   Children <3 years, weight for height >95th percentile.
   Children >3 years BMI for age >95th percentile.

3. **For recommendations for management of overweight children, see Figure 20-1.**[4]

III. ESTIMATING ENERGY NEEDS

A. DEFINITIONS OF ENERGY NEEDS[2]

1. **Basal metabolic rate (BMR):** Rate of energy expenditure after an overnight fast, resting comfortably, supine, awake, and motionless in a thermoneutral environment.
2. **Basal energy expenditure (BEE):** BMR over 24 hours.
3. **Physical activity level (PAL):** Ratio of total to basal daily energy expenditure (TEE/BEE). Describes and accounts for physical activity habits.
4. **Thermic effect of food (TEF):** Increase in energy expenditure elicited by food consumption.
5. **Thermoregulation:** Increase in energy expenditures when ambient temperatures are below the zone of thermoneutrality.
6. **Energy deposition:** Energy requirement for growth.
7. **TEE:** Sum of TEF, physical activity, thermoregulation, and the energy expended in depositing new tissues and/or in producing milk.

B. ESTIMATED ENERGY REQUIREMENTS (EER) UNDER NONSTRESSED CONDITIONS[2]

EER is the dietary energy intake that is predicted to maintain energy balance in a healthy individual. In children, it includes the needs associated with growth. For pregnant and lactating women, it includes the needs associated with the deposition of tissue and secretion of milk. For most healthy infants and children, these equations can be used to determine energy needs.

PAL is the ratio of total to basal daily energy expenditure (TEE/BEE). Describes and accounts for physical activity habits. Activity levels are a subjective determination in children:

Sedentary activity (PAL ≥1.0 or <1.4) reflects the basal energy expenditure, thermic effect of food and the physical activity levels required for independent living.

Low active (PAL ≥1.4 or <1.6) is defined as the equivalent of 30 to 45 minutes of sustained activity.

Active (PAL ≥1.6 or <1.9) is defined as the equivalent of 60 minutes of sustained activity.

Very Active (PAL ≥1.9 or <2.5) is defined as the equivalent of ≥90 minutes of sustained activity.

EQUATIONS

EER for Infants and Young Children

EER (kcal/day) = TEE + energy deposition
0–3 months: (89 × weight [kg] – 100) + 175
4–6 months: (89 × weight [kg] – 100) + 56
7–12 months: (89 × weight [kg] – 100) + 22
13–35 months: (89 × weight [kg] – 100) + 20

EER for Boys

EER (kcal/day) = TEE + energy deposition

Boys 3–8 years: 88.5 – 61.9 × age (yr) + PA × (26.7 × weight [kg] + 903 × height [m]) + 20

Boys 9–18 years: 88.5 – 61.9 × age (yr) + PA × (26.7 × weight [kg] + 903 × height [m]) + 25

PA is the physical activity coefficient:
PA = 1.00 if PAL is estimated to be ≥1.0 or <1.4 (sedentary)
PA = 1.13 if PAL is estimated to be ≥1.4 or <1.6 (low active)
PA = 1.26 if PAL is estimated to be ≥1.6 or <1.9 (active)
PA = 1.42 if PAL is estimated to be ≥1.9 or <2.5 (very active)

EER for Girls

EER (kcal/day) = TEE + energy deposition

Girls 3–8 years: 135.3 – 30.8 × age (yr) + PA × (10 × weight [kg] + 934 × height [m]) + 20

Girls 9–18 years: 135.3 – 30.8 × age (yr) + PA × (10 × weight [kg] + 934 × height [m]) + 25

PA is the physical activity coefficient:
PA = 1.00 if PAL is estimated to be ≥1.0 or <1.4 (sedentary)
PA = 1.16 if PAL is estimated to be ≥1.4 or <1.6 (low active)
PA = 1.31 if PAL is estimated to be ≥1.6 or <1.9 (active)
PA = 1.56 if PAL is estimated to be ≥1.9 or <2.5 (very active)

EER for Pregnancy

EER = adolescent EER + pregnancy energy deposition

14–18 years:

First trimester = adolescent EER + 0 kcal
Second trimester = adolescent EER + 340 kcal
Third trimester = adolescent EER + 452 kcal

EER for lactation

EER = adolescent EER + milk energy output – weight loss

14–18 years:

First 6 months = adolescent EER + 500 – 170
Second 6 months = adolescent EER + 400 – 0

Table 20-1[2] contains the estimated EER for boys and girls of median weight.

TABLE 20-1

EXAMPLE EER FOR BOYS AND GIRLS

Age	Boys EER (kcal/kg/day)			Girls EER (kcal/kg/day)	
0–2 mo	107			104	
3 mo	95			95	
4–35 mo	82			82	
	Median Weight, Boys kg (lb)	**PAL 1 (Sedentary)**	**PAL 4 (Very Active)**	**Median Weight, Girls kg (lb)**	**PAL 1 (Sedentary)**
3 yr	14.3 (31.5)	80	118	13.9 (30.6)	76
4 yr	16.2 (35.7)	74	110	15.8 (34.8)	70
5 yr	18.4 (40.5)	68	103	17.9 (39.4)	65
6 yr	20.7 (45.6)	63	96	20.2 (44.5)	61
7 yr	23.1 (50.9)	59	92	22.8 (50.2)	56
8 yr	25.6 (56.4)	56	87	25.6 (56.4)	52
9 yr	28.6 (63.0)	53	82	29.0 (63.9)	48
10 yr	31.9 (70.3)	49	78	32.9 (72.5)	44
11 yr	35.9 (79.1)	46	74	37.2 (81.9)	41
12 yr	40.5 (89.2)	44	70	41.6 (91.6)	38
13 yr	45.6 (100.4)	42	67	45.8 (100.9)	36
14 yr	51.0 (112.3)	40	64	49.4 (108.8)	34
15 yr	56.3 (124.0)	39	62	52.0 (114.5)	33
16 yr	60.9 (134.1)	38	60	53.9 (118.7)	32
17 yr	64.6 (142.3)	36	58	55.1 (121.4)	31
18 yr	67.2 (148.0)	35	57	56.2 (123.8)	30

Data from Food and Nutrition Board, National Research Council: Dietary Reference Intakes: Energy. Washington, DC, National Academy Press, 2004.

C. ESTIMATED ENERGY REQUIREMENTS (EER) UNDER STRESSED CONDITIONS[2]

It many cases there is little need to provide critically ill patients with more than their basal energy expenditure. Ideally, energy expenditure should be measured in critically ill patients but this requires expensive equipment and may not always be practical.

There are numerous prediction equations available. The following equation is from the Dietary Reference Intakes:

1. Calculation of BEE

For Boys: BEE (kcal/d) = $68 - 43.3 \times$ Age (y) $+ 712 \times$ Height (m) $+ 19.2 \times$ Weight (kg)

For Girls: BEE (kcal/d) = $189 - 17.6 \times$ Age (y) $+ 625 \times$ Height (m) $+ 7.9 \times$ Weight (kg)

Appropriate changes should be made as indicated by real (not fluid) weight gain and signs and symptoms of overfeeding.

D. CATCH-UP GROWTH REQUIREMENT FOR MALNOURISHED INFANTS AND CHILDREN (<3 years of age)[2,5]

Table 20-2 represents the estimated energy needs for infants and children recovering from moderate to severe wasting. Children with severe wasting

TABLE 20-2
ENERGY NEEDS FOR CATCH-UP GROWTH

	Normal Composition of Weight Gain[a]		High Rate of Fat Deposition[b]	
Rate of Gain (g/kg/d)	EE[c] = 80 Energy (kcal/kg/d)	EE = 90 Energy (kcal/kg/d)	EE = 80 Energy (kcal/kg/d)	EE = 90 Energy (kcal/kg/d)
1	83	93	86	96
2	87	97	92	102
5	97	107	110	120
10	113	123	140	150
20	146	156	200	210

[a]Normal composition of weight gain is applicable to the stunted child with normal body composition.
[b]A high rate of fat deposition is applicable to the severely wasted children.
[c]EE, energy expenditure for maintenance and activity. EE of 80 is for preschool children and 90 is for infants.
Data from Dewey KG, Beaton G, Fields C, et al: Protein requirements of infants and children. Eur J Clin Nutr 1996;50:S119–S150; Energy Needs for Catch-up Growth. Food and Nutrition Board, National Research Council: Dietary Reference Intakes: Energy. Washington, DC, National Academy Press, 2004.

will require a higher rate of fat deposition, whereas those with moderate wasting will require a lesser rate.

To determine the caloric needs for catch-up growth, perform the following steps:

1. **Determine the goal weight.**
2. **Determine time period to reach goal weight.**
3. **Calculate difference between goal and actual weight, then divide by actual weight (kg) and the number of days to reach goal.**
4. **Decide composition of weight gain desired (normal versus high rate of fat deposition).**
5. **Determine baseline energy expenditure for maintenance and activity (80 for preschool children or 90 for infants) (see Table 20-2).**[2,5]

Example: A 21-month-old girl, actual weight 7.5 kg, length 77 cm. Goal weight of 9 kg for surgery in 30 days. Activity level is normal, and goal is normal composition of weight gain.

$$9 \text{ kg} - 7.5 \text{ kg} = 1500 \text{ g}/7.5 \text{ kg}/30 \text{ days}$$
$$= 6.7 \text{ g/kg/day to attain goal weight}$$

Goal kcal is 97 – 113 kcal/kg/day.

IV. RECOMMENDED INTAKES FOR INDIVIDUALS

A. DEFINITIONS[6]

Dietary reference intakes (DRIs): Reference values that are quantitative estimates of nutrient intakes. Include EAR, RDA, AI, and UL.

TABLE 20-3
PROTEIN REQUIREMENTS

Age	EAR (g/kg/d)	RDA (g/kg/d)
0–6 mo	1.52 (Adequate Intake)	
7–12 mo	1.1	1.5
1–3 yr	0.88	1.1
4–8 yr	0.76	0.95
9–13 yr	0.76	0.95
14–18 yr, boys	0.73	0.85
14–18 yr, girls	0.71	0.85
Pregnancy	0.88 + 21 g/d	1.1 + 25 g/d
Lactation	1.05 + 21.2 g/d	1.1 + 25 g/d

Data from Food and Nutrition Board, National Research Council: Dietary Reference Intakes for Energy, Carbohydrate, Fiber, Fat, Fatty Acids, Cholesterol, Protein, and Amino Acids (Macronutrients). Washington, DC, National Academy Press, 2002.

Estimated average requirement (EAR): Daily nutrient intake level estimated to meet the requirement of half the healthy individuals in a particular life stage and gender group.

Recommended dietary allowance (RDA): EAR ± 2 standard deviations. The daily nutrient intake level estimated to meet the requirement of 97%–98% of healthy individuals in a particular life stage and gender group.

Adequate intake (AI): Observed range of intakes in a healthy population used when there is not sufficient data to calculate the EAR and RDA.

Tolerable upper intake level (UL): Highest daily nutrient intake level that is likely to pose no risk for adverse health effects to almost all individuals in the general population.

B. PROTEIN (Table 20-3)[7]

C. FAT (Table 20-4)[7]

D. VITAMINS (Table 20-5)[8]

E. MINERALS (Table 20-6)[8]

F. FIBER (Table 20-7)[7]

V. VITAMIN-MINERAL SUPPLEMENTATION[9]

A. VITAMIN D

200 IU per day is recommended for the following:

1. **All breast-fed infants consuming <500 mL/day of vitamin D–fortified formula or milk.**
2. **All non-breast-fed infants ingesting <200 mL/day of vitamin D–fortified formula or milk.**
3. **Children and adolescents who do not get regular sunlight exposure, do not ingest 500 mL/day of vitamin D–fortified milk, or do not take a**

TABLE 20-4

FAT REQUIREMENTS: ADEQUATE INTAKE

Age	Total Fat (g/d)	Linoleic Acid (g/d)	α-Linolenic Acid (g/d)
0–6 mo	31	4.1 (n-6 PUFA)	0.5 (n-3 PUFA)
7–12 mo	30	4.6 (n-6 PUFA)	0.5 (n-3 PUFA)
1–3 yr	*	7	0.7
4–8 yr	*	10	0.9
9–13 yr, boys	*	12	1.2
9–13 yr, girls	*	10	1.0
14–18 yr, boys	*	16	1.6
14–18 yr, girls	*	11	1.1
Pregnancy	*	13	1.4
Lactation	*	13	1.3

*No AI, EAR, or RDA established.

Data from Food and Nutrition Board, National Research Council: Dietary Reference Intakes for Energy, Carbohydrate, Fiber, Fat, Fatty Acids, Cholesterol, Protein, and Amino Acids (Macronutrients). Washington, DC, National Academy Press, 2002.

daily multivitamin supplement containing at least 200 IU of vitamin D.

Generally, an ADC multivitamin such as Tri-Vi-Sol or Vi-Daylin ADC can be used (Table 20-8).

B. FLUORIDE

Supplementation is not needed during the first 6 months of life. Thereafter, 0.25 mg/day is recommended for the exclusively breast-fed infant. Of note, another factor that should be considered is the use of bottled water and home filtration systems. Most bottled water does not contain adequate amounts of fluoride. Some home water treatment systems have the ability to reduce fluoride levels. To avoid fluorosis, it is recommended that children should not use fluoridated toothpaste until reaching the age of 2 years, and then only a small pea-sized amount up to the age of 6 years. See Formulary for complete fluoride recommendations (i.e., in areas where water is not fluoridated).

C. IRON

1. Breast-fed

For full-term breast-fed infants, approximately 1 mg/kg/day is recommended after 4–6 months of age, preferably from iron-fortified cereal or elemental iron if sufficient cereal is not consumed.

For preterm or low-birth-weight breast-fed infants, an iron supplement of 2 mg/kg/day should be given until 12 months of age.

For all infants younger than 12 months, only iron-fortified formula should be used for weaning or supplementing breast milk.

2. Formula-fed

Infants who are formula-fed should receive an iron-fortified formula containing 4–12 mg/L of iron from birth to 12 months.

TABLE 20-5

DIETARY REFERENCE INTAKES: RECOMMENDED INTAKES FOR INDIVIDUALS—VITAMINS

Life Stage Group	Vitamin A[a] (IU)	Vitamin C (mg/d)	Vitamin D[b,c] (IU)	Vitamin E[d] (IU)	Vitamin K (μg/d)	Thiamin (mg/d)	Riboflavin (mg/d)	Niacin (mg/d)[e]	Vitamin B_6 (mg/d)	Folate (μg/d)[f]	Vitamin B_{12} (μg/d)	Pantothenic Acid (mg/d)	Biotin (μg/d)	Choline[g] (mg/d)
Infants														
0–6 mo	**1333**	40*	200	4*	2.0*	0.2*	0.3*	2*	0.1*	65*	0.4*	1.7*	5*	125*
7–12 mo	**1666**	50*	200	5*	2.5*	0.3*	0.4*	4*	0.3*	80*	0.5*	1.8*	6*	150*
Children														
1–3 y	**1000**	**15**	200	**6**	30*	**0.5**	**0.5**	**6**	**0.5**	**150**	0.9	2*	8*	200*
4–8 y	**1333**	**25**	200	**7**	55*	**0.6**	**0.6**	**8**	**0.6**	**200**	1.2	3*	12*	250*
Males														
9–13 y	**2000**	**45**	200	**11**	60*	**0.9**	**0.9**	**12**	**1.0**	**300**	1.8	4*	20*	375*
14–18 y	**3000**	**75**	200	**15**	75*	**1.2**	**1.3**	**16**	**1.3**	**400**	2.4	5*	25*	550*
19–30 y	**3000**	**90**	200	**15**	120*	**1.2**	**1.3**	**16**	**1.3**	**400**	2.4	5*	30*	550*
Females														
9–13 y	**2000**	**45**	200	**11**	60*	**0.9**	**0.9**	**12**	**1.0**	**300**	1.8	4*	20*	375*
14–18 y	**2333**	**65**	200	**15**	75*	**1.0**	**1.0**	**14**	**1.2**	**400**	2.4	5*	25*	400*
19–30 y	**2333**	**75**	200	**15**	90*	**1.1**	**1.1**	**14**	**1.3**	**400**	2.4	5*	30*	425*
Pregnancy														
<18 y	**2500**	**80**	200	**15**	75*	**1.4**	**1.4**	**18**	**1.9**	**600**	2.6	6*	30*	450*
19–30 y	**2567**	**85**	200	**15**	90*	**1.4**	**1.4**	**18**	**1.9**	**600**	2.6	6*	30*	450*
Lactation														
<18 y	**4000**	**115**	200	**19**	75*	**1.4**	**1.6**	**17**	**2.0**	**500**	2.8	7*	35*	550*
19–30 y	**4333**	**120**	200	**19**	90*	**1.4**	**1.6**	**17**	**2.0**	**500**	2.8	7*	35*	550*

This table (taken from the DRI reports, see www.nap.edu) presents Recommended Dietary Allowances (RDAs) in **bold type** and Adequate Intakes (AIs) in ordinary type followed by an asterisk (*), RDAs and AIs may both be used as goals for individual intake. RDAs are set to meet the needs of almost all (97%–98%) individuals in a group. For healthy breast-fed infants, the AI is the mean intake. The AI for other life stage and gender groups is believed to cover needs of all individuals in the group, but lack of data or uncertainty in the data prevent being able to specify with confidence the percentage of individuals covered by this intake.

[a]One IU = 0.3 µg Retinol equivalent.

[b]One µg cholecalciferol = 40 IU vitamin D.

[c]In the absence of adequate exposure to sunlight.

[d]One IU = 1 mg vitamin E.

[e]As niacin equivalents (NE). 1 mg of niacin = 60 mg of tryptophan; 0–6 months = preformed niacin (not NE).

[f]As dietary folate equivalents (DFE). 1 DFE = 1 µg food folate = 0.6 µg of folic acid from fortified food or as a supplement consumed with food = 0.5 µg of a supplement taken on an empty stomach. In view of evidence linking folate intake with neural tube defects in the fetus, it is recommended that all women capable of becoming pregnant consume 400 µg from supplements or fortified foods in addition to intake of food folate from a varied diet. It is assumed that women will continue consuming 400 µg from supplements or fortified food until their pregnancy is confirmed and they enter prenatal care, which ordinarily occurs after the end of the periconceptual period—the critical time for formation of the neural tube.

[g]Although AIs have been set for choline, there are few data to assess whether a dietary supply of choline is needed at all life stages, and it may be that the choline requirement can be met by endogenous synthesis at some of these stages.

Modified from Food and Nutrition Board, National Research Council: Dietary Reference Intakes for Vitamin A, Vitamin K, Arsenic, Boron, Chromium, Copper, Iodine, Iron, Manganese, Molybdenum, Nickel, Silicon, Vanadium, and Zinc. Washington, DC, National Academy Press, 2000.

TABLE 20-6

DIETARY REFERENCE INTAKES: RECOMMENDED INTAKES FOR INDIVIDUALS—ELEMENTS

Life Stage Group	Calcium (mg/d)	Chromium (μg/d)	Copper (μg/d)	Fluoride (mg/d)	Iodine (μg/d)	Iron (mg/d)	Magnesium (mg/d)	Manganese (mg/d)	Molybdenum (μg/d)	Phosphorus (mg/d)	Selenium (μg/d)	Zinc (mg/d)
Infants												
0–6 mo	210*	0.2*	200*	0.01*	110*	0.27*	30*	0.003*	2*	100*	15*	2*
7–12 mo	270*	5.5*	220*	0.5*	130*	**11**	75*	0.6*	3*	275*	20*	**3**
Children												
1–3 yr	500*	11*	**340**	0.7*	**90**	**7**	**80**	1.2*	**17**	**460**	**20**	**3**
4–8 yr	800*	15*	**440**	1.0*	**90**	**10**	**130**	1.5*	**22**	**500**	**30**	**5**
Males												
9–13 yr	1300*	25*	**700**	2*	**120**	**8**	**240**	1.9*	**34**	**1250**	**40**	**8**
14–18 yr	1300*	35*	**890**	3*	**150**	**11**	**410**	2.2*	**43**	**1250**	**55**	**11**
19–30 yr	1000*	35*	**900**	4*	**150**	**8**	**400**	2.3*	**45**	**700**	**55**	**11**
Females												
9–13 yr	1300*	21*	**700**	2*	**120**	**8**	**240**	1.6*	**34**	**1250**	**40**	**8**
14–18 yr	1300*	24*	**890**	3*	**150**	**15**	**360**	1.6*	**43**	**1250**	**55**	**9**
19–30 yr	1000*	25*	**900**	3*	**150**	**18**	**310**	1.8*	**45**	**700**	**55**	**8**
Pregnancy												
<18 yr	1300*	29*	**1000**	3*	**220**	**27**	**400**	2.0*	**50**	**1250**	**60**	**13**
19–30 yr	1000*	30*	**1000**	3*	**220**	**27**	**350**	2.0*	**50**	**700**	**60**	**11**
Lactation												
<18 yr	1300*	44*	**1300**	3*	**290**	**10**	**360**	2.6*	**50**	**1250**	**70**	**14**
19–30 yr	1000*	45*	**1300**	3*	**290**	**9**	**310**	2.6*	**50**	**700**	**70**	**12**

This table presents Recommended Dietary Allowances (RDAs) in **bold type** and Adequate Intakes (AIs) in ordinary type followed by an asterisk (*). RDAs and AIs may both be used as goals for individual intake. RDAs are set to meet the needs of almost all (97%–98%) individuals in a group. For healthy breast-fed infants, the AI is the mean intake. The AI for other life stage and gender groups is believed to cover needs of all individuals in the group, but lack of data of uncertainly in the data prevent being able to specify with confidence the percentage of individuals covered by this intake.

Modified from the Food and Nutrition Board, National Research Council: Dietary Reference Intakes for Vitamin A, Vitamin K, Arsenic, Boron, Chromium, Copper, Iodine, Iron, Manganese, Molybdenum, Nickel, Silicon, Vanadium, and Zinc, Washington, DC, National Academy Press, 2000.

TABLE 20-7

FIBER REQUIREMENTS: ADEQUATE INTAKE

Age	Total Fiber (g/d)
1–3 yr	19
4–8 yr	25
9–13 yr, boys	31
9–13 yr, girls	26
14–18 yr, boys	38
14–18 yr, girls	26
Pregnancy	28
Lactation	29

Data from Food and Nutrition Board, National Research Council: Dietary Reference Intakes for Energy, Carbohydrate, Fiber, Fat, Fatty Acids, Cholesterol, Protein, and Amino Acids (Macronutrients). Washington, DC, National Academy Press, 2002.

TABLE 20-8

INFANT MULTIVITAMIN DROPS ANALYSIS (PER mL)*

	Poly-Vi-Sol/(Flor) [with iron] Vi Daylin/F Multivitamin [with iron]	Tri-Vi-Sol/(Flor) [with iron] Vi-Daylin/(F) ADC [with iron]	ADEK†‡
Vitamin A (IU)	1500	1500	1500
Vitamin D (IU)	400	400	400
Vitamin E (IU)	5	—	40
Vitamin C (mg)	35	35	45
Thiamin (mg)	0.5	—	0.5
Riboflavin (mg)	0.6	—	0.6
Niacin (mg)	8	—	6
Vitamin B_6 (mg)	0.4	—	0.6
Vitamin B_{12} (μg)	2§	—	4
Iron (mg)	[10]	[10]	—
Fluoride (mg)	(0.25)	(0.25)	—

*Standard dose = 1 mL.

†Also contains biotin 15 μg; pantothenic acid 3 mg; zinc 5 mg; β-carotene 1 mg = 1666 IU vitamin A, 100 μg vitamin K.

‡Recommended for use in infants with fat malabsorption such as cystic fibrosis, liver disease.

§Poly-Vi-Sol only.

Formula fed preterm infants should receive an additional 1 mg/kg/day, administered either as iron drops or in a vitamin preparation with iron.

D. EXAMPLES OF MULTIVITAMINS FOR CHILDREN (Table 20-9)

VI. ENTERAL NUTRITION (Tables 20-10 to 20-16)

VII. PARENTERAL NUTRITION (Tables 20-17 to 20-19)

Text continues on p. 583

TABLE 20-9

MULTIVITAMIN TABLETS (ANALYSIS/TABLET)

	Multivitamins				Fat Malabsorption			Prenatal		Powder
	Flintstones Original Bugs Bunny Generic Poly-Vi-Sol/ (Flor) Vi-Daylin/(F) [with iron]	Flintstones + Extra C Sunkist + Extra C Generic + C Bugs Bunny + Extra C	Centrum Jr	Flintstones Complete Generic Complete	ADEK	Source CF	Vitamax	Stuart Natal Plus 3	OBEGYN Prenatal[e]	Phlexy-Vits (7 g packet)
Vitamin A (IU)[a]	2500	2500	5000	5000	4000	9000[b]	5000[c]	3000[d]	5000[f]	2664
Vitamin D (IU)	400	400	400	400	400	400	400	400	400	400
Vitamin E (IU)	15	15	30	30	150	200	200	22	30	13.5
Vitamin K (mcg)	—	—	10	—	150	50	200	—	—	70
Vitamin C (mg)	60	250	60	60	60	100	60	120	120	50
Thiamin (mg)	1.05	1.05	1.5	1.5	1.2	1.5	1.5	1.8	1.7	1.2
Riboflavin (mg)	1.2	1.2	1.7	1.7	1.3	1.7	1.7	4	2	1.4
Niacin (mg)	13.5	13.5	20	20	10	20	20	—	20	20
Vitamin B_6 (mg)	1.05	1.06	2	2	1.5	1.9	2	25	10	1.6
Folate (mcg)	300	300	400	400	200	200	200	1	1	700
Vitamin B_{12} (mcg)	4.5	4.5	6	6	12	6	6	12	12	5
Biotin (mcg)	—	—	45	40	50	100	300	—	300	150
Panathenic acid (mg)	—	—	10	10	10	12	10	—	—	5

Calcium (mg)	—	—	108	100	—	—	—	200	455	1000
Phosphorus (mg)	—	—	50	100	—	—	—	—	—	775
Iron (mg)	[10–15]	—	18	18	—	—	—	27	18	15.1
Iodine (mcg)	—	—	150	150	—	—	—	—	0.15	150
Magnesium (mg)	—	—	40	20	—	—	—	25	150	300
Zinc (mg)	—	—	15	15	1.1	10	7.5	25	25	11.1
Copper (mg)	—	—	2	2	—	—	—	2	2	1.5
Manganese (mg)	—	—	1	—	—	—	—	—	—	1.5
Chromium (mcg)	—	—	20	—	—	—	—	—	—	30
Molybdenum (mcg)	—	—	20	—	—	—	—	—	—	70
Selenium (mcg)	—	—	—	—	—	—	—	—	—	75
β-Carotene (mg)	—	—	—	—	3	—	—	—	—	—
Fluoride (mg)	[0.25, 0.5, 1.0]	—	—	—	—	—	—	—	—	—

[a]Vitamin A as palmitate and 60% β-carotene.
[b]Vitamin A: 3600 IU as retinol and 5400 IU as β-carotene.
[c]Vitamin A as acetate and 50% β-carotene.
[d]Vitamin A as β-carotene.
[e]Contraindicated with kidney stones.
[f]Vitamin A as 50% palmitate and 50% β-carotene.

TABLE 20-10

PREPARATION OF INFANT FORMULAS FOR STANDARD AND SOY FORMULAS*

Formula Type	Caloric Concentration (kcal/oz)	Amount of Formula	Water (oz)
Liquid concentrates (40 kcal/oz)	20	13 oz	13
	24	13 oz	8.5
	26	13 oz	7
	28	13 oz	5.5
	30	13 oz	4.3
Small volume preparation of powder (44 kcal/scoop)	20	1 scoop	2
	24	3 scoops	5
	26	2 scoops	3
	28	7 scoops	10
	30	3 scoops	4

*Does not apply to Enfacare, Neocate, Neosure, Elecare, Enfamil AR should not be concentrated greater than 24 kcal/oz. Use a packed measure for Portagen, Nutramigen, and Pregestimil.

TABLE 20-11

COMMON CALORIC SUPPLEMENTS*

Component	Calories
PROTEIN	
Casec	3.7 kcal/g (0.9 g protein) 17 kcal/tbsp (4 g protein)
CARBOHYDRATE	
Polycose	Powder: 3.8 kcal/g 8 kcal/tsp Liquid: 2.0 kcal/mL, 10 kcal/tsp
FAT	
MCT oil†	7.7 kcal/mL
Vegetable oil	8.3 kcal/mL

*Use these caloric supplements when you want to increase protein or when you have reached the maximum concentration tolerated and wish to further increase caloric density.

†MCT oil is unnecessary unless there is fat malabsorption.

TABLE 20-12a

COMPOSITION OF PEDIATRIC FORMULAS (PER LITER)

Human Milk	kcal/oz (kcal/ml)	Protein Source	Protein g (%kcal)	Fat Source	Fat g (%kcal)	Carbohydrate Source	Carbohydrate g (%kcal)	Na (mEq)	K (mEq)	Ca (mg)	P (mg)	Fe (mg)	Osmolality (mOsm/kg water)	Suggested Uses
Term Human Milk	20 (0.67)	Human milk protein	10.5 (6)	Human milk fat	39 (52)	Lactose	72 (42)	7.7	13.6	279	143	0.3	286	Infants
Preterm Human Milk	20 (0.67)	Human milk protein	14 (8)	Human milk fat	39 (52)	Lactose	66 (40)	10.8	14.6	248	128	1.2	290	Preterm infants

TABLE 20-12b

HUMAN MILK AND FORTIFIERS ANALYSIS (PER LITER)

		Protein		Fat		Carbohydrate								
Formula	kcal/oz (kcal/ml)	Source	g (%kcal)	Source (%)	g (%kcal)	Source (%)	g (%kcal)	Na (mEq)	K (mEq)	Ca (mg)	P (mg)	Fe (mg)	Osmolality (mOsm/kg water)	Suggested Uses
Enfamil Human Milk Fortifier (per pkt) (Mead Johnson)	3.5 (–)	Milk protein isolate Whey protein isolate hydrolysate	0.3 (32)	MCT oil (70) Soy oil (30)	0.25 (63)	Corn syrup solids	<0.1 (5)	0.17	0.19	22.5	12.5	0.36	+9	Fortifier for preterm human milk
Preterm Human Milk + Enfamil Human Milk Fortifier (1 pkt/25 ml)	24 (0.8)	Human milk protein Milk protein isolate Whey protein isolate hydrolysate	26 (13)	Human milk fat MCT oil Soy oil	49 (53)	Lactose Corn syrup solids	70 (34)	17.6	22	1140	630	16	326	Preterm infants
Similac Human Milk Fortifier (per pkt) (Ross)	3.5 (–)	Nonfat milk Whey protein concentrate	0.25 (28)	MCT oil	0.09 (21)	Corn syrup solids	0.45 (51)	0.18	0.4	29	17	0.1	—	Fortifier for preterm human milk

Preterm Human Milk + Similac Human Milk Fortifier (1 pkt/25 ml) (Ross)	24 (0.8)	Human milk protein Nonfat milk Whey protein concentrate	23.5 (12)	Human milk fat MCT oil	41.4 (47)	Lactose Corn syrup solids	82 (42)	16.9	29.9	1381	777	4.6	385	Preterm infants
Similac Natural Care Advance (Ross)	24 (0.8)	Nonfat milk Whey protein concentrate	24.4 (12)	MCT oil (50) Soy oil (30) Coconut oil (18) DHA (0.25) ARA (0.4)	44 (47)	Lactose (50) Corn syrup solids (50)	84 (41)	15	27	1704	941	3	280	Fortifier for preterm human milk
Preterm Human Milk + Similac Natural Care Advance (50 : 50 Ratio)(Ross)	22 (0.74)	Human milk Nonfat milk Whey protein concentrate	19.2 (10)	Human milk fat MCT oil Soy oil Coconut oil DHA ARA	36.7 (47)	Lactose Corn syrup solids	75 (40)	13	21	976	534	2.1	285	Preterm infants

TABLE 20-13a

PRETERM INFANT FORMULAS (PER LITER)

Formula	kcal/oz (kcal/ml)	Protein: Source	Protein: g (%kcal)	Fat: Source (%)	Fat: g (%kcal)	Carbohydrate: Source (%)	Carbohydrate: g (%kcal)	Na (mEq)	K (mEq)	Ca (mg)	P (mg)	Fe (mg)	Osmolality (mOsm/kg water)	Suggested Uses
Enfamil Premature LIPIL (with iron) (Mead Johnson)	20 (0.67)	Nonfat milk Whey protein concentrate	20 (12)	MCT oil (40) Soy oil (30) HO vegetable oil (27) DHA and ARA (3)	34 (44)	Corn syrup solids (60) Lactose (40)	74 (44)	17	17	1100	553	3.3 (12)	240	Preterm infants
Enfamil Premature LIPIL (with iron) (Mead Johnson)	24 (0.8)	Nonfat milk Whey protein concentrate	24 (12)	MCT oil (40) Soy oil (30) HO vegetable oil (27) DHA and ARA (3)	41 (44)	Corn syrup solids (60) Lactose (40)	89 (44)	20	20	1320	664	4 (15)	300	Preterm infants
Similac Special Care Advance (with iron) (Ross)	20 (0.67)	Nonfat milk Whey protein concentrate	20 (12)	MCT oil (50) Soy oil (30) Coconut oil (18) DHA (0.25) ARA (0.4)	37 (47)	Corn syrup solids (50) Lactose (50)	70 (41)	13	22	1217	676	3 (12)	235	Preterm infants
Similac Special Care Advance (with iron) (Ross)	24 (0.8)	Nonfat milk Whey protein concentrate	24 (12)	MCT oil (50) Soy oil (30) Coconut oil (18) DHA (0.25) ARA (0.4)	44 (47)	Corn syrup solids (50) Lactose (50)	84 (41)	15	27	1461	812	3 (14.4)	280	Preterm infants

TABLE 20-13b

POST-DISCHARGE FORMULAS (PER LITER)

Formula	kcal/oz (kcal/ml)	Protein Source	Protein g (%kcal)	Fat Source (%)	Fat g (%kcal)	Carbohydrate Source (%)	Carbohydrate g (%kcal)	Na (mEq)	K (mEq)	Ca (mg)	P (mg)	Fe (mg)	Osmolality (mOsm/kg water)	Suggested Uses
Enfamil EnfaCare LIPIL (Ready to Feed) (Mead Johnson)	22 (0.73)	Nonfat milk Whey protein concentrate	20.7 (11)	HO Vegetable oil (34) Soy oil (29) MCT oil (20) Coconut oil (14) DHA and ARA (3)	39 (47)	Maltodextrin (60) Lactose (40)	77 (42)	11	20	889	489	13	250	Preterm infant discharge formula can be used through 12 months
Similac NeoSure Advance (Ross)	22 (0.73)	Nonfat milk Whey protein concentrate	20.8 (11)	Soy oil (45) Coconut oil (29) MCT oil (25) DHA (0.15) ARA (0.4)	41 (49)	Corn syrup solids (50) Lactose (50)	75 (40)	11	27	781	461	13	250	Preterm infant discharge formula can be used through 12 months

TABLE 20-13c

COW'S MILK BASED FORMULAS (PER LITER)

		Protein		Fat		Carbohydrate								
Formula	kcal/oz (kcal/ml)	Source	g (%kcal)	Source (%)	g (%kcal)	Source	g (%kcal)	Na (mEq)	K (mEq)	Ca (mg)	P (mg)	Fe (mg)	Osmolality (mOsm/kg water)	Suggested Uses
America's Store Brand Infant Formula (PBM Nutritionals)	20 (0.67)	Nonfat milk Whey protein concentrate	15 (11)	Palm or Palm olein oil Coconut oil HO safflower oil or HO sunflower oil Soy oil	36 (48)	Lactose	72 (43)	6.5	14	420	280	12	—	Infants with normal GI tract
America's Store Brand Infant Formula with ARA/DHA (PBM Nutritionals)	20 (0.67)	Nonfat milk Whey protein concentrate	15 (11)	Palm olein oil HO safflower oil or HO sunflower oil Coconut oil Soy oil DHA and ARA	36 (48)	Lactose	72 (43)	6.5	14	420	280	12	—	Infants with normal GI tract
Enfamil with Iron (Mead Johnson)	20 (0.67)	Nonfat milk Whey protein concentrate	14 (8.5)	Palm olein oil (44) Soy oil (19.5) Coconut oil (19.5) HO sunflower oil (14.5)	34 (48)	Lactose	75 (45)	7.8	18.5	250	353	12	265	Infants with normal GI tract

Enfamil LIPIL (with iron) (Mead Johnson)	20 (0.67)	Nonfat milk Whey protein concentrate	14 (8.5)	Palm olein oil (44) Soy oil (19.5) Coconut oil (19.5) HO sunflower oil (14.5) DHA and ARA (2.5)	35 (48)	Lactose	73 (43.5)	7.8	18.5	520	353	4.7 (12)	300	Infants with normal GI tract
Enfamil LIPIL (with iron) (Mead Johnson)	24 (0.8)	Nonfat milk Whey protein concentrate	16.8 (8.5)	Palm olein oil (44) Soy oil (19.5) Coconut oil (19.5) HO sunflower oil (14.5) DHA and ARA (2.5)	42 (48)	Lactose	87.6 (43.5)	9.4	22.2	624	424	5.6 (14.4)	360	Infants with normal GI tract requiring additional calories
Enfamil A.R. LIPIL (Mead Johnson)	20 (0.67)	Nonfat milk	16.7 (10)	Plam olein oil (44) Soy oil (19.5) Coconut oil (19.5) HO sunflower oil (14.5) DHA and ARA (2.5)	34 (46)	Lactose Rich starch Maltodextrin	73 (44)	11.6	18.5	520	353	12	240	Thickened feeding for infants who spit-up frequently

continued

TABLE 20-13c
COW'S MILK BASED FORMULAS (PER LITER)—*cont'd*

Formula	kcal/oz (kcal/ml)	Protein Source	Protein g (%kcal)	Fat Source (%)	Fat g (%kcal)	Carbohydrate Source	Carbohydrate g (%kcal)	Na (mEq)	K (mEq)	Ca (mg)	P (mg)	Fe (mg)	Osmolality (mOsm/kg water)	Suggested Uses
Enfamil LactoFree LIPIL (Mead Johnson)	20 (0.67)	Milk protein isolate	14 (8.5)	Palm olein oil (44) Soy oil (19.5) Coconut oil (19.5) HO sunflower (oil 14.5) DHA and ARA (2.5)	35 (48)	Lactose Rich starch Maltodextrin	73 (43.5)	8.7	18.8	547	367	12	200	Infants with lactose malabsorption
Good Start Supreme (Nestle)	20 (0.67)	Enzymatically hydrolyzed reduced minerals Whey	14.7 (8.8)	Palm olein oil (47) Soy oil (26) Coconut oil (21) HO safflower oil or HO sunflower oil (6)	34 (46)	Lactose (70) Maltodextrin (30)	75 (45)	7.8	18.5	427	240	10	250	Infants with normal GI tract

Good Start Supreme DHA & ARA (Nestle)	20 (0.67)	Enzymatically hydrolyzed reduced minerals Whey	14.7 (8.8)	Palm olein oil (46) Soy oil (26) Coconut oil (20) HO safflower oil or HO sunflower oil (6) DHA (0.32) ARA (0.64)	34 (46)	Lactose (70) Maltodextrin (30)	75 (45)	7.8	19.8	427	240	10	250	Infants with normal GI tract
Good Start Essentials (Nestle)	20 (0.67)	Nonfat milk Reduced minerals Whey protein	14.7 (8.8)	Palm olein oil (47) Soy oil (26) Coconut oil (21) HO safflower oil or HO sunflower oil (6)	34 (46)	Lactose (70) Corn syrup solids (30)	75 (45)	7	18	500	280	10	295	Infants with normal GI tract

continued

TABLE 20-13c

COW'S MILK BASED FORMULAS (PER LITER)—cont'd

		Protein		Fat		Carbohydrate								
Formula	kcal/oz (kcal/ml)	Source	g (%kcal)	Source (%)	g (%kcal)	Source	g (%kcal)	Na (mEq)	K (mEq)	Ca (mg)	P (mg)	Fe (mg)	Osmolality (mOsm/kg water)	Suggested Uses
NAN DHA & ARA (Nestle)	20 (0.67)	Nonfat milk Reduced minerals Whey protein	14.7 (8.8)	Palm olein oil (46) Soy oil (26) Coconut oil (20) HO safflower oil or HO sunflower oil (6) DHA (0.32) ARA (0.64)	34 (46)	Lactose (74) Corn syrup solids (26)	75 (45)	7.8	18.5	500	280	10	295	Infants with normal GI tract
Similac with Iron (low iron) (Ross)	20 (0.67)	Nonfat milk Whey protein concentrate	14 (8)	HO safflower oil (41) Soy oil (30) Coconut oil (29)	36.5 (49)	Lactose	73 (43)	7	18	528	284	12 (4.7)	300	Infants with normal GI tract
Similac Advance (Ross)	20 (0.67)	Nonfat milk Whey protein concentrate	14 (8)	HO safflower oil (41) Soy oil (30) Coconut oil (28) DHA (0.15) ARA (0.4)	36.5 (49)	Lactose	73 (43)	7	18	528	284	12	300	Infants with normal GI tract

Similac Lactose Free (Ross)	20 (0.67)	Milk protein isolate	14.5 (9)	HO safflower oil (41) Soy oil (30) Coconut oil (28) DHA (0.15) ARA (0.4)	36.5 (49)	Maltodextrin (55) Sucrose (45)	72 (43)	8.8	18.5	568	379	12	200	Infants with lactose malabsorption
Similac PM 60/40	20 (0.67)	Whey protein concentrate Na caseinate	15 (9)	Corn oil (50) Coconut oil (38) Soy oil (12)	37.8 (50)	Lactose	69 (41)	7.1	13.8	379	189	4.7	280	Infants who require lower calcium and phosphorus levels
Evaporated Milk Formula 13 oz evaporated whole milk 19 oz water 2 tbsp corn syrup	20 (0.67)	Cow's milk	27 (16)	Butterfat	31 (41)	Lactose Corn syrup	72 (43)	21	32	1066	832	0.8	—	Infants with normal GI tract

TABLE 20-13d

SOY BASED INFANT FORMULAS (PER LITER)

Formula	kcal/oz (kcal/ml)	Protein Source	Protein g (%kcal)	Fat Source (%)	Fat g (%kcal)	Carbohydrate Source	Carbohydrate g (%kcal)	Na (mEq)	K (mEq)	Ca (mg)	P (mg)	Fe (mg)	Osmolality (mOsm/kg water)	Suggested Uses
America's Store Brand Soy Infant Formula (PBM Nutritionals)	20 (0.67)	Soy protein isolate L-Methionine	18 (11)	Palm or Palm olein oil Coconut oil HO sunflower oil or HO safflower oil Soy oil	35 (47)	Corn syrup solids Sucrose	69 (41)	8.7	17.9	600	420	12	—	Infants with cow's milk allergy, galactose mia, or lactose malabsorption
America's Store Brand Soy Infant Formula with ARA/DHA (PBM Nutritionals)	20 (0.67)	Soy protein isolate L-Methionine	18 (11)	Palm or Palm olein oil Coconut oil HO sunflower oil or HO safflower oil Soy oil DHA and ARA	35 (47)	Corn syrup solids Sucrose	69 (41)	8.7	17.9	600	420	12	—	Infants with cow's milk allergy, galactose mia, or lactose malabsorption
Good Start Supreme Soy DHA and ARA (Nestle)	20 (0.67)	Partially hydrolyzed soy protein isolate	16.7 (10)	Palm olein oil (46) Soy oil (26) Coconut oil (20) HO safflower oil or HO sunflower oil (6) DHA (0.32) ARA (0.64)	34 (46)	Corn maltodextrin (79) Sucrose (21)	74 (44)	11.6	19.8	700	420	12	180	Infants with cow's milk allergy, galactose mia, or lactose malabsorption

Isomil Advance (Ross)	20 (0.67)	Soy protein isolate L-Methionine	16.6 (10)	HO Safflower oil (41) Soy oil (30) Coconut oil (28) DHA (0.15) ARA (0.4)	37 (49)	Corn syrup (80) Sucrose (20)	70 (41)	13	19	710	507	12	200	Infants with cow's milk allergy, galactose mia, or lactose malabsorption
Isomil DF (Ross)	20 (0.67)	Soy protein isolate L-Methionine	18 (11)	Soy oil (60) Coconut oil (40)	37 (49)	Corn syrup (60) Sucrose (40) Fiber (soy)	68 (40)	13	19	710	507	12	240	Short term management of diarrhea in infants >6 mo
ProSobee LIPIL (Mead Johnson)	20 (0.67)	Soy protein isolate L-Methionine	16.6 (10)	Palm olein oil (44) Soy oil (19.5) Coconut oil (19.5) HO sunflower oil (14.5) DHA and ARA (2.5)	35.3 (48)	Corn syrup solids	25 (42)	10.4	20.5	700	553	12	200	Infants with cow's milk allergy, galactose mia, or lactose malabsorption

TABLE 20-13e

CASEIN HYDROLYSATE INFANT FORMULAS (PER LITER)

		Protein		Fat		Carbohydrate								
Formula	kcal/oz (kcal/ml)	Source	g (%kcal)	Source (%)	g (%kcal)	Source (%)	g (%kcal)	Na (mEq)	K (mEq)	Ca (mg)	P (mg)	Fe (mg)	Osmolality (mOsm/kg water)	Suggested Uses
Alimentum Advance (Ross)	20 (0.67)	Casein hydrolysate L-Cystine L-Tyrosine L-Tryptophan	18.6 (11)	Safflower oil (38) MCT oil (33) Soy oil (28) DHA (0.15) ARA (0.4)	37.5 (48)	Sucrose (70) Modified tapioca starch (30)	69 (41)	13	20	710	507	12	370	Infants with food allergies, protein or fat malabsorption
Nutramigen made from powder (Mead Johnson)	20 (0.67)	Casein hydrolysate L-Cystine L-Tyrosine L-Tryptophan	18.6 (11)	Palm olein oil (44) Soy oil (19.5) Coconut oil (19.5) HO sunflower oil (14.5) DHA and ARA (2.5)	35.3 (48)	Corn syrup solids (86) Modified corn starch (14)	68.7 (41)	13.6	18.8	627	420	12	300	Infants with food allergies or protein malabsorption
Pregestimil made from powder (Mead Johnson)	20 (0.67)	Casein hydrolysate L-Cystine L-Tyrosine L-Tryptophan	18.6 (11)	MCT oil (55) Soy oil (25) Corn oil (10) HO sunflower oil or HO safflower (10)	37.3 (48)	Corn syrup solid (65) Dextrose (20) Modified corn starch (15)	68 (41)	13.6	18.8	767	500	12.5	330	Infants with food allergies, protein or fat malabsorption
Pregestimil liquid (Mead Johnson)	24 (0.8)	Casein hydrolysate L-Cystine L-Tyrosine L-Tryptophan	22.4 (11)	MCT oil (55) Soy oil (35) HO safflower (10)	44.8 (48)	Corn syrup solids (75) Modified corn starch (25)	81.6 (41)	16.3	22.6	920	600	15	330	Infants with food allergies, protein or fat malabsorption requiring additional calories

TABLE 20-13f

AMINO ACID BASED INFANT FORMULAS (PER LITER)

Formula	kcal/oz (kcal/ml)	Protein Source	Protein g (%kcal)	Fat Source (%)	Fat g (%kcal)	Carbohydrate Source (%)	Carbohydrate g (%kcal)	Na (mEq)	K (mEq)	Ca (mg)	P (mg)	Fe (mg)	Osmolality (mOsm/kg water)	Suggested Uses
EleCare (Ross)	20 (0.67)	Free L-amino acids	20.4 (15)	HO Safflower oil (39) MCT oil (33) Soy oil (28)	32 (42)	Corn syrup solids	72 (43)	13	26	730	548	12	335	Infants with severe food allergies, fat malabsorption
Neocate (SHS)	20 (0.67)	Free L-amino acids	20.7 (12)	HO safflower oil Coconut oil Soy oil	30 (41)	Corn syrup solids	78 (47)	10.8	23.1	827	620	12.3	375	Infants with severe food allergies

TABLE 20-13g
SPECIAL INFANT FORMULAS (PER LITER)

Formula	kcal/oz (kcal/ml)	Protein Source	Protein g (%kcal)	Fat Source (%)	Fat g (%kcal)	Carbohydrate Source (%)	Carbohydrate g (%kcal)	Na (mEq)	K (mEq)	Ca (mg)	P (mg)	Fe (mg)	Osmolality (mOsm/kg water)	Suggested Uses
MJ 3232AProtein Hydrolysate Formula Base (without added carbohydrate) (Mead Johnson)	12.7 (0.42)	Casein hydrolysate L-Cystine L-Tyrosine L-Tryptophan	18.9 (18)	MCT oil (85) Corn oil (15)	28 (55)	Modified tapioca starch	28 (27)	12.4	18.5	621	412	12.4	250	Infants with severe CHO intolerance (CHO must be added)
Portagen (Mead Johnson) (Not recommended for use as an infant formula)	20 (0.67)	Na Caseinate	22.8 (14)	MCT (87) Corn oil (13)	31 (40)	Corn syrup solids (75) Sucrose (25)	74 (46)	15.4	20.6	603	456	12	235	Fat malabsorption, intestinal lymphatic obstruction, chylothorax
RCF (Ross) 13 oz concentrate 52 g carbohydrate 12 oz water	20 (0.67)	Soy protein isolate L-Methionine	20 (12)	HO safflower oil (40) Coconut oil (30) Soy oil (30)	36 (48)	Selected by physician	68 (40)	13	19	710	507	12	168	Infants with severe CHO intolerance (CHO must be added) Can be modified for ketogenic diet

TABLE 20-13h

FOLLOW-UP FORMULAS FOR OLDER INFANTS EATING SOLIDS (PER LITER)

		Protein		Fat		Carbohydrate								
Formula	kcal/oz (kcal/ml)	Source	g (%kcal)	Source (%)	g (%kcal)	Source (%)	g (%kcal)	Na (mEq)	K (mEq)	Ca (mg)	P (mg)	Fe (mg)	Osmolality (mOsm/kg water)	Suggested Uses
America's Store Brand for older infants with ARA/DHA (PBM Nutritionals)	20 (0.67)	Cow's milk protein	18 (11)	Palm or Palm olein oil Coconut oil HO safflower oil or HO sunflower oil Soy oil DHA and ARA	37 (49)	Lactose Corn syrup solids	69 (40)	9.6	21.8	816	579	12	280	Infants >4 mo with normal GI tract
Enfamil Next Step LIPIL (Mead Johnson)	20 (0.67)	Nonfat milk	17.3 (10)	Palm olein oil (44) Soy oil (19.5) Coconut oil (19.5) HO sunflower oil (6) DHA and ARA (2.5)	35.3 (48)	Lactose (55) Corn syrup solids (45)	70 (42)	10.4	22.2	1300	867	13.3	270	Infants 9–24 mo with normal GI tract
Enfamil Next Step ProSobee LIPIL (Mead Johnson)	20 (0.67)	Soy protein L-Methionine	22 (13)	Palm olein oil (44) Soy oil (19.5) Coconut oil (19.5) HO sunflower oil (6) DHA and ARA (3)	29.3 (40)	Corn syrup solids	79 (47)	10.4	20.5	1300	867	13.3	230	Infants 9–24 mo with cow's milk protein allergy, galactosemia, or lactose malabsorption

continued

TABLE 20-13h

FOLLOW-UP FORMULAS FOR OLDER INFANTS EATING SOLIDS (PER LITER)—*cont'd*

		Protein		Fat		Carbohydrate								
Formula	kcal/oz (kcal/ml)	Source	g (%kcal)	Source (%)	g (%kcal)	Source (%)	g (%kcal)	Na (mEq)	K (mEq)	Ca (mg)	P (mg)	Fe (mg)	Osmolality (mOsm/kg water)	Suggested Uses
Good Start 2 Surpreme DHA and ARA (Nestle)	20 (0.67)	Enzymatically hydrolyzed reduced minerals Whey	14.7 (8.8)	Palm olein oil (47) Soy oil (26) Coconut oil (21) HO safflower oil or HO sunflower oil (6) DHA (0.32) ARA (0.64)	34 (46)	Lactose (70) Maltodextrin (30)	74.7 (45)	10.1	18.5	800	450	10	265	Infants 9–24 mo with normal GI tract
Good Start 2 Essentials (Nestle)	20 (0.67)	Nonfat milk	17.3 (10)	Palm olein oil (47) Soy oil (26) Coconut oil (21) HO safflower oil or HO sunflower (oil 6)	27.3 (37)	Corn syrup solids (52) Lactose (30) Corn maltodextrin (18)	88 (53)	11.3	23	800	533	12	325	Infants >4 mo with normal GI tract

Good Start 2 Essentials Soy (Nestle)	20 (0.67)	Soy protein L-Methionine	20.7 (12.4)	Palm olein oil (47) Soy oil (26) Coconut oil (21) HO safflower oil or HO sunflower oil (6)	29.3 (40)	Corn maltodextrin (69) Sucrose (31)	80 (48)	11	20	900	600	12	215	Infants >4 mo with cow's milk protein allergy, galactosemia, or lactose malabsorption
Similac 2 Advance (Ross)	20 (0.67)	Nonfat milk Whey protein concentrate	14 (8)	HO safflower oil (40) Soy oil (30) Coconut oil (28)	37 (49)	Lactose	72 (43)	7	18	798	433	12	300	Infants 9–24 mo with normal GI tract
Similac Isomil 2 Advance (Ross)	20 (0.67)	Soy protein L-Methionine	16.6 (10)	HO safflower oil (40) Soy oil (30) Coconut oil (28) DHA (0.15) ARA (0.4)	37 (49)	Corn syrup solids (80) Sucrose (20)	70 (41)	13	19	913	609	12	200	Infants 9–24 mo with cow's milk protein allergy, galactosemir, or lactose malabsorption

TABLE 20-14a

TODDLER AND YOUNG CHILD 1–10 YEARS (PER LITER)

Formula	kcal/oz (kcal/ml)	Protein Source	Protein g (%kcal)	Fat Source (%)	Fat g (%kcal)	Carbohydrate Source (%)	Carbohydrate g (%kcal)	Na (mEq)	K (mEq)	Ca (mg)	P (mg)	Fe (mg)	Osmolality (mOsm/kg water)	Suggested Uses
Bright Beginnings Soy Pediatric Drink (PBM Products, LLC)	30 (1)	Soy protein isolate	30 (12)	HO safflower oil Soy oil MCT oil	50 (45)	Maltodextrin Sucrose	110 (44)	17	34	970	800	14	350	Children with cow's milk protein allergy or lactose malabsorption
Carnation Instant Breakfast Junior (Nestle)	30 (1)	Nonfat milk	32 (12)	Soybean oil Canola oil	48 (44)	Sugar Modified corn starch Fiber (inulin, fructooligo-saccharides)	108 (44) (7 g fiber)	37	52	1120	1120	14	505	High calorie supplement for children with normal GI tract
Carnation Instant Breakfast Juice Drink (Nestle)	30 (1)	Whey protein concentrate	40 (16)	—	—	High fructose corn syrup Maltodextrin Sucrose Apple and strawberry juice (sweet Berry)	215 (84)	6.7	7	509	1018	9.2	990	Oral supplement for clear liquid nutrition support

Compleat Pediatric (Novartis)	30 (1)	Chicken Na Caseinate Pea puree	38 (15%)	Canola oil MCT oil Chicken fat	39 (35%)	Corn syrup solids Cranberry juice Fruits, vegetables	130 (50)	33	41	1440	1000	13	380	Blenderized tube feeding for children with normal GI tract
Cow's Milk, whole	20 (0.67)	Cow's milk protein	34 (22)	Butter fat	34.5 (49)	Lactose	48 (38)	22	40	1226	956	0.5	285	Normal GI tract
Cow's Milk, 2%	15 (0.51)	Cow's milk protein	34.5 (27)	Butter fat	19.6 (34)	Lactose	49.5 (38)	22	40	1258	979	0.5	—	Normal GI tract
Enfamil Kindercal Beverage (Mead Johnson)	32 (1.06)	Milk protein concentrate	30 (11)	Canola oil (40) HO Sunflower oil (28) Corn oil (20) MCT (12)	44 (37)	Vanilla; sugar (50) Maltodextrin (50) Chocolate; sugar (75) Maltodextrin (25)	135 (52)	16	34	1010	850	10.6	Van 440 Choc 520	Tube feeding and oral supplement for children with normal GI tract
Enfamil Kindercal Beverage with fiber Vanilla (Mead Johnson)	32 (1.06)	Milk protein concentrate	30 (11)	Canola oil (40) HO Sunflower oil (28) Corn oil (20) MCT (12)	44 (37)	Sugar (50) Maltodextrin (45) Fiber (5) (gum arabic and soy fiber)	135 (52) (6.3 g fiber)	16	34	1010	850	10.6	440	Tube feeding and oral supplement for children with normal GI tract

continued

TABLE 20-14a

TODDLER AND YOUNG CHILD 1–10 YEARS (PER LITER)—*cont'd*

Formula	kcal/oz (kcal/ml)	Protein Source	Protein g (%kcal)	Fat Source (%)	Fat g (%kcal)	Carbohydrate Source (%)	Carbohydrate g (%kcal)	Na (mEq)	K (mEq)	Ca (mg)	P (mg)	Fe (mg)	Osmolality (mOsm/kg water)	Suggested Uses
Enfamil Kindercal TF Vanilla (Mead Johnson)	32 (1.06)	Milk protein concentrate	30 (11)	Canola oil (40) HO Sunflower oil (28) Corn oil (20) MCT (12)	44 (37)	Maltodextrin (75) Sugar (25)	135 (52)	16	34	1010	850	10.6	345	Tube feeding for children with normal GI tract
Enfamil Kindercal TF Vanilla with fiber (Mead Johnson)	32 (1.06)	Milk protein concentrate	30 (11)	Canola oil (40) HO Sunflower oil (28) Corn oil (20) MCT (12)	44 (37)	Maltodextrin (75) Sugar (20) Fiber (5) (gum arabic and soy fiber)	135 (52) (6.3 g fiber)	16	34	1010	850	10.6	345	Tube feeding for children with normal GI tract
KetoCal (SHS)	43 (1.44)	Cow's milk protein	30 (8.4)	Soy oil	144 (90)	Corn syrup solids	6 (1.6)	26	55	1600	1300	22	197	Children with intractable epilepsy
Nutren Junior (Nestle)	30 (1)	Milk protein concentrate Whey protein concentrate	30 (12)	Soy oil Canola oil MCT oil	50 (44)	Sucrose Maltodextrin	110 (44)	20	34	1000	800	14	350	Tube feeding and oral supplement for children with normal GI tract

Nutren Junior with fiber (Nestle)	30 (1)	Milk protein concentrate Whey protein concentrate	30 (12)	Soybean oil Canola oil MCT oil	50 (44)	Sucrose Maltodextrin Fiber (pea fiber, oligofructose, inulin)	110 (44) (2.2 g soluble fiber, 3.8 insoluble fiber)	20	34	1000	800	14	350	Tube feeding and oral supplement for children with normal GI tract
Pediasure (Ross)	30 (1)	Na caseinate Whey protein concentrate	30 (12)	HO Safflower oil Soy oil MCT oil	50 (44)	Sugar Corn maltodextrin	110 (44)	16.5	33.5	970	802	14	Van, Straw, Banana Cream 430 Choc, Orange Cream 520	Tube feeding and oral supplement for children with normal GI tract
Pediasure Enteral (Ross)	30 (1)	Milk protein concentrate	30 (12)	HO Safflower oil Soy oil MCT oil	40 (35)	Corn maltodextrin Sugar	133 (53)	16.5	33.5	970	844	14	335	Tube feeding for children with normal GI tract
Pediasure Enteral with fiber (Ross)	30 (1)	Milk protein concentrate	30 (12)	HO Safflower oil Soy oil MCT oil	40 (35)	Corn maltodextrin Sugar Fiber (oat, soy and arabic fiber, fructooligo-saccharides)	138 (53) (8 g fiber)	16.5	33.5	970	844	14	345	Tube feeding for children with normal GI tract

continued

TABLE 20-14a

TODDLER AND YOUNG CHILD 1–10 YEARS (PER LITER)—*cont'd*

Formula	kcal/oz (kcal/ml)	Protein Source	Protein g (%kcal)	Fat Source (%)	Fat g (%kcal)	Carbohydrate Source (%)	Carbohydrate g (%kcal)	Na (mEq)	K (mEq)	Ca (mg)	P (mg)	Fe (mg)	Osmolality (mOsm/kg water)	Suggested Uses
Resource Just for Kids (Novartis)	30 (1)	Na caseinate Ca caseinate Whey protein concentrate	30 (12)	HO Sunflower oil Soy oil MCT oil	50 (44)	Hydrolyzed corn starch Sucrose Fructose (chocolate)	110 (44)	26	29	1140	800	14	Van, Straw 390 Choc 440	Tube feeding and oral supplement for children with normal GI tract
Resource Just for Kids Vanilla with fiber (Novartis)	30 (1)	Na caseinate Ca caseinate Whey protein concentrate	30 (12)	HO Sunflower oil Soy oil MCT oil	50 (44)	Hydrolyzed corn starch Sucrose Fiber (guar gum and soy fiber)	110 (44) (6 g fiber)	26	29	1140	800	14	390	Tube feeding and oral supplement for children with normal GI tract
Resource Just for Kids 1.5 Cal Vanilla (Novartis)	45 (1.5)	Na caseinate Ca caseinate Whey protein concentrate	42 (11)	HO Sunflower oil Soy oil MCT oil	75 (45)	Hydrolyzed corn starch Sucrose	165 (44)	30	33.5	1310	992	14	390	Tube feeding and oral supplement for children with normal GI tract who need additional calories

Resource Just for Kids 1.5 Cal Vanilla with fiber (Novartis)	45 (1.5)	Na caseinate Ca caseinate Whey protein concentrate	42 (11)	HO Sunflower oil Soy oil MCT oil	75 (45)	Hydrolyzed corn starch Sucrose Fiber (guar gum and soy fiber)	165 (44) (9 g fiber)	30	33.5	1310	992	14	405	Tube feeding and oral supplement for children with normal GI tract who need additional calories
Store Brand Milk-based Pediatric Nutritional Drink (PBM Products)	30 (1)	Na caseinate Whey protein concentrate	30 (12)	HO Safflower oil Soy oil MCT oil	50 (45)	Maltodextrin Sucrose	110 (44)	18	34	970	800	14	350	Tube feeding and oral supplement for children with normal GI tract

TABLE 20-14b

MODIFIED PROTEIN PEDIATRIC PRODUCTS AGES 1–10 YEARS (PER LITER)

		Protein		Fat		Carbohydrate								
Formula	kcal/oz (kcal/ml)	Source	g (%kcal)	Source (%)	g (%kcal)	Source (%)	g (%kcal)	Na (mEq)	K (mEq)	Ca (mg)	P (mg)	Fe (mg)	Osmolality (mOsm/kg water)	Suggested Uses
Elecare (Ross)	30 (1)	Free L-amino acids	30 (15)	HO safflower oil (39) MCT oil (33) Soy oil (28)	478.3 (42)	Corn syrup solids	108.5 (43)	20	39	1096	822	18	551	Children with malabsorption or protein allergy
Modulen IBD (Nestle)	30 (1)	Casein (transforming growth factor β2) (TGF-β2)	36 (14)	Milk fat MCT oil Corn oil	46 (42)	Corn syrup Sucrose	108 (44)	14.8	30.8	888	600	10.8	370	Children with Crohn's disease
Neocate Junior Unflavored (SHS)	30 (1)	Free L-amino acids	30 (12)	MCT oil (35) Canola oil HO safflower oil	50 (46)	Corn syrup solids	104 (42)	17.8	35	1130	940	14	607	Children with malabsorption or protein allergy
Neocate Junior Tropical Fruit (SHS)	30 (1)	Free L-amino acids	32 (13)	MCT oil (35) Canola oil HO safflower oil	49 (44)	Corn syrup solids	109 (43)	18.7	36.4	1180	977	14	690	Children with malabsorption or protein allergy

Neocate One + (SHS)	30 (1)	Free L-amino acids	25 (10)	MCT oil (35) Canola oil HO safflower oil	35 (32)	Corn syrup solids	146 (58)	8.7	24	620	620	7.7	610	Children with malabsorption or protein allergy
Pediatric E028 (SHS)	30 (1)	Free L-amino acids	25 (10)	MCT oil (35) Canola oil HO safflower oil	35 (32)	Maltodextrin Sucrose	146 (58)	8.7	23.8	620	620	7.7	820	Children with malabsorption or protein allergy
Pediatric Peptinex DT (Novartis)	30 (1)	Casein hydrolysate Free L-amino acids	30 (12)	MCT oil (50) Soy oil (50)	39 (33)	Maltodextrin Modified corn starch Fiber (guar gum and soy fiber)	138 (55) (6 g fiber)	30	26	1140	1000	14	290	Children with malabsorption
Pepdite One + (SHS)	30 (1)	Hydrolyzed protein (pork, soy) Free L-amino acids	31 (12)	MCT oil (35) Coconut oil HO safflower oil	50 (46)	Corn syrup solids	106 (42)	17.8	35	1130	940	14	Unflavored 430 Banana 440	Children with malabsorption
Peptamen Junior (Nestle)	30 (1)	Enzymatically hydrolyzed whey protein	31 (12)	MCT oil (60) Soy oil Canola oil	38.4 (33)	Maltodextrin Corn starch	138 (55)	20	34	1000	800	14	Unflavored 260 Vanilla 360	Children with malabsorption

continued

TABLE 20-14b

MODIFIED PROTEIN PEDIATRIC PRODUCTS AGES 1–10 YEARS (PER LITER)—*cont'd*

		Protein		Fat		Carbohydrate								
Formula	kcal/oz (kcal/ml)	Source	g (%kcal)	Source (%)	g (%kcal)	Source (%)	g (%kcal)	Na (mEq)	K (mEq)	Ca (mg)	P (mg)	Fe (mg)	Osmolality (mOsm/kg water)	Suggested Uses
Peptamen Junior with Prebio	30 (1)	Enzymatically hydrolyzed whey protein	31 (12)	MCT oil (60) Soy oil Canola oil	38.4 (33)	Maltodextrin Sucrose Corn starch Fiber (oligofructose, inulin)	138 (55)	20	34	1000	800	14	Unflavored 260 Vanilla 360	Children with malabsorption
Pro-Peptide for Kids (Hormel Health Labs)	30 (1)	Hydrolyzed whey protein	31 (12)	Canola oil MCT oil Soy oil	38 (34)	Maltodextrin Sucrose Corn starch	135 (54)	19.6	33	1215	980	24.7	—	Children with malabsorption
Tolerex (Novartis	30 (1)	Free L-amino acids	21 (8)	Safflower oil	1.5 (1)	Maltodextrin Modified corn starch	230 (91)	37	54	1000	1000	18	550	Children with malabsorption, intestinal lymphatic obstruction, chylothorax
Vivonex Pediatric (Novartis)	24 (0.8)	Free L-amino acids	24 (12)	MCT oil Soy oil	24 (25)	Maltodextrin Modified corn starch	130 (63)	20	36	1100	930	12	360	Children with malabsorption

TABLE 20-15a

OLDER CHILDREN AND ADULT STANDARD FORMULAS (PER LITER)

		Protein		Fat		Carbohydrate								
Formula	kcal/oz (kcal/ml)	Source	g (%kcal)	Source (%)	g (%kcal)	Source (%)	g (%kcal)	Na (mEq)	K (mEq)	Ca (mg)	P (mg)	Fe (mg)	Osmolality (mOsm/kg water)	Suggested Uses
Compleat (Novartis)	32 (1.07)	Na caseinate Chicken	48 (18)	Canola oil Chicken	40 (34)	Hydrolyzed corn starch Vegetables Fruits	128 (48)	43	44	760	760	14	340	Blenderized tube feeding for patients with normal GI tract
Ensure (Ross)	32 (1.06)	Ca caseinate Soy protein isolate Whey protein concentrate	35 (14)	HO safflower oil (40) Canola oil (40) Corn oil (20)	24.4 (22)	Sucrose Corn syrup Corn maltodextrin	160 (64)	35	38	1200	1000	18	590	Oral supplement or tube feeding for patients with normal GI tract
Isocal (Novartis)	32 (1.06)	Ca caseinate Na caseinate Soy protein isolate	34 (13)	Soy oil MCT oil (20)	44 (37)	Maltodextrin	135 (50)	23	34	630	530	9.5	270	Tube feeding for patients with normal GI tract
Isocal HN (Novartis)	32 (1.06)	Ca caseinate Na caseinate Soy protein isolate	44 (17)	Soy oil MCT oil (20)	45 (37)	Maltodextrin	124 (46)	40	41	850	850	15	270	Tube feeding for patients with normal GI tract
Jevity 1 Cal (Ross)	32 (1.06)	Ca caseinate Na caseinate Soy protein isolate	44 (17)	HO safflower oil Canola oil MCT oil	35 (29)	Maltodextrin (66) Corn syrup solids (22) Soy fiber (12)	155 (54) (14.4 g fiber)	40	40	910	760	14	300	Tube feeding for patients with normal GI tract

continued

TABLE 20-15a

OLDER CHILDREN AND ADULT STANDARD FORMULAS (PER LITER)—*cont'd*

		Protein		Fat		Carbohydrate								
Formula	kcal/oz (kcal/ml)	Source	g (%kcal)	Source (%)	g (%kcal)	Source (%)	g (%kcal)	Na (mEq)	K (mEq)	Ca (mg)	P (mg)	Fe (mg)	Osmolality (mOsm/kg water)	Suggested Uses
Nutren 1.0 (Nestle)	30 (1)	Ca-K caseinate	40 (16)	Canola oil MCT oil (25) Corn oil	38 (33)	Maltodextrin Corn syrup solids	127 (51)	38	32	668	668	12	Unflavored 315 Vanilla 370	Oral supplement or tube feeding for patients with normal GI tract
Nutren Fiber (Nestle)	30 (1)	Ca-K caseinate	40 (16)	Canola oil MCT oil (25) Corn oil	38 (33)	Maltodextrin Corn syrup solids Fiber (pea and oligofructose and inulin fiber)	127 (51) 14 g fiber)	38	32	668	668	12	Unflavored 330 Vanilla 410	Oral supplement or tube feeding for patients with normal GI tract
Osmolite (Ross)	32 (1.06)	Ca caseinate Na caseinate	37 (14)	HO safflower oil Canola oil MCT oil	35 (29)	Corn maltodextrin	151 (57)	28	26	535	535	10	300	Tube feeding for patients with normal GI tract
Ultracal (Novartis)	32 (1.06)	Milk protein concentrate Casein	45 (17)	Canola oil MCT oil HO sunflower oil Corn oil	39 (33)	Maltodextrin Fiber (microcrystalline cellulose, soy and acacia)	142 (50) (13.6 g fiber)	59	47	1000	1000	18	300	Tube feeding for patients with normal GI tract

TABLE 20-15b

OLDER CHILDEN AND ADULT MODIFIED PROTEIN FORMULAS (PER LITER)

Formula	kcal/oz (kcal/ml)	Protein Source	Protein g (%kcal)	Fat Source (%)	Fat g (%kcal)	Carbohydrate Source (%)	Carbohydrate g (%kcal)	Na (mEq)	K (mEq)	Ca (mg)	P (mg)	Fe (mg)	Osmolality (mOsm/kg water)	Suggested Uses
Crucial (Nestle)	45 (1.5)	Enzymatically hydrolyzed casein L-arginine (15 g)	94 (25)	MCT oil (50) Fish oil (DHA & EPA) Soy oil	67.6 (39)	Maltodextrin	135 (36)	51	48	1000	1000	18	490	High calorie, high protein for immune support and wound healing
Criticare (Novartis)	32 (1.06)	Casein hydrolysate Free L-amino acids	38 (14)	Safflower oil Emulsifiers	5.3 (4.5)	Maltodextrin Modified corn starch	220 (81)	27	34	530	530	9.7	650	Patients with malabsorption
f.a.a. (Nestle)	30 (1)	L-amino acids	50 (20)	Soy oil MCT oil	11.2 (10)	Maltodextrin Corn starch	176 (70)	24.3	38.5	800	700	18	700	Patients with malabsorption
IntensiCal (Novartis)	39 (1.3)	Casein hydrolysate L-arginine	81 (25)	Canola oil MCT oil HO sunflower oil Corn oil Menhaden oil	42 (29)	Maltodextrin Modified corn starch	150 (46)	48	33	1130	1080	18	550	High calorie, high protein for critically ill patients

continued

TABLE 20-15b
OLDER CHILDEN AND ADULT MODIFIED PROTEIN FORMULAS (PER LITER)—*cont'd*

Formula	kcal/oz (kcal/ml)	Protein Source	Protein g (%kcal)	Fat Source (%)	Fat g (%kcal)	Carbohydrate Source (%)	Carbohydrate g (%kcal)	Na (mEq)	K (mEq)	Ca (mg)	P (mg)	Fe (mg)	Osmolality (mOsm/kg water)	Suggested Uses
Optimental (Ross)	30 (1)	Soy protein hydrolysate Partially hydrolyzed Na caseinate L-arginine	51 (21)	Sardine oil/ MCT structured lipid (60) Canola oil (18) Soy oil (18) Emulsifiers (4)	28 (25)	Maltodextrin (56) Sucrose (60) Fructooligo-saccharides (4)	139 (55) (5 g fiber)	46	45	1055	1055	13	540	Oral supplement or tube feeding high calorie, high protein for critically ill patients and/or malabsorption
Peptamen (Nestle)	30 (1)	Enzymatically hydrolyzed whey protein	40 (16)	MCT oil (70) Soy oil	39 (33)	Maltodextrin Corn starch	127 (51)	24	38.5	800	700	18	Unflavored 270 Vanilla 380	Oral supplement or tube feeding for patients with malabsorption
Peptamen with Prebio (Nestle)	30 (1)	Enzymatically hydrolyzed whey protein	40 (16)	MCT oil (70) Soy oil	39 (33)	Maltodextrin Corn starch Fiber (inulin and oligofructose fiber)	127 (51) (4 g fiber)	24	38.5	800	700	18	300	Oral supplement or tube feeding for patients with malabsorption

Peptamen 1.5 (Nestle)	45 (1.5)	Enzymatically hydrolyzed whey protein	67.6 (18)	MCT oil (70) Soy oil	56 (33)	Maltodextrin Corn starch	188 (49)	44	48	1000	1000	27	Unflavored 550 Vanilla 550	Oral supplement or tube feeding for patients with malabsorption requiring additional calories
Peptamen VHP (Nestle)	30 (1)	Enzymatically hydrolyzed whey protein	62.5 (25)	MCT oil (70) Soy oil	39 (33)	Maltodextrin Corn starch	104.5 (42)	24	38.5	800	700	18	Unflavored 270 Vanilla 380	Oral supplement or tube feeding for patients with malabsorption requiring additional protein
Peptinex DT (Novartis)	30 (1)	Casein hydrolysate Free L-amino acids	50 (20)	MCT oil (50) Soy oil (50)	17.4 (15)	Maltodextrin Modified corn starch	164 (65)	44	31	670	670	12	460	Tube feeding for patients with malabsorption
Subdue (Novartis)	30 (1)	Hydrolyzed whey protein concentrate (RTU) Casein hydrolysate (RTH)	50 (20)	MCT oil Canola oil HO sunflower oil Corn oil Milk fat (RTU)	34 (30)	Maltodextrin Modified corn starch Sugar (flavored)	130 (50)	48	41	1100	1050	15.3	RTU Unflavored 330 RTH 440 RTU Flavored 525	Oral supplement or tube feeding for patients with malabsorption

continued

TABLE 20-15b

OLDER CHILDEN AND ADULT MODIFIED PROTEIN FORMULAS (PER LITER)—*cont'd*

		Protein		Fat		Carbohydrate								
Formula	kcal/oz (kcal/ml)	Source	g (%kcal)	Source (%)	g (%kcal)	Source (%)	g (%kcal)	Na (mEq)	K (mEq)	Ca (mg)	P (mg)	Fe (mg)	Osmolality (mOsm/kg water)	Suggested Uses
Subdue Plus (Novartis)	45 (1.5)	Hydrolyzed whey protein concentrate	76 (20)	MCT oil Canola oil HO sunflower oil Corn oil Milk fat	51 (30)	Maltodextrin Modified corn starch	186 (50)	51	51	1390	1310	19	400	Oral supplement or tube feeding for patients with malabsorption requiring additional calories
Vital HN (Ross)	30 (1)	Partially hydrolyzed whey, meat and soy Free L-amino acids	42 (17)	Safflower oil (55) MCT oil (45)	11 (10)	Maltodextrin (>82.5) Sucrose (17) Lactose (<0.5)	185 (74)	25	36	667	667	12	500	Oral supplement or tube feeding for patients with malabsorption
Vivonex Plus (Novartis)	30 (1)	Free L-amino acids	45 (18)	Soy oil	6.7 (6)	Maltodextrin Modified corn starch	190 (76)	27	27	560	560	10	650	Tube feeding for patients with malabsorption
Vivonex T.E.N. (Novartis)	30 (1)	Free L-amino acids	38 (15)	Safflower oil	2.8 (3)	Maltodextrin Modified corn starch	210 (82)	26	24	500	500	9	630	Tube feeding for patients with malabsorption

TABLE 20-15c

OLDER CHILDREN AND ADULT CONCENTRATED CALORIES AND/OR PROTEIN FORMULAS (PER LITER)

		Protein		Fat		Carbohydrate								
Formula	kcal/oz (kcal/ml)	Source	g (%kcal)	Source (%)	g (%kcal)	Source (%)	g (%kcal)	Na (mEq)	K (mEq)	Ca (mg)	P (mg)	Fe (mg)	Osmolality (mOsm/kg water)	Suggested Uses
Deliver 2.0 (Novartis)	60 (2)	Ca caseinate Na caseinate	75 (15)	Soy oil (70) MCT oil (30)	101 (45)	Corn syrup	200 (40)	35	43	1010	1010	18	640	High calorie, high protein oral supplement or tube feeding
Ensure Plus (Ross)	45 (1.5)	Ca caseinate Na caseinate Soy protein isolate	54 (15)	Canola oil (50) Corn oil (25) HO Safflower oil (25)	47.5 (29)	Corn syrup Corn maltodextrin Sucrose	208 (56)	43	47	800	800	18	680	High calorie oral supplement or tube feeding
Ensure Plus HN Vanilla (Ross)	45 (1.5)	Ca caseinate Na caseinate Soy protein isolate	62 (17)	Corn oil	49 (30)	Corn maltodextrin (70) Sucrose (30)	197 (53)	51	46	1041	1041	18.8	650	High calorie, high protein oral supplement or tube feeding
Isocal HN Plus (Novartis)	36 (1.2)	Milk protein concentrate Casein (in RTH only)	54 (18)	Canola oil HO Sunflower oil Corn oil	40 (29)	Maltodextrin	156 (53)	59	47	1000	1000	18	390–400	High calorie, high protein tube feeding

continued

TABLE 20-15c

OLDER CHILDREN AND ADULT CONCENTRATED CALORIES AND/OR PROTEIN FORMULAS (PER LITER)—*cont'd*

		Protein		Fat		Carbohydrate								
Formula	kcal/oz (kcal/ml)	Source	g (%kcal)	Source (%)	g (%kcal)	Source (%)	g (%kcal)	Na (mEq)	K (mEq)	Ca (mg)	P (mg)	Fe (mg)	Osmolality (mOsm/kg water)	Suggested Uses
Jevity 1.2 Car (Ross)	36 (1.2)	Ca caseinate Na caseinate Soy protein isolate	56 (19)	HO safflower oil Canola oil MCT oil	39 (29)	Corn syrup solids (51) Maltodextrin (34) Fiber (soy and oat) (8.5) Fructooligo-saccharides (6.5)	155 (54) (22 g fiber)	59	47	1200	1200	18	450	High calorie, high protein tube feeding
Jevity 1.5 Cal (Ross)	45 (1.5)	Ca caseinate Na caseinate Soy protein isolate	64 (17)	HO safflower oil Canola oil MCT oil	50 (29)	Corn syrup solids (45) Maltodextrin (44) Fiber (soy and oat) (6) Fructooligo-saccharides (5)	216 (54) (22 g fiber)	61	55	1200	1200	18	525	High calorie, high protein tube feeding
Nutren 1.5 (Nestle)	45 (1.5)	Ca-K caseinate	60 (16)	MCT oil (50) Canola oil Corn oil	67.6 (39)	Maltodextrin	169 (45)	51	48	1000	1000	18	Unflavored 430 Vanilla 510	High calorie, high protein oral supplement or tube feeding

Nutren 2.0 (Nestle)	60 (2)	Ca-K caseinate	80 (16)	MCT oil (75) Canola oil Corn oil	104 (45)	Corn syrup solids Maltodextrin Sugar	196 (39)	57	49	1340	1340	24	745	High calorie, high protein oral supplement or tube feeding
Promote (Rose)	30 (1)	Ca caseinate Na caseinate Soy protein isolate	62.5 (25)	HO safflower oil Canola oil MCT oil	26 (23)	Corn maltodextrin (91) Sucrose (9)	130 (52)	44	51	1200	1200	18	340	High protein oral supplement or tube feeding
Promote with fiber (Ross)	30 (1)	Ca caseinate Na caseinate Soy protein isolate	62.5 (25)	HO safflower oil Canola oil MCT oil	28 (25)	Corn maltodextrin (76) Sucrose (12) Fiber (oat and soy) (12)	138 (50)	57	54	1200	1200	18	380	High protein oral supplement or tube feeding
Replete (Nestle)	30 (1)	Ca-K caseinate	62.4 (25)	Canola oil MCT oil (25)	34 (30)	Maltodextrin	113 (45)	38	38	1000	1000	18	Unflavored 300 Vanilla 350	High protein oral supplement or tube feeding

continued

TABLE 20-15c

OLDER CHILDREN AND ADULT CONCENTRATED CALORIES AND/OR PROTEIN FORMULAS (PER LITER)—*cont'd*

		Protein		Fat		Carbohydrate								
Formula	kcal/oz (kcal/ml)	Source	g (%kcal)	Source (%)	g (%kcal)	Source (%)	g (%kcal)	Na (mEq)	K (mEq)	Ca (mg)	P (mg)	Fe (mg)	Osmolality (mOsm/kg water)	Suggested Uses
Replete with fiber (Nestle)	30 (1)	Ca-K caseinate	62.4 (25)	Canola oil MCT oil (25)	34 (30)	Maltodextrin Corn syrup solids Fiber (soy polysaccharides)	113 (45) (14 g fiber)	38	38	1000	1000	18	Unflavored 310 Vanilla 390	High protein oral supplement or tube feeding
TramaCal (Novartis)	45 (1.5)	Ca caseinate Na caseinate	82 (22)	Soy oil MCT oil	68 (40)	Corn syrup Sugar	144 (38)	51	36	750	750	8.9	560	High calorie, high protein oral supplement or tube feeding
Ultracal HN Plus (Novartis)	36 (1.2)	Milk protein concentrate casein (in RTH only)	54 (18)	Canola oil MCT oil HO sunflower oil Corn oil	40 (29)	Maltodextrin Fiber (microcrystalline cellulose, soy, and acacia)	156 (53) (10 g fiber)	59	47	1000	1000	18	370	High calorie, high protein tube feeding

TABLE 20-15d

OLDER CHILDREN AND ADULT SPECIAL FORMULAS (PER LITER)

		Protein		Fat		Carbohydrate								
Formula	kcal/oz (kcal/ml)	Source	g (%kcal)	Source (%)	g (%kcal)	Source (%)	g (%kcal)	Na (mEq)	K (mEq)	Ca (mg)	P (mg)	Fe (mg)	Osmolality (mOsm/kg water)	Suggested Uses
Glucerna (Ross)	30 (1)	Ca caseinate Na caseinate	42 (17)	HO safflower oil Canola oil	55 (49)	Maltodextrin (61) Soy fiber (20) Fructose (19)	96 (34) (14.4 g fiber)	40	40	705	705	13	355	Oral supplement or tube feeding for patients with impaired glucose tolerance
Glytrol (Nestle)	30 (1)	Ca-K caseinate	45 (18)	Canola oil HO safflower oil MCT oil	47.6 (42)	Maltodextrin Modified corn starch Fiber (pea, gum arabic, oligofructose and inulin)	100 (40) (15 g fiber)	32	36	720	720	12.8	280	Oral supplement or tube feeding for patients with impaired glucose tolerance
Lipisorb (Novartis)	40 (1.35)	Ca caseinate Na caseinate	57 (17)	MCT oil Soy oil	57 (35)	Maltodextrin Sugar	161 (48)	59	43	850	850	15.2	630	Patients with fat malabsorption
Magnacal Renal (Novartis)	60 (2)	Ca caseinate Na caseinate	75 (15)	Canola oil HO sunflower oil MCT oil Corn oil	101 (45)	Maltodextrin Sugar	200 (40)	35	32	1010	800	18.2	570	Oral supplement or tube feeding for dialysis patients
Nepro (Ross)	60 (2)	Ca caseinate Na caseinate Mg caseinate Milk protein isolate	70 (14)	HO safflower oil Canola oil	96 (43)	Corn syrup solids Sucrose Fructooligo-saccharides	223 (43)	37	27	1370	605	19	665	Oral supplement or tube feeding for dialysis patients

continued

TABLE 20-15d

OLDER CHILDREN AND ADULT SPECIAL FORMULAS (PER LITER)—*cont'd*

		Protein		Fat		Carbohydrate								
Formula	kcal/oz (kcal/ml)	Source	g (%kcal)	Source (%)	g (%kcal)	Source (%)	g (%kcal)	Na (mEq)	K (mEq)	Ca (mg)	P (mg)	Fe (mg)	Osmolality (mOsm/kg water)	Suggested Uses
NutriRenal (Nestle)	60 (2)	Ca-K caseinate	70 (14)	MCT oil (50) Canola oil Corn oil	104 (46)	Corn syrup solids Maltodextrin Sucrose	204 (40)	32	32	1400	700	24	650	Oral supplement or tube feeding for dialysis patients
Renalcal (Nestle)	60 (2)	Whey protein concentrate Amino acid blend	34.4 (7)	MCT oil (70) Canola oil Corn oil	82.4 (35)	Maltodextrin Corn starch	290 (58)	—	—	—	—	—	600	Oral supplement or tube feeding for patients with acute renal failure not receiving dialysis
Store Brand Diabetic Nutritional Drink (PBM Products)	30 (1)	Caseinates Soy protein isolate	42.5 (20)	HO safflower oil Canola oil	50 (40)	Maltodextrin Fiber (inulin, fiberso1–2)	80 (36)	40	40	705	705	13	335	Oral supplement or tube feeding for patients with impaired glucose tolerance
Suplena (Ross)	60 (2)	Ca caseinate Na caseinate	30 (6)	HO safflower oil Soy oil	96 (43)	Maltodextrin (90) Sugar (10)	255 (51)	34	29	1390	730	19	600	Oral supplement or tube feeding for patients with acute or chronic renal failure not receiving dialysis

TABLE 20-15e

OLDER CHILDREN AND ADULT ORAL SUPPLEMENTS (PER LITER)

Formula	kcal/oz (kcal/ml)	Protein Source	Protein g (%kcal)	Fat Source (%)	Fat g (%kcal)	Carbohydrate Source (%)	Carbohydrate g (%kcal)	Na (mEq)	K (mEq)	Ca (mg)	P (mg)	Fe (mg)	Osmolality (mOsm/kg water)	Suggested Uses
Boost Drink Vanilla (Novartis)	30 (1)	Milk protein concentrate	42 (17)	Canola oil HO sunflower oil Corn oil	17.8 (16)	Corn syrup solids Sugar	173 (67)	24	43	1390	1310	19	610–670	Oral supplement
Boost with fiber (Novartis)	30 (1)	Milk protein concentrate	43 (17)	Canola oil HO sunflower oil Corn oil	17.8 (16)	Corn syrup solids Sugar Fiber (soy, acacia microcrystalline cellulose fibers)	178 (67) (11 g fiber)	31	41	1390	1310	19	480	Oral supplement
Boost Plus (Novartis)	45 (1.5)	Milk protein concentrate Ca caseinate Na caseinate	59 (16)	Canola oil HO sunflower oil Corn oil	58 (34)	Corn syrup solids Sugar	200 (50)	31	41	1390	1310	19	720	High calorie oral supplement
Boost High Protein (Novartis)	30 (1)	Milk protein concentrate Ca caseinate Na caseinate	61 (24)	Canola oil HO sunflower oil Corn oil	23 (21)	Corn syrup solids Sugar	139 (55)	31	41	1390	1310	19	Vanilla, strawberry 540 Chocolate 610	High protein oral supplement
Carnation Instant Breakfast with whole milk (Nestle)	32 (1.06)	Cow's milk protein	49 (18)	Butterfat	30 (26)	Lactose Maltodextrin Sucrose	147 (56)	36	62	1885	1885	17	590	Oral supplement

continued

TABLE 20-15e

OLDER CHILDREN AND ADULT ORAL SUPPLEMENTS (PER LITER)—*cont'd*

		Protein		Fat		Carbohydrate								
Formula	kcal/oz (kcal/ml)	Source	g (%kcal)	Source (%)	g (%kcal)	Source (%)	g (%kcal)	Na (mEq)	K (mEq)	Ca (mg)	P (mg)	Fe (mg)	Osmolality (mOsm/kg water)	Suggested Uses
Carnation Instant Breakfast Lactose Free (Nestle)	30 (1)	Ca caseinate	35 (14)	Canola oil Corn oil	37 (35)	Corn syrup solids Sugar	134 (51)	38	32	500	500	9	480–490	Oral supplement for lactose malabsorpiton
Carnation Instant Breakfast Lactose Free Plus (Nestle)	45 (1.5)	Ca caseinate	52 (14)	Canola oil Corn oil	65 (39)	Corn syrup solids Sugar	176 (47)	51	48	748	748	13.6	620	High calorie oral supplement for lactose malabsorption
Carnation Instant Breakfast VHC (Nestle)	67.5 (2.25)	Ca-K caseinate Isolated soy protein	90 (16)	Canola oil Corn oil	122 (50)	Corn syrup solids Sugar	197 (34)	50	45	1232	1232	22.5	950	High calorie, high protein oral supplement
Enlive (Ross)	37.5 (1.25)	Whey protein isolate	41 (13)	—	—	Maltodextrin (75) Sugar (25)	267 (87)	11.5	4	247	82	11.1	840	Oral clear liquid supplement
NUTRA Shake (Nutra-Balance)	50 (1.67)	Milk protein concentrate Cow's milk protein	50 (12)	Soy oil	50 (27)	Corn syrup	258 (61)	20	45	1667	1250	—	—	High calorie oral supplement
Scandishake with whole milk (Axcan Pharma, Inc)	60 (2)	Cow's milk Na caseinate	43 (9)	Partially hydrogenated vegetable oil Coconut oil Soy oil MCT oil	97 (44)	Maltodextrin Sugar Lactose Corn syrup solids	230 (47)	35	60	N/A	N/A	N/A	N/A	High calorie oral supplement for patients with cystic fibrosis

TABLE 20-16

ORAL REHYDRATION SOLUTIONS

Solution	Kcal/mL (kcal/oz)	Carbohydrate (g/L)	Na (mEq/L)	K (mEq/L)	Osmolality (mOsm/kg H_2O)
CeraLyte-70 (Cera)	0.16 (4.9)	Rice digest 40	70	20	232
CeraLyte-50 (Cera)	0.16 (4.9)	Rice digest, glucose 40	50	20	200
Enfalyte (Mead Johnson)	0.12 (3.7)	Rice syrup solids 30	50	25	200
Oral Rehydration Salts (WHO) (Jianas)	0.06 (2)	Dextrose 20	90	20	330
Pedialyte Unflavored (Ross)	0.1 (3)	Dextrose 25	45	20	250
Rehydralyte (Ross)	0.1 (3)	Dextrose 25	75	20	305

TABLE 20-17

INITIATION AND ADVANCEMENT OF PARENTERAL NUTRITION*

Nutrient	Initial Dose	Advancement	Maximum
Glucose	5%–10%	2.5%–5%/day	12.5% peripheral 18 mg/kg/min (maximum rate of infusion)
Protein	1 g/kg/day	0.5–1 g/kg/day	3 g/kg/day 10%–16% of calories
Fat	0.5–1 g/kg/day	1 g/kg/day	4 g/kg/day 0.17 g/kg/hr (maximum rate of infusion)

*Acceptable osmolarity of parenteral nutrition through a peripheral line varies between 900 and 1050 osm/L by institution. An estimate of the osmolarity of parenteral nutrition can be obtained with the following formula: Estimated osmolarity = (dextrose concentration × 50) + (amino acid concentration × 100) + (mEq of electrolytes × 2). Consult individual pharmacy for hospital limitations.

Modified from Baker RD, Baker SS, Davis AM: Pediatric Parenteral Nutrition. New York, Chapman and Hall, 1997; and Cox JH, Cooning SW: Parenteral nutrition. In Samour PQ, Helm KK, Lang CE (eds): Handbook of Pediatric Nutrition. Gaithersburg. MD, Aspen, 1999.

TABLE 20-18

DAILY PARENTERAL NUTRIENT RECOMMENDATIONS

Component	0–1 yr	1–7 yr	>7 yr
Energy (kcal/kg)	80–120	55–90	55–75
Protein (g/kg)	2–3	1.5–2.5	1.5–2.5
Sodium (mEq/kg)	3–4	2–4	2–4
Potassium (mEq/kg)	2–3	2–3	2–3
Magnesium (mEq/kg)	0.25–1	0.25–1	0.25–1
Calcium (mg/kg)	40–60	10–50	10–50
Phosphorus (mg/kg)	20–45	15–40	15–40
Zinc (mcg/kg)	400 (preterm) 100	100	100 (maximum 4 mg/day)
Copper (μg/kg)	20	20	20 (maximum 1.5 mg/day)
Chromium (μg/kg)	0.2	0.2	0.2 (maximum 15 mg/day)
Manganese (μg/kg)	2–10	2–10	2–10 (maximum 0.8 mg/day)
Selenium (μg/kg)	3	3	3 (maximum 40 mg/day)

Modified from Baker RD. Baker SS, Davis AM: Pediatric Parenteral Nutrition. New York, Chapman and Hail, 1997; and Cox JH, Cooning SW: Parenteral nutrition. In Samour PQ, Helm KK, Lang CE (eds): Handbook of Pediatric Nutrition. Gaithersburg. MD, Aspen, 1999.

TABLE 20-19

MONITORING SCHEDULE FOR PATIENTS RECEIVING PARENTERAL NUTRITION*

Variable	Initial Period†	Later Period‡
GROWTH		
Weight	Daily	2 times/wk
Height	Weekly (infants) Monthly	Monthly
Head circumference (infants)	Weekly	Monthly§
Arm circumference	Monthly	Monthly
Skin-fold thickness	Monthly	Monthly
LABORATORY STUDIES		
Electrolytes and glucose	Daily until stable	Weekly
BUN/creatlnine	2 times/wk	Weekly
Albumin or prealbumin	Weekly	Weekly
Ca^{2+}, Mg^{2+}, P	2 times/wk	Weekly
ALT, AST, Alk P	Weekly	Weekly
Total and direct bilirubin	Weekly	Weekly
CBC	Weekly	Weekly
Triglycerides	With each increase	Weekly
Vitamins	—	As indicated
Trace minerals	—	As indicated

*For patients on long-term parenteral nutrition, monitoring every 2 to 4 weeks is adequate in most cases.

†The period before nutritional goals are reached or during any period of instability.

‡When stability is reached, no changes in nutrient composition.

§Weekly in preterm infants.

Alk P, Alkaline phosphatase; *ALT*, alanine transaminase; *AST*, aspartate transaminase; *BUN*, blood urea nitrogen; *CBC*, complete blood count.

REFERENCES

1. Centers for Disease Control and Prevention (CDC) [Online]. Available: www.cdc.gov/growth.
2. Food and Nutrition Board, National Research Council: Dietary Reference Intakes: Energy. Washington, DC, National Academy Press, 2004.
3. Frankel HM: Body mass index graphics for children. Pediatrics 2004;113(2): 425–426.
4. Barlow SE, Dietz WH: Obesity evaluation and treatment: expert committee recommendations. Pediatrics 1998;102(3):7.
5. Dewey KG, et al: Protein requirements of infants and children. Eur J Clin Nutr 1996;50:S119–S150.
6. Food and Nutrition Board, National Research Council: Dietary Reference Intakes: Applications in Dietary Planning. Washington, DC, National Academy Press, 2003.
7. Food and Nutrition Board, National Research Council: Dietary Reference Intakes for Energy, Carbohydrate, Fiber, Fat, Fatty Acids, Cholesterol, Protein, and Amino Acids (Macronutrients). Washington, DC, National Academy Press, 2002.
8. Food and Nutrition Board, National Research Council: Dietary Reference Intakes for Vitamin A, Vitamin K, Arsenic, Boron, Chromium, Copper, Iodine, Iron, Manganese, Molybdenum, Nickel, Silicon, Vanadium, and Zinc. Washington, DC, National Academy Press, 2000.
9. Kleinman RE (ed), and the Committee on Nutrition of the AAP: Pediatric Nutrition Handbook, 5th ed. Illinois, American Academy of Pediatrics 2004.

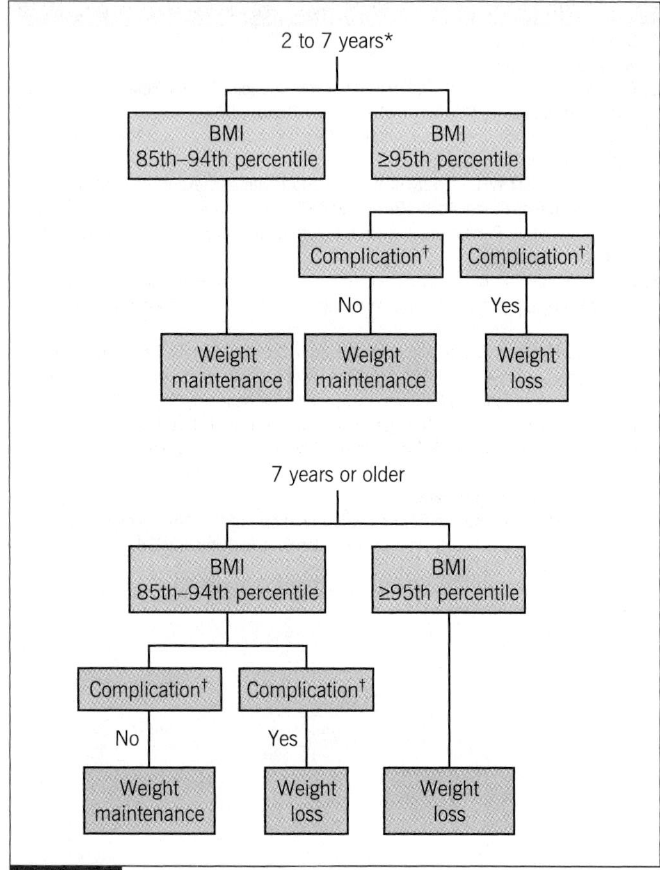

FIG. 20-1

Obesity decision tree. Recommendations for obesity management. *, Indicates that children younger than 2 years should be referred to a pediatric obesity center for treatment. †, Indicates complications such as mild hypertension, dyslipidemias, and insulin resistance. Patients with acute complications, such as pseudotumor cerebri, sleep apnea, obesity hypoventilation syndrome, or orthopedic problems, should be referred to a pediatric obesity center. Weight maintenance implies no change in weight while child grows in height. *(Modified from Barlow SE, Dietz WH: Pediatrics 1998;102[3]:7.)*

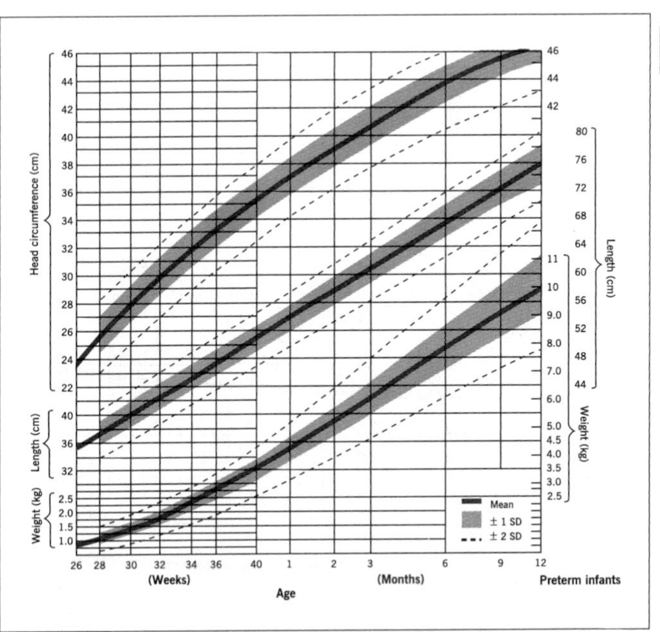

FIG. 20-2

Length, weight, and head circumference for preterm infants. *(Modified from Babson SG, Benda GI: J Pediatr 1976;89:815.)*

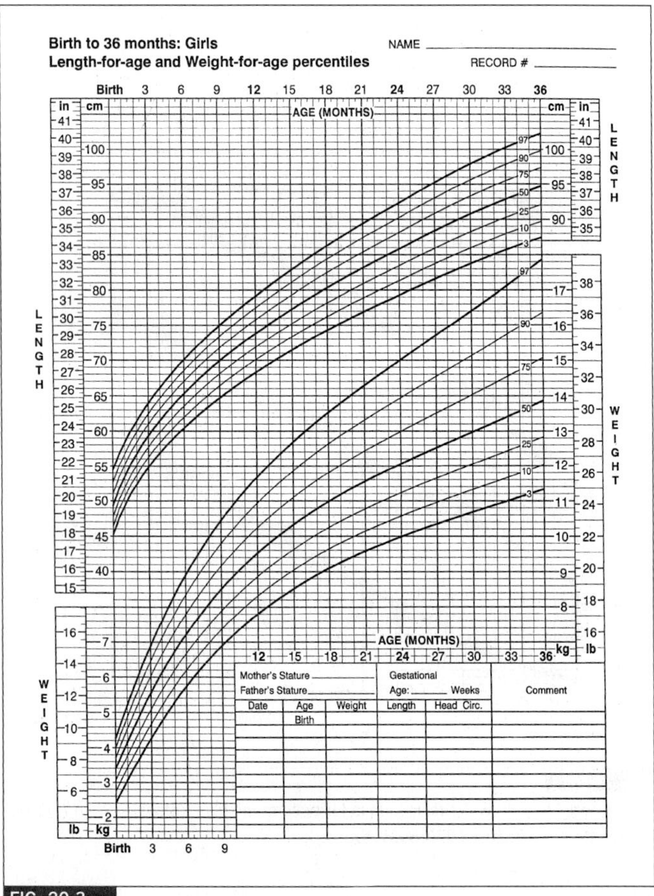

FIG. 20-3

Length and weight for girls, from birth to 36 months. *(Developed by the National Center for Health Statistics in collaboration with the National Center for Chronic Disease Prevention and Health Promotion, 2000.)*

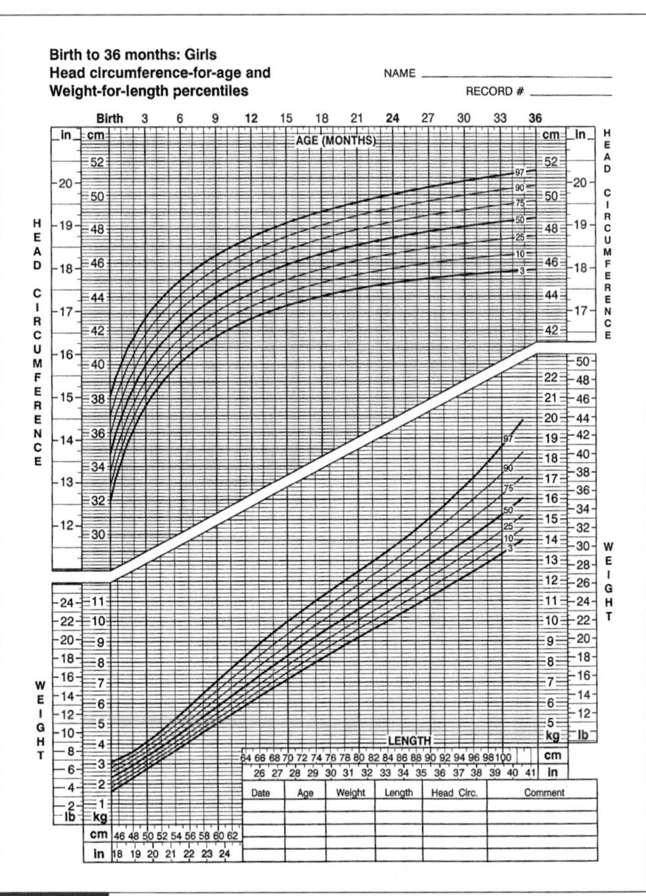

FIG. 20-4

Head circumference and length-to-weight ratio for girls, from birth to 36 months. *(Developed by the National Center for Health Statistics in collaboration with the National Center for Chronic Disease Prevention and Health Promotion, 2000.)*

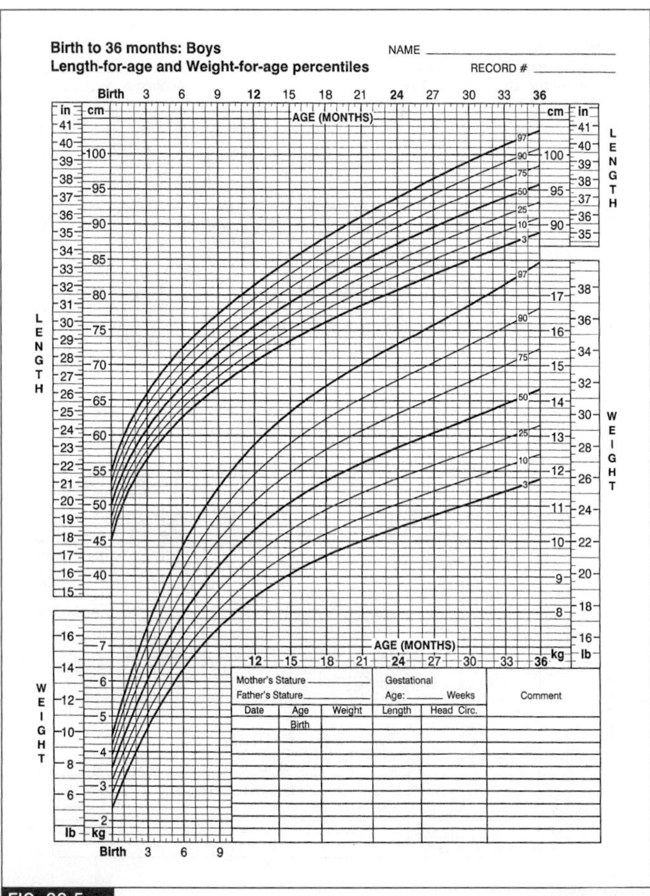

FIG. 20-5

Length and weight for boys, from birth to 36 months. *(Developed by the National Center for Health Statistics in collaboration with the National Center for Chronic Disease Prevention and Health Promotion, 2000.)*

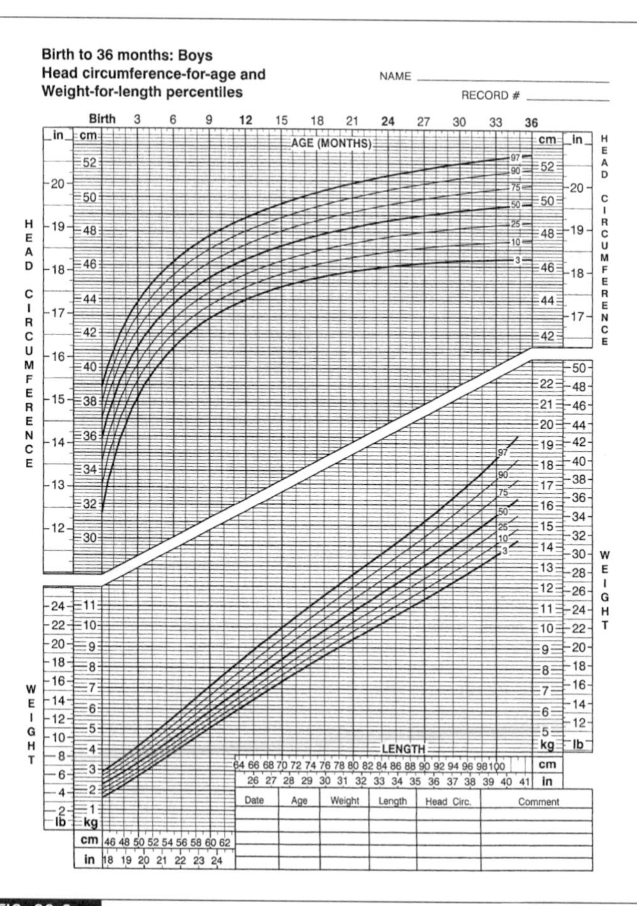

FIG. 20-6

Head circumference and length-to-weight ratio for boys, from birth to 36 months. *(Developed by the National Center for Health Statistics in collaboration with the National Center for Chronic Disease Prevention and Health Promotion, 2000.)*

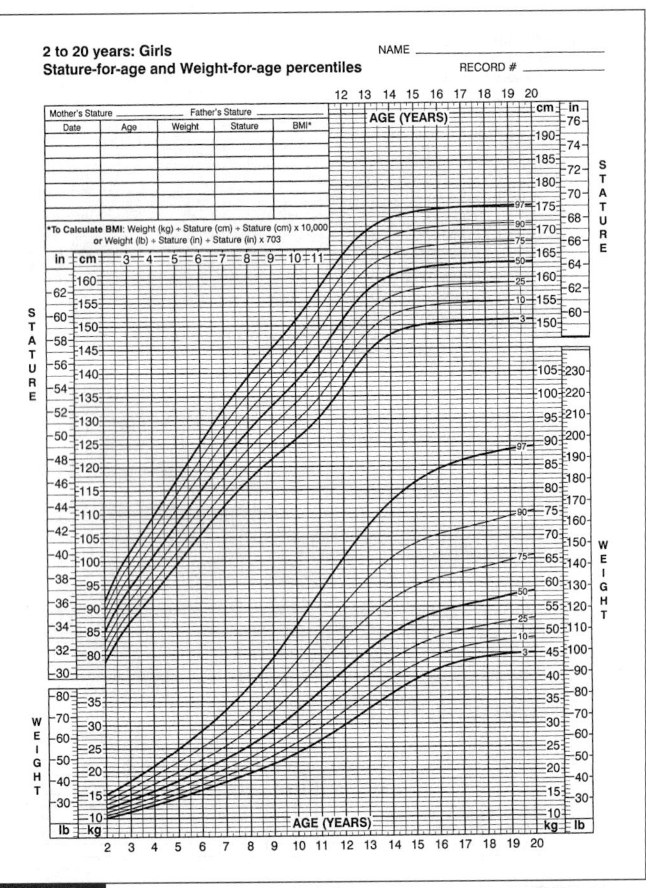

FIG. 20-7

Stature and weight for girls 2 to 20 years. *(Developed by the National Center for Health Statistics in collaboration with the National Center for Chronic Disease Prevention and Health Promotion, 2000.)*

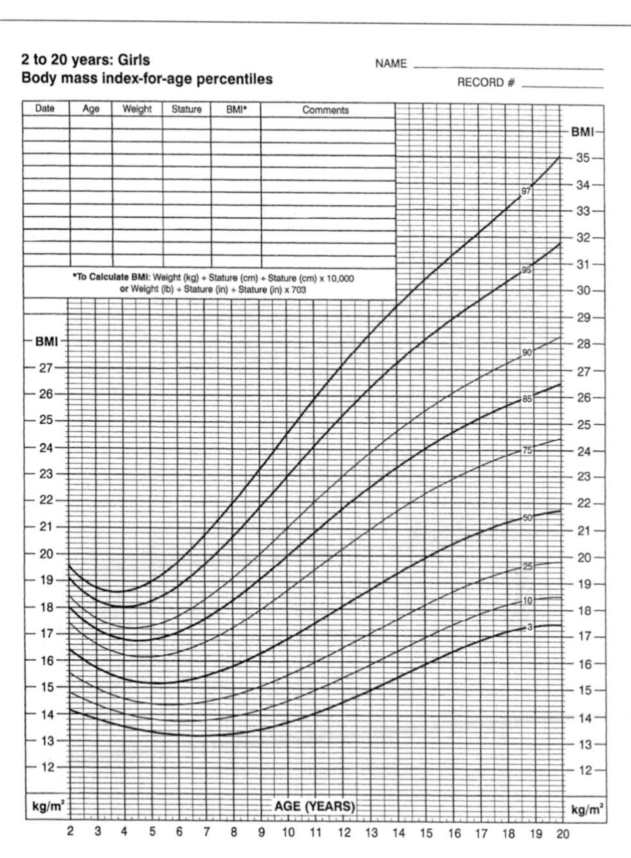

FIG. 20-8

Body mass index for girls 2 to 20 years. *(Developed by the National Center for Health Statistics in collaboration with the National Center for Chronic Disease Prevention and Health Promotion, 2000.)*

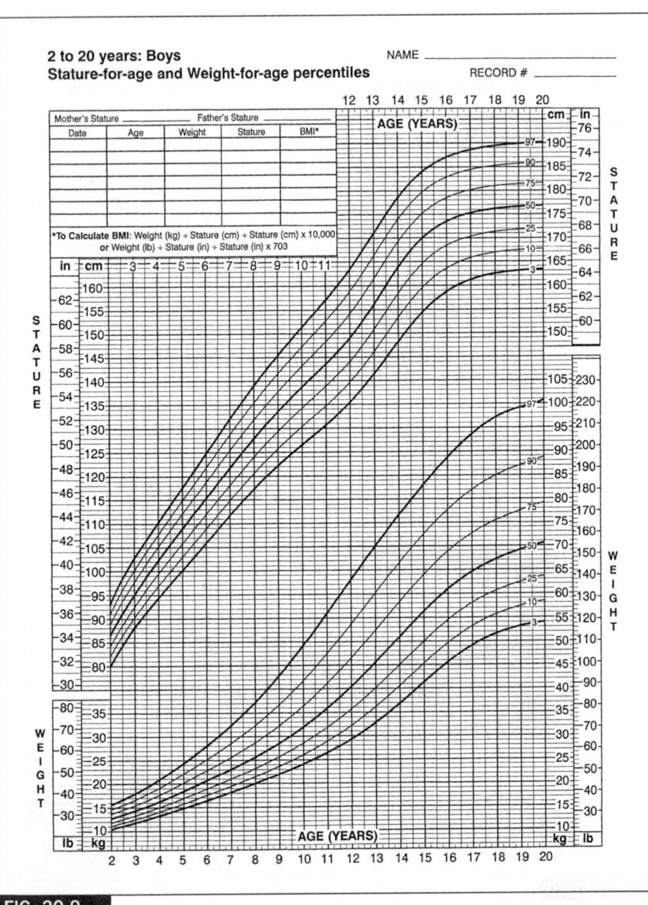

FIG. 20-9

Stature and weight for boys 2 to 20 years. *(Developed by the National Center for Health Statistics in collaboration with the National Center for Chronic Disease Prevention and Health Promotion, 2000.)*

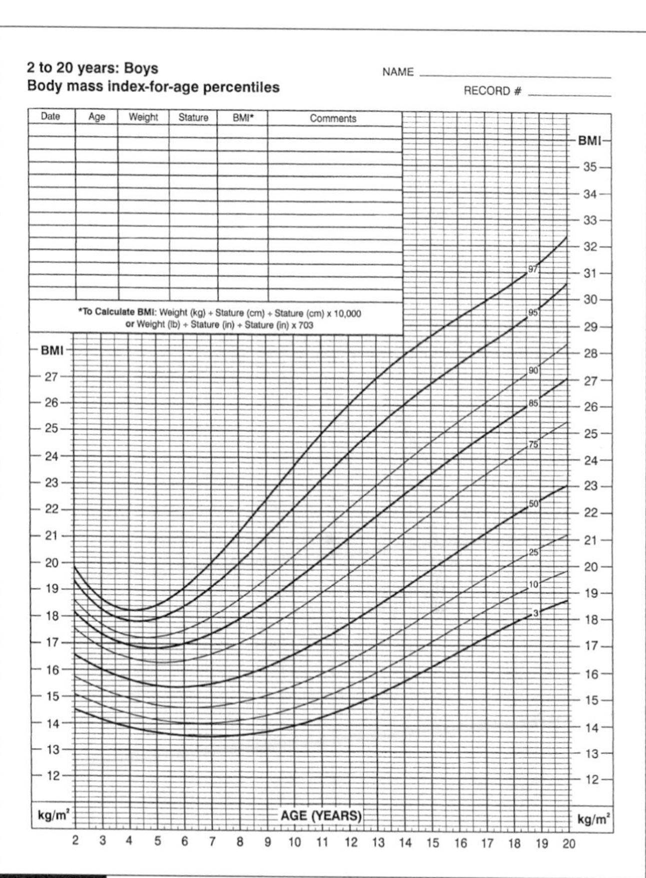

FIG. 20-10

Body mass index for boys 2 to 20 years. *(Developed by the National Center for Health Statistics in collaboration with the National Center for Chronic Disease Prevention and Health Promotion, 2000.)*

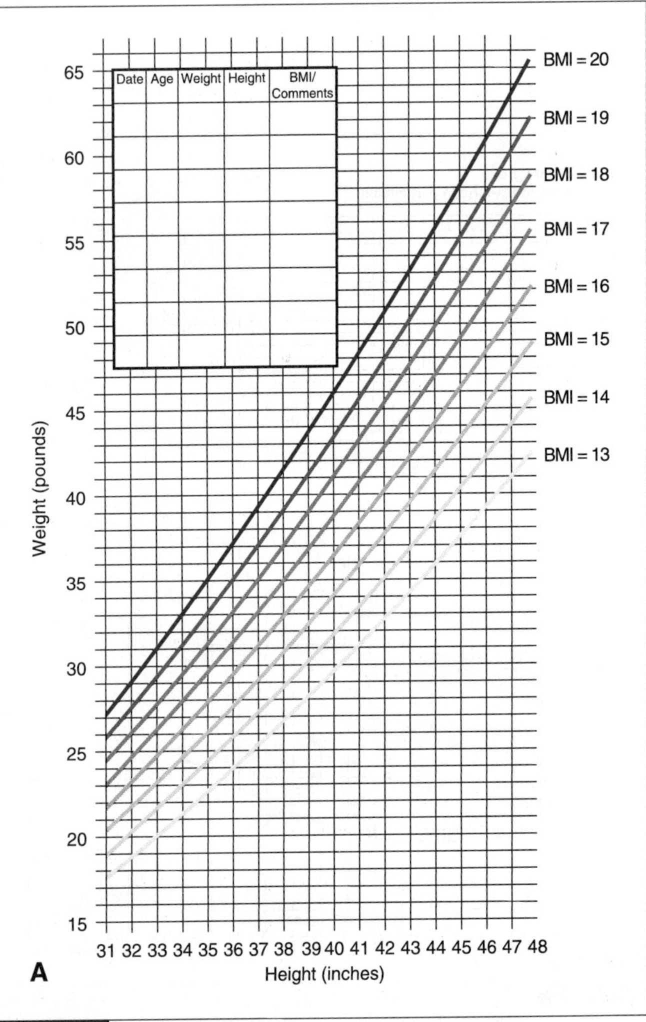

FIG. 20-11

Body mass index. Interplot height (inches) and weight (pounds); note the curved line nearest the intersection of the horizontal and vertical axis, which is the BMI. *A,* Age 2 to 5 years.

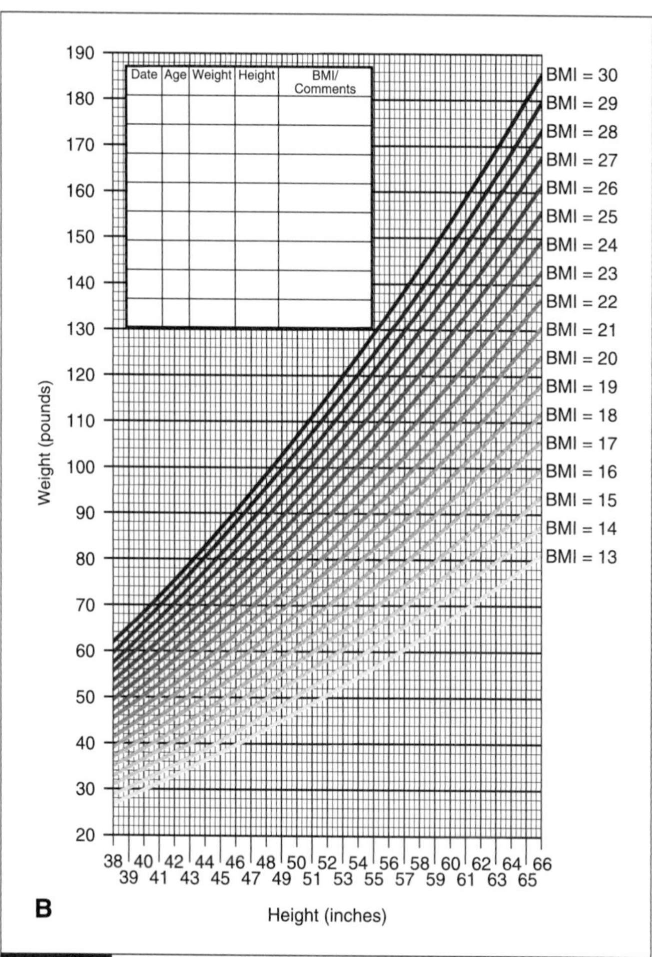

FIG. 20-11

B, Age 5 to 12 years. *(Data from Portland Health Institute, Inc., Portland, Oregon.)*

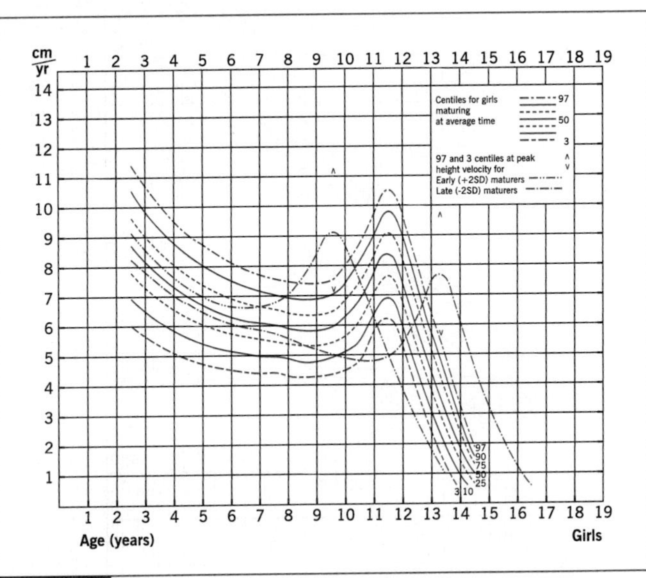

FIG. 20-12

Height velocity for girls 2 to 18 years. *(Modified from Tanner JM, Davis PS: J Pediatr 1985;107:317–329. Courtesy of Castlemead Publications, 1985. Distributed by Serono Laboratories.)*

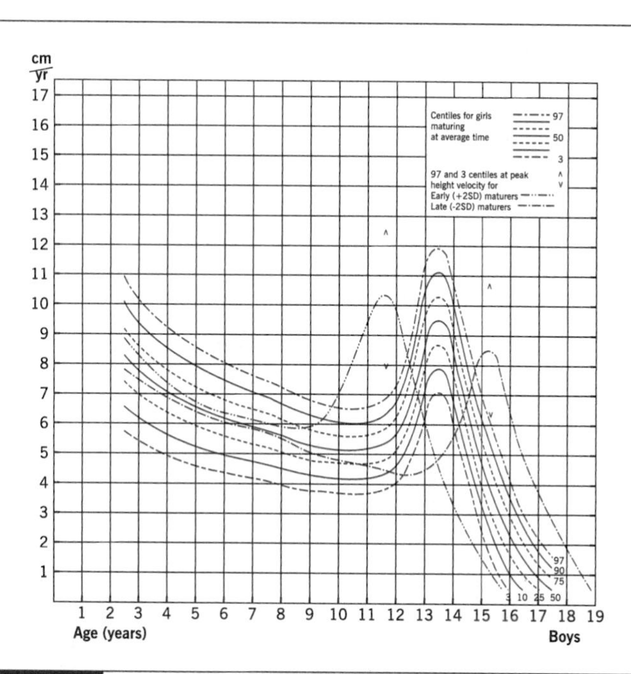

FIG. 20-13

Height velocity for boys 2 to 18 years. *(Modified from Tanner JM, Davis PS: J Pediatr 1985;107:317–329. Courtesy of Castlemead Publications, 1985. Distributed by Serono Laboratories.)*

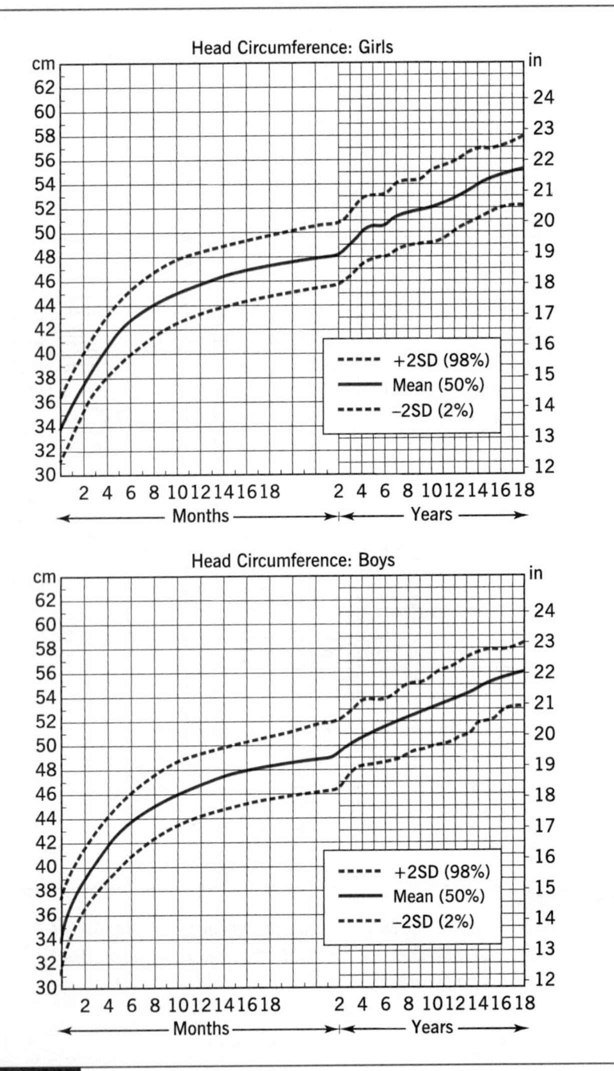

FIG. 20-14

Head circumference for girls and boys 2 to 18 years. *(Modified from Nelhaus G: J Pediatr 1968;48:106.)*

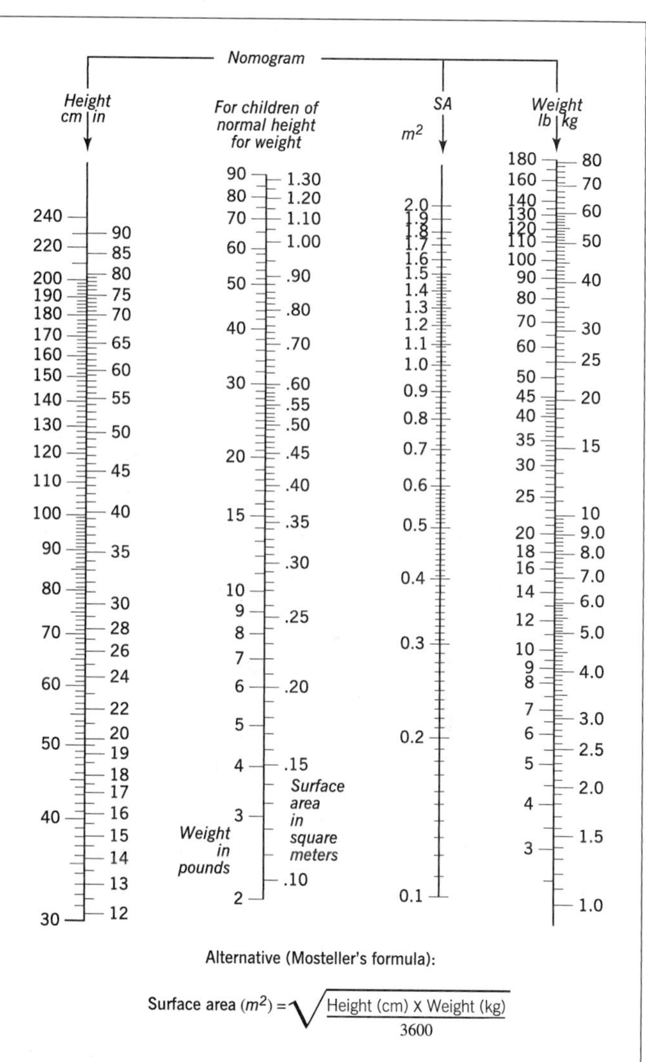

FIG. 20-15

Body surface area nomogram and equation. *(Data from Briars GL, Bailey BJ: Arch Dis Child 1994;70:246–247.)*

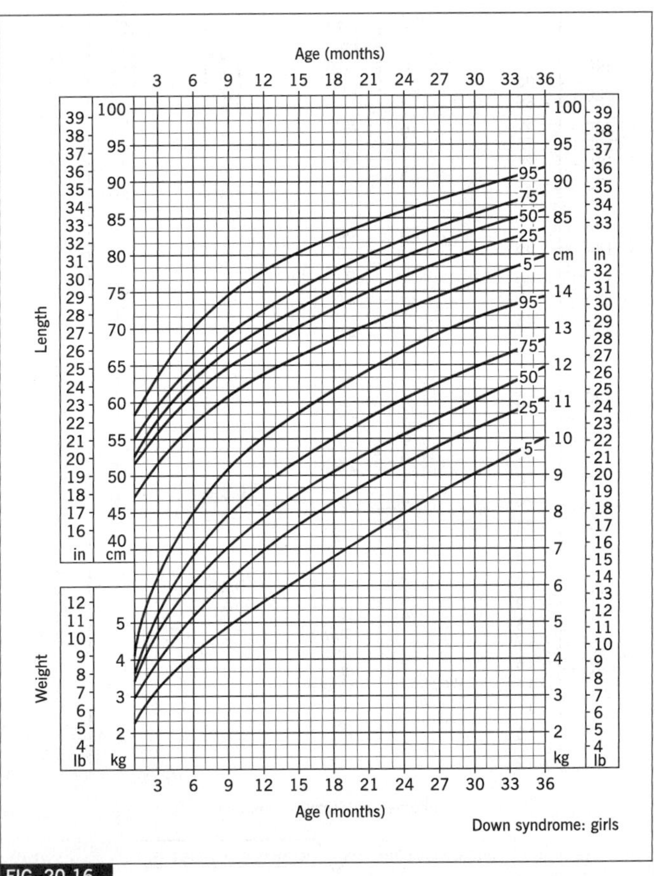

FIG. 20-16

Length and weight for girls with Down syndrome, from birth to 36 months. *(Modified from Cronk C, et al: Pediatrics 1988;81:102–110.)*

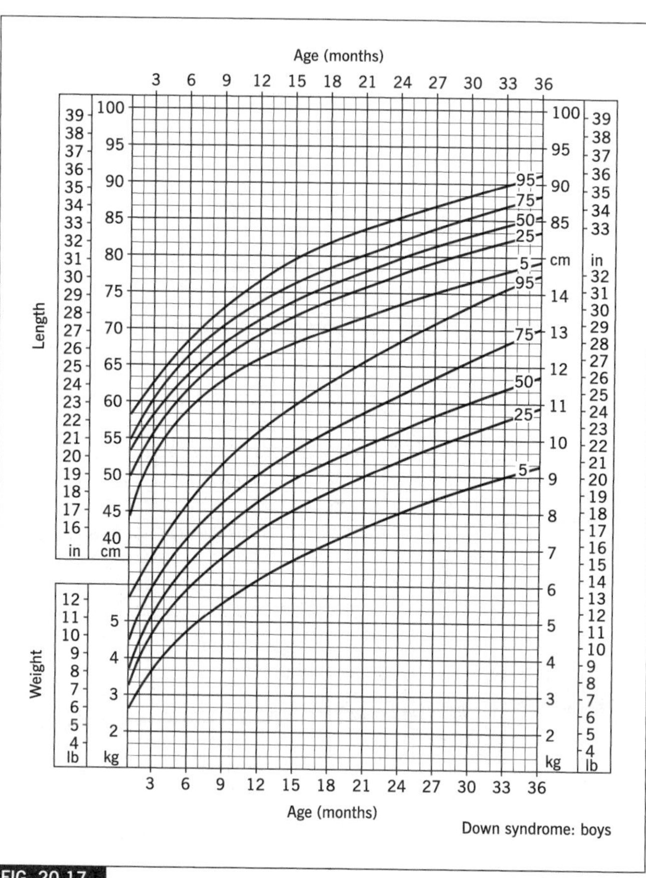

FIG. 20-17

Length and weight for boys with Down syndrome, from birth to 36 months. *(Modified from Cronk C et al: Pediatrics 1988;81:102–110.)*

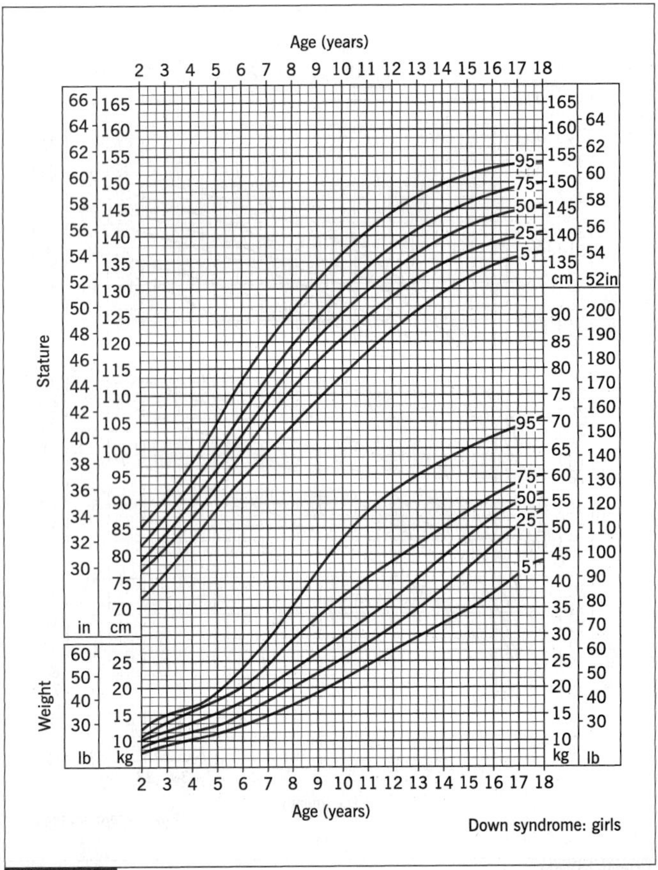

Down syndrome: girls

FIG. 20-18

Stature and weight for girls with Down syndrome 2 to 18 years. *(Modified from Cronk C et al: Pediatrics 1988;81:102–110.)*

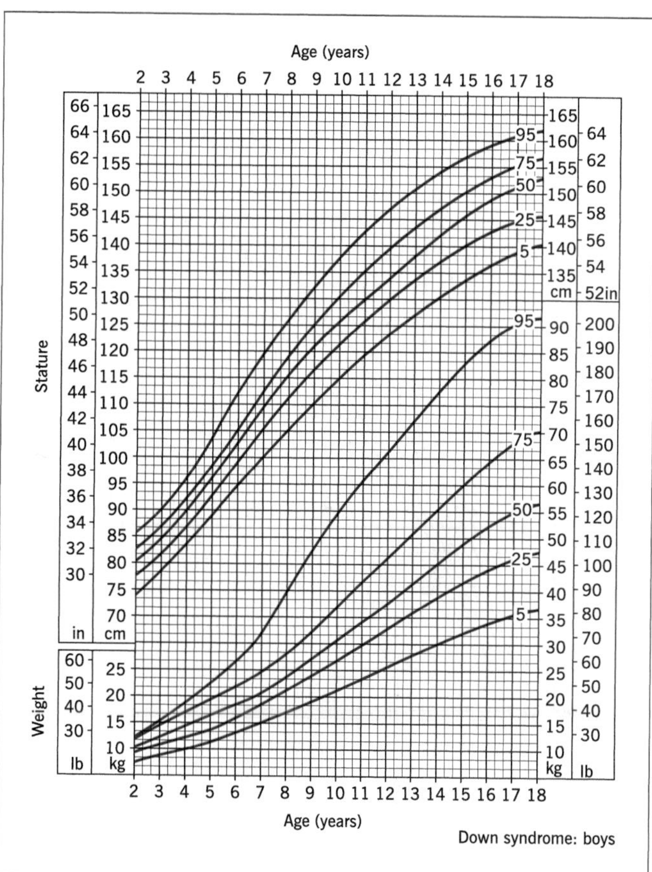

FIG. 20-19

Stature and weight for boys with Down syndrome 2 to 18 years. *(Modified from Cronk C et al: Pediatrics 1988;81:102–110.)*

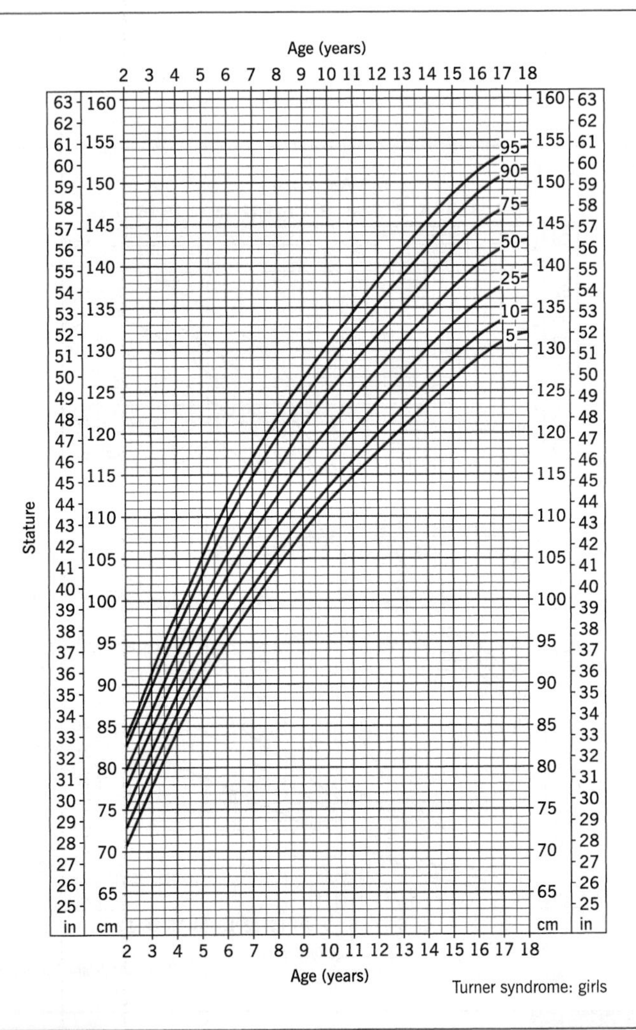

FIG. 20-20

Stature for girls with Turner syndrome 2 to 18 years. *(From Lyon AJ, Preece MA, Grant DB: Arch Dis Child 1985;60:932–935.)*

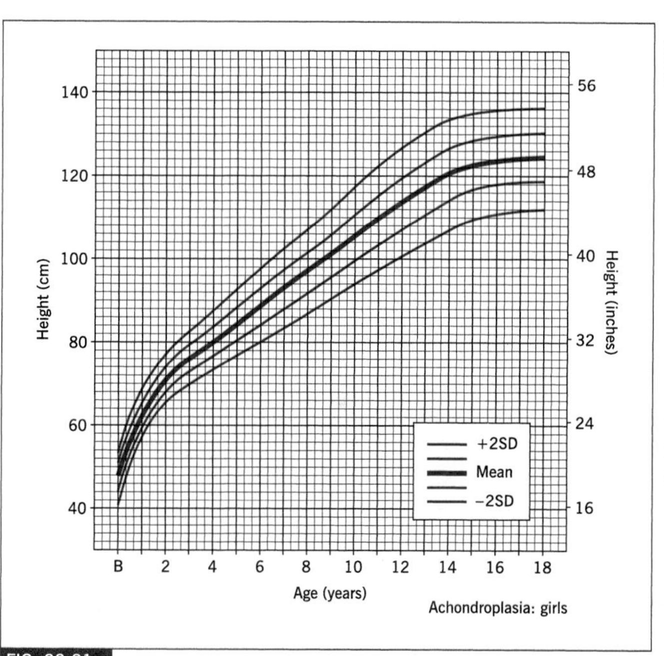

FIG. 20-21

Height for girls with achondroplasia, from birth to 18 years. *(From Horton WA, et al: J Pediatr 1978;93:435–438.)*

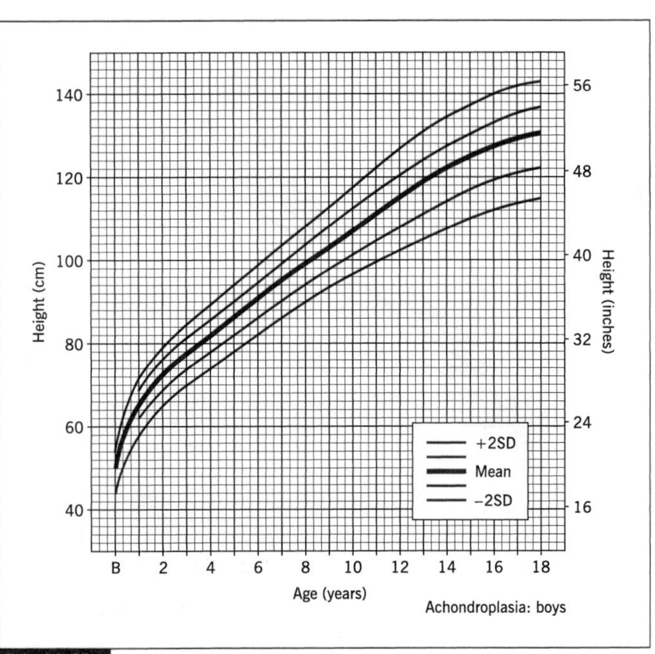

FIG. 20-22

Height for boys with achondroplasia, from birth to 18 years. *(From Horton WA, et al: J Pediatr 1978;93:435–438.)*

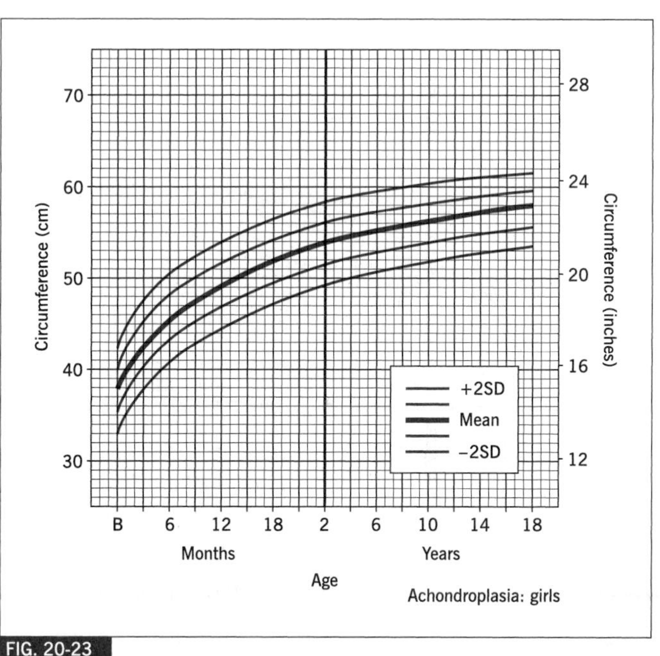

FIG. 20-23

Head circumference for girls with achondroplasia, from birth to 18 years. *(From Horton WA, et al. J Pediatr 1978;93:435–438.)*

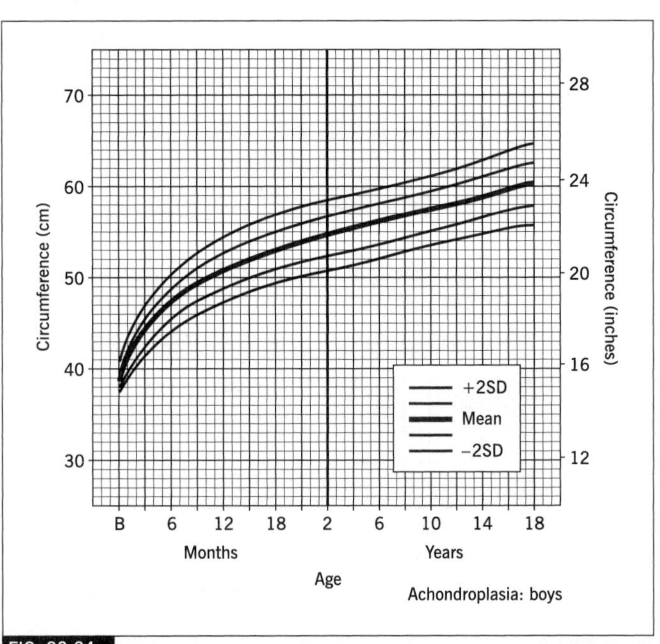

FIG. 20-24

Head circumference for boys with achondroplasia, from birth to 18 years. *(From Horton WA, et al: J Pediatr 1978;93:435–438.)*

Oncology

Jason T. Yustein MD, PhD, and Anthony Caterina, MD

21

I. WEBSITES: RESOURCES FOR PHYSICIANS, PATIENTS, AND FAMILIES

Candlelighters Childhood Cancer Foundation is a nonprofit organization to educate, support, and advocate for families with children with cancer, survivors of cancer, and professionals who care for them: www.candlelighters.org.

Oncology Link provides information regarding individual types of pediatric malignancies: www.Oncolink.org.

Children's Cancer Web is an international directory of childhood resources: www.cancerindex.org.

II. PRESENTING SIGNS AND SYMPTOMS OF PEDIATRIC MALIGNANCIES (Table 21-1)

Note: *Common presenting signs and symptoms of many malignancies include weight loss, failure to thrive, anorexia, malaise, fever, pallor, and lymphadenopathy.*

III. FEVER AND NEUTROPENIA[1,2]

See Figure 21-1.

IV. ONCOLOGIC EMERGENCIES[1,3]

A. TUMOR LYSIS SYNDROME

1. **Etiology:** Lysis of tumor cells before or during early stages of chemotherapy (especially Burkitt lymphoma/leukemia, T-cell acute lymphocytic leukemia [ALL]).
2. **Presentation:** Hyperuricemia, hypocalcemia, hyperkalemia, hyperphosphatemia. Can lead to acute renal failure.
3. **Prevention and management:**

a. Hydration and alkalinization: D_5 0.2 normal saline (NS) + 25 to 50 mEq $NaHCO_3$ (without K^+) at two times the maintenance rate. Keeping urine specific gravity <1.010 and pH 7.0 to 7.5 reduces risk for urate crystal formation. Reduce $NaHCO_3$ if pH >7.5 to avoid calcium phosphate precipitation.

b. Allopurinol (100 mg/m^2 per dose) q8hr by mouth (PO), alternative dosing 10 mg/kg/day divided q8hr by mouth (PO).

c. Check K^+, Ca^{2+}, phosphate, uric acid, and urinalysis frequently.

d. Manage abnormal electrolytes as described in Chapter 10. See Chapter 18 for dialysis indications.

e. Consider stopping alkalinization soon after starting chemotherapy (if uric acid is normal).

TABLE 21-1

COMMON SIGNS AND SYMPTOMS OF PEDIATRIC MALIGNANCIES

Type of Malignancy	Signs/Symptoms
Leukemia	Limp, hepatomegaly, splenomegaly, petechiae/bruising, bone pain, anemia, thrombocytopenia
Lymphoma	Night sweats; pruritus; stridor; persistent respiratory symptoms; GI bleeding; back pain; hepatomegaly; splenomegaly; abdominal, head, neck, or chest mass
Wilms' tumor	Hypertension, abdominal mass, abdominal distention, hematuria
Neuroblastoma	Emesis; diarrhea; hypertension; opsoclonus-myoclonus; periorbital ecchymoses; Horner syndrome; stridor; persistent respiratory symptoms; abdominal, head, neck or chest mass; limp; blue subcutaneous nodules
CNS tumors	Irritability, headache, emesis, seizure, cranial nerve palsies, visual changes, proptosis, ataxia
Testicular tumors	Abdominal pain or tenderness, scrotal swelling or mass
Bone tumors	Limp, back pain, persistent limb pain, fracture
Histiocytic disease	Polyuria, polydipsia, otorrhea, hepatomegaly, splenomegaly, cutaneous lesions, osteolytic lesions, pulmonary infiltrates, anemia, thrombocytopenia
Retinoblastoma	Leukocoria, asymmetric red reflex, orbital inflammation, hyphema, pupil irregularity

Data from Crist WM: Principles of diagnosis. In Behrman RE, Kliegman RM, Jenson NB (eds): Nelson's Textbook of Pediatrics, 17th ed. Philadelphia, WB Saunders, 2004; and Hogarty MD, et al: Oncologic emergencies. In Fleisher G, Ludwig S (eds): Textbook of Pediatric Emergency Medicine. Philadelphia, Lippincott Williams & Wilkins, 2000.

B. SPINAL CORD COMPRESSION

1. **Etiology:** Extension of tumor into spinal cord. Occurs most commonly with brain tumors, sarcomas, leukemia, lymphoma, and neuroblastoma.
2. **Presentation:** Back pain (localized, radicular), weakness, sensory loss, change in bowel or bladder function. Prognosis for recovery based on duration and level of disability at presentation.
3. **Diagnosis:** Magnetic resonance imaging (MRI) or computed tomography (CT) scan of spine. Plain radiograph of spine specific but not sensitive. A plain film of the spine detects only two-thirds of abnormalities.
4. **Management:**

a. In the presence of neurologic abnormalities, immediately start dexamethasone 1 to 2 mg/kg/day IV and obtain an emergent MRI of the spine.

b. With back pain and no neurologic abnormalities, may start dexamethasone, 0.25 to 0.5 mg/kg/day PO divided q6hr and perform MRI of the spine within 24 hours. Be aware that steroids may prevent

Temperature >38.3 C × 1 or >38 C × 2 at least 4 hr apart within 24 hr AND ANC < 500 or ANC > 1000 with expected drop in ANC*
(Alternative definitions include: 1. Low grade fever while on steroids
2. Any ill appearing neutropenic patient regardless of body temperature)
* Absolute Neutrophil Count (ANC) = WBC × (% neutrophils + % bands)

↓

Admit to hospital
History: Ill appearance, recent steroid use or procedures, chills, rigors, respiratory symptoms, mental status changes, myalgias, bone pain.
Physical: Include line sites, incisions, perianal (no rectal), skin, oropharynx.
Labs: CBC with differential, blood cultures (include all central line lumens), urinalysis and urine culture (clean catch, no urine catheters)
As indicated: Blood type and screen, electrolytes, coagulation studies, mucosal surveillance cultures
Respiratory symptoms: chest x-ray
Suspected typhlitis: KUB, abdominal CT

↓

Focus of infection identified?

Yes → See Table 21–2 and modify treatment accordingly → Choose antibiotics based on ...

No → Choose antibiotics based on
1. Local sensitivities and preferences
2. Past culture sensitivities
3. Level of suspicion
For low risk, provide coverage for Gram negative and positive.
For high risk patients, include double coverage for Pseudomonas.

→ Continue to evaluate patient, follow culture results and fever curve. If cultures become positive or new focus identified, modify regimen accordingly.

↓

Does fever resolve within 72 hours?

Yes → Continue antibiotic course for at least 3 more days after resolution and WBC recovery (ANC rising and above 200).

No → Consider
1. Adding a semi-synthetic penicillin (oxacillin, vancomycin) for increased gram positive coverage.
2. Repeating cultures for bacteria and fungus.
3. Adding broader gram negative coverage.
4. Further studies including C-reactive protein, DIC profile, CBC with differential, chest x-ray.
5. If neutropenia expected to be longer than 7 days, consider adding antifungal coverage.

→ Does fever resolve after 72 hours?

Yes → Modify antibiotic regimen based on any positive culture results. If the central line culture is persistently positive, consider removal of the line.

No → If fever persists for 4 to 7 days, consider adding IV amphotericin. If fever persists for 2 days on amphotericin, consider increasing the dose. Modify regimen if any cultures positive, consider removal of hardware.

↓

Any positive cultures?

Yes → Consider sending home on IV/PO antibiotics when ANC > 500 OR > 200 AND WBC recovering.

No → Consider sending home when ANC > 250 measured > 6 hours apart AND WBC recovering.

FIG. 21-1

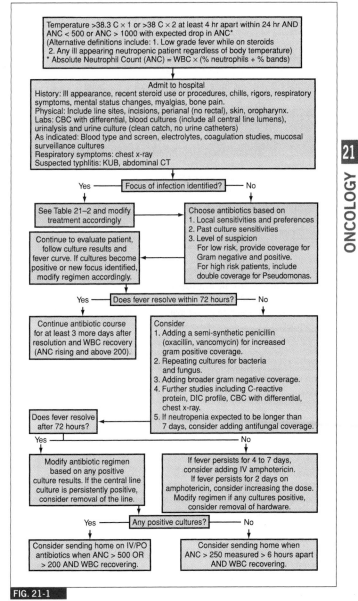

Fever and neutropenia.

diagnosis of lymphoma; therefore, plan diagnostic procedure as soon as possible.

c. If the cause of the tumor is known, emergent radiotherapy or chemotherapy is indicated for sensitive tumors; otherwise, emergent neurosurgery consultation is warranted.

d. If cause of tumor is unknown or debulking may remove most or all of the tumor, surgery is indicated to decompress the spine.

C. INCREASED INTRACRANIAL PRESSURE

1. **Etiology:** Ventricular obstruction, obstruction of cerebrospinal fluid (CSF) flow.
2. **Presentation:** Headaches, irritability, lethargy, emesis (especially if projectile).
3. **Diagnosis:** Obtain CT scan or MRI of the head. MRI is more sensitive for diagnosis of posterior fossa tumors. Evaluate vital signs for Cushing triad, funduscopic exam for papilledema.
4. **Management:**

a. See Chapter 4 for basic ICP management.

b. If tumor is identified, add dexamethasone, 2 mg/kg/day IV divided q6hr.

c. Obtain emergent neurosurgical consultation.

D. CEREBROVASCULAR ACCIDENT

1. **Etiology:** Hyperleukocytosis, coagulopathy, thrombocytopenia, chemotherapy-related (e.g., L-asparaginase–induced hemorrhage or thrombosis).
2. **Diagnosis and management:**

a. Platelet transfusions, fresh-frozen plasma (FFP) as needed to replace factors (e.g., if depleted by L-asparaginase).

b. Brain CT scan with contrast, MRI, magnetic resonance angiography (MRA), or magnetic resonance venography (MRV) if venous thrombosis is suspected.

c. Administer heparin acutely, followed by warfarin, for thromboses (if no venous hemorrhage is observed on MRI).

d. Avoid L-asparaginase.

E. RESPIRATORY DISTRESS AND SUPERIOR VENA CAVA SYNDROME

1. **Etiology:** Hodgkin disease, non-Hodgkin lymphoma (e.g., lymphoblastic lymphoma), ALL (T-lineage), germ cell tumors.
2. **Presentation:** Orthopnea, headaches, facial swelling, dizziness, plethora.
3. **Diagnosis:** Chest radiograph. Consider CT or MRI scan to assess airway. Attempt diagnosis of malignancy (if not known) by the least invasive method possible.
4. **Management:**

a. Control airway.

b. Biopsy (e.g., bone marrow, pleurocentesis, lymph-node biopsy) before therapy if patient can tolerate sedation or general anesthesia.
c. Empiric therapy: Radiotherapy, steroids, cyclophosphamide.

F. HYPERLEUKOCYTOSIS

1. **Etiology:** In acute myeloid leukemia (AML) (especially M4 and M5), hyperleukocytosis occurs with a white blood cell (WBC) count as low as 100,000/mm^3. It occurs in ALL with a WBC count above 300,000/mm^3.
2. **Presentation:** Hypoxia and dyspnea from pulmonary leukostasis, mental status changes, headaches, seizures, papilledema from leukostasis in cerebral vessels; occasionally, gastrointestinal (GI) bleeding, abdominal pain, renal failure, priapism, and tumor lysis syndrome.
3. **Management:**

a. Transfuse platelets as needed to keep count above 20,000/mm^3 (reduce risk for intracranial hemorrhage).
b. Avoid red blood cell (RBC) transfusions because they will raise viscosity (keep hemoglobin ≤10 g/dL). If RBCs are required, consider partial exchange transfusion.
c. Hydration, alkalinization, and allopurinol should be initiated (as discussed in section IV.A).
d. Administer FFP and vitamin K if patient is coagulopathic.
e. Before cytotoxic therapy, consider leukapheresis to lower WBC count if CNS or pulmonary symptoms exist.

V. COMMON COMPLICATIONS OF BONE MARROW TRANSPLANT[1]

A. GRAFT VERSUS HOST DISEASE (GVHD)

1. **Etiology:** Primarily T-cell–mediated reaction to foreign antigen occurs after hematopoietic cell transplant. Risk factors include HLA disparity, radiation therapy, gender disparity, and increasing age.
2. **Presentation:** Usually occurs within 100 days after transplantation. Maculopapular skin rash develops, which can progress to bullous lesions and toxic epidermal necrolysis. Laboratory findings notable for abnormal liver enzymes, especially increased direct bilirubin and elevated alkaline phosphatase. Upper GI symptoms include anorexia, dyspepsia, nausea, and vomiting. Lower GI symptoms include abdominal cramping and diarrhea.
3. **Diagnosis:** Triad of classic rash, abdominal cramping with diarrhea, and rising bilirubin level is suggestive of diagnosis. Tissue biopsy of skin or rectum provides histologic confirmation.
4. **Prevention and management:**

a. Prophylaxis involves T-cell depletion of donor marrow or immunomodulation. Commonly used adjuvants are methotrexate and prednisone.
b. Steroids are first-line treatment. Commonly used second-line agents include tacrolimus, sirolimus, antithymocyte globulin, and

mycophenolate mofetil. Psoralen plus ultraviolet A photophoresis (PUVA) is an alternative for skin GVHD. Pentostatin is useful in treating cutaneous and oral GVHD.

For chronic GVHD, acute therapies are complemented by monoclonal antibodies, such as infliximab (anti-tumor necrosis factor-α). Thalidomide is also useful for chronic GVHD.

B. VENOOCCLUSIVE DISEASE (SINUSOIDAL OBSTRUCTION SYNDROME)

1. **Etiology:** Occlusive fibrosis of terminal intrahepatic venules and sinusoids occurs as a consequence of hematopoietic cell transplantation or high-dose liver radiation. Typically occurs within 3 weeks of the insult. Incidence highest with unmatched, unrelated transplants and lowest with autologous transplantation.
2. **Presentation:** Hepatomegaly, right upper quadrant abdominal pain, jaundice, edema, ascites, and sudden weight gain.
3. **Diagnosis:** Liver ultrasound with Doppler, looking for reversal of portal venous flow, or MRI. Laboratory studies show elevated bilirubin and aminotransferases (ALT, AST). More severe disease will result in elevation of prothrombin time (PT) and a decrease in factor VII levels. A useful but invasive measurement is the portal hepatic venous gradient. A gradient greater than 10 mm Hg is consistent with veno-occlusive disease.
4. **Prevention and management:**

a. Prophylaxis typically includes ursodeoxycholic acid and glutamine. Other preventative measures include T-cell–depleted transplant, low-molecular-weight heparin, and low-dose heparin drip.

b. Treatment commonly includes either defibrotide or alteplase (tissue plasminogen activator) with or without heparin. Fluid and sodium intake should be restricted. Antithrombin infusion may benefit patients with low antithrombin levels. For severe disease, surgical intervention with transjugular intrahepatic portosystemic stent shunt (TIPS) is effective in reducing the portal hepatic venous gradient. Liver transplantation is considered for the most severe cases.

VI. HEMATOLOGIC CARE AND COMPLICATIONS[1]

Note: *Transfuse only irradiated packed RBC (pRBC)/platelets, cytomegalovirus (CMV)-negative or leukofiltered pRBC/platelets for CMV-negative patients. Use leukofiltered pRBC/platelets for those who may undergo bone marrow transplantation (BMT) in the future to prevent alloimmunization, or for those who have had nonhemolytic febrile transfusion reactions.*

A. ANEMIA

1. **Etiology:** Blood loss, chemotherapy, marrow infiltration, hemolysis.
2. **Management:**

a. See Chapter 13 for specific details on pRBC transfusions.

b. Generally, pRBC transfusions in cancer patients are not recommended until hematocrit falls below 20% to 22%, or if the patient is symptomatic.

B. THROMBOCYTOPENIA

1. **Etiology:** Chemotherapy, marrow infiltration, consumptive coagulopathy, medications.
2. **Management:**
   a. See Chapter 13 for specific details on platelet transfusions.
   b. Generally, maintain platelet count above 10,000/mm^3 unless patient is clinically bleeding or febrile, or before procedure (e.g., lumbar puncture or intramuscular [IM] injection requires >50,000/mm^3). Consider maintaining platelet counts at higher levels for patients who have brain tumors or those who have had recent brain surgery.

C. NEUTROPENIA

1. **Etiology:** Chemotherapy, marrow infiltration, radiation.
2. **Management:**
   a. Broad-spectrum antibiotics with concomitant fever (see Fig. 21-1).
   b. Granulocyte colony-stimulating factor (G-CSF) to assist in recovery of neutrophils.
   c. Rarely, use of neutrophil transfusion.

VII. NAUSEA TREATMENT IN CANCER PATIENTS[1]

A. ETIOLOGY

The usual cause of nausea is chemotherapy treatment. Also suspect opiate therapy, GI and central nervous system (CNS) radiotherapy, obstructive abdominal process, CNS mass, certain antibiotics, or hypercalcemia.

B. THERAPY

Hydration plus one or more antinausea medications (see Formulary for dosing):

1. **5-HT$_3$ Antagonists:** Ondansetron, dolasetron, granisetron, or palonosetron. Usually a first-line therapy. Patients may respond preferentially to one of these agents.
2. **Histamine-1 antagonist:** Diphenhydramine.
3. **Serotonin antagonist:** Cyproheptadine. Also, Histamine-1 antagonist used for appetite stimulation.
4. **Steroids:** Dexamethasone. Especially helpful in patients with brain tumor. Synergy of unknown mechanism with 5-HT$_3$ antagonists.
5. **Benzodiazepines:** Lorazepam. Used as an adjunct antiemetic agent.
6. **Metoclopramide:** Use diphenhydramine to reduce extrapyramidal symptoms (EPS).
7. **Phenothiazines:** Promethazine, chlorpromazine. Use diphenhydramine to reduce EPS.
8. **Cannabinoids:** Dronabinol. Can be helpful in resistant cases, especially in patients with large tumor burden. May also be used as an appetite stimulant in malnourished patients.
9. **Substance P and neurokinin-1 receptor antagonist:** Aprepitant.

VIII. ANTIMICROBIAL PROPHYLAXIS IN ONCOLOGY PATIENTS (Table 21-2)

Note: *Treatment length and dosage may vary per protocol.*

IX. GENETICS OF CHILDHOOD CANCER

See Table 21-3.

TABLE 21-2

ANTIMICROBIAL PROPHYLAXIS IN ONCOLOGY PATIENTS

Organism	Medication	Indication
Pneumocystis carinii	TMP-SMX, dapsone, or pentamidine	Chemotherapy and BMT per protocol (usually at least 6 mo after chemotherapy, 12 mo after BMT)
HSV	Acyclovir (dosing is different for zoster, varicella, and mucocutaneous HSV)	After BMT if patient or donor is HSV or CMV positive; recurrent zoster
Candida albicans	Fluconazole or voriconazole	After BMT (usual minimum 28 days)
Gram-positive organisms	Penicillin	After BMT (usually at least 1 mo)

TMP-SMX, trimethoprim-sulfamethoxazole; BMT, bone marrow transplantation; HSV, herpes simplex virus; CMV, cytomegalovirus.

TABLE 21-3

GENETICS OF CHILDHOOD CANCER

Malignancy	Genetic Marker	Function	Significance
ALL, CML	BCR-abl fusion, t(9;22)	Tyrosine kinase	Poor prognosis
Neuroblastoma	myc	Transcription factor	Advanced stage, aggressive More intensive therapy needed
Ewing sarcoma	EWS-FLI1	Transcription factor	Distinguish Ewing sarcoma from other small, round tumors
Osteosarcoma	p53, RB1	Tumor suppressor genes	Increased incidence
	HER2	Growth factor receptor	Poor response to chemotherapy
Wilms tumor	WT1	Transcription factor, tumor suppressor gene	Association with WAGR syndrome

ALL, acute lymphoblastitic leukemia; CML, chronic myelogenous leukemia; RBI, retinoblastoma gene 1; WAGR, Wilms tumor, aniridia, genitourinary anomalies, mental retardation.

REFERENCES

1. Poplack D, Pizzo P: Principles and Practice of Pediatric Oncology, 4th ed. Philadelphia, Lippincott Williams and Wilkins, 2001.
2. Chanock SJ, Pizzo PA: Fever in the neutropenic host. Infect Dis Clin North Am. 1996;10(4):777–796.
3. Kelly KM, Lange B: Oncologic emergencies. Pediatr Clin North Am. 1997;44(4):809–830.

Pulmonology

Ceila E. Loughlin, MD

22

I. WEBSITES

www.lungusa.org (American Lung Association)
www.cff.org (Cystic Fibrosis Foundation)
www.aaaai.org (American Academy of Allergy, Asthma and Immunology)
www.nhlbi.nih.gov (National Asthma Education and Prevention Program)

II. RESPIRATORY PHYSICAL EXAMINATION

A. NORMAL RESPIRATORY RATES (Table 22-1)

B. RESPIRATORY AUSCULTATION (Table 22-2)

III. ASTHMA GUIDELINES (Figs. 22-1 and 22-2)

Asthma is a chronic inflammatory disorder of the airways resulting in recurrent episodes of wheezing, breathlessness, chest tightness, and cough, particularly at night and in early morning.[1] These episodes are usually associated with widespread yet variable airflow obstruction, reversible either spontaneously or with therapy. The inflammation also causes increased airway hyperreactivity to a variety of stimuli (viral infections, cold air, exercise, emotions, as well as environmental allergens and pollutants).

IV. ASTHMA ACTION PLAN (www.nationalasthma.org.au/publications/action)

This is an important educational and therapeutic tool for patients. Patients should leave all visits with a copy of their individual plan.

For management of acute asthma exacerbation and status asthmaticus, see Chapter 1.

V. PULMONARY FUNCTION TESTS

Pulmonary function tests (PFTs) provide objective and reproducible measurements of airway function and lung volumes. PFTs are used to characterize disease, assess severity, and follow response to therapy.

A. PEAK EXPIRATORY FLOW RATE

The peak expiratory flow rate (PEFR) is the maximum flow rate generated during a forced expiratory maneuver. It is useful in following the course of asthma and response to therapy. Compare a patient's PEFR to the previous "personal best" and the normal predicted value (Table 22-3). Normal predicted values vary across different racial groups; therefore, the best indicator of patient condition is comparison to their own personal best. It is important to remember PEFRs are effort dependent and insensitive to small airway function.

TABLE 22-1

NORMAL RESPIRATORY RATES IN CHILDREN

Age (yr)	Respiratory Rate (breaths/min)
0–1*	24–38
1–3	22–30
4–6	20–24
7–9	18–24
10–14	16–22
14–18	14–20

*Slightly higher respiratory rates in the neonatal period (i.e., 40–50 breaths/min) may be normal in the absence of other signs and symptoms.

Data from Bardella IJ: Am Fam Phys 1999;60(6):1743–1750.

TABLE 22-2

RESPIRATORY AUSCULTATION

Sound	Description	Possible Causes
Crackles (rales)	Intermittent, scratchy, bubbly noises	Bronchiolitis, pulmonary edema
	Heard predominantly on inspiration	Pneumonia
	Produced by reopening of airways closed on previous expiration	
Wheezes	Continuous, high-pitched, musical sound	Asthma, bronchiolitis, foreign body
Rhonchi	Continuous, low-pitched, nonmusical sound	Pneumonia, cystic fibrosis
Stridor	High-pitched, harsh, blowing sound Heard predominantly on inspiration	Croup, laryngomalacia, subglottic stenosis, allergic reaction, vocal cord dysfunction

TABLE 22-3

PREDICTED AVERAGE PEAK EXPIRATORY FLOW RATES FOR NORMAL CHILDREN

Height (in & cm)		PEFR (L/min)	Height (in & cm)		PEFR (L/min)
43	109	147	56	142	320
44	112	160	57	145	334
45	114	173	58	147	347
46	117	187	59	150	360
47	119	200	60	152	373
48	122	214	61	155	387
49	124	227	62	157	400
50	127	240	63	160	413
51	130	254	64	163	427
52	132	267	65	165	440
53	135	280	66	168	454
54	137	293	67	170	467
55	140	307			

PEFR, peak expiratory flow rate.

Data from Voter KZ. Pediatr Rev 1996;17(2):53–63.

‡ Classify severity: Clinical features before treatment or adequate control		Medications required to maintain long-term control *
	Symptoms/Day **Symptoms/Night**	**Daily medications**
Step 4 Severe persistent	Continual Frequent	■ Preferred treatment: – High-dose inhaled corticosteroids AND – Long-acting inhaled beta$_2$-agonists AND, if needed, – Corticosteroid tablets or syrup long term (2 mg/kg/day, generally do not exceed 60 mg per day). (Make repeat attempts to reduce systemic corticosteroids and maintain control with high-dose inhaled corticosteroids.)
Step 3 Moderate persistent	Daily >1 night/week	■ Preferred treatment: – Low-dose inhaled corticosteroids and long-acting inhaled beta$_2$-agonists OR – Medium-dose inhaled corticosteroids. ■ Alternative treatment: – Low-dose inhaled corticosteroids and either leukotriene receptor antagonist or theophylline If needed (particularly in patients with recurring severe exacerbations): ■ Preferred treatment: – Medium-dose inhaled corticosteroids and long-acting beta$_2$-agonists. ■ Alternative treatment: – Medium-dose inhaled corticosteroids and either leukotriene receptor antagonist or theophylline.
Step 2 Mild persistent	>2/week but <1x/day >2 nights/month	■ Preferred treatment: – Low-dose inhaled corticosteroids (with nebulizer or MDI with holding chamber with or without face mask or DPI). ■ Alternative treatment: – Cromolyn (nebulizer is preferred or MDI with holding chamber) OR leukotriene receptor antagonist
Step 1 Mild intermittent	≤2 days/week ≤2 nights/month	■ No daily medication needed

*Review treatment every 1 to 6 months; A gradual stepwise reduction in treatment may be possible.
‡Consultation with an asthma specialist is recommended for patients with moderate or severe persistent asthma.

FIG. 22-1

Asthma guidelines for managing infants and young children (age 5 years and younger). MDI, metered dose inhaler; DPI, dry powder inhaler. (Adapted from NAEPP Expert Panel Report: Guidelines for the diagnosis and management of asthma 2002. See www.nhlbi.nih.gov.)

‡ Classify severity: Clinical features before treatment or adequate control		Medications required to maintain long-term control *
	Symptoms/Day Symptoms/Night PEF or FEV_1	Daily medications
Step 4 Severe persistent	Continual ≤60% Frequent	■ Preferred treatment: – High-dose inhaled corticosteroids AND – Long-acting inhaled $beta_2$-agonists AND, if needed, – Corticosteroid tablets or syrup long term (2 mg/kg/day, generally do not exceed 60 mg per day). (Make repeat attempts to reduce systemic corticosteroids and maintain control with high-dose inhaled corticosteroids.)
Step 3 Moderate persistent	Daily >1 night/week >60% – <80%	■ Preferred treatment: – Low-to-medium dose inhaled corticosteroids and long-acting inhaled $beta_2$-agonists ■ Alternative treatment: – Increase inhaled corticosteroids within medium-dose range OR – Low-to-medium dose inhaled corticosteroids and either leukotriene modifier or theophylline. If needed (particularly in patients with recurring severe exacerbations): ■ Preferred treatment: – Increase inhaled corticosteroids within medium-dose range and add long-acting inhaled $beta_2$-agonists. ■ Alternative treatment: –Increase inhaled corticosteroids within medium-dose range and add either leukotriene modifier or theophylline.
Step 2 Mild persistent	>2/week but <1x/day >2 nights/month ≥80%	■ Preferred treatment: – Low-dose inhaled corticosteroids. ■ Alternative treatment: cromolyn, leukotriene modifier, nedocromil, OR sustained release theophylline to serum concentration of 5–15 mcg/mL.
Step 1 Mild intermittent	≤2 days/week ≤2 nights/month ≥80%	■ No daily medication needed. ■ Severe exacerbations may occur, separated by long periods of normal lung function and no symptoms. A course of systemic corticosteroids is recommended.

*Review treatment every 1 to 6 months; A gradual stepwise reduction in treatment may be possible.
‡Consultation with an asthma specialist is recommended for patients with moderate or severe persistent asthma.

FIG. 22-2

Asthma guidelines for managing adults and children older than 5 years. (Adapted from NAEPP Expert Panel Report: Guidelines for the diagnosis and management of asthma 2002. See www.nhlbi.nih.gov.)

B. SPIROMETRY (for children 6 years and older)

Spirometry is the plot of airflow versus time. Measurements are made from a rapid, forceful, and complete expiration from total lung capacity (TLC) to residual volume (RV). Spirometry is usually performed before and after a bronchodilator to assess response to therapy or after bronchial challenge to assess airway hyperreactivity.

1. **Forced vital capacity (FVC):** FVC is the maximum volume of air exhaled from the lungs after a maximum inspiration. Bedside measurement of vital capacity with a handheld spirometer can be useful in confirming or predicting hypoventilation associated with muscle weakness. FVC <15 mL/kg may be an indication for ventilatory support.
2. **Forced expiratory volume in 1 second (FEV_1):** Volume exhaled during the first second of an FVC maneuver. It is the single best measure of airway function.
3. **Forced expiratory flow (FEF_{25-75}):** Mean rate of airflow over the middle half of the FVC between 25% and 75% of FVC. Sensitive to medium and small airway obstruction.

C. FLOW-VOLUME CURVES

Flow-volume curves are the plot of airflow versus lung volume. They are useful in characterizing different patterns of airway obstruction (Fig. 22-3).

D. LUNG VOLUMES

See Figure 22-4.

E. MAXIMAL INSPIRATORY AND EXPIRATORY PRESSURES

Obtained by asking patient to inhale and exhale against a fixed obstruction. Low pressures suggest a neuromuscular problem or submaximal effort. An inspiratory pressure <20 to 25 cm H_2O (negative inspiratory force [NIF]) may be an indication for ventilatory support. A low positive expiratory pressure suggests decreased effectiveness of coughing.

F. INTERPRETATION OF PFTS (Table 22-4)

VI. CYSTIC FIBROSIS[2]

Cystic fibrosis (CF) is an autosomal recessive disorder in which most patients have chronic obstructive pulmonary disease, pancreatic exocrine deficiency, and abnormally high sweat electrolyte concentrations.

A. CLINICAL MANIFESTATIONS OF CYSTIC FIBROSIS BY SYSTEM (Table 22-5)

B. SWEAT CHLORIDE TEST[3]

Normal (1 week to adult) <40 mmol/L

Patients with cystic fibrosis (CF) >60 mmol/L (mmol/L = mEq/L)

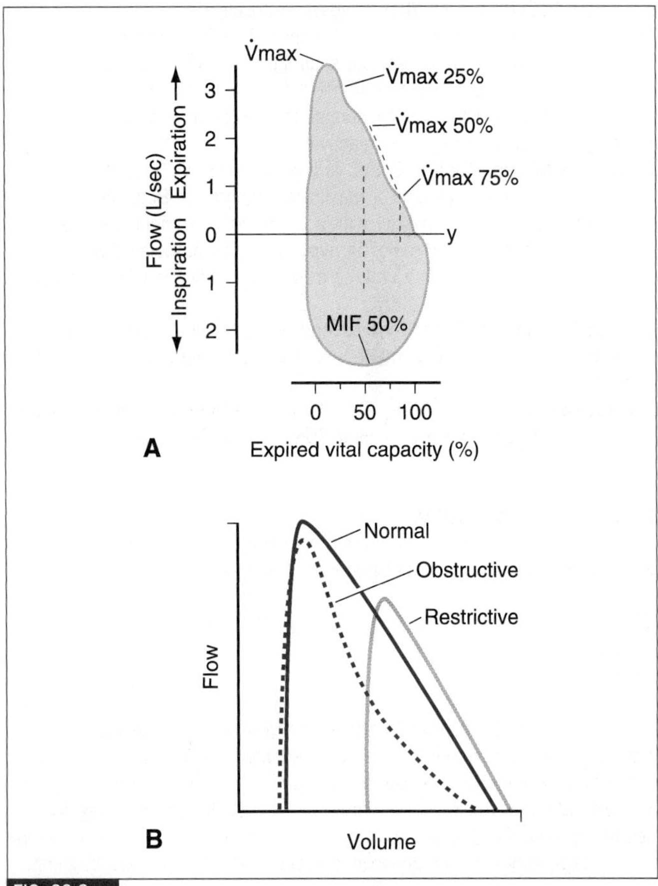

FIG. 22-3

A, Normal flow-volume curve. *B*, Worsening intrathoracic airway obstruction as in asthma or cystic fibrosis. *(B, Data from Baum GL, Wolinsky E: Textbook of Pulmonary Diseases, 5th ed. Boston, Little, Brown, 1994.)*

1. Sweat is obtained through quantitative pilocarpine iontophoresis (>75 mg of sweat must be collected).
2. Results between 40 and 60 mmol/L require repeat testing or other tests for CF including genetic analysis.
3. Normal levels (false-negative results) may be found in patients with CF in the presence of edema and hypoproteinemia or inadequate sweat rate.

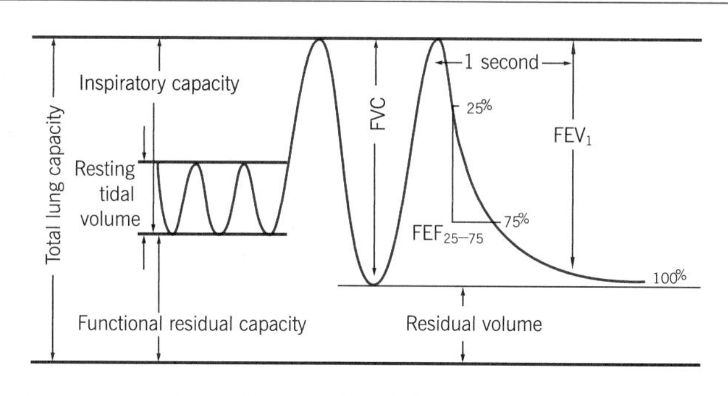

FIG. 22-4
Lung volumes. See text for abbreviations.

TABLE 22-4
INTERPRETATION OF SPIROMETRY AND LUNG VOLUME READINGS

	Obstructive Disease (Asthma, Cystic Fibrosis)	Restrictive Disease (Interstitial Fibrosis, Scoliosis, Neuromuscular Disease)
SPIROMETRY		
FVC[a]	Normal or reduced	Reduced
FEV_1[a]	Reduced	Reduced[d]
FEV_1/FVC[b]	Reduced	Normal
FEF_{25-75}	Reduced	Normal or reduced[d]
PEFR[a]	Normal or reduced	Normal or reduced[d]
LUNG VOLUMES		
TLC[a]	Normal or increased	Reduced
RV[a]	Increased	Reduced
RV/TLC[c]	Increased	Unchanged
FRC	Increased	Reduced

[a]Normal range: ±20% of predicted.
[b]Normal range: >85%.
[c]Normal range: 20 ± 10%.
[d]Reduced proportional to FVC.

4. Elevated chloride levels may be from CF, untreated adrenal insufficiency, glycogen storage disease type I, fucosidosis, hypothyroidism, nephrogenic diabetes insipidus, ectodermal dysplasia, malnutrition, mucopolysaccharidosis, panhypopituitarism, or poor testing technique.

VII. OBSTRUCTIVE SLEEP APNEA SYNDROME (OSAS)

OSAS is a "disorder of breathing during sleep characterized by prolonged partial upper airway obstruction and/or intermittent complete obstruction

TABLE 22-5

MAJOR CLINICAL MANIFESTATIONS OF CYSTIC FIBROSIS BY ORGAN SYSTEM	
Respiratory	Chronic productive cough, hemoptysis
	Bronchiectasis, bronchitis, pneumonia
	Sinusitis
	Nasal polyposis
Gastrointestinal	Meconium ileus
	Rectal prolapse
	Pancreatic insufficiency
	Distal intestinal obstruction syndrome (DIOS)
	Fat-soluble vitamin deficiency (A, D, E, K)
Genitourinary	Infertility (male) and decreased fertility (female)
	Absence of vas deferens
Miscellaneous	Increased sweat electrolytes
	Hypokalemic alkalosis
	Digital clubbing
	Pulmonary hypertrophic osteoarthropathy
	Failure to thrive

(obstructive apnea) that disrupts normal ventilation during sleep and normal sleep patterns."[4] This is to be distinguished from primary snoring (PS), which is snoring without frequent arousals or obstructive apnea. Complications from OSAS include failure to thrive, behavior problems, neurocognitive impairment, cor pulmonale, and disturbed sleep.

A. SYMPTOMS[2]

1. Regular snoring. Usually with intermittent pauses in breathing, snorts, or gasps.
2. Disturbed sleep.
3. Daytime cognitive and/or behavioral problems. Young children rarely present with daytime sleepiness.

B. RISK FACTORS[4]

1. Adenotonsillar hypertrophy.
2. Obesity.
3. Craniofacial anomalies.
4. Central nervous system (CNS) disease, including brainstem dysfunction or compression, cerebral palsy, and neuromuscular disease.

C. WORKUP FOR OSAS[4]

1. Screen for snoring during routine well child care.
2. Referral to specialist for nocturnal polysomnography (sleep study) for patients with history of snoring, risk factors, and/or daytime symptoms.

3. Nocturnal polysomnography is the gold standard for diagnosis of OSAS. This study is able to quantitate abnormalities in ventilation and sleep. Nap studies and overnight oximetry are useful if positive.

D. TREATMENT OPTIONS FOR OSAS

1. Tonsillectomy and adenoidectomy.
2. Continuous positive airway pressure (CPAP) or BiPAP (bilevel positive airway pressure).
   a. Initiation often requires assistance from psychologists and developmental specialists.
   b. Requires follow-up by physician with sleep expertise for pressure titration mask adjustment and monitoring craniofacial development.
   c. Prolonged use of tight-fitting mask may alter the growth and shape of midface region.
3. Weight loss in obese children.
4. Treatment of upper respiratory allergies.

VIII. PULMONARY GAS EXCHANGE

A. ARTERIAL BLOOD GAS

Measurement of arterial blood gas (ABG) is used to assess oxygenation (Pao_2), ventilation (V), $Paco_2$, and acid-base status (pH and HCO_3^-). See Chapter 25 for normal mean ABG values.

B. VENOUS BLOOD GAS

Measurement of venous blood gas (VBG) through peripheral venous samples is strongly affected by the local circulatory and metabolic environment. It can be used to assess acid-base status. $Pvco_2$ averages 6 to 8 mmHg higher than $Paco_2$, and pH is slightly lower.

C. CAPILLARY BLOOD GAS

Correlation of capillary blood gas (CBG) with arterial sampling is generally best for pH, moderate for Pco_2, and worst for Po_2.

D. ANALYSIS OF ACID-BASE DISTURBANCES[5,6]

1. **Pure respiratory acidosis (or alkalosis):** 10 mmHg rise (fall) in $Paco_2$ results in an average 0.08 fall (rise) in pH.
2. **Pure metabolic acidosis (or alkalosis):** 10 mEq/L fall (rise) in HCO_3^- results in an average 0.15 fall (rise) in pH.
3. Determine primary disturbance and then assess for mixed disorder by calculating expected compensatory response (Table 22-6).

E. PULSE OXIMETRY[7,8]

1. **Arterial oxygen saturation:** Noninvasive method of indirectly measuring arterial oxygen saturation (Sao_2). Uses light absorption characteristics of oxygenated and deoxygenated hemoglobin to estimate O_2 saturation.

TABLE 22-6

CALCULATION OF EXPECTED COMPENSATORY RESPONSE

Disturbance	Primary Change	pH	Expected Compensatory Response
Acute respiratory acidosis	↑ $Paco_2$	↓ pH	↑ HCO_3^- by 1 mEq/L for each 10 mmHg rise in $Paco_2$
Acute respiratory alkalosis	↓ $Paco_2$	↑ pH	↓ HCO_3^- by 1–3 mEq/L for each 10 mmHg fall in $Paco_2$
Chronic respiratory acidosis	↑ $Paco_2$	↓ pH	↑ HCO_3^- by 4 mEq/L for each 10 mmHg rise in $Paco_2$
Chronic respiratory alkalosis	↓ $Paco_2$	↑ pH	↓ HCO_3^- by 2–5 mEq/L for each 10 mmHg fall in $Paco_2$
Metabolic acidosis	↓ HCO_3^-	↓ pH	↓ $Paco_2$ by 1 to 1.5 × fall in HCO_3^-
Metabolic alkalosis	↑ HCO_3^-	↑ pH	↑ $Paco_2$ by 0.25–1 × rise in HCO_3^-

Data from Schrier RW: Renal and Electrolyte Disorders, 3rd ed. Boston, Little, Brown, 1986.

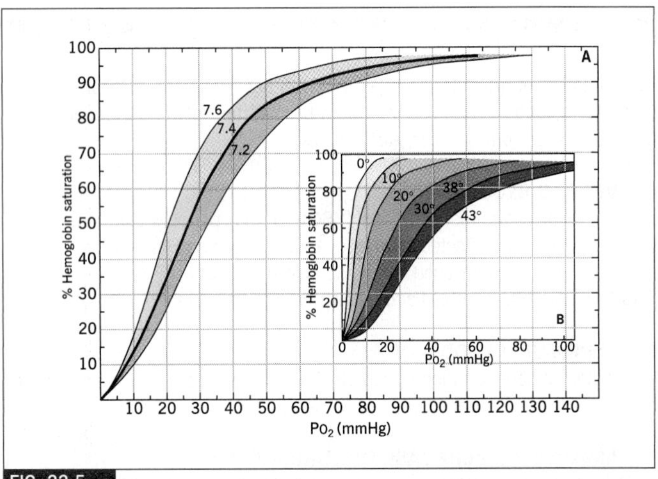

FIG. 22-5

Oxyhemoglobin dissociation curve. *A,* Curve shifts to the left as pH increases. *B*, Curve shifts to the left as temperature decreases. *(Data from Lanbertsten CJ: Transport of oxygen, CO_2, and inert gases by the blood. In Mountcastle VB [ed]: Medical Physiology, 14th ed. St. Louis, Mosby, 1980.)*

2. **The oxyhemoglobin dissociation curve** (Fig. 22-5): This relates O_2 saturation to Pao_2. Increased hemoglobin affinity for oxygen (shift to the left) occurs with alkalemia, hypothermia, hypocapnia, decreased 2,3-diphosphoglycerate (2,3-DPG), increased fetal hemoglobin, and anemia. Decreased hemoglobin affinity for oxygen (shift to the right)

occurs with acidemia, hyperthermia, hypercapnia, and increased 2,3-DPG.

3. **Important uses of pulse oximetry:**
   a. Rapid and continuous assessment of oxygenation in acutely ill patients.
   b. Monitoring of patients requiring oxygen therapy.
   c. Assessment of oxygen requirements during feeding, sleep, and exercise.
   d. Home monitoring of physiologic effects of apnea and bradycardia.
4. **Limitations of pulse oximetry:**
   a. Measures saturation (Sao_2) and not O_2 delivery to tissues. A marginally low saturation may be clinically significant in an anemic patient because a normal O_2 saturation does not ensure a normal O_2-carrying capacity (see oxygen content calculation in Chapter 4).
   b. Unreliable when detection of pulse signal is poor as a result of physiologic conditions (hypothermia, hypovolemia, shock) or movement artifact. The oximeter's pulse rate should match the patient's heart rate to ensure an accurate measurement.
   c. Insensitive to hyperoxia because of the sigmoid shape of the oxyhemoglobin curve.
   d. Sao_2 is artificially increased by carboxyhemoglobin levels >1% to 2% (e.g., in chronic smokers or with smoke inhalation).
   e. Sao_2 is artificially decreased by patient motion, intravenous dyes, such as methylene blue and indocyanine green, and opaque nail polish.
   f. Sao_2 is artificially decreased by methemoglobin levels >1% ; electrosurgical interference or xenon arc surgical lamps may alter accuracy of pulse ox readings.
   g. Sao_2 reading often does not correlate with Pao_2 in sickle cell disease.[9]

22 PULMONOLOGY

F. CAPNOGRAPHY

Capnography measures CO_2 concentration of expired gas by infrared spectroscopy or mass spectroscopy. End-tidal CO_2 ($ETco_2$) correlates with $Paco_2$ (usually within 5 mmHg of $Paco_2$ in healthy subjects). Capnography can be used for demonstrating proper placement of an endotracheal tube, continuous monitoring of CO_2 trends in ventilated patients, and monitoring ventilation during polysomnography.

REFERENCES

1. Kwong KYC, Jones CA: Chronic asthma therapy. Pediatr Rev 1999;20(10):329.
2. Loughin GM, Eigen H: Respiratory Disease in Children: Diagnosis and Management. Baltimore, Williams & Wilkins, 1994.
3. Soldin SJ, Brugnara C, Wong EC: Pediatric Reference Ranges, 4th ed. Washington, DC, AACC Press, 2003.
4. AAP Clinical Practice Guideline: Diagnosis and Management of Childhood Obstructive Sleep Apnea. 2002;109(4):704–712.
5. Schrier RW: Renal and Electrolyte Disorders, 6th ed. Lippincott, Williams and Wilkins, 2002.
6. Brenner BM, Rector FC (eds): The Kidney, Vol. 1, 7th ed. Philadelphia, WB Saunders, 2003.

7. Murray CB, Loughlin GM. Making the most of pulse oximetry. Contemp Pediatr 1995;12(7):45–52, 55–57, 61–62.
8. Lanbertsten CJ: Transport of oxygen, CO_2, and inert gases by the blood. In Mountcastle VB (ed): Medical Physiology, 14th ed. St. Louis, Mosby, 1980.
9. Comber JT, Lopez BL: Examination of pulse oximetry in sickle cell anemia patients presenting to the emergency department in acute vasoocclusive crisis. Am J Emerg Med 1996;14(1):16.

Radiology

Alexander M. Kowal, MD

23

I. HEAD

Most intracranial processes, malformations, and tumors are best imaged with magnetic resonance imaging (MRI). MRI is useful for neurodegenerative and demyelination disorders, diffuse axonal injury detection, neurocutaneous syndromes, structural lesions in focal seizure disorders, and vascular lesions. Compared to computed tomography (CT), MRI is more useful in detecting lesions in the posterior fossa.

A. GERMINAL MATRIX HEMORRHAGE

Premature infants should undergo head ultrasonography (US) to detect intraventricular hemorrhage and periventricular leukomalacia and to screen for hydrocephalus and congenital abnormalities.

B. CONGENITAL MALFORMATIONS

Once detected on US, malformations are further defined with MRI.

C. CONGENITAL INFECTIONS

Congenital infections such as herpes simplex virus (HSV) are best imaged on MRI. Computed tomography (CT) may detect calcifications consistent with toxoplasmosis and cytomegalovirus (CMV) infection.

D. HEAD TRAUMA

Best imaged by non-contrast CT to reveal skull fractures and subdural and epidural hematomas. A head CT should be part of a physical abuse workup. Skull radiography is of limited value. Multiple hemorrhages of various ages are best detected with MRI.

E. VENTRICULOPERITONEAL SHUNT MALFUNCTION

Initial imaging includes a head CT to determine ventricle size. If signs of shunt malfunction are noted, radiographs of the length of the shunt (a shunt series) should follow to look for kinks or disconnections.

F. CRANIOSYNOSTOSIS

Suture examination is best done initially with radiographs of the skull. If there are changes consistent with craniosynostosis, three-dimensional CT reconstructions should then be obtained.

II. EYES

A. ORBITAL CELLULITIS

Best imaged with contrast CT with orbital cuts. To determine whether an infection is preseptal or postseptal, a line is drawn from the medial to the lateral bony walls of the orbit on transverse cuts.

III. SPINE

A. CERVICAL SPINE TRAUMA

After immobilization in a collar, lateral and anteroposterior (AP) radiographs of the cervical spine (C-spine) should be performed in all children who have sustained significant head trauma or deceleration injury or who have undergone unwitnessed trauma. The seventh cervical vertebral body and the C7-T1 junction must be visualized. C-spine injuries are most common from the occiput to C3 in children (especially subluxation at the atlanto-occipital joint or atlantoaxial joint in infants and toddlers) and in the lower C-spine in older children and adults. Flexion-extension films may be helpful, especially in patients with Down syndrome who are at risk for atlantoaxial subluxation. Odontoid views may be helpful in older children with suspected occipitocervical injury (e.g., whiplash).

B. READING C-SPINE FILMS

The following ABCDDS (or ABCDs) mnemonic is useful:

1. **Alignment:** The anterior vertebral body line, posterior vertebral body line, facet line, and spinous process line should each form a continuous line with smooth contour and no step-offs.
2. **Bones:** Assess each bone looking for chips or fractures.
3. **Count:** Must see C7 body in its entirety.
4. **Dens:** Examine for chips or fractures.
5. **Disc spaces:** Should see consistent distance between each vertebral body.
6. **Soft tissue:** Assess for swelling, particularly in the prevertebral area.

C. SCIWORA

Spinal cord injury without radiographic abnormality (SCIWORA) is a functional C-spine injury that cannot be excluded by abnormality on a radiograph; it is thought to be attributable to increased mobility of a child's spine. SCIWORA should be suspected in the setting of normal C-spine images when clinical signs or symptoms (e.g., point tenderness, focal neurologic symptoms) suggest C-spine injury. If neurologic symptoms persist despite normal C-spine and flexion-extension views, MRI is indicated to rule out swelling, contusion, or intramedullary hemorrhage of the cord.

D. SPINAL DYSRAPHISM (e.g., Myelocele, Myelomeningocele)

Initial imaging consists of radiographs. Most often screened for with US. Complications are followed by MRI.

E. SCOLIOSIS

Best evaluated by erect AP spine radiograph. PA views can be used in postpubertal girls to decrease breast radiation dose.

IV. AIRWAY

A. LATERAL RADIOGRAPH

The lateral radiograph of the upper airway is the single most useful film for evaluating a child with stridor. If possible, this view should be obtained on inspiration. A radiologic workup should always include AP and lateral radiographs of the chest, with inclusion of the upper airway on the AP chest radiograph. Diagnosis is based on airway radiologic examination in conjunction with clinical presentation (Table 23-1; Figs. 23-1 and 23-2).

B. VASCULAR RINGS

Vascular rings and other masses that extrinsically obstruct the lower airways can be imaged with contrast-enhanced CT or MRI. Tracheomalacia and intrinsic masses can be studied with bronchoscopy.

C. FOREIGN BODIES

1. **Lower airway foreign bodies:** In the absence of a radiopaque foreign body, radiologic findings include air trapping, hyperinflation, atelectasis, consolidation, pneumothorax, and pneumomediastinum. Further studies should include expiratory films (in a cooperative patient), bilateral decubitus chest films (in an uncooperative patient), or airway fluoroscopy.
2. **Esophageal foreign bodies:** Usually lodged at one of three locations: the thoracic inlet, the level of the aortic arch and left mainstem bronchus, or the gastroesophageal junction. Evaluation should include the following:

a. Lateral airway film.
b. AP film of the chest and abdomen (including the supraclavicular region).
c. Contrast study of the esophagus if other films are normal. If perforation is suspected, use nonionic, water-soluble contrast.

V. CHEST

A. POSTEROANTERIOR AND LATERAL RADIOGRAPHS

PA and lateral radiographs are the first images obtained when studying the chest (Figs. 23-3 and 23-4).

B. PNEUMONIA

Lobar or segmental consolidation and atelectasis are more typical of bacterial infections, whereas hyperinflation, bilateral patchy or streaky densities, and peribronchial thickening are more typical of nonbacterial disease.

C. ATELECTASIS VERSUS INFILTRATE

1. **Atelectasis:** When air is removed from the lung, the tissue collapses, resulting in volume loss on chest radiographs. Air may still remain in

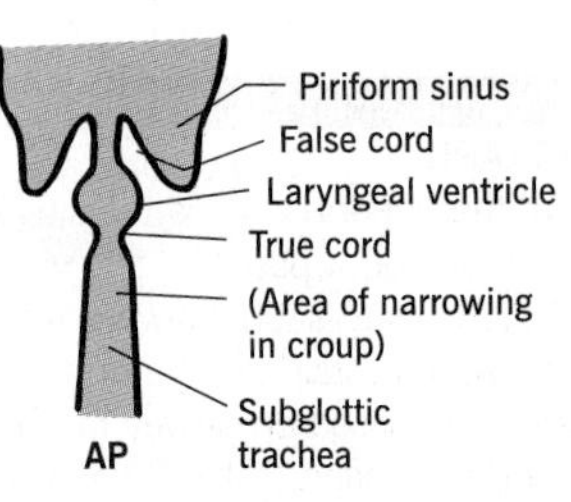

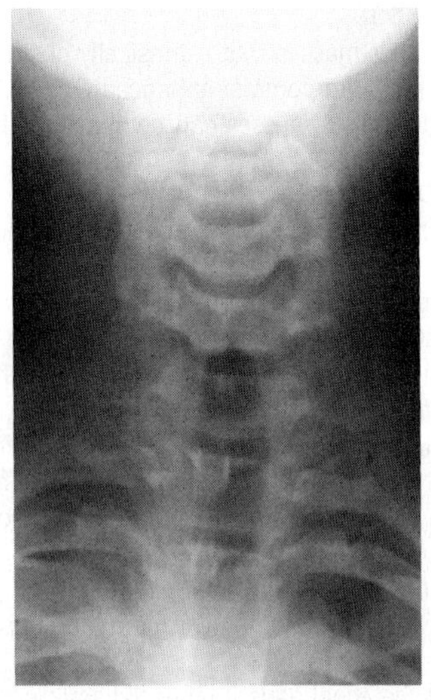

FIG. 23-1
Anteroposterior (AP) neck film with normal anatomy on AP airway view.

TABLE 23-1
DIAGNOSIS OF DISEASES BASED ON AIRWAY RADIOLOGIC EXAMINATION

Diagnosis	Findings on Airway Films
Croup	AP and lateral films with subglottic narrowing ("steeple sign")
Epiglottitis	Enlarged, indistinct epiglottis on lateral film ("thumb print sign")
Vascular ring	AP and lateral films with narrowing; double or right aortic arch
Retropharyngeal abscess or pharyngeal mass	Soft tissue air or persistent enlargement of prevertebral soft tissues; more than half of a vertebral body above C3 and one vertebral body below C3
Immunodeficiency	Absence of adenoidal and tonsillar tissue after age 6 mo

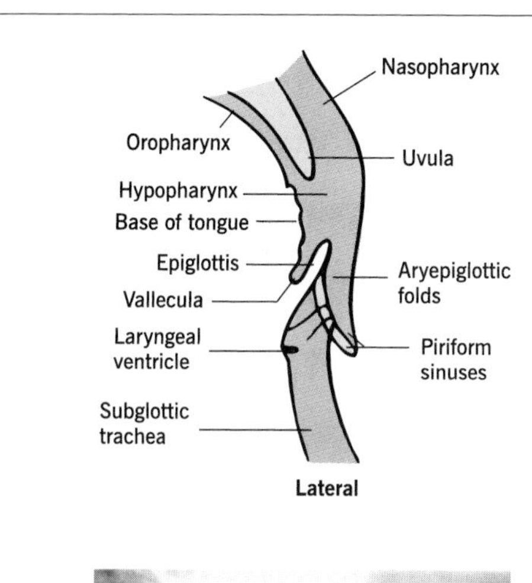

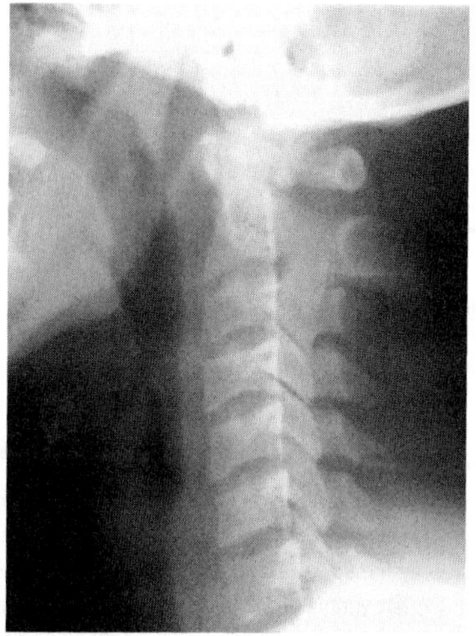

FIG. 23-2
Lateral neck film with normal anatomy on lateral airway view.

the larger bronchi, creating air bronchograms on the radiograph. Collapse and re-expansion can occur quickly.

2. **Infiltrate:** A fluid (blood, pus, edema) that invades one of the compartments of the lung (bronchoalveolar air space or peribronchial interstitial space) is seen as a density on a radiograph. When alveolar

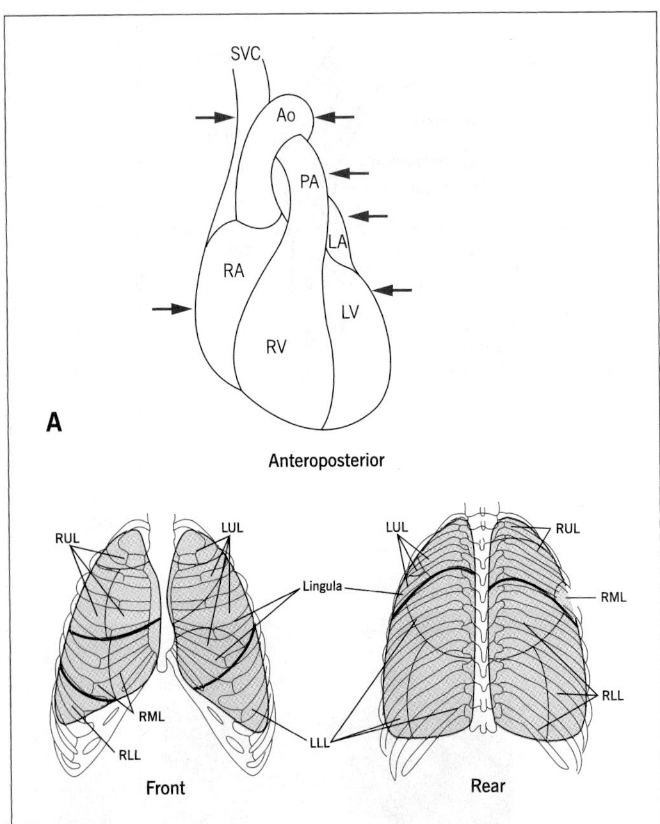

FIG. 23-3

A, Lung and cardiac anatomy on an AP chest radiograph. Divisions within lobes indicate segments matched with x-rays. *Arrows* indicate contours seen on anteroposterior chest x-ray films *(B)*. Ao, aorta; LA, left atrium; LLL, left lower lobe; LUL, left upper lobe; LV, left ventricle; PA, pulmonary artery; RA, right atrium; RLL, right lower lobe; RML, right middle lobe; RUL, right upper lobe; RV, right ventricle; SVC, superior vena cava. *(Heart diagram modified from Kirks DR, et al: Practical Pediatric Imaging: Diagnostic Radiology of Infants and Children, 3rd ed. Philadelphia, Lippincott-Raven, 1998.)*

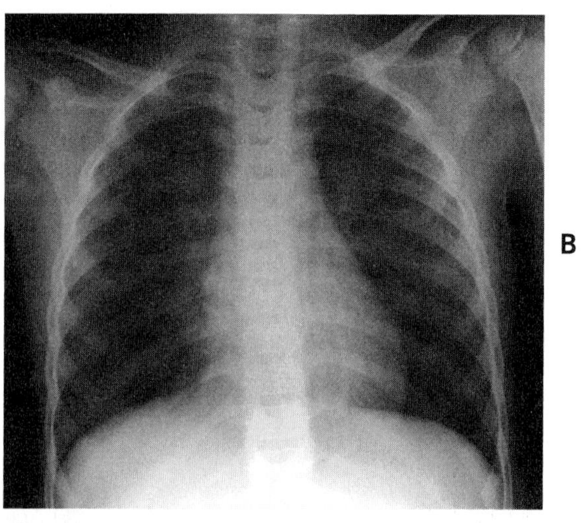

FIG. 23-3—cont'd

air is displaced by fluid, but air remains in the bronchi, the classic pneumonic infiltrate with air bronchograms is seen. When the infiltrate is interstitial, its borders are more vague, and bronchial walls may be thickened. Typically, infiltrates resolve in 2 to 6 weeks.

D. PARAPNEUMONIC EFFUSIONS AND EMPYEMA

PA and lateral radiographs are initially obtained. Lateral decubitus radiographs may also be helpful, followed by either US or contrast-enhanced CT to determine if effusion is loculated, and to mark area for percutaneous drainage.

E. PARENCHYMAL FINDINGS

Parenchymal findings, such as lung abscess, cavitary necrosis, pneumatocele, fungal infections, or lung contusions are best imaged with contrast-enhanced CT.

F. MEDIASTINAL MASSES

Mediastinal masses (thymus, lymphoma, bronchogenic cyst, neuroblastoma, neurofibroma) are initially imaged with radiography, followed by CT or MRI.

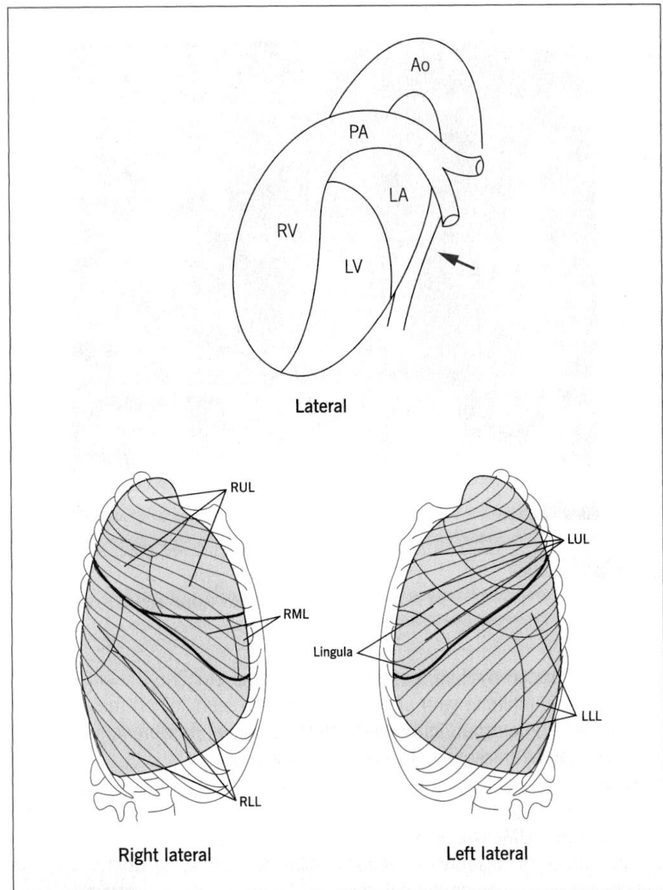

FIG. 23-4

A, Lung and cardiac anatomy on lateral chest radiograph. Divisions within lobes indicate segments matched with x-rays. *Arrows* indicate contours seen on lateral chest x-ray films *(B)*. Ao, aorta; LA, left atrium; LLL, left lower lobe; LUL, left upper lobe; LV, left ventricle; PA, pulmonary artery; RLL, right lower lobe; RML, right middle lobe; RUL, right upper lobe; RV, right ventricle. *(Heart diagram modified from Kirks DR, et al: Practical Pediatric Imaging: Diagnostic Radiology of Infants and Children, 3rd ed. Philadelphia, Lippincott-Raven, 1998.)*

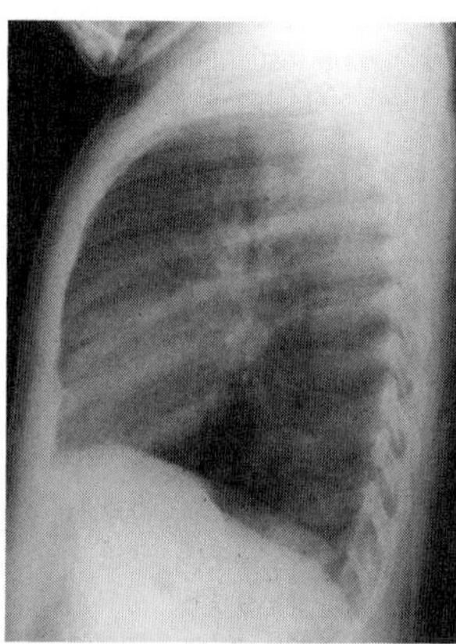

FIG. 23-4—cont'd

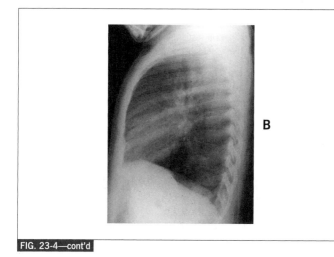

G. CENTRAL LINE PLACEMENT

On chest radiograph, central venous catheters are ideally placed with the catheter tip at the junction of the superior vena cava and right atrium. Some extension into the right atrium is acceptable, but if the catheter is noted to curve to the patient's left on the PA film, the catheter may be positioned in the right ventricle.

H. ENDOTRACHEAL TUBE (ETT) PLACEMENT

On chest radiograph, the end of the ETT should rest approximately midway between the thoracic inlet and carina. The lung fields should show symmetric aeration.

VI. HEART AND VESSELS

A. CONGENITAL HEART DISEASE

Most often and clearly defined by echocardiography, but evaluation of an initial PA and lateral chest radiograph may yield important clues:

1. **Position of the aortic arch**—left or right.
2. **Situs**—noting the position of the apex, stomach bubble, and liver.
3. **Heart size**—with particular attention paid to the lateral chest radiograph.
4. **Pulmonary vascularity**—increased or decreased flow in arteries and veins.

B. VESSELS

Moving blood is detected by ultrasonographic frequency shifts. Color Doppler flow imaging can be used to evaluate deep-vein thrombosis, vascular patency, intracranial blood flow (including transcranial Doppler to screen for ischemic brain injury risk in sickle cell disease), cardiac shunt flow, transplant vascularity, and testicular perfusion in acute scrotum. Power Doppler is particularly sensitive in detecting slow flow in small vessels (e.g., infant testes).

C. VESSEL ABNORMALITIES

Vessel abnormalities can be studied with echocardiography/US, CT, and MRI, which can detect coarctation of the aorta, aortic stenosis, pulmonary artery and vein abnormalities, vascular rings, arteriovenous malformations and hemangiomas, aneurysms, and postoperative complications such as thrombosis and stenosis.

VII. ABDOMEN

A. NEONATAL ENTEROCOLITIS (NEC)

NEC is initially diagnosed and followed by abdominal radiographs, which may show focal dilation, featureless loops, pneumatosis, and portal venous gas.

B. ESOPHAGEAL ATRESIA AND TRACHEOESOPHAGEAL FISTULA (TEF)

These are studied initially with radiographs of the chest, which may reveal the air-distended esophageal atretic pouch, the nasogastric tube curled up in this pouch, or excessive dilation of stomach as a result of fistula communication.

C. HIGH INTESTINAL OBSTRUCTION

Diagnosed with an upper gastrointestinal (UGI) series, during which contrast is ingested and the esophagus, stomach, and duodenum are visualized. Causes include esophageal webs and rings, masses, duodenal atresia or webs, annular pancreas, midgut volvulus, and Ladd bands. UGI can also help evaluate hiatal hernias, varices, gastric outlet obstruction, motility problems, ulcerations, and reflux. During an UGI, identification of the duodenojejunal junction (the ligament of Treitz) helps to diagnose malrotation. Normally, the junction is to the left of the spine, at or above the level of the duodenal bulb.

D. PYLORIC STENOSIS

US will directly visualize the muscle and is the preferred examination. Normally, the pylorus is <15 cm in length and <3 mm in width. Radiographs will show gastric distention. If an UGI is done, delayed gastric emptying and a narrow pyloric channel will be evident.

E. BOWEL OBSTRUCTION

Determination of large or small bowel obstruction is often aided by a supine radiograph, a prone radiograph, and either an upright, supine cross-table lateral or left lateral decubitus film to look for free air and air-fluid levels. Causes of obstruction can include adhesions, appendicitis, incarcerated inguinal hernias, Meckel diverticulum, or intussusception. US can be helpful in thin patients as well as in female patients who have ovarian pathology in their differential for abdominal pain. CT with intravenous (IV), oral, or rectal contrast is more useful with an obese patient or when looking for perforated appendicitis or abscess. Contrast enemas with dilute, water-soluble agents can also be useful in lower intestinal obstruction in the newborn.

F. INTUSSUSCEPTION

On abdominal radiographs, particularly the prone view, findings include minimal gas in the right abdomen and ascending colon. Both US and CT will show alternating rings. Air insufflation is preferred, but contrast enema with fluoroscopic guidance can also reduce an intussusception. These methods are contraindicated if perforation is suspected.

G. MECKEL DIVERTICULUM

Suggested by painless lower gastrointestinal bleeding, Meckel diverticulum is diagnosed by nuclear scintigraphy using ^{99m}Tc-pertechnetate.

H. ABDOMINAL TRAUMA

CT of abdomen and pelvis is done to detect solid organ injury, vascular extravasation, free fluid, bowel wall thickening, and organ laceration.

I. BILIARY ATRESIA

In neonates with jaundice, US is initially done to distinguish biliary atresia from hepatitis. The gallbladder will be small or absent with biliary atresia. Hepatobiliary scintigraphy with ^{99m}Tc iminodiacetate (HIDA) may be helpful.

VIII. GENITOURINARY TRACT

A. URINARY TRACT INFECTION

Initial febrile UTIs in children younger than 5 years require imaging to look for congenital anomalies (e.g., posterior urethral valves, ureterocele), vesicoureteral reflux, baseline renal measurements, and damage to the cortex of the kidneys. Workup first includes US to diagnose hydronephrosis, ureteropelvic junction obstruction, posterior urethral valves, multicystic dysplastic kidneys, chronic pyelonephritis, renal fusion (horseshoe kidney), and renal cysts. A voiding cystourethrogram (VCUG) can then be done to diagnose vesicoureteral reflux, abnormalities of bladder or urethral function and anatomy including ureterocele, and posterior urethral valves. Occasionally, dimercaptosuccinic acid (DMSA) scan is useful in following renal cortical scarring and pyelonephritis.

B. UTERINE AND OVARIAN PATHOLOGY

Transvaginal or transabdominal US should be performed in women whose clinical picture is suspicious for ovarian torsion, tubo-ovarian abscess (TOA), or ectopic pregnancy.

IX. EXTREMITIES

A. TRAUMA

An adequate evaluation requires an AP and a lateral radiograph. Restricting the film to include only the area of interest improves the resolution (e.g., for a thumb injury, ask for an image of the thumb, not the hand). In general, comparison films of the uninvolved extremity are not necessary but may be helpful in several instances, such as the evaluation of joint effusions (particularly the hip), suspected osteomyelitis, or pyarthrosis and/or the evaluation of subtle fractures, especially in areas of multiple ossification centers such as the elbow. See Chapter 4 for the Salter-Harris classification of growth-plate injury. Avulsion injuries tend to occur at the knee and pelvis.

B. STRESS FRACTURES

Occur most often at the tibia, fibula, metatarsals, and calcaneus. Radiography will show a band of sclerosis and new bone formation. Skeletal scintigraphy and CT can be used to make the diagnosis.

C. OSTEOMYELITIS

Tends to occur at the metaphysis of long bones and within flat bones. Radiography will show deep soft tissue swelling and bony changes (which may take 10 days to appear). Skeletal scintigraphy and MRI will often be positive before radiographic changes are noticeable.

D. HIP DISORDERS

Developmental dysplasia of the hip (congenital hip dislocation) is imaged initially with US. Once the femoral heads ossify, radiographs are more helpful. Legg-Calvé-Perthes disease (avascular necrosis of the femoral head) can be imaged with AP and frog-leg lateral hip films as well as MRI and bone scintigraphy. Slipped capital femoral epiphysis (SCFE) will show displacement of the femoral head on frog-leg lateral and AP radiographs.

E. BONE AGE

Obtain a PA view of the left hand and wrist.

F. SKELETAL SURVEY

In cases of suspected child abuse or metastatic oncologic disease, this survey should include a lateral skull film with a C-spine film, an AP chest film (bone technique), oblique views of the ribs, an AP view of the pelvis, an abdominal film (bone technique) with the lateral thoracic and lumbar spine, and AP long-bone films. Classic findings are multiple metaphyseal injuries (especially corner and "bucket-handle" fractures) and other fractures of various ages. In addition, suspicion should be raised by fracture at unusual sites, such as posterior rib fractures or solitary spiral and transverse fractures of the long bones with an inconsistent history of trauma.

REFERENCES

1. Kirks DR, et al: Practical Pediatric Imaging: Diagnostic Radiology of Infants and Children, 3rd ed. Philadelphia, Lippincott-Raven, 1998.
2. Blickman H: Pediatric Radiology: The Requisites, 2nd ed. St. Louis, Mosby, 1998.
3. Donnelly LF: Fundamentals of Pediatric Radiology. Philadelphia, WB Saunders, 2001.

Rheumatology

Susan McFarland, MD

24

I. LABORATORY STUDIES

Laboratory studies used in the diagnosis of rheumatic diseases are usually quite nonspecific for rheumatic diseases and must be put into the context of the full clinical picture. However, once a diagnosis is established, these laboratory studies can be used to follow the clinical course of the rheumatic diseases indicating flares or remission of the disease state.

A. ACUTE PHASE REACTANTS

Acute phase reactants are general markers, which can indicate the presence of inflammation when elevated. However, the elevation is nonspecific because it can result from trauma, infection, rheumatic diseases, and even some cancers.[2] Examples and measures of acute phase reactants include erythrocyte sedimentation rate (ESR), C-reactive protein (CRP), platelet count, ferritin, haptoglobin, fibrinogen, serum amyloid A, and complement.[2,3]

1. **ESR, which is a measure of the rate of fall of red blood cells in anticoagulated blood in a vertical tube, reflects the level of Rouleaux formation caused by acute phase reactants.[2]**

a. Can be falsely lowered in the presence of afibrinogenemia, anemia, and sickle cells since these states will interfere with rouleaux formation.[3]

b. Levels can also vary depending on age, ethnicity, and gender.[2]

c. Following levels over time can be helpful in monitoring the state of rheumatic diseases such as systemic lupus erythematosus (SLE) and juvenile rheumatoid arthritis (JRA).

2. **CRP is an acute phase reactant that can activate the complement pathway and that interacts with phagocytic cells.[2]**

a. Can increase and decrease rapidly because of its short half-life of about 18 hours.[2]

b. Elevations are nonspecific, indicating only presence of inflammation.

   (1) Most active phases of rheumatic diseases can result in an elevation to 1–10 mg/dL.[2]

   (2) Levels of greater than 10mg/dL can be suspicious for a bacterial infection but can also occur in the presence of a systemic vasculitis.[2]

B. AUTOANTIBODIES (Table 24-1)

1. **The positive predictive value of any autoantibody depends on the clinical context;** hence, antibody studies are useful for confirming a clinical suspicion, but are not useful as diagnostic tests in nonsuspicious clinical settings.
2. **An example of an initial general autoantibody screen useful in the evaluation of a child with a possible rheumatologic disorder includes anti-dsDNA (double-stranded DNA), anti-Ro (Robert: SSA), anti-La**

TABLE 24-1

AUTOANTIBODIES AND THEIR ASSOCIATED DISEASE STATES

Autoantibody	Disease State(s)
ANCA-cytoplasmic/PR3*	Wegener granulomatosis
ANCA-perinuclear/MPO*	Microscopic polyangiitis
Anticentromere	CREST syndrome Variant scleroderma
Anti–double-stranded DNA	Systemic lupus erythematosus
Antihistone	Drug-induced systemic lupus erythematosus
Anti-Jo-1	Dermatomyositis Polymyositis
Anti-La	Neonatal lupus syndrome Sjögren syndrome Systemic lupus erythematosus
Antimicrosomal	Chronic active hepatitis Systemic lupus erythematosus
Antimitochondrial	Primary biliary cirrhosis Systemic lupus erythematosus
Anti-RNP	Mixed connective tissue disease Polymyositis Scleroderma Sjögren syndrome Systemic lupus erythematosus
Anti-Ro	Neonatal lupus Sjögren syndrome Systemic lupus erythematosus
Anti-Smith	Systemic lupus erythematosus
Antithyroid	Systemic lupus erythematosus Thyroiditis

*ANCA (antineutrophil cytoplasmic antibody) can be measured by immunofluorescence [cytoplasmic-ANCA (c-ANCA) or perinuclear-ANCA (p-ANCA)] or ELISA methods [Proteinase 3 (PR3) or myeloperoxidase (MPO)].
Data from references 1, 2, and 9.

(Lane: SSB), anti-RNP (ribonucleoprotein), and anti-Sm (Smith). Anti-dsDNA and anti-Sm, for example, are highly specific for SLE.

3. **Antinuclear antibody (ANA) is a nonspecific test for rheumatic disease.**

a. Approximately 60% to 70% of children with a positive ANA have an autoimmune disease,[2] but it can be seen in about 15% to 35% of normal persons.

b. ANA can also be positive in nonrheumatic diseases, such as neoplastic diseases, as well as infections, including mononucleosis, endocarditis, hepatitis, and malaria.[2]

c. Whether or not ANA is positive can be of great importance, particularly in pauciarticular JRA, where it connotes an increased risk of uveitis.

4. Antineutrophil cytoplasmic antibodies (ANCA).

a. Tests that suggest the presence of a vasculitis without immune complex deposition.

b. Can be measured by two methods:

  (1) Immunofluorescence: Positive test resulted as cytoplasmic-ANCA (c-ANCA) or perinuclear-ANCA (p-ANCA).

  (2) Enzyme-linked immunosorbent assay (ELISA): Positive test resulted as proteinase 3 (PR3) or myeloperoxidase (MPO).

c. c-ANCA or PR3 can be seen in Wegener granulomatosis.

d. p-ANCA or MPO can be seen in microscopic polyangiitis (MPA).

C. RHEUMATOID FACTOR (RF)

Antibodies to the Fc portion of immunoglobulin G:[2]

1. Positive RF, like ANA, is not specific for a rheumatic disease, nor does a negative test rule out a rheumatic disease.

2. The presence of RF can suggest immune complex formation and/or deposition.

3. It can occur in multiple states:

a. Rheumatic diseases such as SLE, JRA, and Henoch-Schönlein purpura (HSP).[2]

b. Numerous infections, such as hepatitis B, bacterial endocarditis, tuberculosis, and congenital TORCH infections.[2]

D. COMPLEMENT

The complement system is composed of multiple proteins, which are important in the inflammatory processes involved in fighting infections. Any process that causes an inflammatory response can affect the complement proteins by increasing their synthesis and/or increasing their consumption.

1. Total hemolytic complement level, which is also known as CH_{50}, is a general measure of complement, and is also an acute phase reactant.

a. Increased in the acute phase response of numerous states, which cause inflammation.

b. Useful screening test for homozygous complement deficiency states.[1]

c. Typically becomes decreased in SLE.

2. The two complement proteins that are primarily followed in rheumatic diseases are C3 and C4 because the immunoassays that measure them are the ones that are most widely available.[1] Because levels can be increased or decreased in rheumatic diseases, depending on where one is in the active phase of the disease as well as the severity of the disease, it is more important to follow the complement trend over time rather than an isolated result.

3. Decreased levels of complement proteins can be seen in multiple states.

a. Indicator of immune complex formation, which can occur in the presence of active SLE as well as some vasculitides,[1,2] and in multiple infections including gram-negative sepsis, hepatitis, and pneumococcal infections.[1] Decreased levels are typically a sign of more severe SLE, particularly in regard to renal disease.[1]
b. Severe hepatic failure because complement proteins are primarily made in the liver.
c. Congenital complement deficiency, which can predispose to the development of an autoimmune disease.

4. Increased levels of complement proteins can also be seen in multiple states:[1]

a. Can occur during the active phase of most rheumatic diseases including SLE, JRA, and dermatomyositis.
b. Can be seen in multiple infections as part of the acute phase response, including hepatitis and pneumococcal pneumonia.

E. URINALYSIS

In many rheumatic diseases, obtaining urinalysis is important to rule out renal involvement, including looking for proteinuria, red blood cells (RBCs), or casts. See Chapter 18 for further details regarding urinalysis.

F. SERUM MUSCLE ENZYMES

Muscle enzymes can be elevated in the presence of rheumatic diseases, which cause muscle inflammation, such as dermatomyositis. Such enzymes include creatine kinase, aspartate transaminase (AST), lactate dehydrogenase (LDH), and aldolase.[3]

G. JOINT FLUID ANALYSIS (Table 24-2)

Evaluation of joint fluid in the presence of an effusion, especially in monoarticular disease, is very important.[4] Although an effusion can be seen in rheumatic diseases, it can also be present in other disease processes such as septic arthritis.

II. JUVENILE RHEUMATOID ARTHRITIS (JRA)[1-3,5]

Diagnosing a child with arthritis can be challenging because of the usual young age at onset and varied presentations, from walking with a limp or refusal to walk, irritability, poor growth, or limb discrepancy, besides presenting with joint pain or effusion. Also, the differential diagnosis for arthritis depends on the number of joints involved as well as the acute or chronic nature of the arthritis.[1,3]

A. CLASSICAL DIVISIONS

Classical divisions of JRA are based on the clinical course over the first 6 months of illness[2,3] (Table 24-3). The divisions used here are based on the American College of Rheumatology. There are multiple other

TABLE 24-2
JOINT FLUID ANALYSIS

Disorder	Cells/μL	Glucose*
Trauma	More red cells than white cells; usually <2000 white cells	Normal
Reactive arthritis	3000–10,000 white cells, mostly mononuclear	Normal
Juvenile rheumatoid arthritis and other inflammatory arthritides	5000–60,000 white cells, mostly neutrophils	Usually normal or slightly low
Septic arthritis	>60,000 white cells, >90% neutrophils	Low to normal

*Normal value is 75% or more of serum glucose value.
Data from Hay WW, Hayward AR, Levin MJ, Sondheimer JM: Current Pediatric Diagnosis and Treatment, 15th ed. New York, Lange Medical Books/McGraw-Hill, 2001.

classifications as well as new proposals for changes in the classical divisions.

1. **Pauciarticular JRA.**
2. **Polyarticular JRA.**
3. **Systemic-onset JRA, also referred to as Still's disease.**

B. PAUCIARTICULAR JRA

Pauciarticular JRA, which is the most common type of JRA, accounts for approximately 60% of the cases.[1,3] It is characterized by the involvement of four or fewer joints during the first 6 months of the illness. There are two major subtypes of pauciarticular JRA.

1. **Type I—Female-predominant subtype with a greater than 4:1 female-to-male ratio:**
   a. Peak age of onset is younger than the onset for the male-predominant subtype, being around preschool age.
   b. Laboratory values include positive ANA in greater than 50% of patients, with RF being rarely present.
2. **Type II—Male-predominant subtype with a greater than 20:1 male-to-female ratio:**
   a. Peak age of onset is about 9 to 11 years, with joint involvement starting commonly in the lower extremities in an asymmetric fashion.
   b. Hips are also commonly involved, which is rare in the case of the female-predominant subtype. Sacroiliac and intervertebral joints can become involved in late adolescence.
   c. Unlike the female-predominant subtype, the uveitis is usually acute rather than chronic in nature.
   d. HLA-B27 is usually positive.
   e. Laboratory values usually include a negative ANA and RF.

TABLE 24-3

COMPARISON OF MAJOR DIVISIONS OF JUVENILE RHEUMATOID ARTHRITIS

	Pauciarticular	Polyarticular	Systemic-Onset
Frequency	60%	30%	10%
Number of joints involved during first 6 mo	≤4	≥5	Variable
Gender predominance	Type I: female > male Type II: male > female	Female > male	None
Age predominance	Type I: preschool age; rare >10 yr Type II: 9–11 yr	2–5 yr and 10–18 yr	None
Joints involved	Any but particularly knees and ankles; rare to start in hips	Any but typically larger joints; often symmetric involvement of joints; rare to start in hips	Any, including hips; extra-articular manifestations may precede joint involvement
Extra-articular manifestations	Generally absent except for uveitis	Moderate degree including fever, hepatosplenomegaly, and lymphadenopathy	High-spiking fevers that occur daily or twice daily; hepatosplenomegaly; lymphadenopathy; polyserositis; characteristic rash
Uveitis	20% Significantly higher when ANA positive Type I: chronic uveitis Type II: acute uveitis	5%	Rare
Antinuclear antibody	Low titer common	Low titer common in younger group	Typically absent
Rheumatoid factor	Typically absent	Common in older group	Rare
Destructive arthritis	Rare	>50%	>50%

Data from references 1–3 and 5.

C. POLYARTICULAR JRA

Polyarticular JRA accounts for approximately 30% of the cases of JRA.[1,3] It is characterized by the involvement of five or more joints during the first 6 months of the illness. Like pauciarticular JRA, it can be divided into two subtypes. There is an approximately 5:1 female-to-male ratio. Articular involvement is often unremitting, requiring rehabilitation and/or orthopedic surgery involvement. Polyarticular JRA is associated with mild systemic manifestations, such as fever and malaise.

1. Seronegative for RF, which is the most common subtype:

a. Approximately 25% of the patients are ANA positive.

b. Age of onset is usually less than 10 years, with a peak onset near 1 to 3 years of age.

c. It usually has a more favorable disease course than the RF seropositive subtype, and also responds better to nonsteroidal anti-inflammatory drug (NSAID) therapy.

2. Seropositive for RF:

a. Approximately 50% of the patients are ANA positive.

b. Age of onset is usually older than 10 years.

c. It has a less favorable disease course than the RF-seronegative subtype, requiring more advanced therapies, such as methotrexate, glucocorticoids, cyclosporine, and etanercept.

d. Usually, by the end of the first year of illness, there exists radiographic evidence of destructive arthritis.

D. SYSTEMIC-ONSET JRA

Systemic-onset JRA accounts for approximately 10% of the cases of JRA.[1,3] There is no gender predominance and no peak age of onset. Systemic-onset JRA is differentiated from the other types of JRA due to the predominance of the extra-articular manifestations such as fever and rash, which can precede the onset of articular symptoms and signs by months or longer. Laboratory values usually include a negative ANA and negative RF with leukocytosis, thrombocytosis, and elevated ESR demonstrating the systemic inflammation. Prognosis is variable. However, pericarditis and pleuropericarditis are potentially serious manifestations of systemic-onset JRA.

E. TREATMENT OF ARTHRITIS

1. Pharmacologic agents[1-3,6]:

a. NSAIDS: Usual initial treatment; examples include ibuprofen and naproxen.

b. Corticosteroids: Can be systemic and/or intra-articular.

c. Disease-modifying and cytotoxic drugs: Examples include cyclosporine, hydroxychloroquine, and methotrexate.

d. Biologic immunomodulators: Examples include etanercept.

2. Vaccines: Child with a rheumatologic disease should follow the regular immunization schedule with a few noted exceptions.

a. Live vaccines are contraindicated in children receiving immunosuppressive therapy; typically, vaccinations with live vaccines should wait until at least 3 months after discontinuation of the immunosuppressive agent.[6]
b. Varicella vaccine, therefore, should be given before starting immunosuppressive therapies if patient not previously vaccinated or previously had a documented case of varicella.
c. Influenza vaccine should be given to any patient receiving immunosuppressive therapies[2,6]; if under 10 years old when receiving first influenza vaccine, then patient requires 2 injections 1 month apart to help ensure appropriate coverage.
d. Children with hypocomplementemia as part of their rheumatologic condition are at risk for infections with encapsulated bacteria and might benefit from vaccination with the pneumococcal and meningococcal vaccines.[6]

3. **Prevention or minimization of osteopenia:** Adequate calcium and vitamin D intake and weight-bearing activities.[1,2]
4. **Physical and occupational therapy:** Important in maintaining range of motion of a joint and strength of associated muscle groups as well as in decreasing pain and preventing joint deformity and contractures.[1,2]
5. **Orthopedic surgery is necessary in some cases for pain control, improvement in function, or contractures.**[1,2]

F. UVEITIS

Due to the silent nature of uveitis, routine pediatric ophthalmology screening is recommended for children with pauciarticular and polyarticular JRA. For younger children who are also ANA positive, screening is recommended every 4 months, and it is recommended every 6 months for children who are ANA negative.[3]

III. REACTIVE ARTHRITIS[3]

A. DEFINITION

Reactive arthritis refers to a diverse group of inflammatory arthritides, which follow a bacterial or viral infection particularly involving the respiratory, gastrointestinal, and genitourinary tracts.

1. **Infection typically precedes the development of arthritis by 1 to 4 weeks, with approximately 80% of cases of reactive arthritis being preceded by gastroenteritis.**
2. **Some arthritogenic organisms include *Chlamydia, Yersinia, Salmonella, Shigella, Campylobacter,* parvovirus B19, and enteroviruses.**
3. **Arthritis can be accompanied by constitutional signs and symptoms, including fever, weight loss, and fatigue, as well as dermatologic and ophthalmologic findings.** For example, Reiter syndrome is reactive arthritis in the presence of conjunctivitis and urethritis.

4. **There is a strong association between the presence of HLA-B27 and the susceptibility to developing reactive arthritis following an infection with a bacterial arthritogenic agent.** There is an approximately 65% to 85% frequency of HLA-B27 seen in reactive arthritis.
5. **Laboratory studies can demonstrate evidence of systemic inflammation including leukocytosis, thrombocytosis, and elevated ESR and CRP.** Autoantibodies are typically absent. Stool cultures can be helpful in determining bacteria involved, but a negative culture does not exclude the diagnosis of a reactive arthritis secondary to an enteric organism. Also, joint fluid analysis may be helpful to distinguish a septic arthritis from a reactive arthritis, especially because in the case of *Salmonella*, either a septic or reactive arthritis can develop.
6. **Arthritis can last weeks to months, with eventual development of remission versus development of recurrent episodes.**

B. PHARMACOLOGY

See Pharmacologic Agent section under JRA for treatment options.

IV. SYSTEMIC LUPUS ERYTHEMATOSUS (SLE)

SLE is a multisystem inflammatory disease related to deposition of immune complexes in tissues.

A. AMERICAN COLLEGE OF RHEUMATOLOGY CLASSIFICATION CRITERIA

Must have 4 or more of the 11 criteria (Table 24-4).[7]

B. CLINICAL FEATURES

1. **Females most commonly affected with onset usually between 9 to 15 years of age.**[4]

TABLE 24-4

THE 1982 REVISED CRITERIA FOR CLASSIFICATION OF SYSTEMIC LUPUS ERYTHEMATOSUS[5,7]

CRITERION*	DEFINITION
1. Malar rash	Fixed erythema, flat or raised, over the malar eminences, tending to spare the nasolabial folds
2. Discoid rash	Erythematous raised patches with adherent keratotic scaling and follicular plugging; atrophic scarring may occur in older lesions
3. Photosensitivity	Skin rash as a result of unusual reaction to sunlight, by patient history or physician observation
4. Oral ulcers	Oral or nasopharyngeal ulceration, usually painless, observed by physician
5. Arthritis	Nonerosive arthritis involving 2 or more peripheral joints, characterized by tenderness, swelling, or effusion

continued

TABLE 24-4

THE 1982 REVISED CRITERIA FOR CLASSIFICATION OF SYSTEMIC LUPUS ERYTHEMATOSUS[5,7]—cont'd

CRITERION*	DEFINITION
6. Serositis	(a) Pleuritis—convincing history of pleuritic pain or rubbing heard by a physician or evidence of pleural effusion *or* (b) Pericarditis—documented by ECG or rub or evidence of pericardial effusion
7. Renal disorder	(a) Persistent proteinuria greater than 0.5 grams per day or greater than 3+ if quantitation not performed *or* (b) Cellular casts—may be red cell, hemoglobin, granular, tubular, or mixed
8. Neurologic disorder	(a) Seizures—in the absence of offending drugs or known metabolic derangements; e.g., uremia, ketoacidosis, or electrolyte imbalance *or* (b) Psychosis—in the absence of offending drugs or known metabolic derangements; e.g., uremia, ketoacidosis, or electrolyte imbalance
9. Hematologic disorder	(a) Hemolytic anemia—with reticulocytosis *or* (b) Leukopenia—less than 4,000/mm^3 total on 2 or more occasions *or* (c) Lymphopenia—less than 1,5000/mm^3 on 2 or more occasions *or* (d) Thrombocytopenia—less than 100,000/mm^3 in the absence of offending drugs
10. Immunologic disorder	(a) Positive LE cell preparation *or* (b) Anti-DNA: antibody to native DNA in abnormal titer *or* (c) Anti-Sm: presence of antibody to Sm nuclear antigen *or* (d) False positive serologic test for syphilis known to be positive for at least 6 months and confirmed by *Treponema pallidum* immobilization or fluorescent treponemal antibody absorption test
11. Antinuclear antibody	An abnormal titer of antinuclear antibody by immunofluorescence or an equivalent assay at any point in time and in the absence of drugs known to be associated with "drug-induced lupus" syndrome

*The proposed classification is based on 11 criteria. For the purpose of identifying patients in clinical studies, a person shall be said to have systemic lupus erythematosus if 4 or more of the 11 criteria are present, serially or simultaneously, during any interval of observation.

Data from American College of Rheumatology website, which was adapted from Arthritis Rheum 1982;25:1271–1277.

2. African Americans are more commonly affected than whites.[2]
3. Characterized by periods of exacerbation followed by remission.
4. Renal involvement is the leading cause of death.[4]

C. LABORATORY STUDIES[2,4]

1. Immune leukopenia typically but can have inflammatory leukocytosis.
2. Anemia.
3. Occasionally direct Coombs positive.
4. Immune thrombocytopenia.
5. Elevated acute phase reactants.
6. **Urinalysis with renal involvement:** RBCs, white blood cells (WBCs), casts, and proteinuria.
7. Low complement levels.
8. Autoantibodies (see Table 24-1)[2]:
   (1) Anti-dsDNA can be seen in about 60% of patients with SLE and is highly specific for SLE, with low titers rarely being seen in other inflammatory conditions.
   (2) Anti-Sm is also highly specific for SLE, being seen in about 10% to 30% of patients with SLE.

D. DRUG-INDUCED SLE

Drug-induced SLE can be caused by multiple inciting drugs, including hydralazine, procainamide, isoniazid, chlorpromazine, phenytoin, and carbamazepine,[2] and usually resolves with discontinuation of the drug. Of note, it is often associated with antihistone antibodies.

E. NEONATAL SLE

Maternal autoantibodies, anti-Ro and La, cross the placenta manifesting as discoid lesions with exposure to ultraviolet lights; may also present as thrombocytopenia, hemolytic anemia, or congenital heart block; there is a 25% chance of having another child with neonatal SLE.[2]

V. VASCULITIS

A. DEFINITION

Vasculitis refers to the inflammation of a blood vessel wall. Systemic vasculitis syndromes, although rare, are a concern in childhood. The clinical presentation of a vasculitis condition can be quite variable from a fever of unknown origin to a rash to multisystem failure. Vasculitis can be classified based on the size of the predominant vessels involved (Table 24-5) or by whether it is a primary or secondary vasculitis. There are no definite laboratory tests or radiographic studies in diagnosing a vasculitis with the exception of a biopsy, which is not always possible.

B. HENOCH-SCHÖNLEIN PURPURA (HSP)

1. Most common small vessel vasculitis in children characterized by a nonthrombocytopenic purpuric rash, migratory polyarthritis and

TABLE 24-5

CHILDHOOD VASCULITIS SYNDROMES

Vessel Size	Vasculitis	Clinical and Distinguishing Features
Large arteries	Takayasu arteritis	Aortic arch involved Predominantly seen in young women Third most common vasculitis in pediatrics Hypertension most common sign
Medium-sized arteries	Kawasaki disease	Refer to Chapter 6
	Polyarteritis nodosa	Very rare in the pediatric population Involves small vessels as well, particularly at bifurcations of vessels Cutaneous lesions include livedo reticularis, tender nodules, and purpura Can involve renal, GI and CNS vessels leading to hypertension, abdominal pain, and headaches, but can progress to renal failure, intestinal infarction, and cerebrovascular accidents
Small arterioles and venules	Microscopic polyangiitis	Rare in pediatrics p-ANCA or myeloperoxidase (MPO) Glomerulonephritis
	Henoch-Schönlein purpura	Most common pediatric vasculitis See Section V.B
	Wegener granulomatosis	Rare in pediatrics Also involves medium-sized vessels Affects respiratory tract and kidneys c-ANCA or proteinase 3 (PR3)

Data from references 1–3, 8, and 9.

polyarthralgia, abdominal pain, and glomerulonephritis with widespread deposition of immunoglobulin A (IgA).[2,3,8]

2. Clinical features[3,8,9]:

a. Males most commonly affected with onset usually between 2 and 7 years of age.

b. History of an upper respiratory infection a few weeks preceding onset in one-half to two-thirds of cases.

c. Palpable purpura.
   (1) Most common and frequently presenting feature.
   (2) Evolution of rash starts with urticarial lesions with progression to a macular-papular rash followed by purpuric lesions.
   (3) Distribution typically involves ankles, buttocks, and elbows beginning on the lower extremities but can involve the entire body.
   (4) New lesions can appear for 2 to 4 weeks.

d. Migratory polyarthritis and/or polyarthralgias.
   (1) Presenting feature in one-fourth of cases is a tender and painful periarticular joint swelling.

(2) No joint effusion present.
(3) Ankles and knees most commonly affected.
(4) Usually transient with no permanent deformities.

e. Abdominal pain.
(1) Colicky in nature.
(2) Secondary to hemorrhage and edema of the small intestine, which can result in intussusception in about 2% of cases, which is usually ileoileal in nature.
(3) Stool can be heme positive without obvious signs of intestinal bleeding.

f. Glomerulonephritis.
(1) Renal involvement can occur in one-fourth to one-half of cases, but may develop months after the onset of the rash.
(2) More common in male patients and in older patients.

g. Other features.
(1) Dorsal edema of the feet.

h. Typically self-limited course but may reoccur in a minority of cases.

3. Laboratory studies[3,8]:

a. Normal to elevated platelet count.
b. Normal platelet function tests and bleeding time.
c. Normal coagulation studies.
d. Urinalysis may demonstrate proteinuria and hematuria, but casts are uncommon.
e. IgA levels may be elevated, especially in the acute phase of the disease.
f. Stool hemoccult may be positive.
g. Elevated ASO titer may be present.
h. Throat culture may be positive for group A β-hemolytic streptococcus, which requires treatment with antibiotics.

4. Treatment[8].

a. Maintain adequate hydration.
b. Monitoring vital signs due to gastrointestinal (GI) bleeding and renal involvement.
c. Analgesia for joint pain.
d. Possibly steroids, especially for painful cutaneous edema.

VI. JUVENILE DERMATOMYOSITIS[2-4]

Juvenile dermatomyositis is a rare disease involving small vessel vasculitis of the skin and muscles. Typical clinical features include symmetric proximal muscle pain and/or weakness involving the shoulder and pelvic girdles with a heliotropic rash involving the upper eyelids, and rash to the extensor surfaces of the metacarpophalangeal and proximal interphalangeal joints (Gottron papules). Periorbital edema can also be present, along with nail-fold capillary abnormalities, including aneurysms and drop out. Laboratory studies are significant for elevated muscle enzymes, and the child can be ANA positive; however, acute phase reactants are frequently not elevated. T2-weighted magnetic resonance imaging (MRI) images demonstrate muscle inflammation in the affected muscle groups.

REFERENCES

1. Ruddy S: Kelley's Textbook of Rheumatology, 6th ed. Philadelphia, WB Saunders, 2001.
2. Behrman RE, Kliegman RM: Nelson Essentials of Pediatrics, 4th ed. Philadelphia, WB Saunders, 2002.
3. Cassidy JT, Petty RE: Textbook of Pediatric Rheumatology, 4th ed. Philadelphia, WB Saunders, 2001.
4. Hay WW, Hayward AR, Levin MJ, Sondheimer JM: Current Pediatric Diagnosis and Treatment, 15th ed. New York, Lange Medical Books/McGraw-Hill, 2001.
5. Lehman TJ: JRA sites [Online]. Available: www.UpToDate.com.
6. Milojevic DS, Ilowite NT: Treatment of rheumatic diseases in children: Special considerations. Rheum Dis Clin North Am 2002;28(3):461–482.
7. Tan EM, Cohen AS, Fries JF, et al: The 1982 revised criteria for the classification of systemic lupus erythematosus. Arthritis Rheum 1982;25:1271–1277.
8. Sundel R, Szer I: Vasculitis in childhood. Rheum Dis Clin North Am 2002;28(3):625–654.
9. Gross WL, Trabandt A, Reinhold-Keller E: Diagnosis and evaluation of vasculitis. Rheumatology 2000;39:245–252.

PART III

Reference

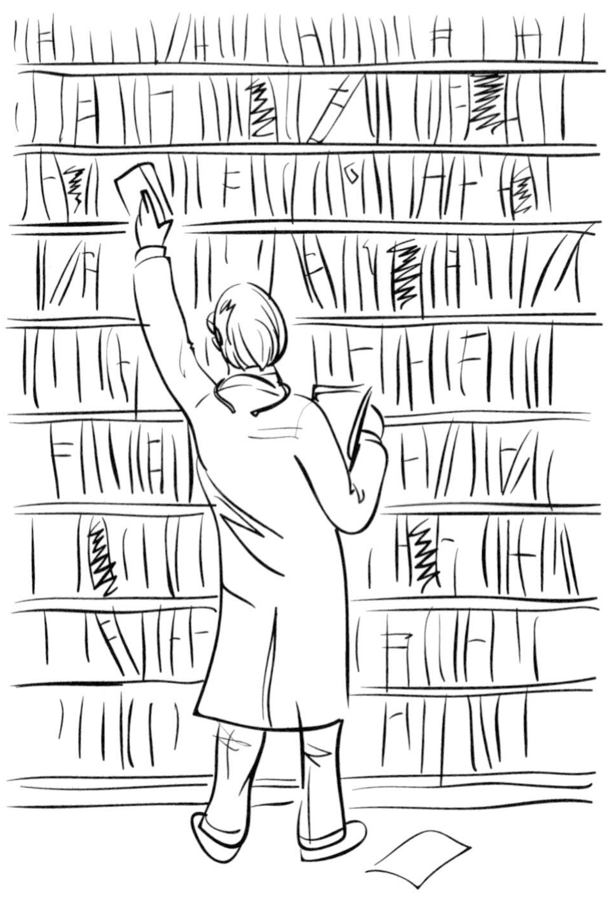

Blood Chemistries and Body Fluids

Jason Robertson, MD

These values are compiled from the published literature[1–6] and from the Johns Hopkins Hospital Department of Laboratory Medicine. Normal values vary with the analytic method used. Consult your laboratory for its analytic method and range of normal values and for less commonly used parameters, which are beyond the scope of this text. Additional normal laboratory values may be found in the Chapters 9, 13, and 14.

25

I. REFERENCE VALUES (Table 25-1)

II. EVALUATION OF BODY FLUIDS

A. EVALUATION OF TRANSUDATE VERSUS EXUDATE (Table 25-2)

B. EVALUATION OF CEREBROSPINAL FLUID (Table 25-3)

C. EVALUATION OF SYNOVIAL FLUID (Table 25-4)

III. CONVERSION FORMULAS

A. TEMPERATURE

1. To convert degrees Celsius to degrees Fahrenheit: ([9/5] × Temperature) + 32.
2. To convert degrees Fahrenheit to degrees Celsius: (Temperature − 32) × (5/9).

B. LENGTH AND WEIGHT

1. Length: To convert inches to centimeters, multiply by 2.54.
2. Weight: To convert pounds to kilograms, divide by 2.2.

REFERENCES

1. Meites S (ed): Pediatric Clinical Chemistry, 2nd and 3rd eds. Washington, DC, American Association for Clinical Chemistry, 1981.
2. Burtis CA, Ashwood ER: Tietz Textbook of Clinical Chemistry, 3rd ed. Philadelphia, WB Saunders, 1999.
3. Soldin SJ, et al: Pediatric Reference Ranges, 3rd ed. Washington, DC, AACC Press, 1999.
4. Lundberg GD: SI unit implementation: The next step. JAMA 1988;260:73.
5. Wallach J: Interpretation of Diagnostic Tests. Boston, Little, Brown, 1992.
6. Berkow R: The Merck Manual of Diagnosis and Therapy. Rahway, NJ, Merck Research Laboratories, 1992.
7. Rogers M: Textbook of Pediatric Intensive Care, 2nd ed. Baltimore, Williams & Wilkins, 1992.

Text continues on p. 672

TABLE 25-1

REFERENCE VALUES[1-6]

	Conventional Units	SI Units
ACID PHOSPHATASE		
(Major sources: prostate and erythrocytes)		
Newborn	7.4–19.4 U/L	7.4–19.4 U/L
2–13 yr	6.4–15.2 U/L	6.4–15.2 U/L
Adult male	0.5–11.0 U/L	0.5–11.0 U/L
Adult female	0.2–9.5 U/L	0.2–9.5 U/L
ALANINE AMINOTRANSFERASE (ALT)		
(Major sources: liver, skeletal muscle, and myocardium)		
Neonate/infant	13–45 U/L	13–45 U/L
Adult male	10–40 U/L	10–40 U/L
Adult female	7–35 U/L	7–35 U/L
ALBUMIN		
(See Proteins)		
ALDOLASE		
(Major sources: skeletal muscle and myocardium)		
10–24 mo	3.4–11.8 U/L	3.4–11.8 U/L
2–16 yr	1.2–8.8 U/L	1.2–8.8 U/L
Adult	1.7–4.9 U/L	1.7–4.9 U/L
ALKALINE PHOSPHATASE		
(Major sources: liver, bone, intestinal mucosa, placenta, and kidney)		
Infant	150–420 U/L	150–420 U/L
2–10 yr	100–320 U/L	100–320 U/L
Adolescent males	100–390 U/L	100–390 U/L
Adolescent females	100–320 U/L	100–320 U/L
Adult	30–120 U/L	30–120 U/L
AMMONIA		
(Heparinized venous specimen on ice analyzed within 30 min)		
Newborn	90–150 μg/dL	64–107 μmol/L
0–2 wk	79–129 μg/dL	56–92 μmol/L
>1 mo	29–70 μg/dL	21–50 μmol/L
Adult	0–50 μg/dL	0–35.7 μmol/L
AMYLASE		
(Major sources: pancreas, salivary glands, and ovaries)		
Newborn	5–65 U/L	5–65 U/L
Adult	27–131 U/L	27–131 U/L
ANTINUCLEAR ANTIBODY (ANA)		
Not significant	<1 : 80	
Likely significant	>1 : 320	
Patterns with clinical correlation:		
Centromere—CREST		
Nucleolar—Scleroderma		
Homogeneous—SLE		

TABLE 25-1

REFERENCE VALUES[1–6]—*cont'd*

	Conventional Units	SI Units
ANTISTREPTOLYSIN O TITER		
(4-fold rise in paired serial specimens is significant)		
Preschool	<1 : 85	
School age	<1 : 170	
Older adult	<1 : 85	
NOTE: Alternatively, values up to 200 Todd units are normal.		
ASPARTATE AMINOTRANSFERASE (AST)		
(Major sources: liver, skeletal muscle, kidney, myocardium, and erythrocytes)		
Newborn	25–75 U/L	25–75 U/L
Infant	15–60 U/L	15–60 U/L
1–3 yr	20–60 U/L	20–60 U/L
4–6 yr	15–50 U/L	15–50 U/L
7–9 yr	15–40 U/L	15–40 U/L
10–11 yr	10–60 U/L	10–60 U/L
12–19 yr	15–45 U/L	15–45 U/L
BICARBONATE		
Newborn	17–24 mEq/L	17–24 mmol/L
2 mo–2 yr	16–24 mEq/L	16–24 mmol/L
>2 yr	22–26 mEq/L	22–26 mmol/L
BILIRUBIN (TOTAL)		
Cord		
Preterm	<2 mg/dL	<34 μmol/L
Term	<2 mg/dL	<34 μmol/L
0–1 days		
Preterm	<8 mg/dL	<137 μmol/L
Term	<8.7 mg/dL	<149 μmol/L
1–2 days		
Preterm	<12 mg/dL	<205 μmol/L
Term	<11.5 mg/dL	<197 μmol/L
3–5 days		
Preterm	<16 mg/dL	<274 μmol/L
Term	<12 mg/dL	<205 μmol/L
Older infant		
Preterm	<2 mg/dL	<34 μmol/L
Term	<1.2 mg/dL	<21 μmol/L
Adult	0.3–1.2 mg/dL	5–21 μmol/L
BILIRUBIN (CONJUGATED)		
Neonate	<0.6 mg/dL	<10 μmol/L
Infants/children	<0.2 mg/dL	<3.4 μmol/L

continued

TABLE 25-1

REFERENCE VALUES[1–6]—*cont'd*

BLOOD GAS, ARTERIAL[7]

	PH	Pao_2 (mmHg)	$Paco_2$ (mmHg)	HCO_3^- (mEq/L)
Newborn (birth)	7.26–7.29	60	55	19
Newborn (>24 hr)	7.37	70	33	20
Infant (1–24 mo)	7.40	90	34	20
Child (7–19 yr)	7.39	96	37	22
Adult (>19 yr)	7.35–7.45	90–110	35–45	22–26

NOTE: Venous blood gases can be used to assess acid-base status, not oxygenation. Pco_2 averages 6–8 mmHg higher than $Paco_2$, and pH is slightly lower. Peripheral venous samples are strongly affected by the local circulatory and metabolic environment. Capillary blood gases correlate best with arterial pH and moderately well with $Paco_2$.

	Conventional Units	SI Units
CALCIUM (TOTAL)		
Preterm	6.2–11 mg/dL	1.6–2.8 mmol/L
Full term <10 days	7.6–10.4 mg/dL	1.9–2.6 mmol/L
10 days–24 mo	9.0–11.0 mg/dL	2.3–2.8 mmol/L
2–12 yr	8.8–10.8 mg/dL	2.2–2.7 mmol/L
Adult	8.6–10 mg/dL	2.2–2.5 mmol/L
CALCIUM (IONIZED)		
Newborn <36 hr	4.20–5.48 mg/dL	1.05–1.37 mmol/L
Newborn 36–84 hr	4.40–5.68 mg/dL	1.10–1.42 mmol/L
1–18 yr	4.80–5.52 mg/dL	1.20–1.38 mmol/L
Adult	4.64–5.28 mg/dL	1.16–1.32 mmol/L
CARBON DIOXIDE (CO_2 CONTENT)		
Cord blood	14–22 mEq/L	14–22 mmol/L
Newborn	13–22 mEq/L	13–22 mmol/L
Premature, 1 wk	14–27 mEq/L	14–27 mmol/L
Infant/child	20–28 mEq/L	20–28 mmol/L
Adult	22–28 mEq/L	22–28 mmol/L
CARBON MONOXIDE (CARBOXYHEMOGLOBIN)		
Nonsmoker	0.5%–1.5% of total hemoglobin	
Smoker	4%–9% of total hemoglobin	
Toxic	20%–50% of total hemoglobin	
Lethal	>50% of total hemoglobin	
CHLORIDE (SERUM)		
Newborn	98–113 mEq/L	98–113 mmol/L
Child/adult	98–107 mEq/L	98–107 mmol/L
CHOLESTEROL		
(see Lipids)		
C-REACTIVE PROTEIN		
(Other laboratories may have different reference values)	0–0.5 mg/dL	

TABLE 25-1
REFERENCE VALUES[1–6]—*cont'd*

	Conventional Units	SI Units
CREATINE KINASE (CREATINE PHOSPHOKINASE)		
(Major sources: myocardium, skeletal muscle, smooth muscle, and brain)		
Newborn	10–200 U/L	10–200 U/L
Man	15–105 U/L	15–105 U/L
Woman	10–80 U/L	10–80 U/L
CREATININE (SERUM)		
Cord	0.6–1.2 mg/dL	53–106 μmol/L
Newborn	0.3–1.0 mg/dL	27–88 μmol/L
Infant	0.2–0.4 mg/dL	18–35 μmol/L
Child	0.3–0.7 mg/dL	27–62 μmol/L
Adolescent	0.5–1.0 mg/dL	44–88 μmol/L
Man	0.7–1.3 mg/dL	62–115 μmol/L
Woman	0.6–1.1 mg/dL	53–97 μmol/L
ERYTHROCYTE SEDIMENTATION RATE (ESR)		
Term neonate	0–4 mm/hr	
Child	4–20 mm/hr	
Adult (male)	1–15 mm/hr	
Adult (female)	4–25 mm/hr	
FERRITIN		
Newborn	25–200 ng/mL	20–200 ng/mL
1 mo	200–600 ng/mL	200–600 ng/mL
2–5 mo	50–200 ng/mL	50–200 ng/mL
6 mo–15 yr	7–140 ng/mL	7–140 ng/mL
Adult male	20–250 ng/mL	20–250 ng/mL
Adult female	10–120 ng/mL	10–120 ng/mL
FIBRINOGEN		
(See Table 13-6, p. 348)		
FOLATE (SERUM)		
Newborn	5–65 ng/mL	11–147 nmol/L
Infant	15–55 ng/mL	34–125 nmol/L
2–16 yr	5–21 ng/mL	11–48 nmol/L
>16 yr	3–20 ng/mL	7–45 nmol/L
FOLATE (RBC)		
Newborn	150–200 ng/mL	340–453 nmol/L
Infant	75–1000 ng/mL	170–2265 nmol/L
2–16 yr	>160 ng/mL	>362 nmol/L
>16 yr	140–628 ng/mL	317–1422 nmol/L
GALACTOSE		
Newborn	0–20 mg/dL	0–1.11 mmol/L
Thereafter	<5 mg/dL	<0.28 mmol/L

continued

TABLE 25-1

REFERENCE VALUES[1–6]—*cont'd*

	Conventional Units	SI Units
γ-GLUTAMYL TRANSFERASE (GGT)		
(Major sources: liver [biliary tree] and kidney)		
Cord	19–270 U/L	19–270 U/L
Preterm	56–233 U/L	56–233 U/L
0–3 wk	0–130 U/L	0–130 U/L
3 wk–3 mo	4–120 U/L	4–120 U/L
3–12 mo boy	5–65 U/L	5–65 U/L
3–12 mo girl	5–35 U/L	5–35 U/L
1–15 yr	0–23 U/L	0–23 U/L
Adult male	11–50 U/L	11–50 U/L
Adult female	7–32 U/L	7–32 U/L
GLUCOSE (SERUM)		
Preterm	20–60 mg/dL	1.1–3.3 mmol/L
Newborn, <1 day	40–60 mg/dL	2.2–3.3 mmol/L
Newborn, >1 day	50–80 mg/dL	2.8–4.5 mmol/L
Child	60–100 mg/dL	3.3–5.6 mmol/L
>16 yr	74–106 mg/dL	4.1–5.9 mmol/L
HAPTOGLOBIN		
Newborn	5–48 mg/dL	50–480 mg/L
>30 days	26–185 mg/dL	260–1850 mg/L
HEMOGLOBIN A_1C	5.0–7.5% total Hgb	
HEMOGLOBIN F [MEAN (SD) % TOTAL HGB]		
1 day	77.0 (7.3)	
5 days	76.8 (5.8)	
3 wk	70.0 (7.3)	
6–9 wk	52.9 (11)	
3–4 mo	23.2 (16)	
6 mo	4.7 (2.2)	
8–11 mo	1.6 (1.0)	
Adult	<2.0	
IRON		
Newborn	100–250 μg/dL	17.9–44.8 μmol/L
Infant	40–100 μg/dL	7.2–17.9 μmol/L
Child	50–120 μg/dL	9.0–21.5 μmol/L
Adult male	65–175 μg/dL	11.6–31.3 μmol/L
Adult female	50–170 μg/dL	9.0–30.4 μmol/L
KETONES (SERUM)		
Quantitative	0.5–3.0 mg/dL	5–30 mg/L
LACTATE		
Capillary blood		
Newborn	<27 mg/dL	0.0–3.0 mmol/L
Child	5–20 mg/dL	0.56–2.25 mmol/L
Venous	5–20 mg/dL	0.5–2.2 mmol/L
Arterial	5–14 mg/dL	0.5–1.6 mmol/L

TABLE 25-1
REFERENCE VALUES[1-6]—*cont'd*

	Conventional Units	SI Units
LACTATE DEHYDROGENASE (AT 37°C)		
(Major sources: myocardium, liver, skeletal muscle, erythrocytes, platelets, and lymph nodes)		
0–4 days	290–775 U/L	290–775 U/L
4–10 days	545–2000 U/L	545–2000 U/L
10 days–24 mo	180–430 U/L	180–430 U/L
24 mo–12 yr	110–295 U/L	110–295 U/L
>12 yr	100–190 U/L	100–190 U/L
LEAD		
(see pp. 35–38)		
Child	<10 μg/dL	<0.48 μmol/L
LIPASE		
0–90 days	10–85 U/L	
3–12 mo	9–128 U/L	
1–11 yr	10–150 U/L	
>11 yr	10–220 U/L	

LIPIDS[8]

	Cholesterol (mg/dL)			LDL (mg/dL)			HDL (mg/dL)
	Desirable	Borderline	High	Desirable	Borderline	High	Desirable
Child/ adolescent	<170	170–199	>200	<110	110–129	>130	45
Adult	<200	200–239	>240	<100	100–159	>160	45

	Conventional Units	SI Units
MAGNESIUM	1.3–2.0 mEq/L	0.65–1.0 mmol/L
METHEMOGLOBIN	<1.5% total Hgb	
OSMOLALITY	275–295 mOsm/kg	275–295 mmol/kg
PHENYLALANINE		
Preterm	2.0–7.5 mg/dL	121–454 μmol/L
Newborn	1.2–3.4 mg/dL	73–206 μmol/L
Adult	0.8–1.8 mg/dL	48–109 μmol/L
PHOSPHORUS		
Newborn	4.5–9.0 mg/dL	1.45–2.91 mmol/L
10 days–24 mo	4.5–6.7 mg/dL	1.45–2.16 mmol/L
24 mo–12 yr	4.5–5.5 mg/dL	1.45–1.78 mmol/L
>12 yr	2.7–4.5 mg/dL	0.87–1.45 mmol/L
PORCELAIN[9]	3.0–9.02 mg/dL	8.20–20.03 mmol/L
POTASSIUM		
Newborn	3.7–5.9 mEq/L	3.7–5.9 mmol/L
Infant	4.1–5.3 mEq/L	4.1–5.3 mmol/L
Child	3.4–4.7 mEq/L	3.4–4.7 mmol/L
Adult	3.5–5.1 mEq/L	3.5–5.1 mmol/L

continued

TABLE 25-1
REFERENCE VALUES[1–6]—*cont'd*

	Conventional Units	SI Units
PREALBUMIN		
Newborn	7–39 mg/dL	
1–6 mo	8–34 mg/dL	
6 mo–4 yr	2–36 mg/dL	
4–6 yr	12–30 mg/dL	
6–19 yr	12–42 mg/dL	
PROTEINS		

Protein Electrophoresis (g/dL)

Age	TP	Albumin	α-1	α-2	β	γ
Cord	4.8–8.0	2.2–4.0	0.3–0.7	0.4–0.9	0.4–1.6	0.8–1.6
Newborn	4.4–7.6	3.2–4.8	0.1–0.3	0.2–0.3	0.3–0.6	0.6–1.2
1 day–1 mo	4.4–7.6	2.5–5.5	0.1–0.3	0.3–1.0	0.2–1.1	0.4–1.3
1–3 mo	3.6–7.4	2.1–4.8	0.1–0.4	0.3–1.1	0.3–1.1	0.2–1.1
4–6 mo	4.2–7.4	2.8–5.0	0.1–0.4	0.3–0.8	0.3–0.8	0.1–0.9
7–12 mo	5.1–7.5	3.2–5.7	0.1–0.6	0.3–1.5	0.4–1.0	0.2–1.2
13–24 mo	3.7–7.5	1.9–5.0	0.1–0.6	0.4–1.4	0.4–1.4	0.4–1.6
25–36 mo	5.3–8.1	3.3–5.8	0.1–0.3	0.4–1.1	0.3–1.2	0.4–1.5
3–5 yr	4.9–8.1	2.9–5.8	0.1–0.4	0.4–1.0	0.5–1.0	0.4–1.7
6–8 yr	6.0–7.9	3.3–5.0	0.1–0.5	0.5–0.8	0.5–0.9	0.7–2.0
9–11 yr	6.0–7.9	3.2–5.0	0.1–0.4	0.7–0.9	0.6–1.0	0.8–2.0
12–16 yr	6.0–7.9	3.2–5.1	0.1–0.4	0.5–1.1	0.5–1.1	0.6–2.0
Adult	6.0–8.0	3.1–5.4	0.1–0.4	0.4–1.1	0.5–1.2	0.7–1.7

	Conventional Units	SI Units
PYRUVATE	0.3–0.9 mg/dL	0.03–0.10 mmol/L
RHEUMATOID FACTOR	<30 U/mL	
SODIUM		
Preterm	130–140 mEq/L	130–140 mmol/L
Older	133–146 mEq/L	133–146 mmol/L
TOTAL IRON-BINDING CAPACITY (TIBC)		
Infant	100–400 μg/dL	17.9–71.6 μmol/L
Adult	250–425 μg/dL	44.8–76.1 μmol/L
TOTAL PROTEIN		
(See Proteins)		
TRANSAMINASE (SGOT)		
(See Aspartate aminotransferase [AST])		
TRANSAMINASE (SGPT)		
(See Alanine aminotransferase [ALT])		
TRANSFERRIN		
Newborn	130–275 mg/dL	1.30–2.75 g/L
3 mo–10 yr	203–360 mg/dL	2.03–3.6 g/L
Adult	215–380 mg/dL	2.15–3.8 g/L

TOTAL TRIGLYCERIDE (mg/dL)[10]

	5th	Mean	75th	90th	95th
Cord	14	34	—	—	84
1–4 yr					
Male	29	56	68	85	99
Female	34	64	74	95	112

TABLE 25-1
REFERENCE VALUES[1–6]—*cont'd*

5–9 yr					
Male	28	52	58	70	85
Female	32	64	74	103	126
10–14 yr					
Male	33	63	74	94	111
Female	39	72	85	104	120
15–19 yr					
Male	38	78	88	125	143
Female	36	73	85	112	126

	Conventional Units	SI Units
TROPONIN-I	0–0.1 μg/L	
UREA NITROGEN		
Premature (<1 week)	3–25 mg/dL	1.1–8.9 mmol/L
Newborn	4–12 mg/dL	1.4–4.3 mmol/L
Infant/child	5–18 mg/dL	1.8–6.4 mmol/L
Adult	6–20 mg/dL	2.1–7.1 mmol/L
URIC ACID		
0–2 yr	2.4–6.4 mg/dL	0.14–0.38 mmol/L
2–12 yr	2.4–5.9 mg/dL	0.14–0.35 mmol/L
12–14 yr	2.4–6.4 mg/dL	0.14–0.38 mmol/L
Adult male	3.5–7.2 mg/dL	0.20–0.43 mmol/L
Adult female	2.4–6.4 mg/dL	0.14–0.38 mmol/L
VITAMIN A		
(Retinol)		
Preterm	13–46 μg/dL	0.46–1.61 μmol/L
Full term	18–50 μg/dL	0.63–1.75 μmol/L
1–6 yr	20–43 μg/dL	0.7–1.5 μmol/L
7–12 yr	20–49 μg/dL	0.9–1.7 μmol/L
13–19 yr	26–72 μg/dL	0.9–2.5 μmol/L
VITAMIN B_1		
(Thiamine)	5.3–7.9 μg/dL	0.16–0.23 μmol/L
VITAMIN B_2		
(Riboflavin)	4–24 μg/dL	106–638 nmol/L
VITAMIN B_{12}		
(Cobalamin)		
Newborn	160–1300 pg/mL	118–959 pmol/L
Child/adult	200–835 pg/mL	148–616 pmol/L
VITAMIN C		
(Ascorbic acid)	0.4–1.5 mg/dL	23–85 μmol/L
VITAMIN D_3		
(1,25-dihydroxy-vitamin D)	16–65 pg/mL	42–169 pmol/L
VITAMIN E		
<11 yr	3–15 mg/L	7.0–35 μmol/L
>11 yr	5–20 mg/L	11.6–46.4 μmol/L
ZINC	70–120 mg/dL	10.7–18.4 mmol/L

TABLE 25-2

EVALUATION OF TRANSUDATE vs. EXUDATE (PLEURAL, PERICARDIAL, OR PERITONEAL FLUID)

Measurement*	Transudate	Exudate†
Specific gravity	<1.016	>1.016
Protein (g/dL)	<3.0	>3.0
Fluid : serum ratio	<0.5	>0.5
LDH (IU)	<200	>200
Fluid : serum ratio (isoenzymes not useful)	<0.6	>0.6
WBCs‡	<1000/mm^3	>1000/mm^3
RBCs	<10,000	Variable
Glucose	Same as serum	Less than serum
pH§	7.4–7.5	<7.4

*Always obtain serum for glucose, LDH, protein, amylase, etc.

†Not required to meet all of the following criteria to be considered an exudate.

‡In peritoneal fluid, WBC > 800/mm^3 suggests peritonitis.

§Collect anaerobically in a heparinized syringe.

LDH, lactate dehydrogenase; *RBCs,* red blood cells; *WBCs,* white blood cells.

Note: Amylase >5000 U/mL or pleural fluid : serum ratio >1 suggests pancreatitis.

TABLE 25-3

EVALUATION OF CEREBROSPINAL FLUID

	WBC Count	Mean % PMNs
Preterm	0–25 WBCs/mm^3	57%
Term	0–22 WBCs/mm^3	61%
Child	0–7 WBCs/mm^3	5%
GLUCOSE		
Preterm	24–63 mg/dL	1.3–3.5 mmol/L
Term	34–119 mg/dL	1.9–6.6 mmol/L
Child	40–80 mg/dL	2.2–4.4 mmol/L
CSF GLUCOSE/BLOOD GLUCOSE		
Preterm	55%–105%	
Term	44%–128%	
Child	50%	
LACTIC ACID DEHYDROGENASE		
Normal range	5–30 U/L (or about 10% of serum value)	
MYELIN BASIC PROTEIN	<4 ng/mL	
OPENING PRESSURE		
(Lateral recumbent)		
Newborn	8–11 cmH_2O	
Infant/child	<20 cmH_2O	
Respiratory variations	0.5–1 cmH_2O	
PROTEIN		
Preterm	65–150 mg/dL	0.65–1.5 g/L
Term	20–170 mg/dL	0.20–1.7 g/L
Child	5–40 mg/dL	0.05–0.40 g/L

CSF, cerebrospinal fluid; PMNs, polymorphonuclear lymphocytes; WBC, white blood cell.

Modified from Oski FA: Principles and Practice of Pediatrics, 3rd ed. Philadelphia, JB Lippincott, 1999.

TABLE 25-4

CHARACTERISTICS OF SYNOVIAL FLUID IN THE RHEUMATIC DISEASES

Group	Condition	Synovial Complement	Color/ Clarity	Viscosity	Mucin Clot	WBC Count	PMN (%)	Miscellaneous Findings
Noninflammatory	Normal	N	Yellow Clear	VH	G	<200	<25	
	Traumatic arthritis	N	Xanthochromic Turbid	H	F–G	<2000	<25	Debris
	Osteoarthritis	N	Yellow Clear	H	F–G	1000	<25	
Inflammatory	Systemic lupus erythematosus	↓	Yellow Clear	N	N	5000	10	Lupus erythematosus cellls
	Rheumatic fever	N–↑	Yellow Cloudy	↓	F	5000	10–50	
	Juvenile rheumatoid arthritis	N–↓	Yellow Cloudy	↓	Poor	15,000–20,000	75	
	Reiter's syndrom	↑	Yellow Opaque	↓	Poor	20,000	80	Reiter's cells
Pyogenic	Tuberculous arthritis	N–↑	Yellow-white Cloudy	↓	Poor	25,000	50–60	Acid-fast bacteria
	Septic arthritis	↑	Serosanguineous Turbid	↓	Poor	50,000–300,000	>75	Low glucose, bacteria

WBC, white blood cell; PMN, polymorphonuclear leukocyte; N, normal; VH, very high; H, high; G, good; F, fair; ↓, decreased; ↑, increased.
From Cassidy JT, Petty RE: Textbook of Pediatric Rheumatology, 4th ed. Philadelphia, WB Saunders, 2001.

8. Summary of NCEP ATP II and ATP III reports: Highlights of the report of the expert panel on blood and cholesterol levels in children and adolescents, 1991, U.S. Department of Health and Human Services. JAMA 1993;269 and 2001.
9. Robertson JW, Shilkofski, NA: Surviving pediatric chief residency at Hopkins: Outwit, outlast, and outplay. Baltimore, 2004–2005.
10. Behrman RE, et al: Nelson Textbook of Pediatrics, 16th ed. Philadelphia, WB Saunders, 2000.

Biostatistics and Evidence-based Medicine

Jason Robertson, MD

I. WEBSITES

www.welch.jhu.edu/internet/ebr.html
www.pedsccm.wustl.edu/EBJ/EB_Resources.html
www.tripdatabase.com
www.cochranelibrary.com
www.guideline.gov/body_home_nf.asp?view=home
www.ncbi.nlm.nih.gov/entrez/query/stastic/clinical.html

II. BIOSTATISTICS FOR MEDICAL LITERATURE

A. STUDY DESIGN COMPARISON (Table 26-1)

B. MEASUREMENTS IN CLINICAL STUDIES (Table 26-2)

1. Prevalence:

a. Proportion of study population who have a disease (at one point or period in time).
b. Number of old cases and new cases divided by total population.
c. In cross-sectional studies (see Table 26-2): (A + B)/(A + B + C + D).

2. Incidence:

a. Number of people in study population who newly develop an outcome (disease) per total study population per given time period.
b. Number of new cases divided by the total population over a given time period (see Table 26-2).
c. For cohort studies and clinical trials: (A + B)/(A + B + C + D).

3. Relative risk (RR):

a. Ratio of incidence of disease among people with risk factor to incidence of disease among people without risk factor.
b. For cohort studies or clinical trials (see Table 26-2): [A/(A + C)]/[B/(B + D)].
c. RR = 1 means no effect of exposure (or treatment) on outcome (or disease). RR <1 indicates exposure or treatment protective against disease. RR >1 indicates exposure/treatment increases probability of outcome/disease.

4. Odds ratio (OR):

a. For case-control studies, ratio of odds of having risk factor in people with disease (A/B) to odds of having risk factor in people without disease (C/D), or (A/B)/(C/D) = (A × D)/(B × C). (See Table 26-2.)
b. Good estimate of RR if disease is rare. OR = 1 means no risk factor–disease association. OR >1 suggests risk factor associated with increased disease, and OR <1 suggests risk factor protective against disease.

TABLE 26-1
STUDY DESIGN COMPARISON

Design Type	Definition	Advantages	Disadvantages
Case-control (often called *retrospective*)	Define diseased subjects (cases) and nondiseased subjects (controls); compare proportion of cases with exposure (risk factor) with proportion of controls with exposure (risk factor).	Good for rare diseases Small sample size Faster (not followed over time) Less expensive	Highest potential for biases (recall, selection and others) Weak evidence for causality No prevalence, PPV, NPV
Cohort (usually prospective; occasionally retrospective)	In study population, define exposed group (with risk factor) and nonexposed group (without risk factor). Over time, compare proportion of exposed group with outcome (disease), with proportion of nonexposed group with outcome (disease).	Defines incidence Stronger evidence for causality Decreases biases (sampling, measurement, reporting)	Expensive Long study times May not be feasible for rare diseases/outcomes Factors related to exposure and outcome may falsely alter effect of exposure on outcome (confounding)
Cross-sectional	In study population, concurrently measure outcome (disease) and risk factor. Compare proportion of diseased group with risk factor, with proportion of nondiseased group with risk factor.	Defines prevalence Short time to complete	Selection bias Weak evidence for causality
Clinical trial (experiment)	In study population, assign (randomly) subjects to receive treatment or receive no treatment. Compare rate of outcome (e.g., disease cure) between treatment and nontreatment groups.	Randomized blinded trial is gold standard Randomization reduces confounding Best evidence for causality	Expensive Risks of experimental treatments in humans Longer time Bad for rare outcomes/diseases

NPV, negative predictive value; PPV, positive predictive value.

TABLE 26-2
GRID FOR CALCULATIONS IN CLINICAL STUDIES

	Exposure or Risk Factor or Treatment	
Disease or Outcome	Positive	Negative
Positive	A	B
Negative	C	D

TABLE 26-3
GRID FOR EVALUATING A CLINICAL TEST

	Disease Status	
Test Result	Positive	Negative
Positive	A (true positive)	B (false positive)
Negative	C (false negative)	D (true negative)

5. **α (Significance level of statistical test):**
a. Probability of finding a statistical association by chance alone when there truly is no association (type I error).
b. Often set at 0.05; low α especially important when interpreting a finding of an association.
6. **Power (of a statistical test):**
a. β = Probability of finding no statistical association when there truly is one (type II error).
b. Power = 1 − β = Probability of finding a statistical association when there truly is one.
c. Power often set at 0.80; high power especially important when interpreting a finding of no association.
7. **Sample size: About number of subjects required in a clinical study to achieve a sufficiently high power and sufficiently low α to obtain a clinically relevant result.**
8. ***p* value:**
a. Probability of a finding by chance alone.
b. If *p* value is less than preset α level (often 0.05), then finding is interpreted as unlikely to be due to chance simply from sampling.
9. **Confidence interval (95%): About 95% probability that the reported interval contains the true value.**

C. MEASUREMENTS FOR EVALUATING A CLINICAL TEST (Table 26-3)

1. **Sensitivity (Sens):**
a. Proportion of all diseased who have positive test (see Table 26-3): A/(A + C).
b. Use highly sensitive test to help exclude a disease. (Low false-negative rate. High likelihood ratio [LR] negative. This is good for screening.)

2. **Specificity (Spec):**
   a. Proportion of all nondiseased who have a negative test (see Table 26-3): D/(B + D).
   b. Use highly specific test to help confirm a disease. (Low false-positive rate. High LR positive.)

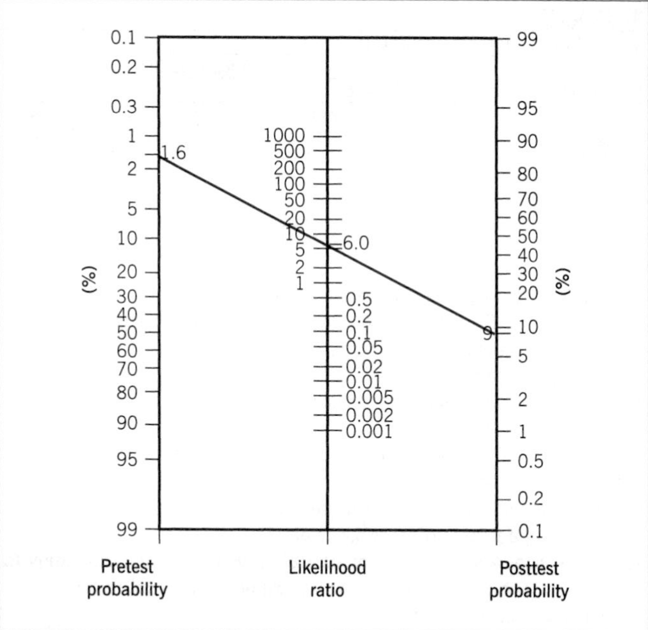

FIG. 26-1

Nomogram for calculating the change in probability by applying tests with known LRs. For example, the prevalence (i.e., pretest probability) of occult bacteremia in a well-appearing 3- to 36-month-old with temperature ≥39°C without source is 1.6%. LR positive for WBC > 20 × 10^9/L is 6.0. For such infants, then, with a WBC >20 × 10^9/L, you can use the nomogram to determine the increased probability from the positive test. Anchor a straight edge at 1.6% on the left pretest probability column and direct the straight edge through the central column at the LR of 6.0. The straight edge will intersect the right column with your answer to give a post-test probability of about 9%. It is then up to you to decide the clinical importance of a 9% probability of bacteremia. *(Data from Fagan TJ: Letter: Nomogram for Bayes theorem. N Engl J Med 1975;293:257; Lee GM, Harper MB: Risk of bacteremia for febrile young children in the post-Haemophilus influenzae type b era. Arch Pediatr Adolesc Med 1998;152:624–628.)*

3. Positive predictive value (PPV):

a. Proportion of all those with positive tests who truly have disease (see Table 26-3): A/(A + B).

b. Increased PPV with higher disease prevalence and higher specificity (and, to a lesser degree, higher sensitivity).

4. Negative predictive value (NPV):

a. Proportion of all those with negative tests who truly do not have disease (see Table 26-3): D/(C + D).

b. Increased NPV with lower prevalence (rarer disease) and higher sensitivity.

5. Likelihood ratio (LR):

a. LR positive: Ability of positive test result to confirm diseased status: LR positive = (Sens)/(1 – Spec).

b. LR negative: Ability of negative test result to confirm nondiseased status: LR negative = (Spec)/(1 – Sens). [Alternative LR negative = (1 – Sens)/Spec.]

c. Good tests have LR ≥10. (Good tests ≤0.1 if using alternative LR-negative formula.) Physical examination findings often have LR of about 2.

d. LR should not be affected by disease prevalence. LR can be used to calculate increase in probability of disease from baseline prevalence with positive test (LR positive) and decrease in probability of disease from baseline prevalence with negative test (using alternative LR negative) for any level of disease prevalence (Fig. 26-1).

Drug Doses

*Carlton Lee, PharmD, MPH, Jason Robertson, MD,
and Nicole Shilkofski, MD*

I. NOTE TO THE READER

The authors have made every attempt to check dosages and medical content for accuracy. Because of the incomplete data on pediatric dosing, many drug dosages will be modified after the publication of this text. We recommend that the reader check product information and published literature for changes in dosing, especially for newer medicines.

II. SAMPLE ENTRY

Pregnancy: Refer to explanation of pregnancy categories (on facing page).

Breast: Refer to explanation of breast-feeding categories (on facing page).

Kidney: Indicates need for caution or need for dose adjustment in renal failure (see also Chapter 30).

How supplied

ACETAZOLAMIDE ← Generic name

Diamox ← **Trade name and other names**

Carbonic anhydrase inhibitor, diuretic ← **Drug category**

Yes 1 C

Tabs: 125, 250 mg
Suspension: 25, 50 mg/mL ← **Mortar and pestle: Indicates need for extemporaneous compounding by a pharmacist**
Capsules (sustained release): 500 mg
Injection (sodium): 500 mg/5 mL
Contains 2.05 mEq Na/500 mg drug

Diuretic (PO, IV)
Child: 5 mg/kg/dose QD–QOD
Adult: 250–375 mg/dose QD–QOD

Glaucoma
Child: 20–40 mg/kg/24 hr ÷ Q6 hr IM/IV; 8–30 mg/kg/24 hr ÷ Q6–8 hr PO
Adult: 1000 mg/24 hr ÷ Q6 hr PO; for rapid decrease in intraocular pressure, administer 500 mg/dose IV

Seizures: 8–30 mg/kg/24 hr ÷ Q6–12 hr PO
Max. dose: 1 g/24 hr

Urine alkalinization: 5 mg/kg/dose PO repeated BID–TID over 24 hr.

Management of hydrocephalus: Start with 20 mg/kg/24 hr ÷ Q8 hr PO/IV; may increase to 100 mg/kg/24 hr up to a **max. dose** of 2 g/24 hr.

Drug dosing

Contraindicated in hepatic failure, severe renal failure (GFR < 10 mL/min), and hypersensitivity to sulfonamides.

$T_{1/2}$: 2–6 hr; **do not use** sustained-release capsules in seizures; IM injection may be painful; bicarbonate replacement therapy may be required during long-term use (see *Citrate* or *Sodium Bicarbonate*).

Possible side effects (more likely with long-term therapy) include GI irritation, paresthesias, sedation, hypokalemia, acidosis, reduced urate secretion, aplastic anemia, polyuria, and development of renal calculi.

May increase toxicity of cyclosporin. Aspirin may increase toxicity of acetazolamide. May decrease the effects of salicylates, lithium, and phenobarbital. False-positive urinary protein may occur with several assays. **Adjust dose in renal failure (see Chapter 30).**

Brief remarks about side effects, drug interactions, precautions, therapeutic monitoring, and other relevant information

III. EXPLANATION OF BREAST-FEEDING CATEGORIES

See sample entry.

1 Compatible
2 Use with caution
3 Unknown with concerns
X Contraindicated
? Safety not established

IV. EXPLANATION OF PREGNANCY CATEGORIES

A Adequate studies in pregnant women have not demonstrated a risk to the fetus in the first trimester of pregnancy, and there is no evidence of risk in later trimesters.

B Animal studies have not demonstrated a risk to the fetus, but there are no adequate studies in pregnant women; or animal studies have shown an adverse effect, but adequate studies in pregnant women have not demonstrated a risk to the fetus during the first trimester of pregnancy, and there is no evidence of risk in later trimesters.

C Animal studies have shown an adverse effect on the fetus, but there are no adequate studies in humans; or there are no animal reproduction studies and no adequate studies in humans.

D There is evidence of human fetal risk, but the potential benefits from the use of the drug in pregnant women may be acceptable despite its potential risks.

X Studies in animals or humans demonstrate fetal abnormalities or adverse reaction; reports indicate evidence of fetal risk. The risk of use in pregnant woman clearly outweighs any possible benefit.

V. DRUG INDEX

Trade name	Generic name
1,25-Dihydroxycholecalciferol	Calcitriol
2-PAM*	Pralidoxime chloride
3TC*	Lamivudine
5-Aminosalicylic acid*	Mesalamine
5-ASA*	Mesalamine
5-FC*	Flucytosine
5-Fluorocytosine*	Flucytosine
9-Fluorohydrocortisone*	Fludrocortisone acetate
A-200	Pyrethrins
Abbokinase	Urokinase
Abelcet	Amphotericin B lipid complex
Accolate	Zafirlukast
AccuNeb (prediluted nebulized solution)	Albuterol
Accutane	Isotretinoin
Acetadote	Acetylcysteine
Acticin	Permethrin
Actigall	Ursodiol
Actiq	Fentanyl

*Common abbreviation or other name (not recommended for use when writing a prescription)

For explanation of icons, see p. 680.

Trade name	Generic name
Activase	Alteplase
Acular, Acular LC, Acular PF	Ketorolac
Adalat, Adalat CC	Nifedipine
Adderall, Adderall XR	Dextroamphetamine ± amphetamine
Adenine arabinoside	Vidarabine
Adenocard	Adenosine
Adrenalin	Epinephrine HCl
Advair Diskus	Fluticasone propionate and salmeterol
Advil	Ibuprofen
Aerobid, Aerobid-M	Flunisolide
Afrin (nasal)	Oxymetazoline
Aftate	Tolnaftate
Akarpine	Pilocarpine HCl
AK-Poly-Bac Ophthalmic	Bacitracin ± polymyxin B
AK-Spore HC Otic	Polymyxin B sulfate, neomycin sulfate, hydrocortisone
AK-Sulf	Sulfacetamide sodium
AKTob	Tobramycin
AK-Tracin Ophthalmic	Bacitracin ± polymyxin B
Albumarc	Albumin, human
Albuminar	Albumin, human
Albutein	Albumin, human
Aldactone	Spironolactone
Aleve [OTC]	Naproxen/naproxen sodium
Allegra	Fexofenadine ± pseudoephedrine
Allehist-1	Clemastine
Allergen Ear Drops	Antipyrine and benzocaine
Alloprim	Allopurinol
Almacone	Aluminum hydroxide with magnesium hydroxide
Alocril	Nedocromil sodium
AlternaGEL	Aluminum hydroxide
Alu-Cap	Aluminum hydroxide
Alu-Tab	Aluminum hydroxide
AmBisome	Amphotericin B, liposomal
Amen	Medroxyprogesterone ± estradiol
Amicar	Aminocaproic acid
Amikin	Amikacin sulfate
Amino-Aqueous	Amiodarone HCl
Aminophyllin	Aminophylline
Aminoxin	Pyridoxine
Amnesteem	Isotretinoin
Amoxil	Amoxicillin
Amphadase	Hyaluronidase
Amphocin	Amphotericin B
Amphojel	Aluminum hydroxide
Amphotec	Amphotericin B cholesteryl sulfate
Anacin	Aspirin

Trade name	Generic name
Anacin-3	Acetaminophen
Anaprox	Naproxen/naproxen sodium
Ancef	Cefazolin
Ancobon	Flucytosine
Anectine	Succinylcholine
Antilirium	Physostigmine salicylate
Antiminth	Pyrantel pamoate
Antizol	Fomepizole
Anzemet	Dolasetron
Apresoline	Hydralazine HCl
Aquachloral Supprettes	Chloral hydrate
Aquasol A	Vitamin A
Aquavit-E	Vitamin E/alpha-tocopherol
ara-A*	Vidarabine
Aralen	Chloroquine HCl/phosphate
Aranesp	Darbepoetin alfa
Aredia	Pamidronate
Aristocort	Triamcinolone
ASA*	Aspirin
Asacol	Mesalamine
Astelin	Azelastine
Atarax	Hydroxyzine
Ativan	Lorazepam
Atretol	Carbamazepine
Atropen	Atropine Sulfate
Atrovent	Ipratropium bromide
Augmentin, Augmentin ES-600, Augmentin XR	Amoxicillin-clavulanic acid
Auro Ear Drops	Carbamide peroxide
Auroto Otic	Antipyrine and benzocaine
Aventyl	Nortriptyline hydrochloride
Avita	Tretinoin
Azactam	Aztreonam
Azasan	Azathioprine
Azmacort	Triamcinolone
Azo-Standard [OTC]	Phenazopyridine HCl
AZT	Zidovudine
Azulfidine, Azulfidine EN-tabs	Sulfasalazine
Baciguent Topical	Bacitracin ± polymyxin B
Bactrim	Co-trimoxazole
Bactroban, Bactroban Nasal	Mupirocin
BAL	Dimercaprol
Beconase, Beconase AQ	Beclomethasone dipropionate
Benadryl	Diphenhydramine
Benzac 5, Benzac 10	Benzoyl peroxide
Benzac AC Wash $2^1/_2$, 5, 10	Benzoyl peroxide
Betatrex	Betamethasone
Biaxin, Biaxin XL	Clarithromycin

*Common abbreviation or other name (not recommended for use when writing a prescription)

For explanation of icons, see p. 680.

Trade name	Generic name
Bicillin C-R, Bicillin C-R 900/300	Penicillin G preparations–Penicillin G benzathine and Penicillin G procaine
Bicillin L-A	Penicillin G preparations–benzathine
Biltricide	Praziquantel
Biocef	Cephalexin
Bleph 10	Sulfacetamide sodium
Brethine	Terbutaline
Brevibloc	Esmolol HCl
Brevoxyl Creamy Wash	Benzoyl peroxide
British anti-Lewisite*	Dimercaprol
Bromfed	Brompheniramine ± pseudoephedrine
Bufferin	Aspirin
Bumex	Bumetanide
Buminate	Albumin, human
Cafcit	Caffeine citrate
Cafergot	Ergotamine tartrate
Calan, Calan SR	Verapamil
Calciferol	Ergocalciferol
Calcijex	Calcitriol
Calcium disodium versenate	EDTA calcium disodium
Camphorated opium tincture	Paregoric
Canasa	Mesalamine
Cancidas	Caspofungin
Capoten	Captopril
Carafate	Sucralfate
Carbatrol	Carbamazepine
Carbic-D	Carbinoxamide with pseudoephedrine
Cardec, Cardec-S	Carbinoxamide with pseudoephedrine
Cardene, Cardene SR	Nicardipine
Cardizem, Cardizem CD, Cardizem LA, Cardizem S	Diltiazem
Carnitor	Carnitine
Catapres, Catapres TTS	Clonidine
Cathflo	Alteplase
Ceclor, Ceclor CD	Cefaclor
Cecon	Ascorbic acid
Cedax	Ceftibuten
Cefizox	Ceftizoxime
Cefobid	Cefoperazone
Cefotan	Cefotetan
Ceftin (PO)	Cefuroxime (IV, IM)/cefuroxime axetil (PO)
Cefzil	Cefprozil
Celestone, Celestone Soluspan	Betamethasone
CellCept	Mycophenolate mofetil
Cephulac	Lactulose
Ceptaz [arginine salt]	Ceftazidime
Cerebyx	Fosphenytoin
Cerumenex	Triethanolamine polypeptide oleate
Chemet	Succimer

*Common abbreviation or other name (not recommended for use when writing a prescription)

Trade name	Generic name
Chibroxin	Norfloxacin
Children's Advil	Ibuprofen
Children's Dramamine	Dimenhydrinate
Children's Motrin	Ibuprofen
Chloromycetin	Chloramphenicol
Chlor-Trimeton	Chlorpheniramine maleate
Chronulac	Lactulose
Ciloxan ophthalmic	Ciprofloxacin
Cipro, Cipro HC Otic, Cipro XR	Ciprofloxacin
Claforan	Cefotaxime
Claravis	Isotretinoin
Clarinex, Clarinex RediTabs	Desloratadine
Claritin, Claritin RediTabs, Claritin-D 12 Hour/24 Hour	Loratadine ± pseudoephedrine
Cleocin, Cleocin-T	Clindamycin
Clopra	Metoclopramide
Cogentin	Benztropine
Colace	Docusate
CoLyte	Polyethylene glycol-electrolyte solution
Compazine	Prochlorperazine
Concerta	Methylphenidate HCl
Copegus	Ribavirin
Cordarone	Amiodarone HCl
Cortef	Hydrocortisone
Cortifoam	Hydrocortisone
Cortisporin Otic	Polymyxin B sulfate, neomycin sulfate, hydrocortisone
Cortone acetate	Cortisone acetate
Coumadin	Warfarin
Covera-HS	Verapamil
Crolom	Cromolyn
Cuprimine	Penicillamine
Curex	Clotrimazole
Curosurf	Surfactant, pulmonary/poractant alfa
Curretab	Medroxyprogesterone ± estradiol
Cutivate	Fluticasone propionate
Cyanoject	Cyanocobalamin/vitamin B_{12}
Cyclogyl	Cyclopentolate
Cyclomydril	Cyclopentolate + phenylephrine
Cycrin	Medroxyprogesterone ± estradiol
Cyomin	Cyanocobalamin/vitamin B_{12}
Cytovene	Ganciclovir
Dantrium	Dantrolene
Daraprim	Pyrimethamine ± sulfadoxine
Dayhist-1	Clemastine
DDAVP	Desmopressin acetate
DDS*	Dapsone

*Common abbreviation or other name (not recommended for use when writing a prescription)

For explanation of icons, see p. 680.

Trade name	Generic name
Debrox	Carbamide peroxide
Decadron	Dexamethasone
Deltasone	Prednisone
Demerol	Meperidine HCl
Deodorized tincture of opium (DTO)	Opium tincture
Depacon	Valproic acid
Depakene	Valproic acid
Depakote, Depakote ER	Divalproex sodium
Depen	Penicillamine
Depo-Medrol	Methyprednisolone
Depo-Provera	Medroxyprogesterone ± estradiol
Desferal	Deferoxamine mesylate
Desquam-E 5, Desquam-E 10	Benzoyl peroxide
Desyrel	Trazodone
Dexedrine, Dexedrine Spansules	Dextroamphetamine ± amphetamine
DexFerrum	Iron dextran
Dextrostat	Dextroamphetamine ± amphetamine
DHT, DHT Intensol	Dihydrotachysterol
Di-5-ASA*	Olsalazine
Diaminodiphenylsufone*	Dapsone
Diamox	Acetazolamide
Diflucan	Fluconazole
Digibind	Digoxin immune FAB (ovine)
Digitek	Digoxin
Dilacor XR	Diltiazem
Dilantin, Dilantin Infatab	Phenytoin
Dilaudid, Dilaudid-HP	Hydromorphone HCl
Di-mesalazine*	Olsalazine
Dimetapp	Brompheniramine ± pseudoephedrine
Dipentum	Olsalazine
Diprolene, Diprolene AF	Betamethasone
Diprosone	Betamethasone
Dispermox	Amoxicillin
Ditropan, Ditropan XL	Oxybutynin chloride
Diurigen	Chlorothiazide
Diuril	Chlorothiazide
DMSA (dimercaptosuccinic acid)*	Succimer
Dobutrex	Dobutamine
Dolophine	Methadone HCl
Dopram	Doxapram HCl
Dramamine	Dimenhydrinate
Drisdol	Ergocalciferol
Dulcolax	Bisacodyl
Duraclon	Clonidine
Duragesic	Fentanyl
Duramist	Oxymetazoline
Duricef	Cefadroxil
Dycill	Dicloxacillin sodium

*Common abbreviation or other name (not recommended for use when writing a prescription)

Trade name	Generic name
Dynacin	Minocycline
Dyrenium	Triamterene
EC-Naprosyn	Naproxen/naproxen sodium
Efidac 24	Chlorpheniramine maleate
Efidac 24-Pseudoephedrine	Pseudoephedrine
Elavil	Amitriptyline
Elidel	Pimecrolimus
Elimite	Permethrin
Elitek	Rasburicase
EMLA	Lidocaine and prilocaine
E-Mycin	Erythromycin preparations
Enbrel	Etanercept
Endocet	Oxycodone and acetaminophen
Enlon	Edrophonium chloride
Enulose	Lactulose
Epitol	Carbamazepine
Epivir, Epivir-HBV	Lamivudine
Epogen	Epoetin alfa
Epsom salts	Magnesium sulfate
Ery-Ped	Erythromycin preparations
Erythrocin	Erythromycin preparations
Erythropoietin	Epoetin alfa
Esidrix	Hydrochlorothiazide
Eskalith, Eskalith CR	Lithium
Exsel (Rx)	Selenium sulfide
Famvir	Famciclovir
Fansidar	Pyrimethamine ± sulfadoxine
Felbatol	Felbamate
Fentanyl Oralet	Fentanyl
Feosol	Iron preparations
Fergon	Iron preparations
Fer-In-Sol	Iron preparations
Feverall	Acetaminophen
Fiberall	Psyllium
FIV-ASA*	Mesalamine
FK506*	Tacrolimus
Flagyl, Flagyl ER	Metronidazole
Fleet Babylax	Glycerin
Fleet Bisacodyl, Fleet Laxative	Bisacodyl
Fleet, Fleet Phospho-soda	Sodium phosphate
Flonase	Fluticasone propionate
Florinef acetate	Fludrocortisone acetate
Flovent, Flovent Rotadisk	Fluticasone propionate
Floxin, Floxin Otic	Ofloxacin
Flumadine	Rimantadine

*Common abbreviation or other name (not recommended for use when writing a prescription)

For explanation of icons, see p. 680.

Trade name	Generic name
Fluohydrisone	Fludrocortisone acetate
Fluoritab	Fluoride
Folvite	Folic acid
Fortaz	Ceftazidime
Foscavir	Foscarnet
Fulvicin P/G, Fulvicin U/F	Griseofulvin
Fungizone	Amphotericin B
Furadantin	Nitrofurantoin
Furomide	Furosemide
Gabitril	Tiagabine
Galzin	Zinc Salts
Gamma benzene hexachloride*	Lindane
Gantrisin	Sulfisoxazole
Garamycin	Gentamicin
Gastrocrom	Cromolyn
Gas-X	Simethicone
G-CSF*	Filgrastim
Gengraf	Cyclosporine, cyclosporine microemulsion
GlucaGen	Glucagon HCl
Glucagon Emergency Kit	Glucagon HCl
Glucophage	Metformin
Gly-Oxide	Carbamide peroxide
GoLYTELY	Polyethylene glycol-electrolyte solution
Grifulvin V	Griseofulvin
Grisactin	Griseofulvin
Gris-PEG	Griseofulvin
Gyne-Lotrimin 3, Gyne-Lotrimin 7	Clotrimazole
H.P. Acthar	Corticotropin
Haldol	Haloperidol
Hexadrol	Dexamethasone
Humatin	Paromomycin sulfate
Hydrocortone	Hydrocortisone
Hydrodiuril	Hydrochlorothiazide
Hydro-Par	Hydrochlorothiazide
Hyperstat IV	Diazoxide
Hytakerol	Dihydrotachysterol
Imitrex	Sumatriptan succinate
Imodium, Imodium AD	Loperamide
Imuran	Azathioprine
Inapsine	Droperidol
Inderal	Propranolol
Indocin, Indocin I.V., Indocin SR	Indomethacin
Infasurf	Surfactant, pulmonary/calfactant
InFed	Iron dextran
INH	Isoniazid
Intal	Cromolyn
Intropin	Dopamine

*Common abbreviation or other name (not recommended for use when writing a prescription)

Trade name	Generic name
Iostat	Potassium iodide
Iquix	Levofloxacin
Isoptin, Isotopin SR	Verapamil
Isopto Carpine	Pilocarpine HCl
Isopto Hyoscine	Scopolamine hydrobromide
Isuprel	Isoproterenol
Kantrex	Kanamycin
Kaopectate	Bismuth subsalicylate
Kayexalate	Sodium polystyrene sulfonate
Keflex	Cephalexin
Kemstro	Baclofen
Kenalog	Triamcinolone
Ketalar	Ketamine
Kionex	Solium polystyrene sulfonate
Klonopin	Clonazepam
Kondremul	Mineral oil
Konsyl	Psyllium
K-PHOS M.F., K-PHOS Neutral, K-PHOS No. 2	Phosphorus supplements
Kytril	Granisetron
Lamictal	Lamotrigine
Laniazid	Isoniazid
Lanoxicaps	Digoxin
Lanoxin	Digoxin
Lariam	Mefloquine HCl
Lasix	Furosemide
Lax-Pills	Senna/sennosides
Levaquin	Levofloxacin
Levocarnitine	Carnitine
Levophed	Norepinephrine bitartrate
Levothroid	Levothyroxine (T4)
Levoxyl	Levothyroxine (T4)
Lioresal	Baclofen
Liquid Pred	Prednisone
Lithobid	Lithium
L-M-X	Lidocaine
LoCHOLEST, LoCHOLEST Light	Cholestyramine
Loniten	Minoxidil
Lorabid	Loracarbef
Lotrimin AF	Clotrimazole
Lotrimin AF	Miconazole
Lovenox	Enoxaparin
Luminal	Phenobarbital
Lunelle	Medroxyprogesterone ± estradiol
Luride	Fluoride
Luvox	Fluvoxamine

For explanation of icons, see p. 680.

Trade name	Generic name
Maalox, Maalox Max, Maalox TC	Aluminum hydroxide with magnesium hydroxide
Macrobid	Nitrofurantoin
Macrodantin	Nitrofurantoin
Mag-200	Magnesium oxide
Mag-Ox 400	Magnesium oxide
Marinol	Dronabinol
Maxipime	Cefepime
Maxivate	Betamethasone
Maxolon	Metoclopramide
Medrol	Methylprednisolone
Mefoxin	Cefoxitin
Mellaril	Thioridazine
Men's Rogaine Extra Strength	Minoxidil
Mephyton	Phytonadione/vitamin K1
Merrem	Meropenem
Mestinon	Pyridostigmine bromide
Metadate CD, Metadate ER	Methylphenidate HCl
Metamucil	Psyllium
Methadose	Methadone HCl
Methylin, Methylin ER	Methylphenidate HCl
MetroCream	Metronidazole
MetroGel, MetroGel-Vaginal	Metronidazole
MetroLotion	Metronidazole
Miacalcin, Miacalcin Nasal Spray	Calcitonin
Micatin	Miconazole
MicroNefrin	Epinephrine, racemic
Milk of Magnesia	Magnesium hydroxide
Minipress	Prazosin HCl
Minocin	Minocycline
Mintezol	Thiabendazole
MiraLax	Polyethylene glycol-electrolyte solution
Monistat	Miconazole
Motrin	Ibuprofen
MS Contin	Morphine sulfate
Mucomyst	Acetylcysteine
Mucosol	Acetylcysteine
Murine Ear Drops	Carbamide peroxide
Myambutol	Ethambutol HCl
Mycelex, Mycelex-7	Clotrimazole
Mycifradin	Neomycin sulfate
Myciguent	Neomycin sulfate
Mycobutin	Rifabutin
Mycostatin	Nystatin
Myfortic	Mycophenolate mofetil
Mykrox	Metolazone
Mylanta Gas	Simethicone

Trade name	Generic name
Mylanta, Mylanta Double Strength	Aluminum hydroxide with magnesium hydroxide
Mylicon	Simethicone
Mysoline	Primidone
Nallpen	Nafcillin
Naprelan	Naproxen/naproxen sodium
Naprosyn	Naproxen/naproxen sodium
Narcan	Naloxone
Nasacort AQ	Triamcinolone
Nasalcrom	Cromolyn
Nasalide	Flunisolide
Nasarel	Flunisolide
Nebcin	Tobramycin
NebuPent	Pentamidine isethionate
Nembutal	Pentobarbital
Neo-Calglucon	Calcium glubionate
Neo-fradin	Neomycin sulfate
Neoral	Cyclosporine, cyclosporine microemulsion
Neosporin, Neosporin GU Irrigant, Neosporin Ophthalmic	Neomycin/polymyxin B/± bacitracin
Neo-Synephrine	Phenylephrine HCl
Neo-Synephrine 12 Hour Nasal	Oxymetazoline
Neo-Tabs	Neomycin sulfate
Nephron	Epinephrine, racemic
Neupogen	Filgrastim
Neurontin	Gabapentin
Neut	Sodium bicarbonate
Neutra-Phos, Neutra-Phos-K	Phosphorus supplements
Niacor	Niacin/vitamin B_3
Niaspan	Niacin/vitamin B_3
Nicolor	Niacin/vitamin B_3
Nicotinic acid	Niacin/vitamin B_3
Niferex	Iron preparations
Nilstat	Nystatin
Nipride	Nitroprusside
Nitro-Bid	Nitroglycerin
Nitro-Dur	Nitroglycerin
Nitrostat	Nitroglycerin
Nix	Permethrin
Nizoral, Nizoral A-D	Ketoconazole
Norcuron	Vecuronium bromide
Noritate	Metronidazole
Normal Serum Albumin (Human)	Albumin, human
Normodyne	Labetalol
Noroxin	Norfloxacin
Norpace	Disopyramide phosphate
Norvasc	Amlodipine
Nostrilla	Oxymetazoline

For explanation of icons, see p. 680.

Trade name	Generic name
NuLYTELY	Polyethylene glycol-electrolyte solution
Nutr-E-sol	Vitamin E/alpha-tocopherol
NVP*	Nevirapine
Nydrazid	Isoniazid
OCL	Polyethylene glycol-electrolyte solution
Ocu Clear (ophthalmic)	Oxymetazoline
Ocuflox	Ofloxacin
Ocusert Pilo	Pilocarpine HCl
Ocusulf-10	Sulfacetamide sodium
Omnicef	Cefdinir
Omnipen	Ampicillin
Opitvar	Azelastine
Opticrom	Cromolyn
Oramorph SR	Morphine sulfate
Orapred	Prednisolone
Orasone	Prednisone
Orazinc	Zinc salts
Oretic	Hydrochlorothiazide
Os-Cal	Calcium carbonate
Osmitrol	Mannitol
Ovide	Malathion
Oxy Trol	Oxybutynin chloride
Oxy-5, Oxy-10	Benzoyl peroxide
Oxycontin	Oxycodone
Pacerone	Amiodarone HCl
Pamelor	Nortriptyline hydrochloride
Panadol	Acetaminophen
Patanol	Olopatadine
Pathocil	Dicloxacillin sodium
Paxil, Paxil CR	Paroxetine
Pediaflor	Fluoride
Pediamycin	Erythromycin preparations
Pediapred	Prednisolone
Pediazole	Erythromycin ethylsuccinate and acetylsulfisoxazole
Pentam 300	Pentamidine isethionate
Pentasa	Mesalamine
Pentothal	Thiopental sodium
Pepcid AC (OTC), Pepcid Complete (OTC)	Famotidine
Pepcid, Pepcid RPD	Famotidine
Pepto-Bismol	Bismuth subsalicylate
Percocet	Oxycodone and acetaminophen
Percodan, Percodan-Demi	Oxycodone and aspirin
Perdiem Fiber	Psyllium
Periactin	Cyproheptadine
Periostat	Doxycycline
Permapen	Penicillin G preparations–benzathine

*Common abbreviation or other name (not recommended for use when writing a prescription)

Trade name	Generic name
Pexeva	Paroxetine
Pfizerpen	Penicillin G preparations—aqueous potassium and sodium
PGE1*	Alprostadil
Phazyme	Simethicone
Phenergan	Promethazine
Phenytek	Phenytoin
Phylocontin	Aminophylline
Pilocar	Pilocarpine HCl
Pima	Potassium iodide
Pin-Rid	Pyrantel pamoate
Pin-X	Pyrantel pamoate
Pipracil	Piperacillin
Pitressin	Vasopressin
Plaquenil	Hydroxychloroquine
Plasbumin	Albumin, human
Polymox	Amoxicillin
Polysporin Ophthalmic, Polysporin Topical	Bacitracin ± polymyxin B
Potassium Phosphate	Phosphorus supplements
Prelone	Prednisolone
Prevacid	Lansoprazole
Prevalite	Cholestyramine
Prilosec, Prilosec OTC	Omeprazole
Primacor	Milrinone
Primaxin IM, Primaxin IV	Imipenem-cilastatin
Principen	Ampicillin
Prinivil	Lisinopril
Procanbid	Procainamide
Procardia, Procardia XL	Nifedipine
Procrit	Epoetin alfa
Proglycem	Diazoxide
Prograf	Tacrolimus
Pronto	Pyrethrins
Prostaglandin E_1*	Alprostadil
Prostigmin	Neostigmine
Prostin VR	Alprostadil
Protonix	Pantoprazole
Protopam	Pralidoxime chloride
Protopic	Tacrolimus
Protostat	Metronidazole
Proventil, Proventil HFA (aerosol inhaler)	Albuterol
Provera	Medroxyprogesterone ± estradiol
Proxigel	Carbamide peroxide
Prozac, Prozac Weekly	Fluoxetine hydrochloride
PTU*	Propylthiouracil
Pulmicort Respules	Budesonide
Pulmicort Turbuhaler	Budesonide
Pulmozyme	Dornase alfa/DNase

*Common abbreviation or other name (not recommended for use when writing a prescription)

For explanation of icons, see p. 680.

Trade name	Generic name
Pyrazinoic acid amide	Pyrazinamide
Pyridium	Phenazopyridine HCl
Pyrinyl	Pyrethrins
Quelicin	Succinylcholine
Questran, Questran Light	Cholestyramine
Quineprox	Hydroxychloroquine
Quinidex	Quinidine
Quixin	Levofloxacin
QVAR	Beclomethasone dipropionate
Rebetol	Ribavirin
Reese's Pinworm	Pyrantel pamoate
Regitine	Phentolamine mesylate
Reglan	Metoclopramide
Relenza	Zanamivir
Renova	Tretinoin
Retin-A, Retin-A Micro	Tretinoin
Retrovir	Zidovudine
Reversol	Edrophonium chloride
Rhinocort, Rhinocort Aqua Nasal Spray	Budesonide
RID	Pyrethrins
Rifadin	Rifampin
Rimactane	Rifampin
Risperdal, Risperdal Consta, Risperdal M-Tab	Risperidone
Ritalin, Ritalin LA, Ritalin SR	Methylphenidate HCl
Robinul	Glycopyrrolate
Rocaltrol	Calcitriol
Rocephin	Ceftriaxone
Rogaine	Minoxidil
Romazicon	Flumazenil
Rondec	Brompheniramine ± pseudoephedrine
Rondec, Rondec TR	Carbinoxamide with pseudoephedrine
Rowasa	Mesalamine
Roxanol	Morphine sulfate
Roxicet	Oxycodone and acetaminophen
Roxicodone	Oxycodone
Roxilox	Oxycodone and acetaminophen
Roxiprin	Oxycodone and aspirin
Rulox	Aluminum hydroxide with magnesium hydroxide
S-2 Inhalant	Epinephrine, racemic
Salagen	Pilocarpine HCl
Salicylazosulfapyridine	Sulfasalazine
Sal-Tropine	Atropine Sulfate
Sandimmune	Cyclosporine, cyclosporine microemulsion
Sandostatin, Sandostatin LAR Depot	Octreotide acetate
Sani-Supp	Glycerin
Sarafem	Fluoxetine hydrochloride

Trade name	Generic name
SAS*	Sulfasalazine
Scopace	Scopolamine hydrobromide
Selsum	Selenium sulfide
Senna-Gen	Senna/sennosides
Senokot	Senna/sennosides
Septra	Co-trimoxazole
Serevent Diskus	Salmeterol
Serutan	Psyllium
Silvadene	Silver sulfadiazine
Singulair	Montelukast
Slo-bid Gyrocap	Theophylline
Slo-Phyllin Gyrocaps	Theophylline
Slow FE	Iron preparations
Sodium Phosphate	Phosphorus supplements
Sofarin	Warfarin
Solu-cortef	Hydrocortisone
Solu-Medrol	Methylprednisolone
Sotret	Isotretinoin
Sporanox	Itraconazole
SPS Suspension	Sodium polystyrene sulfonate
SSD AF Cream, SSD Cream	Silver sulfadiazine
SSKI	Potassium iodide
Stimate	Desmopressin acetate
Strattera	Atomoxetine
Streptase	Streptokinase
Stromectol	Ivermectin
Sublimaze	Fentanyl
Sudafed	Pseudoephedrine
Sulfatrim	Co-trimoxazole
Sumycin	Tetracycline HCl
Sunkist Vitamin C	Ascorbic acid
Suprax	Cefixime
Surfak	Docusate
Survanta	Surfactant, pulmonary/beractant
Symmetrel	Amantadine hydrochloride
Synagis	Palivizumab
Synercid	Quinupristin and dalfopristin
Synthroid	Levothyroxine (T_4)
Tagamet, Tagamet HB [OTC]	Cimetidine
Tambocor	Flecainide acetate
Tamiflu	Oseltamivir phosphate
Tapazole	Methimazole
Tavist	Clemastine
Tazicef	Ceftazidime
Tazidime	Ceftazidime
Tegretol, Tegretol-XR	Carbamazepine
Tempra	Acetaminophen
Tenormin	Atenolol

*Common abbreviation or other name (not recommended for use when writing a prescription)

For explanation of icons, see p. 680.

Trade name	Generic name
Tensilon	Edrophonium chloride
Tequin	Gatifloxacin
Tetrahydrocannabinoid*	Dronabinol
THC*	Dronabinol
TheoDur	Theophylline
Thermazene	Silver sulfadiazine
Thiomalate	Thiamine
Thorazine	Chlorpromazine
Tiazac	Diltiazem
Ticar	Ticarcillin
Tigan	Trimethobenzamide HCl
Tilade	Nedocromil sodium
Timentin	Ticarcillin/clavulanate
Tinactin	Tolnaftate
TMP-SMX*	Co-trimoxazole
TOBI	Tobramycin
Tobrex	Tobramycin
Tofranil, Tofranil-PM	Imipramine
Topamax	Topiramate
Toradol	Ketorolac
Totacillin	Ampicillin
tPA*	Alteplase
Trandate	Labetalol
Transderm Scop	Scopolamine hydrobromide
Triaz	Benzoyl peroxide
Tridil	Nitroglycerin
Trileptal	Oxcarbazepine
Trilisate	Choline magnesium trisalicylate
TriLyte	Polyethylene glycol-electrolyte solution
Trimethoprim-sulfamethoxazole	Co-trimoxazole
Trimox	Amoxicillin
Tri-Nasal	Triamcinolone
Trobicin	Spectinomycin
Tums	Calcium carbonate
Tylenol	Acetaminophen
Tylenol #1, Tylenol #2, Tylenol #3, Tylenol #4	Codeine and acetaminophen
Tylox	Oxycodone and acetaminophen
Unasyn	Ampicillin/sulbactam
Unipen	Nafcillin
Urecholine	Bethanechol chloride
Uro-KP-Neutral	Phosphorus supplements
Urolene Blue	Methylene blue
Uro-Mag	Magnesium oxide
Urso	Ursodiol
Valcyte	Valganciclovir
Valium	Diazepam
Valtrex	Valacyclovir

*Common abbreviation or other name (not recommended for use when writing a prescription)

Trade name	Generic name
Vancenase, Vancenase AQ 84 mcg, Vancenase Pockethaler	Beclomethasone dipropionate
Vancocin	Vancomycin
Vantin	Cefpodoxime proxetil
Vasotec, Vasotec IV	Enalapril maleate, enalaprilat
Veetids	Penicillin V potassium
Velosef	Cephradine
Ventolin, Ventolin HFA (aerosol inhaler)	Albuterol
Verelan, Verelan PM	Verapamil
Vermox	Mebendazole
Versed	Midazolam
VFEND	Voriconazole
Vibramycin	Doxycycline
Vira-A	Vidarabine
Viramune	Nevirapine
Virazole	Ribavirin
Visicol	Sodium phosphate
Visine LR (ophthalmic)	Oxymetazoline
Vistaril	Hydroxyzine
Vistide	Cidofovir
Vitamin B_1	Thiamine
Vitamin B_{12}	Cyanocobalamin/vitamin B_{12}
Vitamin B_2	Riboflavin
Vitamin B_3	Niacin/vitamin B_3
Vitamin B_6	Pyridoxine
Vitamin C	Ascorbic acid
Vitrase	Hyaluronidase
VZIG*	Varicella-zoster immuneglobulin (human)
WinRho-SDF	Rho (D) immune globulin intravenous (human)
Women's Rogaine	Minoxidil
Wycillin	Penicillin G preparations–procaine
Wymox	Amoxicillin
Xopenex	Levalbuterol
Xylocaine	Lidocaine
Zantac, Zantac 75 [OTC]	Ranitidine HCl
Zarontin	Ethosuximide
Zaroxolyn	Metolazone
Zegerid	Omeprazole
Zemuron	Rocuronium
Zestril	Lisinopril
Zinacef (IV)	Cefuroxime (IV, IM)/cefuroxime axetil (PO)
Zincate	Zinc Salts
Zithromax, Zithromax 2-PAK, Zithromax TRI-PAK	Azithromycin
Zofran	Ondansetron
Zolicef	Cefazolin
Zoloft	Sertraline HCl

*Common abbreviation or other name (not recommended for use when writing a prescription)

For explanation of icons, see p. 680.

Trade name	Generic name
Zonegran	Zonisamide
Zosyn	Piperacillin/tazobactam
Zovirax	Acyclovir
Zyloprim	Allopurinol
Zymar	Gatifloxacin
Zyrtec, Zyrtec-D 12 Hour	Cetirizine
Zyvox	Linezolid

VI. DRUG DOSES

ACETAMINOPHEN

Tylenol, Tempra, Panadol, Feverall, Anacin-3, and others

Analgesic, antipyretic

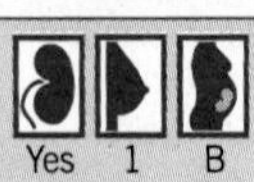

Tabs: 160, 325, 500, 650 mg
Chewable tabs: 80, 160 mg
Infant drops, solution/suspension: 80 mg/0.8 mL
Child suspension/syrup: 160 mg/5 mL
Oral liquid: 160, 166.7 mg/5 mL
Elixir: 160 mg/5 mL
Caplet: 500 mg
Extended-release caplet/geltab: 650 mg
Gelcap: 500 mg
Capsules: 500, 650 mg
Suppositories: 80, 120, 325, 650 mg
(Combination product with Codeine, see *Codeine and Acetaminophen*)

Neonates: 10–15 mg/kg/dose PO/PR Q6–8 hr. Some advocate loading doses of 20–25 mg/kg/dose for PO dosing or 30 mg/kg/dose for PR dosing.
Pediatric: 10–15 mg/kg/dose PO/PR Q4–6 hr. For rectal dosing, some may advocate a 40–45 mg/kg/dose loading dose.
Dosing by age *(PO/PR Q4–6 hr):*

- *0–3 mo:* 40 mg/dose
- *4–11 mo:* 80 mg/dose
- *12–24 mo:* 120 mg/dose
- *2–3 yr:* 160 mg/dose
- *4–5 yr:* 240 mg/dose
- *6–8 yr:* 320 mg/dose
- *9–10 yr:* 400 mg/dose
- *11–12 yr:* 480 mg/dose

Adult: 325–650 mg/dose
Max. dose: 4 g/24 hr, 5 doses/24 hr

Does not possess anti-inflammatory activity. **Use with caution** in patients with known G6PD deficiency.

$T_{1/2}$: 1–3 hr, 2–5 hr in neonates; metabolized in the liver; see Chapter 2, Table 2-3 for management of overdosage.

Continued

ACETAMINOPHEN *continued*

Some preparations contain alcohol (7%–10%) and/or phenylalanine; all suspensions should be shaken before use.

May decrease the activity of lamotrigine and increase the activity of zidovudine. Rifampin and anticholinergic agents (e.g., scopolamine) may decrease the effect of acetaminophen. Increased risk for hepatotoxicity may occur with barbiturates, carbamazepine, phenytoin, carmustine (with high acetaminophen doses), and chronic alcohol use. **Adjust dose in renal failure (see Chapter 30).**

ACETAZOLAMIDE

Diamox

Carbonic anhydrase inhibitor, diuretic

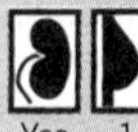

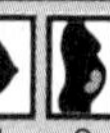

Yes 1 C

Tabs: 125, 250 mg
Suspension: 25, 50 mg/mL
Capsules (sustained release): 500 mg
Injection (sodium): 500 mg/5 mL
Contains 2.05 mEq Na/500 mg drug

Diuretic (PO, IV)
Child: 5 mg/kg/dose QD–QOD
Adult: 250–375 mg/dose QD–QOD

Glaucoma
Child: 20–40 mg/kg/24 hr ÷ Q6 hr IM/IV; 8–30 mg/kg/24 hr ÷ Q6–8 hr PO
Adult: 1000 mg/24 hr ÷ Q6 hr PO; for rapid decrease in intraocular pressure, administer 500 mg/dose IV.

Seizures: 8–30 mg/kg/24 hr ÷ Q6–12 hr PO
Max. dose: 1 g/24 hr

Urine alkalinization: 5 mg/kg/dose PO repeated BID–TID over 24 hr.

Management of hydrocephalus: Start with 20 mg/kg/24 hr ÷ Q8 hr PO/IV; may increase to 100 mg/kg/24 hr up to a **max. dose** of 2 g/24 hr.

Contraindicated in hepatic failure, severe renal failure (GFR <10 mL/min), and hypersensitivity to sulfonamides.

$T_{1/2}$: 2–6 hr; **do not use** sustained-release capsules in seizures; IM injection may be painful; bicarbonate replacement therapy may be required during long-term use (see *Citrate* or *Sodium Bicarbonate*).

Possible side effects (more likely with long-term therapy) include GI irritation, paresthesias, sedation, hypokalemia, acidosis, reduced urate secretion, aplastic anemia, polyuria, and development of renal calculi.

May increase toxicity of cyclosporin. Aspirin may increase toxicity of acetazolamide. May decrease the effects of salicylates, lithium, and phenobarbital. False-positive urinary protein may occur with several assays. **Adjust dose in renal failure (see Chapter 30).**

For explanation of icons, see p. 680.

ACETYLCYSTEINE
Mucomyst, Acetadote
Mucolytic, antidote for acetaminophen toxicity

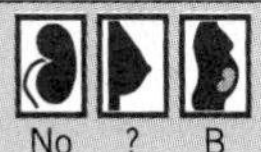
No ? B

Solution: 100 mg/mL (10%) or 200 mg/mL (20%) (4, 10, 30 mL)
Injection (Acetadote): 200 mg/mL (20%) (30 mL)

For acetaminophen poisoning, see Chapter 2, Table 2-3.
Nebulizer:
Children: 3–5 mL of 20% solution (diluted with equal volume of H_2O, or sterile saline to equal 10%), or 6–10 mL of 10% solution; administer TID–QID.
Adolescents: 5–10 mL of 10% or 20% solution; administer TID–QID.
Distal intestinal obstruction syndrome in Cystic Fibrosis:
Adolescents and Adults: 10 mL of 20% solution (diluted in a sweet drink) PO QID with 100 mL of 10% solution PR as an enema QD-QID.

For nebulized use, give inhaled bronchodilator 10–15 min before use and follow with postural drainage and/or suctioning after acetylcysteine administration. Prior hydration is essential for distal intestinal obstruction syndrome treatment.

May induce bronchospasm, stomatitis, drowsiness, rhinorrhea, nausea, vomiting, and hemoptysis.

ACTH

See *Corticotropin*

ACYCLOVIR
Zovirax
Antiviral

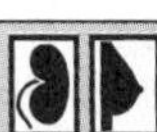
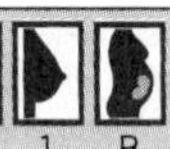
Yes 1 B

Capsules: 200 mg
Tabs: 400, 800 mg
Suspension: 200 mg/5 mL
Ointment: 5% (15 g)
Cream: 5% (2 g)
Injection in powder (with sodium): 500, 1000 mg
Injection in solution (with sodium): 25, 50 mg/mL
Contains 4.2 mEq Na/1 g drug

IMMUNOCOMPETENT:
Neonatal (HSV and HSV encephalitis):
<35 wk postconceptional age: 40 mg/kg/24 hr ÷ Q12 hr IV × 14–21 days
≥35 wk postconceptional age: 60 mg/kg/24 hr ÷ Q8 hr IV × 14–21 days
Mucocutaneous HSV (including genital):
Initial infection:
IV: 15 mg/kg/24 hr or 750 mg/m²/24 hr ÷ Q8 hr × 5–7 days

Continued

ACYCLOVIR *continued*

PO: 1200 mg/24 hr ÷ Q8 hr × 7–10 days with a **max. dose** in children at 80 mg/kg/24 hr ÷ Q6–8 hr

Recurrence:

PO: 1200 mg/24 hr ÷ Q8 hr or 1600 mg/24 hr ÷ Q12 hr × 5 days with a **max. dose** in children at 80 mg/kg/24 hr ÷ Q6–8 hr

Chronic suppressive therapy:

PO: 800–1000 mg/24 hr ÷ 2–5 times/24 hr for up to 1 year with a **max. dose** in children at 80 mg/kg/24 hr ÷ Q6–8 hr

Zoster:

IV: 30 mg/kg/24 hr or 1500 mg/m^2/24 hr ÷ Q8 hr × 7–10 days

PO: 4000 mg/24 hr ÷ 5×/24 hr × 5–7 days for patients ≥ 12 yr

Varicella:

IV: 30 mg/kg/24 hr or 1500 mg/m^2/24 hr ÷ Q8 hr × 7–10 days

PO: 80 mg/kg/24 hr ÷ QID × 5 days (begin treatment at earliest signs/symptoms); **max. dose:** 3200 mg/24 hr

Max. dose of oral acyclovir in children = 80 mg/kg/24 hr

IMMUNOCOMPROMISED:

HSV:

IV: 750–1500 mg/m^2/24 hr ÷ Q8 hr × 7–14 days

PO: 1000 mg/24 hr ÷ 3–5 times/24 hr × 7–14 days

HSV prophylaxis:

IV: 750 mg/m^2/24 hr ÷ Q8 hr during risk period

PO: 600–1000 mg/24 hr ÷ 3–5 times/24 hr during risk period

Varicella or zoster:

IV: 1500 mg/m^2/24 hr ÷ Q8 hr × 7–10 days

PO: 250–600 mg/m^2/dose 4–5 times/24 hr

CMV prophylaxis:

IV: 1500 mg/m^2/24 hr ÷ Q8 hr during risk period

PO: 800–3200 mg/24 hr ÷ Q6–24 hr during risk period

Max. dose of oral acyclovir in children = 80 mg/kg/24 hr

TOPICAL:

Apply 0.5-inch ribbon of 5% ointment for 4-inch square surface area 6 times a day × 7 days.

See most recent edition of the AAP *Red Book* for further details. Oral absorption is unpredictable (15%–30%). Use ideal body weight for obese patients when calculating dosages. Resistant strains of HSV and VZV have been reported in immunocompromised patients (e.g., advanced HIV infection).

Adequate hydration and slow (1 hr) IV administration are essential to prevent crystallization in renal tubules; **dose alteration necessary in patients with impaired renal function (see Chapter 30).**

Can cause renal impairment; has been infrequently associated with headache, vertigo, insomnia, encephalopathy, GI tract irritation, elevated liver function tests, rash, urticaria, arthralgia, fever, and adverse hematologic effects. Probenecid decreases acyclovir renal clearance. Acyclovir may increase the concentration of meperidine and its metabolite, normeperidine.

For explanation of icons, see p. 680.

ADENOSINE

Adenocard

Antiarrhythmic

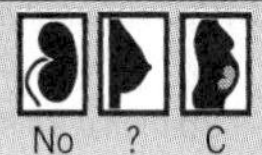

Injection: 3 mg/mL (2, 4 mL)

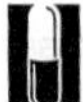

Supraventricular tachycardia:

Children: 0.1–0.2 mg/kg rapid IV push over 1–2 seconds followed by rapid saline flush; may increase dose by 0.05-mg/kg increments every 2 min to **max. dose** of 0.25 mg/kg (up to 12 mg) or until termination of SVT. **Max. single dose:** 12 mg

Adolescents and adults ≥50 kg: 6 mg rapid IV push over 1–2 seconds; if no response after 1–2 min, give 12 mg rapid IV push. May repeat a second 12 mg dose after 1–2 min if required. **Max. single dose:** 12 mg

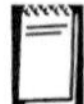

Contraindicated in 2nd and 3rd degree AV block or sick-sinus syndrome unless pacemaker placed. **Use with caution** in combination with digoxin (enhanced depressant effects on SA and AV nodes).

Follow each dose with rapid NS flush. $T_{1/2}$: <10 seconds.

May precipitate bronchoconstriction, especially in asthmatics. Side effects include transient asystole, facial flushing, headache, shortness of breath, dyspnea, nausea, chest pain, and lightheadedness.

Carbamazepine and dipyridamole may increase the effects/toxicity of adenosine. Methylxanthines (e.g., caffeine and theophylline) may decrease the effects of adenosine.

ALBUMIN, HUMAN

Albumarc, Albuminar, Albutein, Buminate, Plasbumin, Normal Serum Albumin (Human), and others

Blood product derivative, plasma volume expander

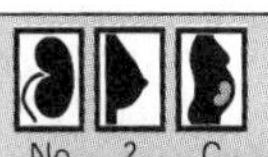

Injection: 5% (50 mg/mL) (50, 250, 500 mL); 25% (250 mg/mL) (20, 50, 100 mL); both concentrations contain 130–160 mEq Na/L

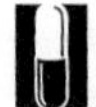

Hypoproteinemia:

Children: 0.5–1 g/kg/dose IV over 30–120 min; repeat Q1–2 days PRN

Adult: 25 g/dose IV over 30–120 min; repeat Q1–2 days PRN

Hypovolemia:

Children: 0.5–1 g/kg/dose IV rapid infusion

Adult: 25 g/dose IV rapid infusion; may repeat PRN

Max. dose: 6 g/kg/24 hr or 250 g/48 hr

Continued

A

FORMULARY

ALBUMIN, HUMAN *continued*

Contraindicated in cases of CHF or severe anemia; rapid infusion may cause fluid overload; hypersensitivity reactions may occur; may cause rapid increase in serum sodium levels.

Caution: 25% concentration contraindicated in preterm infants due to risk for IVH. For infusion, use 5-micron filter or larger. Both 5% and 25% products are isotonic but differ in oncotic effects. Dilutions of the 25% product should be made with D5W or NS; **avoid sterile water.**

ALBUTEROL

Proventil, VoSpire ER (sustained-release tabs), Proventil HFA (aerosol inhaler),Ventolin HFA (aerosol inhaler), AccuNeb (prediluted nebulized solution)

Beta-2-adrenergic agonist

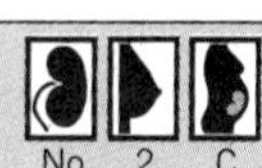

Tabs: 2, 4 mg
Sustained-release tabs: 4, 8 mg
Oral solution: 2 mg/5 mL (473 mL)
Aerosol inhaler: 90 mcg/actuation (200 actuations/inhaler) (17 g)
Nebulization solution: 0.5% (5 mg/mL) (20 mL)
Prediluted nebulized solution: 0.63 mg in 3 mL NS, 1.25 mg in 3 mL NS, and 2.5 mg in 3 mL NS (0.083%)

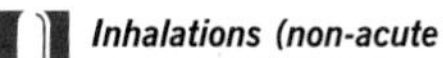

Inhalations (non-acute use):
Aerosol (MDI): 1–2 puffs (90–180 mcg) Q4–6 hr PRN
Nebulization:
<1 yr: 0.05–0.15 mg/kg/dose Q4–6 hr
1–5 yr: 1.25–2.5 mg/dose Q4–6 hr
5–12 yr: 2.5 mg/dose Q4–6 hr
>12 yr: 2.5–5 mg/dose Q6 hr

For use in acute exacerbations more aggressive dosing may be employed.

Oral:
Children <6 yr: 0.3 mg/kg/24 hr PO ÷ TID; **max. dose:** 12 mg/24 hr
6–11 yr: 6 mg/24 hr PO ÷ TID; **max. dose:** 24 mg/24 hr
>12 yr and adults: 2–4 mg/dose PO TID–QID; **max. dose:** 32 mg/24 hr

Inhaled doses may be given more frequently than indicated. In such cases, consider cardiac monitoring and monitoring of serum potassium. Systemic effects are dose related. Please verify the concentration of the nebulization solution used.

Use of oral dosage form is discouraged owing to increased side effects and decreased efficacy compared with inhaled formulations.

Possible side effects include tachycardia, palpitations, tremor, insomnia, nervousness, nausea, and headache.

Use of tube spacers or chambers may enhance efficacy of the metered dose inhalers and have been proved just as effective and sometimes safer than nebulizers. Proventil HFA and Ventolin HFA are CFC-free metered dose inhalers.

For explanation of icons, see p. 666

ALLOPURINOL

Zyloprim, Alloprim, and others

Uric acid lowering agent, xanthine oxidase inhibitor

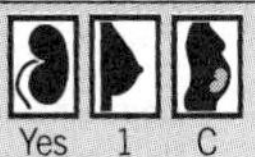

Tabs: 100, 300 mg
Suspension: 20 mg/mL
Injection (Alloprim): 500 mg
Contains ~ 1.45 mEq Na/500 mg drug

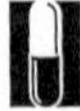

For use in tumor lysis syndrome, see Chapter 21.
Child:
Oral: 10 mg/kg/24 hr PO ÷ BID–QID; **max. dose:** 800 mg/24 hr
Injectable: 200 mg/m²/24 hr IV ÷ Q 6–12 hr; **max. dose:** 600 mg/24 hr
Adult:
Oral: 200–800 mg/24 hr PO ÷ BID–TID
Injectable: 200–400 mg/m²/24 hr IV ÷ Q 6–12 hr; **max. dose:** 600 mg/24 hr

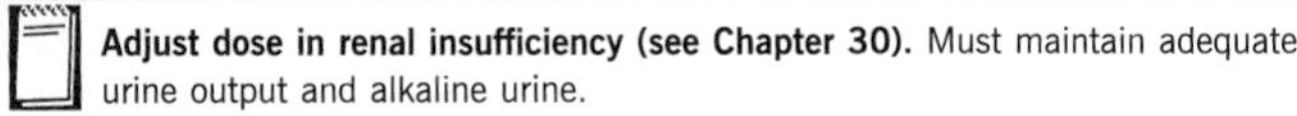

Adjust dose in renal insufficiency (see Chapter 30). Must maintain adequate urine output and alkaline urine.

Drug interactions: increases serum theophylline level; may increase the incidence of rash with ampicillin and amoxicillin; increases risk for toxicity with azathioprine, didanosine, and mercaptopurine; and increases risk for hypersensitivity reactions with ACE inhibitors and thiazide diuretics.

Side effects include rash, neuritis, hepatotoxicity, GI disturbance, bone marrow suppression, and drowsiness.

IV dosage form is very alkaline and must be diluted to a minimum concentration of 6 mg/mL and infused over 30 min.

ALPROSTADIL

Prostin VR, Prostaglandin E_1, PGE_1

Prostaglandin E_1, vasodilator

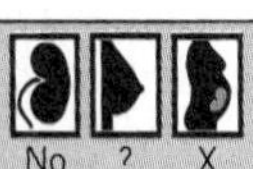

Injection: 500 mcg/mL (contains dehydrated alcohol)

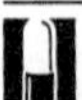

Neonates:
Initial: 0.05–0.1 mcg/kg/min. Advance to 0.2 mcg/kg/min if necessary.
Maintenance: When increase in PaO_2 is noted, decrease immediately to lowest effective dose. Usual dosage range: 0.01–0.4 mcg/kg/min; doses above 0.4 mcg/kg/min not likely to produce additional benefit.
To prepare infusion: See inside front cover.

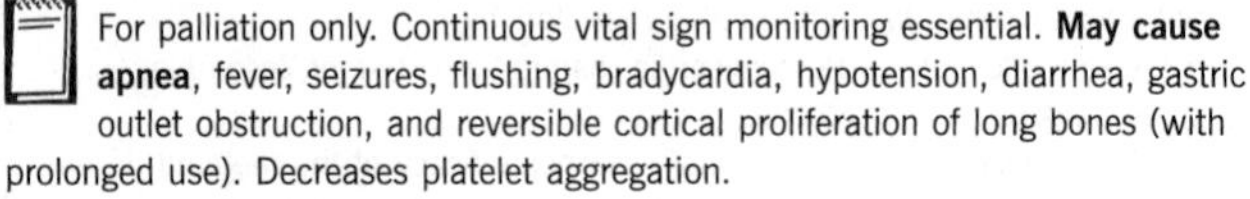

For palliation only. Continuous vital sign monitoring essential. **May cause apnea**, fever, seizures, flushing, bradycardia, hypotension, diarrhea, gastric outlet obstruction, and reversible cortical proliferation of long bones (with prolonged use). Decreases platelet aggregation.

ALTEPLASE

Activase, Cathflo Activase, tPA

Thrombolytic agent, tissue plasminogen activator

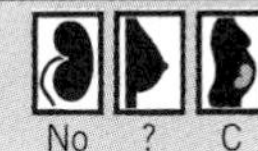

Injection:

Cathflo Activase: 2 mg

Activase: 50 mg (29 million unit), 100 mg (58 million unit)

Contains: L-arginine and polysorbate 80.

Occluded IV catheter:

Aspiration method: Use 1 mg/1 mL concentration as follows:

Weight (Kg)	Single-Lumen CVL	Double-Lumen CVL	Subcutaneous Port
<10	0.5 mg, dilute with normal saline to required volume to fill line	0.5 mg each lumen, dilute with normal saline to required volume to fill line	0.5 mg, dilute with normal saline to 3 mL
≥10	1–2 mg, use required amount to fill lumen (max: 2 mg)	1–2 mg each lumen, use required amount to fill lumen (max: 2 mg) and treat one lumen at a time	2 mg, dilute with normal saline to 3 mL

CVL, Central venous line.

Instill into catheter over 1–2 min and leave in place for 2–4 hours before attempting blood withdrawal. Dose may be repeated once in 24 hours using a longer catheter dwell time. **DO NOT** infuse into patient.

Systemic thrombolytic therapy (use in consultation with a hematologist): 0.1–0.6 mg/kg/hr × 6 hr has been recommended (Chest 2004;126:645–687S). The length of continuous infusion is variable because patients may respond to longer or shorter courses of therapy.

Current use in the pediatric population is limited. May cause bleeding, rash, and increase prothrombin time.

THROMBOLYTIC USE: History of stroke, transient ischemic attacks, other neurologic disease, and hypertension are **contraindications** in adults but considered relative contraindications in children. Monitor fibrinogen, thrombin clotting time, PT, and APTT when used as a thrombolytic.

Newborns have reduced plasminogen levels (~50% of adult values), which decrease the thrombolytic effects of alteplase. Plasminogen supplementation may be necessary.

For explanation of icons, see p. 680.

ALUMINUM HYDROXIDE

Amphojel, Alu-Cap, Alu-Tab, AlternaGEL, and others

Antacid, phosphate binder

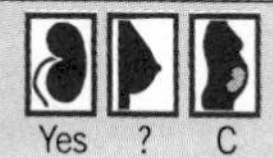

Tabs: 300, 500, 600 mg
Caps: 400 mg
Suspension: 320 mg, 450 mg, 600 mg, 675 mg/5 mL (180, 360, 480 mL)
Each tablet, capsule, and 5 mL suspension contains <0.13 mEq Na.

(mL volume dosages are based on the 320 mg/5 mL suspension concentration):

Peptic ulcer:
Child: 5–15 mL PO Q3–6 hr or 1–3 hr after meals and QHS
Adult: 15–45 mL PO Q3–6 hr or 1–3 hr after meals and QHS

Prophylaxis against GI bleeding:
Neonate: 1 mL/kg/dose PO Q4 hr PRN
Infant: 2–5 mL PO Q1–2 hr
Child: 5–15 mL PO Q1–2 hr
Adult: 30–60 mL PO Q1–2 hr

Hyperphosphatemia:
Child: 50–150 mg/kg/24 hr ÷ Q4–6 hr PO
Adult: 30–40 mL TID–QID PO between meals and QHS

Use with caution in patients with renal failure and upper GI hemorrhage. Interferes with the absorption of several orally administered medications, including digoxin, ethambutol, indomethacin, isoniazid, tetracyclines, quinolones (e.g., ciprofloxacin), and iron. Do not take oral mediations within 1–2 hours of taking aluminum dose unless specified by your physician.

May cause constipation, decreased bowel motility, encephalopathy, and phosphorus depletion.

ALUMINUM HYDROXIDE WITH MAGNESIUM HYDROXIDE

Maalox, Maalox TC, Maalox Max, Mylanta, Mylanta Double Strength, Alamacone, Rulox, and others

Antacid

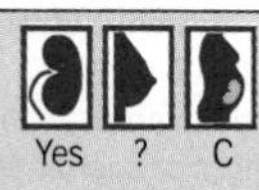

Chewable tabs: (Al $(OH)_3$: Mg $(OH)_2$)
200 mg: 200 mg (Rulox)
200 mg: 200 mg + simethicone 20 mg (Almacone)
Each tablet contains 0.03–0.06 mEq Na.

Suspension:
Maalox: each 5 mL contains 225 mg ALOH, 200 mg MgOH.
Maalox TC: each 5 mL contains 600 mg ALOH, 300 mg MgOH.
Maalox Antacid/Anti-Gas, Mylanta: each 5 mL contains 200 mg ALOH, 200 mg MgOH, and 20 mg simethicone.

Continued

ALUMINUM HYDROXIDE WITH MAGNESIUM HYDROXIDE *continued*

Maalox Max Antacid/Anti-Gas, Mylanta Double Strength: each 5 mL contains 400 mg ALOH, 400 mg MgOH, and 40 mg simethicone.
Maalox Maximum Strength: each 5 mL contains 500 mg ALOH, 450 mg MgOH, and 40 mg simethicone.
Many other combinations exist.
Contains 0.03–0.06 mEq Na/5 mL

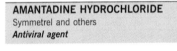

Same as for aluminum hydroxide preparations. **Do not use** combination product for hyperphosphatemia.

May have laxative effect. May cause hypokalemia. **Use with caution** in patients with renal insufficiency (magnesium), gastric outlet obstruction.

Interferes with the absorption of the benzodiazepines, chloroquine, digoxin, phenytoin, quinolones (e.g., ciprofloxacin), tetracyclines, and iron. Do not take oral medications within 1–2 hours of taking antacid dose unless specified by your physician.

AMANTADINE HYDROCHLORIDE

Symmetrel and others
Antiviral agent

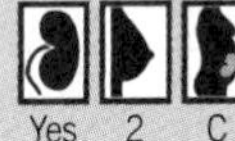

Capsule: 100 mg
Tabs: 100 mg
Syrup: 50 mg/5 mL (480 mL)

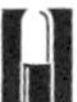

Influenza A prophylaxis and treatment:
1–9 yr: 5 mg/kg/24 hr PO ÷ QD–BID; **max. dose:** 150 mg/24 hr
>9 yr:
<40 kg: 5 mg/kg/24 hr PO ÷ QD–BID; **max. dose:** 200 mg/24 hr
≥40 kg: 200 mg/24 hr ÷ QD–BID

Alternative dosing for influenza A prophylaxis:
Children >20 kg and adults: 100 mg/24 hr PO ÷ QD–BID

Prophylaxis (duration of therapy):
Single exposure: at least 10 days
Repeated/uncontrolled exposure: up to 90 days
Use with influenza A vaccine when possible.

Symptomatic treatment (duration of therapy):
Continue for 24–48 hr after disappearance of symptoms.

Use with caution in patients with liver disease, seizures, renal disease, congestive heart failure, peripheral edema, orthostatic hypotension, or history of recurrent eczematoid rash and in those receiving CNS stimulants. **Dose must be adjusted in patients with renal insufficiency (see Chapter 30).**

May cause dizziness, anxiety, depression, mental status change, rash (livedo reticularis), nausea, orthostatic hypotension, edema, CHF, and urinary retention.

For treatment of influenza A, it is best to initiate therapy immediately after the onset of symptoms (within 2 days).

For explanation of icons, see p. 680.

AMIKACIN SULFATE

Amikin

Antibiotic, aminoglycoside

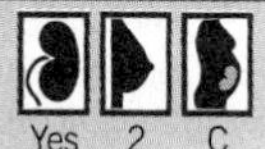

Injection: 50, 250 mg/mL

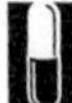

Neonates: See table below.

Postconceptional Age (wk)	Postnatal Age (days)	Dose (mg/kg/dose)	Interval (hr)
≤29*	0–7	18	48
	8–28	15	36
	>28	15	24
30–33	0–7	18	36
	>7	15	24
≥34	0–7	15	24
	>7	15	12–18

*Or significant asphyxia, PDA, indomethacin use, poor cardiac output, reduced renal function.

Infants and children: 15–22.5 mg/kg/24 hr ÷ Q8 hr IV/IM; infants and patients requiring higher doses may receive initial doses of 30 mg/kg/24 hr ÷ Q8 hr IV/IM
Adults: 15 mg/kg/24 hr ÷ Q8–12 hr IV/IM
Initial **max. dose:** 1.5 g/24 hr, then monitor levels

Adjust dose in renal failure (see Chapter 30). Rapidly eliminated in patients with cystic fibrosis or burns, and in febrile neutropenic patients. CNS penetration is poor beyond early infancy.

Therapeutic levels: peak 20–30 mg/L; trough 5–10 mg/L.

Recommended serum sampling time at steady-state: trough within 30 min before the third consecutive dose and peak 30–60 min after the administration of the third consecutive dose.

Peak levels of 25–30 mg/L have been recommended for CNS, pulmonary, bone, life-threatening infections, and in febrile neutropenic patients. Longer dosing intervals may be necessary for neonates receiving indomethacin for PDAs and for all patients with poor cardiac output.

May cause ototoxicity, nephrotoxicity, neuromuscular blockade, and rash. Loop diuretics may potentiate the ototoxicity of all aminoglycoside antibiotics.

AMINOCAPROIC ACID

Amicar and others

Hemostatic agent

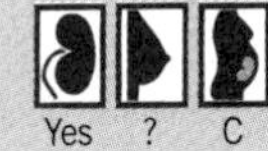

Tabs: 500 mg
Syrup: 250 mg/mL (480 mL) (may contain 0.2% methylparaben and 0.05% propylparaben)
Injection: 250 mg/mL (20 mL) (contains 0.9% benzyl alcohol)

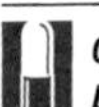

Children:
Loading dose: 100–200 mg/kg IV/PO
Maintenance: 100 mg/kg/dose Q4–6 hr; **max. dose:** 30 g/24 hr

Contraindications: DIC, hematuria. **Use with caution** in patients with cardiac, renal, or hepatic disease. Should not be given with Factor IX Complex concentrates or Anti-Inhibitor Coagulant concentrates because of risk for thrombosis. Dose should be reduced by 75% in oliguria or end-stage renal disease. Hypercoagulation may be produced when given in conjunction with oral contraceptives.

May cause nausea, diarrhea, malaise, weakness, headache, decreased platelet function, hypotension, and false increase in urine amino acids. Elevation of serum potassium may occur, especially in patients with renal impairment.

AMINOPHYLLINE

Aminophyllin, Phylocontin, and others

Bronchodilator, methylxanthine

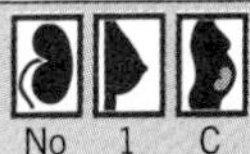

Tabs: 100, 200 mg (79% theophylline)
Liquid (oral): 105 mg/5 mL (240 mL) (86% theophylline)
Injection: 25 mg/mL (79% theophylline)
Sustained-release tablet (Phylocontin): 225 mg (79% theophylline)
NOTE: Pharmacy may dilute IV and oral dosage forms to enhance accuracy of neonatal dosing.

PO:
Infants: (see *Theophylline* and convert to mg of aminophylline)
1–9 yr: 27 mg/kg/24 hr ÷ Q4–6 hr
9–12 yr: 20 mg/kg/24 hr ÷ Q6 hr
12–16 yr: 16 mg/kg/24 hr ÷ Q6 hr
Adults: 12.5 mg/kg/24 hr ÷ Q6 hr

Neonatal apnea:
Loading dose: 5–6 mg/kg IV or PO
Maintenance dose: 1–2 mg/kg/dose Q6–8 hr, IV or PO

IV loading: 6 mg/kg IV over 20 min (each 1.2 mg/kg dose raises the serum theophylline concentration 2 mg/L)

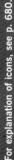

Continued

For explanation of icons, see p. 680.

AMINOPHYLLINE *continued*

IV maintenance: *Continuous IV drip:*

Neonates: 0.2 mg/kg/hr
6 wk–6 mo: 0.5 mg/kg/hr
6 mo–1 yr: 0.6–0.7 mg/kg/hr
1–9 yr: 1–1.2 mg/kg/hr
9–12 yr *and young adult smokers:* 0.9 mg/kg/hr
>12 yr *healthy nonsmokers:* 0.7 mg/kg/hr

The above total daily doses may also be administered IV ÷ Q4–6 hr.

Consider mg of theophylline available when dosing aminophylline.

Monitoring serum levels is essential, especially in infants and young children.

Intermittent dosing for infants and children 1–5 yr may require Q4 hr dosing regimen owing to enhanced metabolism. *Side effects:* restlessness, GI upset, headache, tachycardia, seizures (may occur in absence of other side effects with toxic levels).

Therapeutic level (theophylline): for asthma, 10–20 mg/L; for neonatal apnea, 6–13 mg/L.

Recommended guidelines for obtaining levels:

IV bolus: 30 min after infusion
IV continuous; 12–24 hr after initiation of infusion

PO liquid, immediate-release tab:

Peak: 1 hr after dose
Trough: just before dose

PO sustained-release tab:

Peak: 4 hr after dose
Trough: just before dose

Ideally, obtain levels after steady state has been achieved (after at least 1 day of therapy). See *Theophylline* for drug interactions.

Use in breastfeeding may cause irritability in infant.

AMIODARONE HCL

Cordarone, Pacerone, Amino-Aqueous
Antiarrhythmic, Class III

No 2 D

Tabs: 200, 400 mg
Suspension: 5 mg/mL
Injection: 50 mg/mL (3 mL) (contains 20.2 mg/mL benzyl alcohol and 100 mg/mL polysorbate 80 or Tween 80)
Injection (without benzyl alcohol and polysorbate 80): 15 mg/mL (Amino-Aqueous) (10 mL)
Contains 37% iodine by weight.

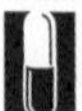

See algorithms in front cover of book for arrest dosing.

Children PO:

<1 yr: 600–800 mg/1.73 m^2/24 hr ÷ Q12–24 hr × 4–14 days and/or until adequate control achieved, then reduce to 200–400 mg/1.73 m^2/24 hr.

Continued

AMIODARONE HCL *continued*

≥1 yr: 10–15 mg/kg/24 hr ÷ Q12–24 hr × 4–14 days and/or until adequate control achieved, then reduce to 5 mg/kg/24 hr ÷ Q12–24 hr if effective.

Children IV (limited data):

5 mg/kg over 30 min followed by a continuous infusion starting at 5 mcg/kg/min; infusion may be increased to a **max. dose** of 10 mcg/kg/min or 20 mg/kg/24 hr.

Adults PO:

Loading dose: 800–1600 mg QD for 1–3 wk

Maintenance: 600–800 mg QD × 1 mo, then 200–400 mg QD

Use lowest effective dose to minimize adverse reactions.

Adults IV:

Loading dose: 150 mg over 10 min (15 mg/min) followed by 360 mg over 6 hr (1 mg/min), followed by a maintenance dose of 0.5 mg/min. Supplemental boluses of 150 mg over 10 min may be given for breakthrough VF or hemodynamically unstable VT, and the maintenance infusion may be increased to suppress the arrhythmia.

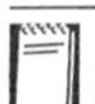

Amiodarone replaces bretylium in the resuscitation algorithm for ventricular fibrillation/pulseless ventricular tachycardia **(see front cover for arrest dosing and back cover for PALS algorithm)**.

Contraindicated in severe sinus node dysfunction, marked sinus bradycardia, second- and third-degree AV block.

Long elimination half-life (40–55 days). Major metabolite is active.

Increases cyclosporine, digoxin, phenytoin, tacrolimus, warfarin, calcium-channel blockers, theophylline, and quinidine levels.

Proposed therapeutic level with chronic oral use: 1–2.5 mg/L.

Asymptomatic corneal microdeposits should appear in all patients. Alters liver enzymes, thyroid function. Pulmonary fibrosis reported in adults. May cause worsening of preexisting arrhythmias with bradycardia and AV block. May also cause hypotension, anorexia, nausea, vomiting, dizziness, paresthesias, ataxia, tremor, SIADH, and hypothyroidism or hyperthyroidism.

Intravenous continuous infusion concentration for peripheral administration **should not exceed** 2 mg/mL and **must be diluted** with D5W. The intravenous dosage form can leach out plasticizers such as DEHP. It is recommended to reduce the potential exposure to plasticizers in pregnant women and children at the toddler stages of development and younger by using alternative methods of IV drug administration. The preservative-free intravenous product is available as an orphan/compassionate use drug from Academic Pharmaceuticals, Inc. at (847) 735-1170.

Oral administration should be consistent with regard to meals because food increases the rate and extent of oral absorption.

For explanation of icons, see p. 680.

AMITRIPTYLINE

Elavil and others

Antidepressant, tricyclic

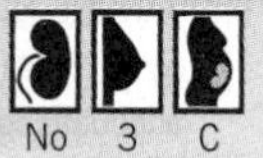

Tabs: 10, 25, 50, 75, 100, 150 mg

Injection: 10 mg/mL (10 mL)

Antidepressant:

Children (PO): Start with 1 mg/kg/24 hr ÷ TID for 3 days; then increase to 1.5 mg/kg/24 hr. Dose may be gradually increased to a **max. dose** of 5 mg/kg/24 hr if needed. Monitor ECG, BP, and heart rate for doses >3 mg/kg/24 hr.

Adolescents (PO): 10 mg TID with 20 mg QHS; dose may be gradually increased up to a **max. dose** of 200 mg/24 hr if needed.

Adults:

PO: 40–100 mg/24 hr ÷ QHS–BID; dose may be gradually increased up to 300 mg/24 hr if needed; gradually decrease dose to lowest effective dose when symptoms are controlled.

IM: 20–30 mg QID (convert to oral therapy as soon as possible)

Augment analgesia for chronic pain:

Initial: 0.1 mg/kg/dose QHS PO; increase as needed and tolerated over 2–3 wk to 0.5–2 mg/kg/dose QHS.

Migraine prophylaxis:

Children: Initial 0.1–0.25 mg/kg/dose QHS PO; increase as needed and tolerated every 2 wk by 0.1–0.25 mg/kg/dose up to a **max. dose** of 2 mg/kg/24 hr or 75 mg/24 hr. For doses >1 mg/kg/24 hr, divide daily dose BID and monitor ECG.

Adults: 25–50 mg/dose QHS PO

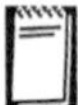

Contraindicated in narrow-angle glaucoma, seizures, severe cardiac disorders, and patients who received MAO inhibitors within 14 days. See Chapter 2 for management of toxic ingestion.

$T_{1/2}$ = 9–25 hr in adults. Maximum antidepressant effects may not occur for 2 wk or more after initiation of therapy. **Do not abruptly discontinue therapy in patients receiving high doses for prolonged periods.**

Therapeutic levels (sum of amitriptyline and nortriptyline): 100–250 ng/mL. Recommended serum sampling time: obtain a single level 8 hr or more after an oral dose (following 4–5 days of continuous dosing).

Side effects include sedation, urinary retention, constipation, dry mouth, dizziness, drowsiness, and arrhythmia. May discolor urine (blue/green). QHS dosing during first weeks of therapy will reduce sedation. Monitor ECG, BP, CBC at start of therapy and with dose changes. Decrease dose if PR interval reaches 0.22 sec, QRS reaches 130% of baseline, HR rises above 140 bpm, or if BP is more than 140/90 mmHg. Tricyclics may cause mania.

AMLODIPINE

Norvasc

Calcium-channel blocker, antihypertensive

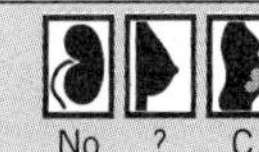

No ? C

Tabs: 2.5, 5, 10 mg
Suspension: 1 mg/mL

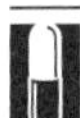

Children:

Hypertension: Start with 0.1 mg/kg/dose PO QD–BID; dosage may be gradually increased to a **max. dose** of 0.6 mg/kg/24 hr up to 20 mg/24 hr.

Adults:

Hypertension: 5–10 mg/dose QD PO; use 2.5 mg/dose QD PO in patients with hepatic insufficiency. **Max. dose:** 10 mg/24 hr

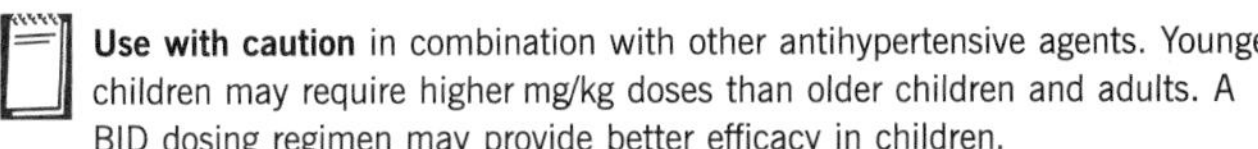

Use with caution in combination with other antihypertensive agents. Younger children may require higher mg/kg doses than older children and adults. A BID dosing regimen may provide better efficacy in children.

Reduce dose in hepatic insufficiency. Allow 5–7 days of continuous initial dose therapy before making dosage adjustments because of the drug's gradual onset of action and lengthy elimination half-life. Amlodipine is a substrate for CYP450 3A4 and should be used with caution with 3A4 inhibitors such as protease inhibitors and azole antifungals (e.g., fluconazole and ketoconazole).

Dose-related side effects include edema, dizziness, flushing, fatigue, and palpitations. Other side effects include headache, nausea, abdominal pain, and somnolence.

AMMONIUM CHLORIDE

Diuretic, urinary acidifying agent

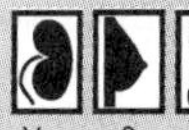

Yes ? B

Tabs: 500 mg
Enteric coated tabs: 486 mg
Injection: 5 mEq/mL (26.75%) (20 mL)
1 mEq = 53 mg

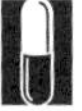

Urinary acidification:

Child: 75 mg/kg/24 hr ÷ Q6 hr PO or IV; **max. dose:** 6 g/24 hr

Adult:

Intravenous: 1.5 g/dose IV Q6 hr; **max. IV dose:** 6 g/24 hr

Oral: 2–3 g/dose PO Q6 hr; **max. PO dose:** 12 g/24 hr

Injection: Dilute to concentration not >0.4 mEq/mL.
Infusion **not to exceed** 50 mg/kg/hr or 1 mEq/kg/hr.

Contraindicated in hepatic or renal insufficiency; **use with caution** in infants. May produce acidosis, hyperammonemia, and GI irritation. Monitor serum chloride level, acid/base status, and ammonia.

Administer oral doses after meals.

For explanation of icons, see p. 680.

AMOXICILLIN

Amoxil, Trimox, Wymox, Polymox, DisperMox, and others
Antibiotic, aminopenicillin

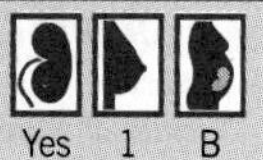

Drops: 50 mg/mL (15, 30 mL)
Suspension: 125, 250 mg/5 mL (80, 100, 150 mL) and 200, 400 mg/5 mL (50, 75, 100 mL)
Caps: 250, 500 mg
Tabs: 500, 875 mg
Chewable tabs: 125, 200, 250, 400 mg
Tabs for oral suspension (DisperMox): 200, 400, 600 mg

Infant ≤3 months: 20–30 mg/kg/24 hr ÷ BID PO
Child:
Standard dose: 25–50 mg/kg/24 hr ÷ BID–TID PO
High dose: 80–90 mg/kg/24 hr ÷ BID PO
Adult: 250–500 mg/dose TID PO
Max. dose: 2–3 g/24 hr
Recurrent otitis media prophylaxis: 20 mg/kg/dose QHS PO
SBE prophylaxis: see Chapter 6.

Renal elimination. **Adjust dose in renal failure (see Chapter 30).** Serum levels about twice those achieved with equal dose of ampicillin. Less GI effects but otherwise similar to ampicillin. Side effects: rash and diarrhea.

High-dose regimen increasingly useful in respiratory infections, acute otitis media and sinusitis, owing to increasing incidence of penicillin-resistant pneumococci. Chewable tablets and DisperMox may contain phenylalanine and **should not** be used by phenyketonurics.

DisperMox oral suspension is prepared by swirling/stirring each tablet thoroughly in about 10 mL of water only. Do not chew or swallow (whole tablets) DisperMox.

AMOXICILLIN-CLAVULANIC ACID

Augmentin, Augmentin ES-600, Augmentin XR
Antibiotic, aminopenicillin with beta-lactamase inhibitor

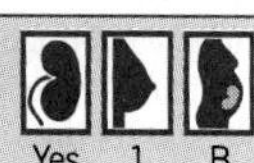

Tabs:
For TID dosing: 250, 500 (with 125 mg clavulanate)
For BID dosing: 875 mg amoxicillin (with 125 mg clavulanate); Augmentin XR: 1 g amoxicillin (with 62.5 mg clavulanate)
Chewable tabs:
For TID dosing: 125, 250 mg amoxicillin (31.25 and 62.5 mg clavulanate, respectively)
For BID dosing: 200, 400 mg amoxicillin (28.5 and 57 mg clavulanate, respectively)

Continued

AMOXICILLIN-CLAVULANIC ACID *continued*

Suspension:

For TID dosing: 125, 250 mg amoxicillin/5mL (31.25 and 62.5 mg clavulanate/5 mL, respectively) (75, 100, 150 mL)

For BID dosing: 200, 400 mg amoxicillin/5 mL (28.5 and 57 mg clavulanate/5 mL, respectively) (50, 75, 100 mL)

Augmentin ES-600: 600 mg amoxicillin/5 mL (42.9 mg clavulanate/5 mL) (50, 75, 100, 150 mL)

Contains 0.63 mEq K^+ per 125 mg clavulanate (Augmentin ES-600 contains 0.23 mEq K^+ per 42.9 mg clavulanate)

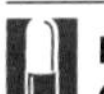

Dosage based on amoxicillin component.

Children <3 mo: 30 mg/kg/24 hr ÷ BID PO (recommended dosage form is 125 mg/5 mL suspension)

Children ≥3 mo:

TID dosing (see remarks):

20–40 mg/kg/24 hr ÷ TID PO

BID dosing (see remarks):

25–45 mg/kg/24 hr ÷ BID PO

Augmentin ES-600:

≥3 mo and <40 kg: 90 mg/kg/24 hr ÷ BID PO × 10 days

Adults: 250–500 mg/dose TID PO or 875 mg/dose BID PO for more severe and respiratory infections

Augmentin XR:

≥16 yr and adults: 2 g BID PO × 10 days for acute bacterial sinusitis or × 7–10 days for community-acquired pneumonia

---

Clavulanic acid extends the activity of amoxicillin to include beta-lactamase–producing strains of *H. influenzae, M. catarrhalis, N. gonorrhoeae,* and some *S. aureus* and may increase the risk for diarrhea. See *Amoxicillin* for additional comments. **Adjust dose in renal failure (see Chapter 30).** Augmentin XR is contraindicated in patients with CrCl <30 mL/min.

The BID dosing schedule is associated with less diarrhea. For BID dosing, the 875-mg tablet, the 200-mg and 400-mg chewable tablets, or the 200-mg/5mL, 400-mg/5mL, or 600-mg/5mL suspension should be used. These BID dosage forms contain phenylalanine and **should not be used** by phenyketonurics. For TID dosing, the 250-mg or 500-mg tablets, the 125-mg or 250-mg chewable tablets, or the 125-mg/5mL or 250-mg/5mL suspension should be used.

Higher doses of 80–90 mg/kg/24 hr (amoxicillin component) have been recommended for resistant strains of *S. pneumoniae* in acute otitis media (use BID formulations containing 7:1 ratio of amoxicillin to clavulanic acid or Augmentin ES-600).

The 250- or 500-mg tablets **cannot be** substituted for Augmentin XR.

For explanation of icons, see p. 680.

AMPHOTERICIN B

Fungizone, Amphocin
Antifungal

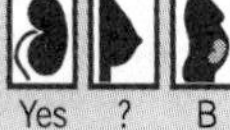

Injection: 50 mg vials
Cream: 3% (20 g)
Lotion: 3% (30 mL)

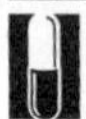

Topical: Apply BID–QID
IV: mix with D5W to concentration 0.1 mg/mL (peripheral administration) or 0.25 mg/mL (central line only). pH >4.2. Infuse over 2–6 hr.
Optional test dose: 0.1 mg/kg/dose IV up to **max. dose** of 1 mg (followed by remaining initial dose).
Initial dose: 0.5–1 mg/kg/24 hr; if test dose **NOT** used, infuse first dose over 6 hr and monitor frequently during the first several hours.
Increment: Increase as tolerated by 0.25–0.5 mg/kg/24 hr QD or QOD.
Usual maintenance:
  QD dosing: 0.5–1 mg/kg/24 hr QD
  QOD dosing: 1.5 mg/kg/dose QOD
Max. dose: 1.5 mg/kg/24 hr
Intrathecal: 25–100 mcg Q48–72 hr. Increase to 500 mcg as tolerated.

Monitor renal, hepatic, electrolyte, and hematologic status closely. Hypercalciuria, hypokalemia, hypomagnesemia, RTA, renal failure, acute hepatic failure, hypotension, and phlebitis may occur. **For dosing information in renal failure, see Chapter 30.**

Common infusion-related reactions include fever, chills, headache, hypotension, nausea, vomiting; may premedicate with acetaminophen and diphenhydramine 30 min before and 4 hr after infusion. Meperidine useful for chills. Hydrocortisone, 1 mg/kg ampho (**max. dose:** 25 mg) added to bottle may help prevent immediate adverse reactions.

Salt loading with 10–15 mL/kg of NS infused before each dose may minimize the risk for nephrotoxicity.

AMPHOTERICIN B CHOLESTERYL SULFATE

Amphotec
Antifungal

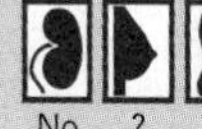
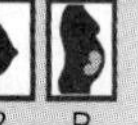

Injection: 50, 100 mg (vials)
(formulated as a 1:1 molar ratio of amphotericin B complexed to cholesteryl sulfate)

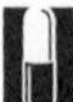

IV: Start at 3–4 mg/kg/24 hr QD; dose may be increased to 6 mg/kg/24 hr if necessary.
  Mix with D5W to concentration 0.16–0.83 mg/mL.

Continued

AMPHOTERICIN B CHOLESTERYL SULFATE *continued*

Test dose: 10 mL of the diluted solution administered over 15–30 min has been recommended.

Infusion rate: Give first dose at 1 mg/kg/hr; if well tolerated, infusion time can be gradually shortened to a minimum of 2 hr.

Monitor renal, hepatic, electrolyte, and hematologic status closely. Thrombocytopenia, tachycardia, hypokalemia, hypomagnesemia, hypocalcemia, hyperglycemia, diarrhea, dyspnea, back pain, and increases in aminotransferases and bilirubin may occur.

Common infusion-related reactions, including fever, chills, rigors, nausea, vomiting, hypotension, and headache, are more frequent with the initial doses; may premedicate with acetaminophen, diphenhydramine, and meperidine (see *Amphotericin B* remarks).

Doses as high as 7.5 mg/kg/24 hr have been used to treat invasive fungal infections in BMT patients.

AMPHOTERICIN B LIPID COMPLEX

Abelcet

Antifungal

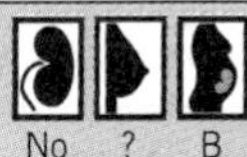

Injection: 5 mg/mL (10, 20 mL)
(formulated as a 1:1 molar ratio of amphotericin B to lipid complex comprising dimyristoylphosphatidylcholine and dimyristoylphosphatidylglycerol)

IV: 2.5–5 mg/kg/24 hr QD

Mix with D5W to concentration 1 mg/mL or 2 mg/mL for fluid-restricted patients.

Infusion rate: 2.5 mg/kg/hr; shake the infusion bag every 2 hr if total infusion time exceeds 2 hr.

Monitor renal, hepatic, electrolyte, and hematologic status closely. Thrombocytopenia, anemia, leukopenia, hypokalemia, hypomagnesemia, diarrhea, respiratory failure, skin rash, and increases in liver enzymes and bilirubin may occur.

Common infusion-related reactions include fever, chills, rigors, nausea, vomiting, hypotension, and headache; may premedicate with acetaminophen, diphenhydramine, and meperidine (see *Amphotericin B* remarks).

For explanation of icons, see p. 680.

AMPHOTERICIN B, LIPOSOMAL
AmBisome
Antifungal

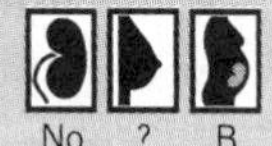
No ? B

Injection: 50 mg (vials)
(formulated in liposomes composed of hydrogenated soy phosphatidylcholine, cholesterol, distearoylphosphatidylglycerol, and alpha-tocopherol)

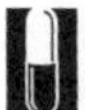

IV: 3–5 mg/kg/24 hr QD
Mix with D5W to concentration 1–2 mg/mL (0.2–0.5 mg/mL may be used for infants and small children).
Infusion rate: Administer dose over 2 hr; infusion may be reduced to 1 hr if well tolerated.

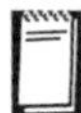

Monitor renal, hepatic, electrolyte, and hematologic status closely. Thrombocytopenia, tachycardia, hypokalemia, hypomagnesemia, hypocalcemia, hyperglycemia, diarrhea, dyspnea, skin rash, low back pain, and increases in liver enzymes and bilirubin may occur.

Common infusion-related reactions include fever, chills, rigors, nausea, vomiting, hypotension, and headache; may premedicate with acetaminophen, diphenhydramine, and meperidine (see *Amphotericin B* remarks).

Doses as high as 6 mg/kg/24 hr have been used in patients with aspergillus. A dose of 6 mg/kg/24 hr is recommended for cryptococcal meningitis in adults with HIV.

AMPICILLIN
Omnipen, Principen, Totacillin, and others
Antibiotic, aminopenicillin

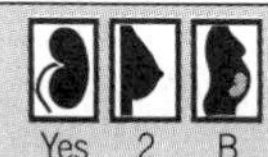
Yes 2 B

Suspension: 125 mg/5 mL (100, 150, 200 mL), 250 mg/5 mL (100, 200 mL)
Caps: 250, 500 mg
Injection: 125, 250, 500 mg; 1, 2, 10 g
Contains 3 mEq Na/1 g IV drug

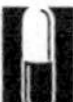

Neonate IM/IV:
<7 days:
- ***<2 kg:*** 50–100 mg/kg/24 hr IM/IV ÷ Q12 hr
- ***≥2 kg:*** 75–150 mg/kg/24 hr IM/IV ÷ Q8 hr

≥7 days:
- ***<1.2 kg:*** 50–100 mg/kg/24 hr ÷ Q12 hr IM/IV
- ***1.2–2 kg:*** 75–150 mg/kg/24 hr ÷ Q8 hr IM/IV
- ***>2 kg:*** 100–200 mg/kg/24 hr ÷ Q6 hr IM/IV

Continued

AMPICILLIN *continued*

Infant/child:

Mild-moderate infections:

IM/IV: 100–200 mg/kg/24 hr ÷ Q6 hr

PO: 50–100 mg/kg/24 hr ÷ Q6 hr; **max. PO dose:** 2–3 g/24 hr

Severe infections: 200–400 mg/kg/24 hr ÷ Q4–6 hr IM/IV

Adult:

IM/IV: 500–3000 mg Q4–6 hr

PO: 250–500 mg Q6 hr

Max IV/IM dose: 12 g/24 hr

SBE prophylaxis: see Chapter 6

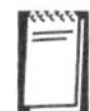

Use higher doses to treat CNS disease. CSF penetration occurs only with inflammed meninges. **Adjust dose in renal failure (see Chapter 30).**

Produces the same side effects as penicillin, with cross-reactivity. Rash commonly seen at 5–10 days, and rash may occur with concurrent EBV infection or allopurinol use. May cause interstitial nephritis, diarrhea, and pseudomembranous enterocolitis. Chloroquine reduces ampicillin's absorption.

AMPICILLIN/SULBACTAM

Unasyn

Antibiotic, aminopenicillin with beta-lactamase inhibitor

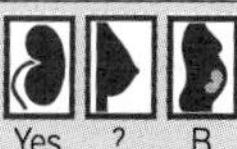

Injection:

1.5 g = ampicillin 1 g + sulbactam 0.5 g

3 g = ampicillin 2 g + sulbactam 1 g

Contains 5 mEq Na per 1.5 g drug combination

Dosage based on ampicillin component:

Infant ≥1 month:

Mild/moderate infections: 100–150 mg/kg/24 hr ÷ Q6 hr IM/IV

Meningitis/severe infections: 200–300 mg/kg/24 hr ÷ Q6 hr IM/IV

Child:

Mild/moderate infections: 100–200 mg/kg/24 hr ÷ Q6 hr IM/IV

Meningitis/severe infections: 200–400 mg/kg/24 hr ÷ Q4–6 hr IM/IV

Adult: 1–2 g Q6–8 hr IM/IV

Max. dose: 8 g ampicillin/24 hr

Similar spectrum of antibacterial activitiy to ampicillin with the added coverage of beta-lactamase–producing organisms. Total sulbactam dose should not exceed 4 g/24 hr.

Adjust dose in renal failure (see Chapter 30). Similar CSF distribution and side effects to ampicillin.

For explanation of icons, see p. 680.

ANTIPYRINE AND BENZOCAINE
Allergen Ear Drops and others
Otic analgesic, cerumenolytic

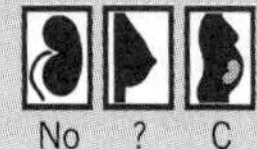
No ? C

Otic solution: antipyrine, 5.4%; benzocaine, 1.4% (15 mL)

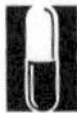
Otic analgesia: fill external ear canal (2–4 drops) Q1–2 hr PRN. After instillation of the solution, a cotton pledget should be moistened with the solution and inserted into the meatus.
Cerumenolytic: fill external ear canal (2–4 drops) TID–QID for 2–3 days

Benzocaine sensitivity may develop. **Contraindicated** if tympanic membrane perforated or PE tubes in place.

ASCORBIC ACID
Vitamin C, Cecon, Sunkist Vitamin C, and others
Water-soluble vitamin

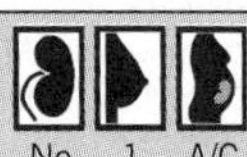
No 1 A/C

Tabs [OTC]: 100, 200, 250, 500 mg, 1, 1.5 g
Chewable tabs (Sunkist Vitamin C) [OTC]: 60, 100, 250, 500, 1000 mg (some may contain aspartame)
Tabs (timed release) [OTC]: 0.5, 1, 1.5 g
Caps [OTC]: 500 mg
Extended-release caps [OTC]: 250, 500 mg
Injection: 250, 500 mg/mL
Solution (Cecon) [OTC]: 100 mg/mL (50 mL)
Liquid [OTC]: 500 mg/5 mL (120, 480 mL)
Lozenges [OTC]: 60 mg
Some products may contain about 5 mEq Na/1 g drug and/or calcium.

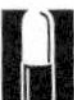
Scurvy (PO/IM/IV/SC):
Children: 100–300 mg/24 hr ÷ QD–BID for at least 2 wk
Adults: 100–250 mg QD–BID for at least 2 wk
U.S. Recommended Daily Allowance (RDA):
See Chapter 20

Adverse reactions: nausea, vomiting, heartburn, flushing, headache, faintness, dizziness, hyperoxaluria. Use high doses with **caution** in G6PD patients. May cause false-negative and false-positive urine glucose determinations with glucose oxidase and cupric sulfate tests, respectively.

Oral dosing is preferred with or without food. IM route is the preferred parenteral route. Protect the injectable dosage form from light.

Pregancy category changes to C if used in doses above the RDA.

ASPIRIN

ASA, Anacin, Bufferin, and various trade names
Nonsteroidal anti-inflammatory agent, antiplatelet agent, analgesic

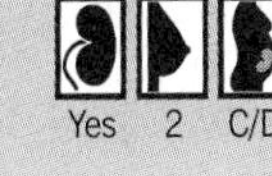

Tabs: 325, 500 mg
Tabs, enteric coated: 81, 165, 325, 500, 650, 975 mg
Tabs, timed release: 81, 325, 650, 800 mg
Tabs, buffered: 325, 500 mg
Tabs, caffeinated: 400 mg ASA + 32 mg caffeine, 500 mg ASA + 32 mg caffeine
Tabs, chewable: 81 mg
Suppository: 60, 80, 120, 125, 200, 300, 325, 600, 650 mg, and 1.2 g

Analgesic/antipyretic: 10–15 mg/kg/dose PO/PR Q4–6 hr up to total 60–80 mg/kg/24 hr
Max. dose: 4 g/24 hr

Anti-inflammatory: 60–100 mg/kg/24 hr PO ÷ Q6–8 hr

Kawasaki disease: 80–100 mg/kg/24 hr PO ÷ QID during febrile phase until defervescence, then decrease to 3–5 mg/kg/24 hr PO QAM. Continue for at least 8 wk or until both platelet count and ESR normal.

Do not use in children <16 yr for treatment of varicella or flu-like symptoms (risk for Reye syndrome), in combination with other nonsteroidal anti-inflammatory drugs, or in severe renal failure. **Use with caution** in bleeding disorders, renal dysfunction, gastritis, and gout. May cause GI upset, allergic reactions, liver toxicity, and decreased platelet aggregation. See Chapter 2 for management of overdose.

Drug interactions: may increase effects of methotrexate, valproic acid, and warfarin, which may lead to toxicity (protein displacement). Buffered dosage forms may decrease absorption of ketoconazole and tetracycline. GI bleeds have been reported with concurrent use of SSRIs (e.g., fluoxetine, paroxetine, sertraline).

Therapeutic levels: antipyretic/analgesic: 30–50 mg/L, anti-inflammatory: 150–300 mg/L. Tinnitus may occur at levels of 200–400 mg/L. Recommended serum sampling time at steady state: obtain trough level just before dose following 1–2 days of continuous dosing. Peak levels obtained 2 hr (for non–sustained-release dosage forms) after a dose may be useful for monitoring toxicity.

Pregnancy category changes to D if full-dose aspirin is used during the third trimester. **Adjust dose in renal failure (see Chapter 30).**

For explanation of icons, see p. 680.

ATENOLOL

Tenormin

Beta-1 selective adrenergic blocker

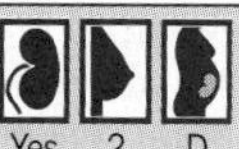

Injection: 0.5 mg/mL (10 mL)
Tab: 25, 50, 100 mg
Suspension: 2 mg/mL 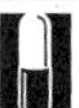

Children: 1–1.2 mg/kg/dose PO QD; **max. dose:** 2 mg/kg/24 hr
Adults:

PO: 25–100 mg/dose PO QD; **max. dose:** 200 mg/24 hr
After myocardial infarction: 5 mg IV × 1 over 5 min and then repeat in 10 min if initial dose tolerated. Then start 50 mg/dose PO Q 12 hr × 2 doses 10 min after last IV dose followed by 100 mg/24 hr PO ÷ QD–BID × 6–9 days. Discontinue atenolol if bradycardia or hypotension requiring treatment or any other untoward effects occur.

Contraindicated in pulmonary edema, cardiogenic shock. May cause bradycardia, hypotension, second- or third-degree AV block, dizziness, fatigue, lethargy, headache. **Use with caution** in diabetes and asthma. Wheezing and dyspnea have occurred when daily dosage exceeds 100 mg/24 hr. Postmarketing evaluation reports a temporal relationship for causing elevated LFTs and/or bilirubin, hallucinations, psoriatic rash, thrombocytopenia, visual disturbances, and dry mouth. **Avoid** abrupt withdrawal of the drug. Does not cross the blood–brain barrier; lower incidence of CNS side effects compared with propranolol. Neonates born to mothers receiving atenolol during labor or while breast-feeding may be at risk for hypoglycemia.

Adjust dose in renal impairment (see Chapter 30). IV administration rate **not to exceed** 1 mg/min.

ATOMOXETINE

Strattera

Norepinephrine reuptake inhibitor, attention deficit hyperactivity disorder agent

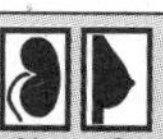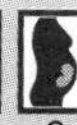

Capsules: 10, 18, 25, 40, 60 mg

≤70 kg (children ≥6 yr and adolescents):
Start with 0.5 mg/kg/24 hr PO QAM and increase after a minimum of 3 days to about 1.2 mg/kg/24 hr PO ÷ QAM or BID (morning and late afternoon/early evening). **Max. daily dose:** 1.4 mg/kg/24 hr or 100 mg, whichever is less

If used with a strong CYP450 2D6 inhibitor (e.g., fluoxetine, paroxetine, quinidine): Maintain above initial dose for 4 wk, and increase to a **maximum** of 1.2 mg/kg/24 hr if symptoms do not improve and initial dose is tolerated.

Continued

ATOMOXETINE *continued*

>70 kg (children and adolescents):

Start with 40 mg PO QAM and increase after a minimum of 3 days to about 80 mg/24 hr PO ÷ QAM or BID (morning and late afternoon/early evening). After 2–4 wk, dose may be increased to a **maximum** of 100 mg/24 hr.

Use with a strong CYP450 2D6 inhibitor (e.g., fluoxetine, paroxetine, quinidine): Maintain above initial dose for 4 wk, and increase to 80 mg/24 hr if symptoms do not improve and initial dose is tolerated.

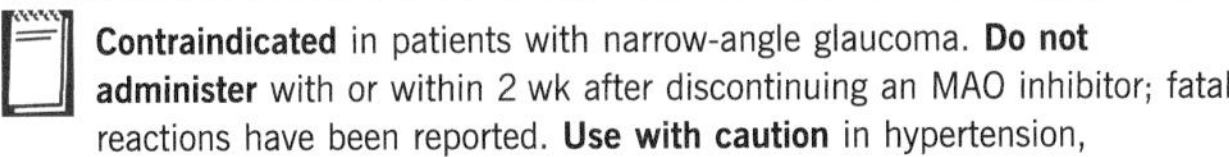

Contraindicated in patients with narrow-angle glaucoma. **Do not administer** with or within 2 wk after discontinuing an MAO inhibitor; fatal reactions have been reported. **Use with caution** in hypertension, tachycardia, cardiovascular or cerebrovascular diseases, or with concurrent albuterol therapy.

Doses >1.2 mg/kg/24 hr in patients ≤70 kg have not been shown to be of additional benefit. Reduce initial and target doses by 50% and 25% for patients with moderate and severe hepatic insufficiency, respectively.

Major side effects include GI discomfort, vomiting, fatigue, anorexia, dizziness, and mood swings. Hypersensitivity reactions, aggression, and irritability have also been reported. Consider interrupting therapy in patients who are not growing or gaining weight satisfactorily.

Doses may be administered with or without food. Atomoxetine can be discontinued without tapering.

ATROPINE SULFATE

Sal-Tropine, AtroPen, and others

Anticholinergic agent

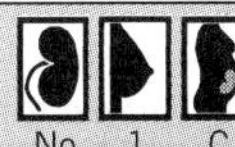

No 1 C

Tabs (Sal-Tropine): 0.4 mg
Injection: 0.05, 0.1, 0.3, 0.4, 0.5, 0.8, 1 mg/mL
Injection (auto-injector as AtroPen): 0.5, 1, 2 mg
Ointment (ophthalmic): 1% (1, 3.5 g)
Solution (ophthalmic): 0.5%, 1%, 2% (1, 2, 5, 15 mL)

Preanesthesia dose (30–60 min preoperation):

Child: 0.01 mg/kg/dose SC/IV/IM; **max. dose:** 0.4 mg/dose; **min. dose:** 0.1 mg/dose; may repeat Q4–6 hr

Adult: 0.5 mg/dose SC/IV/IM

Cardiopulmonary resuscitation:

Child: 0.02 mg/kg/dose IV Q5 min × 2–3 doses PRN; **min. dose:** 0.1 mg; **max. single dose:** 0.5 mg in children, 1 mg in adolescents; **max. total dose:** 1 mg children, 2 mg adolescents

Adult: 0.5–1 mg/dose IV Q5 min; **max. total dose:** 2 mg

Bronchospasm: 0.025–0.05 mg/kg/dose in 2.5 mL NS; **max. dose:** 2.5 mg/dose Q6–8 hr via nebulizer

Continued

For explanation of icons, see p. 680.

ATROPINE SULFATE *continued*

Ophthalmic:

Child: (0.5% solution) 1–2 drops in each eye QD-TID

Adult: (1% solution) 1–2 drops in each eye QD-QID

Organophosphate or carbamate poisoning: see Chapter 2.

Contraindicated in glaucoma, obstructive uropathy, tachycardia, and thyrotoxicosis. **Use with caution** in patients sensitive to sulfites.

Doses <0.1 mg have been associated with paradoxical bradycardia. Side effects include dry mouth, blurred vision, fever, tachycardia, constipation, urinary retention, and CNS signs (dizziness, hallucinations, restlessness, fatigue, headache).

In case of bradycardia, may give via endotracheal tube (dilute with NS to volume of 1–2 mL). Use injectable solution for nebulized use; can be mixed with albuterol for simultaneous administration.

AZATHIOPRINE

Imuran, Azasan, and others

Immunosuppressant

Yes ? D

Suspension: 50 mg/mL

Tabs:

Imuran: 50 mg

Azasan: 25, 50, 75, 100 mg

Injection: 100 mg (20 mL)

Immunosuppression:

Initial: 3–5 mg/kg/24 hr IV/PO QD

Maintenance: 1–3 mg/kg/24 hr IV/PO QD

Toxicity: bone marrow suppression, rash, stomatitis, hepatotoxicity, alopecia, arthralgias, and GI disturbances. Use $\frac{1}{4}$–$\frac{1}{3}$ dose when given with allopurinol.

Severe anemia has been reported when used in combination with captopril or enalapril. Monitor CBC, platelets, total bilirubin, alkaline phosphatase, BUN, and creatinine. **Adjust dose in renal failure (see Chapter 30).**

Administer oral doses with food to minimize GI discomfort.

AZELASTINE

Astelin, Opitvar

Antihistamine

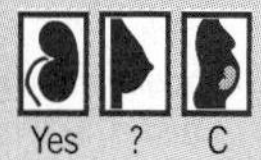

Yes ? C

Nasal spray (Astelin): 1% (137 mcg/spray), 100 actuations (17 mL)

Ophthalmic drops (Opitvar): 0.05% (0.5 mg/mL) (6 mL)

Continued

AZELASTINE *continued*

Seasonal allergic rhinitis:
Children 5–11 yr: 1 spray each nostril BID
≥12 yr and adults: 2 sprays each nostril BID
Ophthalmic:
≥3 yr and adults: instill 1 drop into each affected eye BID

Use with caution in asthmatics. Reduced dosages have been recommended in patients with renal and hepatic dysfunction. Optivar **should not be used** to treat contact lens–related irritation. Soft contact lens users should wait at least 10 min after dose instillation before they insert their lenses.

Drowsiness may occur despite the nasal route of administration (**avoid** concurrent use of alcohol or CNS depressants). Bitter taste, nasal burning, epistaxis may also occur with nasal route. Eye burning and stinging have been reported in about 30% of patients receiving the ophthalmic dosage form.

AZITHROMYCIN

Zithromax, Zithromax TRI-PAK, Zithromax Z-PAK
Antibiotic, macrolide

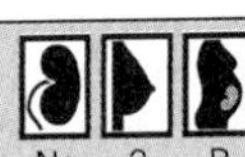
No 2 B

Tabs: 250, 500, 600 mg
TRI-PAK: 500 mg (3s as unit dose pack)
Z-PAK: 250 mg (6s as unit dose pack)
Suspension: 100 mg/5 mL (15 mL), 200 mg/5 mL (15, 22.5, 30 mL)
Oral powder (Sachet): 1 g (3s, 10s)
Injection: 500 mg (10 mL)

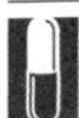

Children:
Otitis media (≥6 mo):
5-day regimen: 10 mg/kg PO day 1 (**not to exceed** 500 mg), followed by 5 mg/kg/24 hr PO QD (**not to exceed** 250 mg/24 hr) on days 2–5
3-day regimen: 10 mg/kg/24 hr PO QD × 3 days (**not to exceed** 500 mg/24 hr)
1-day regimen: 30 mg/kg/24 hr PO ×1 (**not to exceed** 1500 mg/24 hr)
Community acquired pneumonia (≥6 mo): use otitis media 5-day regimen from above.
Pharyngitis/tonsillitis (≥2 yr): 12 mg/kg/24 hr PO QD × 5 days (**not to exceed** 500 mg/24 hr)
M. avium complex prophylaxis:
Daily regimen: 5 mg/kg/24 hr PO QD (**not to exceed** 250 mg/dose)
Weekly regimen: 20 mg/kg/dose PO Q 7 days (**not to exceed** 1200 mg/dose)

Adolescents and adults:
Respiratory tract, skin, and soft tissue infection: 500 mg PO day 1, then 250 mg/24 hr PO on days 2–5
Mild/moderate bacterial COPD exacerbation: above 5-day dosing regimen *OR* 500 mg PO QD × 3 days

Continued

For explanation of icons, see p. 680.

AZITHROMYCIN *continued*

Uncomplicated chlamydial urethritis or cervicitis: single 1 g dose PO
M. avium complex prophylaxis: 1200 mg PO Q 7 days
M. avium complex treatment: 600 mg PO QD with ethambutol 800–1200 mg PO QD ± rifabutin 300 mg PO QD
Acute PID (chlamydia): 500 mg IV QD × 1–2 days followed by 250 mg PO QD to complete a 7–10 day regimen.

Contraindicated in hypersensitivity to macrolides. Can cause increase in hepatic enzymes, cholestatic jaundice, GI discomfort, and pain at injection site (IV use). Compared with other macrolides, less risk for drug interactions. Vomiting, diarrhea, and nausea have been reported at higher frequency in otitis media with 1-day dosing regimen. CNS penetration is poor.

Ethambutol, 15 mg/kg/24 hr (**max. dose:** 900 mg/24 hr) PO QD ± rifabutin 5 mg/kg/24 hr (**max. dose:** 300 mg/24 hr) PO QD is recommended with azithromycin for prevention of recurrence (secondary prophylaxis) of disseminated MAC in children. See www.aidsinfo.nih.gov/guidelines for most current recommendations.

Aluminum- and magnesium-containing antacids decrease absorption. Oral dosage forms (except capsules) may be administered with food. Intravenous administration is over 1–3 hours; do not give as a bolus or IM injection.

AZTREONAM

Azactam
Antibiotic, monobactam

Yes 1 B

Injection: 0.5, 1, 2 g
Each 1 g drug contains about 780 mg L-arginine

Neonates:
30 mg/kg/dose:
- ***<1.2 kg and 0–4 wk age:*** Q12 hr IV/IM
- ***1.2–2 kg and 0–7 days:*** Q12 hr IV/IM
- ***1.2–2 kg and >7 days:*** Q8 hr IV/IM
- ***>2 kg and 0–7 days:*** Q8 hr IV/IM
- ***>2 kg and >7 days:*** Q6 hr IV/IM

Children: 90–120 mg/kg/24 hr ÷ Q6–8 hr IV/IM
Cystic fibrosis: 150–200 mg/kg/24 hr ÷ Q6–8 hr IV/IM
Adults:
Moderate infections: 1–2 g/dose Q8–12 hr IV/IM
Severe infections: 2 g/dose Q6–8 hr IV/IM
Max. dose: 8 g/24 hr

Continued

AZTREONAM *continued*

Typically indicated in multidrug-resistant aerobic gram-negative infections when beta-lactam therapy is contraindicated. Well-absorbed IM. Low cross-allergenicity between aztreonam and other beta-lactams. Adverse reactions: thrombophlebitis, eosinophilia, leukopenia, neutropenia, thrombocytopenia, elevation of liver enzymes, hypotension, seizures, and confusion. Good CNS penetration. **Adjust dose in renal failure (see Chapter 30).**

BACITRACIN ± POLYMYXIN B

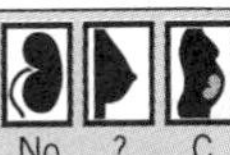

AK-Tracin Ophthalmic, Baciguent Topical, and others; in combination with polymyxin B: AK-Poly-Bac Ophthalmic, Polysporin Ophthalmic, Polysporin Topical, and others

Antibiotic, topical

Ophthalmic ointment: 500 units/g (3.5, 3.75 g)
Topical ointment: 500 units/g (0.9, 15, 30, 120, 454 g)
In combination with polymyxin B:
Ophthalmic ointment: 500 units bacitracin + 10,000 units polymyxin B/g (3.5 g)
Topical ointment: 500 units bacitracin + 10,000 units polymyxin B/g (0.9, 15, 30 g)
Topical powder: 500 units bacitracin + 10,000 units polymyxin B/g (10 g)

BACITRACIN

Children and adults:

Topical: Apply to affected area 1–5 times/24 hr.

Ophthalmic: Apply 0.25–0.5 inch ribbon into the conjunctival sac of the infected eye(s) Q3–12 hr; frequency depends on severity of infection.

BACITRACIN + POLYMYXIN B

Childen and adults:

Topical: Apply ointment or powder to affected area QD–TID.

Ophthalmic: Apply 0.25–0.5 inch ribbon into the conjunctival sac of the infected eye(s) Q3–12 hr; frequency depends on severity of infection.

Hypersensitivity reactions to bacitracin and/or polymyxin B can occur. **Do not use** topical ointment for the eyes. Side effects may include rash, itching, burning, and edema. Ophthalmic dosage form may cause temporary blurred vision and retard corneal healing. For neomycin containing products, see *Neomycin/Polymyxin B/± Bacitracin*.

For explanation of icons, see p. 680.

BACLOFEN

Lioresal, Kemstro, and others

Centrally acting skeletal muscle relaxant

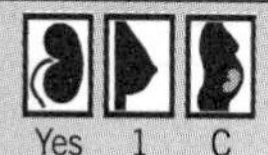

Tabs: 10, 20 mg
Disintegrating tabs (Kemstro): 10, 20 mg
Suspension: 5, 10 mg/mL
Intrathecal Injection: 50 mcg/mL (1 mL), 0.5 mg/mL (20 mL), 2 mg/mL (5 mL)

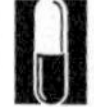

Dosage increments are made at 3-day intervals until desired effect or max. dose is achieved.

Children PO:

≥2 yr: 10–15 mg/24 hr ÷ Q8 hr
Max. dose: <8 yr: 40 mg/24 hr
Max. dose: ≥ 8 yr: 60 mg/24 hr

Adults PO:

5 mg TID; **max. dose:** 80 mg/24 hr

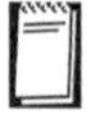

Avoid abrupt withdrawal of drug. **Use with caution** in patients with seizure disorder, impaired renal function. About 70% to 80% of the drug is excreted in the urine unchanged. Administer oral doses with food or milk.

Adverse effects: drowsiness, fatigue, nausea, vertigo, psychiatric disturbances, rash, urinary frequency, and hypotonia. Intrathecal dosing in children is not well established. **Avoid** abrupt withdrawal of intrathecal therapy to prevent potential life-threatening events.

BECLOMETHASONE DIPROPIONATE

QVAR, Beconase, Beconase AQ, Vancenase, Vancenase Pockethaler, Vancenase AQ 84 mcg

Corticosteroid

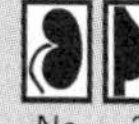
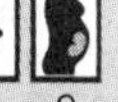

Inhalation, oral:

QVAR: 40 mcg/inhalation (100 inhalations, 7.3 g), 80 mcg/inhalation (100 inhalations, 7.3 g)

Inhalation, nasal:

Beconase or Vancenase: 42 mcg/inhalation (80 inhalations, 6.7 g; 200 inhalations, 16.8 g)
Vancenase Pockethaler: 42 mcg/inhalation (200 metered doses, 7 g)

Spray, aqueous nasal:

Beconase AQ: 42 mcg/inhalation (200 metered doses, 25 g)
Vancenase AQ 84 mcg: 84 mcg/inhalation (120 metered doses, 19 g)

Continued

BECLOMETHASONE DIPROPIONATE *continued*

Oral inhalation (QVAR):
5–11 yr: 40 mcg BID; **max. dose:** 80 mcg BID
≥12 yr and adults:
Corticosteroid naïve: 40–80 mcg BID; **max. dose:** 320 mcg BID
Previous corticosteroid use: 40–160 mcg BID; **max. dose:** 320 mcg BID
Nasal inhalation:
6–12 yr: 1 spray each nostril TID
>12 yr and adults: 1 spray each nostril BID-QID or 2 sprays each nostril BID
Aqueous nasal spray:
>6 yr and adults: 1–2 sprays each nostril BID

Not recommended for children <5 yr with oral inhalation and <6 yr with the nasal administration owing to unknown safety and efficacy. Dose should be titrated to lowest effective dose. **Avoid** using higher than recommended doses.

Monitor for hypothalamic, pituitary, adrenal, or growth suppression and hypercortism. Rinse mouth and gargle with water after oral inhalation; may cause thrush. Consider using with tube spacers for oral inhalation.

BENZOYL PEROXIDE

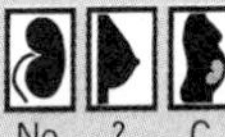

Benzac AC Wash $2^1/_2$, 5, 10; Benzac 5,10; Brevoxyl Creamy Wash, Desquam-E 5, Desquam-E 10, Oxy-5, Oxy-10, Triaz, and various other names
Topical acne product

Liquid wash: 2.5% (240 mL), 5% (120, 150, 240 mL), 10%* (120, 150, 240 mL)
Liquid cream wash: 4% (170 g), 8% (170 g)
Bar: 5%* (113 g), 10%* (106, 113 g)
Lotion: 4% (297 units), 5% (30 units), 8% (297 units), 10% (30 units)
Mask:
Cleanser: 3.5%* (125 mL)
Treatment: 5%* (60 g)
Cream: 5%* (18 g), 10%* (18, 28 g)
Gel: 2.5% (45, 60, 90, 113 g), 3% (42.5 g), 4% (42.5, 90 g), 5% (42.5, 60, 85, 90, 113.4 g), 6% (42.5%), 7% (45, 90 g), 8% (42.5, 90 g), 9% (42.5 g), 10% (42.5, 60, 85, 90, 113.4 g)
NOTE: Some preparations may contain alcohol.
Combination product with erythromycin (Benzamycin and others):
Gel: 30 mg erythromycin and 50 mg benzoyl peroxide per g (23.3 g) (some preparations may contain 20% alcohol)
Combination product with clindamycin (BenzaClin, Duac):
Gel: 10 mg clindamycin and 50 mg benzoyl peroxide per g (25, 45 g)

* Available over the counter without a prescription.

Continued

For explanation of icons, see p. 680.

BENZOYL PEROXIDE *continued*

Children and adults:
Cleanser, liquid wash, or bar: Wet affected area before application. Apply and wash QD–BID; rinse thoroughly and pat dry. Modify dose frequency or concentration to control the amount of drying or peeling.
Lotion, cream, or gel: Cleanse skin and apply small amounts over affected areas QD initially; increase frequency to BID–TID if needed. Modify dose frequency or concentration to control drying or peeling.
Combination products:
Benzamycin and BenzaClin: apply BID (morning and evening) to affected areas after washing and drying skin.
Duac: apply QHS to affected areas after washing and drying skin.

Contraindicated in known history of hypersensitivity to product's components (benzoyl peroxide, clindamycin, or erythromycin). **Avoid** contact with mucous membranes and eyes. May cause skin irritation, stinging, dryness, peeling, erythema, edema, and contact dermatitis. Concurrent use with tretinoin (Retin-A) will increase risk for skin irritation. Products containing clindamycin and erythromycin should not be used in combination. Any single application resulting in excessive stinging or burning may be removed with mild soap and water. Lotion, cream, and gel dosage forms should be applied to dry skin.

BENZTROPINE

Cogentin
Anticholinergic agent, drug induced dystonic reaction antidote, anti-Parkinson's agent

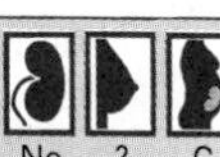

Injection: 1 mg/mL (2 mL)
Tabs: 0.5, 1, 2 mg

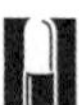

Drug-induced extrapyramidal symptoms:
>3 yr: 0.02–0.05 mg/kg/dose QD–BID PO/IM/IV
Adults: 1–4 mg/dose QD–BID PO/IM/IV

Contraindicated in myasthenia gravis, GI/GU obstruction, untreated narrow-angle glaucoma, and peptic ulcer. Use IV route **only** when PO and IM routes are not feasible. May cause anticholinergic side effects, especially constipation and dry mouth. Drug interactions include potentiation of CNS depressant effects when used with CNS depressants, enhancement of CNS side effects of amantadine, and inhibition of the response of neuroleptics.

Onset of action: 15 min for IV/IM and 1 hr for PO.

Oral doses should be administered with food to decrease GI upset.

BERACTANT

See *Surfactant, pulmonary*

BETAMETHASONE

Celestone, Celestone Soluspan, Betatrex, Diprolene, Diprolene AF, Diprosone, Maxivate, and others
Corticosteroid

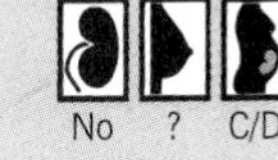

Betamethasone base (Celestone):
- **Tabs:** 0.6 mg
- **Syrup:** 0.6 mg/5 mL (120 mL)

Na phosphate (Celestone phosphate):
- **Injection solution:** 3 mg/mL (5 mL)

Na phosphate and acetate (Celestone Soluspan):
- **Injection suspension:** 6 mg/mL (3 mg/mL Na phosphate + 3 mg/mL betamethasone acetate) (5 mL)

Dipropionate:
- **Topical aerosol:** 0.1% (85g) with 10% isopropyl alcohol
- **Topical cream:** 0.05% (15, 45, 60 g)
- **Topical lotion:** 0.05% (20, 30, 60 mL)
- **Topical ointment:** 0.05% (15, 45 g)

Valerate:
- **Topical cream:** 0.05%, 0.1% (15, 45 g)
- **Topical foam:** 1.2 mg/g (50, 100 g); may contain 60.4% ethanol, cetyl alcohol, stearyl alcohol
- **Topical lotion:** 0.1% (60 mL); may contain 47.5% isopropyl alcohol
- **Topical ointment:** 0.1% (15, 45 g)

Dipropionate augmented (Diprolene and Diprolene AF):
- **Topical cream:** 0.05% (15, 45 g)
- **Topical gel:** 0.05% (15, 50 g)
- **Topical lotion:** 0.05% (30, 60 mL) with 30% isopropyl alcohol
- **Topical ointment:** 0.05% (15, 45, 50 g)

All dosages should be adjusted based on patient response and severity of condition.

Anti-inflammatory:

Children:
- ***Oral:*** 0.0175–0.25 mg/kg/24 hr or 0.5-7.5 mg/m²/24 hr ÷ Q6–8 hr
- ***IM:*** 0.0175–0.125 mg/kg/24 hr or 0.5-7.5 mg/m²/24 hr ÷ Q6–12 hr

Adolescents and adults:
- ***Oral:*** 2.4–4.8 mg/24 hr ÷ Q6–12 hr; may range from 0.6–7.2 mg/24 hr depending on disease being treated
- ***IM:*** 0.5–9 mg/24 hr ÷ Q12–24 hr
- ***Topical (see remarks):***
  - ***Valerate and dipropionate forms:***
  - ***Children and adults:*** apply to affected areas QD–BID
  - ***Dipropionate augmented forms:***
  - ***≥13 yr–adult:*** apply to affected areas QD–BID

Continued

For explanation of icons, see p. 680.

BETAMETHASONE *continued*

Max. dose: 14 days and
Cream and ointment: 45 g/wk
Gel: 50 g/wk
Lotion: 50 mL/wk

Use with caution in hypothyroidism, cirrhosis, and ulcerative colitis. See Chapter 29 for relative steroid potencies and doses based on body surface area. Betamethasone is inadequate when used alone for adrenocortical insufficiency because of its minimal mineralocorticoid properties. Like all steroids, may cause hypertension, pseudotumor cerebri, acne, Cushing syndrome, adrenal axis suppression, GI bleeding, hyperglycemia, and osteoporosis.

Na phosphate and acetate injectable suspension recommended for IM, intra-articular, intrasynovial, intralesional, soft tissue use **only**; but **not** for IV use. **Topical betamethasone dipropionate augmented (Diprolene and Diprolene AF) is not recommended in children ≤12 yr owing to the higher risk for adrenal suppression.**

Used in premature labor to stimulate fetal lung maturation. Pregnancy category changes to D if used in first trimester.

BETHANECHOL CHLORIDE

Urecholine and other brand names
Cholinergic agent

No ? C

Tabs: 5, 10, 25, 50 mg
Suspension: 1, 5 mg/mL
Injection: 5 mg/mL

Children:
Abdominal distention/urinary retention: 0.6 mg/kg/24 hr ÷ Q6–8 hr PO
Gastroesophageal reflux: 0.1–0.2 mg/kg/dose 30 min–1 hr before meals and QHS PO; **max. dose:** 4 doses/24 hr

Adults:
Urinary retention: 10–50 mg Q6–12 hr PO

Contraindicated in asthma, mechanical GI or GU obstruction, peptic ulcer disease, hyperthyroidism, cardiac disease, and seizure disorder. May cause hypotension, nausea, bronchospasm, salivation, flushing, and abdominal cramps. **Warning: severe hypotension may occur when given with ganglionic blockers (trimethaphan). Atropine is the antidote.**

BICITRA

See *Citrate Mixtures*

B

BISACODYL

Dulcolax, Fleet Laxative, Fleet Bisacodyl, and various other names
Laxative, stimulant

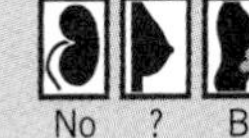

Tabs (enteric coated): 5 mg
Suppository: 10 mg
Enema: 10 mg/30 mL (37.5 mL)

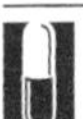

Oral:
Child: 0.3 mg/kg/24 hr or 5–10 mg to be given 6 hr before desired effect; **max. dose:** 30 mg/24 hr
Adult (>12 yr): 5–15 mg to be given 6 hr before desired effect; **max. dose:** 30 mg/24 hr
Rectal (as a single dose):
<2 yr: 5 mg
2–11 yr: 5–10 mg
>11 yr: 10 mg

Do not chew or crush tablets; do not give within 1 hr of antacids or milk. **Do not use** in newborn period. May cause abdominal cramps, nausea, vomiting, and rectal irritation. Oral usually effective within 6–10 hr; rectal usually effective within 15–60 min.

BISMUTH SUBSALICYLATE

Pepto-Bismol, Kaopectate, and others
Antidiarrheal, gastrointestinal ulcer agent

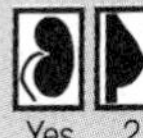
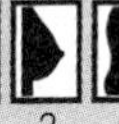
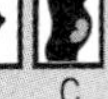

Liquid: 130 mg/15 mL (240 mL), 262 mg/15 mL (120, 240, 360, 480 mL), 524 mg/15 mL (120, 240, 360 mL)
Caplet: 262 mg
Chewable tabs: 262 mg
Contains 102 mg salicylate per 262 mg tablet; or 129 mg salicylate per 15 mL of the 262 mg/15 mL suspension.

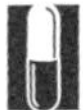

Diarrhea:
Children: 100 mg/kg/24 hr ÷ 5 equal doses for 5 days; **max. dose:** 4.19 g/24 hr
Dosage by age: give following dose Q 30 min to 1 hr PRN up to a **max. dose** of 8 doses/24 hr:
3–5 yr: 87.3 mg (1/3 tablet or 5 mL of 262 mg/15 mL)
6–8 yr: 174.7 mg (2/3 tablet or 10 mL of 262 mg/15 mL)

Continued

FORMULARY

For explanation of icons, see p. 680.

BISMUTH SUBSALICYLATE *continued*

9–11 yr: 262 mg (1 tablet or 15 mL of 262 mg/15 mL)
≥12 yr–adults: 524 mg (2 tablets or 30 mL of 262 mg/15 mL)

***H. pylori* gastric infection** (in combination with ampicillin and metronidazole or with tetracycline and metronidazole for adults; doses not well established for children):

<10 yr: 262 mg PO QID × 6 wk
≥10 yr–adults: 524 mg PO QID × 6 wk

Generally **not recommended** in children <16 yr with chicken pox or flu-like symptoms (risk for Reye syndrome), in combination with other nonsteroidal anti-inflammatory drugs, or in severe renal failure. **Use with caution** in bleeding disorders, renal dysfunction, gastritis, and gout. May cause darkening of tongue and/or black stools, GI upset, impaction, and decreased platelet aggregation.

Drug combination appears to have antisecretory and antimicrobial effects with some anti-inflammatory effects. Absorption of bismuth is negligible, whereas about 80% of the salicylate is absorbed. Decreases absorption of tetracycline.

BROMPHENIRAMINE + PSEUDOEPHEDRINE

Bromfed, Dimetapp, Rondec, and various other names
Antihistamine + decongestant

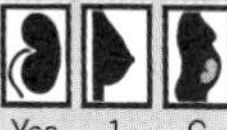

Drops: brompheniramine 5 mg + pseudoephedrine 62.5 mg/5 mL (30 mL), brompheniramine 5 mg + pseudoephedrine 75 mg/5 mL (30 mL)
Elixir: brompheniramine 1 mg + pseudoephedrine 15 mg/5 mL (118, 237, 473 mL), brompheniramine 2 mg + pseudoephedrine 30 mg/5 mL (480 mL), brompheniramine 4 mg + pseudoephedrine 30 mg/5 mL (473 mL), brompheniramine 4 mg + pseudoephedrine 45 mg (118, 473 mL), brompheniramine 4 mg + pseudoephedrine 60 mg/5 mL (473 mL)
Tabs: Brompheniramine 4 mg + pseudoephedrine 60 mg
Extended-released capsules: brompheniramine 6 mg + pseudoephedrine 60 mg, brompheniramine 12 mg + pseudoephedrine 120 mg

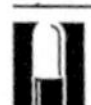

All doses based on brompheniramine component
Oral, drops:

1–3 mo: 0.25 mg QID up to a **max. dose** of 1 mg/24 hr
≥3–6 mo: 0.5 mg QID up to a **max. dose** of 2 mg/24 hr
≥6–12 mo: 0.75 mg QID up to a **max. dose** of 3 mg/24 hr
≥12–24 mo: 1 mg QID up to a **max. dose** of 4 mg/24 hr

Oral, elixir:

Children 6–11 yr: 2 mg Q4 hr up to a **max. dose** of 4 doses in 24 hours.
≥12 yr and adult: 4 mg Q4 hr up to a **max. dose** of 4 doses in 24 hours.

Oral, tablet:

Children 6–11 yr: ½ tab QID; **max. dose** of 8 mg/24 hr
≥12 yr and adult: 1 tab QID; **max. dose** of 16 mg/24 hr

Continued

BROMPHENIRAMINE + PSEUDOEPHEDRINE *continued*

Extended-released capsules:

Children 6–11 yr:

Product containing 6 mg brompheniramine: 1 cap BID

≥12 yr and adult:

Product containing 6 mg brompheniramine: 2 caps BID

Product containing 12 mg brompheniramine: 1 cap BID

Generally **not recommended** for treating URIs for infants. No proven benefit for infants or young children with URIs. **Contraindicated** in narrow-angle glaucoma, bladder neck obstruction, and asthma, and with concurrent use of MAO inhibitors. In addition, pseudoephedrine product is **contraindicated** in severe hypertension, coronary artery disease, diabetes mellitus, and thyroid disease. Discontinue use 48 hours before allergy skin testing.

Both products may cause drowsiness, fatigue, CNS excitation, xerostomia, blurred vision, and wheezing. The combination products have been reformulated without phenylpropanolamine (PPA) as the decongestant. PPA has been associated with an increased risk for hemorrhagic strokes.

Dosage adjustment may be necessary in renal failure for patients receiving the combination product because pseudoephedrine and its metabolite are significantly excreted in the urine.

BUDESONIDE

Pulmicort Respules, Pulmicort Turbuhaler, Rhinocort, Rhinocort Aqua Nasal Spray

Corticosteroid

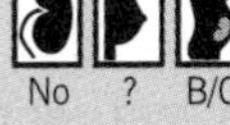

Nasal aerosol (Rhinocort): 32 mcg/actuation (7 g, delivers about 200 sprays)
Nasal spray (Rhinocort Aqua): 32 mcg/actuation (10 mL, delivers about 120 sprays)
Nebulized inhalation suspension: 0.25 mg/2 mL, 0.5 mg/2 mL (30's)
Oral inhaler: 200 mcg/metered dose (1 inhaler delivers about 200 doses)

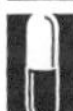

Nebulized inhalation suspension:

Children 1–8 yr:

No prior steroid use: 0.5 mg/24 hr ÷ QD–BID; **max. dose:** 0.5 mg/24 hr
Prior inhaled steroid use: 0.5 mg/24 hr ÷ QD–BID; **max. dose:** 1 mg/24 hr
Prior oral steroid use: 1 mg/24 hr ÷ QD–BID; **max. dose:** 1 mg/24 hr

Oral inhalation:

Children ≥6 yr: Start at 1 inhalation (200 mcg) BID and increase, as needed, up to a **max. dose** of 4 inhalations/24 hr.

Adult:

No prior steroid use: 1–2 inhalations BID; **max. dose:** 4 inhalations/24 hr
Prior inhaled steriod use: start at 1–2 inhalations BID and increase, as needed, up to a **max. dose** of 8 inhalations/24 hr.
Prior oral steroid use: start at 2–4 inhalations BID; **max. dose:** 8 inhalations/24 hr.

Continued

For explanation of icons, see p. 680.

BUDESONIDE *continued*

Nasal inhalation (≥6 yr):

Aerosol: (initial): 2 sprays in each nostril QAM and QHS or 4 sprays in each nostril QAM. Reduce dose gradually to the lowest effective dose after resolution of symptoms.

Spray: (initial): 1 spray in each nostril QD. Increase dose as needed up to maximum dose.

Max. nasal spray dose: *6–11 yr:* 128 mcg/24 hr (4 sprays/24 hr); *≥12 yr:* 256 mcg/24 hr (8 sprays/24 hr)

Reduce maintenance dose to as low as possible to control symptoms. May cause pharyngitis, cough, epistaxis, nasal irritation, and HPA-axis suppression. Rinse mouth after each use via the oral inhalation route. Nebulized budesonide has been shown effective in mild to moderate croup at doses of 2 mg × 1 [N Engl J Med 1994, 331(5):285].

Significant hepatic impairment may increase systemic exposure of budesonide.

Onset of action for oral inhalation and nebulized suspension is within 1 day and 2–8 days, respectively, with peak effects at 1–2 wk and 4–6 wk, respectively.

For nasal use, onset of action is seen after 1 day with peak effects after 3–7 days of therapy. Discontinue therapy if no improvement in nasal symptoms after 3 wk of continuous therapy.

Pregnancy codes are B for oral inhalation and C for nasal inhalation.

BUMETANIDE

Bumex

Loop diuretic

No ? C/D

Tabs: 0.5, 1, 2 mg

Injection: 0.25 mg/mL (some preparations may contain 1% benzyl alcohol)

Neonates and infants (see remarks): *PO/IM/IV*

≤6 mo: 0.01–0.05 mg/kg/dose QD–QOD

Infants and children: *PO/IM/IV*

>6 mo: 0.015–0.1 mg/kg/dose QD–QOD; **max. dose:** 10 mg/24 hr

Adults:

PO: 0.5–2 mg/dose QD-BID

IM/IV: 0.5–1 mg over 1–2 min. May give additional doses Q2–3 hr PRN

Usual max. dose (PO/IM/IV): 10 mg/24 hr

Cross-allergenicity may occur in patients allergic to sulfonamides. Dosage reduction may be necessary in patients with hepatic dysfunction. Administer oral doses with food.

Side effects include cramps, dizziness, hypotension, headache, electrolyte losses (hypokalemia, hypocalcemia, hyponatremia, hypochloremia), and encephalopathy. May also lead to metabolic alkalosis.

Continued

BUMETANIDE *continued*

Drug elimination has been reported to be slower in neonates with respiratory disorders compared to neonates without. May displace bilirubin in critically ill neonates. Maximal diuretic effect for infants ≤6 mo has been reported at 0.04 mg/kg/dose, with greater efficacy seen at lower dosages.

Pregnancy category changes to D if used in pregnancy-induced hypertension.

CAFFEINE CITRATE

Cafcit

Methylxanthine, respiratory stimulant

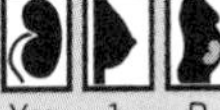
Yes 1 B

Injection: 20 mg/mL (3 mL)
Oral liquid: 20 mg/mL (3 mL), also available as powder for compounding
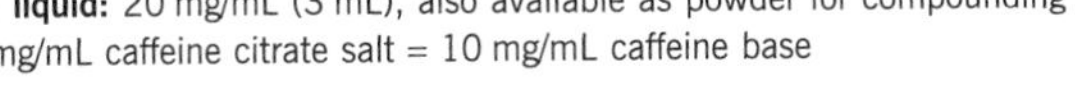
20 mg/mL caffeine citrate salt = 10 mg/mL caffeine base

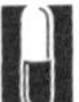

Doses expressed in mg of caffeine citrate
Neonatal apnea:
Loading dose: 10–20 mg/kg IV/PO × 1
Maintenance dose: 5–10 mg/kg/dose PO/IV QD, to begin 24 hr after loading dose

Avoid use in symptomatic cardiac arrhythmias. Do not use caffeine benzoate formulation because it has been associated with kernicterus in neonates. **Use with caution** in impaired renal or hepatic function.

Therapeutic levels: 5–25 mg/L. Cardiovascular, neurologic, or GI toxicity reported at serum levels >50 mg/L. Recommended serum sampling time: obtain trough level within 30 min before a dose. Steady-state is typically achieved 3 wk after the initiation of therapy. Levels obtained before steady state are useful for preventing toxicity.

CALCITONIN

Miacalcin, Miacalcin Nasal Spray

Hypercalcemia antidote, antiosteoporotic

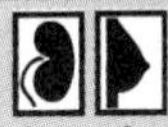
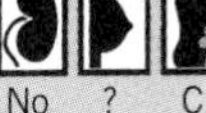
No ? C

Injection:
Salmon: 200 U/mL (2 mL); contains phenol
Nasal spray:
Salmon: 200 U/metered dose (2 mL, provides 14 doses)

Ostegenesis imperfecta:
6 mo–15 yr (salmon calcitonin): 2 U/kg/dose IM/SC 3 times per week with oral calcium supplements

Continued

For explanation of icons, see p. 680.

CALCITONIN *continued*

Hypercalcemia (adult doses):

Salmon calcitonin: start with 4 U/kg/dose IM/SC Q12 hr; if response is unsatisfactory after 1 or 2 days, increase dose to 8 U/kg/dose Q12 hr. If response remains unsatisfactory after 2 more days, increase to a **max. dose** of 8 U/kg/dose Q6 hr.

Paget's disease (adult doses):

Salmon calcitonin:

IM/SC: start with 100 U QD initially, followed by a usual maintenance dose of 50 U QD *OR* 50–100 U Q 1–3 days.

Intranasal: 1–2 sprays (200–400 U) QD

Contraindicated in patients sensitive to salmon protein or gelatin. If using salmon calcitonin product, prepare a 10-U/mL dilution with normal saline and administer 0.1 mL intradermally as a skin test (observe for 15 min). Nausea, abdominal pain, flushing, and inflammation at the injection site have been reported with IM/SC route of administration. Nasal irritation, rhinitis, and epistaxis may occur with use of the nasal spray. If the injection volume exceeds 2 mL, use IM route and multiple sites of injection.

CALCITRIOL

1,25-dihydroxycholecalciferol, Rocaltrol, Calcijex

Active form vitamin D, fat soluble

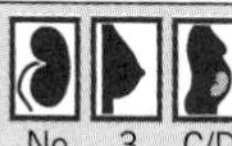

Caps: 0.25, 0.5 mcg

Oral solution: 1 mcg/mL (15 mL)

Injection (Calcijex): 1, 2 mcg/mL (1 mL)

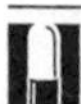

Renal failure (see remarks):

Children:

Oral: Suggested dose range 0.01–0.05 mcg/kg/24 hr. Titrate in 0.005–0.01 mcg/kg/24 hr increments Q4–8 wk based on clinical response.

IV: 0.01–0.05 mcg/kg/dose given 3 times per week

Adults:

Oral initial: 0.25 mcg/dose PO QD–QOD

Oral increment: 0.25 mcg/dose PO Q4–8 wk. Usual dose is 0.5–1 mcg/24 hr.

IV: 0.5 mcg/24 hr given 3 times per week. Usual dose is 0.5–3 mcg/24 hr given 3 times per week.

Hypoparathyroidism:

For children >1 yr and adults, initial dose is 0.25 mcg/dose PO QD. May increase daily dosage by 0.25 mcg at 2- to 4-week intervals. Usual maintenance dosage as follows:

<1 yr: 0.04–0.08 mcg/kg/dose PO QD

1–5 yr: 0.25–0.75 mcg/dose PO QD

>6 yr and adults: 0.5–2 mcg/dose PO QD

Continued

CALCITRIOL *continued*

Most potent vitamin D metabolite available. Monitor serum calcium and phosphorus and PTH in dialysis patients. **Avoid** concomitant use of Mg^{2+}-containing antacids. IV dosing applies if patient is undergoing hemodialysis. A mean weekly IV dose of 1–1.4 mcg has been reported in 13- to 18-year-old patients with ESRD.

Contraindicated in patients with hypercalcemia, vitamin D toxicity. Side effects include weakness, headache, vomiting, constipation, hypotonia, polydipsia, polyuria, myalgia, metastatic calcification, etc. Allergic reaction has been reported.

Pregnancy category changes to D if used in doses above the recommended daily allowance.

CALCIUM CARBONATE

Tums, Os-Cal, and others; 40% Elemental Ca

Calcium supplement, antacid

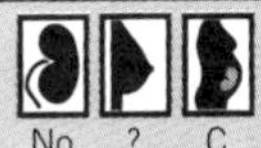

No ? C

Tabs, chewable: 500, 750, 1000, 1250 mg
Tabs: 650, 1250, 1500 mg
Suspension: 1250 mg/5 mL
Caps: 125, 364, 1250 mg
Powder: 454 g
Each 1000 mg of salt contains 20 mEq elemental Ca (400 mg elemental Ca)

Doses expressed in mg of elemental calcium. To convert to mg of salt, divide elemental dose by 0.4.

Hypocalcemia:

Neonate: 50–150 mg/kg/24 hr ÷ Q4–6 hr PO; **max. dose:** 1 g/24 hr
Child: 45–65 mg/kg/24 hr PO ÷ QID
Adult: 1–2 g/24 hr PO ÷ TID-QID

Side effects: Constipation, hypercalcemia, hypophosphatemia, hypomagnesemia, nausea, vomiting, headache, and confusion. May reduce absorption of tetracycline, iron, and effectiveness of polystyrene sulfonate. May potentiate effects of digoxin. Some products may contain trace amounts of Na. Administer each dose with meals or with lots of fluid.

CALCIUM CHLORIDE

27% Elemental Ca

Calcium supplement

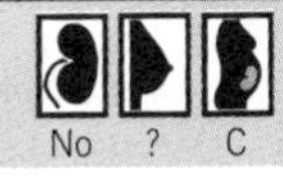

No ? C

Injection: 100 mg/mL (10%) (1.36 mEq Ca/mL); 1 g of salt contains 13.6 mEq (273 mg) elemental Ca.

Continued

For explanation of icons, see p. 680.

CALCIUM CHLORIDE *continued*

Doses expressed in mg of CaCl
Cardiac arrest:
Infant/child: 20 mg/kg/dose IV Q10 min PRN
Adult: 250–500 mg/dose IV Q10 min PRN or 2–4 mg/kg/dose Q10 min PRN

MAXIMUM IV ADMINISTRATION RATES:
IV push: **Do not exceed** 100 mg/min.
IV infusion: **Do not exceed** 45–90 mg/kg/hr with a **maximum concentration** of 20 mg/mL.

Use IV with extreme caution. Extravasation may lead to necrosis. Hyaluronidase may be helpful for extravasation. Central-line administration is preferred IV route of administration. **Do not use** scalp veins. **Do not administer** via IM or SC route. Not recommended for asystole and electromechanical dissociation.

Rapid IV infusion associated with bradycardia, hypotension, and peripheral vasodilation. May cause hyperchloremic acidosis.

CALCIUM GLUBIONATE
Neo-Calglucon; 6.4% Elemental Ca
Calcium supplement

No ? C

Syrup: 1.8 g/5 mL (480 mL) (1.2 mEq Ca/mL); 1 g of salt contains 3.2 mEq (64 mg) elemental Ca.

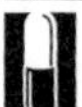

Doses expressed in mg calcium glubionate
Neonatal hypocalcemia: 1200 mg/kg/24 hr PO ÷ Q4–6 hr
Maintenance:
Infant/child: 600–2000 mg/kg/24 hr PO ÷ QID; **max. dose:** 9 g/24 hr
Adult: 6–18 g/24 hr PO ÷ QID

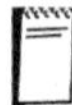

Side effects include GI irritation, dizziness, and headache. Best absorbed when given before meals. Absorption inhibited by high phosphate load. High osmotic load of syrup (20% sucrose) may cause diarrhea.

CALCIUM GLUCEPTATE
(8.2% Elemental Ca)
Calcium supplement

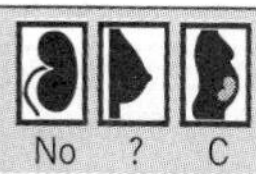

Injection: 220 mg/mL (22%) (0.9 mEq Ca/mL); 1 g of salt contains 4.1 mEq (82 mg) elemental Ca.

Continued

CALCIUM GLUCEPTATE *continued*

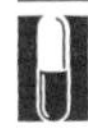

Doses expressed in mg of calcium gluceptate

Hypocalcemia:

Child: 200–500 mg/kg/24 hr IV ÷ Q6 hr

Adult: 500–1100 mg/dose IV as needed

Cardiac arrest:

Child: 110 mg/kg/dose IV Q10 min

MAXIMUM IV ADMINISTRATION RATES:

IV push: **Do not exceed** 100 mg/min.

IV infusion: **Do not exceed** 150–300 mg/kg/hr with a **maximum concentration** of 55 mg/mL.

See *Calcium gluconate*

CALCIUM GLUCONATE

9% Elemental Ca

Calcium supplement

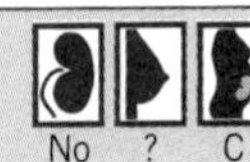

No ? C

Tabs: 500, 650, 975, 1000 mg

Powder for oral suspension: 3852.2 mg (346.7 mg elemental)/15 mL (454 g)

Injection: 100 mg/mL (10%) (0.45 mEq Ca^{2+}/mL)

1 g of salt contains 4.5 mEq (90 mg) elemental Ca.

Doses expressed in mg calcium gluconate

Maintenance/hypocalcemia:

Neonate: IV: 200–800 mg/kg/24 hr ÷ Q6 hr

Infant:

IV: 200–500 mg/kg/24 hr ÷ Q6 hr

PO: 400–800 mg/kg/24 hr ÷ Q6 hr

Child: 200–500 mg/kg/24 hr IV or PO ÷ Q6 hr

Adult: 5–15 g/24 hr IV or PO ÷ Q6 hr

For cardiac arrest:

Infant and child: 100 mg/kg/dose IV Q10 min

Adult: 500–800 mg/dose IV Q10 min

Max. dose: 3 g/dose

MAXIMUM IV ADMINISTRATION RATES:

IV push: **Do not exceed** 100 mg/min.

IV infusion: **Do not exceed** 120–240 mg/kg/hr with a **maximum concentration** of 50 mg/mL.

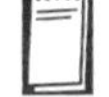

Avoid peripheral infusion as extravasation may cause tissue necrosis. IV infusion associated with hypotension and bradycardia. Also associated with arrhythmias in digitalized patients. May precipitate when used with bicarbonate. **Do not use** scalp veins.

Do not administer IM or SC.

For explanation of icons, see p. 680.

CALCIUM LACTATE
13% Elemental Ca
Calcium supplement

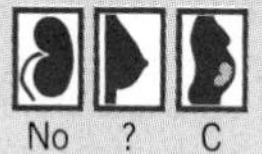

Tabs: 650, 769.2 mg
Caps: 500 mg
1 g salt contains 6.5 mEq (130 mg) elemental Ca.

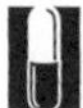

Doses expressed in mg of calcium lactate
Infant: 400–500 mg/kg/24 hr PO ÷ Q4–6 hr
Child: 500 mg/kg/24 hr PO ÷ Q6–8 hr
Adult: 1.5–3 g PO Q8 hr
Max. dose: 9 g/24 hr

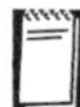

Give with meals. **Do not** dissolve tablets in milk.

CALFACTANT

See *Surfactant, pulmonary*

CAPTOPRIL
Capoten
Angiotensin-converting enzyme inhibitor, antihypertensive

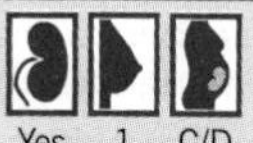

Tabs: 12.5, 25, 50, 100 mg
Suspension: 0.75, 1 mg/mL

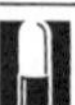

Neonate: 0.1–0.4 mg/kg/24 hr PO ÷ Q6–8 hr
Infant: Initially 0.15–0.3 mg/kg/dose; titrate upward if needed; **max. dose:** 6 mg/kg/24 hr ÷ QD–QID.
Child: Initially 0.3–0.5 mg/kg/dose Q8 hr; titrate upward if needed; **max. dose:** 6 mg/kg/24 hr ÷ BID–QID.
Adolescent and adult: Initially 12.5–25 mg/dose PO BID–TID; increase weekly if necessary by 25 mg/dose to **max. dose:** 450 mg/24 hr.

Onset within 15–30 min of administration. Peak effect within 1–2 hr. **Adjust dose with renal failure (see Chapter 30).** Should be administered on an empty stomach 1 hr before or 2 hr after meals. Titrate to minimal effective dose.

Use with caution in collagen vascular disease and concomitant potassium-sparing diuretics. **Avoid use** with dialysis with high-flux membranes since anaphylactoid reactions have been reported. May cause rash, proteinuria, neutropenia, cough, angioedema (head, neck, and intestinal), hyperkalemia,

Continued

CAPTOPRIL *continued*

hypotension, or diminution of taste perception (with long-term use). Known to decrease aldosterone and increase renin production.

Pregnancy category is a C during the first trimester but changes to a D for the second and third trimester (fetal injury and death have been reported).

CARBAMAZEPINE

Atretol, Epitol, Tegretol, Tegretol-XR, Carbatrol

Anticonvulsant

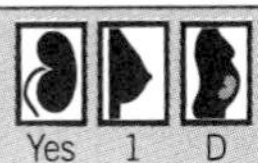

Tabs: 200 mg
Chewable tabs: 100 mg
Extended-release tabs (Tegretol-XR): 100, 200, 400 mg
Extended-release caps: 200, 300 mg
Suspension: 100 mg/5 mL (450 mL)

See remarks regarding dosing intervals and dosage forms:

<6 yr:
Initial: 10–20 mg/kg/24 hr PO ÷ BID-TID (QID for suspension)
Increment: Q5–7 days up to 35 mg/kg/24 hr PO

6–12 yr:
Initial: 10 mg/kg/24 hr PO ÷ BID up to **max. dose:** 100 mg/dose BID
Increment: 100 mg/24 hr at 1 wk intervals (÷ TID-QID) until desired response is obtained
Maintenance: 20–30 mg/kg/24 hr PO ÷ BID-QID; usual maintenance dose is 400–800 mg/24 hr; **max. dose:** 1000 mg/24 hr

>12 yr:
Initial: 200 mg PO BID
Increment: 200 mg/24 hr at 1 wk intervals (÷ BID–QID) until desired response is obtained
Maintenance: 800–1200 mg/24 hr PO ÷ BID–QID

Max. dose:
Child 12–15 yr: 1000 mg/24 hr
Child >15 yr: 1200 mg/24 hr
Adult: 1.6–2.4 g/24 hr

Contraindicated for patients taking MAO inhibitors or who are sensitive to tricyclic antidepressants. Should not be used in combination with clozapine because of increased risk for bone marrow suppression and agranulocytosis. Erythromycin, diltiazem, verapamil, cefixime, cimetidine, itraconazole, and INH may increase serum levels. Carbamazepine may decrease activity of warfarin, doxycycline, oral contraceptives, cyclosporine, theophylline, phenytoin, benzodiazepines, ethosuximide, and valproic acid.

Suggested dosing intervals for specific dosage forms: extended-release tabs or caps (BID); chewable and immediate release tablets (BID–TID); suspension (QID). Doses may be administered with food. **Do not** crush or chew extended release dosage forms. Shake bottle well before dispensing oral suspension dosage form, and **do not** administer simultaneously with other liquid medicines or diluents.

Continued

For explanation of icons, see p. 680.

CARBAMAZEPINE *continued*

Drug metabolism typically increases after the first month of therapy owing to hepatic autoinduction.

Therapeutic blood levels: 4–12 mg/L. Recommended serum sampling time: obtain trough level within 30 min before an oral dose. Steady state is typically achieved 1 month after the initiation of therapy (following enzymatic autoinduction). Levels obtained before steady state are useful for preventing toxicity. Blood levels of 7–10 mg/L have been recommended for bipolar disorders.

Side effects include sedation, dizziness, diplopia, aplastic anemia, neutropenia, urinary retention, nausea, SIADH, and Stevens-Johnson syndrome. Pretreatment CBCs and LFTs are suggested. Patient should be monitored for hematologic and hepatic toxicity. **Adjust dose in renal impairment (see Chapter 30).**

See Chapter 2 for management of ingestions.

CARBAMIDE PEROXIDE

Debrox, Murine Ear Drops, Auro Ear Drops, Gly-Oxide, Proxigel, and others

Ceruminolytic, topical oral analgesic

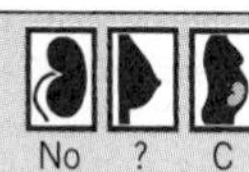

Otic solution (OTC): 6.5% (15, 30 mL)
Oral gel (OTC) [Proxigel]: 10% (36 g)
Oral liquid (OTC) [Gly-Oxide]: 10% (15, 60 mL)

Ceruminolytic:

<12 yr: Tilt head sideways and instill 1–5 drops (according to patient size) into affected ear, and keep drops in ear for several minutes. Remove wax by gently flushing the ear with warm water, using a soft rubber bulb ear syringe. Dose may be repeated BID PRN for **up to** 4 days.

≥12 yr: Following the same instructions from above, instill 5–10 drops into affected ear BID PRN for **up to** 4 days.

Oral analgesic (see remarks):

Liquid:

≥3 yr (able to follow instructions): Instill several drops to affected area and expectorate after 2–3 min *OR* place 10 drops on tongue and mix with saliva, swish for several minutes and expectorate. Administer QID, after meals and QHS, for **up to** 7 days.

Gel:

Child and adult: Gently massage on affected area QID for **up to** 7 days.

Contraindicated if tympanic membrane perforated; following otic surgery; ear discharge, drainage, pain, irritation or rash; or PE tubes in place. Prolonged use of the oral product may result in fungal overgrowth.

Tip of applicator should not enter ear canal when used as a ceruminolytic.

Do not rinse the mouth or drink for at least 5 min when using oral preparations.

CARBINOXAMINE WITH PSEUDOEPHEDRINE

Rondec, Rondec TR, Carbic-D, Cardec, Cardec-S, and others

Antihistamine with decongestant

Yes ? C

Oral drops:

Rondec: carbinoxamine 1 mg + pseudoephedrine 15 mg/1 mL (30 mL)

Others: carbinoxamine 2 mg + pseudoephedrine 25 mg/1 mL (30 mL)

Oral solution:

Carbic-D: carbinoxamine 2 mg + pseudoephedrine 30 mg/5 mL (480 mL)

Cardec-S and others: carbinoxamine 4 mg + pseudoephedrine 60 mg/5 mL (480 mL)

Cardec: carbinoxamine 5 mg + pseudoephedrine 75 mg/5 mL (30 mL)

Tabs:

Rondec and others: carbinoxamine 4 mg + pseudoephedrine 60 mg

Extended-release tabs:

Rondec TR and others: carbinoxamine 8 mg + pseudoephedrine 120 mg

---

Child (PO): carbinoxamine at 0.2–0.4 mg/kg/24 hr and pseudoephedrine at 4 mg/kg/24 hr; alternative oral dosing of carbinoxamine by age:

1–3 mo: 0.25–0.5 mg QID
3–6 mo: 0.5–1 mg QID
6–12 mo: 0.75–1.5 mg QID
12–24 mo: 1–2 mg QID
24 mo–6 yr: 2 mg QID
≥6 yr and adult: 4 mg QID for immediate release products *OR* 8 mg BID for extended release tabs

---

Contraindicated in acute asthma, hypersensitivity with other ethanolamine antihistamines, MAO inhibitors, severe hypertension, narrow-angle glaucoma, severe coronary artery disease, and urinary retention. **Be aware of the corresponding amount of pseudoephedrine**. See *Pseudoephedrine* for additional remarks.

May cause drowsiness, vertigo, dry mucus membranes, and headache. Contact dermatitis and CNS excitation have been reported.

Do not crush or chew extended release tablets.

For explanation of icons, see p. 680.

CARNITINE
Levocarnitine, Carnitor
L-Carnitine

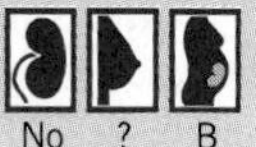

Tabs: 330, 500 mg
Caps: 250 mg
Oral solution: 100 mg/mL (118 mL)
Injection: 200 mg/mL (5mL) (preservative free)

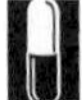

Primary carnitine deficiency:
Oral:
Child: 50–100 mg/kg/24 hr PO ÷ Q8–12 hr; increase slowly as needed and tolerated to **max. dose** of 3 g/24 hr.
Adult: 330 mg to 1 g/dose BID–TID PO
IV:
Child and adult: 50 mg/kg as loading dose; may follow with 50 mg/kg/24 hr IV infusion; maintenance: 50 mg/kg/24 hr ÷ Q4–6 hr; increase to **max. dose** of 300 mg/kg/24 hr if needed.

May cause nausea, vomiting, abdominal cramps, diarrhea, and body odor. Seizures have been reported in patients with or without a history of seizures. Give bolus IV infusion over 2–3 min.

CASPOFUNGIN
Cancidas
Antifungal

No ? C

Injection: 50, 70 mg

Children (pharmacokinetic data in 2–17 yr with oncologic fever and neutropenia, see remarks):
50 mg/m²/dose IV QD; **max. dose:** 50 mg/dose
Adolescents and adults (see remarks):
Loading dose: 70 mg IV × 1
Maintenance dose:
Usual: 50 mg IV QD. If tolerated and response is inadequate, may increase to 70 mg IV QD.
Hepatic insufficiency: 35 mg IV QD
Concomitant rifampin: 70 mg IV QD

Currently used as a second-line agent for candidiasis and aspergillosis. **Use with caution** in hepatic impairment and concomitant enzyme-inducing drugs. Higher maintenance doses (70 mg QD in adults) may be necessary for concomitant use of enzyme inducers such as carbamazepine, dexamethasone, phenytoin, nevirapine, or efavirenz. May cause fever, facial swelling, rash, nausea/vomiting, headache, infusion-site phlebitis, and LFT elevation.

Continued

CASPOFUNGIN *continued*

Use with cyclosporine may cause transient increase in LFTs and caspofungin level elevations. May decrease tacrolimus levels.

Administer doses by slow IV infusion over 1 hour. **Do not** mix or coinfuse with other medications, and **avoid** using dextrose-containing diluents (e.g., D5W).

CEFACLOR

Ceclor, Ceclor CD, and others

Antibiotic, cephalosporin (second generation)

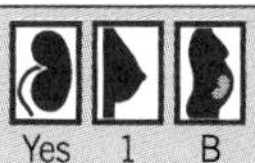

Caps: 250, 500 mg
Extended-release tabs (Ceclor CD): 375, 500 mg
Suspension: 125 mg/5 mL (75, 150 mL); 187 mg/5 mL (50, 100 mL); 250 mg/5 mL (75, 150 mL); 375 mg/5 mL (50, 100 mL)

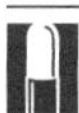

Infant and child: 20–40 mg/kg/24 hr PO ÷ Q8 hr; **max. dose:** 2 g/24 hr (Q12 hr dosage interval optional in otitis media or pharyngitis)
Adult: 250–500 mg/dose PO Q8 hr; **max. dose:** 4 g/24 hr
Extended-release tablets: 375–500 mg/dose PO Q12 hr

Use with caution in patients with penicillin allergy or renal impairment. Side effects include elevated liver function tests, bone marrow suppression, and moniliasis. May cause positive Coombs test or false-positive test for urinary glucose. Serum sickness reactions have been reported in patients receiving multiple courses of cefaclor.

Do not crush, cut, or chew extended-release tablets. Extended-release tablets are **not recommended** for children. **Adjust dose in renal failure (see Chapter 30).**

CEFADROXIL

Duricef and others

Antibiotic, cephalosporin (first generation)

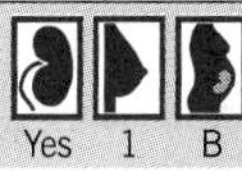

Suspension: 125, 250, 500 mg/5 mL (50, 75, 100 mL)
Tabs: 1 g
Caps: 500 mg

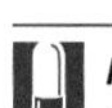

Infant and child: 30 mg/kg/24 hr PO ÷ Q12 hr (daily dose may be administered QD for group A beta-hemolytic streptococci pharyngitis/tonsillitis); **max. dose:** 2 g/24 hr
Adolescent and adult: 1–2 g/24 hr PO ÷ Q12–24 hr (administer Q12 hr for complicated UTIs); **max. dose:** 2 g/24 hr

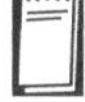

See *Cephalexin.* Side effects include nausea, vomiting, pseudomembranous colitis, pruritus, neutropenia, vaginitis, and candidiasis. **Adjust dose in renal failure (see Chapter 30).**

For explanation of icons, see p. 680.

CEFAZOLIN

Ancef, Zolicef, and others

Antibiotic, cephalosporin (first generation)

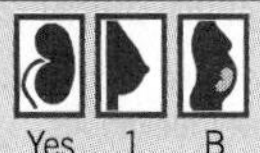

Injection: 0.5, 1, 5, 10, 20 g
Frozen injection: 500 mg/50 mL 5% dextrose, 1 g/50 mL 5% dextrose (iso-osmotic solutions)
Contains 2.1 mEq Na/g drug

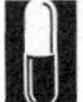

Neonate IM, IV:
Postnatal age ≤7 days: 40 mg/kg/24 hr ÷ Q12 hr
Postnatal age >7 days:
≤2000 g: 40 mg/kg/24 hr ÷ Q12 hr
>2000 g: 60 mg/kg/24 hr ÷ Q8 hr
Infant >1 mo/child: 50–100 mg/kg/24 hr ÷ Q8 hr IV/IM; **max. dose:** 6 g/24 hr
Adult: 2–6 g/24 hr ÷ Q6–8 hr IV/IM; **max. dose:** 12 g/24 hr

See *Cephalexin.* **Use with caution** in renal impairment or in penicillin-allergic patients. Does not penetrate well into CSF. May cause phlebitis, leukopenia, thrombocytopenia, transient liver enzyme elevation, false-positive urine-reducing substance (Clinitest) and Coombs test. **Adjust dose in renal failure (see Chapter 30).**

CEFDINIR

Omnicef

Antibiotic, cephalosporin (third generation)

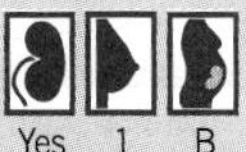

Caps: 300 mg
Suspension: 125 mg/5 mL, 250 mg/5 mL (60, 100 mL)

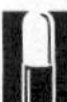

6 mo–12 yr:
Otitis media, sinusitis, pharyngitis/tonsillitis: 14 mg/kg/24 hr PO ÷ Q12–24 hr; **max. dose**: 600 mg/24 hr
Uncomplicated skin infections: 14 mg/kg/24 hr PO ÷ Q12 hr; **max. dose**: 600 mg/24 hr
≥13 yr and adult:
Bronchitis, sinusitis, pharyngitis/tonsillitis: 600 mg/24 hr PO ÷ Q12–24 hr
Community-acquired pneumonia, uncomplicated skin infections: 600 mg/24 hr PO ÷ Q12 hr

Use with caution in penicillin-allergic patients or in presence of renal impairment. Good gram-positive cocci activity. May cause diarrhea and false-positive urine-reducing substance (Clinitest) and Coombs test. Eosinophilia and abnormal liver function tests have been reported with higher than usual doses.

Once-daily dosing has not been evaluated in pneumonia and skin infections. **Avoid** concomitant administration with iron and iron-containing vitamins and

Continued

CEFDINIR *continued*

antacids containing aluminum or magnesium (space by 2 hr apart) to reduce the risk for decreasing antibiotic's absorption. Doses may be taken without regard to food. **Adjust dose in renal failure (see Chapter 30).**

CEFEPIME
Maxipime
Antibiotic, cephalosporin (fourth generation)

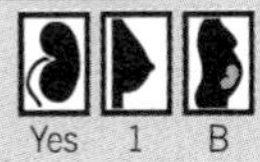

Injection: 0.5, 1, 2 g
Each 1 g drug contains 725 mg L-arginine.

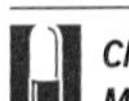

Child ≥2 mo: 100 mg/kg/24 hr ÷ Q12 hr IV/IM
Meningitis, fever, with neutropenia or serious infections: 150 mg/kg/24 hr ÷ Q8 hr IV/IM
Max. dose: 6 g/24 hr
Cystic fibrosis: 150 mg/kg/24 hr ÷ Q8 hr IV/IM, up to a **max. dose** of 6 g/24 hr
Adult: 1–4 g/24 hr ÷ Q12 hr IV/IM
Severe infections: 6 g/24 hr ÷ Q8 hr IV/IM
Max. dose: 6 g/24 hr

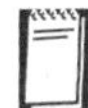

Use with caution in patients with penicillin allergy or renal impairment. Good activity against *P. aeruginosa* and other gram-negative bacteria plus most gram-positive bacteria (*S. aureus*). May cause thrombophlebitis, gastrointestinal discomfort, transient increases in liver enzymes, false-positive urine-reducing substance (Clinitest), and Coombs test. Encephalopathy, myoclonus, seizures, transient leukopenia, neutropenia, agranulocytosis, and thrombocytopenia have been reported. **Adjust dose in renal failure (see Chapter 30).**

CEFIXIME
Suprax
Antibiotic, cephalosporin (third generation)

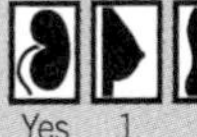

Tabs: 400 mg
Suspension: 100 mg/5 mL (50, 75, 100 mL)

Infant and child: 8 mg/kg/24 hr ÷ Q12–24 hr PO; **max. dose**: 400 mg/24 hr
Adolescent/adult: 400 mg/24 hr ÷ Q12–24 hr PO
Uncomplicated cervical, urethral, or rectal infections due to N. gonorrhoeae: 400 mg × 1 PO

Use with caution in patients with penicillin allergy or renal failure. Adverse reactions include diarrhea, abdominal pain, nausea, and headaches. May increase carbamazepine serum concentrations. **Do not use** tablets for the treatment of otitis media owing to reduced bioavailability. May cause false-positive urine-reducing substance (Clinitest), Coombs test, and nitroprusside test for ketones. **Adjust dose in renal failure (see Chapter 30).**

For explanation of icons, see p. 680.

CEFOPERAZONE
Cefobid
Antibiotic, cephalosporin (third generation)

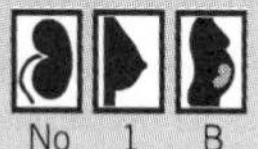

Injection: 1, 2, 10 g
Contains: 1.5 mEq Na/g drug

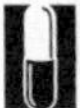

Infant and child: 100–150 mg/kg/24 hr ÷ Q8–12 hr IV/IM
Adult: 2–4 g/24 hr ÷ Q12 hr IV/IM
Maximum doses:
Usual: 12 g/24 hr
Hepatic disease and/or biliary obstruction: 4 g/24 hr
Mixed hepatic and renal impairment: 1–2 g/24 hr

Use with caution in penicillin-allergic patients or in patients with hepatic failure or biliary obstruction. Drug is extensively excreted in bile. May cause disulfiram-like reaction with ethanol and false-positive urine-reducing substance (Clinitest) and Coombs test. Bleeding and bruising may occur, especially in patients with vitamin K deficiency. Does not penetrate well into CSF.

Doses up to 16 g/24 hr administered by continuous IV infusion have been used in immunocompromised adults without complications (steady-state serum level of 150 mcg/mL).

CEFOTAXIME
Claforan
Antibiotic, cephalosporin (third generation)

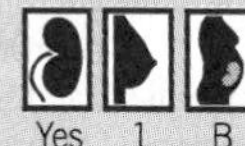

Injection: 0.5, 1, 2, 10 g
Frozen injection: 1 g/50 mL 3.4% dextrose, 2 g/50 mL 1.4% dextrose (iso-osmotic solutions)
Contains 2.2 mEq Na/g drug.

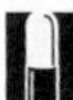

Neonate: IV/IM:
Postnatal age ≤7 days:
<2000 g: 100 mg/kg/24 hr ÷ Q12 hr
≥2000 g: 100–150 mg/kg/24 hr ÷ Q8–12 hr
Postnatal age >7 days:
<1200 g: 100 mg/kg/24 hr ÷ Q12 hr
1200–2000 g: 150 mg/kg/24 hr ÷ Q8 hr
>2000 g: 150–200 mg/kg/24 hr ÷ Q6–8 hr
Infant and child (1 mo–12 yr) (<50 kg): 100–200 mg/kg/24 hr ÷ Q6–8 hr IV/IM (see remarks)
Meningitis: 200 mg/kg/24 hr ÷ Q6 hr IV/IM (see remarks)
Max. dose: 12 g/24 hr
Adult (≥50 kg): 1–2 g/dose Q6–8 hr IV/IM
Severe infection: 2 g/dose Q4–6 hr IV/IM
Max. dose: 12 g/24 hr
Uncomplicated gonorrhea: 0.5–1 g × 1 IM

Continued

CEFOTAXIME *continued*

Use with caution in penicillin-allergy and renal impairment (reduce dosage). Toxicities similar to other cephalosporins: allergy, neutropenia, thrombocytopenia, eosinophilia, false-positive urine-reducing substance (Clinitest) and Coombs test, elevated BUN, creatinine, and liver enzymes.

Good CNS penetration. Doses of 225–300 mg/kg/24 hr ÷ Q6–8 hr, in combination with vancomycin (60 mg/kg/24 hr), have been recommended for meningitis because of penicillin-resistant pneumococci. Doses of 150–225 mg/kg/24 hr ÷ Q6–8 hr have been recommended for infections outside the CSF because of penicillin-resistant pneumococci. **Adjust dose in renal failure (see Chapter 30).**

CEFOTETAN

Cefotan

Antibiotic, cephalosporin (second generation)

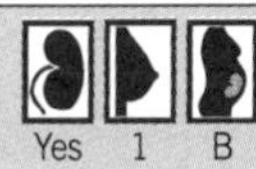

Frozen injection: 1 g/50 mL 3.8% dextrose, 2 g/50 mL 2.2% dextrose (iso-osmotic solutions)

Contains 3.5 mEq Na/g drug.

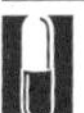

Infant and child: 40–80 mg/kg/24 hr ÷ Q12 hr IV/IM

Adolescent and adult: 2–6 g/24 hr ÷ Q12 hr IV/IM

PID: 2 g Q12 hr IV × 24–48 after clinical improvement with doxycycline, 100 mg Q12 hr PO/IV × 14 days

Max. dose: 6 g/24 hr

Use with caution in penicillin-allergic patients or in presence of renal impairment. Has good anaerobic activity. May cause disulfiram-like reaction with ethanol, false-positive urine-reducing substance (Clinitest), and false elevations of serum and urine creatinine (Jaffe method). Hemolytic anemia has been reported. CSF penetration is poor. **Adjust dose in renal failure (see Chapter 30).**

CEFOXITIN

Mefoxin

Antibiotic, cephalosporin (second generation)

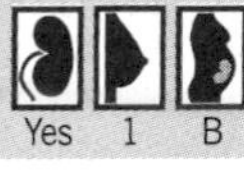

Injection: 1, 2, 10 g

Frozen injection: 1 g/50 mL 4% dextrose, 2 g/50 mL 2.2% dextrose (iso-osmotic solutions)

Contains 2.3 mEq Na/g drug.

Infant and child: 80–160 mg/kg/24 hr ÷ Q4–8 hr IM/IV

Adult: 4–12 g/24 hr ÷ Q6–8 hr IM/IV

PID: 2 g IV Q6h × 24–48 hr after clinical improvement with doxycycline 100 mg Q12 hr PO/IV × 14 days

Max. dose: 12 g/24 hr

Continued

For explanation of icons, see p. 680.

CEFOXITIN *continued*

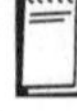

Use with caution in penicillin-allergic patients or in presence of renal impairment. Has good anaerobic activity. May cause false-positive urine-reducing substance (Clinitest and other copper-reduction method tests), and false elevations of serum and urine creatinine. CSF penetration is poor. **Adjust dose in renal failure (see Chapter 30).**

CEFPODOXIME PROXETIL

Vantin

Antibiotic, cephalosporin (third generation)

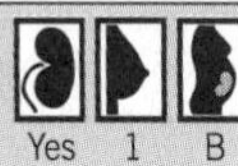

Tabs: 100, 200 mg
Suspension: 50, 100 mg/5 mL (50, 75, 100 mL)

2 mo–12 yr:
Otitis media: 10 mg/kg/24 hr PO ÷ Q12–24 hr; **max. dose:** 400 mg/24 hr
Pharyngitis/tonsillitis: 10 mg/kg/24 hr PO ÷ Q12 hr; **max. dose:** 200 mg/24 hr
Acute maxillary sinusitis: 10 mg/kg/24 hr PO ÷ Q12 hr; **max. dose:** 400 mg/24 hr

≥13 yr–adult: 200–800 mg/24 hr PO ÷ Q12 hr
Uncomplicated gonorrhea: 200 mg PO × 1

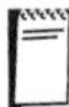

Use with caution in penicillin-allergic patients or in presence of renal impairment. May cause diarrhea, nausea, vomiting, vaginal candidiasis, and false-positive Coombs test.

Tablets should be administered with food to enhance absorption. Suspension may be administered without regard to food. High doses of antacids or H_2 blockers may reduce absorption. **Adjust dose in renal failure (see Chapter 30).**

CEFPROZIL

Cefzil

Antibiotic, cephalosporin (second generation)

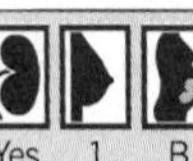

Tabs: 250, 500 mg
Suspension: 125 mg/5 mL, 250 mg/5 mL (50, 75, 100 mL) (contains aspartame and phenylalanine)

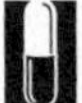

Otitis media:
6 mo–12 yr: 30 mg/kg/24 hr PO ÷ Q12 hr
Pharyngitis/tonsillitis:
2–12 yr: 15 mg/kg/24 hr PO ÷ Q12 hr

Acute sinusitis:
6 mo–12 yr: 15–30 mg/kg/24 hr PO ÷ Q12–24 hr

Uncomplicated skin infections:
2–12 yr: 20 mg/kg/24 hr PO ÷ Q24 hr

Other:
≥13 yr and adult: 500–1000 mg/24 hr PO ÷ Q12–24 hr

Max. dose: 1 g/24 hr

Continued

CEFPROZIL *continued*

Use with caution in penicillin-allergic patients or in presence of renal impairment. Oral suspension contains aspartame and phenylalanine and should not be used by phenylketonurics. May cause nausea, vomiting, diarrhea, liver enzyme elevations, and false-positive urine-reducing substance (Clinitest and other copper-reduction method tests) and Coombs test. Absorption is not affected by food. **Adjust dose in renal failure (see Chapter 30).**

CEFTAZIDIME

Fortaz, Tazidime, Tazicef, Ceptaz (arginine salt)
Antibiotic, cephalosporin (third generation)

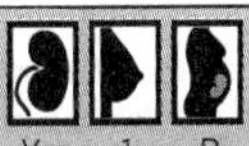

Injection: 0.5, 1, 2, 6, 10 g
Frozen injection: 1 g/50 mL 4.4% dextrose, 2 g/50 mL 3.2% dextrose (iso-osmotic solutions)
(Fortaz, Tazicef, Tazidime contains 2.3 mEq Na/g drug)
(Ceptaz contains 349 mg L-arginine/g drug)

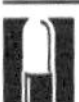

Neonate: IV/IM:
Postnatal age ≤7 days: 100 mg/kg/24 hr ÷ Q12 hr
Postnatal age >7 days:
<1200 g: 100 mg/kg/24 hr ÷ Q12 hr
≥1200 g: 150 mg/kg/24 hr ÷ Q8 hr
Infant and child: 90–150 mg/kg/24 hr ÷ Q8 hr IV/IM; **max. dose:** 6 g/24 hr
Cystic fibrosis and meningitis: 150 mg/kg/24 hr ÷ Q8 hr IV/IM; **max. dose:** 6 g/24 hr
Adult: 2–6 g/24 hr ÷ Q8–12 hr IV/IM; **max. dose:** 6 g/24 hr

Use with caution in penicillin-allergic patients or in presence of renal impairment. Good *Pseudomonas* species coverage and CSF penetration. May cause rash, liver enzyme elevations, and false-positive urine-reducing substance and Coombs test. **Adjust dose in renal failure (see Chapter 30).**

CEFTIBUTEN

Cedax
Antibiotic, cephalosporin (third generation)

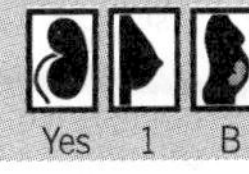

Suspension: 90 mg/5 mL (30, 60, 90, 120 mL); 180 mg/5 mL (30, 60, 120 mL)
Caps: 400 mg

Child:
Otitis media and pharyngitis/tonsillitis: 9 mg/kg/24 hr PO QD; **max. dose:** 400 mg/24 hr
≥12 yr: 400 mg PO QD; **max. dose:** 400 mg/24 hr

Use with caution in penicillin-allergic patients or in presence of renal impairment. May cause GI symptoms and elevations in eosinophils and BUN. Suspension should be administered 2 hr before or 1 hr after a meal. **Adjust dose in renal failure (see Chapter 30).**

For explanation of icons, see p. 680.

CEFTIZOXIME
Cefizox
Antibiotic, cephalosporin (third generation)

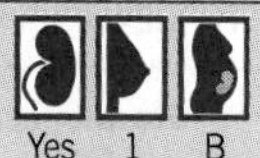

Injection: 0.5, 1, 2, 10 g
Frozen injection: 1 g/50 mL 3.8% dextrose, 2 g/50 mL 1.9% dextrose (iso-osmotic solutions)
Contains 2.6 mEq Na/g drug.

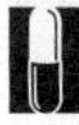

Infant >1 mo and <6 mo: 100–200 mg/kg/24 hr ÷ Q6–8 hr IV/IM
Infant ≥6 mo and child: 150–200 mg/kg/24 hr ÷ Q6–8 hr IV/IM; **max. dose:** 12 g/24 hr
Adult: 2–12 g/24 hr ÷ Q8–12 hr IV/IM; **max. dose:** 12 g/24 hr
Uncomplicated gonorrhea: 1 g IM × 1

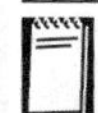

Use with caution in penicillin-allergic patients or in presence of renal impairment. May cause liver enzyme elevation, false-positive urine-reducing substances (Clinitest). Good CNS penetration. **Adjust dose in renal failure (see Chapter 30).**

CEFTRIAXONE
Rocephin
Antibiotic, cephalosporin (third generation)

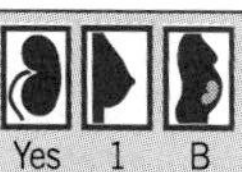

Injection: 0.25, 0.5, 1, 2, 10 g
Frozen injection: 1 g/50 mL 3.8% dextrose, 2 g/50 mL 2.4% dextrose (iso-osmotic solutions)
Intramuscular kit with 1% lidocaine diluent: 0.5, 1 g
Contains 3.6 mEq Na/g drug.

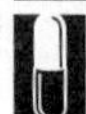

Neonate:
Gonococcal ophthalmia or prophylaxis: 25–50 mg/kg/dose IM/IV × 1; **max. dose**: 125 mg/dose
Infant and child: 50–75 mg/kg/24 hr ÷ Q12–24 hr IM/IV; **max. dose:** 2 g/24 hr (see remarks)
Meningitis (including penicillin resistant pneumococci): 100 mg/kg/24 hr IM/IV ÷ Q12 hr; **max. dose:** 4 g/24 hr
Acute otitis media: 50 mg/kg IM × 1; **max. dose:** 1g
Adult: 1–2 g/dose Q12–24 hr IV/IM; **max. dose:** 4 g/24 hr
Uncomplicated gonorrhea or chancroid: 250 mg IM × 1

Continued

CEFTRIAXONE *continued*

Use with caution in penicillin-allergic patients or in presence of renal impairment. May cause reversible cholelithiasis, sludging in gallbladder, and jaundice.

Use with caution in neonates and continuous dosing because of risk for hyperbilirubinemia. Consider using an alternative third-generation cephalosporin with similar activity.

80–100 mg/kg/24 hr ÷ Q12–24 hr has been recommended for infections outside the CSF due to penicillin-resistant pneumococci.

For IM injections, dilute drug with either sterile water for injection or 1% lidocaine to a concentration of 250 or 350 mg/mL (250 mg/mL has lower incidence of injection site reactions). See *Lidocaine* for additional remarks.

CEFUROXIME (IV, IM)/CEFUROXIME AXETIL (PO)

IV: Zinacef; PO: Ceftin

Antibiotic, cephalosporin (second generation)

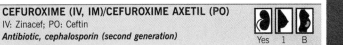

Injection: 0.75, 1.5, 7.5 g
Frozen injection: 750 mg/50 mL 2.8% dextrose, 1.5 g/50 mL water (iso-osmotic solutions)
Injectable dosage forms contain 2.4 mEq Na/g drug.
Tabs: 125, 250, 500 mg
Suspension: 125, 250 mg/5 mL (50, 100 mL)

IM/IV:
Neonate: 20–60 mg/kg/24 hr ÷ Q12 hr
Infant (>3 mo)/child: 75–150 mg/kg/24 hr ÷ Q8 hr;
Max. dose: 6 g/24 hr
Adult: 750–1500 mg/dose Q8 hr;
Max. dose: 9 g/24 hr

PO:
Child (3 mo–12 yr):
Pharyngitis:
Suspension: 20 mg/kg/24 hr ÷ Q12 hr; **max. dose:** 500 mg/24 hr
Tab: 125 mg Q12 hr
Otitis media, impetigo, and maxillary sinusitis:
Suspension: 30 mg/kg/24 hr ÷ Q12 hr; **max. dose:** 1 g/24 hr
Tab: 250 mg Q12 hr
Adult: 250–500 mg BID
Max. dose: 1 g/24 hr

Continued

For explanation of icons, see p. 680.

CEFUROXIME (IV, IM)/CEFUROXIME AXETIL (PO) *continued*

Use with caution in penicillin-allergic patients or in presence of renal impairment. May cause GI discomfort; thrombophlebitis at the infusion site; false-positive urine-reducing substance (Clinitest and other copper-reduction method tests) and Coombs test; and may interfere with serum and urine creatinine determinations by the alkaline picrate method. **Not recommended** for meningitis.

Tablets and suspension are **NOT** bioequivalent and are **NOT** substitutable on a mg/mg basis. Administer suspension with food. Concurrent use of antacids, H_2 blockers, and proton pump inhibitors may decrease oral absorption. **Adjust dose in renal failure (see Chapter 30).**

CEPHALEXIN

Keflex, Biocef, and others

Antibiotic, cephalosporin (first generation)

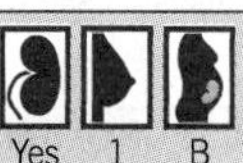

Tabs: 250, 500 mg
Caps: 250, 500 mg
Suspension: 125 mg/5 mL, 250 mg/5 mL (100, 200 mL)

Infant and child (see remarks): 25–100 mg/kg/24 hr PO ÷ Q6 hr
Adult: 1–4 g/24 hr PO ÷ Q6 hr
Max. dose: 4 g/24 hr

Some cross-reactivity with penicillins. **Use with caution** in renal insufficiency. May cause GI discomfort; false-positive urine-reducing substance (Clinitest and other copper-reduction method tests) and Coombs test; false elevation of serum theophylline levels (HPLC method); and false urinary protein test. May increase the effects of metformin.

Administer doses on an empty stomach, 2 hr before or 1 hr after meals. Less frequent dosing (Q8–12 hr) can be used for uncomplicated infections.

Total daily dose may be divided Q12 hr for streptococcal pharyngitis (>1 yr) and for skin or skin structure infections.

Adjust dose in renal failure (see Chapter 30).

CEPHRADINE

Velosef and others

Antibiotic, cephalosporin (first generation)

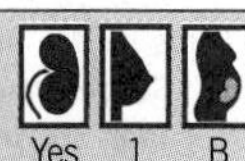

Suspension: 125 mg/5 mL, 250 mg/5 mL (100, 200 mL)
Caps: 250, 500 mg
Injection: 0.25, 0.5, 1, 2 g (6 mEq Na/1g)

Infant (≥9 mo) and child: PO: 25–50 mg/kg/24 hr ÷ Q6–12 hr
Adult: PO: 1–4 g/24 hr ÷ Q6–12 hr
Max. dose: 4 g/24 hr

Continued

CEPHRADINE *continued*

Use with caution in penicillin-allergic patients and in those with renal insufficiency. **Does not** penetrate well into CSF. May cause GI discomfort; transient eosinophilia; interfere with serum and urine creatinine assays and theophylline assays (HPLC method); and cause false-positive urinary protein and urine-reducing substances (Clinitest).

Adjust dose in renal failure (see Chapter 30).

CETIRIZINE

Zyrtec, Zyrtec-D 12 Hour

Antihistamine, less sedating

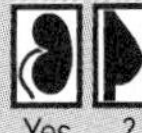
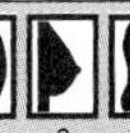
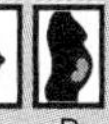

Yes ? B

Syrup: 5 mg/5 mL (120, 473 mL)
Tabs and chewable tabs: 5, 10 mg
Extended-release tabs in combination with pseudoephedrine (PE):
Zyrtec-D 12 Hour: 5 mg cetirizine + 120 mg PE

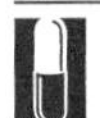

Cetirizine (see remarks):
6 mo and < 2 yr: 2.5 mg PO QD; dose may be increased for child 12–23 mo to a **max. dose** of 2.5 mg PO Q12 hr.
2–5 yr: initial dose: 2.5 mg PO QD; if needed, may increase dose to a **max. dose** of 5 mg/24 hr.
≥6 yr–adult: 5–10 mg PO QD

Extended-release tabs of cetirizine and pseudoephedrine:
≥12 yr and adult:
Zyrtec-D 12 Hour: 1 tablet PO BID

May cause headache, pharyngitis, GI symptoms, dry mouth, and sedation. Aggressive reactions and convulsions have been reported. Has **NOT** been implicated in causing cardiac arrhythmias when used with other drugs that are metabolized by hepatic microsomal enzymes (e.g., ketoconazole, erythromycin).

In hepatic impairment, the following doses have been recommended:
<6 yr: use is **not recommended.**
6 yr–adult: 5 mg PO QD

Doses may be administered regardless to food. For Zyrtec-D 12 Hour, see *Pseudoephedrine* for additional remarks. **Dosage adjustment is recommended in renal impairment (see Chapter 30).**

CHARCOAL, ACTIVATED

See *Chapter 2*

For explanation of icons, see p. 680.

CHLORAL HYDRATE

Aquachloral Supprettes and others

Sedative, hypnotic

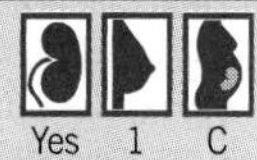

Caps: 500 mg
Syrup: 250, 500 mg/5 mL
Suppository: 324, 500, 648 mg

Child:

Sedative: 25–50 mg/kg/24 hr PO/PR ÷ Q6–8 hr; **max. dose:** 500 mg/dose

Sedation for procedures: 25–100 mg/kg/dose PO/PR; **max. dose:** 1 g/dose (infant); 2 g/dose (child)

Adult:

Sedative: 250 mg/dose TID PO/PR

Hypnotic: 500–1000 mg/dose PO/PR; **max. dose:** 2 g/24 hr

Contraindicated in patients with hepatic or renal disease. Use with caution in combination with IV furosemide (vasodilation) or warfarin (potentiates warfarin). May cause GI irritation, paradoxical excitement, hypotension, and myocardial/respiratory depression. Chronic administration in neonates can lead to accumulation of active metabolites. Requires same monitoring as other sedatives.

Not analgesic. Peak effects occur within 30–60 min. **Do not exceed** 2 wk of chronic use. **Avoid use** in moderate to severe renal failure. Sudden withdrawal may cause delirium tremens.

For additional information, see Chapter 28.

CHLORAMPHENICOL

Chloromycetin and others

Antibiotic

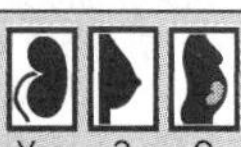

Injection: 1 g (2.25 mEq Na/1g)

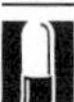

Neonate IV:

Loading dose: 20 mg/kg

Maintenance dose (first dose should be given 12 hr after loading dose):

≤7 days: 25 mg/kg/24 hr QD

>7 days:

≤2 kg: 25 mg/kg/24 hr QD

>2 kg: 50 mg/kg/24 hr ÷ Q12 hr

Infant/child/adult: 50–75 mg/kg/24 hr IV ÷ Q6 hr

Meningitis: 75–100 mg/kg/24 hr IV ÷ Q6 hr

Max. dose: 4 g/24 hr

Dose recommendations are just guidelines for therapy; monitoring of blood levels is essential in neonates and infants. Follow hematologic status for dose-related or idiosyncratic marrow suppression. "Gray baby" syndrome may be seen with levels >50 mg/L. **Use with caution** in G6PD deficiency, renal or hepatic dysfunction, and neonates.

Continued

CHLORAMPHENICOL *continued*

Concomitant use of phenobarbital and rifampin may lower chloramphenicol serum levels. Phenytoin may increase chloramphenicol serum levels. Chloramphenicol may increase phenytoin levels, reduce metabolism of oral anticoagulants, and decrease absorption of vitamin B_{12}.

Therapeutic levels: 15–25 mg/L for meningitis; 10–20 mg/L for other infections. Trough: 5–15 mg/L for meningitis; 5–10 mg/L for other infections. Recommended serum sampling time: trough (IV/PO) within 30 min before next dose; peak (IV) 30 min after the end of infusion; peak (PO) 2 hr after oral administration. Time to achieve steady state: 2–3 days for newborns; 12–24 hr for children and adults.

NOTE: higher serum levels may be achieved using the oral rather than the IV route.

CHLOROQUINE HCL/PHOSPHATE

Aralen and others

Amebicide, antimalarial

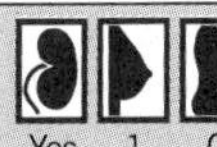

Tabs: 250, 500 mg as phosphate (150, 300 mg base, respectively)
Suspension: 16.67 mg/mL as phosphate (10 mg/mL base)
Injection: 50 mg/mL as HCl (40 mg/mL base) (5 mL)

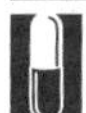

Doses expressed in mg of chloroquine base:

Malaria prophylaxis (start 1 wk before exposure and continue for 4 wk after leaving endemic area):

Child: 5 mg/kg/dose PO Q wk; **max. dose**: 300 mg/dose
Adult: 300 mg/dose PO Q wk

Malaria treatment (chloroquine sensitive strains):

For treatment of malaria, consult with ID specialist or see the latest edition of the AAP *Red Book*. For IV use, consider safer alternatives such as quinidine or quinine.

Child: 10 mg/kg/dose (**max. dose:** 600 mg/dose) PO × 1; followed by 5 mg/kg/dose (**max. dose:** 300 mg/dose) 6 hr later and then once daily for 2 days

Adult: 600 mg/dose PO × 1; followed by 300 mg/dose 6 hr later and then once daily for 2 days

Use with caution in liver disease, preexisting auditory damage or seizures, G6PD deficiency, or concomitant hepatotoxic drugs. May cause nausea, vomiting, blurred vision, retinal and corneal changes, headaches, confusion, skeletal muscle weakness, and hair depigmentation.

Antacids, ampicillin, and kaolin may decrease the absorption of chloroquine (allow 4-hr interval between these and chloroquine). May increase serum cyclosporin levels. **Adjust dose in renal failure (see Chapter 30).**

For explanation of icons, see p. 680.

CHLOROTHIAZIDE

Diuril, Diurigen, and others
Thiazide diuretic

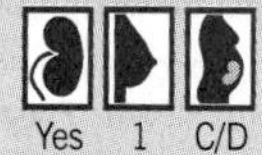
Yes 1 C/D

Tabs: 250, 500 mg
Suspension: 250 mg/5 mL (237 mL)
Injection: 500 mg (5 mEq Na/1g)

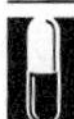

<6 mo: 20–40 mg/kg/24 hr ÷ Q12 hr PO/IV; alternatively, lower IV doses of 2–8 mg/kg/24 hr ÷ Q12 hr may be used.

≥6 mo: 20 mg/kg/24 hr ÷ Q12 hr PO/IV; alternatively, lower IV doses of 4 mg/kg/24 hr ÷ Q12-24 hr may be used.

Max. PO dose:
≤2 yr: 375 mg/24 hr
2–12 yr: 1 g/24 hr

Adult: 500–2000 mg/24 hr ÷ Q12-24 hr PO/IV; alternative IV dosing, some may respond to intermittent dosing on alternate days or on 3–5 days each week.

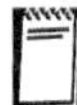

Use with caution in liver and severe renal disease. May increase serum calcium, bilirubin, glucose, and uric acid. May cause alkalosis, pancreatitis, dizziness, hypokalemia, and hypomagnesemia.

Avoid IM or SC administration.

Pregnancy category changes to D if used in pregnancy-induced hypertension.

CHLORPHENIRAMINE MALEATE/ DEXCHLORPHENIRAMINE MALEATE

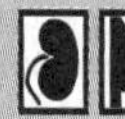
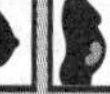
No ? B

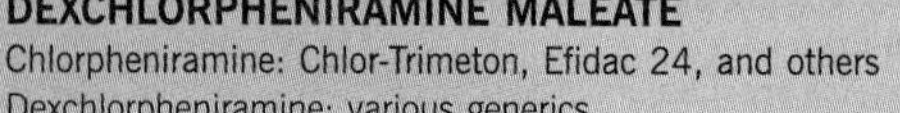

Chlorpheniramine: Chlor-Trimeton, Efidac 24, and others
Dexchlorpheniramine: various generics
Antihistamine

Chlorpheniramine maleate:
Tabs: 4 mg
Chewable tabs: 2 mg
Sustained-release caps and tabs: 8, 12 mg
Combined immediate and sustained-release tabs (Efidac 24): 16 mg (4 mg immediate and 12 mg sustained)
Syrup: 2 mg/5 mL (473 mL) (contains 5% alcohol)

Dexchlorpheniramine maleate:
Sustained-release tabs: 4, 6 mg
Oral solution: 2mg/5 mL (473 mL)

Chlorpheniramine maleate dosing:
Child: 0.35 mg/kg/24 hr PO ÷ Q4–6 hr or dose based on age below
2–6 yr: 1 mg/dose PO Q4–6 hr; **max. dose:** 6 mg/24 hr
6–11 yr: 2 mg/dose PO Q4–6 hr; **max. dose:** 12 mg/24 hr
Sustained release (6–12 yr): 8 mg/dose PO Q12 hr

Continued

CHLORHENIRAMINE MALEATE/DEXCHLORPHENIRAMINE MALEATE *continued*

≥12 yr–adult: 4 mg/dose Q4–6 hr PO; **max. dose:** 24 mg/24 hr
Sustained release: 8–12 mg PO Q 12 hr
Efidac 24: 16 mg PO Q24 hr; **max. dose:** 16 mg/24 hr

Dexchlorpheniramine maleate dosing:
2–5 yr: 0.5 mg/dose PO Q4–6hr; **max. dose:** 3 mg/24 hr
6–11 yr: 1 mg/dose PO Q4–6 hr; **max. dose:** 6 mg/24 hr
Sustained release: 4 mg PO QHS
≥12 yr–adult:
Sustained release: 4–6 mg PO QHS or Q8–10 hr; **max. dose:** 12 mg/24 hr

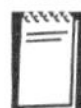

Use with caution in asthma. May cause sedation, dry mouth, blurred vision, urinary retention, polyuria, and disturbed coordination. Young children may be paradoxically excited.

NOTE: Dexchlorpheniramine maleate doses are 50% of chlorpheniramine maleate; it does not possess any significant advantages over other antihistamines.

Doses may be administered PRN. Administer oral doses with food. Sustained-release forms are **NOT** recommended in children <6 yr and should **NOT** be crushed, chewed, or dissolved.

CHLORPROMAZINE

Thorazine and others
Antiemetic, antipsychotic, phenothiazine derivative

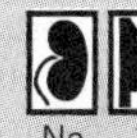
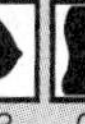

No 3 C

Tabs: 10, 25, 50, 100, 200 mg
Extended-release caps: 30, 75, 150 mg
Syrup: 10 mg/5 mL (120 mL)
Suppository: 25, 100 mg
Oral concentrate: 30 mg/mL (120 mL), 100 mg/mL (240 mL)
Injection: 25 mg/mL (contains 2% benzyl alcohol)

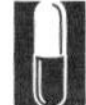

Psychosis:
Child >6 mo:
IM/IV: 2.5–4 mg/kg/24 hr ÷ Q6–8 hr
PO: 2.5–6 mg/kg/24 hr ÷ Q4–6 hr
PR: 1 mg/kg/dose Q6–8 hr
Max. IM/IV dose:
<5 yr: 40 mg/24 hr
5–12 yr: 75 mg/24 hr

Adult:
IM/IV: Initial: 25 mg; repeat with 25–50 mg/dose, if needed, Q1–4 hr up to a **max. dose** of 400 mg/dose Q4–6 hr
PO: 10–25 mg/dose Q4–6 hr; **max. dose**: 2 g/24 hr

Antiemetic:
Child (≥6 mo):
IV/IM: 0.55 mg/kg/dose Q6–8 hr PRN

Continued

For explanation of icons, see p. 680.

CHLORPROMAZINE *continued*

Max. IM/IV dose:
<5 yr: 40 mg/24 hr
5–12 yr: 75 mg/24 hr
PO: 0.55 mg/kg/dose Q4–6 hr PRN
PR: 1.1 mg/kg/dose Q6–8 hr PRN

Adult:
IV/IM: 25–50 mg/dose Q4–6 hr PRN
PO: 10–25 mg/dose Q4–6 hr PRN
PR: 50–100 mg/dose Q6–8 hr PRN

Adverse effects include drowsiness, jaundice, lowered seizure threshold, extrapyramidal/anticholinergic symptoms, hypotension (more with IV), arrhythmias, agranulocytosis, and neuroleptic malignant syndrome. May potentiate effect of narcotics, sedatives, and other drugs. Monitor BP closely. ECG changes include prolonged PR interval, flattened T waves, and ST depression. **Do not administer** oral liquid dosage form simultaneously with carbamazepine oral suspension because an orange rubbery precipitate may form.

CHOLESTYRAMINE

Questran, Questran Light, LoCHOLEST, LoCHOLEST Light, Prevalite, and others
Antilipemic, binding resin

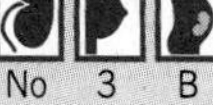
No 3 B

Questran, LoCHOLEST, and others: 4 g anhydrous resin per 9 g powder (9, 378 g)
Questran Light: 4 g anhydrous resin per 5 g powder with aspartame (5, 5.7, 210, 231, 239 g)
LoCHOLEST Light: 4 g anhydrous resin per 5.7 g powder with aspartame (5.7, 240 g)
Prevalite: 4 g anhydrous resin per 5.5 g powder with aspartame (5.5, 231 g)

All doses based in terms of anhydrous resin. Titrate dose based on response and tolerance.

Child: 240 mg/kg/24 hr ÷ TID; doses normally do not exceed 8 g/24 hr. Give PO as slurry in water, juice, or milk before meals.

Adult: 3–4 g of cholestyramine BID-QID

Max. dose: 32 g/24 hr

In addition to the use for managing hypercholesterolemia, drug may be used for itching associated with elevated bile acids and diarrheal disorders associated with excess fecal bile acids or *Clostridium difficile* (pseudomembranous colitis). May cause constipation, abdominal distention, vomiting, vitamin deficiencies (A, D, E, K), and rash. Hyperchloremic acidosis may occur with prolonged use.

Give other oral medications 4–6 hr after cholestyramine or 1 hr before dose to avoid decreased absorption.

CHOLINE MAGNESIUM TRISALICYLATE

Trilisate and others

Nonsteroidal antiinflammatory agent

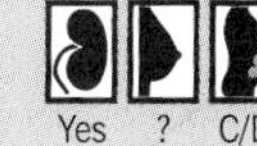

Combination of choline salicylate and magnesium salicylate (1:1.24 ratio, respectively); strengths expressed in terms of mg salicylate:
Tabs: 500, 750, 1000 mg
Liquid: 500 mg/5 mL (237 mL)

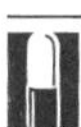

Dose based on total salicylate content.
Child: 30–60 mg/kg/24 hr PO ÷ TID–QID
Adult: 500 mg–1.5 g/dose PO QD–TID

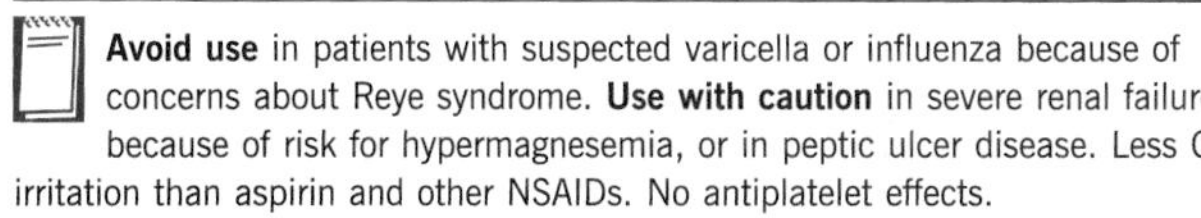

Avoid use in patients with suspected varicella or influenza because of concerns about Reye syndrome. **Use with caution** in severe renal failure because of risk for hypermagnesemia, or in peptic ulcer disease. Less GI irritation than aspirin and other NSAIDs. No antiplatelet effects.

Pregnancy category changes to D if used during the third trimester.

Therapeutic salicylate levels—see *Aspirin*. 500 mg choline magnesium trisalicylate is equivalent to 650 mg aspirin.

CIDOFOVIR

Vistide

Antiviral

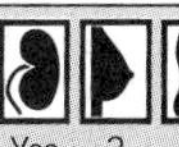

Injection: 75 mg/mL (5 mL)

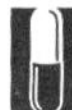

Safety and efficacy have not been established in children.
CMV retinitis:
Induction: 5 mg/kg IV × 1 with probenecid and hydration
Maintenance: 3 mg/kg IV Q7 days with probenecid and hydration
Adenovirus infection after bone marrow transplantation (limited data):
5 mg/kg/dose IV once weekly × 3, followed by 5 mg/kg/dose IV once every 2 wk. Administer oral probenecid 1–1.25 g/m^2/dose (rounded to the nearest 250-mg interval) 3 hr before and 1 hr and 8 hr after each dose of cidofovir. Also give IV normal saline at 3 times maintenance fluid 1 hr before and 1 hr after cidofovir, followed by 2 times maintenance fluid for an additional 2 hr.

Contraindicated in hypersensitivity to probenecid or sulfa-containing drugs, sCr >1.5 mg/dL, CrCl ≤55 mL/min, urine protein ≥100 mg/dL (2+ proteinuria), and concomitant nephrotoxic drugs. **Renal impairment is the major dose-limiting toxicity.** IV NS prehydration and probenecid must be used to reduce risk for nephrotoxicity. May also cause nausea, vomiting, headache, rash, metabolic acidosis, uveitis, decreased intraocular pressure, and neutropenia.

Reduce dose to 3 mg/kg if sCr increases 0.3–0.4 mg/dL from baseline. Discontinue therapy if sCr increases >0.5 mg/dL from baseline or development of >3+ proteinuria.

Administer doses via IV infusion over 1 hr at a concentration ≤8 mg/mL.

For explanation of icons, see p. 680.

CIMETIDINE

Tagamet, Tagamet HB [OTC], and others

Histamine-2 antagonist

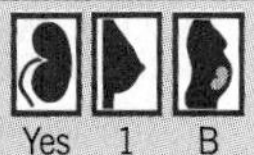

Tabs: 100 (OTC), 200, 300, 400, 800 mg
Syrup: 300 mg/5 mL (240, 470 mL) (contains 2.8% alcohol)
Injection: 150 mg/mL
Premixed injection: 300 mg in 50 mL normal saline

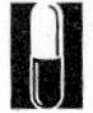

Neonate: 5–20 mg/kg/24 hr IM/PO/IV ÷ Q6–12 hr
Infant: 10–20 mg/kg/24 hr IM/PO/IV ÷ Q6–12 hr
Child: 20–40 mg/kg/24 hr IM/PO/IV ÷ Q6 hr
Adult:
PO: 300 mg/dose QID or 400 mg/dose BID or 800 mg/dose QHS
IV/IM: 300 mg/dose Q6 hr; **max. dose:** 2400 mg/24 hr
Continuous IV infusion: 150 mg IV × 1 followed by 37.5 mg/hr; infusions have ranged from 40–600 mg/hr with a mean rate of 160 mg/hr.
Ulcer prophylaxis: 400–800 mg PO QHS

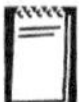

Diarrhea, rash, myalgia, confusion, neutropenia, gynecomastia, elevated liver function tests, or dizziness may occur.

Increases levels and effects of many hepatically metabolized drugs (i.e., theophylline, phenytoin, lidocaine, diazepam, warfarin). Cimetidine may decrease the absorption of iron, ketoconazole, and tetracyclines. **Adjust dose in renal failure (see Chapter 30).**

CIPROFLOXACIN

Cipro, Cipro XR, Ciloxan ophthalmic, Cipro HC Otic

Antibiotic, quinolone

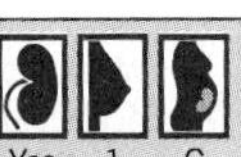

Tabs: 100, 250, 500, 750 mg
Extended-release tabs (Cipro XR): 500, 1000 mg
Oral suspension: 250, 500 mg/5 mL (100 mL)
Injection: 10 mg/mL (20, 40 mL)
Premixed injection: 200 mg/100 mL 5% dextrose, 400 mg/100 mL 5% dextrose (iso-osmotic solutions)
Ophthalmic solution: 3.5 mg/mL (2.5, 5 mL)
Ophthalmic ointment: 3.3 mg/g (3.5 g)
Otitic suspension (Cipro HC Otic): 2 mg/mL ciprofloxacin + 10 mg/mL hydrocortisone (10 mL)

Continued

CIPROFLOXACIN *continued*

Child:
PO: 20–30 mg/kg/24 hr ÷ Q12 hr; **max. dose:** 1.5 g/24 hr
IV: 10–20 mg/kg/24 hr ÷ Q12 hr; **max. dose:** 800 mg/24 hr
Cystic fibrosis:
PO: 40 mg/kg/24 hr ÷ Q12 hr; **max. dose:** 2 g/24 hr
IV: 30 mg/kg/24 hr ÷ Q8 hr; **max. dose:** 1.2 g/24 hr
Anthrax (see remarks):
Inhalational/systemic/cutaneous: start with 20–30 mg/kg/24 hr ÷ Q12 hr IV (**max. dose:** 800 mg/24 hr), and convert to oral dosing with clinical improvement at 20–30 mg/kg/24 hr ÷ Q12 hr PO (**max. dose:** 1 g/24 hr). Duration of therapy: 60 days (IV and PO combined)
Postexposure prophylaxis: 20–30 mg/kg/24 hr ÷ Q12 hr PO × 60 days; **max. dose:** 1 g/24 hr

Adult:
PO:
Immediate release: 250–750 mg/dose Q12 hr
Extended release (Cipro XR):
Uncomplicated UTI/cystitis: 500 mg/dose Q24 hr
Complicated UTI/uncomplicated pyelonephritis: 1000 mg/dose Q24 hr
IV: 200–400 mg/dose Q12 hr
Anthrax (see remarks):
Inhalational/systemic/cutaneous: start with 400 mg/dose Q12 hr IV, and convert to oral dosing with clinical improvement at 500 mg/dose Q12 hr PO. Duration of therapy: 60 days (IV and PO combined)
Postexposure prophylaxis: 500 mg/dose Q12 hr PO × 60 days

Ophthalmic solution: 1–2 drops Q2 hr while awake × 2 days, then 1–2 gtts Q4 hr while awake × 5 days
Ophthalmic ointment: apply 0.5-inch ribbon TID × 2, then BID × 5 days.
Otic:
>1 yr and adult: 3 drops to affected ear(s) BID × 7 days

Can cause GI upset, renal failure, and seizures. GI symptoms, headache, restlessness, and rash are common side effects. **Use with caution** in children <18 yr. Like other quinolones, tendon rupture can occur during or after therapy. **Do not use** otic suspension with perforated tympanic membranes.

Combination antimicrobial therapy is recommended for anthrax. For penicillin-susceptible strains, consider changing to high-dose amoxicillin (25–35 mg/kg/dose TID PO). See www.bt.cdc.gov for the latest information.

Ciprofloxacin can increase effects and/or toxicity of theophylline, warfarin, and cyclosporine.

Do not administer antacids or other divalent salts with or within 2–4 hr of oral ciprofloxacin dose. **Adjust dose in renal failure (see Chapter 30).**

For explanation of icons, see p. 680.

CITRATE MIXTURES

Alkalinizing agent, electrolyte supplement

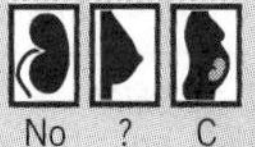

No ? C

Each mL contains (mEq):

	Na	K	Citrate or HCO_3^-
Polycitra or Cytra-3 (120, 480 mL)	1	1	2
Polycitra-LC or Cytra-LC (120, 480 mL)*	1	1	2
Polycitra-K or Cytra-K (120, 480 mL)	0	2	2
Bicitra or Cytra-2 (15, 30, 120, 480 mL)	1	0	1
Oracit (15, 30, 500 mL)	1	0	1

*LC, low calorie (contains no sucrose, sorbitol, or glycerin).

Dilute in water or juice, and administer doses after meals and at bedtime. All mEq doses based on citrate.

Child: 5–15 mL/dose Q6–8 hr PO or 2–3 mEq/kg/24 hr PO ÷ Q6–8 hr

Adult: 15–30 mL/dose Q6–8 hr PO or 100–200 mEq/24 hr ÷ Q6–8 hr

Contraindicated in severe renal impairment and acute dehydration. **Use with caution** in patients already receiving potassium supplements and in those who are sodium restricted. May have laxative effect and cause hypocalcemia and metabolic alkalosis.

Adjust dose to maintain desired pH. 1 mEq of citrate is equivalent to 1 mEq HCO_3 in patients with normal hepatic function.

CLARITHROMYCIN

Biaxin, Biaxin XL

Antibiotic, macrolide

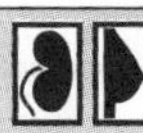 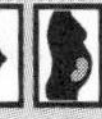 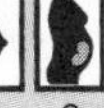

Yes 2 C

Film tablets: 250, 500 mg
Extended-release tablets: 500 mg
Granules for suspension: 125, 250 mg/5 mL (50, 100 mL)

Child:

Acute otitis media, pharyngitis/tonsillitis, pneumonia, acute maxillary sinusitis, or uncomplicated skin infections: 15 mg/kg/24 hr PO ÷ Q12 hr

M. avium complex prophylaxis (first episode and recurrence): 15 mg/kg/24 hr PO ÷ Q12 hr

Max. dose: 1 g/24 hr

Continued

CLARITHROMYCIN *continued*

Adult:

Pharyngitis/tonsillitis, acute maxillary sinusitis, bronchitis, pneumonia, or uncomplicated skin infections:

Immediate release: 250–500 mg/dose Q12 hr PO

Biaxin XL: 1000 mg Q24 hr PO (currently not indicated for pharyngitis/tonsillitis or uncomplicated skin infections)

M. avium complex prophylaxis (1st episode and recurrence): 500 mg/dose Q12 hr PO

Contraindicated in patients allergic to erythromycin. As with other macrolides, clarithromycin has been associated with QT prolongation and ventricular arrhythmias, including ventricular tachycardia and torsades de pointes. May cause cardiac arrhythmias in patients also receiving cisapride. Side effects: diarrhea, nausea, abnormal taste, dyspepsia, abdominal discomfort (less than erythromycin but greater than azithromycin), and headache. Rare cases of anaphylaxis, Stevens-Johnson, and toxic epidermal necrolysis have been reported. May increase carbamazepine, theophylline, cyclosporin, and tacrolimus levels.

Adjust dose in renal failure (see Chapter 30). Doses, regardless of dosage form, may be administered with food.

CLEMASTINE

Tavist, Allehist-1, Dayhist-1, and others

Antihistamine

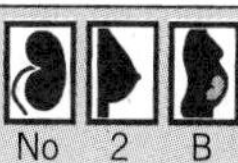

Available as clemastine fumarate salt:

Tabs: 1.34 mg (1 mg base) [OTC], 2.68 mg (2 mg base)

Syrup: 0.67 mg/5 mL (0.5 mg/5 mL base) (120 mL) (contains 5.5% alcohol)

Doses expressed as clemastine base

Infant and child <6yr: 0.05 mg/kg/24 hr ÷ BID–TID PO; **max. dose:** 1 mg/24 hr

6–12 yr: 0.5 mg BID PO; **max. dose**: 3 mg/24 hr

>12 yr and adult: 1 mg BID PO; if needed, may increase dose up to a **max. dose** of 6 mg/24 hr

Contraindicated in narrow-angle glaucoma, bladder neck obstruction, and stenosing peptic ulcer. May cause dizziness, drowsiness, dry mouth, and constipation. Doses may be taken with food.

For explanation of icons, see p. 680.

CLINDAMYCIN
Cleocin-T, Cleocin, and others
Antibiotic

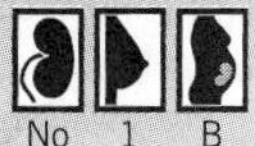

Caps: 75, 150, 300 mg
Oral solution: 75 mg/5 mL (100 mL)
Injection: 150 mg/mL (contains 9.45 mg/mL benzyl alcohol)
Solution, topical: 1% (30, 60, 480 mL)
Gel, topical: 1% (7.5, 30, 42, 60, 77 g)
Lotion, topical: 1% (60 mL)
Vaginal cream: 2% (40 g)
Vaginal suppository: 100 mg (3s)

Neonate: IV/IM: *5 mg/kg/dose*
≤7 days:
≤2 kg: Q12 hr
>2 kg: Q8 hr
>7 days:
<1.2 kg: Q12 hr
1.2–2 kg: Q8 hr
>2 kg: Q6 hr
Child:
PO: 10–30 mg/kg/24 hr ÷ Q6–8 hr
IM/IV: 25–40 mg/kg/24 hr ÷ Q6–8 hr
Adult:
PO: 150–450 mg/dose Q6–8 hr; **max. dose:** 1.8 g/24 hr
IM/IV: 1200–1800 mg/24 hr IM/IV ÷ Q6–12 hr; **max. dose:** 4.8 g/24 hr
Topical: apply to affected area BID.
Bacterial vaginosis:
Suppositories: 100 mg/dose QHS × 3 days
Vaginal cream (2%): 1 applicator dose (5 g) QHS for 3 or 7 days in nonpregnant patients and for 7 days in pregnant patients in second and third trimester

Not indicated in meningitis; CSF penetration is poor. Pseudomembranous colitis may occur up to several weeks after cessation of therapy. May cause diarrhea, rash, Stevens-Johnson syndrome, granulocytopenia, thrombocytopenia, or sterile abscess at injection site.

Clindamycin may increase the neuromuscular blocking effects of tubocurarine, pancuronium. **Do not exceed** IV infusion rate of 30 mg/min because hypotension and cardiac arrest have been reported with rapid infusions.

C

CLONAZEPAM
Klonopin
Benzodiazepine

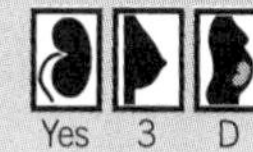

Tabs: 0.5, 1, 2 mg
Disintegrating oral tabs: 0.125, 0.25, 0.5, 1, 2 mg
Suspension: 100 mcg/mL

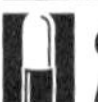

Child <10 yr or <30 kg:
Initial: 0.01–0.03 mg/kg/24 hr ÷ Q8 hr PO
Increment: 0.25–0.5 mg/24 hr Q3 days, up to **max. maintenance dose** of 0.1–0.2 mg/kg/24 hr ÷ Q8 hr
Child ≥10 yr or ≥30 kg and adult:
Initial: 1.5 mg/24 hr PO ÷ TID
Increment: 0.5–1 mg/24 hr Q3 days; **max. dose:** 20 mg/24 hr

Contraindicated in severe liver disease and acute narrow-angle glaucoma. Drowsiness, behavior changes, increased bronchial secretions, GI, CV, GU, and hematopoietic toxicity (thrombocytopenia, leukopenia) may occur. **Use with caution** in patients with renal impairment. **Do not** discontinue abruptly. $T_{1/2}$ = 24–36 hr.

Therapeutic levels: 20–80 ng/mL. Recommended serum sampling time: obtain trough level within 30 min before an oral dose. Steady state is typically achieved after 5–8 days of continuous therapy using the same dose.

Carbamazepine, phenytoin, and phenobarbital may decrease clonazepam levels and effect. Drugs that inhibit cytochrome P-450 3A4 isoenzymes (e.g., erythromycin) may increase clonazepam levels and effects/toxicity.

CLONIDINE
Catapres, Catapres TTS, Duraclon
Central alpha-adrenergic agonist, antihypertensive

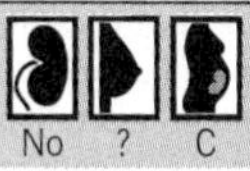

Tabs: 0.1, 0.2, 0.3 mg
Transdermal patch (Catapres TTS): 0.1, 0.2, 0.3 mg/24 hr (7-day patch)
Injection, epidural (Duraclon): 100, 500 mcg/mL (preservative free, 10 mL)

Hypertension:
Child (PO): 5–7 mcg/kg/24 hr PO ÷ Q6–12 hr; if needed, increase at 5–7 day intervals to 5–25 mcg/kg/24 hr PO ÷ Q6 hr; **max. dose:** 0.9 mg/24 hr
Adult (PO): 0.1 mg BID initially; increase in 0.1 mg/24 hr increments at weekly intervals until desired response is achieved (usual range: 0.1–0.8 mg/24 hr ÷ BID), **max. dose:** 2.4 mg/24 hr
Transdermal patch:
Child: conversion to patch only after establishing an optimal oral dose first.

Continued

FORMULARY For explanation of icons, see p. 680.

CLONIDINE *continued*

Adult: Initial 0.1 mg/24 hr patch for first week. May increase dose by 0.1 mg/24 hr at 1–2 wk intervals PRN. Usual range: 0.1–0.3 mg/24 hr. Each patch lasts for 7 days. Doses >0.6 mg/24 hr do not provide additional benefit.

ADHD:

Child: Start with 0.05 mg QHS PO; if needed, increase by 0.05 mg every 3–7 days up to a **max. dose** of 0.4 mg/24 hr. Titrated doses may be divided TID–QID.

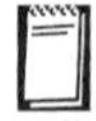

Side effects: dry mouth, dizziness, drowsiness, fatigue, constipation, anorexia, arrhythmias, and local skin reactions with patch. **Do not abruptly discontinue;** signs of sympathetic overactivity may occur; taper gradually over >1 wk.

Beta-blockers may exacerbate rebound hypertension during and following the withdrawal of clonidine. If patient is receiving both clonidine and a beta-blocker and clonidine is to be discontinued, the beta-blocker should be withdrawn several days before tapering the clonidine. If converting from clonidine to a beta-blocker, introduce the beta-blocker several days after discontinuing clonidine (following taper).

$T_{1/2}$: 44–72 hr (neonate), 6–20 hr (adult). Onset of action (antihypertensive): 0.5–1 hr for oral route, 2–3 days for transdermal route.

CLOTRIMAZOLE

Lotrimin AF, Cruex, Gyne-Lotrimin 3, Gyne-Lotrimin 7, Mycelex, Mycelex-7, and others

Antifungal

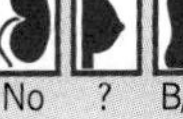

Oral troche: 10 mg
Cream, topical (OTC): 1% (12, 15, 24, 30, 45 g)
Solution, topical (OTC): 1% (10, 30 mL)
Lotion, topical (OTC): 1% (20 mL)
Vaginal suppository (OTC): 200 mg
Vaginal cream: 1% (OTC) (15, 30, 45 g), 2% (OTC) (21 g)
Combination packs:

Mycelex-7 Combination Pack (OTC): Vaginal suppository 100 mg (7) and vaginal cream 1% (7 g)

Gyne-Lotrimin 3 Combination Pack (OTC): Vaginal suppository 200 mg (3) and vaginal cream 1% (7 g)

Topical: Apply to skin BID × 4–8 wk.

Vaginal candidiasis: *(vaginal suppositories)*

100 mg/dose QHS × 7 days, or
200 mg/dose QHS × 3 days, or
1 applicator dose (5 g) of 1% vaginal cream QHS × 7–14 days, or
1 applicator dose of 2% vaginal cream QHS × 3 days

Thrush:

>3 yr–adult: dissolve slowly (15–30 min) one troche in the mouth 5 times/ 24 hr × 14 days

Continued

CLOTRIMAZOLE *continued*

May cause erythema, blistering, or urticaria with topical use. Liver enzyme elevation, nausea, and vomiting may occur with troches.

Pregnancy code is a B for topical and vaginal dosage forms and C for troches.

CODEINE
Various brands
Narcotic, analgesic, antitussive

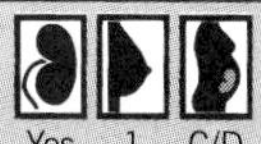

Tabs: 15, 30, 60 mg
Injection: 30, 60 mg/mL
Oral solution: 15 mg/5 mL (500 mL)

Analgesic:
Child: 0.5–1 mg/kg/dose Q4–6 hr IM, SC, or PO; **max. dose:** 60 mg/dose
Adult: 15–60 mg/dose Q4–6 hr IM, SC, or PO

Antitussive (all doses PRN): 1–1.5 mg/kg/24 hr ÷ Q4–6 hr; alternatively dose by age:
- ***2–6 yr:*** 2.5–5 mg/dose Q4–6 hr; **max. dose:** 30 mg/24 hr
- ***6–12 yr:*** 5–10 mg/dose Q4–6 hr; **max. dose:** 60 mg/24 hr
- ***≥12 yr and adult:*** 10–20 mg/dose Q4–6 hr; **max. dose:** 120 mg/24 hr

Do not use in children <2 yrs old as antitussive. **Not intended** for IV use, owing to large histamine release and cardiovascular effects. Side effects: CNS and respiratory depression, constipation, cramping, hypotension, and pruritus. May be habit forming.

For analgesia, use with acetaminophen orally. **See Chapter 28 for equianalgesic dosing. Adjust dose in renal failure (see Chapter 30).**

Pregnancy risk factor changes to D if used for prolonged periods or in high doses at term.

CODEINE AND ACETAMINOPHEN
Tylenol #1, #2, #3, #4, and others
Narcotic analgesic combination product

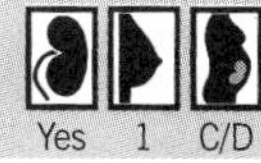

Elixir (7% alcohol and saccharin), suspension, solution: acetaminophen 120 mg and codeine 12 mg/5 mL (120, 473 mL)
Tabs (all containing 300 mg acetaminophen per tab):
- Tylenol #2: 15 mg codeine
- Tylenol #3: 30 mg codeine
- Tylenol #4: 60 mg codeine

Continued

For explanation of icons, see p. 680.

CODEINE AND ACETAMINOPHEN *continued*

See *Acetaminophen* and *Codeine* for additional dosing information:
Child: 0.5–1 mg codeine/kg/dose PO Q4–6 hr PRN
Using elixir:
3–6 yr: 5 mL (12 mg codeine and 120 mg acetaminophen) PO Q6–8 hr PRN
7–12 yr: 10 mL (24 mg codeine and 240 mg acetaminophen) PO Q6–8 hr PRN
≥12 yr: 15 mL (36 mg codeine and 360 mg acetaminophen) PO Q4 hr PRN
Adult: 1–2 tablets PO Q4 hr PRN; **max. codeine dose:** 120 mg/24 hr, **max. acetaminophen dose:** 4 g/24 hr

See *Acetaminophen* and *Codeine*. Pregnancy category is C (changes to D if used for prolonged periods or in high doses at term) for codeine.

Do not use combination product in renal impairment because codeine requires dosage adjustment; consider using each drug separately with proper dose adjustments.

CORTICOTROPIN

H. P. Acthar
Adrenocorticotropic hormone

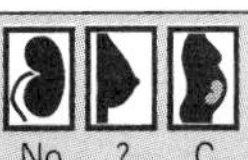

Injection, repository gel: 80 U/mL (5 mL)
1 unit = 1 mg

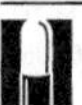

Antiinflammatory:
0.8 U/kg/24 hr ÷ Q12–24 hr IM
Infantile spasms: many regimens exist.
20–40 U/24 hr IM QD × 6 wk or 150 U/m^2/24hr ÷ BID for 2 wk; followed by a gradual taper

Contraindicated in acute psychoses, CHF, Cushing disease, TB, peptic ulcer, ocular herpes, fungal infections, recent surgery, and sensitivity to porcine products. **Repository gel dosage form is only for IM route.**

Hypersensitivity reactions may occur. Similar adverse effects as corticosteroids.

CORTISONE ACETATE

Cortone acetate and others

Corticosteroid

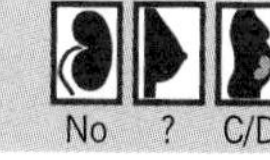

Tabs: 5, 10, 25 mg

Antiinflammatory/immunosuppressive:
PO: 2.5–10 mg/kg/24 hr ÷ Q6–8 hr

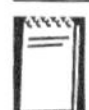

May produce glucose intolerance, Cushing syndrome, edema, hypertension, adrenal suppression, cataracts, hypokalemia, skin atrophy, peptic ulcer, osteoporosis, and growth suppression.

Pregnancy category changes to D if used in the first trimester.

CO-TRIMOXAZOLE

Trimethoprim-sulfamethoxazole, TMP-SMX; Bactrim, Septra, Sulfatrim, and others

Antibiotic, sulfonamide derivative

Yes 1 C/D

Tabs (reg. strength): 80 mg TMP/400 mg SMX
Tabs (double strength): 160 mg TMP/800 mg SMX
Suspension: 40 mg TMP/200 mg SMX per 5 mL (20, 100, 150, 200, 480 mL)
Injection: 16 mg TMP/mL and 80 mg SMX/mL; some preparations may contain propylene glycol and benzyl alcohol (5, 10, 20, 30 mL).

Doses based on TMP component
Minor infections (PO or IV):
Child: 8–10 mg/kg/24 hr ÷ BID
Adult (>40 kg): 160 mg/dose BID
UTI prophylaxis: 2–4 mg/kg/24 hr PO QD
Severe infections and Pneumocystis carinii pneumonitis (PO or IV): 20 mg/kg/24 hr ÷ Q6–8 hr
Pneumocystis prophylaxis (PO or IV): 5–10 mg/kg/24 hr ÷ BID or 150 mg/m^2/24 hr ÷ BID for 3 consecutive days/wk; **max. dose:** 320 mg/24 hr

Not recommended for use with infants <2 mo. **Contraindicated** in patients with sulfonamide or trimethoprim hypersensitivity or megaloblastic anemia due to folate deficiency. May cause kernicterus in newborns; may cause blood dyscrasias, crystalluria, glossitis, renal or hepatic injury, GI irritation, rash, Stevens-Johnson syndrome, hemolysis in patients with G6PD deficiency. Hyperkalemia may appear in HIV/AIDS patients. **Do not use drug at term during pregnancy.** Pregnancy category changes to D if administered near term. **Use with caution** in renal and hepatic impairment.

Reduce dose in renal impairment (see Chapter 30). See Chapter 16 for PCP prophylaxis guidelines.

For explanation of icons, see p. 680.

CROMOLYN

Intal, Nasalcrom, Gastrocrom, Crolom, Opticrom

Antiallergic agent

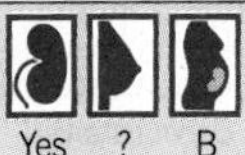

Nebulized solution: 10 mg/mL (2 mL)
Aerosol inhaler: 800 mcg/spray (112 inhalations, 8.1 g; 200 inhalations, 14.2 g)
Oral concentrate: 100 mg/5 mL
Ophthalmic solution: 4% (2.5, 10, 15 mL)
Nasal spray (OTC): 4% (5.2 mg/spray) (100 sprays, 13 mL; 200 sprays, 26 mL)

Nebulization: 20 mg Q6–8 hr
Nasal: 1 spray each nostril TID-QID
Aerosol inhaler:
- ***Child:*** 1–2 puffs TID-QID
- ***Adult:*** 2–4 puffs TID-QID

Ophthalmic: 1–2 gtts 4–6 times/24 hr
Food allergy/inflammatory bowel disease:
- ***>2 yr and <12 yr:*** 100 mg PO QID; give 15–20 min AC and QHS; **max. dose:** 40 mg/kg/24 hr
- ***≥12 yr and adult:*** 200–400 mg PO QID; give 15–20 min AC and QHS

Systemic mastocytosis:
- ***<2 yr:*** 20 mg/kg/24 hr ÷ QID PO; **max. dose:** 30 mg/kg/24 hr
- ***2–12 yr:*** 100 mg PO QID; **max. dose:** 40 mg/kg/24 hr
- ***Adult:*** 200 mg PO QID

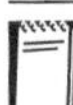
May cause rash, cough, bronchospasm, and nasal congestion. May cause headache and diarrhea with oral use. **Use with caution** in patients with renal or hepatic dysfunction.

Therapeutic response often occurs within 2 wk; however, a 4- to 6-wk trial may be needed to determine maximum benefit. For exercise induced asthma, give no longer than 1 hour before activity. Oral concentrate can only be diluted in water. Nebulized solution can be mixed with albuterol nebs.

CYANOCOBALAMIN/VITAMIN B_{12}

Cyanoject, Cyomin, vitamin B_{12}, and others

Vitamin (synthetic), water soluble

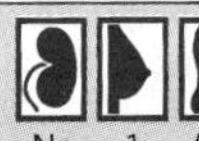

Tabs (OTC): 50, 100, 250, 500, 1000, 5000 mcg
Lozenges (OTC): 100, 250, 500 mcg
Injection: 1000 mcg/mL; some preparations may contain benzyl alcohol.

U.S. RDA: *see Chapter 20.*
Vitamin B_{12} deficiency, treatment (administered IM or deep SC):
- ***Child:*** 100 mcg/24 hr × 10–15 days
  - ***Maintenance:*** at least 60 mcg/month
- ***Adult:*** 30–100 mcg/24 hr × 5–10 days
  - ***Maintenance:*** 100–200 mcg/month

Continued

CYANOCOBALAMIN/VITAMIN B_{12} *continued*

Pernicious anemia (administered IM or deep SC):

Child: 30–50 mcg/24 hr for at least 14 days to total dose of 1000 mcg

Maintenance: 100 mcg/month

Adult: 100 mcg/24 hr × 7 days, followed by 100 mcg/dose QOD × 14 days, then 100 mcg/dose Q 3–4 days until remission is complete.

Maintenance: 100 mcg/month

Contraindicated in optic nerve atrophy. May cause hypokalemia, hypersensitivity, pruritus, and vascular thrombosis. Pregnancy category changes to C if used in doses above the RDA.

Prolonged use of acid-suppressing medications may reduce cyanocobalamin oral absorption.

Protect product from light. Oral route of administration is generally **not recommended** for pernicious anemia and B_{12} deficiency because of poor absorption. IV route of administration is **not recommended** because of a more rapid elimination. **See Chapter 20 for multivitamin preparations.**

CYCLOPENTOLATE

Cyclogyl and others

Anticholinergic, mydriatic agent

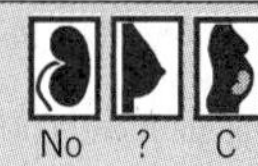

Ophthalmic solution: 0.5%, 1%, 2% (2, 5, 15 mL)

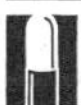

Infant: 1 drop of 0.5% OU 10–30 min before exam; use of cyclopentolate/phenylephrine (Cyclomydril) may be preferred due to lower cyclopentolate concentration.

Child: 1 drop of 0.5–1% OU, followed by repeat drop, if necessary, in 5 min

Adult: 1 drop of 1% OU followed by another drop OU in 5 min; use 2% solution for heavily pigmented iris.

Do not use in narrow-angle glaucoma. May cause a burning sensation, behavioral disturbance, tachycardia, and loss of visual accommodation. To minimize absorption, apply pressure over nasolacrimal sac for at least 2 min. CNS and cardiovascular side effects are common with the 2% solution in children. **Avoid** feeding infants within 4 hr of dosing to prevent potential feeding intolerance.

Onset of action: 15–60 min. Observe patient closely for at least 30 min after dose.

For explanation of icons, see p. 680.

CYCLOPENTOLATE WITH PHENYLEPHRINE

Cyclomydril

Anticholinergic/sympathomimetic, mydriatic agent

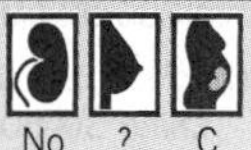

Ophthalmic solution: 0.2% cyclopentolate/1% phenylephrine (2, 5 mL)

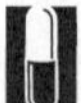
1 drop OU Q5–10 min; **max. dose:** 3 drops per eye

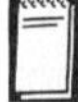
Used to induce mydriasis. See cyclopentolate for additional comments.

CYCLOSPORINE, CYCLOSPORINE MICROEMULSION

Sandimmune, Gengraf, Neoral, and others

Immunosuppressant

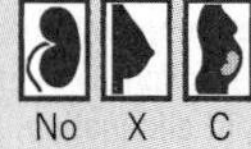

Injection: 50 mg/mL; contains 32.9% alcohol and 650 mg/mL polyoxyethylated castor oil
Oral solution: 100 mg/mL (50 mL); contains 12.5% alcohol
Caps: 25, 100 mg; contains 12.7% alcohol
Neoral cap: 25, 100 mg
Neoral solution: 100 mg/mL (50 mL)
Neoral products contain 11.9% alcohol

Neoral manufacturer recommends a 1:1 conversion ratio with Sandimmune. Due to its better absorption, however, lower doses of Neoral may be required. Exact dosing may vary depending on transplant type.

Oral: 15 mg/kg/24 hr as a single dose given 4–12 hr pretransplantation; give same daily dose for 1–2 wk posttransplantation, then reduce by 5% per wk to 3–10 mg/kg/24 hr ÷ Q12–24 hr.

IV: 5–6 mg/kg/24 hr as a single dose given 4–12 hr pretransplantation; administer over 2–6 hr; give same daily dose posttransplantation until patient able to tolerate oral form.

May cause nephrotoxicity, hepatotoxicity, hypomagnesemia, hyperkalemia, hyperuricemia, hypertension, hirsutism, acne, GI symptoms, tremor, leukopenia, sinusitis, gingival hyperplasia, and headache. Encephalopathy, convulsions, vision and movement disturbances, and impaired consciousness have been reported, especially in liver transplant recipients. **Use caution** with concomitant use of other nephrotoxic drugs such as amphotericin B, aminoglycosides, nonsteroidal antiinflammatory drugs, and tacrolimus.

Plasma concentrations increased with the use of fluconazole, ketoconazole, itraconazole, erythromycin, clarithromycin, diltiazem, verapamil, nicardipine, carvedilol, and corticosteroids. Plasma concentrations decreased with the use of carbamazepine, nafcillin, rifampin, phenobarbital, octreotide, and phenytoin. Cyclosporine is a substrate for CYP450 3A4.

Continued

CYCLOSPORINE, CYCLOSPORINE MICROEMULSION *continued*

Children may require dosages 2–3 times higher than adults. Plasma half-life 6–24 hr.

Monitor trough levels (just before a dose at steady state). Steady state is generally achieved after 3–5 days of continuous dosing. Interpretation will vary based on treatment protocol and assay methodology (RIA monoclonal vs. RIA polyclonal vs. HPLC) as well as whole blood vs. serum sample.

CYPROHEPTADINE

Periactin and others

Antihistamine

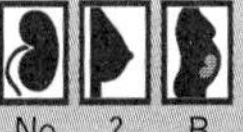

Tabs: 4 mg

Syrup: 2 mg/5 mL (473 mL); contains 5% alcohol

Antihistaminic uses:

Child: 0.25 mg/kg/24 hr or 8 mg/m^2/24 hr ÷ Q8–12 hr PO or by age:

2–6 yr: 2 mg Q8–12 hr PO; **max. dose:** 12 mg/24 hr

7–14 yr: 4 mg Q8–12 hr PO; **max. dose:** 16 mg/24 hr

Adult: Start with 12 mg/24 hr ÷ TID PO; dosage range: 12–32 mg/24 hr ÷ TID PO; **max. dose:** 0.5 mg/kg/24 hr

Migraine prophylaxis: 0.25–0.4 mg/kg/24 hr ÷ BID–TID PO up to following **max. doses:**

2–6 yr: 12 mg/24 hr

7–14 yr: 16 mg/24 hr

Adult: 0.5 mg/kg/24 hr

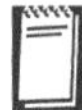

Contraindicated in neonates, patients currently taking MAO inhibitors, and patients suffering from asthma, glaucoma, or GI/GU obstruction. May produce anticholinergic side effects including appetite stimulation. Consider reducing dosage with hepatic insufficiency.

Allow 4 to 8 wk of continuous therapy for assessing efficacy in migraine prophylaxis.

DANTROLENE

Dantrium

Skeletal muscle relaxant

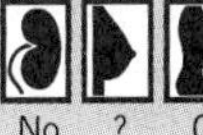

Cap: 25, 50, 100 mg

Injection: 20 mg (3 gm mannitol/20 mg drug)

Suspension: 5 mg/mL

Chronic spasticity:

Child (<5 yr):

Initial: 0.5 mg/kg/dose PO BID

Continued

For explanation of icons, see p. 680.

DANTROLENE *continued*

Increment: increase frequency to TID–QID at 4- to 7-day intervals, then increase doses by 0.5 mg/kg/dose

Max. dose: 3 mg/kg/dose PO BID–QID, up to 400 mg/24 hr

Malignant hyperthermia:

Prevention:

PO: 4–8 mg/kg/24 hr ÷ Q6 hr × 1–2 days before surgery

IV: 2.5 mg/kg over 1 hr beginning 1.25 hr before anesthesia, additional doses PRN

Treatment: 1 mg/kg IV, repeat PRN to **maximum cumulative dose** of 10 mg/kg, then continue 4–8 mg/kg/24 hr PO ÷ Q6 hr for 1–3 days.

Contraindicated in active hepatic disease. Monitor transaminases for hepatotoxicity. **Use with caution** in children with cardiac or pulmonary impairment. May cause change in sensorium, weakness, diarrhea, constipation, incontinence, and enuresis.

Avoid unnecessary exposure of medication to sunlight. **Avoid** extravasation into tissues. A decrease in spasticity sufficient to allow daily function should be therapeutic goal. Discontinue if benefits are not evident in 45 days.

DAPSONE

Diaminodiphenylsulfone, DDS

Antibiotic, sulfone derivative

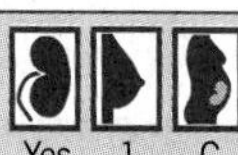

Tabs: 25, 100 mg

Suspension: 2 mg/mL 

Pneumocystis carinii prophylaxis:

Child ≥1 mo: 2 mg/kg/24 hr PO QD; **max. dose:** 100 mg/24 hr

Adult: 100 mg/24 hr PO ÷ QD–BID; other combination regimens with pyrimethamine and leucovorin can be used. (See http://www.hivatis.org/trtgdlns.html# Opportunistic.)

Leprosy (See www.who.int/lep/disease/disease.htm for latest recommendations including combination regimens such as rifampin ± clofazimine):

Child: 1–2 mg/kg/24 hr PO QD; **max. dose:** 100 mg/24 hr

Adult: 50–100 mg PO QD

Patients with HIV, glutathione deficiency, or G6PD deficiency may be at increased risk for developing methemoglobinemia. Side effects include hemolytic anemia (dose related), agranulocytosis, methemoglobinemia, aplastic anemia, nausea, vomiting, hyperbilirubinemia, headache, nephrotic syndrome, and hypersensitivity reaction (sulfone syndrome).

Didanosine, rifabutin, and rifampin decrease dapsone levels. Trimethoprim increases dapsone levels. Pyrimethamine, nitrofurantoin, and primaquine increase risk for hematologic side effects.

Suspension may not be absorbed as well as tablets.

DARBEPOETIN ALFA

Aranesp

Erythropoiesis stimulating protein

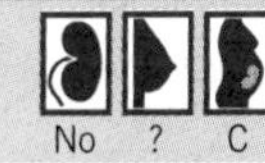

Injection (in either an albumin (2.5 mg/mL) or polysorbate (0.05 mg/mL) solution): 25, 40, 60, 100, 200, 300, 500 mcg/mL (1 mL)

Single-dose prefilled injection syringe (27 gauge, $\frac{1}{2}$-inch needle) with 2.5 mg/mL albumin: 60 mcg/0.3 mL, 100 mcg/0.5 mL, 150 mcg/0.3 mL, 200 mcg/0.4 mL, 300 mcg/0.6 mL, 500 mcg/1 mL

Adult:

Anemia in chronic renal failure: Start with 0.45 mcg/kg/dose IV/SC once weekly and adjust dose accordingly:

DARBEPOETIN ALFA DOSE ADJUSTMENT IN CHRONIC RENAL FAILURE

Response to Dose	Dose Adjustment
<1 g/dL increase in hemoglobin and below target range after 4 wk of therapy	Increase dose by 25% not more frequently than once monthly
>1 g/dL increase in hemoglobin in any 2-wk period or if hemoglobin >12 g/dL	Decrease dose by 25%
Hemoglobin continues to increase despite dosage reduction	Discontinue therapy; reinitiate therapy at a 25% lower dose after the hemoglobin starts to decrease

Anemia associated with chemotherapy (patients with nonmyeloid malignancies): start with 2.25 mcg/kg/dose SC once weekly and adjust dose accordingly:

DARBEPOETIN ALFA DOSE ADJUSTMENT IN CHEMOTHERAPY PATIENTS

Response to Dose	Dose Adjustment
<1 g/dL increase in hemoglobin after 6 wk of therapy	Increase dose to 4.5 mcg/kg/dose SQ once weekly
>1 g/dL increase in hemoglobin in any 2-wk period or if hemoglobin >12 g/dL	Decrease dose by 25%
Hemoglobin >13 g/dL	Hold dose until hemoglobin falls to 12 g/dL and reinitiate therapy at a dose 25% less the previous dose

Continued

For explanation of icons, see p. 680.

DARBEPOETIN ALFA *continued*

Conversion from epoetin alfa to darbepoetin alfa:

Previous Weekly Epoetin Alfa Dose (units/week)[1]	Weekly Darbepoetin Alfa Dose (mcg/week) Administered SC/IV Once Weekly[2]
<2,500	6.25
2,500–4,999	12.5
5,000–10,999	25
11,000–17,999	40
18,000–33,999	60
34,000–89,999	100
≥90,000	200

1. 200 units of epoetin alfa is equivalent to 1 mcg darbepoetin alfa.
2. If patient was receiving epoetin alfa once weekly, darbepoetin alfa should be administered once every 2 weeks.

Contraindicated in uncontrolled hypertension and patients hypersensitive to albumin/polysorbate 80 or epoetin alfa. Darbepoetin alfa is **not intended** for patients requiring acute correction of anemia. **Use with caution** in seizures and liver disease. Evaluate serum iron, ferritin, and TIBC; concurrent iron supplementation may be necessary.

May cause edema, fatigue, GI disturbances, headache, blood pressure changes, fever, cardiac arrhythmia/arrest, infections, and myalgia in chronic renal failure patients. May cause fatigue, fever, edema, dizziness, headache, GI disturbances, arthralgia/myalgia, and rash in chemotherapy patients. Monitor hemoglobin, BP, serum chemistries, and reticulocyte count.

Targeted hemoglobin in adults is 9-12 g/dL. Increases in dose should not be made more frequently than once a month. For IV administration, infuse over 1–3 min.

DEFEROXAMINE MESYLATE

Desferal

Chelating agent

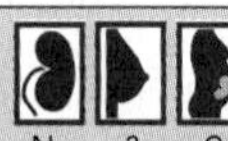

Injection: 500, 2000 mg

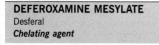

Acute iron poisoning *(see remarks):*

Child:

- *IV:* 15 mg/kg/hr
- *IM:* 50 mg/kg/dose Q6 hr
- **Max. dose:** 6 g/24 hr

Adult:

- *IV:* 15 mg/kg/hr
- *IM:* 1 g × 1, then 0.5 g Q4 hr × 2; may repeat 0.5 g Q4–12 hr
- **Max. dose:** 6 g/24 hr

Continued

DEFEROXAMINE MESLATE *continued*

Chronic iron overload *(see remarks):*

Child:

IV: 15 mg/kg/hr; **max. dose:** 6 g/24 hr

SC: 20–40 mg/kg/dose QD as infusion over 8–12 hr; **max. dose:** 2 g/24 hr

Adult:

IM: 0.5–1 g/dose QD

SC: 1–2 g/dose QD as infusion over 8–24 hr

Contraindicated in anuria. Not approved for use in primary hemochromatosis. May cause flushing, erythema, urticaria, hypotension, tachycardia, diarrhea, leg cramps, fever, cataracts, hearing loss, nausea, and vomiting. Iron mobilization may be poor in children <3 yr.

High doses and concomitant low ferritin levels have also been associated with growth retardation. Growth velocity may resume to pretreatment levels by reducing the dosage. Acute respiratory distress syndrome has been reported following treatment with prolonged infusions or high doses in patients with acute iron intoxication or thalassemia. Toxicity risk has been reported with infusions >8 mg/kg/hr for >4 days for thalassemia; and with infusions of 15 mg/kg/hr for >1 day for acute iron toxicity. Pulmonary toxicity was not seen in 193 courses administered to 13 children with thalassemia at a rate of 15 mg/kg/hr for 48 hrs.

Maximum IV infusion rate: 15 mg/kg/hr. SC route is via a portable controlled-infusion device and is **not recommended** in acute iron poisoning.

DESLORATADINE

Clarinex, Clarinex RediTabs

Antihistamine, less sedating

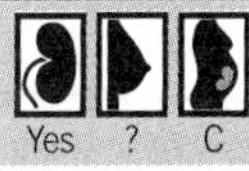

Tabs: 5 mg

Disintegrating tabs (RediTabs): 5 mg; contains 1.75 mg phenylalanine

---

2–5 yr: 1.25 mg PO QD

6–11 yr: 2.5 mg PO QD

≥12 yr and adult: 5 mg PO QD

Liver or renal impairment: administer age-appropriate dose QOD

Contraindicated in loratadine hypersensitivity. **Use with caution** in liver or renal disease (reduce dosage), glaucoma, prostatic hypertrophy, and urinary retention, and with other CNS depressants or anticholinergic drugs. Has **not** been implicated in causing cardiac arrhythmias when used with medications metabolized by hepatic microsomal enzymes (e.g., ketoconazole, erythromycin). May cause somnolence, fatigue, liver enzyme elevation, dizziness, tachycardia, palpitations, and other anticholinergic effects. Individuals with slow metabolism (reported as 7% of population and 20% of African Americans from a clinical trial) may be susceptible to dose-related adverse effects.

Doses may be administered regardless to food. For use of RediTabs, place tablet on tongue and allow it to disintegrate in the mouth with or without water.

For explanation of icons, see p. 680.

DESMOPRESSIN ACETATE

DDAVP, Stimate, and others

Vasopressin analogue, synthetic; hemostatic agent

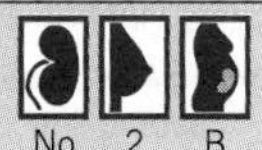

Tabs: 0.1, 0.2 mg

Nasal solution (with rhinal tube): DDAVP, 100 mcg/mL (2.5 mL); contains 9 mg NaCl/mL

Injection: 4 mcg/mL (1, 10 mL); contains 9 mg NaCl/mL

Nasal spray:

100 mcg/mL, 10 mcg/spray (50 sprays, 5 mL); contains 7.5 mg NaCl/Ml

Stimate: 1500 mcg/mL, 150 mcg/spray (25 sprays, 2.5 mL); contains 9 mg NaCl/mL

Conversion: 100 mcg = 400 IU arginine vasopressin

Diabetes insipidus:

Oral:

Child: Start with 0.05 mg/dose BID; titrate to effect; usual dose range: 0.1–0.8 mg/24 hr.

Adult: Start with 0.05 mg/dose BID; titrate dose to effect; usual dose range: 0.1–1.2 mg/24 hr ÷ BID–TID.

Intranasal:

3 mo–12 yr: 5–30 mcg/24 hr ÷ QD–BID

Adult: 10–40 mcg/24 hr ÷ QD–TID; titrate dose to achieve control of excessive thirst and urination. Morning and evening doses should be adjusted separately for diurnal rhythm of water turnover.

IV/SC:

≥12 yr and adult: 2–4 mcg/24 hr ÷ BID

Hemophilia A and von Willebrand's disease *(see remarks):*

Intranasal: 2–4 mcg/kg/dose

IV: 0.2–0.4 mcg/kg/dose over 15–30 min

Nocturnal enuresis (>6 yr):

Oral: 0.2 mg at bedtime, titrated to a **max. dose** of 0.6 mg to achieve desired effect

Intranasal: 20 mcg at bedtime, range 10–40 mcg; divide dose by 2, and administer each one-half dose in each nostril.

Use with caution in hypertension and coronary artery disease. May cause headache, nausea, seizures, blood pressure changes, hyponatremia, nasal congestion, abdominal cramps, and hypertension.

Injection may be used SC or IV at about 10% of intranasal dose. Adjust fluid intake to decrease risk for water intoxication.

If switching stabilized patient from intranasal route to IV/SC route, use 10% of intranasal dose. Peak effects: 1–5 hr with intranasal route; 1.5–3 hr with IV route; and 2–7 hr with PO route.

For hemophilia A and von Willebrand's disease administer dose intranasally, 2 hr before procedure; IV, 30 min before procedure.

DEXAMETHASONE

Decadron, Hexadrol, and other brand names

Corticosteroid

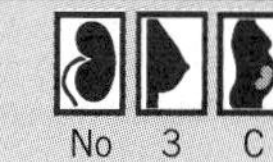

Tabs: 0.25, 0.5, 0.75, 1, 1.5, 2, 4, 6 mg
Injection (sodium phosphate salt): 4, 10, 20, 24 mg/mL (some preparations contain benzyl alcohol or methyl/propyl parabens)
IM injection (acetate salt): 8, 16 mg/mL
Elixir: 0.5 mg/5 mL (some preparations contain 5% alcohol)
Oral solution: 0.1, 1 mg/mL (some preparations contain 30% alcohol)
Ophthalmic ointment: 0.05% (3.5 g)
Ophthalmic solution: 0.1% (5 mL)
Ophthalmic suspension: 0.1% (5, 15 mL)

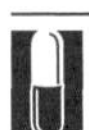

Airway edema: 0.5–2 mg/kg/24 hr IV/IM ÷ Q6 hr (begin 24 hr before extubation and continue for 4–6 doses after extubation)
Croup: 0.6 mg/kg/dose PO/IV/IM × 1 (use sodium phosphate injection)

Antiemetic:
- ***Initial:*** 10 mg/m²/dose IV; **max. dose:** 20 mg
- ***Subsequent:*** 5 mg/m²/dose Q6 hr IV

Antiinflammatory:
- ***Child:*** 0.08–0.3 mg/kg/24 hr PO, IV, IM ÷ Q6–12 hr
- ***Adult:*** 0.75–9 mg/24 hr PO, IV, IM ÷ Q6–12 hr

Brain tumor associated cerebral edema:
- ***Loading dose:*** 1–2 mg/kg/dose IV/IM × 1
- ***Maintenance:*** 1–1.5 mg/kg/24 hr ÷ Q4–6 hr; **max. dose:** 16 mg/24 hr

Spinal cord compression with neurological abnormalities:
- ***Child:*** 2 mg/kg/24 hr IV ÷ Q6 hr

Hib meningitis:
- ***>6 wk:*** 0.6 mg/kg/24 hr IV ÷ Q6 hr × 2 days; initiate before or with the first dose of antibiotic.

Ophthalmic use (child and adult):
- ***Ointment:*** Apply a thin coating of ointment to the conjunctival sac of the affected eye(s) TID–QID. When a favorable response is achieved, reduce daily dosage to BID and later to QD as a maintenance dose sufficient to control symptoms.
- ***Solution:*** Instill 1 to 2 drops into the conjunctival sac of the affected eye(s) Q1 hr during the day and Q2 hr during the night as initial therapy. When a favorable response is achieved, reduce dosage to 1 drop Q4 hr. Further dose reduction to 1 drop TID–QID may be sufficient to control symptoms.
- ***Suspension:*** Shake well before using. Instill 1–2 drops in the conjunctival sac of the affected eye(s). For severe disease, drops may be Q1 hr, being tapered to discontinuation as inflammation subsides. For mild disease, drops may be used ≤4 to 6 times/24 hr.

Continued

For explanation of icons, see p. 680.

DEXAMETHASONE *continued*

Not recommended for systemic therapy in the prevention or treatment of chronic lung disease in infants with very-low-birthweight because of increase risk for adverse events (Pediatrics 2002;109[2]:330–338). Dexamethasone is a substrate of CYP450 3A3/4.

Toxicity: same as for prednisone without mineralocorticoid effects. **Contraindicated** in active untreated infections and fungal, viral, and mycobacterial ocular infections. **Use with caution** in corneal/scleral thinning and glaucoma. Use ophthalmic preparation only in consultation with an ophthalmologist. Ophthalmic solution/suspension may be used in otitis externa.

Use in meningitis (other than Hib) is controversial. Consult ID specialist or latest edition of *Red Book.*

Oral peak serum levels occur 1–2 hr and within 8 hr following IM administration. For other uses, doses based on body surface area, and dose equivalence to other steroids, see Chapter 29; Table 29-3.

DEXTROAMPHETAMINE ± AMPHETAMINE

Dexedrine, Dextrostat, Dexedrine Spansules, and many other brand names; in combination with amphetamine—Adderall, Adderall XR

CNS stimulant

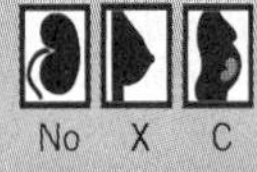

Tabs: 5, 10 mg
Sustained-release caps (Dexedrine Spansules): 5, 10, 15 mg
In combination with amphetamine (Adderall): Available as 1:1:1:1 mixture of dextroamphetamine sulfate, dextroamphetamine saccharate, amphetamine aspartate, and amphetamine sulfate salts; for example, the 5 mg tablet contains: 1.25 mg dextroamphetamine sulfate, 1.25 mg dextroamphetamine saccharate, 1.25 mg amphetamine aspartate, and 1.25 mg amphetamine sulfate.
Tabs: 5, 7.5, 10, 12.5, 15, 20, 30 mg
Caps, extended release (Adderall XR): 5, 10, 15, 20, 25, 30 mg

Dosages are in terms of mg of dextroamphetamine when using Dexedrine (dextroamphetamine alone) OR in terms of mg of the total dextroamphetamine and amphetamine salts when using Adderall.

Attention deficit/hyperactivity disorder:

3–5 yr: 2.5 mg/24 hr QAM; increase by 2.5 mg/24 hr at weekly intervals to a **max. dose** of 40 mg/24 hr ÷ QD–TID.

≥6 yr: 5 mg/24 hr QAM; increase by 5 mg/24 hr at weekly intervals to a **max. dose** of 40 mg/24 hr ÷ QD–TID.

Narcolepsy:

6–12 yr: 5 mg/24 hr ÷ QD–TID; increase by 5 mg/24 hr at weekly intervals to a **max. dose** of 60 mg/24 hr.

>12 yr: 10 mg/24 hr ÷ QD–TID; increase by 10 mg/24 hr at weekly intervals to a **max. dose** of 60 mg/24 hr.

Continued

DEXTROAMPHETAMINE ± AMPHETAMINE *continued*

Use with caution in presence of hypertension or cardiovascular disease. **Do not give** with MAO inhibitors or general anesthetics. **Not recommended** for <3 yr. Medication should generally not be used in children <5 yr old because diagnosis of ADHD in this age group is extremely difficult (use in consultation with a specialist). Interrupt administration occasionally to determine need for continued therapy. Many side effects, including insomnia (avoid dose administration within 6 hr of bedtime), restlessness, anorexia, psychosis, headache, vomiting, abdominal cramps, dry mouth, and growth failure. Tolerance develops. (Same guidelines as for methylphenidate apply). Sudden death and serious cardiovascular effects (e.g., MI and cardiomyopathy) have been reported with misuse of amphetamines.

DIAZEPAM

Valium and others

Benzodiazepine; anxiolytic, anticonvulsant

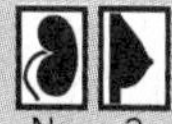
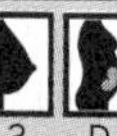
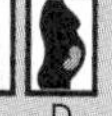

No 3 D

Tabs: 2, 5, 10 mg
Oral solution: 1 mg/mL, 5 mg/mL (contains 19% alcohol)
Injection: 5 mg/mL (contains 40% propylene glycol, 10% alcohol, and 1.5% benzyl alcohol)
Pediatric rectal gel (Diastat): 2.5, 5, 10 mg (5 mg/mL concentration with 4.4 cm rectal tip delivery system; contains 10% alcohol, 1.5% benzyl alcohol, and propylene glycol)
Adult rectal gel (Diastat): 10, 15, 20 mg (5 mg/mL concentration with 6 cm rectal tip delivery system; contains 10% alcohol, 1.5% benzyl alcohol, and propylene glycol)

Sedative/muscle relaxant:
Child:
IM or IV: 0.04–0.2 mg/kg/dose Q2–4 hr
Max. dose: 0.6 mg/kg within an 8-hr period
PO: 0.12–0.8 mg/kg/24 hr ÷ Q6–8 hr
Adult:
IM or IV: 2–10 mg/dose Q3–4 hr PRN
PO: 2–10 mg/dose Q6–12 hr PRN

Status epilepticus:
Neonate: 0.3–0.75 mg/kg/dose IV Q15–30 min × 2–3 doses
>1 mo: 0.2–0.5 mg/kg/dose IV Q15–30 min
Max. total dose: <5 yr: 5 mg; ≥ 5yr: 10 mg
Adult: 5–10 mg/dose IV Q10–15 min
Max. total dose: 30 mg
Rectal dose (using IV dosage form): 0.5 mg/kg/dose followed by 0.25 mg/kg/dose in 10 min PRN
Rectal gel: all doses rounded to the nearest available dosage strength; repeat dose in 4–12 hr PRN.
2–5 yr: 0.5 mg/kg/dose
6–11 yr: 0.3 mg/kg/dose
≥12 yr: 0.2 mg/kg/dose

Continued

For explanation of icons, see p. 680.

DIAZEPAM *continued*

Hypotension and respiratory depression may occur. **Use with caution** in glaucoma, shock, and depression. **Do not use** in combination with protease inhibitors. Concurrent use with CNS depressants, cimetidine, erythromycin, itraconazole, and valproic acid may enhance the effects of diazepam.

Administer the conventional IV product undiluted no faster than 2 mg/min. **Do not** mix with IV fluids.

In status epilepticus, diazepam must be followed by long-acting anticonvulsants. Onset of anticonvulsant effect: 1–3 min with IV route; 2–10 min with rectal route. For management of status epilepticus, see Table 1-4. For management of neonatal seizures, see Chapter 19.

DIAZOXIDE

Hyperstat IV, Proglycem

Antihypertensive agent, antihypoglycemic agent

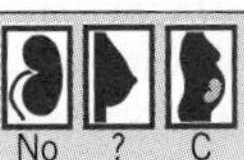

Injection: 15 mg/mL (20 mL)
Suspension: 50 mg/mL (30 mL); contains 7.25% alcohol

Hypertensive crisis: 1–3 mg/kg IV up to a **max. dose** of 150 mg/dose; repeat Q5–15 min PRN, then Q4–24 hr

Hyperinsulinemic hypoglycemia (due to insulin-producing tumors):

Newborn and infant: 8–15 mg/kg/24 hr ÷ Q8–12 hr PO

Child and adult: 3–8 mg/kg/24 hr ÷ Q8–12 hr PO (start at lowest dose)

May cause hyponatremia, salt and water retention, GI disturbances, ketoacidosis, rash, hyperuricemia, weakness, hypertrichosis, and arrhythmias. Monitor BP closely for hypotension. Hyperglycemia occurs in most patients. Hypoglycemia should be treated initially with IV glucose; diazoxide should be introduced only if refractory to glucose infusion.

Peak antihypertensive effect with IV administration occurs within 5 min, with a duration of 3–12 hr. Hyperglycemic effect with PO administration occurs within 1 hr, with a duration of 8 hr.

DICLOXACILLIN SODIUM

Dycill, Pathocil, and others

Antibiotic, penicillin (penicillinase resistant)

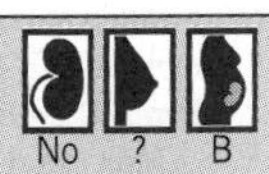

Caps: 250, 500 mg; contains 0.6 mEq Na/250 mg.

Child (<40 kg) *(see remarks):*

Mild/moderate infections: 12.5–25 mg/kg/24 hr PO ÷ Q6 hr

Severe infections: 50–100 mg/kg/24 hr PO ÷ Q6 hr

Adult (≥40 kg): 125–500 mg/dose PO Q6 hr; **max. dose:** 4 g/24 hr

Continued

DICLOXACILLIN SODIUM *continued*

Contraindicated in patients with a history of penicillin allergy. **Use with caution** in cephalosporin hypersensitivity. May cause nausea, vomiting, and diarrhea.

Limited experience in neonates and very young infants. Higher doses (50–100 mg/kg/24 hr) are indicated following IV therapy for osteomyelitis.

Administer 1–2 hr before meals or 2 hr after meals.

DIGOXIN

Lanoxin, Lanoxicaps, Digitek

Antiarrhythmic agent, inotrope

Yes 1 C

Caps: 50, 100, 200 mcg
Tabs: 125, 250 mcg
Elixir: 50 mcg/mL (60 mL); may contain 10% alcohol
Injection: 100, 250 mcg/mL; may contain propylene glycol and alcohol

Digitalizing: total digitalizing dose (TDD) and maintenance doses in mcg/kg/24 hr (see table below):

DIGOXIN DIGITALIZING AND MAINTENANCE DOSES

	Total Digitalizing Dose		Daily Maintenance	
Age	*PO*	*IV/IM*	*PO*	*IV/IM*
Premature	20	15	5	3–4
Full term	30	20	8–10	6–8
<2 yr	40–50	30–40	10–12	7.5–9
2–10 yr	30–40	20–30	8–10	6–8
>10 yr and <100 kg	10–15	8–12	2.5–5	2–3

Initial: ½ TDD, then ¼ TDD Q8–18 hr × 2 doses; obtain ECG 6 hr after dose to assess for toxicity.

Maintenance:

<10 yr: Give maintenance dose ÷ BID
≥10 yr: Give maintenance dose QD

Contraindicated in patients with ventricular dysrhythmias. **Use with caution** in renal failure and with adenosine (enhanced depressant effects on SA and AV nodes). May cause AV block or dysrhythmias. In the patient treated with digoxin, cardioversion or calcium infusion may lead to ventricular fibrillation (pretreatment with lidocaine may prevent this). Decreased serum potassium and magnesium or increased magnesium and calcium may increase risk for digoxin toxicity. For signs and symptoms of toxicity, see Chapter 2.

Continued

For explanation of icons, see p. 680.

DIGOXIN *continued*

Excreted via the kidney; **adjust dose in renal failure (see Chapter 30).** Therapeutic concentration: 0.8–2 ng/mL. Higher doses may be required for supraventricular tachycardia. Neonates, pregnant women, and patients with renal, hepatic, or heart failure may have falsely elevated digoxin levels, owing to the presence of digoxin-like substances.

$T_{1/2}$: Premature infants, 61–170 hr; full-term neonates, 35–45 hr; infants, 18–25 hr; and children, 35 hr

Recommended serum sampling at steady state: Obtain a single level from 6 hr postdose to just before the next scheduled dose following 5–8 days of continuous dosing. Levels obtained before steady state may be useful in preventing toxicity.

DIGOXIN IMMUNE FAB (OVINE)

Digibind

Antidigoxin antibody

No ? C

Injection: 38 mg

First, determine total body digoxin load (TBL):

TBL(mg) = serum digoxin level (ng/mL) × 5.6 × wt (kg) ÷ 1000, **OR**

TBL (mg) = mg digoxin ingested × 0.8

Then, calculate digoxin immune Fab dose:

Dose in number of digoxin immune Fab vials: # vials = TBL ÷ 0.5

Infuse IV over 15–30 min (through 0.22-micron filter).

Contraindicated if hypersensitivity to sheep products, or if renal or cardiac failure. May cause rapidly developing severe hypokalemia, decreased cardiac output, rash, and edema. Digoxin therapy may be reinstituted in 3–7 days, when toxicity has been corrected. See Chapter 2 for additional information.

DIHYDROTACHYSTEROL

DHT, DHT Intensol

Fat-soluble vitamin D analog

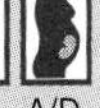

No ? A/D

Solution (DHT Intensol): 0.2 mg/mL (20% alcohol) (30 mL)
Tabs: 0.125, 0.2, 0.4 mg
1 mg = 120,000 IU vitamin D_2

Hypoparathyroidism:
Neonate: 0.05–0.1 mg/24 hr PO
Infant/young child: initial, 1–5 mg/24 hr PO × 4 days, then 0.5–1.5 mg/24 hr PO
Older child/adult: initial, 0.75–2.5 mg/24 hr PO × 4 days, then 0.2–1.5 mg/24 hr PO

Continued

DIHYDROTACHYSTEROL *continued*

Nutritional rickets: 0.5 mg × 1 PO, or 13–50 mcg/24 hr PO QD until healing
Renal osteodystrophy:
Child/adolescent: 0.1–0.5 mg/24 hr PO
Adult: 0.1–0.6 mg/24 hr PO

Use with caution in patients with renal stones, renal failure, and heart disease. Monitor serum Ca^{2+} and PO_4. Toxicities include hypercalcemia or hypervitaminosis D. May cause nausea, vomiting, anorexia, and renal damage.

Activated by 25-hydroxylation in liver; does not require 1-hydroxylation in kidney. More potent than vitamin D_2 but more rapidly inactivated (half-life is hours vs. weeks). Titrate dose with patient response. Oral Ca^{2+} supplementation may be required.

Pregnancy category changes to D if used in doses above RDA.

DILTIAZEM

Cardizem, Cardizem SR, Cardizem CD, Cardizem LA, Dilacor XR, Tiazac, and others
Calcium-channel blocker, antihypertensive

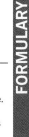

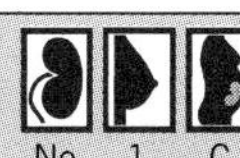

Tabs: 30, 60, 90, 120 mg
Extended-release tabs:
Cardizem LA: 120, 180, 240, 300, 360, 420 mg
Extended-release caps:
Cardizem SR: 60, 90, 120 mg
Cardizem CD: 120, 180, 240, 300, 360 mg
Dilacor XR: 120, 180, 240 mg
Tiazac: 120, 180, 240, 300, 360, 420 mg
Injection: 5 mg/mL (5, 10 mL)

Child: 1.5–2 mg/kg/24 hr PO ÷ TID–QID; **max. dose:** 3.5 mg/kg/24 hr, **alternative maximum dose** of 6 mg/kg/24 up to 360 mg/24 hr has been recommended
Adolescent:
Immediate release: 30–120 mg/dose PO TID–QID; usual range 180–360 mg/24 hr
Extended release: 120–300 mg/24 hr PO ÷ QD–BID (BID dosing with Cardizem SR; QD dosing with Cardizem CD, Cardizem LA, Dilacor XR, Tiazac); **max. dose:** 540 mg/24 hr

Contraindicated in acute MI with pulmonary congestion, second- or third-degree heart block, and sick sinus syndrome. Dizziness, headache, edema, nausea, vomiting, heart block, and arrhythmias may occur.

Diltiazem is a substrate and inhibitor of the cytochrome P-450 3A4 enzyme system. May increase levels and/or effect of buspirone, cyclosporine, carbamazepine, fentanyl, digoxin, quinidine, tacrolimus, benzodiazepines, and beta-blockers. Cimetidine may increase diltiazem serum levels. Rifampin may decrease diltiazem serum levels.

Maximum antihypertensive effect seen within 2 wk.

For explanation of icons, see p. 680.

DIMENHYDRINATE

Dramamine, Children's Dramamine, and other brand names

Antiemetic, antihistamine

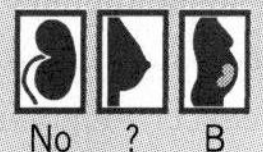
No ? B

Tabs (OTC): 50 mg
Chewable tabs (OTC): 50 mg (contains 1.5 mg phenylalanine)
Solution (OTC): 12.5 mg/4 mL, 12.5 mg/5 mL, 15.62 mg/5 mL (some preparations may contain 5% alcohol)
Injection: 50 mg/mL (benzyl alcohol and propylene glycol)

Child (<12 yr): 5 mg/kg/24 hr ÷ Q6 hr PO/IM/IV; alternative oral dosing by age:
2–5 yr: 12.5–25 mg/dose Q6–8 hr PRN PO with the **max. dosage** below
6–12 yr: 25–50 mg/dose Q6–8 hr PRN PO with the **max. dosage** below
Adult: 50–100 mg/dose Q4–6 hr PRN PO/IM/IV
Max. PO doses:
2–5 yr: 75 mg/24 hr
6–12 yr: 150 mg/24 hr
Adult: 400 mg/24 hr
Max. IM dose: 300 mg/24 hr

Causes drowsiness and anticholinergic side effects. May mask vestibular symptoms and cause CNS excitation in young children. Caution when taken with ototoxic agents or history of seizures. Use should be limited to management of prolonged vomiting of known etiology. **Not recommended** in children <2 yr. Toxicity resembles anticholinergic poisoning.

DIMERCAPROL

BAL, British anti-Lewisite

Heavy-metal chelator (arsenic, gold, mercury, lead)

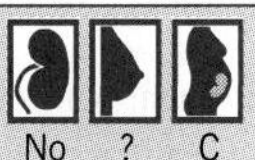
No ? C

Injection (in oil): 100 mg/mL; contains benzyl benzoate and peanut oil (3 mL)

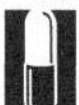

Give all injections deep IM.
Lead poisoning:
Acute severe encephalopathy (lead level >70 mcg/dL): 4 mg/kg/dose Q4 hr × 2–7 days with the addition of Ca-EDTA (given at separate site) at the time of the second dose.
Less severe poisoning: 4 mg/kg × 1, then 3 mg/kg/dose Q4 hr × 2–7 days.
Arsenic or gold poisoning:
Days 1 and 2: 2.5–3 mg/kg/dose Q6 hr
Day 3: 2.5–3 mg/kg/dose Q12 hr
Days 4 to 14: 2.5–3 mg/kg/dose Q24 hr
Mercury poisoning: 5 mg/kg × 1, then 2.5 mg/kg/dose QD–BID × 10 days

Contraindicated in hepatic or renal insufficiency. May cause hypertension, tachycardia, GI disturbance, headache, fever (30% of children), nephrotoxicity, transient neutropenia. Symptoms are usually relieved by antihistamines. Urine should be kept alkaline to protect the kidneys. **Use with caution** in patients with G6PD deficiency. **Do not use** concomitantly with iron.

DIPHENHYDRAMINE
Benadryl and other brand names
Antihistamine

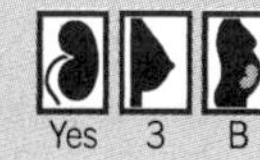

Elixir (OTC): 12.5 mg/5 mL; may contain 5.6% alcohol
Syrup: 12.5 mg/5 mL; some may contain 5% alcohol
Liquid (OTC): 12.5 mg/5 mL
Caps/tabs (OTC): 25, 50 mg
Chewable tabs (OTC): 12.5 mg (aspartame, phenylalanine)
Injection: 50 mg/mL
Cream (OTC): 1, 2% (30 g)
Lotion (OTC): 1% (75, 180 mL)
Topical gel (OTC): 1, 2% (118 g)
Topical spray (OTC): 1% (120 mL)

Child: 5 mg/kg/24 hr ÷ Q6 hr PO/IM/IV
Max. dose: 300 mg/24 hr
Adult: 10–50 mg/dose Q4–8 hr PO/IM/IV
Max. dose: 400 mg/24 hr
For anaphylaxis or phenothiazine overdose: 1–2 mg/kg IV slowly.

Contraindicated with concurrent MAO inhibitor use, acute attacks of asthma, and GI or urinary obstruction. **Use with caution** in infants and young children, and **do not use** in neonates because of potential CNS effects. Side effects include sedation, nausea, vomiting, xerostomia, blurred vision, and other reactions common to antihistamines. CNS side effects more common than GI disturbances. May cause paradoxical excitement in children. **Adjust dose in renal failure (see Chapter 30).**

DISOPYRAMIDE PHOSPHATE
Norpace and others
Antiarrhythmic agent, class Ia

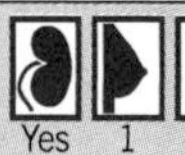
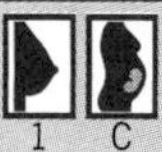

Caps: 100, 150 mg
Extended-release caps (CR): 100, 150 mg
Suspension: 1 mg/mL, 10 mg/mL

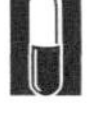

<1 yr: 10–30 mg/kg/24 hr ÷ Q6 hr PO
1–4 yr: 10–20 mg/kg/24 hr ÷ Q6 hr PO
4–12 yr: 10–15 mg/kg/24 hr ÷ Q6 hr PO
12–18 yr: 6–15 mg/kg/24 hr ÷ Q6 hr PO
Adult:
<50 kg: 100 mg/dose Q6 hr PO or 200 mg (extended-release) Q12 hr PO
≥50 kg: 150 mg/dose Q6 hr PO or 300 mg (extended-release) Q12 hr PO
Max. dose: 1.6 g/24 hr

Continued

For explanation of icons, see p. 680.

DISOPYRAMIODE PHOSPHATE *continued*

Contraindicated in second- or third-degree heart block. May cause decreased cardiac output. Anticholinergic effects may occur. Causes dose-related AV block, wide QRS, increased QTc, ventricular dysrhythmias. **Adjust dose in renal or hepatic failure (see Chapter 30).**

Drug is metabolized by cytochrome P450 3A4 isoenzyme. Clarithromycin and erythromycin may increase serum levels. Phenytoin, phenobarbital, and rifampin may decrease serum levels. Therapeutic levels: 3–7 mg/L.

Use limited in neurally mediated syncope.

DIVALPROEX SODIUM

Depakote, Depakote ER

Anticonvulsant

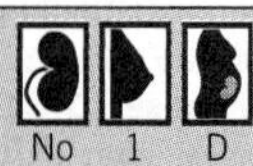

Delayed-release tabs: 125, 250, 500 mg
Extended-release tabs (Depakote ER): 250, 500 mg
Sprinkle caps: 125 mg

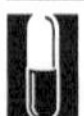

Dose: see *Valproic Acid*

Remarks: see **Valproic Acid.** Preferred over valproic acid for patients on ketogenic diet. Depakote ER is prescribed by a once daily interval; whereas Depakote is typically prescribed BID. Depakote and Depakote ER are not bioequivalent; see package insert for dose conversion.

DOBUTAMINE

Dobutrex

Sympathomimetic agent

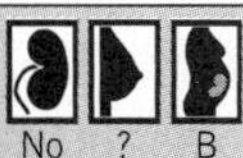

Injection: 12.5 mg/mL (contains sulfites) (20 mL)
Prediluted in D5W: 0.5 mg/mL (500 mL), 1 mg/mL (250, 500 mL), 2 mg/mL (250 mL), 4 mg/mL (250 mL)

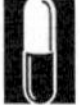

Continuous IV infusion: 2.5–15 mcg/kg/min;
Max. dose: 40 mcg/kg/min
To prepare infusion: see inside front cover.

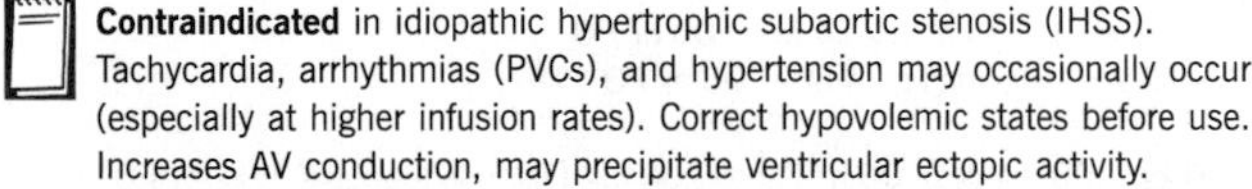

Contraindicated in idiopathic hypertrophic subaortic stenosis (IHSS). Tachycardia, arrhythmias (PVCs), and hypertension may occasionally occur (especially at higher infusion rates). Correct hypovolemic states before use. Increases AV conduction, may precipitate ventricular ectopic activity.

Dobutamine has been shown to increase cardiac output and systemic pressure in pediatric patients of every age group. However, in premature neonates, dobutamine is less effective than dopamine in raising systemic blood pressure without causing undue tachycardia, and dobutamine has not been shown to provide any added benefit when given to such infants already receiving optimal infusions of dopamine.

Monitor BP and vital signs. $T_{1/2}$: 2 min. Peak effects in 10–20 min.

DOCUSATE
Colace, Surfak, and others
Stool softener, laxative

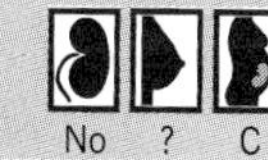
No ? C

Available as docusate sodium:
Caps (OTC): 50, 100, 250 mg
Tabs (OTC): 100 mg
Syrup (OTC): 16.7 mg/5 mL, 20 mg/5 mL; may contain alcohol
Oral liquid (OTC): 10 mg/mL; contains 1 mg/mL sodium
Available as docusate calcium:
Caps (Surfak; OTC): 240 mg

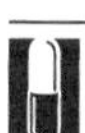

PO (take with liquids):
<3 yr: 10–40 mg/24 hr ÷ QD–QID
3–6 yr: 20–60 mg/24 hr ÷ QD–QID
6–12 yr: 40–150 mg/24 hr ÷ QD–QID
>12 yr: 50–400 mg/24 hr ÷ QD–QID
Rectal: *older child and adult:* add 50–100 mg of oral liquid (not syrup) to enema fluid.

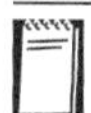

Oral dosage effective only after 1–3 days of therapy. Incidence of side effects is exceedingly low. Oral liquid is bitter; give with milk, fruit juice, or formula to mask taste.

A few drops of the 10 mg/mL oral liquid may be used in the ear as a ceruminolytic. Effect is usually seen within 15 min.

DOLASETRON
Anzemet
Antiemetic agent, 5-HT$_3$ antagonist

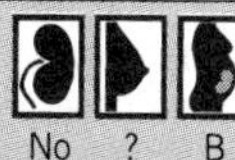
No ? B

Injection: 20 mg/mL (0.625, 5, 25 mL)
Tabs: 25, 50 mg

Chemotherapy-induced nausea and vomiting:
2 yr–adult: 1.8 mg/kg/dose IV/PO up to a **max. dose** of 100 mg. Administer IV doses 30 min before chemotherapy, and administer PO doses 60 min before chemotherapy.

Postoperative nausea and vomiting prevention:
2–16 yr:
IV: 0.35 mg/kg/dose (**max. dose:** 12.5 mg) 15 min before cessation of anesthesia or at onset of nausea and vomiting
PO: 1.2 mg/kg/dose (**max. dose:** 100 mg) 2 hr before surgery

Continued

For explanation of icons, see p. 680.

DOLASETRON *continued*

Adult:

IV: 12.5 mg/dose 15 min before cessation of anesthesia or at onset of nausea and vomiting

PO: 100 mg/dose 2 hr before surgery

May cause hypotension and prolongation of cardiac conduction intervals, particularly QTc interval. Common side effects include dizziness, headache, sedation, blurred vision, fever, chills, and sleep disorders.

Avoid concurrent use with other drugs that increase QTc interval (e.g., erythromycin, cisapride). Drug is a substrate for CYP450 2D6 and 3A3/4 isoenzymes; concomitant use of enzyme inhibitors (e.g., cimetidine) may increase risk for side effects, and use of enzyme inducers (e.g., rifampin) may decrease dolasetron efficacy.

IV doses may be administered undiluted over 30 sec.

DOPAMINE

Intropin and others

Sympathomimetic agent

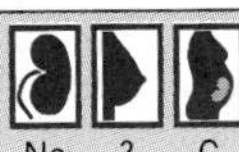

Injection: 40, 80, 160 mg/mL (5, 10, 20 mL)
Prediluted in D5W: 0.8, 1.6, 3.2 mg/mL (250, 500 mL)

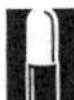

Low dose: 2–5 mcg/kg/min IV; increases renal blood flow; minimal effect on heart rate and cardiac output

Intermediate dose: 5–15 mcg/kg/min IV; increases heart rate, cardiac contractility, cardiac output, and to a lesser extent, renal blood flow

High dose: >20 mcg/kg/min IV; alpha-adrenergic effects are prominent; decreases renal perfusion

Max. dose recommended: 20–50 mcg/kg/min IV

To prepare infusion: see inside front cover.

Do not use in pheochromocytoma, tachyarrhythmias, or hypovolemia. Monitor vital signs and blood pressure continuously. Correct hypovolemic states.

Tachyarrhythmias, ectopic beats, hypertension, vasoconstriction, and vomiting may occur. **Use with caution** with phenytoin because hypotension and bradycardia may be exacerbated.

Newborn infants may be more sensitive to the vasoconstrictive effects of dopamine. Children <2 yr clear dopamine faster and exhibit high variability in neonates.

Should be administered through a central line or large vein. Extravasation may cause tissue necrosis; treat with phentolamine. **Do not administer** into an umbilical arterial catheter.

DORNASE ALFA/DNASE

Pulmozyme

Inhaled mucolytic

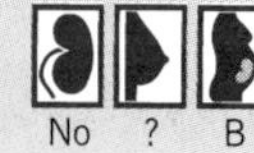

Inhalation solution: 1 mg/mL (2.5 mL)

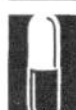

Child >5 yr and adult: 2.5 mg via nebulizer QD. Some patients may benefit from 2.5 mg BID.

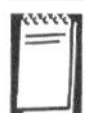

Contraindicated in patients with hypersensitivity to epoetin alfa. Voice alteration, pharyngitis, laryngitis may result. These are generally reversible without dose adjustment.

Do not mix with other nebulized drugs. A beta-agonist may be useful before administration to enhance drug distribution. Chest physiotherapy should be incorporated into treatment regimen. Use of the Sidestream nebulizer cup can significantly reduce the medication administration time.

DOXAPRAM HCL

Dopram

CNS stimulant

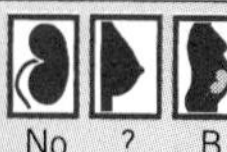

Injection: 20 mg/mL (20 mL); contains 0.9% benzyl alcohol

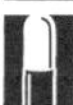

Methylxanthine-refractory neonatal apnea: load with 2.5–3 mg/kg over 15 min, followed by a continuous infusion of 1 mg/kg/hr titrated to the lowest effective dose; **max. dose:** 2.5 mg/kg/hr.

Hypertension occurs with higher doses (>1.5 mg/kg/hr). May also cause tachycardia, arrhythmias, seizure, hyperreflexia, hyperpyrexia, abdominal distension, bloody stools, and sweating. Avoid extravasation into tissues.

Do not use with general anesthetic agents that can sensitize the heart to catecholamines (e.g., halothane, cyclopropane, and enflurane) to reduce the risk for cardiac arrhythmias, including ventricular tachycardia and ventricular fibrillation. **Do not initiate** doxapram until the general anesthetic agent has been completely excreted.

For explanation of icons, see p. 680.

DOXYCYCLINE

Vibramycin, Periostat, and others

Antibiotic, tetracycline derivative

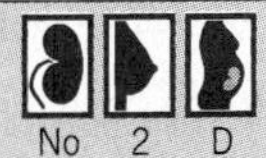

Caps: 20 (Periostat), 50, 75, 100 mg
Tabs: 20 (Periostat), 50, 100 mg
Syrup: 50 mg/5 mL (60 mL)
Suspension: 25 mg/5 mL (60 mL)
Injection: 100, 200 mg

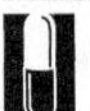

Initial:
- ***≤45 kg:*** 2.2 mg/kg/dose BID PO/IV × 1 day to **max. dose** of 200 mg/24 hr
- ***>45 kg:*** 100 mg/dose BID PO/IV × 1 day

Maintenance:
- ***≤45 kg:*** 2.2–4.4 mg/kg/dose QD–BID PO/IV
- ***>45 kg:*** 100–200 mg/24 hr ÷ QD–BID PO/IV

Max. adult dose: 300 mg/24 hr
PID: see Chapter 16.
Anthrax (inhalation/systemic/cutaneous; see remarks): Initiate therapy with IV route, and convert to PO route when clinically appropriate. Duration of therapy is 60 days (IV and PO combined):
- ***≤8 yr or ≤45 kg:*** 2.2 mg/kg/dose BID IV/PO; **max. dose:** 200 mg/24 hr
- ***>8 yr or >45 kg:*** 100 mg/dose BID IV/PO

Malaria prophylaxis (start 1–2 days before exposure and continue for 4 wk after leaving endemic area):
- ***>8 yr:*** 2 mg/kg/24 hr PO QD; **max. dose:** 100 mg/24 hr
- ***Adult:*** 100 mg PO QD

Periodontitis:
- ***Adult:*** 20 mg BID PO × ≤9 mo

Use with caution in hepatic and renal disease. May cause increased intracranial pressure. Generally **not recommended** for use in children <8 yr owing to risk for tooth enamel hypoplasia and discoloration. However, the AAP *Red Book* recommends doxycycline as the drug of choice for rickettsial disease regardless of age. May cause GI symptoms, photosensitivity, hemolytic anemia, rash and hypersensitivity reactions.

Doxycycline is approved for the treatment of anthrax (*Bacillus anthracis*) in combination with one or two other antimicrobials. If meningitis is suspected, consider using an alternative agent because of poor CNS penetration. Consider changing to high-dose amoxicillin (25–35 mg/kg/dose TID PO) for penicillin susceptible strains. See www.bt.cdc.gov for the latest information.

Rifampin, barbiturates, phenytoin, and carbamazepine may increase clearance of doxycycline. Doxycycline may enhance the hypoprothrombinemic effect of warfarin. See *Tetracycline* for additional drug/food interactions and comments.

Infuse IV over 1–4 hr. Avoid prolonged exposure to direct sunlight.

For periodontitis, take capsules ≥1 hr before meals, and take tablets ≥1 hr before or 2 hr after meals.

DRONABINOL
Tetrahydrocannabinol, THC, Marinol
Antiemetic

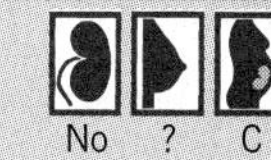
No ? C

Caps: 2.5, 5, 10 mg (contains sesame oil)

Antiemetic:
Child and adult (PO): 5 mg/m^2/dose 1–3 hr before chemotherapy, then Q2–4 hr up to a **max. dose** 6 doses/24 hr; doses may be gradually increased by 2.5 mg/m^2/dose increments up to a **max. dose** of 15 mg/m^2/dose if needed and tolerated.

Appetite stimulant:
Adult (PO): 2.5 mg BID 1 hr before lunch and dinner; if not tolerated, reduce dose to 2.5 mg QHS.
Max. dose: 20 mg/24 hr (**use caution** when increasing doses because of increased risk for dose-related adverse reactions at higher dosages)

Contraindicated in patients with history of substance abuse, mental illness, and allergy to sesame oil. **Use with caution** in heart disease, seizures, and hepatic disease (reduce dose if severe). Side effects: euphoria, dizziness, difficulty concentrating, anxiety, mood change, sedation, hallucinations, ataxia, paresthesia, hypotension, excessively increased appetite, and habit forming potential.

Onset of action: 0.5–1 hr. Duration of psychoactive effects, 4–6 hr; appetite stimulation, 24 hr.

DROPERIDOL
Inapsine
Sedative, antiemetic

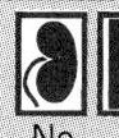
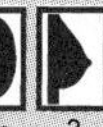
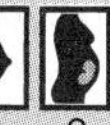
No ? C

Injection: 2.5 mg/mL

Antiemetic/sedation:
Child: 0.03–0.07 mg/kg/dose IM or IV over 2–5 min; if needed, may give 0.1–0.15 mg/kg/dose; initial **max. dose:** 0.1 mg/kg/dose and subsequent **max. dose:** 2.5 mg/dose.
Dosage interval:
Antiemetic: PRN Q4–6 hr
Sedation: Repeat dose in 15–30 min if necessary.

Adult: 2.5–5 mg IM or IV over 2–5 min; **initial max. dose** is 2.5 mg.
Dosage interval:
Antiemetic: PRN Q3–4 hr
Sedation: Repeat dose in 15–30 min if necessary.

Continued

For explanation of icons, see p. 680.

DROPERIDOL *continued*

Side effects include hypotension, tachycardia, extrapyramidal side effects such as dystonia, feeling of motor restlessness, laryngospasm, and bronchospasm. May lower seizure threshold. **Fatal arrhythmias and QT interval prolongation have been associated with use.**

Onset in 3–10 min. Peak effects within 10–30 min. Duration of 2–4 hr. Often given as adjunct to other agents.

EDROPHONIUM CHLORIDE

Tensilon, Enlon, Reversol

Anticholinesterase agent, antidote for neuromuscular blockade

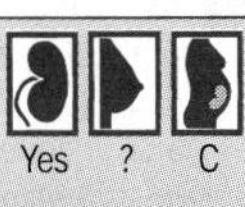

Injection: 10 mg/mL (1, 10, 15 mL) (contains 0.45% phenol and 0.2% sulfite)

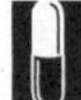

Test for myasthenia gravis (IV):

Neonate: 0.1 mg single dose

Infant and child:

Initial: 0.04 mg/kg/dose × 1

Max. dose: 1 mg for <34 kg, 2 mg for ≥34 kg

If no response after 1 min, may give 0.16 mg/kg/dose for a total of 0.2 mg/kg.

Total max. dose: 5 mg for <34 kg, 10 mg for ≥34 kg

Adult: 2 mg test dose IV; if no reaction, give 8 mg after 45 sec.

May precipitate cholinergic crisis, arrhythmias, and bronchospasm. Keep atropine available in syringe and have resuscitation equipment ready. Hypersensitivity to test dose (fasciculations or intestinal cramping) is indication to stop giving drug. **Contraindicated** in GI or GU obstruction or arrhythmias. Dose may need to be reduced in chronic renal failure.

Short duration of action with IV route (5–10 min). **Antidote:** atropine, 0.01–0.04 mg/kg/dose.

EDTA CALCIUM DISODIUM

Calcium disodium versenate

Chelating agent, antidote for lead toxicity

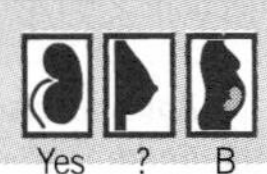

Injection: 200 mg/mL (5 mL)

Lead poisoning:

Lead level >70 mcg/dL (use with dimercaprol): initiate at the time of the second dimercaprol dose and treat for 3–5 days. May repeat a course as needed after 2–4 days of no EDTA.

IM: 1000–1500 mg/m²/24 hr ÷ Q4 hr

IV: 1000–1500 mg/m²/24 hr as an 8–24 hour infusion or divided Q12 hr

Use 1500 mg/m²/24 hr for 5 days in the presence of encephalopathy.

Lead level 20–70 mcg/dL: 1000 mg/m²/24 hr IV as an 8–24 hr infusion OR intermittent dosing divided Q12 hr × 5 days. May repeat a course as needed after 2–4 days of no EDTA.

Max. daily dose: 75 mg/kg/24 hr

Continued

EDTA CALCIUM DISODIUM *continued*

May cause renal tubular necrosis. **Do not use** if anuric. Dosage reduction is recommended with mild renal disease. Follow urinalysis and renal function. Monitor ECG continuously for arrhythmia when giving IV. Rapid IV infusion may cause sudden increase in intracranial pressure in patients with cerebral edema. May cause zinc and copper deficiency. Monitor Ca^{2+} and PO_4.

IM route preferred. Give IM with 0.5% procaine.

EMLA

See *Lidocaine* and *Prilocaine*

ENALAPRIL MALEATE, ENALAPRILAT

Vasotec, Vasotec IV, and others

Angiotensin-converting enzyme inhibitor, antihypertensive

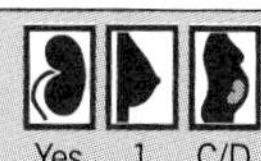

Tabs: 2.5, 5, 10, 20 mg (Enalapril)
Oral suspension: 1 mg/mL 
Injection: 1.25 mg/mL (Enalaprilat); contains benzyl alcohol

Infant and child:
PO: 0.1 mg/kg/24 hr up to 5 mg/24 hr ÷ QD–BID; increase PRN over 2 wk.
Max. dose: 0.5 mg/kg/24 hr up to 40 mg/24 hr
IV: 0.005–0.01 mg/kg/dose Q8–24 hr

Adult:
PO: 2.5–5 mg/24 hr QD initially to **max. dose** of 40 mg/24 hr ÷ QD–BID
IV: 0.625–1.25 mg/dose IV Q6 hr

Use with caution in bilateral renal artery stenosis. **Avoid** use with dialysis with high-flux membranes because anaphylactoid reactions have been reported. Side effects: nausea, diarrhea, headache, dizziness, hyperkalemia, hypoglycemia, hypotension, and hypersensitivity. Cough is a reported side effect of ACE inhibitors.

Enalapril (PO) is converted to its active form (Enalaprilat) by the liver. Administer IV over 5 min. **Adjust dose in renal impairment (see Chapter 30).**

Pregnancy category is C during the first trimester but changes to D during the second and third trimesters (fetal injury and death have been reported).

ENOXAPARIN

Lovenox

Anticoagulant, low-molecular-weight heparin

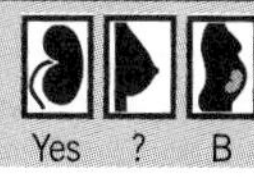

Injection: 100 mg/mL (3 mL); contains 15 mg/mL benzyl alcohol
Injection (prefilled syringes with 27-gauge × ½-inch needle): 30 mg/0.3 mL, 40 mg/0.4 mL, 60 mg/0.6 mL, 80 mg/0.8 mL, 100 mg/1 mL, 120 mg/0.8 mL, 150 mg/1 mL
Approximate anti-factor Xa activity: 100 IU per 1 mg

Continued

For explanation of icons, see p. 680.

ENOXAPARIN *continued*

DVT treatment:

Infant <2 mo: 1.5 mg/kg/dose Q12 hr SC

Infant ≥2 mo–adult: 1 mg/kg/dose Q12 hr SC; alternatively, 1.5 mg/kg/dose Q24 hr SC can be used in adults.

Dosage adjustment to achieve target anti-factor Xa levels of 0.5–1 units/mL (see table below):

Anti–Factor Xa Level (units/mL)	Hold Next Dose?	Dose Change	Repeat Anti–Factor Xa Level?
<0.35	No	Increase by 25%	4 hr post next new dose
0.35–0.49	No	Increase by 10%	4 hr post next new dose
0.5–1	No	No	Next day, then 1 week later at 4 hr post dose
1.1–1.5	No	Decrease by 20%	4 hr post next new dose
1.6–2	3 hr	Decrease by 30%	4 hr post next new dose
>2	Until anti–factor Xa reaches 0.5 units/mL (levels can be measured Q12 hr until it reaches ≤0.5 units/mL)	When anti–factor Xa reaches 0.5 units/mL, dose may be restarted at a dose 40% less than originally prescribed.	4 hr post next new dose

DVT prophylaxis:

Infant <2 mo: 0.75 mg/kg/dose Q12 hr SC

Infant ≥2 mo–child 18 yr: 0.5 mg/kg/dose Q12 hr SC

Adult:

Knee or hip replacement surgery: 30 mg BID SC × 7–14 days; initiate therapy 12–24 hr after surgery provided hemostasis is established. Alternatively for hip replacement surgery, 40 mg QD SC × 7–14 days initially up to 3 wk thereafter; initiate therapy 9–15 hr before surgery.

Abdominal surgery: 40 mg QD SC × 7–12 days initiated 2 hr before surgery.

Inhibits thrombosis by inactivating factor Xa without significantly affecting bleeding time, platelet function, PT, or APTT at recommended doses. Dosages of enoxaparin, heparin, or other low-molecular-weight heparins cannot be used interchangeably on a unit-for-unit (or mg-for-mg) basis because of differences in pharmacokinetics and activity. Peak anti–factor Xa activity is achieved 4 hr after a dose.

Contraindicated in major bleeding and drug-induced thrombocytopenia. **Use with caution** in uncontrolled arterial hypertension, bleeding diathesis, history of recurrent GI ulcers, diabetic retinopathy, and severe renal dysfunction (reduce dose

Continued

ENOXAPARIN *continued*

by increasing the dosage interval from Q12 hr to Q24 hr if GFR <30 mL/min). Concurrent use with spinal or epidural anesthesia or spinal puncture has resulted in long-term or permanent paralysis; potential benefits must be weighed against the risks. May cause fever, confusion, edema, nausea, hemorrhage, thrombocytopenia, hypochromic anemia, and pain/erythema at injection site. Protamine sulfate is the antidote; 1 mg protamine sulfate neutralizes 1 mg enoxaparin.

Recommended anti–factor Xa levels obtained 4 hr after subcutaneous dose:

DVT treatment: 0.5–1 units/mL

DVT prophylaxis: 0.2–0.4 units/mL

Administer by deep SC injection by having the patient lie down. Alternate administration between the left and right anterolateral and left and right posterolateral abdominal wall. See package insert for detailed SC administration recommendations. To minimize bruising, do not rub the injection site. IV or IM route of administration is **not recommended.**

For additional information, see Chest 2004;126:645S–687S.

EPINEPHRINE HCL

Adrenalin and others

Sympathomimetic agent

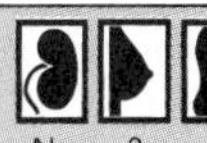
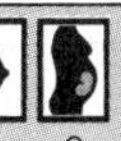

No ? C

1:1000 (aqueous):

Injection: 1 mg/mL (1, 30 mL)

1:200 (Sus-Phrine suspension):

Injection: 5 mg/mL (0.3, 5 mL)

1:10,000 (aqueous):

Injection: 0.1 mg/mL (10 mL prefilled syringes and vials)

EpiPen: 0.3 mg autoinjection (2 mL of 1:1000 solution)

EpiPen Jr: 0.15 mg autoinjection (2 mL of 1:2000 solution)

Aerosol: 0.22 mg epinephrine base/spray (15, 22.5 mL)

Oral inhalation solution: 0.1% (1mg/mL or 1:1000) (30 mL), 1% (10 mg/mL or 1:100) (7.5 mL)

Ophthalmic solution: 0.5%, 1%, 2% (15 mL)

Some preparations may contain sulfites.

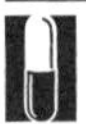

Cardiac uses:

Neonate:

Asystole and bradycardia: 0.01–0.03 mg/kg of 1:10,000 solution (0.1–0.3 mL/kg) IV/ET Q3–5 min

Infant and child:

Bradycardia/asystole and pulseless arrest: see inside front cover and algorithms

Bradycardia, asystole, and pulseless arrest *(see remarks):*

First dose: 0.01 mg/kg of 1:10,000 solution (0.1 mL/kg) IO/IV; **max. dose:** 1 mg (10 mL). **Subsequent doses should be the same.** High dose epinephrine after failure of standard dose has not been shown to be effective (see remarks). Must circulate drug with CPR. For ET route see below.

All ET doses: 0.1 mg/kg of 1:1000 solution (0.1 mL/kg) ET Q3–5 min.

Continued

For explanation of icons, see p. 680.

EPINEPHRINE HCL *continued*

Adult:
Asystole: 1–5 mg IV/ET Q3–5 min
IV drip (all ages): 0.1–1 mcg/kg/min; titrate to effect; to prepare infusion, see inside front cover.

Respiratory uses:
Bronchodilator:
1:1000 (aqueous):
Infant and child: 0.01 mL/kg/dose SC (**max. single dose** 0.5 mL); repeat Q15 min × 3–4 doses or Q4 hr PRN
Adult: 0.3–0.5 mL/dose
1:200 (Sus-Phrine suspension)
Infant and child: 0.005 mL/kg/dose SC (**max. single dose** 0.15 mL); repeat Q8–12 hr PRN
Adult: 0.1–0.3 mL/dose SC Q6 hr PRN
Inhalation: 1–2 puffs Q4 hr PRN
Nebulization (alternative to racemic epinephrine): 0.5 mL/kg of 1:1000 solution diluted in 3 mL NS; **max. doses:** ≤4 yr: 2.5 mL/dose; >4 yr: 5 mL/dose

Hypersensitivity reactions (see remarks for IV dosing):
Child: 0.01 mg/kg/dose IM/SC up to a **max. dose** of 0.5 mg/dose Q20 min–4 hr PRN. IM delivery may be superior in anaphylaxis (see remarks). If using EpiPen or EpiPen Jr, administer only via the IM route using the following dosage:
<30 kg: 0.15 mg
≥30 kg: 0.3 mg
Adult: Start with 0.1–0.5 mg IM/SC Q20 min–4 hr PRN; doses may be increased if necessary to a **single max. dose** of 1 mg.

High-dose rescue therapy for in-hospital cardiac arrest in children after failure of an initial standard dose has been reported to be of no benefit compared with standard dose. In fact, data suggest high dose therapy may be worse than standard dose therapy in some patients. (N Engl J Med 2004;350: 1722–1730).

Hypersensitivity reactions: For bronchial asthma and certain allergic manifestations (e.g., angioedema, urticaria, serum sickness, anaphylactic shock), use epinephrine SC. Patients with anaphylaxis may benefit from IM administration. The adult IV dose for hypersensitivity reactions or to relieve bronchospasm usually ranges from 0.1 to 0.25 mg injected slowly over 5–10 min Q5–15 min as needed. Neonates may be given a dose of 0.01 mg/kg body weight; for the infant, 0.05 mg is an adequate initial dose, and this may be repeated at 20- to 30-min intervals in the management of asthma attacks.

May produce arrhythmias, tachycardia, hypertension, headaches, nervousness, nausea, vomiting. Necrosis may occur at site of repeated local injection.

Concomitant use of noncardiac selective beta-blockers or tricyclic antidepressants may enhance epinephrine's pressor response. Chlorpromazine may reverse the pressor response.

ETT doses should be diluted with NS to a volume of 3–5 mL before administration. Follow with several positive pressure ventilations.

EpiPen and EpiPen Jr should be administered IM into the anterolateral aspect of the thigh.

EPINEPHRINE, RACEMIC

MicroNefrin, Nephron, S-2 Inhalant

Sympathomimetic agent

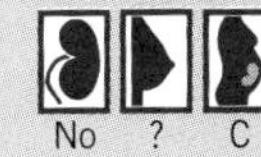

Solution: 2.25% (1.25% epinephrine base) (15, 30 mL)
Contains sulfites

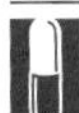

<4 yr:
Croup (using 2.25% solution): 0.05 mL/kg/dose up to a **max. dose** of 0.5 mL/dose diluted to 3 mL with NS. Given via nebulizer over 15 min PRN but not more frequently than Q1–2 hr.
≥4 yr: 0.5 mL/dose via nebulizer over 15 min Q 3–4 hr PRN

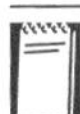

Tachyarrhythmias, headache, nausea, palpitations reported. Rebound symptoms may occur. Cardiorespiratory monitoring should be considered if administered more frequently than Q1–2 hr.

EPOETIN ALFA

Erythropoietin, Epogen, Procrit

Recombinant human erythropoietin

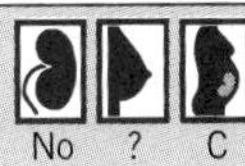

Injection (single-dose, preservative-free vials): 2000, 3000, 4000, 10,000, 40,000 U/mL (1 mL)
Injection (multidose vials): 10,000 U/mL (2 mL), 20,000 U/mL (1 mL); contains 1% benzyl alcohol
All dosage forms contain 2.5 mg albumin per 1 mL.

Renal failure: *SC/IV*
Initial: 50–100 U/kg 3 times per week; may increase dose if hematocrit does not rise by 5–6 points after 8 wk; maintenance doses are individualized.

AZT-treated HIV patients: *SC/IV*
100 U/kg/dose 3 times per wk × 8 wk; the dose may be increased by 50–100 U/kg/dose given 3 times per wk; **max. dose:** 300 U/kg/dose given 3 times per wk.

Anemia of prematurity:
25–100 U/kg/dose SC 3 times per week; alternatively, 200–400 U/kg/dose IV/SC 3–5 times per week for 2–6 wk (**total dose per wk** is 600–1400 U/kg)

Evaluate serum iron, ferritin, TIBC before therapy. Iron supplementation recommended during therapy unless iron stores are already in excess. Monitor Hct, BP, clotting times, platelets, BUN, serum creatinine. Peak effect in 2–3 wk. Reduce dose when target Hct is reached or when Hct increases >4 points in any 2-wk period. May cause hypertension, seizure, hypersensitivity reactions, headache, edema, dizziness. SC route provides sustained serum levels compared with IV route.

For explanation of icons, see p. 680.

ERGOCALCIFEROL

Drisdol, Calciferol

Vitamin D_2

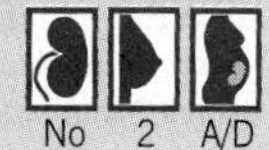

Caps/tabs: 50,000 IU (1.25 mg)
Injection: 500,000 IU/mL (1 mL)
Drops (OTC): 8000 IU/mL (200 mcg/mL) (60 mL)
1 mg = 40,000 IU vitamin D activity

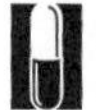

Dietary supplementation:
Preterm: 400–800 IU/24 hr PO
Infant/child: 400 IU/24 hr PO; please refer to Chapter 20 for details.

Renal failure:
Child: 4000–40,000 IU/24 hr PO
Adult: 20,000 IU/24 hr PO

Vitamin D–dependent rickets:
Child: 3000–5000 IU/24 hr PO; **max. dose:** 60,000 IU/24 hr
Adult: 10,000–60,000 IU/24 hr PO; some may require 500,000 IU/24 hr.

Nutritional rickets:
Adult and child with normal GI absorption: 2000–5000 IU/24 hr PO × 6–12 week
Malabsorption:
Child: 10,000–25,000 IU/24 hr PO
Adult: 10,000–300,000 IU/24 hr PO

Vitamin D–resistant rickets (with phosphate supplementation):
Child: initial dose 40,000–80,000 IU/24 hr PO; increase daily dose by 10,000–20,000 IU PO Q3–4 mo if needed.
Adult: 10,000–60,000 IU/24 hr PO

Hypoparathyroidism (with calcium supplementation):
Child: 50,000–200,000 IU/24 hr PO
Adult: 25,000–200,000 IU/24 hr PO

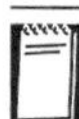

Monitor serum Ca^{2+}, PO_4, and alkaline phosphate. Serum Ca^{2+}, PO_4 product should be <70 mg/dL to avoid ectopic calcification. Titrate dosage to patient response. Watch for symptoms of hypercalcemia: weakness, diarrhea, polyuria, metastatic calcification, and nephrocalcinosis. Vitamin D_2 is activated by 25-hydroxylation in liver and 1-hydroxylation in kidneys.

Oral route is preferred. May use IM route in cases of fat malabsorption. **Injectable for IM administration only.**

Pregnancy category changes to D if used in doses above the RDA.

ERGOTAMINE TARTRATE

Cafergot and others

Ergot alkaloid

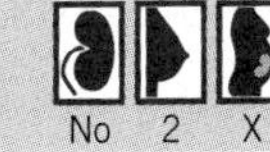

Tabs: 1 mg and 100 mg caffeine
Sublingual tabs: 2 mg
Suppository: 2 mg and 100 mg caffeine
Drug also available in combinations with belladonna alkaloids and/or phenobarbital.

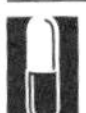

Older child and adolescent:
PO/SL: 1 mg at onset of migraine attack, then 1 mg Q30 min PRN up to **max. dose** of 3 mg per attack.

Adult:
PO/SL: 2 mg at onset of migraine attack, then 1–2 mg Q30 min up to 6 mg per attack; **do not exceed** 10 mg per week.
Suppository: 2 mg at first sign of attack; follow with second dose (2 mg) after 1 hr, **max. dose** 4 mg per attack, **not to exceed** 10 mg/week.

Use with caution in renal or hepatic disease. May cause paresthesias, GI disturbance, angina-like pain, rebound headache with abrupt withdrawal, or muscle cramps. **Contraindicated** in pregnancy and breast-feeding. Concurrent administration with protease inhibitors, clarithromycin, erythromycin, or other CYP450 3A4 inhibitors is **not recommended** owing to risk for ergotism (nausea, vomiting, vasospastic ischemia).

ERYTHROMYCIN ETHYLSUCCINATE AND ACETYLSULFISOXAZOLE

Pediazole, Eryzole, and others

Antibiotic, macrolide + sulfonamide derivative

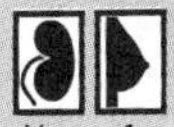

Suspension: 200 mg erythromycin and 600 mg sulfa/5 mL (100, 150, 200, 250 mL)

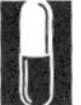

Otitis media: 50 mg/kg/24 hr (as erythromycin) and 150 mg/kg/24 hr (as sulfa) ÷ Q6 hr PO, or give 1.25 mL/kg/24 hr ÷ Q6 hr PO.
Max. dose: 2 g erythromycin, 6 g sulfisoxasole/24 hr

See adverse effects of erythromycin and sulfisoxazole. **Not recommended** in infants <2 mo. **Do not use** in renal impairment because dosage adjustments are inconsistent for sulfisoxazole and erythromycin.
Pregnancy category changes to D if administered near term.

For explanation of icons, see p. 680.

ERYTHROMYCIN PREPARATIONS
Erythrocin, Pediamycin, E-Mycin, Ery-Ped, and others
Antibiotic, macrolide

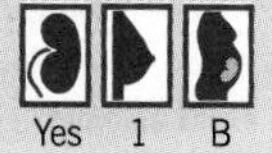
Yes 1 B

Erythromycin base:
- **Tabs:** 250, 333, 500 mg
- **Delayed-release tabs:** 250, 333, 500 mg
- **Delayed-release caps:** 250 mg
- **Topical ointment:** 2% (25 g)
- **Topical gel:** 2% (30, 60 g)
- **Topical solution:** 1.5%, 2% (60 mL)
- **Topical swab:** 2% (60s)
- **Ophthalmic ointment:** 0.5% (1, 3.5 g)

Erythromycin ethyl succinate (EES):
- **Suspension:** 200, 400 mg/5 mL (100, 480 mL)
- **Oral drops:** 100 mg/2.5 mL (50 mL)
- **Chewable tabs:** 200 mg
- **Tabs:** 400 mg

Erythromycin estolate:
- **Suspension:** 125, 250 mg/5 mL (480 mL)

Erythromycin stearate:
- **Tabs:** 250, 500 mg

Erythromycin gluceptate:
- **Injection:** 1000 mg

Erythromycin lactobionate:
- **Injection:** 500, 1000 mg

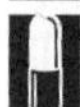

Oral:
Neonate:
- ***<1.2 kg:*** 20 mg/kg/24 hr ÷ Q12 hr PO
- ***≥1.2 kg:***
  - ***0–7 days:*** 20 mg/kg/24 hr ÷ Q12 hr PO
  - ***>7 days:*** 30 mg/kg/24 hr ÷ Q8 hr PO
- ***Chlamydial conjunctivitis and pneumonia:*** 50 mg/kg/24 hr ÷ Q6 hr PO × 14 days.

Child: 30–50 mg/kg/24 hr ÷ Q6–8 hr; **max. dose:** 2 g/24 hr
Adult: 1–4 g/24 hr ÷ Q6 hr; **max. dose:** 4 g/24 hr

Parenteral:
- ***Child:*** 20–50 mg/kg/24 hr ÷ Q6 hr IV
- ***Adult:*** 15–20 mg/kg/24 hr ÷ Q6 hr IV
- **Max. dose:** 4 g/24 hr

Rheumatic fever prophylaxis: 500 mg/24 hr ÷ Q12 hr PO
Ophthalmic: Apply 0.5-inch ribbon to affected eye BID–QID.
Pertussis: Estolate salt: 50 mg/kg/24 hr ÷ Q6 hr PO × 14 days
Preoperative bowel prep: 20 mg/kg/dose PO erythromycin base × 3 doses, with neomycin, 1 day before surgery
Prokinetic agent: 20 mg/kg/24 hr PO ÷ TID–QID (QAC or QAC and QHS)

Continued

ERYTHROMYCIN PREPARATIONS *continued*

Avoid IM route (pain, necrosis). GI side effects common (nausea, vomiting, abdominal cramps). **Use with caution** in liver disease. Estolate may cause cholestatic jaundice, although hepatotoxicity is uncommon (2% of reported cases). Inhibits CYP450 isoenzymes. May produce elevated digoxin, theophylline, carbamazepine, clozapine, cyclosporine, and methylprednisolone levels. **Contraindicated** in combination with cisapride. Hypertrophic pyloric stenosis in neonates receiving prophylactic therapy for pertussis and life-threatening episodes of ventricular tachycardia associated with prolonged QTc interval have been reported.

Oral therapy should replace IV as soon as possible. Give oral doses after meals. Because of different absorption characteristics, higher oral doses of EES are needed to achieve therapeutic effects. May produce false-positive urinary catecholamines. Formulations of IV lactobionate dosage form may contain benzyl alcohol. **Adjust dose in renal failure (see Chapter 30).**

ERYTHROPOIETIN

See *Epoetin Alfa*

ESMOLOL HCL

Brevibloc

Beta-1-selective adrenergic blocking agent, antihypertensive agent, class II antiarrhythmic

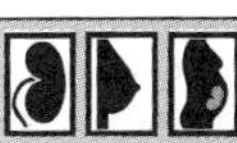

Injection: 10 mg/mL (10 mL), 20 mg/mL (5 mL), 250 mg/mL (10 mL); 250 mg/mL concentration contains 25% alcohol and 25% propylene glycol.
Injection, premixed infusion in iso-osmotic sodium chloride: 10 mg/mL (250 mL), 20 mg/mL (100 mL)

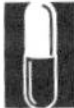

Titrate to individual response (limited information).
Loading dose: 100–500 mcg/kg IV over 1 min
Maintenance dose: 25–100 mcg/kg/min as infusion
If inadequate response, may readminister loading dose above, and/or increase maintenance dose by 25–50 mcg/kg/min in increments of Q5–10 min.
Usual maintenance dose range: 50–500 mcg/kg/min; dosages as high as 1000 mcg/kg/min have been administered.

$T_{1/2}$ = 9 min. May cause bronchospasm, congestive heart failure, hypotension (at doses >200 mcg/kg/min), nausea, and vomiting. May increase digoxin level by 10%–20%. Morphine may increase esmolol level by 46%.

Do not administer the 250 mg/mL concentration undiluted; concentration for administration is typically ≤10 mg/mL; however, 20 mg/mL has been administered in pediatric patients. **Administer only in a monitored setting.**

For explanation of icons, see p. 680.

ETANERCEPT

Enbrel

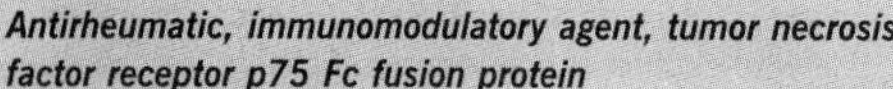

Antirheumatic, immunomodulatory agent, tumor necrosis factor receptor p75 Fc fusion protein

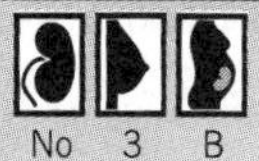

No 3 B

Injection: 25 mg with diluent (1 mL bacteriostatic water containing 0.9% benzyl alcohol)
Contains mannitol, sucrose, tromethamine.

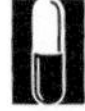

Child 4–17 yr: 0.4 mg/kg/dose SC twice weekly administered 72–96 hr apart; **max. dose:** 25 mg
Adult: 25 mg SC twice weekly administered 72–96 hr apart

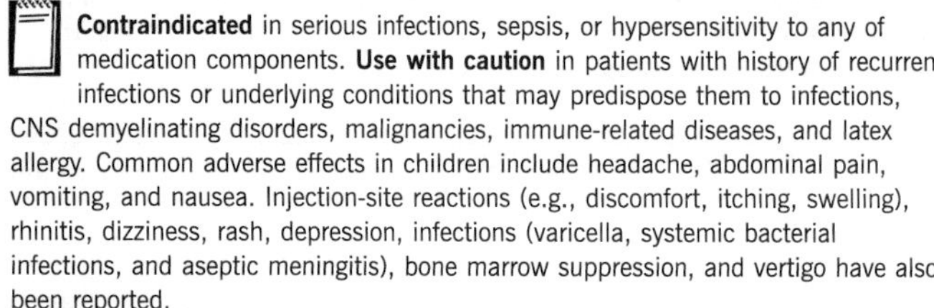

Contraindicated in serious infections, sepsis, or hypersensitivity to any of medication components. **Use with caution** in patients with history of recurrent infections or underlying conditions that may predispose them to infections, CNS demyelinating disorders, malignancies, immune-related diseases, and latex allergy. Common adverse effects in children include headache, abdominal pain, vomiting, and nausea. Injection-site reactions (e.g., discomfort, itching, swelling), rhinitis, dizziness, rash, depression, infections (varicella, systemic bacterial infections, and aseptic meningitis), bone marrow suppression, and vertigo have also been reported.

Do not administer live vaccines concurrently with this drug. In JRA, it is recommended that the patient be brought up to date with all immunizations in agreement with current immunization guidelines prior to initiating therapy.

Onset of action is 1–4 wk, with peak effects usually within 3 mo.

Patients must be properly instructed on preparing and administering the medication. Drug requires reconstitution by gently swirling its contents with the supplied diluent (**do not shake or vigorously agitate**) because some foaming will occur. Reconstituted solutions should be clear and colorless and used within 6 hr.

Drug is administered subcutaneously by rotating injection sites (thigh, abdomen, or upper arm). Administer new injections ≥1 inch from an old site and never where the skin is tender, bruised, red, or hard.

ETHAMBUTOL HCL

Myambutol

Antituberculosis drug

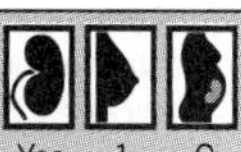

Yes 1 C

Tabs: 100, 400 mg

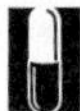

Tuberculosis:
Infant, child, adolescent, and adult: 15–25 mg/kg/dose PO QD or 50 mg/kg/dose PO twice weekly
Max. dose: 2.5 g/24 hr

Continued

ETHAMBUTOL HCL *continued*

Nontuberculous mycobacterial infection:

Child, adolescent, and adult: 15–25 mg/kg/24 hr PO; **max. dose:** 1 g/24 hr

M. avium complex prophylaxis in AIDS *(use in combination with other medications):*

Infant, child, adolescent, and adult: 15 mg/kg/dose PO QD; **max. dose:** 900 mg/dose

May cause reversible optic neuritis, especially with larger doses. Obtain baseline ophthalmologic studies before beginning therapy and then monthly. Follow visual acuity, visual fields, and (red-green) color vision. **Do not use** in children whose visual acuity cannot be assessed. **Discontinue** if any visual deterioration occurs. Monitor uric acid, liver function, heme status, and renal function. May cause GI disturbances. Coadministration with aluminum hydroxide can reduce ethambutol's absorption; space administration by 4 hr. Give with food. **Adjust dose with renal failure (see Chapter 30).**

ETHOSUXIMIDE

Zarontin

Anticonvulsant

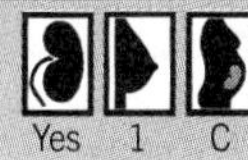

Caps: 250 mg

Syrup: 250 mg/5 mL

Child:

Oral:

≤6 yr: initial: 15 mg/kg/24 hr ÷ BID; **max. dose:** 500 mg/24 hr; increase as needed Q4–7 days. Usual maintenance dose: 15–40 mg/kg/24 hr ÷ BID

>6 yr and adult: 250 mg BID; increase by 250 mg/24 hr as needed Q4–7 days; usual maintenance dose: 20–40 mg/kg/24 hr ÷ BID

Max. dose: 1500 mg/24 hr

Use with caution in hepatic and renal disease. Ataxia, anorexia, drowsiness, sleep disturbances, rashes, and blood dyscrasias are rare idiosyncratic reactions. May cause lupus-like syndrome; may increase frequency of grand mal seizures in patients with mixed-type seizures. Drug of choice for absence seizures. Carbamazepine, phenytoin, primidone, phenobarbital, valproic acid, nevirapine, and ritonavir may decrease ethosuximide levels.

Therapeutic levels: 40–100 mg/L. $T_{1/2}$ = 24–42 hr. Recommended serum sampling time at steady state: obtain trough level within 30 min before the next scheduled dose after 5–10 days of continuous dosing.

To minimize GI distress, may administer with food or milk. Abrupt withdrawal of drug may precipitate absence status.

For explanation of icons, see p. 680.

FAMCICLOVIR
Famvir
Antiviral

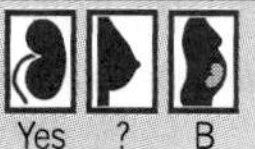

Tabs: 125, 250, 500 mg

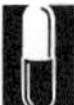

Adolescents:
Genital herpes: 250 mg Q8 hr PO × 7-10 days
Episodic recurrent genital herpes: 125 mg Q12 hr PO × 5 days
Daily suppressive therapy: 125-250 mg Q12 hr PO up to 1 year, then reassess HSV recurrence.

Adult:
Herpes zoster: 500 mg Q8 hr PO × 7 days; initiate therapy promptly as soon as diagnosis is made.
Genital herpes simplex: 125 mg Q12 hr PO × 5 days
Suppression of recurrent genital herpes: 250 mg Q12 hr PO up to 1 year
Recurrent mucocutaneous herpes in HIV: 500 mg Q12 hr PO × 7 days

Drug is converted to its active form (penciclovir). Better absorption than PO acyclovir. May cause headache, diarrhea, nausea, and abdominal pain.

Concomitant use with probenecid and other drugs eliminated by active tubular secretion may result in decreased penciclovir clearance. **Reduce dose in renal impairment (see Chapter 30).**

Safety and efficacy in suppression of recurrent genital herpes **have not been established** beyond 1 year. May be administered with or without food.

FAMOTIDINE
Pepcid, Pepcid AC [OTC], Pepcid Complete [OTC], Pepcid RPD
Histamine-2 receptor antagonist

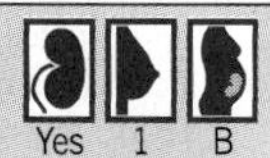

Injection: 10 mg/mL (2, 4, 20 mL); multidose vials contain 0.9% benzyl alcohol.
Premixed injection: 20 mg/50 mL in iso-osmotic sodium chloride
Liquid: 40 mg/5 mL (contains parabens)
Tabs: 10 (OTC), 20, 40 mg
Gel caps: 10 mg (OTC)
Disintegrating oral tabs: 20, 40 mg; contains aspartame
Chewable tabs: 10 mg (OTC); contains aspartame

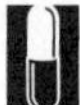

Neonate: 0.5 mg/kg/dose IV Q 24 hr
≥3 mo–1 yr (GERD): 0.5 mg/kg/dose PO Q 12 hr
Child:
IV: initial: 0.6–0.8 mg/kg/24 hr ÷ Q8–12 hr up to a **max. dose** of 40 mg/24 hr
PO: initial: 1–1.2 mg/kg/24 hr ÷ Q8–12 hr up to a **max. dose** of 40 mg/24 hr

Continued

FAMOTIDINE *continued*

Peptic ulcer: 0.5 mg/kg/24 hr PO QHS or ÷ Q 12 hr up to a **max. dose** of 40 mg/24 hr
GERD: 1 mg/kg/24 hr PO ÷ Q 12 hr up to a **max. dose** of 80 mg/24 hr

Adolescent and adult:

Duodenal ulcer:
PO: 20 mg BID or 40 mg QHS × 4–8 wk, then maintenance therapy at 20 mg QHS
IV: 20 mg BID

Esophagitis and GERD: 20 mg BID PO

A Q12-hr dosage interval is generally recommended; however, infants and young children may require a Q8-hr interval because of enhanced elimination. Headaches, dizziness, constipation, diarrhea, and drowsiness have occurred.

Adjust dosages in severe renal failure (see Chapter 30).

Shake oral suspension well before each use. Disintegrating oral tablets should be placed on the tongue to be disintegrated and subsequently swallowed. Doses may be administered with or without food.

FELBAMATE

Felbatol
Anticonvulsant

Yes ? C

Tabs: 400, 600 mg
Suspension: 600 mg/5 mL

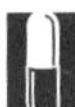

Lennox-Gastaut for child 2–14 yr (adjunctive therapy):
Start at 15 mg/kg/24 hr PO ÷ TID-QID; increase dosage by 15 mg/kg/24 hr increments at weekly intervals up to a **max. dose** of 45 mg/kg/24 hr or 3600 mg/24 hr. See remarks.

Child ≥14 yr–adult:

Adjunctive therapy: start at 1200 mg/24 hr PO ÷ TID–QID; increase dosage by 1200 mg/24 hr at weekly intervals up to a **max. dose** of 3600 mg/24 hr. See remarks.

Monotherapy (as initial therapy): start at 1200 mg/24 hr PO ÷ TID–QID. Increase dose under close clinical supervision at 600 mg increments Q2 wk to 2400 mg/24 hr. **Max. dose:** 3600 mg/24 hr.

Conversion to monotherapy: start at 1200 mg/24 hr ÷ PO TID–QID for 2 wk; then increase to 2400 mg/24 hr for 1 wk. At wk 3, increase to 3600 mg/24 hr. See remarks for dose-reduction instructions of other antiepileptic drugs.

Drug should be prescribed under strict supervision by a specialist. **Contraindicated** in blood dyscrasias or hepatic dysfunction (prior or current) and hypersensitivity to meprobamate. Aplastic anemia and hepatic failure leading to death have been associated with drug. May cause headache, fatigue, anxiety, GI disturbances, gingival hyperplasia, increased liver enzymes, and bone marrow suppression. **Obtain serum levels of concurrent anticonvulsants.** Monitor

Continued

For explanation of icons, see p. 680.

FELBAMATE *continued*

liver enzymes, bilirubin, CBC with differential, and platelets at baseline every 1–2 wk. **Doses should be decreased by 50% in renally impaired patients.**

When initiating adjunctive therapy (all ages), doses of other antiepileptic drugs (AEDs) are reduced by 20% to control plasma levels of concurrent phenytoin, valproic acid, phenobarbital, and carbamazepine. Further reductions of concomitant AEDs dosage may be necessary to minimize side effects caused by drug interactions.

When converting to monotherapy, reduce other AEDs by one third at start of felbamate therapy. Then, after 2 wk and at the start of increasing the felbamate dosage, reduce other AEDs by an additional one third. At wk 3, continue to reduce other AEDs as clinically indicated.

Carbamazepine levels may be decreased, whereas phenytoin and valproic acid levels may be increased. Phenytoin and carbamazepine may increase felbamate clearance; valproic acid may decrease its clearance.

Doses can be administered with or without food.

FENTANYL

Sublimaze, Duragesic, Fentanyl Oralet, Actiq, and others

Narcotic; analgesic, sedative

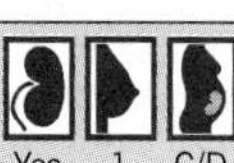

Injection: 50 mcg/mL
SR patch (Duragesic): 25, 50, 75, 100 mcg/hr
Oralet lozenge:
Fentanyl Oralet: 100, 200, 300, 400 mcg
Actiq: 200, 400, 600, 800, 1200, 1600 mcg

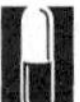

Titrate dose to effect.

IV/IM: 1–2 mcg/kg/dose Q30–60 min PRN

Continuous IV infusion: 1 mcg/kg/hr; titrate to effect; usual infusion range 1–3 mcg/kg/hr

To prepare infusion, use the following formula:

$$50 \times \frac{\text{Desired dose (mcg/kg/hr)}}{\text{Desired infusion rate (mL/hr)}} \times \text{Wt (kg)} = \frac{\text{mcg fentanyl}}{\text{50 mL fluid}}$$

PO (Fentanyl Oralet): Sedation: 5–15 mcg/kg/dose up to **max. dose** of 400 mcg/dose

Transdermal: Safety and efficacy have not been established in pediatrics.

See Chapter 28, Tables 28-16 and 28-17 for equianalgesic dosing and for PCA dosing.

Use with caution in bradycardia, respiratory depression, and increased intracranial pressure. **Adjust dose in renal failure (see Chapter 30).** Highly lipophilic and may deposit into fat tissue. IV onset of action 1–2 min with peak effects in 10 min. IV duration of action 30–60 min. Give IV dose over 3–5 min. Rapid infusion may cause respiratory depression and chest wall rigidity. Respiratory depression may persist beyond the period of analgesia. Transdermal onset of action 6–8 hr with a 72-hr duration of action. Fentanyl Oralet is **contraindicated** in children <10 kg. Actiq is indicated only for the management of breakthrough cancer pain. See Chapter 28 for pharmacodynamic information with transmucosal and transdermal routes.

Continued

FENTANYL *continued*

Fentanyl is a substrate for the cytochrome P-450 3A4 enzyme. Be aware of medications that inhibit or induce this enzyme because it may increase or decrease the effects of fentanyl, respectively.

Pregnancy category changes to D if drug is used for prolonged periods or in high doses at term.

FERROUS SULFATE

See *Iron Preparations*

FEXOFENADINE ± PSEUDOEPHEDRINE

Allegra, Allegra-D 12 Hour

Antihistamine, less sedating ± decongestant

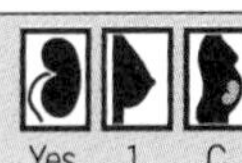

Tabs: 30, 60, 180 mg
Caps: 60 mg
Extended-release tabs in combination with pseudoephedrine (PE):
Allegra-D 12 Hour: 60 mg fexofenadine + 120 mg pseudoephedrine

Fexofenadine:
6–11 yr: 30 mg PO BID
≥12 yr–adult: 60 mg PO BID; 180 mg PO QD may be used in seasonal rhinitis.

Extended-release tabs of fexofenadine and pseudoephedrine:
≥12 yr–adult:
Allegra-D 12 Hour: 1 tablet PO BID

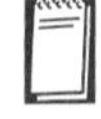

May cause drowsiness, fatigue, headache, dyspepsia, nausea, and dysmenorrhea. Has **not** been implicated in causing cardiac arrhythmias when used with other drugs that are metabolized by hepatic microsomal enzymes (e.g., ketoconazole, erythromycin). **Reduce dose to 30 mg PO QD for child 6–11 yr and 60 mg PO QD for ≥12 yr if CrCl <40 mL/min.** For use of Allegra-D 12 Hour and decreased renal function, an initial dose of 1 tablet PO QD is recommended.

Medication as the single agent may be administered with or without food. **Do not administer** antacids with or within 2 hr of fexofenadine dose. The extended-release combination product should be swallowed whole without food.

FILGRASTIM

Neupogen, G-CSF

Colony-stimulating factor

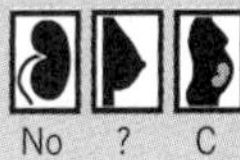

Injection: 300 mcg/mL (1, 1.6 mL)
Injection, prefilled syringes with 27-gauge ½-inch needles: 600 mcg/mL (0.5, 0.8 mL)
All dosage forms are preservative free.

Continued

For explanation of icons, see p. 680.

FILGRASTIM *continued*

IV/SC: 5–10 mcg/kg/dose QD × 14 days or until ANC >10,000/mm^3. Dosage may be increased by 5 mcg/kg/24 hr if desired effect is not achieved within 7 days.

Discontinue therapy when ANC >10,000/mm^3.

Individual protocols may direct dosing. May cause bone pain, fever, and rash. Monitor CBC, uric acid, and LFTs. **Use with caution** in patients with malignancies with myeloid characteristics. **Contraindicated** for patients sensitive to *E. coli*–derived proteins.

SC routes of administration are preferred because of prolonged serum levels over IV route. If used via IV route and G-CSF final concentration <15 mcg/mL, add 2 mg albumin/1 mL of IV fluid to prevent drug adsorption to the IV administration set.

FLECAINIDE ACETATE

Tambocor

Antiarrhythmic, class Ic

Yes 1 C

Tabs: 50, 100, 150 mg

Suspension: 5, 20 mg/mL

Child: Initial: 1–3 mg/kg/24 hr ÷ Q8 hr PO; usual range: 3–6 mg/kg/24 hr ÷ Q8 hr PO, monitor serum levels to adjust dose if needed.

Adult:

Sustained V tach: 100 mg PO Q12 hr; may increase by 50 mg Q12 hr every 4 days to **max. dose** of 600 mg/24 hr.

Paroxysmal SVT/paroxysmal AF: 50 mg PO Q12 hr; may increase dose by 50 mg Q12 hr every 4 days to **max. dose** of 300 mg/24 hr.

May aggravate LV failure, sinus bradycardia, preexisting ventricular arrhythmias. May cause AV block, dizziness, blurred vision, dyspnea, nausea, headache, and increased PR or QRS intervals. **Reserve for life-threatening cases.**

Flecainide is a substrate for the cytochrome P-450 2D6 enzyme. Be aware of medications that inhibit or induce this enzyme for it may increase or decrease the effects of flecainide, respectively.

Therapeutic trough level: 0.2–1 mg/L. Recommended serum sampling time at steady state: Obtain trough level within 30 min before next scheduled dose after 2–3 days of continuous dosing for children; after 3–5 days for adults. **Adjust dose in renal failure (see Chapter 30).**

FLUCONAZOLE
Diflucan
Antifungal agent

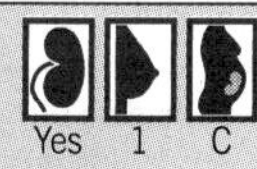

Tabs: 50, 100, 150, 200 mg
Injection: 2 mg/mL (100, 200 mL); contains 9 mEq Na/2 mg drug
Oral suspension: 10 mg/mL (35 mL), 40 mg/mL (35 mL)

Neonate:
Loading dose: 12 mg/kg IV/PO
Maintenance dose: 6 mg/kg IV/PO with the following dosing intervals (see table below)

Postconceptional Age (wk)	Postnatal Age (days)	Dosing Interval (hr) and Time (hr) to Start First Maintenance Dose After Load
≤29	0–14	72
	>14	48
30–36	0–14	48
	>14	24
37–44	0–7	48
	>7	24
≥45	>0	24

Child (IV/PO):

Indication	Loading Dose	Maintenance Dose to Begin 24 hr after Loading Dose
Oropharyngeal candidiasis	6 mg/kg	3 mg/kg
Esophageal candidiasis	12 mg/kg	6 mg/kg
Systemic candidiasis and cryptococcal meningitis	12 mg/kg	6–12 mg/kg

Max. dose: 12 mg/kg/24 hr

Adult:

Oropharyngeal and esophageal candidiasis: loading dose of 200 mg PO/IV followed by 100 mg QD 24 hr after; doses up to **max. dose** of 400 mg/24 hr should be used for esophageal candidiasis
Systemic candidiasis and cryptococcal meningitis: loading dose of 400 mg PO/IV, followed by 200–800 mg QD 24 hr later
Bone marrow transplantation prophylaxis: 400 mg PO/IV Q24hr
Vaginal candidiasis: 150 mg PO × 1

Continued

For explanation of icons, see p. 680.

FLUCONAZOLE *continued*

Cardiac arrhythmias may occur when used with cisapride. Concomitant administration of fluconazole with cisapride is **contraindicated.** May cause nausea, headache, rash, vomiting, abdominal pain, hepatitis, cholestasis, and diarrhea. Neutropenia, agranulocytosis, and thrombocytopenia have been reported.

Inhibits CYP450 2C9/10 and CYP 450 3A3/4 (weak inhibitor). May increase effects, toxicity, or levels of cyclosporine, midazolam, phenytoin, rifabutin, tacrolimus, theophylline, warfarin, oral hypoglycemics, and AZT. Rifampin increases fluconazole metabolism. **Adjust dose in renal failure (see Chapter 30).**

FLUCYTOSINE

Ancobon, 5-FC, 5-Fluorocytosine

Antifungal agent

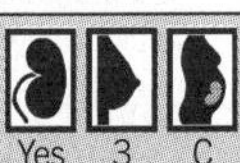

Caps: 250, 500 mg

Oral liquid: 10 mg/mL

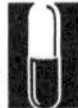

Neonate: 80–160 mg/kg/24 hr ÷ Q6 hr PO

Child and adult: 50–150 mg/kg/24 hr ÷ Q6 hr PO

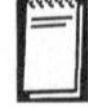

Monitor CBC, BUN, serum creatinine, alkaline phosphatase, AST, and ALT. Common side effects: nausea, vomiting, diarrhea, rash, CNS disturbance, anemia, leukopenia, and thrombocytopenia.

Therapeutic levels: 25–100 mg/L. Recommended serum sampling time at steady state: Obtain peak level 2–4 hr after oral dose following 4 days of continuous dosing. Peak levels of 40–60 mg/L have been recommended for systemic candidiasis. Prolonged levels above 100 mg/L can increase risk for bone marrow suppression. Bone marrow suppression in immunosuppressed patients can be irreversible and fatal.

Flucytosine interferes with creatinine assay tests using the dry-slide enzymatic method (Kodak Ektachem analyzer). **Adjust dose in renal failure (see Chapter 30).**

FLUDROCORTISONE ACETATE

Florinef acetate, 9-Fluorohydrocortisone, Fluohydrisone

Corticosteroid

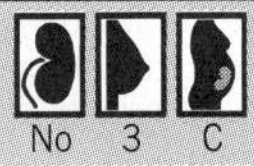

Tabs: 0.1 mg

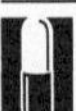

Infant and child: 0.05–0.1 mg/24 hr QD PO

Congenital adrenal hyperplasia: 0.05–0.3 mg/24 hr QD PO

Adult: 0.05–0.2 mg/24 hr QD PO

Contraindicated in CHF and systemic fungal infections. Has primarily mineralocorticoid activity. May cause hypertension, hypokalemia, acne, rash, bruising, headaches, GI ulcers, and growth suppression.

Continued

FLUDROCORTISONE ACETATE *continued*

Monitor BP and serum electrolytes. See Chapter 29 for steroid potency comparison.

Drug interactions: Drug's hypokalemic effects may induce digoxin toxicity; phenytoin and rifampin may increase fludrocortisone metabolism.

Doses of 0.2–2 mg/24 hr have been used in the management of severe orthostatic hypotension in adults.

FLUMAZENIL

Romazicon

Benzodiazepine antidote

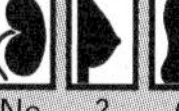

No ? C

Injection: 0.1 mg/mL (5, 10 mL)

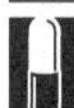

Child, IV: *reversal of benzodiazepine sedation:*

Initial dose: 0.01 mg/kg (**max. dose:** 0.2 mg) given over 15 sec, then 0.01 mg/kg (**max. dose:** 0.2 mg) given Q1 min to a **max. total cumulative dose** of 0.05 mg/kg or 1 mg, whichever is lower. Usual total dose: 0.08–1 mg (average 0.65 mg). Doses may be repeated in 20 min up to a **max. dose** of 3 mg in 1 hr.

Does not reverse narcotics. Onset of benzodiazepine reversal occurs in 1–3 min. Reversal effects of flumazenil ($T_{1/2}$ approximately 1 hr) may wear off sooner than benzodiazepine effects. If patient does not respond after cumulative 1- to 3-mg dose, suspect agent other than benzodiazepines.

May precipitate seizures, especially in patients taking benzodiazepines for seizure control or in patients with tricyclic antidepressant overdose. Fear, panic attacks in patients with history of panic disorders have been reported.

See Chapter 2 for complete management of suspected ingestions.

FLUNISOLIDE

Nasalide, Nasarel, AeroBid, AeroBid-M

Corticosteroid

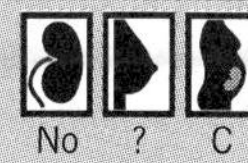

No ? C

Nasal solution: 25 mcg/spray (200 sprays/bottle) (25 mL)

Oral aerosol inhaler: 250 mcg/dose (100 doses/inhaler) (7 g); AeroBid-M contains menthol flavoring.

For all dosage forms, reduce to lowest effective maintenance dose to control symptoms.

Nasal solution:

Child (6–14 yr):

Initial: 1 spray per nostril TID or 2 sprays per nostril BID; **max. dose:** 4 sprays per nostril/24 hr

Continued

For explanation of icons, see p. 680.

FLUNISOLIDE *continued*

Adult:

Initial: 2 sprays per nostril BID; **max. dose:** 8 sprays per nostril/24 hr

Inhaler:

Child (6–15 yr): 2 puffs BID

Adult: 2 puffs BID

Max. dose: 8 puffs/24 hr

Stop gradually after 3 wk if no clinical improvement is seen. May cause a reduction in growth velocity. Shake inhaler well before use. Spacer devices may enhance drug delivery of inhaled form. Rinse mouth after administering drug by inhaler to prevent thrush. Patients using nasal solution should clear nasal passages before use.

FLUORIDE

Luride, Fluoritab, Pediaflor, and others

Mineral

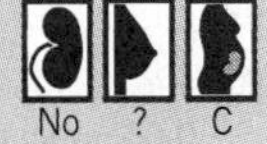

Concentrations and strengths based on fluoride ion:

Drops: 0.125 mg/drop, 0.25 mg/drop, 0.5 mg/mL

Oral solution: 0.2 mg/mL

Chewable tabs: 0.25, 0.5, 1 mg

Tabs: 1 mg

Lozenges: 1 mg

See Chapter 20 for fluoride-containing multivitamins.

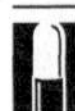

All doses/24 hr (see table below): Recommendations from American Academy of Pediatrics and American Dental Association.

	Concentration of Fluoride in Drinking Water (ppm)		
Age	*<0.3*	*0.3–0.6*	*>0.6*
Birth–6 mo	0	0	0
6 mo–3 yr	0.25 mg	0	0
3–6 yr	0.5 mg	0.25 mg	0
6–16 yr	1 mg	0.5 mg	0

Contraindicated in areas where drinking water fluoridation is >0.7 ppm. **Acute overdose:** GI distress, salivation, CNS irritability, tetany, seizures, hypocalcemia, hypoglycemia, cardiorespiratory failure. Chronic excess use may result in mottled teeth or bone changes.

Take with food, but **NOT** milk, to minimize GI upset. The doses have been decreased owing to concerns over dental fluorosis.

FLUOXETINE HYDROCHLORIDE

Prozac, Sarafem, Prozac Weekly

Antidepressant, selective serotonin reuptake inhibitor

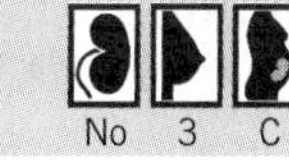

Liquid: 20 mg/5 mL; contains 0.23% alcohol
Caps: 10, 20, 40 mg
Delayed-released caps (Prozac Weekly): 90 mg
Tabs: 10 mg

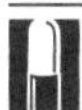

Depression:

Child, 8–18 yr: Start at 10–20 mg QD PO. If started on 10 mg/24 hr, may increase dose to 20 mg/24 hr after 1 wk. Use lower 10 mg/24 hr initial dose for lower-weight children; if needed, increase to 20 mg/24 hr after several weeks.

Adult: Start at 20 mg QD PO. May increase after several weeks by 20 mg/24 hr increments to **max. dose** of 80 mg/24 hr. Doses >20 mg/24 hr should be divided BID.

Obsessive-compulsive disorder:

Child, 7–18 yr:

Lower-weight child: Start at 10 mg QD PO. May increase after several weeks. Usual dose range: 20–30 mg/24 hr. There is very minimal experience with doses >20 mg/24 hr and no experience with doses >60 mg/24 hr.

Higher-weight child and adolescent: Start at 10 mg QD PO and increase dose to 20 mg/24 hr after 2 wk. May further increase dose after several weeks. Usual dose range: 20–60 mg/24 hr.

Bulimia:

Adult: 60 mg QAM PO; it is recommended to titrate up to this dose over several days.

Premenstrual dysphoric disorder:

Adult: Start at 20 mg QD PO using the Sarafem product. **Max. dose:** 80 mg/24 hr. Systematic evaluation has shown that efficacy is maintained for periods of 6 mo at a dose of 20 mg/24 hr. Reassess patients periodically to determine the need for continued treatment.

Contraindicated in patients taking MAO inhibitors due to possibility of seizures, hyperpyrexia, and coma. May increase the effects of tricyclic antidepressants. May cause headache, insomnia, nervousness, drowsiness, GI disturbance, and weight loss. Increased bleeding diathesis with unaltered prothrombin time may occur with warfarin. Monitor for clinical worsening of depression and suicidal ideation/behavior following the initiation of therapy or after dose changes.

May displace other highly protein-bound drugs. Inhibits CYP450 2C19, 2D6, and 3A3/4 drug metabolism isoenzymes that may increase the effects or toxicity of drugs metabolized by these enzymes.

Delayed-release capsule is currently indicated for depression and is dosed at 90 mg Q7 days. It is unknown whether weekly dosing provides the same protection from relapse as does daily dosing.

For explanation of icons, see p. 680.

FLUTICASONE PROPIONATE

Flonase, Cutivate, Flovent, Flovent Rotadisk

Corticosteroid

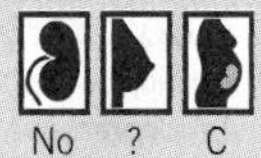

Nasal spray (Flonase): 50 mcg/actuation (16 g = 120 doses)
Topical cream (Cutivate): 0.05% (15, 30, 60 g)
Topical ointment (Cutivate): 0.005% (15, 30, 60 g)
Aerosol inhaler (MDI) (Flovent): 44 mcg/actuation, 110 mcg/actuation, 220 mcg/actuation (7.9 g = 60 doses/inhaler, 13 g = 120 doses/inhaler)
Dry-powder inhalation (DPI): (all strengths come in a package of 15 Rotadisk's; each Rotadisk provides 4 doses for a total of 60 doses per package):
50 mcg/dose, 100 mcg/dose, 250mcg/dose

Intranasal (allergic rhinitis):
≥4 yr and adolescent: 1 spray (50 mcg) per nostril QD. Dose can be increased to 2 sprays (100 mcg) per nostril QD if inadequate response or severe symptoms. Reduce to 1 spray per nostril QD once symptoms are controlled.
Max. dose: 2 sprays (100 mcg) per nostril/24 hr.
Adults: Initial 200 mcg/24 hr [2 sprays (100 mcg) per nostril QD; **OR** 1 spray (50 mcg) per nostril BID]. Reduce to 1 spray per nostril QD once symptoms are controlled. **Max. dose:** 2 sprays (100 mcg) per nostril/24 hr.
Oral inhalation: **Divide all 24-hr doses BID.** If desired response is not seen after 2 wk of starting therapy, increase dosage. Then reduce to the lowest effective dose when asthma symptoms are controlled. Administration of MDI with aerochamber enhances drug delivery.
Converting from other asthma regimens (see table below).

CONVERSION FROM OTHER ASTHMA REGIMENS TO FLUTICASONE

Age	Previous Use of Bronchodilators Only (max. dose)	Previous Use of Inhaled Corticosteroid (max. dose)	Previous Use of Oral Corticosteroid (max. dose)
Children (4–11 yr)	MDI: 88 mcg/24 hr (176 mcg/24 hr)	MDI: 88 mcg/24 hr (176 mcg/24 hr)	Dose not available
	DPI: 100 mcg/24 hr (200 mcg/24 hr)	DPI: 100 mcg/24 hr (200 mcg/24 hr)	
≥12 yr and adults	MDI: 176 mcg/24 hr (880 mcg/24 hr)	MDI: 176–440 mcg/24 hr (880 mcg/24 hr)	MDI: 1760 mcg/24 hr (1760 mcg/24 hr)
	DPI: 200 mcg/24 hr (1000 mcg/24 hr)	DPI: 200–500 mcg/24 hr (1000 mcg/24 hr)	DPI: 2000 mcg/24 hr (2000 mcg/24 hr)

MDI, metered dose inhaler; DPI, dry powder inhaler.

Continued

FLUTICASONE PROPIONATE *continued*

Topical:

≥3 mo and adults: Apply to affected areas BID; then reduce to a less potent topical agent when symptoms are controlled. See Chapter 29 for topical steroid comparisons.

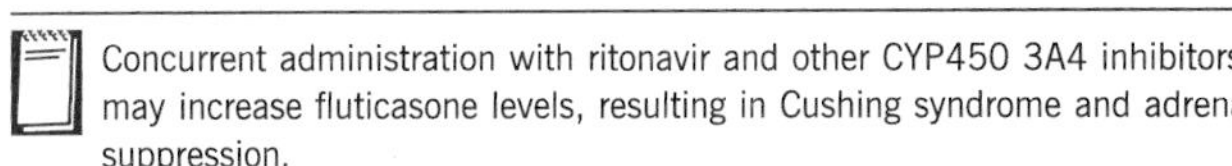

Concurrent administration with ritonavir and other CYP450 3A4 inhibitors may increase fluticasone levels, resulting in Cushing syndrome and adrenal suppression.

Intranasal: Clear nasal passages before use. May cause epistaxis and nasal irritation, which are usually transient. Taste and smell alterations, rare hypersensitivity reactions (angioedema, pruritus, urticaria, wheezing, dyspnea), and nasal septal perforation have been reported in postmarketing studies.

Oral inhalation: Rinse mouth after each use. May cause dysphonia, oral thrush, and dermatitis. Compared with beclomethasone, it has been shown to have less of an effect on suppressing linear growth in asthmatic children. Eosinophilic conditions may occur with the withdrawal or decrease of oral corticosteroids after the initiation of inhaled fluticasone.

Topical use: Avoid application/contact to face, eyes, and open skin. Occlusive dressings are not recommended.

FLUTICASONE PROPIONATE AND SALMETEROL

Advair Diskus

Corticosteroid and long-acting beta-2-adrenergic agonist

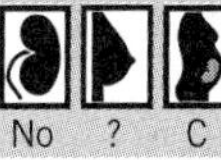

No ? C

Dry-powder inhalation (DPI; Diskus):

100 mcg fluticasone propionate + 50 mcg salmeterol per inhalation (28, 60 inhalations)

250 mcg fluticasone propionate + 50 mcg salmeterol per inhalation (28, 60 inhalations)

500 mcg fluticasone propionate + 50 mcg salmeterol per inhalation (28, 60 inhalations)

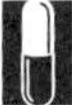

Asthma (without prior inhaled steroid use):

4 yr–adult: Start with one inhalation BID of 100 mcg fluticasone propionate + 50 mcg salmeterol.

Continued

For explanation of icons, see p. 680.

FLUTICASONE PROPIONATE AND SALMETEROL *continued*

Asthma (conversion from other inhaled steroids; see table below):

Inhaled Corticosteroid	Current Daily Dose	Recommended Strength of Fluticasone Propionate + Salmeterol Diskus Administered at One Inhalation BID
Beclomethasone dipropionate	≤420 mcg	100 mcg + 50 mcg
	462–840 mcg	250 mcg + 50 mcg
Budesonide	≤400 mcg	100 mcg + 50 mcg
	800–1200 mcg	250 mcg + 50 mcg
	1600 mcg	500 mcg + 50 mcg
Flunisolide	≤1000 mcg	100 mcg + 50 mcg
	1250–2000 mcg	250 mcg + 50 mcg
Fluticasone propionate aerosol (MDI)	≤176 mcg	100 mcg + 50 mcg
	440 mcg	250 mcg + 50 mcg
	660–880 mcg	500 mcg + 50 mcg
Fluticasone propionate dry powder (DPI)	≤200 mcg	100 mcg + 50 mcg
	500 mcg	250 mcg + 50 mcg
	1000 mcg	500 mcg + 50 mcg
Triamcinolone	≤1000 mcg	100 mcg + 50 mcg
	1100–1600 mcg	250 mcg + 50 mcg

MDI, metered dose inhaler; DPI, dry powder inhaler.

Max. dose: one inhalation BID of 500 mcg fluticasone propionate + 50 mcg salmeterol

See *Fluticasone Propionate* and *Salmeterol* for remarks. Titrate to the lowest effective strength after asthma is adequately controlled. Proper patient education including dosage administration technique is essential; see patient package insert for detailed instructions. Rinse mouth after each use.

FLUVOXAMINE

Luvox and others

Antidepressant, selective serotonin reuptake inhibitor

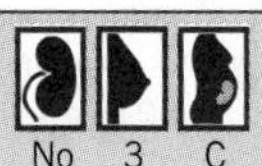

Tabs: 25, 50, 100 mg

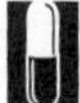

Obsessive-compulsive disorder:

>8 yr: Start at 25 mg PO QHS. Dose may be increased by 25 mg/24 hr Q 4–7 days up to a **max. dose** of 200 mg/24 hr. Total daily doses >50 mg/24 hr should be divided BID.

Adult: Start at 50 mg PO QHS. Dose may be increased by 50 mg/24 hr Q4–7 days up to a **max. dose** of 300 mg/24 hr. Total daily doses >100 mg/24 hr should be divided BID.

Continued

FLUVOXAMINE *continued*

Contraindicated with coadministration of cisapride, pimozide, thioridazine, or MAO inhibitors. **Use with caution** in hepatic disease; drug is extensively metabolized by the liver. Monitor for clinical worsening of depression and suicidal ideation/behavior following the initiation of therapy or after dose changes.

Inhibits CYP450 1A2, 2C19, 2D6, and 3A3/4, which may increase the effects or toxicity of drugs metabolized by these enzymes. Dose-related use of thioridazine with fluvoxamine may cause prolongation of QT interval and serious arrhythmias. May increase warfarin plasma levels by 98% and prolong PT. May increase toxicity and/or levels of theophylline, caffeine, and tricyclic antidepressants. Side effects include: headache, insomnia, somnolence, nausea, diarrhea, dyspepsia, and dry mouth.

Titrate to lowest effective dose.

FOLIC ACID

Folvite and others

Water-soluble vitamin

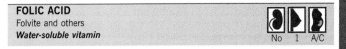

No 1 A/C

Tabs: 0.4, 0.8, 1 mg
Oral solution: 50 mcg/mL, 1 mg/mL
Injection: 5 mg/mL; contains 1.5% benzyl alcohol

For RDA, see Chapter 20.
Folic acid deficiency PO, IM, IV, SC (see table below):

Infants	Children (1–10 yr)	Adults (>11 yr)
INITIAL DOSE		
15 mcg/kg/dose; **max. dose:** 50 mcg/24 hr	1 mg/dose	1 mg/dose
MAINTENANCE		
30–45 mcg/24 hr QD	0.1–0.4 mg/24 hr QD	0.5 mg/24 hr QD; pregnant/lactating women: 0.8 mg/24 hr QD

Normal levels: see Chapter 20. May mask hematologic effects of vitamin B_{12} deficiency but will not prevent progression of neurologic abnormalities. High-dose folic acid may decrease the absorption of phenytoin.

Women of child-bearing age considering pregnancy should take at least 0.4 mg QD before and during pregnancy to reduce risk for neural tube defects in the fetus. Pregnancy category changes to C if used in doses above the RDA.

For explanation of icons, see p. 680.

FOMEPIZOLE
Antizol
Antidote for ethylene glycol or methanol toxicity

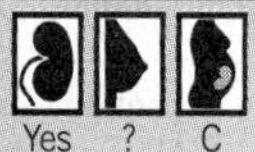

Injection: 1 g/mL (1.5 mL)

Adults not requiring hemodialysis (IV, all doses administered over 30 min):
Load: 15 mg/kg/dose × 1
Maintenance: 10 mg/kg/dose Q12 hr × 4 doses, then 15 mg/kg/dose Q12 hr until ethylene glycol level decreases to < 20 mg/dL and the patient is asymptomatic with normal pH

Adults requiring hemodialysis (IV following the above recommended doses at the intervals indicated below. Fomepizole is removed by dialysis. All doses administered over 30 min.):

Dosing at the beginning of hemodialysis:
If <6 hr since last fomepizole dose: **DO NOT** administer dose.
If ≥6 hr since last fomepizole dose: administer next scheduled dose.

Dosing during hemodialysis: administer Q 4 hr.

Dosing at the time hemodialysis is completed (based on the time between last dose and end of hemodialysis):
<1 hr: **DO NOT** administer dose at end of hemodialysis.
1–3 hr: administer one half of next scheduled dose.
>3 hr: administer next scheduled dose.

Maintenance dose off hemodialysis: give next scheduled dose 12 hr from last dose administered.

Works by competitively inhibiting alcohol dehydrogenase. Safety and efficacy in pediatrics have not been established. **Contraindicated** in hypersensitivity to any components or other pyrazole compounds. Most frequent side effects include headache, nausea, and dizziness. Fomepizole is extensively eliminated by the kidneys (**use with caution in renal failure**) and removed by hemodialysis.

Drug product may solidify at temperatures <25° C (77° F); vial can be liquefied by running it under warm water (efficacy, safety, and stability are not affected). All doses must be diluted with at least 100 mL of D5W or NS to prevent vein irritation.

FOSCARNET
Foscavir
Antiviral agent

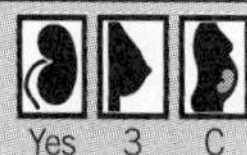

Injection: 24 mg/mL (250, 500 mL)

Adolescents and adults, IV:
CMV retinitis:
Induction: 180 mg/kg/24 hr ÷ Q8 hr × 14–21 days
Maintenance: 90–120 mg/kg/24 hr QD

Continued

FOSCARNET *continued*

Adolescents and adults, IV:

Acyclovir-resistant herpes simplex: 40 mg/kg/dose Q8 hr or 40–60 mg/kg/dose Q12 hr for up to 3 wk or until lesions heal

Use with caution in patients with renal insufficiency. **Discontinue** use in adults if serum Cr ≥2.9 mg/dL. **Adjust dose in renal failure (see Chapter 30).**

May cause peripheral neuropathy, seizures, hallucinations, GI disturbance, increased LFTs, hypertension, chest pain, ECG abnormalities, coughing, dyspnea, bronchospasm, and renal failure (adequate hydration and avoiding nephrotoxic medications may reduce risk). Hypocalcemia (increased risk if given with pentamidine), hypokalemia, and hypomagnesemia may also occur.

FOSPHENYTOIN

Cerebyx

Anticonvulsant

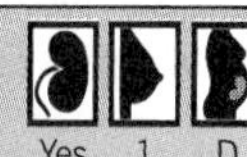

Injection: 50 mg phenytoin equivalent (75 mg fosphenytoin)/1 mL (2, 10 mL)
1 mg phenytoin equivalent provides 0.0037 mmol phosphate.

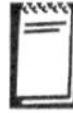

All doses are expressed as phenytoin sodium equivalents (PE):

***Child:* see phenytoin and use the conversion of 1 mg phenytoin = 1 mg PE.**

Adult:

Loading dose:

Status epilepticus: 15–20 mg PE/kg IV

Nonemergent loading: 10–20 mg PE/kg IV/IM

Initial maintenance dose: 4–6 mg PE/kg/24 hr IV/IM

All doses should be prescribed and dispensed in terms of mg phenytoin sodium equivalents (PE) to avoid medication errors. Safety in pediatrics has not been fully established.

Use with caution in patients with porphyria; consider amount of phosphate delivered by fosphenytoin in patients with phosphate restrictions. Drug is also metabolized to liberate small amounts of formaldehyde, which is considered clinically insignificant with short-term use (e.g., 1 wk). Side effects: hypokalemia (with rapid IV administration), slurred speech, dizziness, ataxia, rash, exfoliative dermatitis, nystagmus, diplopia, and tinnitus. Increased unbound phenytoin concentrations may occur in patients with renal disease or hypoalbuminemia; measure “free” or “unbound” phenytoin levels in these patients.

Abrupt withdrawal may cause status epilepticus. BP and ECG monitoring should be present during IV loading dose administration. **Maximum IV infusion rate:** 3 mg PE/kg/min up to a **maximum** of 150 mg PE/min. Administer IM via 1 or 2 injection sites; IM route is **not recommended** in status epilepticus.

Therapeutic levels: 10–20 mg/L (free and bound phenytoin) **OR** 1–2 mg/L (free only). Recommended peak serum sampling times: 4 hr following an IM dose or 2 hr following an IV dose.

See phenytoin remarks for drug interactions. Drug is more safely administered via peripheral IV than phenytoin.

For explanation of icons, see p. 680.

FUROSEMIDE
Lasix and others
Loop diuretic

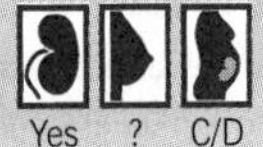

Tabs: 20, 40, 80 mg
Injection: 10 mg/mL (2, 4, 10 mL)
Oral liquid: 10 mg/mL (contains 11.5% alcohol) (60, 120 mL), 40 mg/5 mL (contains 0.2% alcohol) (5, 10, 500 mL)

IM, IV:
Neonate: 0.5–1 mg/kg/dose Q8–24 hr; **max. IV dose:** 2 mg/kg/dose
Infant and child: 0.5–2 mg/kg/dose Q6–12 hr
Adult: 20–40 mg/24 hr div Q6–12 hr; **max. dose:** 600 mg/24 hr or 80 mg/dose

PO:
Neonate: Bioavailability by this route is poor; doses of 1–4 mg/kg/dose QD to BID have been used
Infant and child: 1–6 mg/kg/dose Q12–24 hrs
Adult: 20–80 mg/dose Q6–24 hours; **max. dose:** 600 mg/24 hr

Continuous IV infusion:
Infant and child: 0.05 mg/kg/hour; titrate to clinical effect
Adult: 0.1 mg/kg/hour; titrate to effect; **max. dose:** 0.4 mg/kg/hour

Contraindicated in anuria and hepatic coma. **Use with caution** in hepatic disease. Ototoxicity may occur in presence of renal disease, especially when used with aminoglycosides. May cause hypokalemia, alkalosis, dehydration, hyperuricemia, and increased calcium excretion. Prolonged use in premature infants may result in nephrocalcinosis.

Furosemide-resistant edema in pediatric patients may benefit with the addition of metolazone. Some of these patients may have an exaggerated response leading to hypovolemia, tachycardia, and orthostatic hypotension requiring fluid replacement. Severe hypokalemia has been reported with a tendency for diuresis persisting for up to 24 hr after discontinuing metolazone.

Max. rate of administration of intermittent IV dose: 0.5 mg/kg/min.

Pregnancy category changes to D if used in pregnancy-induced hypertension.

GABAPENTIN
Neurontin
Anticonvulsant

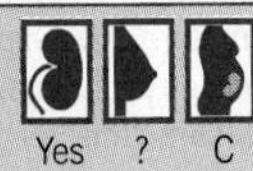

Caps: 100, 300, 400 mg
Tabs: 600, 800 mg
Oral solution: 250 mg/5 mL (480 mL)

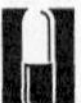

Seizures:
3–12 yr (PO, see remarks):
Day 1: 10–15 mg/kg/24 hr ÷ TID, then gradually titrate dose upward to the following dosages over a 3-day period:

Continued

GABAPENTIN *continued*

3–4 yr: 40 mg/kg/24 hr ÷ TID
≥5–12 yr: 25–35 mg/kg/24 hr ÷ TID
Dosages up to 50 mg/kg/24 hr have been well tolerated.

>12 yr and adult (PO, see remarks): Start with 300 mg TID; if needed, increase dose up to 1800 mg/24 hr ÷ TID. Usual effective doses: 900–1800 mg/24 hr ÷ TID. Doses as high as 3.6 g/24 hr have been tolerated.

Neuropathic pain:

Child (PO; limited data):
Day 1: 5 mg/kg/dose at bedtime
Day 2: 5 mg/kg/dose BID
Day 3: 5 mg/kg/dose TID; then titrate dose to effect. Usual dosage range: 8–35 mg/kg/24 hr

Adult (PO):
Day 1: 300 mg at bedtime
Day 2: 300 mg BID
Day 3: 300 mg TID; then titrate dose to effect. Usual dosage range: 1800–2400 mg/24 hr; **max. dose:** 3600 mg/24 hr.

Generally used as adjunctive therapy for partial and secondary generalized seizures and for neuropathic pain. Side effects include somnolence, dizziness, ataxia, fatigue, and nystagmus. **Do not withdraw medication abruptly.** Drug is not metabolized by the liver and is primarily excreted in the urine unchanged.

May be taken with or without food. In TID dosing schedule, interval between doses **should not exceed** 12 hr. **Adjust dose in renal impairment (see Chapter 30).**

GANCICLOVIR

Cytovene
Antiviral agent

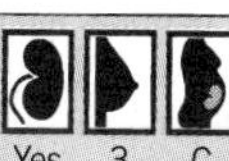

Injection: 500 mg; contains 4 mEq Na per 1 g drug
Caps: 250, 500 mg
Oral solution: 25, 100 mg/mL

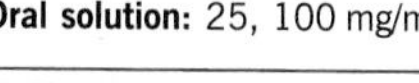

Cytomegalovirus (CMV) infections:

Child >3 mo and adult:
Induction therapy (duration 14–21 days): 10 mg/kg/24 hr ÷ Q12 hr IV
IV maintenance therapy: 5 mg/kg/dose QD IV or 6 mg/kg/dose QD IV for 5 days/wk
Oral maintenance therapy following induction:
6 mo–16 yr: 30 mg/kg/dose PO Q8 hr with food
Adult: 1000 mg PO TID with food

Prevention of CMV in transplant recipients:

Child and adult:
Induction therapy (duration 7–14 days): 10 mg/kg/24 hr ÷ Q12 hr IV
IV maintenance therapy: 5 mg/kg/dose QD IV or 6 mg/kg/dose QD IV for 5 days/wk for 100-120 days post-transplant
Oral maintenance therapy: see oral doses from above.

Continued

For explanation of icons, see p. 680.

GANCICLOVIR *continued*

Prevention of CMV in HIV-infected individuals:

Infant and child:

IV: 5 mg/kg/dose QD

PO: 30 mg/kg/dose Q8 hr with food

Adolescent and adult:

IV: 5–6 mg/kg/dose QD for 5–7 days/wk

PO: 1000–1500 mg PO TID with food

Limited experience with use in children <12 yr old. Use with extreme caution. **Reduce dose in renal failure (see Chapter 30).** Oral absorption is poor; consider the more bioavailable prodrug, valganciclovir, in adult patients. Common side effects: neutropenia, thrombocytopenia, retinal detachment, confusion. Drug reactions alleviated with dose reduction or temporary interruption. Ganciclovir may increase didanosine and zidovudine levels, whereas didanosine and zidovudine may decrease ganciclovir levels.

Minimum dilution is 10 mg/mL and should be infused IV over ≥1 hr. IM and SC administration are **contraindicated** because of high pH (pH = 11).

GATIFLOXACIN

Tequin, Zymar

Antibiotic, quinolone

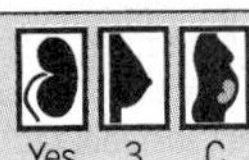

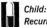

Tabs: 200, 400 mg

Injection: 10 mg/mL (20, 40 mL)

Ready-to-use injection in D5W: 2 mg/mL (100, 200 mL)

Ophthalmic solution (Zymar): 0.3% (2.5, 5 mL)

Child:

Recurrent/nonresponsive acute otitis media: 10 mg/kg/dose (**max. dose:** 600 mg/dose) PO QD × 10 days

Adult:

Community-acquired pneumonia: 400 mg IV/PO QD × 7–14 days

Skin/skin structure infection, pyelonephritis, and complicated UTI: 400 mg IV/PO QD × 7–10 days

Uncomplicated UTI: 400 mg IV/PO × 1, or 200 mg IV/PO QD × 3 days

Gonorrhea: 400 mg IV/PO × 1

Conjunctivitis:

≥1 yr–adult: Instill 1 drop to affected eye(s) Q2 hr while awake (up to 8 × daily) for the first 2 days, then 1 drop up to QID while awake on days 3–7.

Contraindicated in hypersensitivity to other quinolones. **Avoid** in patients with history of QTc prolongation and patients taking QTc prolonging drugs. **Use with caution** in diabetes, seizures, and children <18 yr. May cause GI disturbances, dizziness, headache, and vaginitis. Like other quinolones, tendon rupture can occur during or after therapy. **Adjust dose in renal failure (see Chapter 30).**

Continued

GATIFLOXACIN *continued*

Commonly observed side effects from two pediatric otitis media trials (414 patients) included vomiting, diarrhea, diaper rash, and maculopapular rash. No articular toxicity was observed.

Infuse IV over 1 hr. **Do not administer** antacids or other divalent salts with or within 4 hr of oral gatifloxacin dose; otherwise, may be administered with or without food.

GSCF

See *Filgrastim*

GENTAMICIN

Garamycin and others

Antibiotic, aminoglycoside

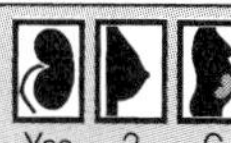

Injection: 10 mg/mL (2 mL), 40 mg/mL (2, 20 mL)
Ophthalmic ointment: 0.3% (3.5 g)
Ophthalmic drops: 0.3% (1, 5, 15 mL)
Topical ointment: 0.1% (15, 30 g)
Topical cream: 0.1% (15 g)

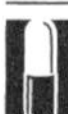

Parenteral (IM or IV):
Neonate/infant (see table below):

Postconceptional Age (wk)	Postnatal Age (days)	Dose (mg/kg/dose)	Interval (hr)
≤29*	0–7	5	48
	8–28	4	36
	>28	4	24
30–33	0–7	4.5	36
	>7	4	24
≥34	0–7	4	24
	>7	4	12–18

*Or significant asphyxia, PDA, indomethacin use, poor cardiac output, reduced renal function.

Child: 7.5 mg/kg/24 hr ÷ Q8 hr
Adult: 3–6 mg/kg/24 hr ÷ Q8 hr
Cystic fibrosis: 7.5–10.5 mg/kg/24 hr ÷ Q8 hr
Intrathecal/intraventricular (use preservative-free product only):
>3 mo: 1–2 mg QD
Adult: 4–8 mg QD
Ophthalmic ointment: apply Q8–12 hr
Ophthalmic drops: 1–2 drops Q2–4 hr

Continued

For explanation of icons, see p. 680.

GENTAMICIN *continued*

Use with caution in patients receiving anesthetics or neuromuscular blocking agents and in patients with neuromuscular disorders. May cause nephrotoxicity and ototoxicity. Ototoxicity may be potentiated with the use of loop diuretics. Eliminated more quickly in patients with cystic fibrosis, neutropenia, and burns. **Adjust dose in renal failure (see Chapter 30).** Monitor peak and trough levels.

Therapeutic peak levels:
- 6–10 mg/L general
- 8–10 mg/L in pulmonary infections, cystic fibrosis, neutropenia, osteomyelitis, and severe sepsis

Therapeutic trough levels: <2 mg/L. Recommended serum sampling time at steady state: trough within 30 min before the third consecutive dose and peak 30–60 min after the administration of the third consecutive dose.

GLUCAGON HCL

GlucaGen, Glucagon Emergency Kit

Antihypoglycemic agent

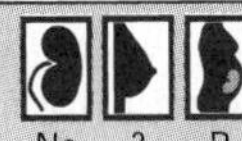

Injection: 1 mg vial (requires reconstitution)
1 unit = 1 mg

Hypoglycemia, IM, IV, SC:
Neonate, infant, and child <20 kg: 0.5 mg/dose (or 0.02–0.03 mg/kg/dose) Q20 min PRN
Child ≥20 kg and adult: 1 mg/dose Q20 min PRN

For beta-blocker and calcium-channel blocker overdose, see Chapter 2.

Drug product is genetically engineered and identical to human glucagon. High doses have cardiac stimulatory effect and have had some success in beta-blocker and calcium-channel blocker overdose. May cause nausea, vomiting, urticaria, and respiratory distress. **Do not delay** glucose infusion; dose for hypoglycemia is 2–4 mL/kg of dextrose 25%.

Onset of action: IM: 8–10 min; IV: 1 min. Duration of action: IM: 12–27 min; IV: 9–17 min.

GLYCERIN

Fleet Babylax, Sani-Supp, and others

Osmotic laxative

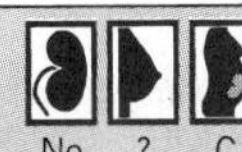

Rectal solution: 4 mL per application (6 doses), 7.5 mL per application (4 doses)

Suppository:
- Infant/pediatric (10s, 12s, 24s, 25s, 50s)
- Adult (10s, 12s, 18s, 24s, 25s, 48s, 50s)

Continued

GLYCERIN *continued*

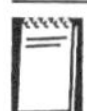

Constipation:
Neonate: 0.5 mL/kg/dose rectal solution PR as an enema QD–BID PRN or half of infant suppository PR QD PRN
Child <6 yr: 2–5 mL rectal solution PR as an enema or 1 infant suppository PR QD–BID PRN
>6 yr–adult: 5–15 mL rectal solution PR as an enema or 1 adult suppository PR QD–BID PRN

Onset of action: 15–30 min. May cause rectal irritation, abdominal pain, bloating, and dizziness. Insert suppository high into rectum, and retain for 15 min.

GLYCOPYRROLATE

Robinul
Anticholinergic agent

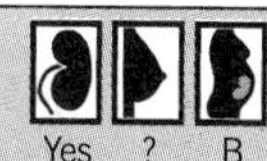

Tabs: 1, 2 mg
Injection: 0.2 mg/mL (1, 2, 5, 20 mL); some multidose vials contain 0.9% benzyl alcohol.

Respiratory antisecretory:
IM/IV:
Children: 0.004–0.01 mg/kg/dose Q4–8 hr
Adults: 0.1–0.2 mg/dose Q4–8 hr
Max. dose: 0.2 mg/dose or 0.8 mg/24 hr
Oral:
Child: 0.04–0.1 mg/kg/dose Q4–8 hr
Adult: 1–2 mg/dose BID–TID
Reverse neuromuscular blockade:
Child and adult: 0.2 mg IV for every 1 mg neostigmine or 5 mg pyridostigmine

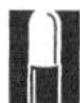

Use with caution in hepatic and renal disease, ulcerative colitis, asthma, glaucoma, ileus, or urinary retention. Atropine-like side effects: tachycardia, nausea, constipation, confusion, blurred vision, and dry mouth. These may be potentiated if given with other drugs with anticholinergic properties. IV dosage form may be used orally.

Onset of action: PO: within 1 hr; IM/SC: 15–30 min; IV: 1 min. Duration of antisialagogue effect: PO: 8–12 hr; IM/SC/IV: 7 hr.

For explanation of icons, see p. 680.

GRANISETRON

Kytril

Antiemetic agent, 5-HT$_3$ antagonist

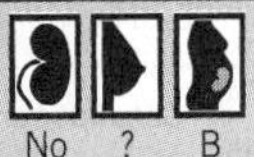

No ? B

Injection: 0.1 mg/mL (1 mL), 1 mg/mL (1, 4 mL); 4 mL vials contain benzyl alcohol
Tabs: 1 mg
Oral liquid: 0.2 mg/mL (30 mL); contains sodium benzoate

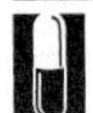

Chemotherapy-induced nausea and vomiting:

IV:

Child ≥2 yr and adult: 10–20 mcg/kg/dose 15–60 min before chemotherapy; the same dose may be repeated 2–3 times at ≥10-min intervals following chemotherapy (within 24 hr after chemotherapy) as a treatment regimen. Alternatively, a single 40 mcg/kg/dose 15–60 min before chemotherapy has been used.

PO:

Adult: 2 mg/24 hr ÷ QD–BID; initiate first dose 1 hr before chemotherapy

Postoperative nausea and vomiting prevention (dosed before anesthesia or immediately before anesthesia reversal) and treatment (IV):

≥4 yr: 40 mg/kg/dose (**max. dose:** 1 mg) × 1

Adult: 1 mg × 1

Radiation-induced nausea and vomiting prevention:

Adult: 2 mg QD PO administered within 1 hr of radiation.

Use with caution in liver disease. May cause hypertension, hypotension, arrhythmias, agitation, and insomnia. Inducers or inhibitors of the cytochrome P-450 3A3/4 drug-metabolizing enzymes may increase or decrease, respectively, the drug's clearance.

Onset of action: IV: 4–10 min. Duration of action: IV: ≤24 hr.

GRISEOFULVIN

Grifulvin V, Grisactin, Fulvicin U/F, Fulvicin P/G, Gris-PEG, and others

Antifungal agent

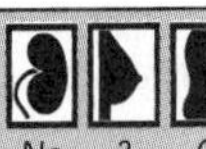

No ? C

Microsize:

Tabs (Fulvicin U/F): 250, 500 mg

Oral suspension (Grifulvin V): 125 mg/5 mL (120 mL); contains 0.2% alcohol and propylene glycol

Ultramicrosize:

Tabs (Fulvicin P/G, Gris-PEG): 125, 165, 250, 330 mg

250 mg ultra is approximately 500 mg micro.

Continued

GRISEOFULVIN *continued*

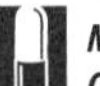

Microsize:

Child >2 yr: 20–25 mg/kg/24 hr PO ÷ QD-BID; give with milk, eggs, fatty foods.

Adult: 500–1000 mg/24 hr PO ÷ QD–BID

Max. dose: 1 g/24 hr

Ultramicrosize:

Child >2 yr: 10–15 mg/kg/24 hr PO ÷ QD–BID

Adult: 330–750 mg/24 hr PO ÷ QD–BID

Max. dose: 750 mg/24 hr

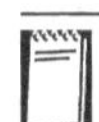

Contraindicated in porphyria and hepatic disease. Monitor hematologic, renal, and hepatic function. May cause leukopenia, rash, headache, paresthesias, and GI symptoms. Possible cross-reactivity in penicillin-allergic patients. Usual treatment period is 8 wk for tinea capitis and 4–6 mo for tinea unguium. Photosensitivity reactions may occur. May reduce effectiveness or decrease level of oral contraceptives, warfarin, and cyclosporin. Induces CYP450 1A2 isoenzyme. Phenobarbital may enhance clearance of griseofulvin. Coadministration with fatty meals will increase the drug's absorption.

HALOPERIDOL

Haldol and others

Antipsychotic agent

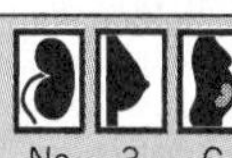

Injection (IM use only):

Lactate: 5 mg/mL (1, 10 mL)

Decanoate (long acting): 50, 100 mg/mL (1, 5 mL); in sesame oil with 1.2% benzyl alcohol

Tabs: 0.5, 1, 2, 5, 10, 20 mg

Solution: 2 mg/mL

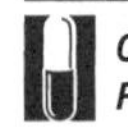

Child 3–12 yr:

PO: initial dose at 0.025–0.05 mg/kg/24 hr ÷ BID-TID. If necessary, increase daily dosage by 0.25–0.5 mg/24 hr Q5–7 days PRN up to a **max. dose** of 0.15 mg/kg/24 hr. Usual maintenance doses for specific indications include the following:

Agitation: 0.01–0.03 mg/kg/24 hr QD PO

Psychosis: 0.05–0.15 mg/kg/24 hr ÷ BID–TID PO

Tourette syndrome: 0.05–0.075 mg/kg/24 hr ÷ BID–TID PO; may increase daily dose by 0.5 mg Q5–7 days.

IM, as lactate, for 6–12 yr: 1–3 mg/dose Q4–8 hr; **max. dose:** 0.15 mg/kg/24 hr

>12 yr:

Acute agitation: 2–5 mg/dose IM as lactate or 1–15 mg/dose PO; repeat in 1 hr PRN.

Psychosis: 2–5 mg/dose Q4–8 hr IM PRN or 1–15 mg/24 hr ÷ BID–TID PO

Tourette syndrome: 0.5–2 mg/dose BID–TID PO

Continued

For explanation of icons, see p. 680.

HALOPERIDOL *continued*

Use with caution in patients with cardiac disease because of the risk for hypotension and in patients with epilepsy because the drug lowers the seizure threshold. Extrapyramidal symptoms, drowsiness, headache, tachycardia, ECG changes, nausea, and vomiting can occur.

Drug is metabolized by cytochrome P-450. May also inhibit cytochrome P-450 isoenzymes. Serotonin-specific reuptake inhibitors (e.g., fluoxetine) may increase levels and effects of haloperidol. Carbamazepine and phenobarbital may decrease levels and effects of haloperidol.

Acutely aggravated patients may require doses as often as Q60 min. **Decanoate salt is given every 3–4 wk in doses that are 10–15 times the individual patient's stabilized oral dose.**

HEPARIN SODIUM

Various trade names

Anticoagulant

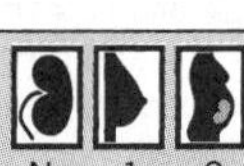

Injection:

Porcine intestinal mucosa: 1000, 2000, 2500, 5000, 7500, 10,000, 20,000, 40,000 U/mL (some products may be preservative-free; multidosed vials contain benzyl alcohol)

Lock flush solution (porcine based): 1, 10, 100 U/mL (some products may be preservative-free or contain benzyl alcohol)

Injection for IV infusion (porcine based):

D5W: 40 U/mL (500 mL), 50 U/mL (250, 500 mL), 100 U/mL (100, 250 mL); contains bisulfite

NS (0.9% NaCl): 2 U/mL (500, 1000 mL);

0.45% NaCl: 50 U/mL (250, 500 mL), 100 U/mL (250 mL)

120 U = approximately 1 mg

Anticoagulation (see Table 13-9 for dosage adjustments):

Infant and child:

Initial: 75–100 U/kg IV bolus

Maintenance IV infusion (preferred):

<1 yr: 28 U/kg/hr

≥1 yr: 20 U/kg/hr; use 18 U/kg/hr for older children.

Maintenance intermittent: 75–100 U/kg/dose Q4 hr IV

Adult:

Initial: 50–100 U/kg IV bolus

Maintenance: 15–25 U/kg/hr as IV infusion or 75–125 U/kg/dose Q4 hr IV

See remarks.

DVT prophylaxis:

Adult: 5000 U/dose SC Q8–12 hr until ambulatory

Heparin flush (dose should be less than heparinizing dose):

Younger child: lower doses should be used to avoid systemic heparinization.

Continued

HEPARIN SODIUM *continued*

Older child and adult:

Peripheral IV: 1–2 mL of 10 U/mL solution Q4 hr
Central lines: 2–3 mL of 100 U/mL solution Q24 hr
TPN (central line) and arterial line: add heparin to make final concentration of 0.5–1 U/mL.

Adjust dose to give PTT 1.5–2.5 times control value. PTT is best measured 6–8 hr after initiation or changes in infusion rate. For intermittent injection, PTT is measured 3.5–4 hr after injection. Toxicities: bleeding, allergy, alopecia, thrombocytopenia.

Use preservative-free heparin in neonates. **NOTE:** heparin flush doses may alter PTT in small patients; consider using more dilute heparin in these cases.

Antidote: Protamine sulfate (1 mg per 100 U heparin in previous 4 hr). For low-molecular-weight heparin, see *Enoxaparin*.

HYALURONIDASE

Amphadase, Vitrase
Antidote, extravasation

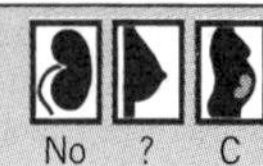

Injection (Amphadase): 150 U/mL (1 mL); bovine source containing thimerosal
Powder for injection (Vitrase): 6200 U; ovine source
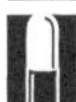 Pharmacy can make a 15-U/mL dilution.

Infant and child: dilute to 15 U/mL; give 1 mL (15U) by injecting 5 separate injections of 0.2 mL (3U) at borders of extravasation site SC or intradermally using a 25- or 26-gauge needle. Alternatively, a 150 U/mL concentration has been used with the same dosing instructions.

Contraindicated in dopamine and alpha-agonist extravasation and hypersensitivity to the respective product sources (bovine or ovine). May cause urticaria. Patients receiving large amounts of salicylates, cortisone, ACTH, estrogens, or antihistamines may decrease the effects of hyaluronidase (larger doses may be necessary). Administer as early as possible (minutes to 1 hour) after IV extravasation.

HYDRALAZINE HYDROCHLORIDE

Apresoline and others
Antihypertensive, vasodilator

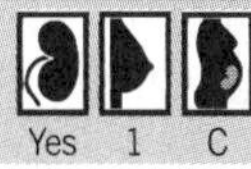

Tabs: 10, 25, 50, 100 mg
Injection: 20 mg/mL
Oral liquid: 1.25, 2, 4 mg/mL
Some dosage forms may contain tartrazines or sulfites.

Continued

For explanation of icons, see p. 680.

HYDRALAZINE HYDROCHLORIDE *continued*

Hypertensive crisis (may result in severe and prolonged hypotension, see Chapter 4, Table 4-7 for alternatives):

Child: 0.1–0.2 mg/kg/dose IM or IV Q4–6 hr PRN; **max. dose:** 20 mg/dose. Usual IV/IM dosage range is 1.7–3.5 mg/kg/24 hr.

Adult: 10–40 mg IM or IV Q4–6 hr PRN

Chronic hypertension:

Infant and child: start at 0.75–1 mg/kg/24 hr PO ÷ Q6–12 hr (**max. dose:** 25 mg/dose). If necessary, increase dose over 3–4 wk up to a **max. dose** of 5 mg/kg/24 hr for infants and 7.5 mg/kg/24 hr for children; or 200 mg/24 hr.

Adult: 10–50 mg/dose PO QID; **max. dose:** 300 mg/24 hr

Use with caution in severe renal and cardiac disease. Slow acetylators, patients receiving high-dose chronic therapy, and those with renal insufficiency are at highest risk for lupus-like syndrome (generally reversible). May cause reflex tachycardia, palpitations, dizziness, headaches, and GI discomfort. MAO inhibitors and beta-blockers may increase hypotensive effects. Indomethacin may decrease hypotensive effects.

Drug undergoes first pass metabolism. Onset of action: PO: 20–30 min; IV: 5–20 min. Duration of action: PO: 2–4 hr; IV: 2–6 hr. **Adjust dose in renal failure (see Chapter 30).**

HYDROCHLOROTHIAZIDE

Esidrix, Hydro-Par, Hydrodiuril, Oretic, and others

Diuretic, thiazide

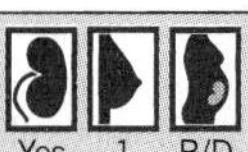

Tabs: 25, 50, 100 mg
Caps: 12.5 mg
Solution: 10 mg/mL (500 mL)

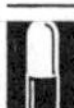

Neonate and infant <6 mo: 2–4 mg/kg/24 hr ÷ BID PO; **max. dose:** 37.5 mg/24 hr

≥6 mo and child: 2 mg/kg/24 hr ÷ BID PO; **max. dose:** 100 mg/24 hr

Adult: 12.5–100 mg/24 hr ÷ QD–BID PO; **max. dose:** 200 mg/24 hr

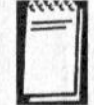

See *Chlorothiazide.* May cause fluid and electrolyte imbalances and hyperuricemia. Drug may not be effective when creatinine clearance is less than 25–50 mL/min.

Hydrochlorothiazide is also available in combination with potassium-sparing diuretics (e.g., spironolactone), ACE inhibitors, angiotensin II receptor antagonists, hydralazine, methyldopa, reserpine, and beta-blockers.

Pregnancy category is a D if used in pregnancy-induced hypertension.

HYDROCORTISONE

Solu-Cortef, Hydrocortone, Cortef, Cortifoam, and others

Corticosteroid

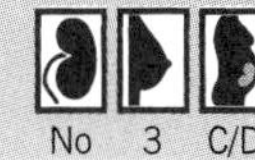

Hydrocortisone base

Tabs: 5, 10, 20 mg
Rectal cream: 1%, 2.5%
Topical ointment: 0.5%, 1%, 2.5%
Topical cream: 0.5%, 1%, 2.5%
Topical lotion: 0.25%, 0.5%, 1%, 2%, 2.5%

Cypionate (Cortef)

Oral suspension: 10 mg/5 mL (120 mL)

Na phosphate (Hydrocortone phosphate)

Injection: 50 mg/mL (2, 10 mL); contains sulfites and parabens

Na succinate (Solu-Cortef)

Injection: 100, 250, 500, 1000 mg/vial; contains benzyl alcohol

Acetate (Hydrocortone)

Injection: 25, 50 mg/mL; may contain 0.9% benzyl alcohol
Topical ointment: 1%
Topical cream: 0.5%, 1%, 2.5%
Rectal cream: 1%, 2.5%
Suppository: 25, 30 mg
Rectal foam aerosol (Cortifoam): 10% (90 mg/dose) (15 g)

Status asthmaticus:
Child:
Load (optional): 4–8 mg/kg/dose IV; **max. dose:** 250 mg
Maintenance: 8 mg/kg/24 hr ÷ Q6 hr IV
Adult: 100–500 mg/dose Q6 hr IV

Physiologic replacement: see Chapter 29 for dosing

Antiinflammatory/immunosuppressive:
Child:
PO: 2.5–10 mg/kg/24 hr ÷ Q6–8 hr
IM/IV: 1–5 mg/kg/24 hr ÷ Q12–24 hr
Adolescent and adult:
PO/IM/IV: 15–240 mg/dose Q12 hr

Acute adrenal insufficiency: see Chapters 9 and 29 for dosing

Topical use:
Child and adult: apply to affected areas TID–QID

For doses based on body surface area and topical preparations, see Chapter 29, Table 29-1. Na succinate used for IV, IM dosing. Na phosphate may be given IM, SC, or IV. **Acetate form recommended for intra-articular, intralesional, soft tissue use only, but not for IV use.**

See Chapter 29 for topical steroid comparisons. Pregnancy category changes to D if used in first trimester.

For explanation of icons, see p. 680.

HYDROMORPHONE HCL

Dilaudid, Dilaudid-HP, and others

Narcotic, analgesic

Yes ? B/D

Tabs: 2, 4, 8 mg
Injection: 1, 2, 4, 10 mg/mL (may contain benzyl alcohol and/or parabens)
Powder for injection: 250 mg
Suppository: 3 mg
Oral liquid: 1 mg/mL

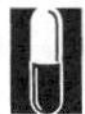

Analgesia, titrate to effect:

Child:

IV: 0.015 mg/kg/dose Q4–6 hr PRN

PO: 0.03–0.08 mg/kg/dose Q4–6 hr PRN; **max. dose:** 5 mg/dose

Adolescent and adult:

IM, IV, SC: 1–2 mg/dose Q4–6 hr PRN

PO: 1–4 mg/dose Q4–6 hr PRN

Refer to Table 28-16 for equianalgesic doses and Table 28-17 for patient-controlled analgesia dosing. Less pruritus than morphine. Similar profile of side effects to other narcotics. **Use with caution** in infants and young children, and **do not use** in neonates because of potential CNS effects. Dose reduction recommended in renal insufficiency or severe hepatic impairment. Pregnancy category changes to D if used for prolonged periods or in high doses at term.

HYDROXYCHLOROQUINE

Plaquenil, Quineprox

Antimalarial, antirheumatic agent

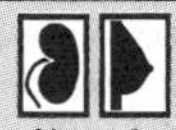
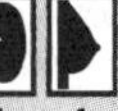
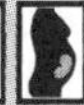

No 1 C

Tabs: 200 mg (155 mg base)
Oral suspension: 25 mg/mL (19.375 mg/mL base)

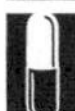

Doses expressed in mg of hydroxychloroquine base.

Malaria prophylaxis (start 1 wk before exposure and continue for 4 wk after leaving endemic area):

Child: 5 mg/kg/dose PO once weekly; **max. dose:** 310 mg

Adult: 310 mg PO once weekly

Malaria treatment (acute uncomplicated cases):

For treatment of malaria, consult with ID specialist or see the latest edition of the AAP *Red Book.*

Child: 10 mg/kg/dose (**max. dose:** 620 mg) PO × 1 followed by 5 mg/kg/dose (**max. dose:** 310 mg) 6 hr later. Then 5 mg/kg/dose (**max. dose:** 310 mg) Q24 hr × 2 doses starting 24 hr after the first dose.

Adult: 620 mg PO × 1 followed by 310 mg 6 hr later. Then 310 mg Q24 hr × 2 doses starting 24 hr after the first dose.

Juvenile rheumatoid arthritis or systemic lupus erythematosus:

Child: 2.325–3.875 mg/kg/24 hr PO ÷ QD-BID; **max. dose:** 310 mg/24 hr

Continued

HYDROXYCHOROQUINE *continued*

Contraindicated in psoriasis, porphyria, retinal or visual field changes, and 4-aminoquinoline hypersensitivity. **Use with caution** in liver disease, G6PD deficiency, concomitant hepatotoxic drugs, renal impairment, metabolic acidosis, or hematologic disorders.

Long-term use in children is **not recommended.** May cause headaches, myopathy, GI disturbances, skin and mucosal pigmentation, agranulocytosis, visual disturbances, and increased digoxin serum levels.

For SLE and JRA, lower doses can be used in combination with other immunosuppressive agents.

HYDROXYZINE

Atarax, Vistaril, and others

Antihistamine, anxiolytic, antiemetic

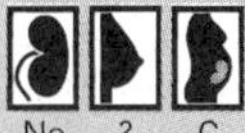

Tabs (HCl): 10, 25, 50, 100 mg
Caps (pamoate): 25, 50, 100 mg
Syrup (HCl): 10 mg/5 mL (118, 473 mL)
Oral suspension (pamoate): 25 mg/5 mL (120, 473 mL)
Injection (HCl): 25, 50 mg/mL; may contain benzyl alcohol.
NOTE: pamoate and HCl salts are equivalent in regard to mg of hydroxyzine.

Oral:
Child: 2 mg/kg/24 hr ÷ Q6–8 hr
Adult: 25–100 mg/dose Q4–6 hr PRN; **max. dose:** 600 mg/24 hr

IM:
Child: 0.5–1 mg/kg/dose Q4–6 hr PRN
Adult: 25–100 mg/dose Q4–6 hr PRN; **max. dose:** 600 mg/24 hr

May potentiate barbiturates, meperidine, and other CNS depressants. May cause dry mouth, drowsiness, tremor, convulsions, blurred vision, and hypotension. May cause pain at injection site.

Onset of action within 15–30 min. Duration of action: 4–6 hr. **IV administration is not recommended.**

IBUPROFEN

Motrin, Advil, Children's Advil, Children's Motrin, and others

Nonsteroidal antiinflammatory agent

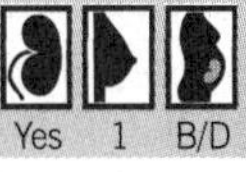

Oral suspension (OTC): 100 mg/5 mL (60, 120, 480 mL)
Oral drops (OTC): 40 mg/mL (7.5, 15 mL)
Chewable tabs (OTC): 50, 100 mg
Caplets (OTC): 100, 200 mg
Tabs: 100 (OTC), 200 (OTC), 400, 600, 800 mg
Capsules (OTC): 200 mg

Continued

For explanation of icons, see p. 680.

IBUPROFEN *continued*

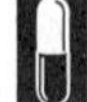

Child:
Analgesic/antipyretic: 5–10 mg/kg/dose Q6–8 hr PO; **max. dose:** 40 mg/kg/24 hr PO
JRA: 30–50 mg/kg/24 hr ÷ Q6 hr PO; **max. dose:** 2400 mg/24 hr

Adult:
Inflammatory disease: 400–800 mg/dose Q6–8 hr PO
Pain/fever/dysmenorrhea: 200–400 mg/dose Q4–6 hr PRN PO
Max. dose: 800 mg/dose or 3200 mg/24 hr

Contraindicated with active GI bleeding and ulcer disease. **Use caution** with aspirin hypersensitivity, hepatic or renal insufficiency, or dehydration, and in patients receiving anticoagulants. GI distress (lessened with milk), rashes, ocular problems, granulocytopenia, and anemia may occur. Inhibits platelet aggregation. Consumption of more than three alcoholic beverages per day may increase risk for GI bleeding.

May increase serum levels and effects of digoxin, methotrexate, and lithium. May decrease the effects of antihypertensives, furosemide, and thiazide diuretics.

Pregnancy category changes to D if used in third trimester or near delivery.

IMIPENEM-CILASTATIN

Primaxin IV, Primaxin IM
Antibiotic, carbapenem

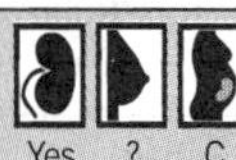

Injection:
Primaxin IV: 250, 500 mg; contains 3.2 mEq Na/g drug
Primaxin IM: 500, 750 mg; contains 2.8 mEq Na/g drug

Neonate:
0–4 wk & <1.2 kg: 50 mg/kg/24 hr ÷ Q12 hr IV
<1 wk & ≥1.2 kg: 50 mg/kg/24 hr ÷ Q12 hr IV
≥1 wk & ≥1.2 kg: 75 mg/kg/24 hr ÷ Q8 hr IV

Child (4 wk–3 mo): 100 mg/kg/24hr ÷ Q6 hr IV

Child (>3 mo): 60–100 mg/kg/24 hr ÷ Q6 hr IV; **max. dose:** 4 g/24 hr
Cystic fibrosis: 90 mg/kg/24 hr ÷ Q6 hr IV; **max. dose:** 4 g/24 hr

Adult:
IV: 250–1000 mg/dose Q6–8 hr; **max. dose:** 4 g/24 hr or 50 mg/kg/24 hr, whichever is less
IM: 500–750 mg/dose Q12 hr

For IV use, give slowly over 30–60 min. Adverse effects: pruritus, urticaria, GI symptoms, seizures, dizziness, hypotension, elevated LFTs, blood dyscrasias, and penicillin allergy. CSF penetration is variable but best with inflamed meninges.

Do not administer with probenecid (increases imipenem/cilastatin levels) or ganciclovir (increases risk for seizures). **Adjust dose in renal insufficiency (see Chapter 30).**

IMIPRAMINE

Tofranil, Tofranil-PM, and others
Antidepressant, tricyclic

No 3 D

Tabs (as HCl salt): 10, 25, 50 mg
Caps (Tofranil-PM, as pamoate salt): 75, 100, 125, 150 mg

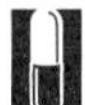

Antidepressant:

Child:

Initial: 1.5 mg/kg/24 hr ÷ TID PO; increase 1–1.5 mg/kg/24 hr Q3–4 days to a **max. dose** of 5 mg/kg/24 hr.

Adolescent:

Initial: 25–50 mg/24 hr ÷ QD-TID PO; **max. dose:** 200 mg/24 hr. Dosages exceeding 100 mg/24 hr are generally not necessary.

Adult:

Initial: 75–100 mg/24 hr ÷ TID PO

Maintenance: 50–300 mg/24 hr QHS PO; **max. dose:** 300 mg/24 hr

Enuresis (≥6 yr):

Initial: 10–25 mg QHS PO

Increment: 10–25 mg/dose at 1- to 2-wk intervals until **max. dose** for age or desired effect achieved. Continue × 2–3 mo, then taper slowly.

Max. dose:

6–12 yr: 50 mg/24 hr

12–14 yr: 75 mg/24 hr

Augment analgesia for chronic pain:

Initial: 0.2–0.4 mg/kg/dose QHS PO; increase 50% every 2–3 days to a **max. dose** of 1–3 mg/kg/dose QHS PO.

Contraindicated in narrow-angle glaucoma and patients who used MAO inhibitors within 14 days. See Chapter 2 for management of toxic ingestion.

Side effects include sedation, urinary retention, constipation, dry mouth, dizziness, drowsiness, and arrhythmia. QHS dosing during first weeks of therapy will reduce sedation. Monitor ECG, BP, CBC at start of therapy and with dose changes. Tricyclics may cause mania.

Therapeutic reference range (sum of imipramine and desipramine) = 150–250 ng/mL. Levels >1000 ng/mL are toxic, however, toxicity may occur at >300 ng/mL.

Recommended serum sampling times at steady state: obtain trough level within 30 min before the next scheduled dose after 5–7 days of continuous therapy. Carbamazepine may reduce imipramine levels; cimetidine, fluoxetine, fluvoxamine, labetalol, and quinidine may increase imipramine levels.

Onset of antidepressant effects: 1–3 weeks. **Do not discontinue abruptly** in patients receiving long-term high-dose therapy.

For explanation of icons, see p. 680.

IMMUNE GLOBULIN

Immune globulins

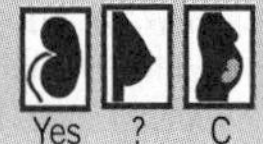

IM preparations

BayGam: 150–180 mg/mL (2, 10 mL)

IV preparations in solution

Gamunex: 10% solution

Gamimune-N: 5%, 10% solution

Venoglobulin S: 5%, 10% solution

IV preparations in powder for reconstitution

Gammagard S/D: 2.5, 5, 10 g; dilute to 5% or 10%

Gammar-P IV: 1, 2.5, 5, 10 g (contains 1 g sucrose per 1 g Ig); dilute to 5%

Iveegam: 5 g; dilute to 5%

Panglobulin: 6, 12 g (contains 1.67 g sucrose per 1 g Ig); dilute to 3%, 6%, or 12%

Polygam S/D: 2.5, 5, 10 g; dilute to 5% or 10%

See indications and doses in Chapter 14.

General guidelines for administration (see package insert of specific products): begin infusion at 0.01 mL/kg/min; double rate every 15–30 min, up to a **maximum** of 0.08 mL/kg/min. If adverse reactions occur, stop infusion until side effects subside, and may restart at rate that was previously tolerated.

May cause flushing, chills, fever, headache, and hypotension. Hypersensitivity reaction may occur when IV form is administered rapidly. Gamimune-N contains maltose and may cause an osmotic diuresis. May cause **anaphylaxis** in IgA-deficient patients owing to varied amounts of IgA. Some products are IgA depleted. Consult a pharmacist.

Intravenous preparations containing sucrose **should not be infused** at a rate such that the amount of sucrose exceeds 3 mg/kg/min to decrease risk for renal dysfunction, including acute renal failure.

Delay some immunizations after IVIG administration (see 2003 Red Book for details).

INDOMETHACIN

Indocin, Indocin SR, Indocin I.V., and others

Nonsteroidal antiinflammatory agent

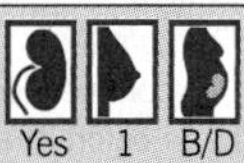

Caps: 25, 50 mg

Sustained-release caps (Indocin SR): 75 mg

Oral suspension: 25 mg/5 mL (237 mL)

Injection (Indocin I.V.): 1 mg

Suppositories: 50 mg (30s)

Continued

INDOMETHACIN *continued*

Antiinflammatory/rheumatoid arthritis:

≥2 yr: start at 1–2 mg/kg/24 hr ÷ BID–QID PO; **max. dose:** the lesser of 4 mg/kg/24 hr or 200 mg/24 hr

Adult: 50–150 mg/24 hr ÷ BID–QID PO; **max. dose:** 200 mg/24 hr

Closure of ductus arteriosus:

Infuse intravenously over 20–30 min:

	Dose (mg/kg/dose Q12–24 hr)		
Age	*#1*	*#2*	*#3*
<48 hr	0.2	0.1	0.1
2–7 days	0.2	0.2	0.2
>7 days	0.2	0.25	0.25

In infants <1500 g, 0.1–0.2 mg/kg/dose IV Q24 hr may be given for an additional 3–5 days.

Intraventricular hemorrhage prophylaxis: 0.1 mg/kg/dose IV Q24 hr × 3 doses, initiated at 6–12 hr of age (give in consultation with a neonatologist).

Contraindicated in active bleeding, coagulation defects, necrotizing enterocolitis, and renal insufficiency. May cause (especially in neonates) decreased urine output, platelet dysfunction, and decreased GI blood flow and reduce the antihypertensive effects of beta-blockers, hydralazine, and ACE inhibitors. **Fatal hepatitis reported in treatment of JRA.** Monitor renal and hepatic function before and during use.

Reduction in cerebral blood flow associated with rapid IV infusion; infuse all IV doses over 20–30 min.

Sustained-release capsules are dosed QD–BID. Pregnancy category changes to D if used for >48 hr or after 34 wk gestation or close to delivery.

INSULIN PREPARATIONS

Pancreatic hormone

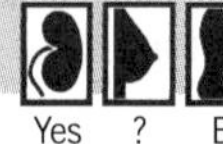

Yes ? B

Many preparations, at concentrations of 40, 100, 500 U/mL

Diluted concentrations of 1 U/mL or 10 U/mL may be necessary for neonates and infants.

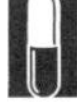

Insulin preparations: see Chapter 29, Table 29-4.

Hyperkalemia: see Chapter 10, Figure 10-2.

DKA: see Chapter 9, Figure 9-1.

When using insulin drip with new IV tubing, fill the tubing with the insulin infusion solution and wait for 30 min (before connecting tubing to the patient). Then flush the line and connect the IV line to the patient to start the infusion. This will ensure proper drug delivery. **Adjust dose in renal failure (see Chapter 30).**

For explanation of icons, see p. 680.

IODIDE

See *Potassium Iodide*

IPECAC

Various generic brands
Emetic agent

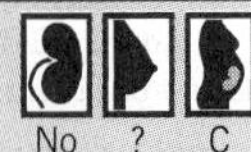

Syrup: 70 mg/mL (15, 30 mL); contains 1.5%–2% alcohol

See Chapter 2 for indications.
All doses are administered × 1 and may be repeated once if vomiting does not occur within 20–30 min. If vomiting does not occur within 30–45 min after the second dose, perform gastric lavage:

6–12 mo: 5–10 mL ipecac followed by 10–20 mL/kg water
1–12 yr: 15 mL ipecac followed by 10–20 mL/kg or 120–240 mL water
≥12 yr and adults: 15–30 mL ipecac followed by 200–300 mL of water

---

Do not administer if patient is unconscious or has potential for decline in mental status, lacks a gag reflex, has seizures, or has ingested corrosives, strong acids or bases, volatile oils. May cause GI irritation, cardiotoxicity, and myopathy. **Do not use** ipecac fluid extract because it is 14 times more potent. **Do not administer** with milk or carbonated beverages.

Onset of action: 15–30 min. Duration of action: 20 min to 1 hr.

IPRATROPIUM BROMIDE

Atrovent
Anticholinergic agent

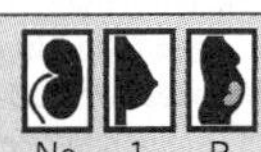

Aerosol: 18 mcg/dose (200 actuations per canister, 14 g)
Nebulized solution: 0.02% (500 mcg/2.5 mL, 25s, 60s)
Nasal spray: 0.03% (21 mcg per actuation, 30 mL); 0.06% (42 mcg per actuation, 15 mL)
In combination with albuterol (DuoNeb):
Nebulized solution: 0.5 mg ipratropium bromide and 2.5 mg albuterol in 3 mL (30s, 60s)

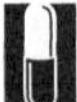

Acute use in the ED or ICU:
Nebulizer treatments:
<12 yr: 250 mcg/dose Q20 min × 3, then Q2–4 hr PRN
≥12 yr: 500 mcg/dose Q30 min × 3, then Q2–4 hr PRN

Inhaler:
Child and adult: 4–8 puffs Q2–4 hr PRN

Continued

IPRATROPIUM BROMIDE *continued*

Nonacute use:

Inhaler:

<12 yr: 1–2 puffs Q6 hr

≥12 yr: 2–3 puffs Q6 hr up to 12 puffs/24 hr

Nebulized treatments:

Infant and child: 250 mcg/dose Q6–8 hr

>12 yr and adult: 250–500 mcg/dose Q6–8 hr

Nasal spray:

Allergic and nonallergic rhinitis:

>6 yr and adult: 2 sprays of 0.03% strength (42 mcg) per nostril BID–TID

Rhinitis associated with common cold:

>5 yr and adult: 2 sprays of 0.06% strength (84 mcg) per nostril TID–QID × 4 days; administer TID for children 5–11 yr.

Contraindicated in soy or peanut allergy (for aerosol inhaler) and atropine hypersensitivity. **Use with caution** in narrow-angle glaucoma or bladder neck obstruction, although ipratropium has fewer anticholinergic systemic effects than atropine. May cause anxiety, dizziness, headache, GI discomfort, and cough with inhaler or nebulized use. Epistaxis, nasal congestion, and dry mouth/throat have been reported with the nasal spray. Reversible anisocoria may occur with unintentional aerosolization of drug to the eyes, particularly with mask nebulizers. Proven efficacy of nebulized solution in pediatrics is currently limited to reactive airway disease management in the emergency room and intensive care unit areas.

Bronchodilation onset of action is 1–3 min with peak effects within 1.5–2 hr and duration of action of 4–6 hr.

Shake inhaler well before use with spacer. Nebulized solution may be mixed with albuterol (or use DuoNeb).

Breast-feeding safety **extrapolated** from safety of atropine.

IRON DEXTRAN

InFed, DexFerrum

Parenteral iron

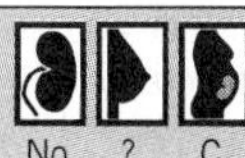

No ? C

Injection: 50 mg/mL (50 mg elemental Fe/mL) (2 mL)

Products containing phenol 0.5% are only for IM administration; products containing sodium chloride 0.9% can be administered via the IM or IV route.

Inject test dose (see remarks).

Iron-deficiency anemia: Total replacement dose of iron dextran (mL) = 0.0476 × lean body wt (kg) × (desired Hgb [g/dL] – measured Hgb [g/dL]) + 1 mL per 5-kg lean body weight (up to **max. dose** of 14 mL).

Acute blood loss: Total replacement dose of iron dextran (mL) = 0.02 × blood loss (mL) × hematocrit expressed as decimal fraction. Assumes 1 mL of RBC = 1 mg elemental iron.

If no reaction to test dose, give remainder of replacement dose ÷ over 2–3 daily doses.

Continued

FORMULARY

For explanation of icons, see p. 680.

IRON DEXTRAN *continued*

Max. daily (IM) dose:

<5 kg: 0.5 mL (25 mg)
5–10 kg: 1 mL (50 mg)
>10 kg: 2 mL (100 mg)

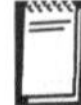

Oral therapy with iron salts is preferred; injectable routes are painful. Numerous adverse effects including anaphylaxis, fever, hypotension, rash, myalgias, and arthralgias.

Use Z-track technique for IM administration. **Inject test dose:** 25 mg (12.5 mg for infants) IV over at least 5 min. May begin treatment dose after 1 hr. **Max. rate of IV infusion:** 50 mg/min. For IV infusion, diluting in NS may lower the incidence of phlebitis. Direct IV push administration is **not recommended. Not recommended** in infants <4 mo. Compatible with parenteral nutrition solutions.

Other forms of parenteral iron such as Ferrlecit (ferric gluconate) and Venofer (iron sucrose) may be useful in combination with erythropoietin in hemodialysis patients who have anemia of chronic renal failure.

IRON PREPARATIONS

Fergon, Fer-In-Sol, Feosol, Niferex, Slow FE, and others
Oral iron supplements

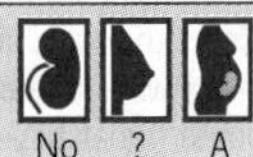

Ferrous sulfate (20% elemental Fe):

Drops (Fer-In-Sol): 75 mg (15 mg Fe)/0.6 mL (50 mL); 125 mg (25 mg Fe)/ 1 mL (50 mL)
Elixir (Feosol): 220 mg (44 mg Fe)/5 mL (5% alcohol)
Tabs: 300 mg (60 mg Fe), 324 mg (65 mg Fe), 325 mg (65 mg Fe)

Ferrous gluconate (12% elemental Fe):

Tabs: 240 mg (27 mg Fe, as Fergon), 300 mg (34 mg Fe), 324 mg (37 mg Fe), 325 mg (38 mg Fe)

Ferrous sulfate, exsiccated/dried (30% elemental Fe):

Tabs: 187 mg (60 mg Fe), 200 mg (65 mg Fe)
Extended-release tabs (Slow FE): 160 mg (50 mg Fe)

Ferrous fumarate (33% elemental Fe):

Tabs: 200 mg (66 mg Fe), 324 mg (106 mg Fe), 325 mg (106 mg Fe), 350 mg (115 mg Fe)
Chewable tabs: 100 mg (33 mg Fe)

Polysaccharide-iron complex and ferrous bis-glycinate chelate (Niferex) (expressed in mg elemental Fe):

Caps: 60, 150 mg; 150 mg strength contains 50 mg vitamin C.
Elixir: 100 mg/5 mL (10% alcohol)

Iron-deficiency anemia:

Premature infant: 2–4 mg elemental Fe/kg/24 hr ÷ QD-BID PO; **max. dose:** 15 mg elemental Fe/24 hr
Child: 3–6 mg elemental Fe/kg/24 hr ÷ QD–TID PO
Adult: 60 mg elemental Fe BID–QID

Prophylaxis:

Child: Give dose below PO ÷ QD-TID.

Premature: 2 mg elemental Fe/kg/24 hr; **max. dose:** 15 mg elemental Fe/24 hr

Continued

IRON PREPARATIONS *continued*

Full-term: 1–2 mg elemental Fe/kg/24 hr; **max. dose:** 15 mg elemental Fe/24 hr

Adult: 60 mg elemental Fe/24 hr PO ÷ QD-BID

Iron preparations are variably absorbed. Less GI irritation when given with or after meals. Vitamin C, 200 mg per 30 mg iron, may enhance absorption.

Liquid iron preparations may stain teeth. Give with dropper or drink through straw. May produce constipation, dark stools (false-positive guaiac is controversial), nausea, and epigastric pain. Iron and tetracycline inhibit each other's absorption. Antacids may decrease iron absorption.

ISONIAZID

INH, Nydrazid, Laniazid, and others

Antituberculous agent

Yes 1 C

Tabs: 100, 300 mg

Syrup: 50 mg/5 mL (473 mL)

Injection: 100 mg/mL (10 mL)

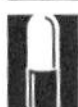

See most recent edition of the AAP *Red Book* for details and length of therapy.

Prophylaxis:

Infant and child: 10 mg/kg (**max. dose:** 300 mg) PO QD. After 1 month of daily therapy and in cases in which daily compliance cannot be ensured, may change to 20–40 mg/kg (**max. dose:** 900 mg) per dose PO, given twice weekly.

Adult: 300 mg PO QD

Treatment:

Infant and child: 10–15 mg/kg (**max. dose:** 300 mg) PO QD or 20–30 mg/kg (**max. dose:** 900 mg) per dose twice weekly with rifampin for uncomplicated pulmonary tuberculosis in compliant patients. Additional drugs are necessary in complicated disease.

Adult: 5 mg/kg (**max. dose:** 300 mg) PO QD or 15 mg/kg (**max. dose:** 900 mg) per dose twice weekly with rifampin. Additional drugs are necessary in complicated disease.

For INH-resistant TB: Discuss with Health Dept., or consult ID specialist.

Should not be used alone for treatment. Peripheral neuropathy, optic neuritis, seizures, encephalopathy, psychosis, and hepatic side effects may occur with higher doses, especially in combination with rifampin. Follow LFTs monthly. Supplemental pyridoxine (1–2 mg/kg/24 hr) is recommended. May cause false-positive urine glucose test.

Inhibits CYP450 1A2, 2C9, 2C19, and 3A3/4 microsomal enzymes; decrease dose of carbamazepine, diazepam, phenytoin, and prednisone. Also a substrate and inducer of CYP450 2E1.

May be given IM (same as oral doses) when oral therapy is not possible. Administer oral doses 1 hr before and 2 hr after meals. **Adjust dose in renal failure (see Chapter 30).**

For explanation of icons, see p. 680.

ISOPROTERENOL
Isuprel and others
Adrenergic agonist

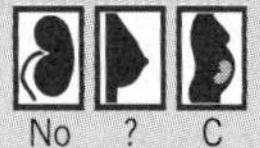
No ? C

Isoproterenol HCl:

Injection, prefilled syringes: 0.02 mg/mL (10 mL); contains sulfites

Injection: 0.2 mg/mL (1, 5 mL); contains sulfites

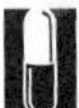

NOTE: The dosage units for adults are in mcg/min, compared to mcg/kg/min for children.

IV infusion:

Child: 0.05–2 mcg/kg/min; start at minimum dose and increase every 5–10 min by 0.1 mcg/kg/min until desired effect or onset of toxicity; **max. dose:** 2 mcg/kg/min

Adult: 2–20 mcg/min

See inside front cover for preparation of infusion.

Use with caution in CHF, ischemia, or aortic stenosis. May cause flushing, ventricular arrhythmias, profound hypotension, anxiety, and myocardial ischemia. Monitor heart rate, respiratory rate, and blood pressure. **Not for treatment** of asystole or for use in cardiac arrests, unless bradycardia is due to heart block.

Continuous infusion for bronchodilatation must be gradually tapered over a 24- to 48-hr period to prevent rebound bronchospasm. Tolerance may occur with prolonged use. Clinical deterioration, myocardial necrosis, CHF, and death have been reported with continuous infusion use in refractory asthmatic children.

ISOTRETINOIN
Accutane, Amnesteem, Claravis, Sotret
Retinoic acid, vitamin A derivative

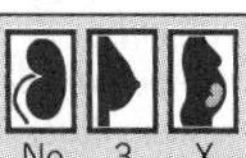
No 3 X

Caps: 10, 20, 40 mg; may contain soybean oil, EDTA, and parabens

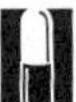

Cystic acne: 0.5–2 mg/kg/24 hr ÷ BID PO × 15–20 wk

Dosages as low as 0.05 mg/kg/24 hr have been reported to be beneficial.

Contraindicated during pregnancy; known teratogen. Use with caution in females during childbearing years. May cause conjunctivitis, xerosis, pruritus, photosensitivity reactions (**avoid** expose to sunlight and use sunscreen), epistaxis, anemia, hyperlipidemia, pseudotumor cerebri (especially in combination with tetracyclines; **avoid** this combination), cheilitis, bone pain, muscle aches, skeletal changes, lethargy, nausea, vomiting, elevated ESR, mental depression, aggressive or violent behavior, and psychosis.

Continued

ISOTRETINOIN *continued*

To avoid additive toxic effects, **do not** take vitamin A concomitantly. Increases clearance of carbamazepine. Hormonal birth control (oral, injectable, and implantable) failures have been reported with concurrent use. Monitor CBC, ESR, triglycerides, and LFTs.

To prescribe Accutane, prescribers must first register with the manufacturer's System to Manage Accutane Related Teratogenicity (SMART) program (1-800-937-6243).

ITRACONAZOLE

Sporanox

Antifungal agent

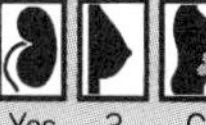

Caps: 100 mg
Oral solution: 10 mg/mL (150 mL)
Injection: 10 mg/mL (25 mL)

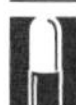

Child (limited data): 3–5 mg/kg/24 hr PO ÷ QD–BID; dosages as high as 5–10 mg/kg/24 hr have been used for aspergillus prophylaxis in chronic granulomatous disease.

Prophylaxis for recurrence of opportunistic disease in HIV:

Cryptococcus neoformans: 2–5 mg/kg/dose PO Q12–24 hr

Histoplasma capsulatum or Coccidioides immitis: 2–5 mg/kg/dose PO Q12–48 hr

Adults:

Blastomycosis and nonmeningeal histoplasmosis:

PO: 200 mg QD up to a **max. dose** of 400 mg/24 hr ÷ BID (**max. dose:** 200 mg/dose)

IV: 400 mg/24 hr ÷ BID × 2 days, followed by 200 mg QD; switch to oral therapy as soon as possible.

Aspergillosis and severe infections:

PO: 600 mg/24 hr ÷ TID × 3–4 days, followed by 200–400 mg/24 hr ÷ BID; **max. dose:** 600 mg/24 hr ÷ TID

IV: 400 mg/24 hr ÷ BID × 2 days, followed by 200 mg QD; switch to oral therapy as soon as possible.

Empiric therapy in febrile, neutropenic patients: 400 mg/24 hr IV ÷ BID × 2 days, followed by 200 mg QD for up to 14 days; continue with the oral solution at 200 mg PO BID until resolution.

Oral solution and capsule dosage form should **NOT** be used interchangeably; oral solution is more bioavailable. Only the oral solution has been demonstrated effective for oral and/or esophageal candidiasis. **Use with caution** in hepatic impairment. May cause GI symptoms, headaches, rash, liver enzyme elevation, hepatitis, and hypokalemia.

Like ketoconazole, it inhibits the activity of the cytochrome P-450 3A4 drug metabolizing isoenzyme. Thus, the coadministration of cisapride, pimozide, quinidine, triazolam, and midazolam is **contraindicated.** See remarks in *Ketoconazole* for additional drug interaction information.

Continued

For explanation of icons, see p. 680.

ITRACONAZOLE *continued*

IV dosage form should **not** be used in patients with GFR <30 mL/min because the hydoxypropyl-beta-cyclodextrin excipient has reduced clearance in patients with renal failure. IV form should be diluted with NS (not compatible with D5W or LR) and infused over 1 hr.

Administer oral solution on an empty stomach, but administer capsules with food. Achlorhydria reduces absorption of the drug.

IVERMECTIN
Stromectol
Antihelminthic

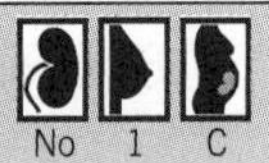

Tabs: 3, 6 mg

Cutaneous larva migrans, or strongyloidiasis: 0.2 mg/kg/dose PO QD × 1–2 days; dosing by body weight (see first table below):
Scabies: 0.2 mg/kg/dose PO × 1; dosing by body weight (see table below):

CUTANEOUS LARVA MIGRANS, SCABIES, STRONGYLOIDIASIS

Weight (kg)	Oral Dose
15–24	3 mg
25–35	6 mg
36–50	9 mg
51–65	12 mg
66–79	15 mg
≥80	0.2 mg/kg

Onchocerciasis: 0.15 mg/kg PO × 1; dosing by body weight (see table below):

ONCHOCERCIASIS

Weight (kg)	Single Oral Dose
15–25	3 mg
26–44	6 mg
45–64	9 mg
65–84	12 mg
≥85	0.15 mg/kg

Dose may be repeated every 6–12 mo until asymptomatic.

Continued

IVERMECTIN *continued*

Adverse reactions experienced in strongyloidiasis include diarrhea, nausea, vomiting, pruritus, rash, dizziness, and drowsiness.

Adverse reactions experienced in onchocerciasis include cutaneous or systemic allergic/inflammatory reactions of varying severity (Mazzotti reaction) and ophthalmologic reactions. Specific reactions may include arthralgia/synovitis, lymph node enlargement and tenderness, pruritus, edema, fever, orthostatic hypotension, and tachycardia. Therapy for postural hypotension may include oral hydration, recumbency, IV normal saline, and/or IV steroids. Antihistamines and/or aspirin has been used for most mild to moderate cases.

KANAMYCIN

Kantrex and others

Antibiotic, aminoglycoside

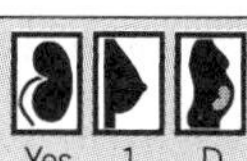

Caps: 500 mg
Injection: 37.5, 250, 333, 500 mg/mL; may contain sulfites

Neonatal IV/IM administration (see table below):

Birth Weight (kg)	<7 Days	≥7 Days
<2	15 mg/kg/24 hr ÷ Q12 hr	22.5 mg/kg/24 hr ÷ Q8 hr
≥2	20 mg/kg/24 hr ÷ Q12 hr	30 mg/kg/24 hr ÷ Q8 hr

Infant and child: IM/IV: 15–30 mg/kg/24 hr ÷ Q8–12 hr
Adult: IV/IM: 15 mg/kg/24 hr ÷ Q8–12 hr
PO administration for GI bacterial overgrowth: 150–250 mg/kg/24 hr ÷ Q6 hr; **max. dose:** 4 g/24 hr

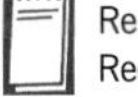

Renal toxicity and ototoxicity may occur. Give over 30 min if IV route is used. Reduce dosage frequency with renal impairment. Poorly absorbed orally; PO used to treat GI bacterial overgrowth.

Therapeutic levels: peak: 15–30 mg/L; trough: <5–10 mg/L. Recommended serum sampling time at steady state: trough within 30 min before third consecutive dose and peak 30–60 min after administration of third consecutive dose. **Adjust dose in renal failure (see Chapter 30).**

For explanation of icons, see p. 680.

KETAMINE
Ketalar and others
General anesthetic

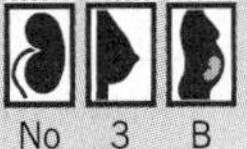
No 3 B

Injection: 10 mg/mL (20 mL), 50 mg/mL (10 mL), 100 mg/mL (5 mL); contains benzethonium chloride

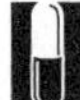
Child:
Sedation:
PO: 5 mg/kg × 1
IV (see remarks): 0.25–0.5 mg/kg
IM: 1.5–2 mg/kg × 1
Adult:
Analgesia with sedation:
IV (see remarks): 0.2–1 mg/kg
IM: 0.5–4 mg/kg

Contraindicated in elevated ICP, hypertension, aneurysms, thyrotoxicosis, CHF, angina, and psychotic disorders. May cause hypertension, hypotension, emergence reactions, tachycardia, laryngospasm, respiratory depression, and stimulation of salivary secretions. Intravenous use may induce general anesthesia. Benzodiazepine may be added to prevent emergence phenomenon. Anticholinergic agent may be added to decrease hypersalivation. Rate of IV infusion should **not exceed** 0.5 mg/kg/min and should **not be administered** in less than 60 sec. For additional information including onset and duration of action, see Chapter 28, Table 28-10.

KETOCONAZOLE
Nizoral, Nizoral A-D, and others
Antifungal agent

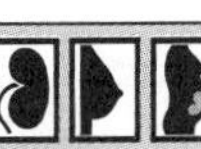
No 1 C

Tabs: 200 mg
Suspension: 100 mg/5 mL
Cream: 2% (15, 30, 60 g)
Shampoo: 1% (Nizoral A-D, OTC) (120, 210 mL), 2% (120 mL)

Oral:
Child ≥2 yr: 3.3–6.6 mg/kg/24 hr QD
Adult: 200–400 mg/24 hr QD
Max. dose: 800 mg/24 hr ÷ BID
Topical: 1–2 applications/24 hr
Shampoo: Twice weekly for 4 wk with at least 3 days between applications; intermittently as needed to maintain control
Suppressive therapy against mucocutaneous candidiasis in HIV:
Child: 5–10 mg/kg/24 hr ÷ QD–BID PO; **max. dose:** 800 mg/24 hr ÷ BID
Adolescent and adult: 200 mg/dose QD PO

Continued

KETOCONAZOLE *continued*

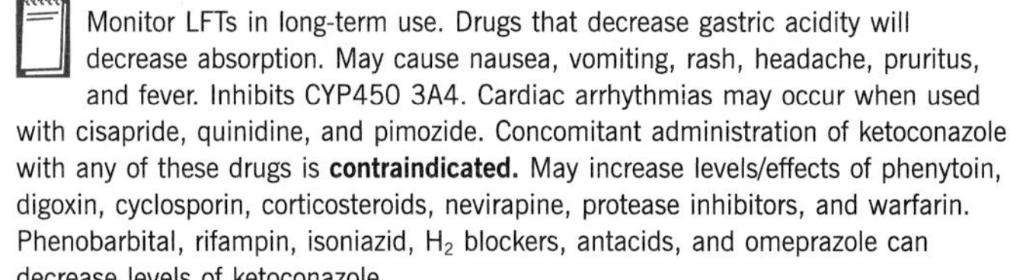

Monitor LFTs in long-term use. Drugs that decrease gastric acidity will decrease absorption. May cause nausea, vomiting, rash, headache, pruritus, and fever. Inhibits CYP450 3A4. Cardiac arrhythmias may occur when used with cisapride, quinidine, and pimozide. Concomitant administration of ketoconazole with any of these drugs is **contraindicated.** May increase levels/effects of phenytoin, digoxin, cyclosporin, corticosteroids, nevirapine, protease inhibitors, and warfarin. Phenobarbital, rifampin, isoniazid, H_2 blockers, antacids, and omeprazole can decrease levels of ketoconazole.

Administering oral doses with food or acidic beverages and 2 hr before antacids will increase absorption.

To use shampoo, wet hair and scalp with water, apply sufficient amount to scalp, and gently massage for about 1 min. Rinse hair thoroughly, reapply shampoo, and leave on the scalp for an additional 3 min; then rinse.

KETOROLAC

Toradol, Acular, Acular LC, Acular PF

Nonsteroidal antiinflammatory agent

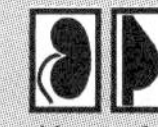
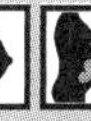
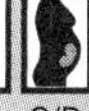

Yes 1 C/D

Injection: 15 mg/mL (1 mL), 30 mg/mL (1, 2 mL); contains 10% alcohol
Tabs: 10 mg
Ophthalmic:

Acular: 0.5% (3, 5, 10 mL)
Acular PF: 0.5% (0.4 mL); preservative-free
Acular LC: 0.4% (5 mL)

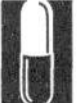

IM/IV:

Child: 0.5 mg/kg/dose IM/IV Q6 hr. **Max. dose:** 30 mg Q6 hr or 120 mg/24 hr
Adult: 30 mg IM/IV Q6 hr. **Max. dose:** 120 mg/24 hr

PO:

Child >50 kg and adult: 10 mg PRN Q6 hr; **max. dose:** 40 mg/24 hr

Ophthalmic (see remarks):

≥3 yr–adult: 1 drop in each affected eye QID

Ketorolac therapy is not to exceed 5 days (IM, IV, PO). Consider adding acid blocker therapy with systemic use. May cause GI bleeding, nausea, dyspepsia, drowsiness, decreased platelet function, and interstitial nephritis. **Not recommended** in patients at increased risk for bleeding. **Do not use** in hepatic or renal failure.

Use Acular PF for incisional refractive surgery and Acular LC for corneal refractive surgery. Duration of therapy for ophthalmic use: 14 days after cataracts surgery up to 4 days after corneal refractive surgery, and up to 3 days after incisional refractive surgery.

Pregnancy category changes to a D if used in the third trimester.

For explanation of icons, see p. 680.

LABETALOL

Normodyne, Trandate, and others

Adrenergic antagonist (alpha and beta), antihypertensive

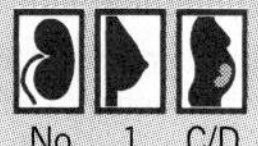

Tabs: 100, 200, 300 mg
Injection: 5 mg/mL (20, 40 mL); contains parabens
Oral suspension: 10, 40 mg/mL 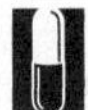

Child:
PO: Initial: 4 mg/kg/24 hr ÷ BID. May increase up to 40 mg/kg/24 hr
IV: Hypertensive emergency (start at lowest dose and titrate to effect; see Chapter 4):
Intermittent dose: 0.2–1 mg/kg/dose Q10 min PRN; **max. dose:** 20 mg/dose
Infusion: 0.4–1 mg/kg/hr, to a **max. dose** of 3 mg/kg/hr; may initiate with a 0.2–1 mg/kg bolus; **max. bolus:** 20 mg.

Adult:
PO: 100 mg BID, increase by 100 mg/dose Q2–3 days PRN to a **max. dose** of 2.4 g/24 hr. *Usual range:* 200–800 mg/24hr ÷ BID
IV: Hypertensive emergency (start at lowest dose and titrate to effect):
Intermittent dose: 20–80 mg/dose (begin with 20 mg) Q10 min PRN; **max. dose:** 300 mg total dose
Infusion: 2 mg/min, increase to titrate to response.

Contraindicated in asthma, pulmonary edema, cardiogenic shock, and heart block. May cause orthostatic hypotension, edema, CHF, bradycardia, AV conduction disturbances, bronchospasm, urinary retention, and skin tingling. **Use with caution** in hepatic disease and diabetes; liver function test elevation, hepatic necrosis, hepatitis, and cholestatic jaundice have been reported.

Patient should remain supine for up to 3 hr after IV administration. Pregnancy category changes to D if used in second or third trimesters.

Onset of action: PO: 1–4 hr; IV: 5–15 min

LACTULOSE

Cephulac, Chronulac, Enulose, and others

Ammonium detoxicant, hyperosmotic laxative

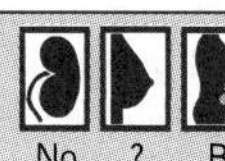

Syrup: 10 g/15 mL; contains galactose, lactose, and other sugars

Chronic constipation:
Child: 7.5 mL/24 hr PO after breakfast
Adult: 15–30 mL/24 hr PO QD to a **max. dose** of 60 mL/24 hr

Portal systemic encephalopathy (adjust dose to produce 2–3 soft stools/day):
Infant: 2.5–10 mL/24 hr PO ÷ TID–QID
Child: 40–90 mL/24 hr PO ÷ TID–QID

Continued

LACTULOSE *continued*

Adult: 30–45 mL/dose PO TID–QID; acute episodes 30–45 mL Q1–2 hr until 2–3 soft stools/day
Rectal (adult): 300 mL diluted in 700 mL water or NS in 30–60 min retention enema; may give Q4–6 hr

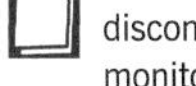

Contraindicated in galactosemia. **Use with caution** in diabetes mellitus. GI discomfort and diarrhea may occur. For portal systemic encephalopathy, monitor serum ammonia, serum potassium, and fluid status.

Adjust dose to achieve 2–3 soft stools per day. **Do not use** with antacids.

LAMIVUDINE

Epivir, Epivir-HBV, 3TC
Antiviral agent, nucleoside analogue reverse transcriptase inhibitor

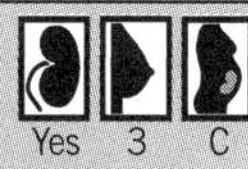

Tabs: 100 mg (Epivir-HBV), 150, 300 mg
Oral solution: 5 mg/mL (Epivir-HBV), 10 mg/mL; contains propylene glycol

HIV: See www.aidsinfo.nih.gov/guidelines
Chronic hepatitis B (see remarks):
2–17 yr: 3 mg/kg/dose PO QD up to a **max. dose** of 100 mg/dose
Adult: 100 mg/dose PO QD

See aidsinfo.nih.gov/guidelines for remarks for use in HIV.

May cause headache, fatigue, GI disturbances, rash, and myalgia/arthralgia. Lactic acidosis, severe hepatomegaly with steatosis, post-treatment exacerbations of hepatitis B and ALT elevations, pancreatitis, and emergence of resistant viral strains have been reported. Concomitant use with cotrimoxazole (TMP/SMX) may result in increased lamivudine levels.

Use Epivir-HBV product for chronic hepatitis B indication. Safety and effectiveness beyond 1 yr have not been determined. Patients with both HIV and hepatitis B should use the higher HIV doses along with an appropriate combination regimen.

May be administered with food. **Adjust dose in renal impairment (see Chapter 30).**

LAMOTRIGINE

Lamictal
Anticonvulsant

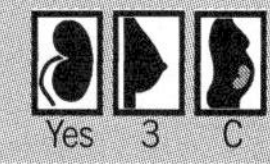

Chewable tabs: 2, 5, 25 mg
Tabs: 25, 100, 150, 200 mg
Oral suspension: 1 mg/mL

Continued

For explanation of icons, see p. 680.

LAMOTRIGINE *continued*

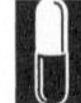

Child 2–12 yr (see remarks):

WITH enzyme-inducing antiepileptic drugs (AEDs) WITHOUT valproic acid:

Weeks 1 and 2: 0.6 mg/kg/24 hr PO ÷ BID; rounded down to the nearest whole tablet

Weeks 3 and 4: 1.2 mg/kg/24 hr PO ÷ BID; rounded down to the nearest whole tablet

Usual maintenance dose: 5–15 mg/kg/24 hr PO ÷ BID titrate to effect; to achieve the usual maintenance dose, increase doses Q1–2 wk by 1.2 mg/kg/24 hr (rounded down to the nearest whole tablet) as needed

Max. dose: 400 mg/24 hr ÷ BID

WITH AEDs WITH valproic acid:

Weeks 1 and 2: 0.15 mg/kg/24 hr PO ÷ QD–BID; rounded down to the nearest whole tablet (see table below)

Weeks 3 and 4: 0.3 mg/kg/24 hr PO ÷ QD–BID; rounded down to the nearest whole tablet (see table below)

Weight (kg)	Weeks 1 & 2	Weeks 3 & 4
6.7–14	2 mg QOD	2 mg QD
14.1–27	2 mg QD	4 mg/24 hr ÷ QD–BID
27.1–34	4 mg/24 hr ÷ QD–BID	8 mg/24 hr ÷ QD–BID
34.1–40	5 mg QD	10 mg/24 hr ÷ QD–BID

Usual maintenance dose: 1–5 mg/kg/24 hr PO ÷ QD–BID titrate to effect; to achieve the usual maintenance dose, increase doses Q1–2 wk by 0.3 mg/kg/24 hr (rounded down to the nearest whole tablet) as needed. If adding lamotrigine with valproic acid alone, usual maintenance dose is 1–3 mg/kg/24 hr.

Max. dose: 200 mg/24 hr

>12 yr and adult:

WITHOUT valproic acid:

Weeks 1 and 2: 50 mg QD PO

Weeks 3 and 4: 50 mg BID PO

Usual maintenance dose: 300–500 mg/24 hr ÷ BID PO titrate to effect; to achieve the usual maintenance dose, increase doses Q1–2 wk by 100 mg/24 hr as needed. Doses as high as 700 mg/24 hr ÷ BID have been used.

WITH valproic acid:

Weeks 1 and 2: 25 mg QOD PO

Weeks 3 and 4: 25 mg QD PO

Usual maintenance dose: 100–400 mg/24 hr ÷ QD–BID PO titrate to effect; to achieve the usual maintenance dose, increase doses Q1–2 wk by 25–50 mg/24 hr as needed. If adding lamotrigine to valproic acid alone, usual maintenance dose is 100–200 mg/kg/24 hr.

Continued

LAMOTRIGINE *continued*

Converting from a single enzyme inducing AED to lamotrigine monotherapy (titrate lamotrigine to maintenance dose, then gradually withdraw enzyme inducing AED by 20% decrements over a 4-wk period):

Weeks 1 and 2: 50 mg QD PO

Weeks 3 and 4: 50 mg BID PO

Usual maintenance dose: 500 mg/24 hr ÷ BID PO titrate to effect; to achieve the usual maintenance dose, increase doses Q1–2 wk by 100 mg/24 hr as needed.

Enzyme-inducing AEDs include carbamazepine, phenytoin, and phenobarbital. Stevens-Johnson syndrome, toxic epidermal necrolysis, and other potentially life-threatening rashes have been reported in children and adults (incidence higher in children). May cause fatigue, drowsiness, ataxia, rash (especially with valproic acid), headache, nausea, vomiting, and abdominal pain. Diplopia, nystagmus, and alopecia have also been reported.

Reduce maintenance dose in renal failure. Reduce all doses (initial, escalation, and maintenance) in liver dysfunction defined by the Child-Pugh grading system as follows:

Grade B: moderate dysfunction, decrease dose by ~50%.

Grade C: severe dysfunction, decrease dose by ~75%.

Withdrawal symptoms may occur if discontinued suddenly. A stepwise dose reduction over ≥2 wk (~50% per week) is recommended unless safety concerns require a more rapid withdrawal.

Acetaminophen, carbamazepine, oral contraceptives, phenobarbital, phenytoin, and rifampin may decrease levels of lamotrigine. Valproic acid may increase levels.

LANSOPRAZOLE

Prevacid

Gastric acid pump inhibitor

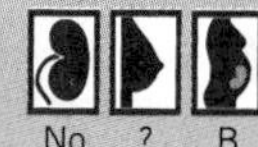

Caps, delayed release: 15, 30 mg

Tabs, disintegrating delayed release: 15, 30 mg; contains aspartame

Granules for delayed release oral suspension: 15, 30 mg packets (30s)

Oral suspension: 3 mg/mL; contains ~0.3 mEq sodium bicarbonate per 1 mg drug

---

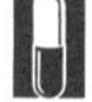

1–11 yr (short-term treatment of GERD and erosive esophagitis, for up to 8 wk):

<10 kg: 7.5 mg PO QD

11–30 kg: 15 mg PO QD–BID; dosage may be increased to 30 mg PO BID after ≥2 wk of therapy without response at a lower dose.

>30 kg: 30 mg PO QD–BID

Continued

For explanation of icons, see p. 680.

LANSOPRAZOLE *continued*

12 yr–adult:

GERD: 15 mg PO QD for up to 8 wk; use 30 mg PO QD for erosive esophagitis.
Duodenal ulcer: 15 mg PO QD × 4 wk
Gastric ulcer: 30 mg PO QD for up to 8 wk
Hypersecretory conditions: 60 mg PO QD; dosage may be increased up to 90 mg PO BID.

Common side effects include GI discomfort, headache, fatigue, rash, and taste perversion. Drug is a substrate for CYP450 2C19 and 3A3/4. May decrease absorption of itraconazole, ketoconazole, iron salts, and ampicillin esters; and increase the effects of warfarin. Theophylline clearance may be enhanced. Reduce dose in severe hepatic impairment. May be used in combination with clarithromycin and amoxicillin for *H. pylori* infections.

Administer all oral doses before meals and 30 min before sucralfate. **Do not** crush or chew the granules (all dosage forms). Capsule may be opened, and intact granules may be administered in an acidic beverage (e.g., apple or cranberry juice) or apple sauce. The extemporaneously compounded oral suspension may be less bioavailable owing to the loss of the enteric coating.

LEVALBUTEROL

Xopenex
Beta-2 adrenergic agonist

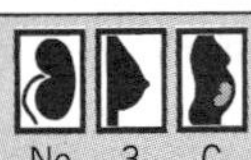

Prediluted nebulized solution: 0.31 mg in 3 mL, 0.63 mg in 3 mL, 1.25 mg in 3 mL (24s)

<6 yr: see remarks
6–11 yr: start at 0.31 mg inhaled TID (Q6–8 hr) PRN; dose may be increased to 0.63 mg TID PRN.
≥12 yr and adult: start at 0.63 mg inhaled TID (Q6–8 hr) PRN; dose may be increased to 1.25 mg inhaled TID PRN.
For use in acute exacerbations, more aggressive dosing may be employed.

R-isomer of racemic albuterol. Side effects include tachycardia, palpitations, tremor, insomnia, nervousness, nausea, and headache.

Current clinical data in children indicate levalbuterol is as effective as albuterol with fewer cardiac side effects at equipotent doses (0.31–0.63 mg levalbuterol ~2.5 mg albuterol). Limited data from a single-dose, randomized, double-blind crossover study in children 2–11 yr indicate that 0.16- to 1.25-mg inhalations were used safely with clinical improvement.

More frequent dosing may be necessary in asthma exacerbation.

LEVOFLOXACIN

Levaquin, Quixin, Iquix

Antibiotic, quinolone

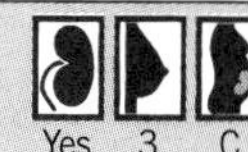

Tabs: 250, 500, 750 mg
Oral suspension: 50 mg/mL
Injection: 25 mg/mL (20, 30 mL)
Prediluted injection in D5W: 250 mg/50 mL, 500 mg/100 mL, 750 mg/150 mL
Ophthalmic drops:
Quixin: 0.5% (2.5, 5 mL)
Iquix: 1.5% (5 mL)

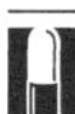

Adult:
Community acquired pneumonia: 500 mg PO/IV Q24 hr × 7–14 days; or 750 mg PO/IV Q24 hr × 5 days
Complicated UTI/pyelonephritis: 250 PO/IV Q24 hr × 10 days
Uncomplicated UTI: 250 mg PO/IV Q24 hr × 3 days
Uncomplicated skin/skin structure infection: 500 mg PO/IV Q24 hr × 7–10 days

Conjunctivitis:
≥1 yr and adult: Instill 1–2 drops of the 0.5% solution to affected eye(s) Q2 hr up to 8 times/24 hr while awake for the first 2 days, then Q4 hr up to 4 times/24 hr while awake for the next 5 days.

Corneal ulcer:
≥6 yr and adult: Instill 1–2 drops of the 1.5% solution to affected eye(s) Q30 min–2 hr while awake and 4 and 6 hr after retiring for the first 3 days, then Q1–4 hr while awake.

Contraindicated in hypersensitivity to other quinolones. Avoid in patients with history of QTc prolongation or taking QTc prolonging drugs, and excessive sunlight exposure. **Use with caution** in diabetes, seizures, and children <18 yr. May cause GI disturbances, headache, and blurred vision with the ophthalmic solution. Like other quinolones, tendon rupture can occur during or after therapy. **Adjust dose in renal failure (see Chapter 30).**

Infuse IV over 1–1.5 hr; avoid IV push or rapid infusion because of risk for hypotension. **Do not administer** antacids or other divalent salts with or within 2 hr of oral levofloxacin dose; otherwise, may administer with or without food.

LEVOTHYROXINE (T_4)

Synthroid, Levothroid, Levoxyl, and others

Thyroid product

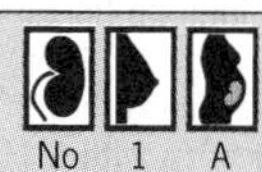

Tabs: 25, 50, 75, 88, 100, 112, 125, 137, 150, 175, 200, 300 mcg
Injection: 200, 500 mcg
Oral suspension: 25 mcg/mL

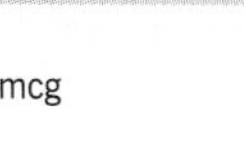

Continued

FORMULARY

For explanation of icons, see p. 680.

LEVOTHYROXINE (T_4) *continued*

Child: PO dosing:
0–6 mo: 8–10 mcg/kg/dose QD
6–12 mo: 6–8 mcg/kg/dose QD
1–5 yr: 5–6 mcg/kg/dose QD
6–12 yr: 4–5 mcg/kg/dose QD
>12 yr: 2–3 mcg/kg/dose QD
IM/IV dose: 50%–75% of oral dose QD
Adult:
PO:
Initial: 12.5–50 mcg/dose QD
Increment: Increase by 25–50 mcg/24 hr at intervals of Q2–4 wk until euthyroid
Usual adult dose: 100–200 mcg/24 hr
IM/IV dose: 50% of oral dose QD
Myxedema coma or stupor: 200–500 mcg IV × 1, then 75–100 mcg IV QD; convert to oral therapy once patient is stabilized.

Contraindications include acute MI, thyrotoxicosis, and uncorrected adrenal insufficiency. May cause hyperthyroidism, rash, growth disturbances, hypertension, arrhythmias, diarrhea, and weight loss. Pseudotumor cerebri has been reported in children. Overtreatment may cause craniosynostosis in infants and premature closure of the epiphyses in children.

Total replacement dose may be used in children unless there is evidence of cardiac disease; in that case, begin with one fourth of maintenance and increase weekly. Titrate dosage with clinical status and serum T_4 and TSH. Increases the effects of warfarin. Phenytoin, rifampin, and carbamazepine may decrease levothyroxine levels.

100 mcg levothyroxine = 65 mg thyroid USP. Administer oral doses on an empty stomach. Excreted in low levels in breast milk; preponderance of evidence suggests no clinically significant effect in infants.

LIDOCAINE

Xylocaine, L-M-X, and others
Antiarrhythmic class Ib, local anesthetic

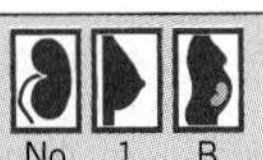

Injection: 0.5%, 1%, 1.5%, 2%, 4%, 10%, 20% (1% sol = 10 mg/mL)
IV infusion (in D5W): 0.4% (4 mg/mL) (250, 500 mL); 0.8% (8 mg/mL) (250, 500 mL)
Injection with 1:50,000 epi: 2%
Injection with 1:100,000 epi: 1%, 2%
Injection with 1:200,000 epi: 0.5%, 1%, 1.5%, 2%
Ointment: 2.5% (37.5 g), 5% (50 g)
Cream, topical: 3% (30 g), 4% (L-M-X) [OTC] (5, 15, 30 g); may contain benzyl alcohol
Cream, rectal: 5% (30 g); contains benzyl alcohol
Jelly: 2% (5, 10, 20, 30 mL)

Continued

LIDOCAINE *continued*

Liquid (topical): 2.5% (7.5 mL)
Liquid (viscous): 2% (20, 100 mL)
Solution (topical): 2% (180 mL), 4% (50 mL)
Topical spray: 0.5% (60 mL), 9.6% (13 mL)
Topical 2.5% (with 2.5% prilocaine): See *Lidocaine and Prilocaine.*

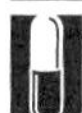

Anesthetic:
Injection:
Without epinephrine: **max. dose** of 4.5 mg/kg/dose (up to 300 mg)
With epinephrine: **max. dose** of 7 mg/kg/dose (up to 500 mg); do not repeat within 2 hr.
Topical: 3 mg/kg/dose no more frequently than Q2 hr

Antiarrhythmic: Bolus with 1 mg/kg/dose slowly IV; may repeat in 10–15 min × 2; **max. total dose** 3–5 mg/kg within the first hour.
ETT dose = 2–2.5 × IV dose

Continuous infusion: 20–50 mcg/kg/min IV (**do not exceed** 20 mcg/kg/min for patients with shock or CHF); see inside cover for infusion preparation.

Oral use:
Adult: 15 mL swish and spit Q3 hr PRN up to a **max. dose** of 8 doses/24 hr.

Contraindicated in Stokes-Adams attacks, SA, AV, or intraventricular heart block without a pacemaker. Side effects include hypotension, asystole, seizures, and respiratory arrest.

CYP450 2D6 and 3A3/4 substrate. **Decrease dose** in hepatic failure or decreased cardiac output. **Do not use** topically for teething. Prolonged infusion may result in toxic accumulation of lidocaine, especially in infants. **Do not use** epinephrine-containing solutions for treatment of arrhythmias.

Therapeutic levels 1.5–5 mg/L. Toxicity occurs at >7 mg/L. Toxicity in neonates may occur at >5 mg/L. Elimination $T_{1/2}$: premature infant: 3.2 hr, adult: 1.5–2 hr.

LIDOCAINE AND PRILOCAINE

EMLA, Eutectic mixture of lidocaine and prilocaine
Topical analgesic

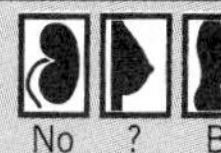

Cream: lidocaine 2.5% + prilocaine 2.5%; 5 g kit (with dressings); 30 g tube
Topical anesthetic disc: lidocaine 2.5% + prilocaine 2.5%; 1 g (contact surface ~10 cm^2) (box of 2s or 10s)

See Chapter 28, general use information.
Newborn ≥37 weeks' gestation, child, and adult:
Minor procedures: 2.5 g/site for at least 60 min
Painful procedures: 2 g/10 cm^2 of skin for at least 2 hr
See following table for maximum dose and application information.

Continued

For explanation of icons, see p. 680.

LIDOCAINE AND PRILOCAINE *continued*

Age and Weight	Maximum Total EMLA Dose	Maximum Application Area	Maximum Application Time
Birth–3 mo or <5 kg	1 g	10 cm^2	1 hr
3–12 mo and >5 kg*	2 g	20 cm^2	4 hr
1–6 yr and >10 kg	10 g	100 cm^2	4 hr
7–12 yr and >20 kg	20 g	200 cm^2	4 hr

*If patient is >3 months old and is not >5 kg, use the maximum total dose that corresponds to the patient's weight.

Should not be used in neonates <37 weeks' gestation nor in infants <12 mo receiving treatment with methemoglobin-inducing agents (e.g., sulfa drugs, acetaminophen, nitrofurantoin, nitroglycerin, nitroprusside, phenobarbital, phenytoin). **Use with caution** in patients with G6PD deficiency and in patients with renal and hepatic impairment. Prilocaine has been associated with methemoglobinemia. Long duration of application, large treatment area, small patients, or impaired elimination may result in high blood levels.

Apply topically to intact skin and cover with occlusive dressing, **avoiding** mucous membranes or the eyes. Wipe cream off before procedure.

LINDANE

Various brands, Gamma benzene hexachloride

Scabicidal agent, pediculicide

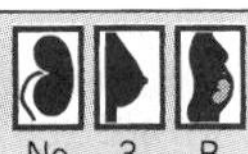

Shampoo: 1% (60, 473 mL)
Lotion: 1% (60, 473 mL)

Scabies: Apply thin layer of lotion to skin. Bathe and rinse off medication in adults after 8–12 hr; children 6–8 hr. May repeat × 1 in 7 days PRN.

Pediculosis capitis: Apply 15–30 mL of shampoo, lather for 4–5 min, rinse hair and comb with fine comb to remove nits. May repeat × 1 in 7 days PRN.

Pediculosis pubis: May use lotion or shampoo (applied locally) as above.

Contraindicated in seizure disorders. Avoid contact with face, urethral meatus, damaged skin, or mucous membranes. Systemically absorbed. Risk for toxic effects is greater in young children; use other agents (permethrin) in infants, young children, and during pregnancy. Lindane is considered second-line therapy owing to side-effect risk. May cause a rash; rarely may cause seizures or aplastic anemia. For scabies, change clothing and bed sheets after starting treatment and treat family members. For pediculosis pubis, treat sexual contacts.

LINEZOLID

Zyvox

Antibiotic, oxazolidinone

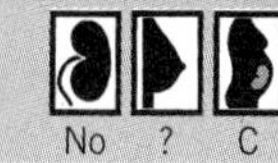

Tabs: 400, 600 mg

Oral suspension: 100 mg/5 mL (150 mL); contains phenylalanine and sodium benzoate

Injection: 2 mg/mL (100, 200, 300 mL)

Injection, premixed: 200 mg in 100 mL, 400 mg in 200 mL, 600 mg in 300 mL

Neonate <7 days: 10 mg/kg/dose IV/PO Q12 hr; if response is suboptimal, increase dose to 10 mg/kg/dose Q8 hr.

Neonate ≥7 days–11 yr:

Pneumonia, bacteremia, complicated skin/skin structure infections, Vancomycin-resistant *E. faecium:* 10 mg/kg/dose IV/PO Q8 hr

Uncomplicated skin/skin structure infections:

<5 yr: 10 mg/kg/dose IV/PO Q8 hr

5–11 yr: 10 mg/kg/dose IV/PO Q12 hr

Adult:

MRSA infections: 600 mg Q12 hr IV/PO

Vancomycin-resistant E. faecium: 600 mg Q12 hr IV/PO × 14–28 days

Community-acquired and nosocomial pneumonia; and bacteremia: 600 mg Q12 hr IV/PO × 10–14 days

Uncomplicated skin infections: 400 mg Q12 hr PO × 10–14 days

Most common side effects include diarrhea, headache, and nausea. Anemia, leukopenia, pancytopenia, and thrombocytopenia may occur in patients who are at risk for myelosuppression and who receive regimens >2 wk. Complete blood count monitoring is recommended in these individuals. Pseudomembranous colitis and neuropathy (peripheral and optic) have also been reported.

Avoid use with SSRIs (e.g., fluoxetine, paroxetine), tricyclic antidepressants, venlafaxine, and trazodone; may cause serotonin syndrome. **Use caution** when using adrenergic (epinephrine, pseudoephedrine) agents or consuming large amounts of foods and beverages containing tyramine; may increase blood pressure. Dosing information in severe hepatic failure and renal impairment with multidoses have not been completed.

Protect all dosage forms from light and moisture. Oral suspension product must be gently mixed by inverting the bottle 3–5 times before each use (**do not shake**). All oral doses may be administered with or without food.

For explanation of icons, see p. 680.

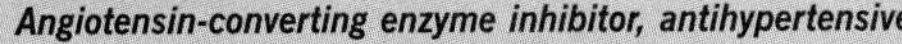

LISINOPRIL
Prinivil, Zestril, and others
Angiotensin-converting enzyme inhibitor, antihypertensive

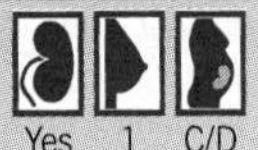

Tabs: 2.5, 5, 10, 20, 30, 40 mg
Oral suspension: 1 mg/mL

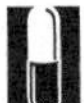

Hypertension:
6–16 yr: Start with 0.07 mg/kg/dose PO QD; **max. initial dose:** 5 mg/dose. If needed, titrate dose upward to doses up to 0.61 mg/kg/24 hr or 40 mg/24 hr (higher doses have not been evaluated).
Adult: Start with 10 mg PO QD. Usual dosage range: 20–40 mg/24 hr. **Max. dose:** 80 mg/24 hr

Contraindicated in hypersensitivity and history of angioedema with other ACE inhibitors. **Avoid** use with dialysis with high-flux membranes because anaphylactoid reactions have been reported. **Use with caution** in aortic or bilateral renal artery stenosis. Side effects include cough, dizziness, headache, hyperkalemia, hypotension, rash, and GI disturbances. **Adjust dose in renal impairment (see Chapter 30).**

Use lower initial dose if using with a diuretic. Onset of action: 1 hr with maximal effect in 6–8 hr. Pregnancy category is C during the first trimester but changes to a D for the second and third trimesters.

LITHIUM
Eskalith, Eskalith CR, Lithobid, and others
Antimanic agent

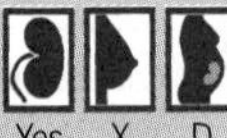

Carbonate:
300 mg carbonate = 8.12 mEq lithium
Caps: 150, 300, 600 mg
Tabs: 300 mg
Controlled-release tabs (Eskalith CR): 450 mg
Slow-release tabs (Lithobid): 300 mg

Citrate:
Syrup: 8 mEq/5 mL (5, 10, 480 mL); 5 mL is equivalent to 300 mg lithium carbonate.

Child:
Initial: 15–60 mg/kg/24 hr ÷ TID–QID PO. Adjust as needed (weekly) to achieve therapeutic levels.
Adolescent: 600–1800 mg/24 hr ÷ TID–QID PO (divided BID using controlled/slow-release tablets)
Adult:
Initial: 300 mg TID PO. Adjust as needed to achieve therapeutic levels. Usual dose is about 300 mg TID–QID. **Max. dose:** 2.4 g/24 hr or 900–1800 mg/24 hr with controlled/slow-released tablets.

Continued

LITHIUM *continued*

Contraindicated in severe cardiovascular or renal disease. Decreased sodium intake or increased sodium wasting will increase lithium levels. May cause goiter, nephrogenic diabetes insipidus, hypothyroidism, arrhythmias, or sedation at therapeutic doses. Coadministration with thiazide diuretics, metronidazole, ACE inhibitors, or nonsteroidal anti-inflammatory drugs may increase risk for lithium toxicity. Iodine may increase risk for hypothyroidism. If used in combination with haloperidol, closely monitor neurologic toxicities because an encephalopathic syndrome followed by irreversible brain damage has been reported.

Therapeutic levels: 0.6–1.5 mEq/L. In either acute or chronic toxicity, confusion, and somnolence may be seen at levels of 2–2.5 mEq/L. **Seizures or death** may occur at levels >2.5 mEq/L. Recommended serum sampling: trough level within 30 min before the next scheduled dose. Steady state is achieved within 4–6 days of continuous dosing. **Adjust dose in renal failure (see Chapter 30).**

LOPERAMIDE

Imodium, Imodium AD, and others

Antidiarrheal

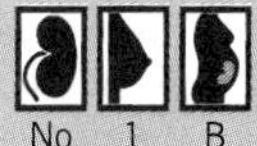

Caps: 2 mg
Tabs: 2 mg
Caplets: 2 mg
Liquid: 1 mg/5 mL; may contain 0.5% alcohol (60, 120 mL)
In combination with simethicone:
Chewable tab: 2 mg loperamide and 125 mg simethicone

Active diarrhea:
Child (initial doses within the first 24 hr):
2–5 yr (13–20 kg): 1 mg PO TID
6–8 yr (20–30 kg): 2 mg PO BID
9–12 yr (>30 kg): 2 mg PO TID
Max. single dose: 2 mg
Follow initial day's dose with 0.1 mg/kg/dose after each loose stool (not to exceed the above initial doses).
Adult: 4 mg/dose × 1, followed by 2 mg/dose after each stool up to **max. dose** of 16 mg/24 hr
Chronic diarrhea:
Child: 0.08–0.24 mg/kg/24 hr ÷ BID–TID; **max. dose:** 2 mg/dose

Contraindicated in acute dysentery. Rare hypersensitivity reaction including anaphylactic shock has been reported. May cause nausea, rash, vomiting, constipation, cramps, dry mouth, CNS depression, and rash. **Avoid** use in children <2 yr because of reports of necrotizing enterocolitis. **Discontinue use if no clinical improvement is observed within 48 hr.** Naloxone may be administered for CNS depression.

For explanation of icons, see p. 680.

LORACARBEF
Lorabid
Antibiotic, carbacephem

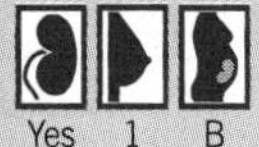

Oral suspension: 100 mg/5 mL, 200 mg/5 mL (50, 75, 100 mL)
Caps: 200, 400 mg

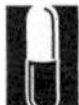

Infant and child (6 mo–12 yr):
Acute otitis media, sinusitis: 30 mg/kg/24 hr ÷ Q12 hr PO × 10 days
Pharyngitis, impetigo, skin/soft tissue infection: 15 mg/kg/24 hr ÷ Q12 hr PO × 7–10 days
≥13 yr and adult:
Uncomplicated cystitis: 200 mg PO Q24 hr × 7 days
Sinusitis, uncomplicated pyelonephritis: 400 mg PO Q12 hr × 10–14 days
Pharyngitis, skin/soft tissue infection: 200 mg PO Q12 hr × 7–10 days
Lower respiratory infections: 200–400 mg PO Q12 hr × 7 days

Use with caution in penicillin-allergic patients. **Adjust dose in renal impairment (see Chapter 30).** Use suspension for acute otitis media because of higher peak plasma levels. Adverse effects similar to other orally administered beta-lactam antibiotics. Administer on an empty stomach 1 hr before or 2 hr after meals.

LORATADINE ± PSEUDOEPHEDRINE
Claritin, Claritin RediTabs, Claritin-D 12 Hour, Claritin-D 24 Hour
Antihistamine, less sedating ± decongestant

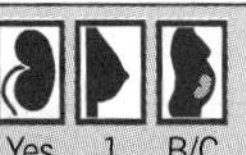

Tabs (OTC): 10 mg
Disintegrating tabs (RediTabs) (OTC): 10 mg
Syrup (OTC): 1 mg/mL (480 mL)
Timed-release tabs in combination with pseudoephedrine (PE):
Claritin-D 12 Hour (OTC): 5 mg loratadine + 120 mg PE
Claritin-D 24 Hour (OTC): 10 mg loratadine + 240 mg PE

Loratadine:
2–5 yr: 5 mg PO QD
≥6 yr and adult: 10 mg PO QD
Timed-release tabs of loratadine and pseudoephedrine:
≥12 yr and adult:
Claritin-D 12 Hour: 1 tablet PO BID
Claritin-D 24 Hour: 1 tablet PO QD

May cause drowsiness, fatigue, dry mouth, headache, bronchospasms, palpitations, dermatitis, and dizziness. Has not been implicated in causing cardiac arrhythmias when used with other drugs that are metabolized by hepatic microsomal enzymes (e.g., ketoconazole, erythromycin). May be administered safely in patients who have allergic rhinitis and asthma.

Continued

LORATADINE ± PSEUDOEPHEDRINE *continued*

In hepatic and renal function impairment (GFR <30 mL/min), prolong loratadine (single-agent) dosage interval to QOD. For timed-release tablets of the combination product (loratadine + pseudoephedrine), prolong dosage interval in renal impairment (GFR <30 mL/min) as follows: Claritin-D 12 Hour: 1 tablet PO QD; Claritin-D 24 Hour: 1 tablet PO QOD. **Do not use** the combination product in hepatic impairment because drugs cannot be individually titrated. **Adjust dose in renal failure (see Chapter 30).**

Administer doses on an empty stomach. For use of RediTabs, place tablet on tongue and allow it to disintegrate in the mouth with or without water. For Claritin-D, also see remarks for *Pseudoephedrine.*

Pregnancy category is B for loratadine and C for the combination product.

LORAZEPAM
Ativan and others
Benzodiazepine anticonvulsant

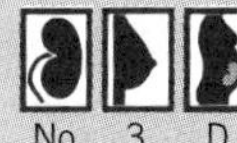

Tabs: 0.5, 1, 2, mg
Injection: 2, 4 mg/mL (each contains 2% benzyl alcohol and propylene glycol)
Oral solution: 2 mg/mL (30 mL); alcohol and dye free

Status epilepticus:

Neonate, infant, child, and adolescent:
0.05–0.1 mg/kg/dose IV over 2–5 min. May repeat 0.05 mg/kg × 1 in 10–15 min.
Max. dose: 2 mg/dose.

Adult:
4 mg/dose given slowly over 2–5 min. May repeat in 10–15 min. Usual total **max. dose** in 12-hr period is 8 mg.

Antiemetic adjunct therapy:

Child:
0.02–0.05 mg/kg/dose IV Q6 hr PRN
Max. single dose: 2 mg

Anxiolytic/sedation:

Child:
0.05 mg/kg/dose Q4–8 hr PO/IV; **max. dose:** 2 mg/dose
May also give IM for preprocedure sedation.

Adult:
1–10 mg/24 hr PO ÷ BID–TID

Contraindicated in narrow-angle glaucoma and severe hypotension. May cause respiratory depression, especially in combination with other sedatives. May also cause sedation, dizziness, mild ataxia, mood changes, rash, and GI symptoms. Significant respiratory depression and/or hypotension have been reported when used in combination with loxapine.

Injectable product may be given rectally. Benzyl alcohol and propylene glycol may be toxic to newborns at high doses.

Onset of action for sedation: PO, 20–30 min; IM, 30–60 min; IV, 1–5 min. Duration of action: 6–8 hr. **Flumazenil is the antidote.**

For explanation of icons, see p. 680.

LOW-MOLECULAR-WEIGHT HEPARIN

See *Enoxaparin*

MAGNESIUM CITRATE

Various, 16.17% Elemental Mg
Laxative/cathartic

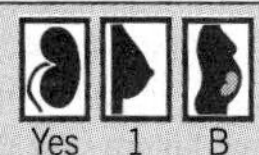

Solution: 1.75 g/30 mL (300 mL); 5 mL = 3.9–4.7 mEq Mg

Child:
<6 yr: 2–4 mL/kg/24 hr PO ÷ QD–BID
6–12 yr: 100–150 mL/24 hr PO ÷ QD–BID
>12 yr: 150–300 mL/24 hr PO ÷ QD–BID

Use with caution in renal insufficiency and patients receiving digoxin. May cause hypermagnesemia, diarrhea, muscle weakness, hypotension, and respiratory depression. Up to about 30% of dose is absorbed. May decrease absorption of H_2 antagonists, phenytoin, iron salts, tetracycline, steroids, benzodiazepines, and quinolone antibiotics.

MAGNESIUM HYDROXIDE

Milk of Magnesia, 41.69% Elemental Mg
Antacid, laxative

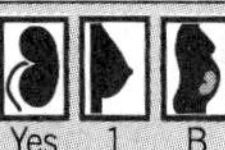

Liquid: 400 mg/5 mL (Milk of Magnesia)
Concentrated liquid: 800 mg/5 mL (Milk of Magnesia concentrate)
Chewable tabs: 311 mg
400 mg magnesium hydroxide is equivalent to 166.76 mg elemental magnesium.
Combination product with aluminum hydroxide: See *Aluminum Hydroxide.*

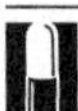

All doses based on 400 mg/5 mL magnesium hydroxide.
Laxative:
Child:
Dose/24 hr ÷ QD–QID PO
<2 yr: 0.5 mL/kg
2–5 yr: 5–15 mL
6–12 yr: 15–30 mL
≥12 yr: 30–60 mL

Continued

MAGNESIUM HYDROXIDE *continued*

Antacid:

Child:

Liquid: 2.5–5 mL/dose QD–QID PO
Tabs: 311 mg QD–QID PO

Adult:

Liquid: 5–15 mL/dose QD–QID PO
Concentrated liquid: 2.5–7.5 mL/dose QD–QID PO
Tabs: 622–1244 mg/dose QD–QID PO

See *Magnesium Citrate*

MAGNESIUM OXIDE

Mag-200, Mag-Ox 400, Uro-Mag, and others
60.32% Elemental Mg
Oral magnesium salt

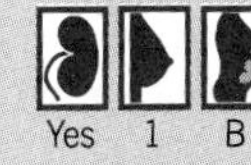

Tabs: 200, 400 mg
Caps (Uro-Mag): 140 mg
400 mg magnesium oxide is equivalent to 241.3 mg elemental Mg or 20 mEq Mg.

Doses expressed in magnesium oxide salt.
Magnesium supplementation:
Child: 5–10 mg/kg/24 hr ÷ TID–QID PO
Adult: 400–800 mg/24 hr ÷ BID–QID PO

Hypomagnesemia:
Child: 65–130 mg/kg/24 hr ÷ QID PO
Adult: 2000 mg/24 hr ÷ QID PO

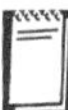

See *Magnesium Citrate*. For dietary recommended intake RDA for magnesium, see Chapter 20.

MAGNESIUM SULFATE

Epsom salts and others
9.9% Elemental Mg
Magnesium salt

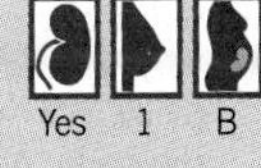

Injection: 100 mg/mL (0.8 mEq/mL), 125 mg/mL (1 mEq/mL), 500 mg/mL (4 mEq/mL)
Injection, prediluted ready to use: 40 mg/mL (0.325 mEq/mL) (100, 500, 1000 mL); 80 mg/mL (0.65 mEq/mL) (50 mL)
Granules: approximately 40 mEq Mg per 5 g (240 g)
500 mg magnesium sulfate is equivalent to 49.3 mg elemental Mg or 4.1 mEq Mg.

Continued

For explanation of icons, see p. 680.

MAGNESIUM SULFATE *continued*

All doses expressed in magnesium sulfate salt.
Cathartic:
Child: 0.25 g/kg/dose PO Q4–6 hr
Adult: 10–30 g/dose PO Q4–6 hr

Hypomagnesemia or hypocalcemia:
IV/IM: 25–50 mg/kg/dose Q4–6 hr × 3–4 doses; repeat PRN. Max. single dose: 2 g
PO: 100–200 mg/kg/dose QID PO

Daily maintenance:
30–60 mg/kg/24 hr or 0.25–0.5 mEq/kg/24 hr IV
Max. dose: 1 g/24 hr

Adjunctive therapy for moderate to severe reactive airway disease exacerbation (bronchodilation):
Child: 25–75 mg/kg/dose (**max. dose:** 2 g) × 1 IV over 20 min
Adult: 2 g/dose × 1 IV over 20 min

When given IV, **beware** of hypotension, respiratory depression, complete heart block, and/or hypermagnesemia. Calcium gluconate (IV) should be available as **antidote. Use with caution** in patients with renal insufficiency and with patients on digoxin. **Serum level–dependent toxicity** includes the following: >3 mg/dL: CNS depression; >5 mg/dL: decreased deep tendon reflexes, flushing, somnolence; and >12 mg/dL: respiratory paralysis, heart block.

Max. IV intermittent infusion rate: 1 mEq/kg/hr or 125 mg $MgSO_4$ salt/kg/hr

MALATHION

Ovide

Pediculicide

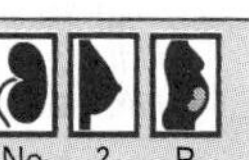

Lotion: 0.5% (59 mL); contains 79% isopropyl alcohol, terpinol, dipentene, and pine needle oil

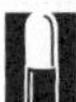

Pediculosis capitis:
≥6 yr and adult: Sprinkle sufficient amounts of lotion onto dry hair, and rub gently until the scalp is fully wet (pay special attention to the back of head and neck). Allow the hair to dry naturally; do not use hair dryer. After 8–12 hr, wash the hair with a nonmedicated shampoo, rinse, and use a fine-toothed comb to remove dead lice and eggs. If lice are still present, a second dose may be administered in 7–9 days.

Contraindicated in neonates. **Do not** expose lotion and wet hair to open flame or electric heat, including hair dyers, because it contains flammable ingredients. For external use only. Launder bedding and clothing. **Avoid** contact with eyes; flush eyes immediately with water if accidental exposure. May cause scalp irritation.

MANNITOL

Osmitrol and others

Osmotic diuretic

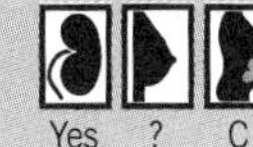

Injection: 50, 100, 150, 200, 250 mg/mL (5%, 10%, 15%, 20%, 25%)

Anuria/oliguria:

Test dose to assess renal function: 0.2 g/kg/dose IV; **max. dose:** 12.5 g over 3–5 min. If there is no diuresis within 2 hr, discontinue mannitol.

Initial: 0.5–1 g/kg/dose

Maintenance: 0.25–0.5 g/kg/dose Q4–6 hr IV

Cerebral edema:

0.25 g/kg/dose IV over 20–30 min. May increase gradually to 1 g/kg/dose if needed. (May give furosemide 1 mg/kg concurrently or 5 min before mannitol.)

Contraindicated in severe renal disease, active intracranial bleed, dehydration, and pulmonary edema. May cause circulatory overload and electrolyte disturbances. For hyperosmolar therapy, keep serum osmolality at 310–320 mOsm/kg.

Caution: may crystallize with concentration ≥20%; use in-line filter. May cause hypovolemia, headache, and polydipsia. Reduction in ICP occurs in 15 min and lasts 3–6 hr.

MEBENDAZOLE

Vermox

Anthelmintic

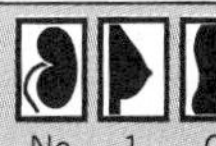

Chewable tabs: 100 mg (may be swallowed whole or chewed) (boxes of 12s, 60s)

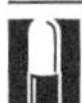

Child and adult:

Pinworms (Enterobius):

100 mg PO × 1, repeat in 2 wk if not cured.

Hookworms, roundworms (Ascaris), and whipworm (Trichuris):

100 mg PO BID × 3 days. Repeat in 3–4 wk if not cured. Alternatively, may administer 500 mg PO × 1.

Capillariasis:

200 mg PO BID × 20 days

See latest edition of the AAP *Red Book* for additional information.

Experience in children <2 yr is limited. May cause diarrhea and abdominal cramping in cases of massive infection. LFT elevations and hepatitis have been reported with prolonged courses; monitor hepatic function with prolonged therapy. Family may need to be treated as a group. Therapeutic effect may be decreased if administered to patients receiving carbamazepine or phenytoin. Administer with food.

For explanation of icons, see p. 680.

MEDROXYPROGESTERONE ± ESTRADIOL

Amen, Curretab, Cycrin, Provera, and Depo-Provera;
in combination with estradiol: Lunelle
Contraceptive, progestin

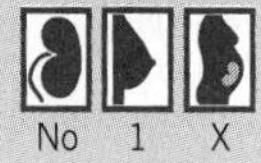

Tabs: 2.5, 5, 10 mg
Injection, suspension as acetate (Depo-Provera; for IM use only): 150 mg/mL (1 mL), 400 mg/mL (1, 2.5, 10 mL)
In combination with estradiol (Lunelle):
Injection, suspension: 25 mg medroxyprogesterone acetate and 5 mg estradiol cypionate per 0.5 mL (0.5 mL); contains 4.28 mg Na/0.5 mL drug

---

Adolescent and adult:
Contraception: 150 mg IM Q 3 mo; initiate therapy during the first 5 days after onset of a normal menstrual period, within 5 days postpartum if not breast-feeding or if breast-feeding, at 6 wk postpartum.
Amenorrhea: 5–10 mg PO QD × 5–10 days
Abnormal uterine bleeding: 5–10 mg PO QD × 5–10 days initiated on the 16th or 21st day of the menstrual cycle
In combination with estradiol (Lunelle):
Contraception: 0.5 ml IM Q month (28–30 days; not to exceed 33 days); initiate therapy during the first 5 days after onset of a normal menstrual period, no earlier than 4 wk postpartum if not breast-feeding or if breast-feeding, at 6 wk postpartum.

Consider patient's risk for osteoporosis because of the potential for decrease in bone mineral density. **Contraindicated** in pregnancy, breast or genital cancer, liver disease, missed abortion, thrombophlebitis, thromboembolic disorders, cerebral vascular disease, and undiagnosed vaginal bleeding. **Use with caution** in patients with family history of breast cancer, depression, diabetes, and fluid retention. May cause dizziness, headache, insomnia, fatigue, nausea, weight increase, appetite changes, amenorrhea, and breakthrough bleeding. Cholestatic jaundice and increased intracranial pressure have been reported.

Aminoglutethimide may decrease medroxyprogesterone levels. May alter thyroid and liver function tests, prothrombin time, factors VII, VIII, IX and X, and metyrapone test.

Injection is for IM use only. Shake IM injection vial well before use. Administer oral doses with food.

Estradiol concerns: use with caution in smoking, hypertriglyceridemia, hypertension, and thrombosis.

M

MEFLOQUINE HCL

Lariam

Antimalarial

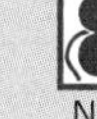
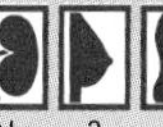
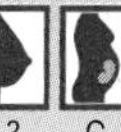

No ? C

Tabs: 250 mg (228 mg base)

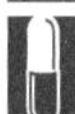

Doses expressed in mg mefloquine HCl salt.

Malaria prophylaxis (start 1 wk before exposure and continue for 4 wk after leaving endemic area):

Child (PO, administered Q weekly):

<10 kg: 5 mg/kg

10–19 kg: 62.5 mg (1/4 tablet)

20–30 kg: 125 mg (1/2 tablet)

31–45 kg: 187.5 mg (3/4 tablet)

>45 kg: 250 mg (1 tablet)

Adult: 250 mg PO Q weekly

Malaria treatment:

<45 kg: 15 mg/kg × 1 PO followed by 10 mg/kg × 1 PO 8–12 hr later

Adult: 750 mg × 1 PO followed by 500 mg × 1 PO 12 hr later

See latest edition of the AAP *Red Book* for additional information.

Contraindicated in active or recent history of depression, anxiety disorders, psychosis or schizophrenia, seizures, or hypersensitivity to quinine or quinidine. **Use with caution** in cardiac dysrhythmias and neurologic disease. May cause dizziness, headache, syncope, seizures, ocular abnormalities, GI symptoms, leukopenia, and thrombocytopenia. Monitor liver enzymes and ocular exams for therapies longer than 1 yr. Mefloquine may reduce valproic acid levels. ECG abnormalities may occur when used in combination with quinine, quinidine, chloroquine, halofantrine, and beta-blockers. If any of the aforementioned antimalarial drugs is used in the initial treatment of severe malaria, initiate mefloquine at least 12 hr after the last dose of any of these drugs.

Do not take on an empty stomach. Administer with at least 240 mL (8 oz) water. Treatment failures in children may be related to vomiting of administered dose. If vomiting occurs less than 30 min after the dose, administer a second full dose. If vomiting occurs 30–60 min after the dose, administer an additional half-dose. If vomiting continues, monitor patient closely and consider alternative therapy.

MEPERIDINE HCL

Demerol and others

Narcotic, analgesic

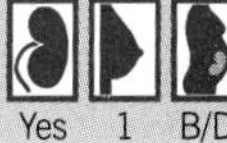

Yes 1 B/D

Tabs: 50, 100 mg

Syrup: 50 mg/5 mL

Injection: 25, 50, 75, and 100 mg/mL

Continued

FORMULARY

For explanation of icons, see p. 680.

MEPERIDINE HCL *continued*

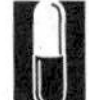

PO, IM, IV, and SC:
Child:
1–1.5 mg/kg/dose Q3–4 hr PRN
Max. dose: 100 mg
Adult:
50–150 mg/dose Q3–4 hr PRN

See Chapter 28 for details of use and equianalgesic dosing. **Contraindicated** in cardiac arrhythmias, asthma, and increased ICP. Potentiated by MAO inhibitors, tricyclic antidepressants, cimetidine, ritonavir, phenothiazines, and other CNS-acting agents. Phenytoin may increase the clearance of meperidine. Meperidine may increase the adverse effects of isoniazid. May cause nausea, vomiting, respiratory depression, smooth muscle spasm, pruritus, palpitations, hypotension, constipation, and lethargy.

Drug is metabolized by the liver, and its metabolite (normeperidine) is renally eliminated. **Caution** in renal and hepatic failure, sickle cell disease, and seizure disorders, accumulation of normeperidine metabolite may precipitate seizures. Acyclovir may increase the concentration of meperidine and its metabolite, normeperidine.

Adjust dose in renal failure (see Chapter 30). Pregnancy category changes to D if used for prolonged periods or in high doses at term. Onset of action: PO/IM/SC, 10–15 min; IV, 5 min.

MEROPENEM
Merrem
Carbapenem antibiotic

Yes ? B

Injection: 0.5, 1 g
Contains 3.92 mEq Na/g drug

Neonate: 20 mg/kg/dose IV using the following dosage intervals:
<7 days old: Q12 hr
≥7 days old:
1.2 –2 kg: Q 12 hr
>2 kg: Q8 hr
Infant >3 mo and child:
Mild to moderate infections: 60 mg/kg/24 hr IV ÷ Q8 hr
Meningitis and severe infections: 120 mg/kg/24 hr IV ÷ Q8 hr
Max. dose: 6 g/24 hr
Adult:
Mild to moderate infections: 1.5–3 g/24 hr IV ÷ Q8 hr
Meningitis and severe infections: 6 g/24 hr IV ÷ Q8 hr

Contraindicated in patients sensitive to carbapenems or with a history of anaphylaxis to beta-lactam antibiotics. Drug penetrates well into the CSF. May cause diarrhea, rash, nausea, vomiting, oral moniliasis, glossitis, pain and irritation at the IV injection site, and headache. Hepatic enzyme and bilirubin elevation, leukopenia, and neutropenia have been reported. **Adjust dose in renal impairment (see Chapter 30).**

MESALAMINE

Asacol, Canasa, Pentasa, Rowasa, FIV-ASA, 5-aminosalicylic acid, 5-ASA
Salicylate, GI antiinflammatory agent

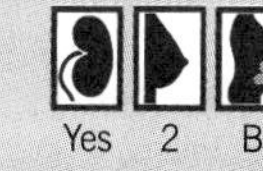

Caps, controlled release (Pentasa): 250, 500 mg
Tabs, delayed release (Asacol): 400 mg
Suppository (Canasa, FIV-ASA): 500, 1000 mg (30s)
Rectal suspension (Rowasa): 4 g/60 mL (7s, 28s); contains sulfites and sodium benzoate

Child:
Caps, controlled release: 50 mg/kg/24 hr ÷ Q6–12 hr PO
Tabs, delayed release: 50 mg/kg/24 hr ÷ Q8–12 hr PO

Adult:
Caps, controlled release: 1 g QID PO up to 8 wk
Tabs, delayed release: 800 mg TID PO for 6 wk; for ulcerative colitis remission, use 1.6 g/24 hr ÷ BID-QID PO up to 6 mo.
Suppository: 500 mg BID PR × 3–6 wk; may increase dose to TID if inadequate response for 2 wk. Alternately, 1000 mg QHS PR may be used. Retain each dose in the rectum for 1–3 hr or longer.
Rectal suspension: 60 mL (4 g) QHS × 3–6 wk, retaining each dose for about 8 hr; lie on left side during administration to improve delivery to the sigmoid colon.

Generally not recommended in children <16 yr with chicken pox or flu-like symptoms (risk of Reye syndrome). **Contraindicated** in active peptic ulcer disease, severe renal failure, and salicylate hypersensitivity. Rectal suspension should not be used in patients with history of sulfite allergy. **Use with caution** in sulfasalazine hypersensitivity, renal insufficiency, pyloric stenosis, and concurrent thrombolytics. May cause headache, GI discomfort, pancreatitis, pericarditis, and Stevens-Johnson syndrome.

Do not administer with lactulose or other medications that can lower intestinal pH. Oral capsules are designed to release medication throughout the GI tract, and oral tablets release medication at the terminal ileus and beyond. 400 mg PO mesalamine is equivalent to 1 g sulfasalazine PO. Tablets should be swallowed whole.

METFORMIN

Glucophage, Glucophage XL, Riomet, and others
Antidiabetic, biguanide

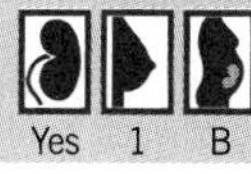

Tabs: 500, 850, 1000 mg
Tabs, extended release (Glucophage XL): 500, 750 mg
Oral suspension: 100 mg/mL (118, 473 mL); contains saccharin

Continued

For explanation of icons, see p. 680.

METFORMIN *continued*

Administer all doses with meals (e.g., BID: morning and evening meals)

Child (10–16 yr): (see remarks): Start with 500 mg BID; may increase dose weekly by 500 mg/24 hr in 2 divided doses up to a **max. dose** of 2000 mg/24 hr.

Adult (see remarks):

500-mg tabs: Start with 500 mg PO BID; may increase dose weekly by 500 mg/24 hr in 2 divided doses up to a **max. dose** of 2500 mg/24 hr. Administer 2500 mg/24 hr doses by dividing daily dose TID with meals.

850-mg tabs: Start with 850 mg PO QD with morning meal; may increase by 850 mg every 2 wk up to a **max. dose** of 2550 mg/24 hr (first dosage increment: 850 mg PO BID; second dosage increment: 850 mg PO TID).

Extended-release tabs: Start with 500 mg PO QD with evening meal; may increase by 500 mg every wk up to a **max. dose** of 2000 mg/24 hr (2000 mg PO QD or 1000 mg PO BID). If a dose >2000 mg is needed, switch to nonextended-release tablets in divided doses and increase to a **max. dose** of 2550 mg/24 hr.

Contraindicated in renal impairment, CHF, metabolic acidosis, and during radiology studies using iodinated contrast media. **Use with caution** when transferring patients from chlorpropamide therapy (potential hypoglycemia risk), excessive alcohol intake, hypoxemia, dehydration, surgical procedures, hepatic disease, anemia, and thyroid disease.

Fatal lactic acidosis (diarrhea; severe muscle pain, cramping; shallow and fast breathing; unusual weakness and sleepiness) and decrease in vitamin B_{12} levels have been reported. May cause GI discomfort (~50% incidence), anorexia, and vomiting. Transient abdominal discomfort or diarrhea has been reported in 40% of pediatric patients. Cimetidine, furosemide, and nifedipine may increase the effects/toxicity of metformin. In addition to monitoring serum glucose and glycosylated hemoglobin, monitor renal function and hematologic parameters (baseline and annual).

Adult patients initiated on 500 mg PO BID may also have their dose increased to 850 mg PO BID after 2 wk.

COMBINATION THERAPY WITH SULFONYLUREAS: If patient has not responded to 4 wk of maximum doses of metformin monotherapy, consider gradual addition of an oral sulfonylurea with continued maximum metformin dosing (even if failure with sulfonylurea has occurred). Attempt to identify the minimum effective dosage for each drug (metformin and sulfonylurea) because the combination can increase risk for sulfonylurea induced hypoglycemia. If patient does not respond to 1–3 mo of combination therapy with maximum metformin doses, consider discontinuing combination therapy and initiating insulin therapy.

Administer all doses with food.

METHADONE HCL

Dolophine, Methadose, and others

Narcotic, analgesic

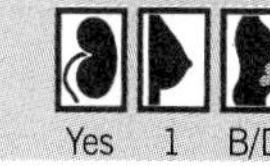

Yes 1 B/D

Tabs: 5, 10 mg
Tabs (dispersible): 40 mg
Solution: 5 mg/5 mL, 10 mg/5 mL; contains 8% alcohol
Concentrated solution: 10 mg/mL
Injection: 10 mg/mL (20 mL), contains 0.5% chlorobutanol

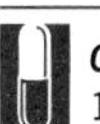

Child: 0.7 mg/kg/24 hr ÷ Q4–6 hr PRN pain PO, SC, IM, or IV. **Max. dose:** 10 mg/dose

Adult: 2.5–10 mg/dose Q3–4 hr PRN pain PO, SC, IM, or IV.

Detoxification or maintenance: see package insert.

May cause respiratory depression, sedation, increased intracranial pressure, hypotension, and bradycardia. Average $T_{1/2}$: children, 19 hr; adults, 35 hr. Oral duration of action is 6–8 hr initially and 22–48 hr after repeated doses. Respiratory effects last longer than analgesia. Accumulation may occur with continuous use making it necessary to adjust dose. Nevirapine may decrease serum levels of methadone. Methadone is a substrate for CYP450 3A3/4, 2D6, 1A2; and inhibitor of 2D6.

See Chapter 28 for equianalgesic dosing and onset of action. **Adjust dose in renal insufficiency (see Chapter 30).** Pregnancy category changes to D if used for prolonged period or in high doses at term.

METHIMAZOLE

Tapazole

Antithyroid agent

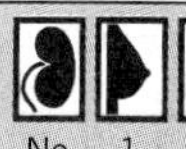

No 1 D

Tabs: 5, 10 mg

Hyperthyroidism:

Child:

- ***Initial:*** 0.4–0.7 mg/kg/24 hr or 15–20 mg/m²/24 hr PO ÷ Q8 hr
- ***Maintenance:*** 1/3–2/3 of initial dose PO ÷ Q8 hr
- **Max. dose:** 30 mg/24 hr

Adult:

- ***Initial:*** 15–60 mg/24 hr PO ÷ TID
- ***Maintenance:*** 5–15 mg/24 hr PO ÷ TID

Readily crosses placental membranes and distributes into breast milk (AAP considers it to be compatible with breast-feeding). Blood dyscrasias, dermatitis, hepatitis, arthralgia, CNS reactions, pruritus, nephritis, hypoprothrombinemia, agranulocytosis, headache, fever, and hypothyroidism may occur.

Continued

For explanation of icons, see p. 680.

METHIMAZOLE *continued*

May increase the effects of oral anticoagulants. When correcting hyperthyroidism, existing beta-blocker, digoxin, and theophylline doses may need to be reduced to avoid potential toxicities.

Switch to maintenance dose when patient is euthyroid.

Administer all doses with food.

METHYLDOPA

Various brand names

Central alpha-adrenergic blocker, antihypertensive

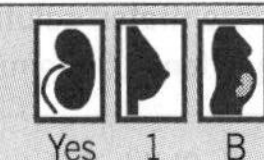

Tabs: 250, 500 mg
Injection: 50 mg/mL; contains bisulfites
Suspension: 50 mg/ mL 

Hypertension:
Child: 10 mg/kg/24 hr ÷ Q6–12 hr PO; increase PRN Q2 days. **Max. dose:** 65 mg/kg/24 hr or 3 g/24 hr, whichever is less.
Adult: 250 mg/dose BID–TID PO. Increase PRN Q2 days to **max. dose** of 3 g/24 hr.
Hypertensive crisis:
Child: 2–4 mg/kg/dose IV to a **max. dose** of 5–10 mg/kg/dose IV Q6–8 hr. **Max. dose** (whichever is less): 65 mg/kg/24 hr or 3 g/24 hr.
Adult: 250–1000 mg IV Q6–8 hr. **Max. dose:** 4 g/24 hr

Contraindicated in pheochromocytoma and active liver disease. **Use with caution** if patient is receiving haloperidol, propranolol, lithium, sympathomimetics. Positive Coombs test rarely associated with hemolytic anemia. Fever, leukopenia, sedation, memory impairment, hepatitis, GI disturbances, orthostatic hypotension, black tongue, and gynecomastia may occur. May interfere with lab tests for creatinine, urinary catecholamines, uric acid, and AST.

Do not co-administer oral doses with iron; decreases methyldopa bioavailability. **Adjust dose in renal failure (see Chapter 30).**

METHYLENE BLUE

Urolene Blue and others

Antidote, drug-induced methemoglobinemia, and cyanide toxicity

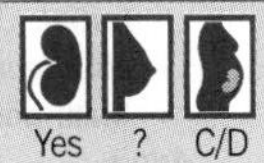

Tabs: 65 mg
Injection: 10 mg/mL (1%) (1, 10 mL)

Methemoglobinemia:
Child and adult:
1–2 mg/kg/dose or 25–50 mg/m^2/dose IV over 5 min. May repeat in 1 hr if needed.

Continued

METHYLENE BLUE *continued*

At high doses, may cause methemoglobinemia. **Avoid** subcutaneous or intrathecal routes of administration. **Use with caution** in G6PD deficiency or renal insufficiency. May cause nausea, vomiting, dizziness, headache, diaphoresis, stained skin, and abdominal pain. Causes blue-green discoloration of urine and feces. Pregnancy category changes to D if injected intra-amniotically.

METHYLPHENIDATE HCL

Ritalin, Methylin, Metadate ER, Methylin ER, Concerta, Ritalin SR, Metadate CD, Ritalin LA, and others

CNS stimulant

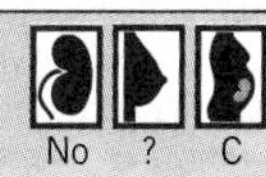

Tabs: 5, 10, 20 mg
Chewable tabs: 2.5, 5, 10 mg
Extended-release tabs:
8-hr duration (Metadate ER, Methylin ER): 10, 20 mg
24-hr duration (Concerta): 18, 27, 36, 54 mg
Sustained-release tabs:
8-hr duration (Ritalin SR): 20 mg
Extended-release caps:
24-hr duration (Metadate CD, Ritalin LA): 10, 20, 30, 40 mg

Attention deficit/hyperactivity disorder:
≥6 yr:
Initial: 0.3 mg/kg/dose (or 2.5–5 mg/dose) given before breakfast and lunch. May increase by 0.1 mg/kg/dose PO (or 5–10 mg/24 hr) weekly until maintenance dose achieved. May give extra afternoon dose if needed.
Maintenance dose range: 0.3–1 mg/kg/24 hr
Max. dose: 2 mg/kg/24 hr or 60 mg/24 hr

Once-daily dosing (Concerta), ≥6 yr:
Patients new to methylphenidate: Start with 18 mg PO QAM, dosage may be increased at weekly intervals at 18-mg increments up to the following **max. dose:**
6–12 yr: 54 mg/24 hr
13–17 yr: 72 mg/24 hr **not to exceed** 2 mg/kg/24 hr
Patients currently receiving methylphenidate: see table below.

RECOMMENDED DOSE CONVERSION FROM METHYLPHENIDATE REGIMENS TO CONCERTA

Previous Methylphenidate Daily Dose	Recommended Concerta Dose
5 mg PO BID–TID or 20 mg SR PO QD	18 mg PO QAM
10 mg PO BID–TID or 40 mg SR PO QD	36 mg PO QAM
15 mg PO BID–TID or 60 mg SR PO QD	54 mg PO QAM

After a week of receiving the above-recommended Concerta dose, dose may be increased in 18-mg increments at weekly intervals up to a **maximum** of 54 mg/24 hr for 6–12 yr and 72 mg/24 hr (not to exceed 2 mg/kg/24 hr) for 13–17 yr.

Continued

For explanation of icons, see p. 680.

METHYLPHENIDATE HCL *continued*

Contraindicated in glaucoma, anxiety disorders, motor tics, and Tourette syndrome. Medication should generally not be used in children <5 yr because diagnosis of ADHD in this age group is extremely difficult and should be only done in consultation with a specialist. **Use with caution** in patients with hypertension and epilepsy. Insomnia, weight loss, anorexia, rash, nausea, emesis, abdominal pain, hypertension or hypotension, tachycardia, arrhythmias, palpitations, restlessness, headaches, fever, tremor, and thrombocytopenia may occur. Abnormal liver function, cerebral arteritis and/or occlusion, leukopenia and/or anemia, transient depressed mood, and scalp hair loss have been reported. High doses may slow growth by appetite suppression.

May increase serum concentrations of tricyclic antidepressants, phenytoin, phenobarbital, and warfarin. Effect of methylphenidate may be potentiated by MAO inhibitors.

Extended- and sustained-release dosage forms have either an 8- or 24-hr dosage interval (see above). Concerta dosage form delivers 22.2% of its dose as an immediate release product with the remaining amounts as an extended release product (e.g., 18 mg strength: 4 mg as immediate release and 14 mg as extended release).

METHYLPREDNISOLONE

Medrol, Solu-Medrol, Depo-Medrol, and others
Corticosteroid

No 3 C

Tabs: 2, 4, 8, 16, 24, 32 mg
Tabs, dose pack: 4 mg (21s)
Injection, Na succinate (Solu-Medrol): 40, 125, 500, 1000, 2000 mg (IV/IM use)
Injection, Acetate (Depo-Medrol): 20, 40, 80 mg/mL (IM repository)

Antiinflammatory/immunosuppressive:
PO/IM/IV: 0.5–1.7 mg/kg/24 hr ÷ Q6–12 hr
Status asthmaticus:
Child: IM/IV:
Loading dose: 2 mg/kg/dose × 1
Maintenance: 2 mg/kg/24 hr ÷ Q6 hr
Adults: 10–250 mg/dose Q4–6 hr IM/IV
Acute spinal cord injury:
30 mg/kg IV over 15 min followed in 45 min by a continuous infusion of 5.4 mg/kg/hr × 23 hr

See Chapter 29 for relative steroid potencies and doses based on body surface area. **Not all** practitioners use loading dose for status asthmaticus. Acetate form may be used for intra-articular and intralesional injection; it should not be given IV. Like all steroids, may cause hypertension, pseudotumor cerebri, acne, Cushing syndrome, adrenal axis suppression, GI bleeding, hyperglycemia, and osteoporosis.

Barbiturates, phenytoin, and rifampin may enhance methylprednisolone clearance. Erythromycin, itraconazole, and ketoconazole may increase methylprednisone levels. Methylprednisolone may increase cyclosporine and tacrolimus levels.

METOCLOPRAMIDE

Reglan, Clopra, Maxolon, and others

Antiemetic, prokinetic agent

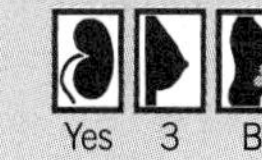

Tabs: 5, 10 mg
Injection: 5 mg/mL
Syrup (sugar-free): 5 mg/5 mL; some may contain sodium benzoate.

Gastroesophageal reflux (GER) or GI dysmotility:

Infant and child: 0.1–0.2 mg/kg/dose up to QID IV/IM/PO; **max. dose:** 0.8 mg/kg/24 hr

Adult: 10–15 mg/dose QAC and QHS IV/IM/PO

Antiemetic:

1–2 mg/kg/dose Q2–6 hr IV/IM/PO. Premedicate with diphenhydramine to reduce EPS.

Postoperative nausea and vomiting:

Child: 0.1–0.2 mg/kg/dose Q6–8 hr PRN IV

>14 yr and adult: 10 mg Q6–8 hr PRN IV

Contraindicated in GI obstruction, seizure disorder, pheochromocytoma, or in patients receiving drugs likely to cause extrapyramidal symptoms (EPS). May cause EPS, especially at higher doses. Sedation, headache, anxiety, depression, leukopenia, and diarrhea may occur. Rare occurrences of neuroleptic malignant syndrome has been reported.

For GER, give 30 min before meals and at bedtime. Reduce dose in renal impairment (see Chapter 30).

METOLAZONE

Zaroxolyn, Mykrox, and others

Diuretic, thiazide-like

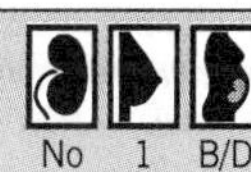

Tabs: 0.5 (Mykrox), 2.5, 5, 10 mg
Oral suspension: 1 mg/mL

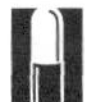

Dosage based on Zaroxolyn (for Mykrox or oral suspension, see remarks)

Child: 0.2–0.4 mg/kg/24 hr ÷ QD–BID PO

Adult:

Hypertension: 2.5–5 mg QD PO

Edema: 5–20 mg QD PO

Contraindicated in patients with anuria, hepatic coma, or hypersensitivity to sulfonamides or thiazides. Electrolyte imbalance, GI disturbance, hyperglycemia, marrow suppression, chills, hyperuricemia, chest pain, hepatitis, and rash may occur. Mykrox and oral suspension have increased bioavailability; therefore, lower doses may be necessary when using these dosage forms.

Continued

For explanation of icons, see p. 680.

METOLAZONE *continued*

More effective than thiazide diuretics in impaired renal function; may be effective in GFRs as low as 20 mL/min. Furosemide-resistant edema in pediatric patients may benefit with the addition of metolazone.

Pregnancy category changes to D if used for pregnancy induced hypertension.

METRONIDAZOLE

Flagyl, Flagyl ER, Protostat, MetroGel, MetroLotion, MetroCream, Noritate, MetroGel-Vaginal, and others
Antibiotic, antiprotozoal

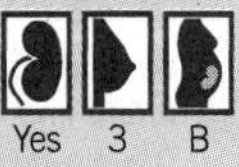

Tabs: 250, 500 mg
Tabs, extended release (Flagyl ER): 750 mg
Caps: 375 mg
Oral suspension: 20 mg/mL or 50 mg/mL 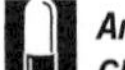
Injection: 500 mg; contains 830 mg mannitol/g drug
Ready-to-use injection: 5 mg/mL (100 mL); contains 28 mEq Na/g drug
Gel, topical (MetroGel): 0.75% (28, 45 g)
Lotion (MetroLotion): 0.75% (59 mL); contains benzyl alcohol
Cream, topical:
- **MetroCream:** 0.75% (45 g); contains benzyl alcohol
- **Noritate:** 1% (30 g)

Gel, vaginal (MetroGel-Vaginal): 0.75% (70 g with 5 applicators)

Amebiasis:
- ***Child:*** 35–50 mg/kg/24 hr PO ÷ TID × 10 days
- ***Adult:*** 750 mg/dose PO TID × 10 days

Anaerobic infection:
- ***Neonate: PO/IV:***
- ***<7 days:***
  - ***<1.2 kg:*** 7.5 mg/kg/dose Q48 hr
  - ***1.2–2 kg:*** 7.5 mg/kg/dose Q24 hr
  - ***≥2 kg:*** 15 mg/kg/24 hr ÷ Q12 hr
- ***≥7 days:***
  - ***<1.2 kg:*** 7.5 mg/kg Q24 hr
  - ***1.2–2 kg:*** 15 mg/kg/24 hr ÷ Q12 hr
  - ***≥2 kg:*** 30 mg/kg/24 hr ÷ Q12 hr
- ***Infant/child/adult:***
  - ***IV/PO:*** 30 mg/kg/24 hr ÷ Q6 hr
  - **Max. dose:** 4 g/24 hr

Bacterial vaginosis:
- ***Adolescent and adult:***
- ***PO:*** 500 mg BID × 7 days or 2 g × 1 dose
- ***Vaginal:*** 5 g (1 applicator-full) BID × 5 days

Giardiasis:
- ***Child:*** 15 mg/kg/24 hr PO ÷ TID × 5 days
- ***Adult:*** 250 mg PO TID × 5 days

Continued

METRONIDAZOLE *continued*

Trichomoniasis: treat sexual contacts.

Child: 15 mg/kg/24 hr PO ÷ TID × 7 days

Adolescent/adult: 2 g PO × 1 or 250 mg PO TID or 375 mg PO BID × 7 days

C. difficile infection (IV may be less efficacious):

Child: 30 mg/kg/24 hr ÷ Q6 hr PO/IV x 10 days

Adult: 250–500 mg TID-QID PO × 10–14 days, or 500 mg Q8 hr IV × 10–14 days

H. pylori infection:

Use in combination with amoxicillin and bismuth subsalicylate.

Child: 15–20 mg/kg/24 hr ÷ BID PO × 4 wk

Adult: 250–500 mg TID PO × 14 days

Inflammatory bowel disease (as alternative to sulfasalazine):

Adult: 400 mg BID PO

Topical use: apply to affected areas BID.

Avoid use in first-trimester pregnancy. **Use with caution** in patients with CNS disease, blood dyscrasias, severe liver or **renal disease (GFR <10 mL/min)**, see Chapter 30. Nausea, diarrhea, urticaria, dry mouth, leukopenia, vertigo, metallic taste, and peripheral neuropathy may occur. Candidiasis may worsen. May discolor urine. Patients **should not** ingest alcohol for 24–48 hr after dose (disulfiram-type reaction).

May increase levels or toxicity of phenytoin, lithium, and warfarin. Phenobarbital and rifampin may increase metronidazole metabolism.

IV infusion must be given slowly over 1 hr. For intravenous use in all ages, some references recommend a 15 mg/kg loading dose.

MICONAZOLE

Monistat and others; topical products: Micatin, Lotrimin AF, and others

Antifungal agent

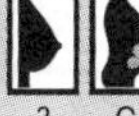

Cream (OTC): 2% (15, 30, 90 g)
Lotion (OTC): 2% (30, 60 mL)
Ointment (OTC): 2% (28.4 g)
Topical solution (OTC): 2% with alcohol (7.4, 29.6 mL)
Vaginal cream (OTC): 2% (15, 25, 45 g)
Vaginal suppository (OTC): 100 mg (7s), 200 mg (3s)
Powder (OTC): 2% (70, 90 g)
Spray, liquid (OTC): 2% (105 mL); contains alcohol
Spray, powder (OTC): 2% (85, 90, 100 g); contains alcohol

Topical: Apply BID × 2–4 wk

Vaginal: 1 applicator full of cream or 100 mg suppository QHS × 7 days or 200 mg suppository QHS × 3 days

Continued

For explanation of icons, see p. 680.

MICONAZOLE *continued*

Use with caution in hypersensitivity to other imidazole antifungal agents (e.g., clotrimazole, ketoconazole). Side effects include pruritus, rash, burning, phlebitis, headaches, and pelvic cramps.

Drug is a substrate and inhibitor of the CYP450 3A3/4 isoenzymes. Vaginal use with concomitant warfarin use has also been reported to increase warfarin's effect. Vegetable oil base in vaginal suppositories may interact with latex products (e.g., condoms and diaphragms); consider switching to the vaginal cream.

MIDAZOLAM

Versed

Benzodiazepine

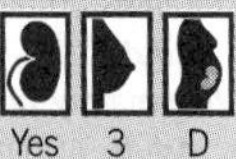

Yes 3 D

Injection: 1, 5 mg/mL; some preparations contain 1% benzyl alcohol.
Oral syrup: 2 mg/mL

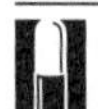

Titrate to effect under controlled conditions.
See Chapter 28, for additional routes of administration.

Sedation for procedures:

Child:

IV:

6 mo–5 yr: 0.05–0.1 mg/kg/dose over 2–3 min. May repeat dose PRN in 2–3 min intervals up to a **max. total dose** of 6 mg. A total dose up to 0.6 mg/kg may be necessary for desired effect.

6–12 yr: 0.025–0.05 mg/kg/dose over 2–3 min. May repeat dose PRN in 2–3 min intervals up to a **max. total dose** of 10 mg. A total dose up to 0.4 mg/kg may be necessary for desired effect.

>12–16 yr: Use adult dose; up to **max. total dose** of 10 mg.

PO:

≥6 mo: 0.25–0.5 mg/kg/dose × 1; **max. dose:** 20 mg. Younger patients (6 mo–5 yr) may require higher doses of 1 mg/kg/dose whereas, older patients (6–15 yr) may require only 0.25 mg/kg/dose. Use 0.25 mg/kg/dose for patients with cardiac or respiratory compromise, concurrent CNS depressive drug, or high-risk surgery.

Adult:

IV: 0.5–2 mg/dose over 2 min. May repeat PRN in 2–3 min intervals until desired effect. *Usual total dose:* 2.5–5 mg. **Max. total dose:** 10 mg.

Sedation with mechanical ventilation:

Intermittent:

Infant and child: 0.05–0.15 mg/kg/dose Q1–2 hr PRN

Continuous IV infusion (initial doses, titrate to effect):

Neonate:

<32 weeks' gestation: 0.5 mcg/kg/min

≥32 weeks' gestation: 1 mcg/kg/min

Infant and child: 1–2 mcg/kg/min

See inside front cover for infusion preparation.

Continued

MIDAZOLAM *continued*

Refractory status epilepticus:

≥2 mo and child: Load with 0.15 mg/kg IV × 1 followed by a continuous infusion of 1 mcg/kg/min, and titrate dose upward Q5 min to effect (mean dose of 2.3 mcg/kg/min with a range of 1–18 mcg/kg/min has been reported).

See inside front cover for infusion preparation.

Contraindicated in patients with narrow-angle glaucoma and shock. Causes respiratory depression, hypotension, and bradycardia. Cardiovascular monitoring is recommended. Use lower doses or reduce dose when given in combination with narcotics or in patients with respiratory compromise.

Drug is a substrate for CYP450 3A4. Serum concentrations may be increased by cimetidine, clarithromycin, diltiazem, erythromycin, itraconazole, ketoconazole, and protease inhibitors. Sedative effects may be antagonized by theophylline. Effects can be reversed by flumazenil. For pharmacodynamic information, see Chapter 28. **Adjust dose in renal failure (see Chapter 30).**

MILRINONE

Primacor

Inotrope

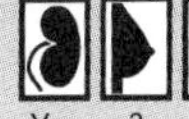
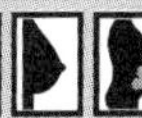

Yes ? C

Injection: 1 mg/mL (5, 10, 20 mL)
Premixed injection in D5W: 200 mcg/mL (100, 200 mL)

Child (limited data): 50 mcg/kg IV bolus over 15 min, followed by a continuous infusion of 0.5–1 mcg/kg/min and titrate to effect.

Adult: 50 mcg/kg IV bolus over 10 min, followed by a continuous infusion of 0.375–0.75 mcg/kg/min and titrate to effect.

Contraindicated in severe aortic stenosis, severe pulmonic stenosis, and acute MI. May cause headache, dysrhythmias, hypotension, hypokalemia, nausea, vomiting, anorexia, abdominal pain, hepatotoxicity, and thrombocytopenia. Pediatric patients may require higher mcg/kg/min doses because of a faster elimination $T_{1/2}$ and larger volume of distribution, when compared with adults. Hemodynamic effects can last up to 3–5 hr after discontinuation of infusion in children. Reduce dose in renal impairment.

MINERAL OIL

Kondremul and others

Laxative, lubricant

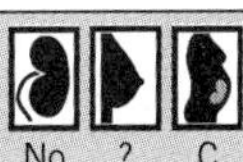

No ? C

Liquid, oral (OTC): 180, 480 mL
Emulsion, oral (Kondremul; OTC): 480 mL
Rectal liquid (OTC): 133 mL

Continued

For explanation of icons, see p. 680.

MINERAL OIL *continued*

Child 5–11 yr:
Oral liquid: 5–15 mL/24 hr ÷ QD–TID PO
Oral emulsion (Kondremul): 10–25 mL/24 hr ÷ QD–TID PO
Rectal: 30–60 mL as single dose

Child ≥12 yr and adult:
Oral liquid: 15–45 mL/24 hr ÷ QD–TID PO
Oral emulsion (Kondremul): 30–75 mL/24 hr ÷ QD–TID PO
Rectal: 60–150 mL as single dose

May cause lipid pneumonitis via aspiration, diarrhea, and cramps. Use as a laxative **should not exceed** >1 wk. Onset of action is about 6–8 hr. Higher doses may be necessary to achieve desired effect. Do not give QHS dose, and **use with caution** in children <5 yr to minimize risk for aspiration. May impair the absorption of fat-soluble vitamins, calcium, phosphorus, oral contraceptives, and warfarin. Emulsified preparations are more palatable and are dosed differently than the oral liquid preparation.

For disimpaction, doses up to 1 ounce (30 mL) per year of age (**max. dose** of 240 mL) BID can be given.

MINOCYCLINE

Minocin, Dynacin, and others
Antibiotic, tetracycline derivative

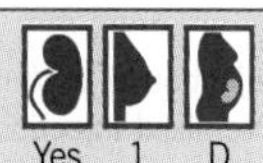

Tabs: 50, 75, 100 mg
Caps: 50, 75, 100 mg
Caps (pellet filled): 50, 100 mg
Oral suspension: 50 mg/5 mL (60 mL); contains 5% alcohol
Injection: 100 mg

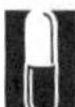

Child (8–12 yr): 4 mg/kg/dose × 1 PO/IV, then 2 mg/kg/dose Q12 hr PO/IV; **max. dose:** 200 mg/24 hr
Adolescent and adult: 200 mg/dose × 1 PO/IV, then 100 mg Q12 hr PO/IV
Acne: 50 mg PO QD–TID
Chlamydia trachomatis/Ureaplasma urealyticum: 100 mg PO Q12 hr × 7 days

Use with caution in renal failure, lower dosage may be necessary. Nausea, vomiting, allergy, increased intracranial pressure, photophobia, and injury to developing teeth may occur. Hepatitis, including autoimmune hepatitis, and liver failure have been reported. High incidence of vestibular dysfunction (30%–90%). May be administered with food but **NOT** with milk or dairy products. See *Tetracycline* for additional drug/food interactions and comments.

MINOXIDIL

Loniten, Rogaine, Women's Rogaine, Men's Rogaine Extra Strength, and others

Antihypertensive agent, hair growth stimulant

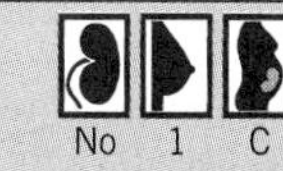

Tabs: 2.5, 10 mg

Topical solution:

Rogaine, Women's Rogaine (OTC): 2% (60 mL)

Men's Rogaine Extra Strength (OTC): 5% (60 mL); contains 30% alcohol

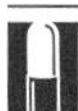

Child <12 yr:

Start with 0.2 mg/kg/24 hr PO QD; **max. dose:** 5 mg/24 hr. Dose may be increased in increments of 0.1–0.2 mg/kg/24 hr at 3-day intervals. Usual effective range: 0.25–1 mg/kg/24 hr PO ÷ QD-BID; **max. dose:** 5 mg/kg/24 hr up to 50 mg/24 hr.

≥12 yr and adult:

Oral: Start with 5 mg QD. Dose may be gradually increased at 3-day intervals. Usual effective range: 10–40 mg/24 hr ÷ QD–BID; **max. dose:** 100 mg/24 hr.

Topical (alopecia): Apply 1 mL to the total affected areas of the scalp BID (QAM and QHS); **max. dose:** 2 mL/24 hr.

Contraindicated in acute MI, dissecting aortic aneurysm, and pheochromocytoma. Concurrent use with a beta-blocker and diuretic is recommended to prevent reflex tachycardia and reduce water retention, respectively. May cause drowsiness, dizziness, CHF, pulmonary edema, pericardial effusion, pericarditis, thrombocytopenia, leukopenia, Stevens-Johnson syndrome, and hypertrichosis (reversible) with systemic use. Concurrent use of guanethidine may cause profound orthostatic hypotension; use with other antihypertensive agents may cause additive hypotension. Antihypertensive onset of action within 30 min and peak effects within 2–8 hr.

TOPICAL USE: Local irritation, contact dermatitis may occur. **Do not use** in conjunction with other topical agents, including topical corticosteroids, retinoids, or petrolatum or agents that are known to enhance cutaneous drug absorption. Onset of hair growth (topical use) is 4 mo. The 5% solution is flammable.

MONTELUKAST

Singulair

Antiasthmatic, antiallergy, leukotriene receptor antagonist

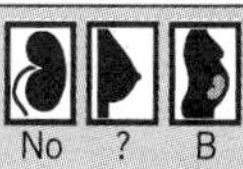

Chewable tabs: 4, 5 mg; contains phenylalanine

Tabs: 10 mg

Oral granules: 4 mg per packet

Continued

For explanation of icons, see p. 680.

MONTELUKAST *continued*

Asthma and seasonal allergic rhinitis:
Child (2–5 yr): Chew 4 mg (chewable tablet) QHS
Child (6–14 yr): Chew 5 mg (chewable tablet) QHS
>15 yr and adult: 10 mg PO QHS

Chewable tablet dosage form is **contraindicated** in phenylketonuric patients. Side effects include headache, abdominal pain, dyspepsia, fatigue, dizziness, cough, and elevated liver enzymes. Diarrhea, eosinophilia, hypersensitivity reactions, pharyngitis, nausea, otitis, sinusitis, and viral infections have been reported in children. Drug is a substrate for CYP450 3A4 and 2C9. Phenobarbital and rifampin may induce hepatic metabolism to increase the clearance of montelukast.

Doses may administered with or without food.

MORPHINE SULFATE

Roxanol, MS Contin, Oramorph SR, and many others
Narcotic, analgesic

Yes 2 C/D

Oral solution: 10 mg/5 mL, 20 mg/5 mL
Concentrated oral solution: 100 mg/5 mL
Caps/tabs: 15, 30 mg
Controlled-release tabs (MS Contin, Oramorph SR): 15, 30, 60, 100, 200 mg
Extended-release tabs: 15, 30, 60, 100 mg
Soluble tabs: 10, 15, 30 mg
Extended-release caps: 30, 60, 90, 120 mg
Sustained-release pellets in caps: 20, 30, 50, 60, 100 mg
Rectal suppository: 5, 10, 20, 30 mg
Injection: 0.5, 1, 2, 4, 5, 8, 10, 15, 25, 50 mg/mL

Titrate to effect.
Analgesia/tetralogy (cyanotic) spells:
Neonate: 0.05–0.2 mg/kg/dose IM, slow IV, SC Q4 hr
Neonatal opiate withdrawal: 0.08–0.2 mg/dose Q3–4 hr PRN
Infant and child:
PO: 0.2–0.5 mg/kg/dose Q4–6 hr PRN (immediate release) or 0.3–0.6 mg/kg/dose Q12 hr PRN (controlled release)
IM/IV/SC: 0.1–0.2 mg/kg/dose Q2–4 hr PRN; **max. dose:** 15 mg/dose
Adult:
PO: 10–30 mg Q4 hr PRN (immediate release) or 15–30 mg Q8–12 hr PRN (controlled release)
IM/IV/SC: 2–15 mg/dose Q2–6 hr PRN
Continuous IV infusion (dosing ranges, titrate to effect):
Neonate: 0.01–0.02 mg/kg/hr
Infant and child:
Postoperative pain: 0.01–0.04 mg/kg/hr
Sickle cell and cancer: 0.04–0.07 mg/kg/hr
Adult: 0.8–10 mg/hr

To prepare infusion for neonates, infants, and children, use the following formula:

$$50 \times \frac{\text{Desired dose (mg/kg/hr)}}{\text{Desired infusion rate (mL/hr)}} \times \text{Wt (kg)} = \frac{\text{mg morphine}}{\text{50 mL fluid}}$$

Continued

MORPHINE SULFATE *continued*

Dependence, CNS and respiratory depression, nausea, vomiting, urinary retention, constipation, hypotension, bradycardia, increased ICP, miosis, biliary spasm, and allergy may occur. **Naloxone may be used to reverse effects, especially respiratory depression.** Causes histamine release, resulting in itching and possible bronchospasm. Low-dose naloxone infusion may be used for itching. Inflammatory masses (e.g., granulomas) have been reported with continuous infusions via indwelling intrathecal catheters.

See Chapter 28 for equianalgesic dosing. Pregnancy category changes to D if used for prolonged periods or in higher doses at term. Rectal dosing is same as oral dosing but is not recommended because of poor absorption.

Controlled/sustained-release oral tablets must be administered whole. Controlled-released oral capsules may be opened and the entire contents sprinkled on applesauce immediately before ingestion. **Adjust dose in renal failure (see Chapter 30).**

MUPIROCIN

Bactroban, Bactroban Nasal, and others

Topical antibiotic

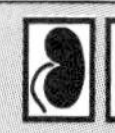
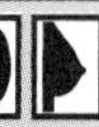
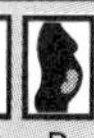
No ? B

Ointment: 2% (15, 22, 30 g); contains polyethylene glycol
Cream: 2% (15, 30 g); contains benzyl alcohol
Nasal ointment: 2% (1 g), as calcium salt

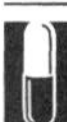

Topical: Apply small amount TID to affected area × 5–14 days.
Intranasal: Apply small amount intranasally 2–4 times/24 hr for 5–14 days.

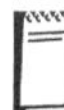

Avoid contact with the eyes. **Do not use** topical ointment preparation on open wounds owing to concerns about systemic absorption of polyethylene glycol. May cause minor local irritation.

If clinical response is not apparent in 3–5 days with topical use, reevaluate infection. Intranasal administration may be used to eliminate carriage of *S. aureus,* including MRSA.

MYCOPHENOLATE MOFETIL

CellCept, Myfortic

Immunosuppressant agent

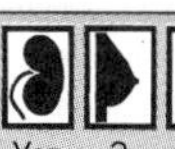
Yes 3 C

Caps: 250 mg
Tabs: 500 mg
Delayed-released tabs (Myfortic): 180, 360 mg
Oral suspension: 200 mg/mL (225 mL); contains phenylalanine (0.56 mg/mL) and methylparabens
Injection: 500 mg

Continued

For explanation of icons, see p. 680.

MYCOPHENOLATE MOFETIL *continued*

Child (see remarks):
Caps, tabs, or suspension: 600 mg/m²/dose PO BID up to a **max. dose** of 2000 mg/24 hr; alternatively, patients with body surface areas ≥1.25 m² may be dosed as follows:
1.25–1.5 m²: 750 mg PO BID
>1.5 m²: 1000 mg PO BID
Delayed-release tabs (Myfortic): 400 mg/m²/dose PO BID; **max. dose:** 720 mg BID; alternatively, patients with body surface areas ≥1.19 m² may be dosed as follows:
1.19–1.58 m²: 540 mg PO BID
>1.58 m²: 720 mg PO BID
Adult (in combination with corticosteroids and cyclosporine):
IV: 2000–3000 mg/24 hr ÷ BID
Oral:
Caps, tabs, or suspension: 2000–3000 mg/24 hr PO ÷ BID
Delayed-release tabs (Myfortic): 720 mg PO BID

Check specific transplantation protocol for specific dosage. Mycophenolate mofetil is a prodrug for mycophenolic acid. Because of differences in absorption, the delayed-release tablets should **not** be interchanged with the other oral dosage forms on an equivalent mg-to-mg basis.

Common side effects may include headache, hypertension, diarrhea, vomiting, bone marrow suppression, anemia, fever, opportunistic infections, and sepsis. May also increase the risk for lymphomas or other malignancies.

Use with caution in patients with active GI disease or renal impairment (GFR <25 mL/min/1.73 m²) outside of the immediate post-transplantation period. In adults with renal impairment, **avoid** doses >2 g/24 hr and observe carefully. No dose adjustment is needed for patients experiencing delayed graft function postoperatively.

Drug interactions: (1) Displacement of phenytoin or theophylline from protein-binding sites will decrease total serum levels and increase free serum levels of these drugs. Salicylates displace mycophenolate to increase free levels of mycophenolate. (2) Competition for renal tubular secretion results in increased serum levels of acyclovir, ganciclovir, probenecid, and mycophenolate (when any of these are used together). (3) **Avoid** live and live attenuated vaccines (including influenza); decreases vaccine effectiveness.

Administer oral doses on an empty stomach. Cholestyramine and antacid use may decrease mycophenolic acid levels. Infuse intravenous doses over 2 hr. Oral suspension may be administered via NG tube with a minimum size of 8 French.

NAFCILLIN

Unipen, Nallpen, and others
Antibiotic, penicillin (penicillinase resistant)

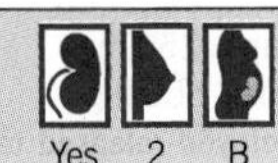

Caps: 250 mg
Injection: 1, 2, 10 g; contains 2.9 mEq Na/g drug
Injection, premixed in iso-osmotic dextrose: 1 g in 50 mL, 2 g in 100 mL

Continued

NAFCILLIN *continued*

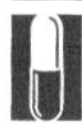

Neonate: IM/IV
≤7 days:
<2 kg: 50 mg/kg/24 hr ÷ Q12 hr
≥2 kg: 75 mg/kg/24 hr ÷ Q8 hr
>7 days:
<1.2 kg: 50 mg/kg/24 hr ÷ Q12 hr
1.2–2 kg: 75 mg/kg/24 hr ÷ Q8 hr
≥2 kg: 100 mg/kg/24 hr ÷ Q6 hr
Infant and child:
PO: 50–100 mg/kg/24 hr ÷ Q6 hr
IM/IV: (mild to moderate infections): 50–100 mg/kg/24 hr ÷ Q6 hr
(severe infections): 100–200 mg/kg/24 hr ÷ Q4–6 hr
Max. dose: 12 g/24 hr
Adult:
PO: 250–1000 mg Q4–6 hr
IV: 500–2000 mg Q4–6 hr
IM: 500 mg Q4–6 hr
Max. dose: 12 g/24 hr

Allergic cross-sensitivity with penicillin. **Oral route not recommended owing to unpredictable absorption.** High incidence of phlebitis with IV dosing. CSF penetration is poor unless meninges are inflamed. **Use with caution** in patients with combined renal and hepatic impairment (reduce dose by 33%–50%). Nafcillin may increase elimination of warfarin. Acute interstitial nephritis is rare. May cause rash and bone marrow suppression.

NALOXONE

Narcan and others
Narcotic antagonist

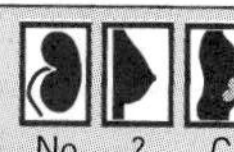

Injection: 0.4 mg/mL (1, 10 mL), 1 mg/mL (2, 10 mL); some preparations may contain parabens.
Neonatal injection: 0.02 mg/mL (2 ml)

Opiate intoxication (see remarks):
Neonate, infant, child <20 kg: **IM/IV/SC/ETT:** 0.1 mg/kg/dose. May repeat PRN Q2–3 min.
Child ≥20 kg or >5 yr: 2 mg/dose. May repeat PRN Q2–3 min.
Continuous infusion (child and adult): 0.005 mg/kg loading dose followed by infusion of 0.0025 mg/kg/hr has been recommended. A range of 0.0025–0.16 mg/kg/hr has been reported. Taper gradually to avoid relapse.
Adult: 0.4–2 mg/dose. May repeat PRN Q2–3 min. Use 0.1- to 0.2-mg increments in opiate-dependent patients.

Short duration of action may necessitate multiple doses. For severe intoxication, doses of 0.2 mg/kg may be required. If no response is achieved after a cumulative dose of 10 mg, reevaluate diagnosis. **In the nonarrest**

Continued

For explanation of icons, see p. 680.

NALOXONE *continued*

situation, use the lowest dose effective (may start at 0.001 mg/kg/dose). See Chapter 28 for additional information.

Will produce narcotic withdrawal syndrome in patients with chronic dependence. **Use with caution** in patients with chronic cardiac disease. Abrupt reversal of narcotic depression may result in nausea, vomiting, diaphoresis, tachycardia, hypertension, and tremulousness.

May be used simultaneously with opiates at lower dosages (~0.25–2 mcg/kg/hr) to abate opiate-related side effects. The neonatal concentration (0.02 mg/mL) is no longer recommended in most instances owing to large volumes of administration (2 mg = 100 mL).

NAPROXEN/NAPROXEN SODIUM

Naprosyn, Anaprox, EC-Naprosyn, Naprelan, Aleve [OTC], and others
Nonsteroidal antiinflammatory agent

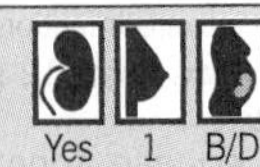

Naproxen:

Tabs: 250, 375, 500 mg
Delayed-release tabs (EC-Naprosyn): 375, 500 mg
Oral suspension: 125 mg/5 mL; contains 0.34 mEq Na/1 mL and parabens

Naproxen sodium:

Tabs:
Aleve: 220 mg (200-mg base); contains 0.87 mEq Na
Anaprox: 275 mg (250-mg base), 550 mg (500-mg base); contains 1 mEq, 2 mEq Na, respectively
Controlled-release tabs (Naprelan): 412.5 mg (375-mg base), 550 mg (500-mg base)

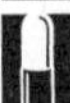

All doses based on naproxen base
Child >2 yr:
Analgesia: 5–7 mg/kg/dose Q8–12 hr PO
JRA: 10–20 mg/kg/24 hr ÷ Q12 hr PO
Usual max. dose: 1250 mg/24 hr

Rheumatoid arthritis, ankylosing spondylitis:
Adult:
Immediate-release forms: 250–500 mg BID PO
Delayed-release tabs (EC-Naprosyn): 375–500 mg BID PO
Controlled-release tabs (Naprelan): 750–1000 mg QD PO; **max. dose:** 1500 mg/24 hr

Dysmenorrhea:
500 mg × 1, then 250 mg Q6–8 hr PO; **max. dose:** 1250 mg/24 hr

May cause GI bleeding, thrombocytopenia, heartburn, headache, drowsiness, vertigo, and tinnitus. **Use with caution** in patients with GI disease, cardiac disease, renal or hepatic impairment, and those receiving anticoagulants. See *Ibuprofen* for other side effects.

Pregnancy category changes to D if used in the third trimester or near delivery. Administer doses with food or milk to reduce GI discomfort.

NEDOCROMIL SODIUM

Tilade, Alocril

Antiallergic agent

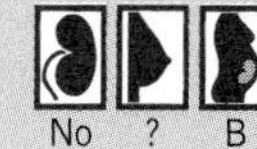

Aerosol inhaler: 1.75 mg/actuation (112 actuations/inhaler, 16.2 g)
Ophthalmic solution (Alocril): 2% (5 mL)

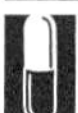

Child ≥6 yr and adult:
2 puffs QID. May reduce dosage to BID–TID once clinical response is obtained.

Ophthalmic use:
≥3 yr–adult: 1–2 drops to affected eye(s) BID

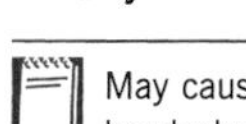

May cause dry mouth/pharyngitis, unpleasant taste, cough, nausea, headache, and rhinitis. Therapeutic response often occurs within 2 wk; however, a 4- to 6-wk trial may be needed to determine maximum benefit.

Use spacer device with MDI to improve drug delivery. Shake MDI well before each use. When using a new canister of drug or if canister has not been used for >7 days, prime the MDI with three actuations before use.
For ophthalmic use, remove contact lens.

NEOMYCIN SULFATE

Mycifradin, Neo-fradin, Neo-Tabs, Myciguent, and others

Antibiotic, aminoglycoside; ammonium detoxicant

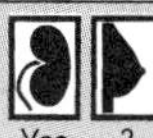
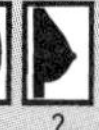
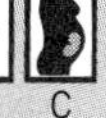

Tabs (Neo-Tabs): 500 mg
Oral solution (Mycifradin, Neo-fradin): 125 mg/5 mL; contains parabens
Ointment (Myciguent): 0.5% (15, 30 g)

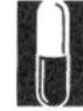

Diarrhea:
Preterm and newborn: 50 mg/kg/24 hr ÷ Q6 hr PO

Hepatic encephalopathy:
Infant and child: 50–100 mg/kg/24 hr ÷ Q6–8 hr PO × 5–6 days. **Max. dose:** 12 g/24 hr
Adult: 4–12 g/24 hr ÷ Q4–6 hr PO × 5–6 days

Bowel prep:
Child: 90 mg/kg/24 hr PO ÷ Q4 hr × 2–3 days
Adult: 1 g Q1 hr PO × 4 doses, then 1 g Q4 hr PO × 5 doses. (Many other regimens exist.)

Topical: Apply QD–TID to infected area.

Contraindicated in ulcerative bowel disease or intestinal obstruction. Monitor for nephrotoxicity and ototoxicity. Oral absorption is limited, but levels may accumulate. Consider dosage reduction in the presence of renal failure. May cause itching, redness, edema, colitis, candidiasis, or poor wound healing if applied topically.

For explanation of icons, see p. 680.

NEOMYCIN/POLYMYXIN B/± BACITRACIN

Neosporin GU Irrigant, Neosporin, Neosporin Ophthalmic, and others

Topical antibiotic

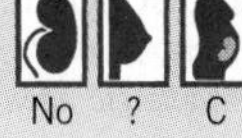
No ? C

Solution, genitourinary irrigant: 40 mg neomycin sulfate, 200,000 U polymyxin B/mL (1, 20 mL); multidose vial contains methylparabens.

In combination with bacitracin:

Ointment, topical (Neosporin) (OTC): 3.5 mg neomycin sulfate, 400 U bacitracin, 5000 U polymyxin B/g (0.9, 14, 28 g)

Ointment, ophthalmic (Neosporin Ophthalmic): 3.5 mg neomycin sulfate, 400 U bacitracin, 10,000 U polymyxin B/g (3.5 g)

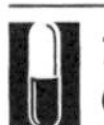

Topical: Apply to minor wounds and burns QD–TID.

Ophthalmic: Apply small amount to conjunctiva Q3–4 hr × 7–10 days, depending on the severity of infection.

Bladder irrigation:

Adults: Mix 1 mL in 1000 mL NS and administer via a 3-way catheter at a rate adjusted to the patient's urine output. **Do not exceed** 10 days of continuous use.

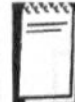

Do not use for extended periods. May cause superinfection, delayed healing. See *Neomycin Sulfate*. Ophthalmic preparation may cause stinging and sensitivity to bright light. **Avoid** use of bladder irrigant in patients with defects in the bladder mucosa or wall.

NEOSTIGMINE

Prostigmin and others

Anticholinesterase (cholinergic) agent

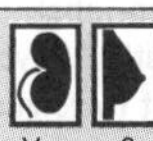
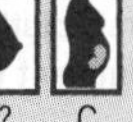
Yes ? C

Tabs: 15 mg (bromide)

Injection: 0.25, 0.5, 1 mg/mL (methylsulfate); may contain parabens or phenol

Myasthenia gravis-diagnosis: use with atropine (see comments).

Child: 0.025–0.04 mg/kg IM × 1

Adult: 0.02 mg/kg IM × 1

Treatment:

Child:

IM/IV/SC: 0.01–0.04 mg/kg/dose Q2–3 hr PRN

PO: 2 mg/kg/24 hr ÷ Q3–4 hr

Adult:

IM/IV/SC: 0.5–2.5 mg/dose Q1–3 hr PRN

PO: 15 mg/dose TID. May increase every 1–2 days. Dosage requirements may vary from 15–375 mg/24 hr.

Continued

NEOSTIGMINE *continued*

Reversal of nondepolarizing neuromuscular blocking agents: Administer with atropine or glycopyrrolate.

Infant: 0.025–0.1 mg/kg/dose IV
Child: 0.025–0.08 mg/kg/dose IV
Adult: 0.5–2.5 mg/dose IV
Max. dose: 5 mg/dose

Contraindicated in GI and urinary obstruction. **Caution** in asthmatics. May cause cholinergic crisis, bronchospasm, salivation, nausea, vomiting, diarrhea, miosis, diaphoresis, lacrimation, bradycardia, hypotension, fatigue, confusion, respiratory depression, and seizures. Titrate for each patient, but **avoid** excessive cholinergic effects.

For diagnosis of myasthenia gravis (MG), administer atropine, 0.011 mg/kg/dose IV immediately before or IM (0.011 mg/kg/dose) 30 min before neostigmine. For treatment of MG, patients may need higher doses of neostigmine at times of greatest fatigue.

Antidote: Atropine 0.01–0.04 mg/kg/dose. Atropine and epinephrine should be available in the event of a hypersensitivity reaction.

Adjust dose in renal failure (see Chapter 30).

NEVIRAPINE

Viramune, NVP

Antiviral, non-nucleoside reverse transcriptase inhibitor

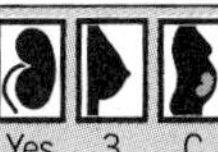

Tabs: 200 mg
Oral suspension: 10 mg/mL (240 mL); contains parabens

HIV: See www.aidsinfo.nih.gov/guidelines
Prevention of vertical transmission: see Chapter 16

See www.aidsinfo.nih.gov/guidelines for additional remarks.
Use with caution in patients with hepatic or renal dysfunction. Most frequent side effects include skin rash (may be life-threatening, including Stevens-Johnson syndrome), fever, abnormal liver function tests, headache, and nausea. **Discontinue therapy** if a severe rash or a rash with fever, blistering, oral lesions, conjunctivitis, or muscle aches occur. **Life-threatening** hepatotoxicity has been reported primarily during the first 12 wk of therapy. Patients with increased serum transaminase or a history of hepatitis B or C infection before nevirapine are at greater risk for hepatotoxicity. Women, including pregnant women, with CD4 counts >250 cell/mm^3 are at risk for hepatotoxicity. Monitor liver function tests and CBCs.

Nevirapine induces the CYP450 3A4 drug metabolizing isoenzyme to cause an autoinduction of its own metabolism within the first 2–4 wk of therapy and has the potential to interact with many drugs. **Carefully review the patients' drug profile for other drug interactions each time nevirapine is initiated or when a new drug is added to a regimen containing nevirapine.**

Doses can be administered with food and concurrently with didanosine.

For explanation of icons, see p. 680.

NIACIN/VITAMIN B_3

Niacor, Niaspan, Nicolar, Nicotinic acid, Vitamin B_3, and others
Vitamin, water soluble

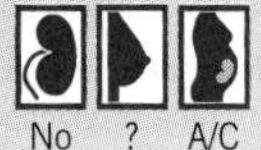
No ? A/C

Tabs (OTC): 50, 100, 250, 500 mg
Timed or extended-release tabs (OTC): 250, 500, 750, 1000 mg
Timed or extended-release caps: 125, 250, 400, 500 mg
Elixir: 50 mg/5 mL (473 mL); contains 10% alcohol

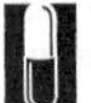

U.S. RDA: see Chapter 20
Pellagra PO:
Child: 50–100 mg/dose TID
Adult: 50–100 mg/dose TID–QID
Max. dose: 500 mg/24 hr

Contraindicated in hepatic dysfunction, active peptic ulcer, and severe hypotension. Adverse reactions of flushing, pruritus, or GI distress may occur with PO administration. May cause hyperglycemia, hyperuricemia, blurred vision, abnormal liver function tests, dizziness, and headaches. May cause false-positive urine catecholamines (fluorometric methods) and urine glucose (Benedict's reagent).

Pregnancy category changes to C if used in doses above the RDA or for typical doses used for lipid disorders. See Chapter 20 for multivitamin preparations.

NICARDIPINE

Cardene, Cardene SR, and others
Calcium-channel blocker, antihypertensive

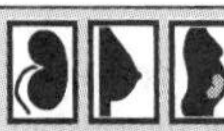
Yes 3 C

Caps (immediate release): 20, 30 mg
Sustained-release caps: 30, 45, 60 mg
Injection: 2.5 mg/mL (10 mL)

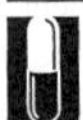

Child (see remarks):
Hypertension:
Continuous IV infusion: 0.5–5 mcg/kg/min

Adult:
Hypertension:
Oral:
Immediate release: 20 mg PO TID, dose may be increased after 3 days to 40 mg PO TID if needed.
Sustained release: 30 mg PO BID, dose may be increased after 3 days to 60 mg PO BID if needed.
Continuous IV infusion: Start at 5 mg/hr, increase dose as needed by 2.5 mg/hr Q5–15 min up to a **max. dose** of 15 mg/hr. Following attainment of desired BP, decrease infusion to 3 mg/hr and adjust rate as needed to maintain desired response.

Continued

NICARDIPINE *continued*

Reported use in children has been limited to a small number of preterm infants, infants, and children. **Contraindicated** in advanced aortic stenosis. **Use with caution** in hepatic or renal dysfunction by carefully titrating dose. The drug undergoes significant first-pass metabolism through the liver and is excreted in the urine (60%). May cause headache, dizziness, asthenia, peripheral edema, and GI symptoms. **See nifedipine for drug and food interactions.** Onset of action for PO administration is 20 min with peak effects in 0.5–2 hr. IV onset of action is 1 min. Duration of action following a single IV or PO dose is 3 hr. For additional information, see Chapter 4.

NIFEDIPINE

Adalat, Adalat CC, Procardia, Procardia XL, and others
Calcium-channel blocker, antihypertensive

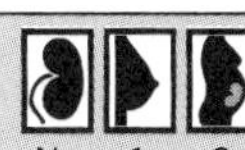

Caps (Adalat, Procardia): 10 mg (0.34 mL), 20 mg (0.45 mL)
Sustained-release tabs (Adalat CC, Procardia XL): 30, 60, 90 mg

Child (see remarks for precautions):
Hypertensive urgency: 0.25–0.5 mg/kg/dose Q4–6 hr PRN PO/SL. **Max. dose:** 10 mg/dose or 3 mg/kg/24 hr
Hypertension:
Sustained-release: Start with 0.25–0.5 mg/kg/24 hr ÷ Q12–24 hr. May increase to **max. dose:** 3 mg/kg/24 hr up to 120 mg/24 hr.
Hypertrophic cardiomyopathy: 0.5–0.9 mg/kg/24 hr ÷ Q6–8 hr PO/SL

Adult:
Hypertension:
Caps: Start with 10 mg/dose PO TID. May increase to 30 mg/dose PO TID–QID. **Max. dose:** 180 mg/24 hr
Sustained-release: Start with 30–60 mg PO QD. May increase to **max. dose:** 120 mg/24 hr.

Use of immediate-release dosage form in children is controversial and has been abandoned by some. **Use with caution** in children with acute CNS injury due to increased risk for stroke, seizure, and altered level of consciousness. To prevent rapid decrease in blood pressure in children, an initial dose of ≤0.25 mg/kg is recommended.

Use with caution in patients with CHF and aortic stenosis. May cause severe hypotension, peripheral edema, flushing, tachycardia, headaches, dizziness, nausea, palpitations, and syncope. Although overall use in adults has been abandoned, the immediate-release dosage form is **contraindicated** in adults with severe obstructive coronary artery disease or recent MI, and hypertensive emergencies.

Nifedipine is a substrate for CYP450 3A3/4 and 3A5-7. **Do not administer** with grapefruit juice; may increase bioavailability and effects. Itraconazole and ketoconazole may increase nifedipine levels/effects. Nifedipine may increase

Continued

For explanation of icons, see p. 680.

NIFEDIPINE *continued*

phenytoin, cyclosporine, and digoxin levels. For hypertensive emergencies, see Chapter 4.

For sublingual administration, capsule must be punctured and liquid expressed into mouth. A small amount is absorbed via the SL route. Most effects are due to swallowing and oral absorption. **Do not** crush or chew sustained-release tablet dosage form.

NITROFURANTOIN

Furadantin, Macrodantin, Macrobid, and others

Antibiotic

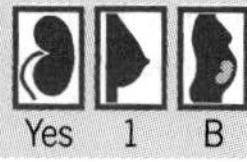

Caps (macrocrystals; Macrodantin): 25, 50, 100 mg
Caps (dual-release; Macrobid): 100 mg (25 mg macrocrystal/75 mg monohydrate)
Oral suspension (Furadantin): 25 mg/5 mL (470 mL); contains saccharin

Child (>1 mo):
Treatment: 5–7 mg/kg/24 hr ÷ Q6 hr PO; **max. dose:** 400 mg/24 hr
UTI prophylaxis: 1–2 mg/kg/dose QHS PO; **max. dose:** 100 mg/24 hr
Adult:
Macrocrystals: 50–100 mg/dose Q6 hr PO
Dual-release: 100 mg/dose Q12 hr PO
UTI prophylaxis (macrocrystals): 50–100 mg/dose PO QHS

Contraindicated in severe renal disease, G6PD deficiency, infants <1 mo of age, and pregnant women at term. May cause nausea, hypersensitivity reactions, vomiting, cholestatic jaundice, headache, hepatotoxicity, polyneuropathy, and hemolytic anemia. Causes false-positive urine glucose with Clinitest. Administer doses with food or milk.

NITROGLYCERIN

Tridil, Nitro-Bid, Nitrostat, Nitro-Dur, and others

Vasodilator, antihypertensive

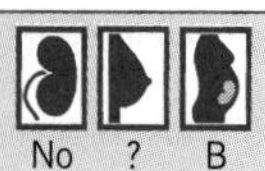

Injection: 0.5, 5 mg/mL; may contain alcohol or propylene glycol.
Prediluted injection in D5W: 100 mcg/mL (250, 500 mL), 200 mcg/mL (250 mL), 400 mcg/mL (250, 500 mL)
Sublingual tabs: 0.3, 0.4, 0.6 mg
Buccal tabs (controlled-release): 2, 3 mg
Sustained-release caps: 2.5, 6.5, 9 mg
Ointment, topical: 2% (30, 60 g)
Patch: 2.5 mg/24 hr (0.1 mg/hr), 5 mg/24 hr (0.2 mg/hr), 7.5 mg/24 hr (0.3 mg/hr), 10 mg/24 hr (0.4 mg/hr), 15 mg/24 hr (0.6 mg/hr), 20 mg/24 hr (0.8 mg/hr)
Spray, translingual: 0.4 mg per metered spray (14.48 g, delivers 200 doses per canister)

Continued

NITROGLYCERIN *continued*

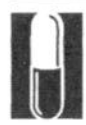

Child:

Continuous IV infusion: Begin with 0.25–0.5 mcg/kg/min; may increase by 0.5–1 mcg/kg/min Q3–5 min PRN. Usual dose: 1–5 mcg/kg/min. **Max. dose:** 20 mcg/kg/min.

Adult:

Continuous IV infusion: 5 mcg/min IV, then increase Q3–5 min PRN by 5 mcg/min up to 20 mcg/min. If no response, increase by 10 mcg/min Q3–5 min PRN up to a **max. dose** of 200 mcg/min.

To prepare infusion: see inside front cover.

NOTE: The dosage units for adults are in mcg/min; compared with mcg/kg/min for children.

Sublingual: 0.2–0.6 mg Q5 min. **Maximum** of three doses in 15 min.
Oral: 2.5–9 mg BID-TID; up to 26 mg QID
Ointment: Apply 1–2 inches Q8 hr, up to 4–5 inches Q4 hr.
Patch: 0.2–0.4 mg/hr initially, then titrate to 0.4–0.8 mg/hr; apply new patch daily (tolerance is minimized by removing patch for 10–12 hr/24 hr).

Contraindicated in glaucoma and severe anemia. In small doses (1–2 mcg/kg/min) acts mainly on systemic veins and decreases preload. At 3–5 mcg/kg/min acts on systemic arterioles to decrease resistance. May cause headache, flushing, GI upset, blurred vision, and methemoglobinemia. **Use with caution** in severe renal impairment, increased ICP, and hepatic failure. IV nitroglycerin may antagonize anticoagulant effect of heparin.

Decrease dose gradually in patients receiving drug for prolonged periods to **avoid** withdrawal reaction. Must use polypropylene infusion sets to avoid adsorption of drug to plastic tubing.

Onset (duration) of action: IV: 1–2 min (3–5 min); sublingual: 1–3 min (30–60 min); PO sustained-release: 40 min (4–8 hr); topical ointment: 20–60 min (2–12 hr); and transdermal patch: 40–60 min (18–24 hr)

NITROPRUSSIDE

Nipride and others

Vasodilator, antihypertensive

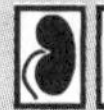
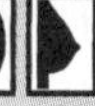
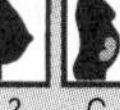

Yes ? C

Injection: 25 mg/mL (2 mL)
Powder for injection: 50 mg

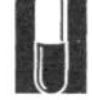

Child and adult: IV, continuous infusion
Dose: Start at 0.3–0.5 mcg/kg/min, titrate to effect. Usual dose is 3–4 mcg/kg/min. **Max. dose:** 10 mcg/kg/min.

To prepare infusion: see inside front cover.

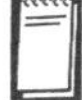

Contraindicated in patients with decreased cerebral perfusion and in situations of compensatory hypertension (increased ICP). Monitor for hypotension and acidosis. Dilute with D5W and protect from light.

Continued

For explanation of icons, see p. 680.

NITROPRUSSIDE *continued*

Nitroprusside is nonenzymatically converted to cyanide, which is converted to thiocyanate. Cyanide may produce metabolic acidosis and methemoglobinemia; thiocyanate may produce psychosis and seizures. Monitor thiocyanate levels if used for >48 hr or if dose ≥4 mcg/kg/min. **Thiocyanate levels should be <50 mg/L.** Monitor **cyanide levels (toxic levels >2 mcg/mL)** in patients with hepatic dysfunction and thiocyanate levels in patients with renal dysfunction.
Onset of action is 2 min with a 1- to 10-min duration of effect.

NOREPINEPHRINE BITARTRATE
Levophed and others
Adrenergic agonist

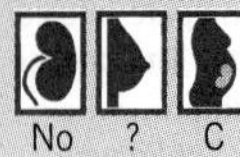

Injection: 1 mg/mL as norepinephrine base (4 mL); contains sulfites

Child: Continuous IV infusion doses as norepinephrine base. Start at 0.05–0.1 mcg/kg/min. Titrate to effect. **Max. dose:** 2 mcg/kg/min.
To prepare infusion: see inside front cover.
Adult: Continuous IV infusion doses as norepinephrine base. Start at 4 mcg/min and titrate to effect. Usual dosage range: 8–12 mcg/min.
NOTE: The dosage units for adults are in mcg/min; compared with mcg/kg/min for children.

May cause cardiac arrhythmias, hypertension, hypersensitivity, headaches, vomiting, uterine contractions, and organ ischemia. May cause decreased renal blood flow and urine output. **Avoid** extravasation into tissues; may cause severe tissue necrosis. If this occurs, treat locally with phentolamine.

NORFLOXACIN
Noroxin, Chibroxin
Antibiotic, quinolone

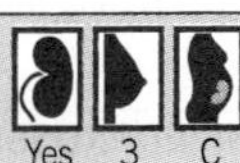

Tabs: 400 mg
Ophthalmic drops (Chibroxin): 3 mg/mL (5 mL)

Child:
UTI (limited data in children 5 mo–19 yr): 9–14 mg/kg/24 hr PO ÷ Q12 hr; **max. dose:** 800 mg/24 hr. For UTI prophylaxis, give 2–6 mg/kg/24 hr.

Adult:
UTI: 400 mg PO Q12 hr (× 7–10 days for uncomplicated cases and × 10–21 days for complicated cases)
Prostatitis: 400 mg PO Q12 hr × 28 days
N. gonorrhoeae (uncomplicated): 800 mg PO × 1

Ophthalmic
≥1 yr–adult: 1–2 drops QID × ≤7 days. May give up to Q2 hr for severe infections during the first day of therapy.

Continued

NORFLOXACIN *continued*

Like other quinolones, there is concern regarding development of arthropathy, which has been shown in immature animals. Norfloxacin does **NOT** adequately treat chlamydia coinfections. UTI dosing can be used for BK virus nephropathy in immunocompromised patients. **Use with caution** in children <18 yr. Inhibits CYP450 1A2. May increase serum theophylline levels. May prolong PT in patients on warfarin. See *Ciprofloxacin* for common side effects and drug interactions. QTc prolongation, peripheral neuropathy, and tendon rupture have been reported.

Ophthalmic dosage form may cause local burning or discomfort, photophobia, and bitter taste. Administer oral doses on an empty stomach.

Adjust dose in renal failure with systemic use (see Chapter 30).

NORTRIPTYLINE HYDROCHLORIDE

Pamelor, Aventyl, and others

Antidepressant, tricyclic

No 3 D

Caps: 10, 25, 50, 75 mg; may contain benzyl alcohol, EDTA
Oral solution: 10 mg/5 mL; contains up to 4% alcohol

Depression:
Child 6–12 yr: 1–3 mg/kg/24 hr ÷ TID–QID PO or 10–20 mg/24 hr ÷ TID–QID PO
Adolescent: 1–3 mg/kg/24 hr ÷ TID–QID PO or 30–50 mg/24 hr ÷ TID–QID PO
Adult: 75–100 mg/24 hr ÷ TID–QID PO
Max. dose: 150 mg/24 hr

Nocturnal enuresis:
6–7 yr (20–25 kg): 10 mg PO QHS
8–11 yr (26–35 kg): 10–20 mg PO QHS
>11 yr (36–54 kg): 25–35 mg PO QHS

See *Imipramine* for contraindications and common side effects. Less CNS and anticholinergic side effects than amitriptyline. Lower doses and slower dose titration are recommended in hepatic impairment. Therapeutic antidepressant effects occur in 7–21 days. **Do not** discontinue abruptly. Nortriptyline is a substrate for the cytochrome P450 1A2 and 2D6 drug metabolizing enzymes.

Therapeutic nortriptyline levels for depression: 50–150 ng/mL. Recommended serum sampling time: obtain a single level 8 or more hr after an oral dose (following 4 days of continuous dosing for children and after 9–10 days for adults).

Administer with food to decrease GI upset.

For explanation of icons, see p. 680.

NYSTATIN

Mycostatin, Nilstat, and others
Antifungal agent

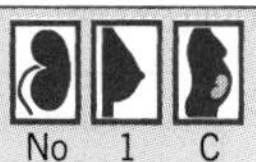

Tabs: 500,000 U
Troches/pastilles: 200,000 U
Oral suspension: 100,000 U/mL (5, 60, 480 mL)
Cream/ointment: 100,000 U/g (15, 30 g)
Topical powder: 100,000 U/g (15, 30 g)
Vaginal tabs: 100,000 U (15s)

Oral:
Preterm infant: 0.5 mL (50,000 U) to each side of mouth QID
Term infant: 1 mL (100,000 U) to each side of mouth QID
Child/adult:
Suspension: 4–6 mL (400,000–600,000 U) swish and swallow QID.
Troche: 200,000–400,000 U 4–5×/24 hr
Vaginal: 1 tab QHS × 14 days
Topical: Apply to affected areas BID–QID.

May produce diarrhea and GI side effects. Treat until 48–72 hr after resolution of symptoms. Drug is poorly absorbed through the GI tract. **Do not** swallow troches whole (allow to dissolve slowly). Oral suspension should be swished about the mouth and retained in the mouth as long as possible before swallowing.

OCTREOTIDE ACETATE

Sandostatin, Sandostatin LAR Depot
Somatostatin analog, antisecretory agent

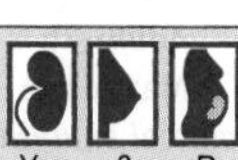

Injection (amps): 0.05, 0.1, 0.5 mg/mL (1 mL)
Injection (multidose vials): 0.2, 1 mg/mL (5 mL)
Injection, microspheres for suspension (Sandostatin LAR Depot): 10, 20, 30 mg

Infant and child (limited data):
Intractable diarrhea (IV/SC): 1–10 mcg/kg/24 hr ÷ Q12–24 hr. Dose may be increased within the recommended range by 0.3 mcg/kg/dose every 3 days as needed.
Max. dose: 1500 mcg/24 hr

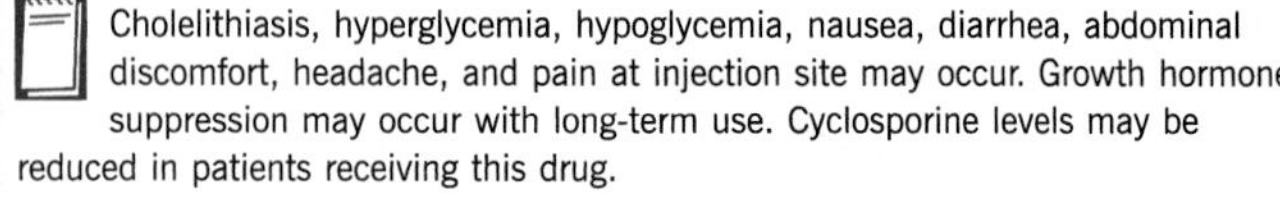

Cholelithiasis, hyperglycemia, hypoglycemia, nausea, diarrhea, abdominal discomfort, headache, and pain at injection site may occur. Growth hormone suppression may occur with long-term use. Cyclosporine levels may be reduced in patients receiving this drug.

Continued

OCTREOTIDE ACETATE *continued*

Patients with severe renal failure requiring dialysis may require dosage adjustments due to an increase in half-life. The effects of hepatic dysfunction on octreotide have not been evaluated.

Sandostatin LAR Depot is administered once every 4 wk **only** by the IM route and is currently indicated for use in adults who have been stabilized on IV/SC therapy. See package insert for details.

OFLOXACIN

Floxin, Floxin Otic, Ocuflox

Antibiotic, quinolone

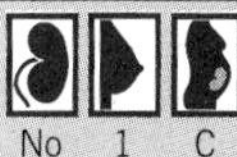

Otic solution (Floxin Otic): 0.3% (5, 10 mL)
Ophthalmic solution (Ocuflox): 0.3% (1, 5, 10 mL)
Tabs: 200, 300, 400 mg
Prediluted injection in D5W: 200 mg/50 mL, 400 mg/100 mL

Otitic use:

Otitis externa:

1–12 yr: 5 drops to affected ear(s) BID × 10 days
≥12 yr: 10 drops to affected ear(s) BID × 10 days

Chronic suppurative otitis media:

≥12 yr: 10 drops to affected ear(s) BID × 14 days

Acute otitis media with tympanostomy tubes:

1–12 yr: 5 drops to affected ear(s) BID × 10 days

Ophthalmic use:

>1 yr: 1–2 drops to affected eye(s) Q2–4 hr × 2 days, then QID for an additional 5 days

Uncomplicated gonorrhea (see remarks):

Adult: 400 mg PO × 1, plus treatment for chlamydia

PID (see remarks):

Adult: 400 mg PO BID × 10–14 days in combination with metronidazole

Pruritus, local irritation, taste perversion, dizziness, earache have been reported with otic use. Ocular burning/discomfort is frequent with ophthalmic use. Consult with ophthalmology in corneal ulcers.

When using otic solution, warm solution by holding the bottle in the hand for 1–2 min. Cold solutions may result in dizziness. For otitis externa, patient should lie with affected ear upward before instillation and remain in the same position after dose administration for 5 min to enhance drug delivery. For acute otitis media with tympanostomy tubes, patient should lie in the same position before instillation, and the tragus should be pumped 4 times after the dose to assist in drug delivery to the middle ear.

Systemic use of ofloxacin is typically replaced by levofloxacin. Levofloxacin is the S-isomer of ofloxacin with a more favorable side-effect profile than ofloxacin. See *Levofloxacin*.

For explanation of icons, see p. 680.

OLOPATADINE
Patanol
Antihistamine

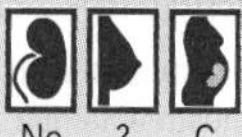
No ? C

Ophthalmic solution: 0.1% (5 mL)

Allergic conjunctivitis:
≥3 yr and adult: 1–2 drops in affected eye(s) BID (spaced 6–8 hr apart)

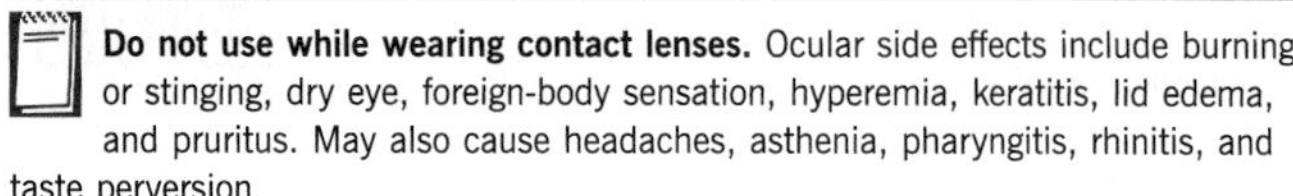
Do not use while wearing contact lenses. Ocular side effects include burning or stinging, dry eye, foreign-body sensation, hyperemia, keratitis, lid edema, and pruritus. May also cause headaches, asthenia, pharyngitis, rhinitis, and taste perversion.

OLSALAZINE
Dipentum, Di-mesalazine, Di-5-ASA
Salicylate, GI antiinflammatory agent

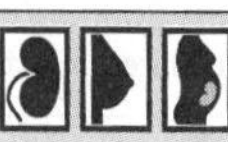
Yes 2 C

Caps: 250 mg

Ulcerative colitis:
Child: see remarks.
Adult: 500 mg PO BID

Drug is converted to 5-aminosalicylic acid (mesalamine) by colonic bacteria. 1 g olsalazine generally delivers 0.9 g of mesalamine to the colon. Only 1%–3% of olsalazine is systemically absorbed.

Contraindicated in salicylate hypersensitivity. **Use with caution** in severe liver disease, renal dysfunction, sulfasalazine hypersensitivity, and bronchial asthma. Diarrhea is the most common side effect. May also cause GI discomfort, headaches, rash, dizziness, and increased PT with warfarin use. Pancreatitis in children and hepatotoxicity has been reported. Monitor urinalysis and renal function.

Administer all doses with food to enhance efficacy.

Use in children (2–18 yr) has been limited to a trial where olsalazine 30 mg/kg/24 hr (**max. dose:** 2 g/24 hr) was found to be less efficacious than sulfasalazine 60 mg/kg/24 hr (**max. dose:** 4 g/24 hr) in treating mild/moderate ulcerative colitis. This may suggest inadequate dosing in this trial; additional studies are needed.

OMEPRAZOLE

Prilosec, Prilosec OTC, Zegerid, and others

Gastric acid pump inhibitor

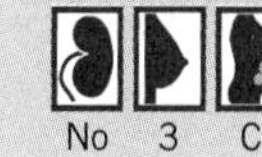

Caps, sustained release: 10, 20 (OTC), 40 mg
Powder for oral suspension (Zegerid): 20, 40 mg packets (30s); each packet (regardless of strength) contains 1680 mg (20 mEq) sodium bicarbonate
Oral suspension: 2 mg/mL ; contains ~0.5 mEq sodium bicarbonate per 1 mg drug

Child:

Esophagitis, GERD, or ulcers: 1 mg/kg/24 hr PO ÷ QD–BID. Reported effective range: 0.2–3.5 mg/kg/24 hr. Children 1–6 yr may require higher doses due to enhanced drug clearance.

Alternative dosing for patients ≥2 yr:

<20 kg: 10 mg PO QD
≥20 kg: 20 mg PO QD

Adult:

Duodenal ulcer or GERD: 20 mg/dose PO QD × 4–8 wk; may give up to 12 wk for erosive esophagitis.

Gastric ulcer: 40 mg/24 hr PO ÷ QD-BID × 4–8 wk

Pathologic hypersecretory conditions: Start with 60 mg/24 hr PO QD. If needed, dose may be increased up to 120 mg/24 hr PO ÷ TID. Daily doses >80 mg should be administered in divided doses.

Common side effects: headache, diarrhea, nausea, and vomiting. Allergic reactions including anaphylaxis have been reported. Drug induces CYP450 1A2 (decreases theophylline levels) and is also a substrate and inhibitor of CYP450 2C19. Increases $T_{1/2}$ of citalopram, diazepam, phenytoin, and warfarin. May decrease absorption of itraconazole, ketoconazole, iron salts, and ampicillin esters. May be used in combination with clarithromycin and amoxicillin for *H. pylori* infections.

Administer all doses before meals. Administer 30 min before sucralfate. Capsules contain enteric-coated granules to ensure bioavailability. **Do not** chew or crush capsule. For doses unable to be divided by 10 mg, capsule may be opened, and intact pellets may be administered in an acidic beverage (e.g., apple juice, cranberry juice) or apple sauce. The extemporaneously compounded oral suspension product may be less bioavailable owing to the loss of the enteric coating.

For explanation of icons, see p. 680.

ONDANSETRON

Zofran

Antiemetic agent, 5-HT_3 antagonist

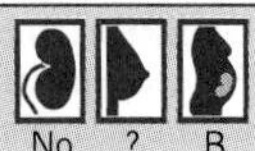

Injection: 2 mg/mL (2, 20 mL); contains parabens
Premixed injection in D5W: 32 mg/50 mL
Tabs: 4, 8, 24 mg
Tabs, orally disintegrating: 4, 8 mg; contains aspartame
Oral solution: 4 mg/5 mL (50 mL); contains sodium benzoate

Preventing nausea and vomiting associated with chemotherapy:
Oral (give initial dose 30 min before chemotherapy):
Child, dose based on body surface area:
- ***<0.3 m²:*** 1 mg TID PRN nausea
- ***0.3–0.6 m²:*** 2 mg TID PRN nausea
- ***0.6–1 m²:*** 3 mg TID PRN nausea
- ***>1 m²:*** 4–8 mg TID PRN nausea

Dose based on age:
- ***<4 yr:*** Use dose based on body surface area from above.
- ***4–11 yr:*** 4 mg TID PRN nausea
- ***≥12 yr and adult:*** 8 mg TID PRN nausea

IV: Child and adult:
Moderately emetogenic drugs: 0.15 mg/kg/dose at 30 min before, 4 and 8 hr after emetogenic drugs. Then same dose Q4 hr PRN.
Highly emetogenic drugs: 0.45 mg/kg/dose (**max. dose:** 32 mg/dose) 30 min before emetogenic drugs. Then 0.15 mg/kg/dose Q4 hr PRN.

Preventing nausea and vomiting associated with surgery *(see remarks):*
IV/IM (administered before anesthesia over 2–5 min.):
Child (2–12 yr):
- ***≤40 kg:*** 0.1 mg/kg/dose × 1
- ***>40 kg:*** 4 mg × 1

Adult: 4 mg × 1
PO:
Adult: 16 mg × 1, one hour prior to induction of anesthesia

Preventing nausea and vomiting associated with radiation therapy (adult):
Total-body irradiation: 8 mg PO 1–2 hr before radiation QD
Single high-dose fraction radiation to abdomen: 8 mg PO 1–2 hr before radiation with subsequent doses Q8 hr after 1st dose × 1–2 days after completion of radiation
Daily fractionated radiation to abdomen: 8 mg PO 1–2 hr before radiation with subsequent doses Q8 hr after first dose for each day radiation is given

Bronchospasm, tachycardia, hypokalemia, seizures, headaches, lightheadedness, constipation, diarrhea, and transient increases in AST, ALT, and bilirubin may occur. Data limited for use in children <3 yr.

Ondansetron is a substrate for cytochrome P-450 1A2, 2D6, 2E1, and 3A3/4 drug-metabolizing enzymes. It is likely that the inhibition/loss of one of the above enzymes will be compensated by others and may result in insignificant changes to ondansetron's elimination. Ondansetron's elimination may be affected by

Continued

ONDANSETRON *continued*

cytochrome P-450 enzyme inducers. Follow theophylline, phenytoin, or warfarin levels closely, if used in combination.

Additional postoperative doses for controlling nausea and vomiting may not provide any benefits.

In severe hepatic impairment, extend dosage interval up to QD and limit **max. dose** to 8 mg/dose.

Administer orally disintegrating tablet by placing it on the tongue and swallowing it with or without taking liquids.

OPIUM TINCTURE

Deodorized tincture of opium

Narcotic, analgesic

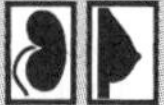
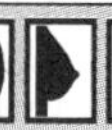
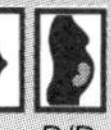

No 2 B/D

Oral liquid: 10% opium. Contains 17%–21% alcohol (1 mL equivalent to 10 mg morphine)

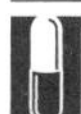

Dilute 25-fold with water to make a final concentration of 0.4 mg/mL morphine equivalent.

Neonatal opiate withdrawal:

Start with 0.08–0.12 mg (or 0.2–0.3 mL)/dose Q3–4 hr, increase dose by 0.02 mg (or 0.05 mL)/dose Q3–4 hr until symptoms abate; **max. dose:** 0.28 mg (or 0.7 mL)/dose.

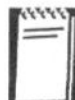

Use 25-fold dilution to treat neonatal abstinence syndrome (NAS). Follow neonatal abstinence scores. **Doses for the dilution are equivalent to paregoric doses.** Morphine may also be used to treat NAS. May cause respiratory depression, hypotension, bradycardia, and CNS depression. Pregnancy category changes to D if used for prolonged periods or in high doses at term.

OSELTAMIVIR PHOSPHATE

Tamiflu

Antiviral

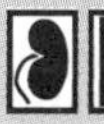
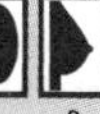
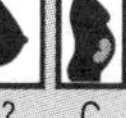

Yes ? C

Caps: 75 mg

Oral suspension: 12 mg/mL (100 mL); contains saccharin and sodium benzoate

Treatment of influenza (initiate therapy within 2 days of onset of symptoms):

Child ≥1 yr: see table below.

Weight (kg)	Dosage for 5 Days	Volume of Oral Suspension
≤15	30 mg PO BID	2.5 mL
>15–23	45 mg PO BID	3.75 mL
>23–40	60 mg PO BID	5 mL
>40	75 mg PO BID	6.25 mL

Continued

For explanation of icons, see p. 680.

OSELTAMIVIR PHOSPHATE *continued*

Treatment of influenza (initiate therapy within 2 days of onset of symptoms):

≥12 yr and adult: 75 mg PO BID × 5 days

Prophylaxis of influenza (see remarks):

≥13 yr and adult: 75 mg PO QD for a minimum of 7 days and up to 6 wk; initiate therapy within 2 days of exposure.

Currently indicated for the treatment of influenza A and B strains. **Do not use** in children <1 yr due to concerns of fatalities related to excessive CNS penetration in 7-day old rats. Nausea and vomiting generally occur within the first 2 days and are the most common adverse effects. Insomnia, vertigo, seizures, arrhythmias, rash, and toxic epidermal necrolysis have also been reported. Reduce dosage treatment dose if GFR is 10–30 mL/min by increasing the dosage interval to QD × 5 days (e.g., 75 mg PO QD × 5 days for ≥12yr and adult).

PROPHYLAXIS USE: Oseltamivir is **not** a substitute for annual flu vaccination. Safety and efficacy have been demonstrated for ≤6 wk; duration of protection lasts for as long as dosing is continued. Adjust prophylaxis dose if GFR is 10–30 mL/min by increasing the dosage interval to QOD (e.g., 75 mg PO QOD for ≥13 yr and adult).

Dosage adjustments in hepatic impairment, severe renal disease, and dialysis have not been established for either treatment or prophylaxis use. The safety and efficacy of repeated treatment or prophylaxis courses have not been evaluated. Doses may be administered with or without food.

OXACILLIN

Various generic brands

Antibiotic, penicillin (penicillinase resistant)

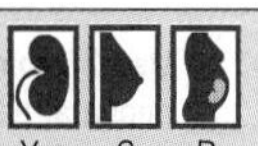

Oral solution: 250 mg/5 mL (100 mL); contains 0.8 mEq Na per 250 mg drug and may contain saccharin

Injection: 0.5, 1, 2, 10 g

Injection, premixed in iso-osmotic dextrose: 1 g/50 mL, 2 g/50 mL

Injectable products contain 2.8–3.1 mEq Na per 1 g drug.

Neonate, IM/IV: doses are the same as for nafcillin.

Infant and child:

Oral: 50–100 mg/kg/24 hr ÷ Q6 hr

IM/IV: 100–200 mg/kg/24 hr ÷ Q4–6 hr

Max. dose: 12 g/24 hr

Adult:

Oral: 500–1000 mg/dose Q4–6 hr

IM/IV: 250–2000 mg/dose Q4–6 hr

Side effects include allergy, diarrhea, nausea, vomiting, leukopenia, and hepatotoxicity. CSF penetration is poor unless meninges are inflamed. Acute interstitial nephritis has been reported. Hematuria and azotemia have occurred in neonates and infants with high doses. Use the lower end of the usual dosage range for patients with creatinine clearances <10 mL/min. Oral form should be administered on an empty stomach. **Adjust dose in renal failure (see Chapter 30).**

OXCARBAZEPINE

Trileptal

Anticonvulsant

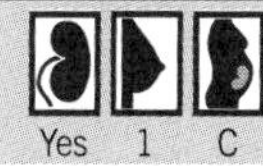

Tabs: 150, 300, 600 mg

Oral suspension: 300 mg/5 mL (250 mL); contains saccharin and ethanol

Child (4–16 yr, see remarks):

Adjunctive therapy: Start with 8–10 mg/kg/24 hr PO ÷ BID up to a **max. dose** of 600 mg/24 hr. Then gradually increase the dose over a 2-week period to the following maintenance doses:

20–29 kg: 900 mg/24 hr PO ÷ BID

29.1–39 kg: 1200 mg/24 hr PO ÷ BID

>39 kg: 1800 mg/24 hr PO ÷ BID

Conversion to monotherapy: Start with 8–10 mg/kg/24 hr PO ÷ BID and simultaneously initiate dosage reduction of concomitant AEDs and withdrawal completely over 3–6 wk. Dose may be increased at weekly intervals, as clinically indicated, by a **maximum** of 10 mg/kg/24 hr to achieve the recommended monotherapy maintenance dose as described below (see table).

Initiation of monotherapy: Start with 8–10 mg/kg/24 hr PO ÷ BID. Then increase by 5 mg/kg/24 hr every 3 days up to the recommended monotherapy maintenance dose as described below:

RECOMMENDED MONOTHERAPY MAINTENANCE DOSES FOR CHILDREN BY WEIGHT

Weight (kg)	Daily oral maintenance dose (mg/24hr) administered as a BID schedule
20	600–900
25–30	900–1200
35–40	900–1500
45	900–1800
50–55	1200–1800
60–65	1200–2100
70	1500–2100

Adult:

Adjunctive therapy: Start with 600 mg/24 hr PO ÷ BID. Dose may be increased at weekly intervals, as clinically indicated, by a **maximum** of 600 mg/24 hr. Usual maintenance dose is 1200 mg/24 hr PO ÷ BID. Doses ≥2400 mg/24 hr are generally not well tolerated due to CNS side effects.

Conversion to monotherapy: Start with 600 mg/24 hr PO ÷ BID and simultaneously initiate dosage reduction of concomitant AEDs. Dose may be increased at weekly intervals, as clinically indicated, by a **maximum** of 600 mg/24 hr to achieve a dose of 2400 mg/24 hr PO ÷ BID. Concomitant AEDs should be terminated gradually over about 3–6 wk.

Initiation of monotherapy: Start with 600 mg/24 hr PO ÷ BID. Then increase by 300 mg/24 hr every 3 days up to 1200 mg/24 hr PO ÷ BID.

Continued

For explanation of icons, see p. 680.

OXCARBAZEPINE *continued*

Clinically significant hyponatremia may occur; generally seen within the first 3 mo of therapy. May also cause headache, dizziness, drowsiness, ataxia, fatigue, nystagmus, urticaria, diplopia, abnormal gait, and GI discomfort. About 25% to 30% of patients with carbamazepine hypersensitivity will experience a cross-reaction with oxcarbazepine.

Inhibits CYP450 2C19 and induces CYP450 3A4/5 drug-metabolizing enzymes. Carbamazepine, phenobarbital, phenytoin, valproic acid, and verapamil may decrease oxcarbazepine levels. Oxcarbazepine may increase phenobarbital and phenytoin levels. Oxcarbazepine can decrease the effects of oral contraceptives, felodipine, and lamotrigine.

A median pediatric maintenance dose of 31 mg/kg/24 hr (range, 6–51 mg/kg/24 hr) was achieved in a clinical trial. Adjust dosage if GFR <30 mL/min by administering 50% of the normal starting dose (**max. dose:** 300 mg/24 hr) followed by a slower than normal increase in dose if necessary. No dosage adjustment is required in mild/moderate hepatic impairment.

Doses may be administered with or without food.

OXYBUTYNIN CHLORIDE

Ditropan, Ditropan XL, Oxytrol, and others
Anticholinergic agent, antispasmodic

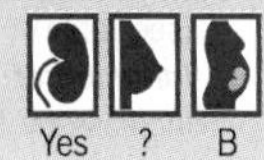

Tabs: 5 mg
Tabs, extended release (Ditropan XL): 5, 10, 15 mg
Syrup: 1 mg/mL (473 mL); contains parabens
Transdermal system (Oxytrol): delivers 3.9 mg/24 hr (8s); contains 36 mg per system

Child ≤5 yr: 0.2 mg/kg/dose BID–QID PO; **max. dose:** 15 mg/24 hr
Child >5 yr: 5 mg/dose BID–TID PO; **max. dose:** 15 mg/24 hr
Adult:
- ***Immediate release:*** 5 mg/dose BID–QID PO
- ***Extended release (Ditropan XL):*** 5–10 mg/dose QD PO up to a **max. dose** of 30 mg/dose QD PO
- ***Transdermal system:*** 1 patch (3.9 mg/24 hr) every 3–4 days (twice weekly)

Use with caution in hepatic or renal disease, hyperthyroidism, IBD, or cardiovascular disease. Anticholinergic side effects may occur, including drowsiness and hallucinations. **Contraindicated** in glaucoma, GI obstruction, megacolon, myasthenia gravis, severe colitis, hypovolemia, and GU obstruction. Oxybutynin is a CYP450 3A4 substrate; inhibitors and inducers of CYP450 3A4 may increase and decrease the effects of oxybutynin, respectively.

Dosage adjustments for the extended-release dosage form are at weekly intervals. **Do not** crush, chew, or divide the extended-release tablets. Apply transdermal system on dry intact skin on the abdomen, hip, or buttock by rotating the site and avoiding same site application within 7 days.

OXYCODONE

Roxicodone, OxyContin, and others

Narcotic, analgesic

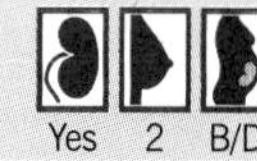
Yes 2 B/D

Solution: 1 mg/mL (5, 500 mL); contains alcohol
Concentrated solution: 20 mg/mL (30 mL); contains saccharin
Tabs: 5, 15, 30 mg
Controlled-release tabs (OxyContin): 10, 20, 40, 80, 160 mg (80 and 160 mg strengths for opioid-tolerant patients only)
Caps: 5 mg

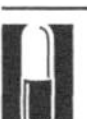

Dose based upon oxycodone salt:
Child: 0.05–0.15 mg/kg/dose Q4–6 hr PRN up to 5 mg/dose PO
Adult: 5–10 mg Q4–6 hr PRN PO; see remarks for use of controlled release tablets.

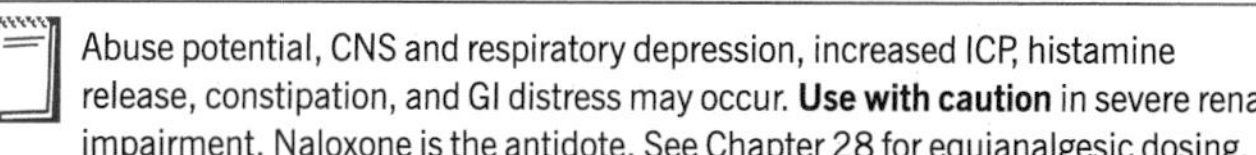

Abuse potential, CNS and respiratory depression, increased ICP, histamine release, constipation, and GI distress may occur. **Use with caution** in severe renal impairment. Naloxone is the antidote. See Chapter 28 for equianalgesic dosing. Check dosages of acetaminophen or aspirin when using combination products (e.g., Tylox, Percodan). Aspirin is not recommended in children because of concerns about Reye syndrome. Oxycodone is metabolized by the cytochrome P-450 2D6 isoenzyme.

When using controlled-release tablets (OxyContin), determine patient's total 24-hr requirements and divide by 2 to administer on a Q12 hr dosing interval. OxyContin 80 mg and 160 mg tablets are **USED ONLY** for opioid-tolerant patients; these strengths can cause fatal respiratory depression in opioid-naïve patients. Controlled-release dosage form **should not** be used as a PRN analgesic and must be swallowed whole.

Pregnancy category changes to D if used for prolonged periods or in high doses at term.

OXYCODONE AND ACETAMINOPHEN

Tylox, Roxilox, Percocet, Endocet, Roxicet, and others

Combination analgesic with a narcotic

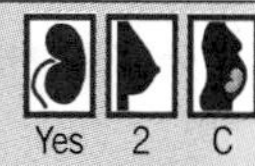
Yes 2 C

Capsule (Tylox, Roxilox)/caplet: oxycodone HCl 5 mg + acetaminophen 500 mg
Tabs (Percocet, Endocet):
Most common strength: oxycodone HCl 5 mg + acetaminophen 325 mg
Other strengths:
Oxycodone HCl 2.5 mg + acetaminophen 325 mg
Oxycodone HCl 7.5 mg + acetaminophen 325 mg or 500 mg
Oxycodone HCl 10 mg + acetaminophen 325 mg or 650 mg
Oral solution (Roxicet): oxycodone HCl 5 mg + acetaminophen 325 mg/5 mL (5, 500 mL); contains 0.4% alcohol and saccharin

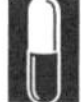

Dose based on amount of oxycodone and acetaminophen.

See *Oxycodone* and *Acetaminophen*.

For explanation of icons, see p. 680.

OXYCODONE AND ASPIRIN

Percodan, Roxiprin, Percodan-Demi, and others

Combination analgesic (narcotic and salicylate)

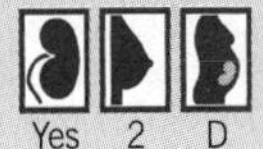

Tabs:

(Percodan or Roxiprin): oxycodone HCl 4.5 mg, oxycodone terephthalate 0.38 mg, and aspirin 325 mg

(Percodan-Demi): oxycodone HCl 2.25 mg, oxycodone terephthalate 0.19 mg, and aspirin 325 mg

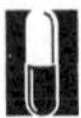

Dose based on amount of oxycodone (combined salts) and aspirin.

See *Oxycodone* and *Aspirin*. **Do not use** in children <16 yr because of risk for Reye syndrome.

OXYMETAZOLINE

Nasal: Afrin, Duramist, Neo-Synephrine 12-Hour Nasal, Nostrilla, and others

Ophthalmic: Ocu Clear, Visine LR

Nasal decongestant, vasoconstrictor

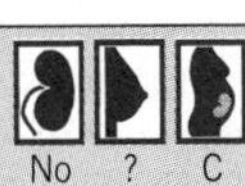

Nasal spray (OTC): 0.05% (15, 30 mL)

Ophthalmic drops (OTC): 0.025% (15, 30 mL)

Nasal decongestant (not to exceed 3 days in duration):

≥6 yr–adult: 2–3 sprays or 2–3 drops or 1–2 metered sprays (Nostrilla) in each nostril BID

Ophthalmic:

≥6 yr–adult: Instill 1–2 drops in the affected eye(s) Q6 hr.

Contraindicated in patients on MAO inhibitor therapy. Rebound nasal congestion may occur with excessive use (>3 days) via the nasal route.

Systemic absorption may occur with either route of administration. Headache, dizziness, hypertension, transient burning, stinging, dryness, nasal mucosa ulceration, sneezing, blurred vision, and mydriasis have occurred. **Do not use** ophthalmic solution if it changes color or becomes cloudy.

PALIVIZUMAB

Synagis

Monoclonal antibody

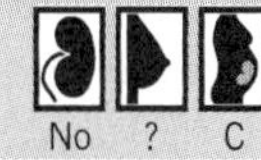

Injection: 50, 100 mg

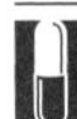

RSV prophylaxis (see Chapter 15 and latest edition of AAP *Red Book* for most recent indications):

≤2 yr with chronic lung disease, premature infants (≤28 weeks' gestation) <12 mo of age, premature infants (29–32 weeks' gestation) <6 mo of age, or hemodynamically significant cyanotic and acyanotic congenital heart disease: 15 mg/kg/dose IM Q monthly just before and during the RSV season.

RSV season is typically November through April in the northern hemisphere but may begin earlier or persist later in certain communities. **Use with caution** in patients with thrombocytopenia or any coagulation disorder because of IM route of administration. IM is currently the only route of administration. The following adverse effects have been reported at slightly higher incidences when compared with placebo: rhinitis, rash, pain, increased liver enzymes, pharyngitis, cough, wheeze, diarrhea, vomiting, conjunctivitis, and anemia.

Does not interfere with the response to routine childhood vaccines. Palivizumab is currently indicated for RSV prophylaxis only and has not been evaluated in immunocompromised children.

Each dose should be administered IM in the anterolateral aspect of the thigh. It is recommended to divide doses with total injection volumes >1 mL. **Avoid** injection in the gluteal muscle because of risk for damage to the sciatic nerve. Reconstitute each vial with 1 mL sterile water for injection, and gently swirl the contents. Dose should be administered within 6 hr of reconstitution.

PAMIDRONATE

Aredia and others

Bisphosphonate derivative, hypercalcemia antidote

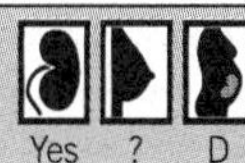

Injection: 3, 6, 9 mg/mL (10 mL); contains mannitol
Injection, powder: 30, 90 mg; contains mannitol

Hypercalcemia *(dose may be repeated after 7 days; see remarks):*

Child (limited data; see J Clin Oncol 1999;17(6):1960):

- ***Mild hypercalcemia:*** 0.5–1 mg/kg/dose IV × 1
- ***Severe hypercalcemia:*** 1.5–2 mg/kg/dose IV × 1

Adult:

- ***Corrected serum Ca^{2+} 12–13.5 mg/dL:*** 60 mg IV × 1 over 4 hr **OR** 90 mg IV × 1 over 24 hr
- ***Corrected serum Ca^{2+} >13.5 mg/dL:*** 90 mg IV × 1 over 24 hr

Continued

For explanation of icons, see p. 680.

PAMIDRONATE *continued*

Osteogenesis imperfecta *(limited data):*

Child: 0.5–1 mg/kg/dose IV QD × 3 days; may be repeated in 4–6 mo

Paget disease:

Adult: 30 mg IV over 4 hr QD × 3 days

May cause headache, hypertension, GI discomfort, uveitis, hyperpyrexia, and decrease in serum calcium, phosphorus, potassium, and magnesium. Renal failure and osteonecrosis of the jaw have been reported. **Use caution** in renal impairment and with other nephrotoxic drugs. Maintain adequate hydration and urinary output during treatment. Longer infusion times (2–24 hr) may decrease the risk for renal toxicity, especially in patients with renal insufficiency.

USE IN HYPERCALCEMIA: correct serum Ca^{2+} for low serum albumin (a change in serum albumin of 1 g/dL changes serum Ca^{2+} in the same direction by 0.8 mg/dL). Local redness, swelling, induration, or pain on palpation at the catheter site is common in patients receiving a 90-mg dose. Seizures have been reported.

PANCREATIC ENZYMES

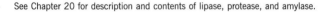

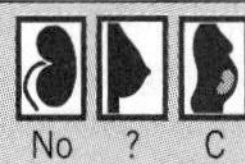

See Chapter 20 for description and contents of lipase, protease, and amylase.

Initial doses: (actual requirements are patient specific)

Enteric-coated microspheres and microtabs:

Infant: 2000–4000 U lipase per 120 mL formula or per breast-feeding

Child <4 yr: 1000 U lipase/kg/meal

Child ≥4 yr and adult: 500 U lipase/kg/meal

Max. dose: 2500 U lipase/kg/meal

The total daily dose should include approximately three meals and two to three snacks per day. Snack doses are approximately half of meal doses.

May cause occult GI bleeding, allergic reactions to porcine proteins, and hyperuricemia and hyperuricosuria with high doses. Dose should be titrated to eliminate diarrhea and to minimize steatorrhea. **Do not** chew microspheres or microtabs. Concurrent administration with H_2 antagonists or gastric acid pump inhibitors may enhance enzyme efficacy. Doses higher than 6000 U lipase/kg/meal have been associated with colonic strictures in children <12 yr. Powder dosage form is **not preferred** because of potential GI mucosal ulceration. **Avoid** use of generic pancreatic enzyme products because they been associated with treatment failures.

PANCURONIUM BROMIDE

Various generic brands

Nondepolarizing neuromuscular blocking agent

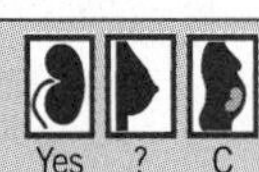

Injection: 1, 2 mg/mL (contains benzyl alcohol)

Continued

PANCURONIUM BROMIDE *continued*

Neonate:
Initial: 0.02 mg/kg/dose IV
Maintenance: 0.05–0.1 mg/kg/dose Q0.5–4 hr PRN

1 mo–adult:
Initial: 0.04–0.1 mg/kg/dose IV
Maintenance: 0.015–0.1 mg/kg/dose IV Q30–60 min
Continuous IV infusion: 0.1 mg/kg/hr

Onset of action is 1–2 min. May cause tachycardia, salivation, and wheezing. Drug effects may be accentuated by hypothermia, acidosis, neonatal age, decreased renal function, halothane, succinylcholine, hypokalemia, hyponatremia, hypocalcemia, clindamycin, tetracycline, and aminoglycoside antibiotics. Drug effects may be antagonized by alkalosis, hypercalcemia, peripheral neuropathies, diabetes mellitus, demyelinating lesions, carbamazepine, phenytoin, theophylline, anticholinesterases (e.g., neostigmine, pyridostigmine), and azathioprine.

Reversal agent is neostigmine (coadminister with atropine or glycopyrrolate). **Avoid** use in severe renal impairment (Creatinine clearance <10 mL/min).

PANTOPRAZOLE
Protonix
Gastric acid pump inhibitor

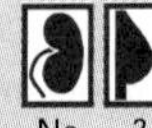
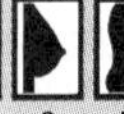
No ? B

Tabs, enteric coated: 20, 40 mg
Injection: 40 mg; contains edetate sodium
Oral suspension: 2 mg/mL ; contains 0.25 mEq sodium bicarbonate per 1 mg drug

Child:
GERD with erosive esophagitis *(limited data):* 0.5–1 mg/kg/dose PO QD × 28 days; dosed as 20 mg PO QD in 15 children 6–13 yr weighing 20–40 kg
IV (data limited to pharmacokinetic trials): Single doses ranging from 0.32–1.88 mg/kg/dose have been reported from three separate trials (total *N*=31; 0.01–16.4 yr). Patients with Systemic Inflammatory Response Syndrome (SIRS) cleared the drug slower, resulting in higher $T_{1/2}$ and AUC, than patients without. Despite limited data, 1–2 mg/kg/24 hr ÷ Q12–24 hr have been used. Additional studies are needed.

Adult:
GERD: 40 mg PO QD × 8–16 wk or 40 mg IV QD × 7–10 days
Peptic ulcer: 40–80 mg PO QD × 4–8 wk
Hypersecretory conditions:
PO: 40 mg BID; dose may be increased as needed up to 240 mg/24 hr.
IV: 80 mg Q12 hr IV; dose may be increased as needed to Q8 hr (240 mg/24 hr). Therapy >6 days at 240 mg/24 hr has not been evaluated.

Convert from IV to PO therapy as soon as patient is able to tolerate PO. Common side effects include diarrhea and headache. May cause transient elevation in LFTs. May decrease the absorption of itraconazole, ketoconazole, iron salts, and ampicillin esters.

Continued

For explanation of icons, see p. 680.

PANTOPRAZOLE *continued*

All oral doses may be taken with or without food. **Do not** crush or chew tablets. The extemporaneously compounded oral suspension may be less bioavailable owing to the loss of the enteric coating.

For IV infusion, doses may be administered over 15 min at a concentration of 0.4–0.8 mg/mL or over 2 min at a concentration of 4 mg/mL. Midazolam and zinc are **not compatible** with the IV dosage form. Parenteral routes other than IV are **not recommended.**

PAREGORIC

Camphorated opium tincture

Narcotic, analgesic

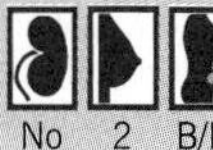

No 2 B/D

Camphorated tincture: 2 mg (morphine equivalent)/5 mL (contains 45% alcohol and may contain benzoic acid or camphor) (473 mL)

Dosages based on mg morphine equivalent.

Analgesia:

Child: 0.1–0.2 mg/kg (or 0.25–0.5 mL/kg)/dose PO QD–QID

Adult: 2–4 mg (or 5–10 mL)/dose PO QD–QID

Neonatal opiate withdrawal:

Start with 0.08–0.12 mg (or 0.2–0.3 mL)/dose Q3–4 hr, increase dose by 0.02 mg (or 0.05 mL)/dose Q3–4 hr until symptoms abate; **max. dose:** 0.28 mg (or 0.7 mL)/dose.

Morphine or DTO is preferred over paregoric because of excipients found in paregoric. Each 5 mL paregoric contains 2 mg morphine equivalent, 0.02 mL anise oil, 20 mg benzoic acid, 20 mg camphor, 0.2 mL glycerin, and alcohol. The final concentration of morphine equivalent is 0.4 mg/mL. This is 25-fold less potent than undiluted deodorized tincture of opium (DTO: 10 mg morphine equivalent/mL). **If using DTO to treat neonatal abstinence, must dilute 25-fold before use.** Similar side effects to morphine. After symptoms are controlled for several days, dose for opiate withdrawal should be decreased gradually over a 2- to 4-wk period (e.g., by 10% Q2–3 days). Monitor neonatal abstinence scores for NAS. Pregnancy category changes to D if used for prolonged periods or in high doses.

PAROMOMYCIN SULFATE

Humatin

Amebicide, antibiotic (aminoglycoside)

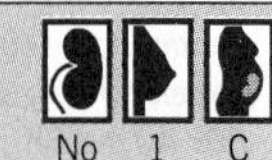

No 1 C

Caps: 250 mg

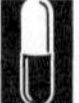

Intestinal amebiasis (Entamoeba histolytica), Dientamoeba fragilis, and Giardia lamblia infection:

Child and adult: 25–35 mg/kg/24 hr PO ÷ Q8 hr × 7 days

Continued

PAROMOMYCIN SULFATE *continued*

Tapeworm *(see comments):*
  Child: 11 mg/kg/dose PO Q15 min × 4 doses
  Adult: 1 g PO Q15 min × 4 doses
Tapeworm (Hymenolepis nana):
  Child and adult: 45 mg/kg/dose PO QD × 5–7 days
Cryptosporidial diarrhea:
  Adult: 1.5–2.25 g/24 hr PO ÷ 3–6 × daily. Duration varies from 10–14 days to 4–8 wk. Maintenance therapy has also been used. Alternatively, 1 g PO BID × 12 wk in conjunction with azithromycin, 600 mg PO QD × 4 wk, has been used in patients with AIDS.

Tapeworms affected by short-duration therapy include *T. saginata, T. solium, D. latum,* and *D. caninum.* Drug is poorly absorbed and therefore not indicated for sole treatment of extraintestinal amebiasis. Side effects include GI disturbance, hematuria, rash, ototoxicity, and hypocholesterolemia. May decrease the effects of digoxin.

PAROXETINE

Paxil, Pexeva, Paxil CR, and others
Antidepressant, selective serotonin reuptake inhibitor

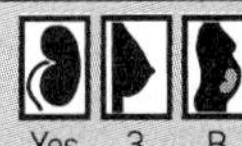
Yes 3 B

Tabs: 10, 20, 30, 40 mg
Controlled-release tabs (Paxil CR): 12.5, 25, 37.5 mg
Oral suspension: 10 mg/5 mL (250 mL); contains saccharin and parabens

---

Child:
Depression (limited data from two studies):
  <14 yr *(mean age, 10.7 ± 2 yr):* Start with 10 mg PO QD. If needed, adjust upward. A mean dose of 16.2 mg/24 hr was used for an average of 8.4 mo in an open-label trial (N = 45). Additional studies are needed.
  12–18 yr *(mean age, 14.8 ± 1.6 yr):* Start with 20 mg PO QAM. If needed, increase dose to 30 mg/24 hr ÷ BID after 5 wk of the initial dose or to 40 mg/24 hr ÷ BID after 6–8 wk of the initial dose. 48% of patients (N = 93) responded at the initial dose level. Mean optimal daily dose: 28 ± 8.54 mg. Additional studies are needed.
Obsessive-compulsive disorder *(limited data, based on a 12-wk open-label trial of 20 children 8–17 yr; mean age, 11.1 ± 2.5 yr):* Start with 10 mg PO QD. If needed, adjust upward by increasing dose no more than 10 mg Q2 wk up to a **max. dose** of 60 mg/24 hr. A mean dose of 41.1 mg/24 hr was used, resulting with a ≥30% reduction in OCD symptom severity (CY-BOCS score).
Social anxiety disorder (8–17 yr): Start with 10 mg PO QD. If needed, increase dose by 10 mg/24 hr no more frequently than Q7 days up to a **max. dose** of 50 mg/24 hr.

Adult:
  Depression: Start with 20 mg PO QAM × 4 wk. If no clinical improvement, increase dose by 10 mg/24 hr Q7 days PRN up to a **max. dose** of 50 mg/24 hr.

Continued

For explanation of icons, see p. 680.

PAROXETINE *continued*

Paxil CR: Start with 25 mg PO QAM × 4 wk. If no improvement, increase dose by 12.5 mg/24 hr Q7 days PRN up to a **max. dose** of 62.5 mg/24 hr.
Obsessive-compulsive disorder: Start with 20 mg PO QD; increase dose by 10 mg/24 hr Q7 days PRN up to a **max. dose** of 60 mg/24 hr. Usual dose is 40 mg PO QD.
Panic disorder: Start with 10 mg PO QAM; increase dose by 10 mg/24 hr Q7 days PRN up to a **max. dose** of 60 mg/24 hr.
Paxil CR: Start with 12.5 mg PO QAM; increase dose by 12.5 mg/24 hr Q7 days PRN up to a **max. dose** of 75 mg/24 hr.

Contraindicated in patients taking MAO inhibitors, within 14 days of discontinuing MAO inhibitors, or thioridazine. Common side effects include anxiety, nausea, anorexia, and decreased appetite. Monitor for clinical worsening of depression and suicidal ideation/behavior following the initiation of therapy or after dose changes.

May increase the effects/toxicity of tricyclic antidepressants, theophylline, and warfarin. Cimetidine, ritonavir, MAO inhibitors (fatal serotonin syndrome), dextromethorphan, phenothiazines, and type 1C antiarrhythmics may increase the effect/toxicity of paroxetine. Weakness, hyperreflexia, and poor coordination have been reported when taken with sumatriptan.

Patients with severe renal or hepatic impairment should initiate therapy at 10 mg/24 hr and increase dose as needed up to a **max. dose** of 40 mg/24 hr. **Do not discontinue therapy abruptly;** may cause sweating, dizziness, confusion and tremor. May be taken with or without food.

PENICILLAMINE

Cuprimine, Depen
Heavy-metal chelator

Yes ? D

Tabs: 250 mg
Caps: 125, 250 mg
Oral suspension: 50 mg/mL

Lead chelation therapy (third-line therapy):
Child: 30–40 mg/kg/24 hr or 600–750 mg/m²/24 hr PO ÷ TID–QID; **max. dose:** 1.5 g/24 hr
Adult: 1–1.5 g/24 hr PO ÷ BID–TID
Durations of treatment vary from 1–6 mo.

Wilson disease *(see remarks for titration information):*
Infant and child: 20 mg/kg/24 hr PO ÷ BID–QID; **max. dose:** 1 g/24 hr
Adult: 250 mg/dose PO QID; **max. dose:** 2 g/24 hr

Arsenic poisoning:
100 mg/kg/24 hr PO ÷ Q6 hr × 5 days; **max. dose:** 1 g/24 hr

Cystinuria *(see remarks for titration information):*
Infant and young child: 30 mg/kg/24 hr ÷ QID PO; **max. dose:** 4 g/24 hr
Older child and adult: 1–4 g/24 hr ÷ QID PO

Continued

PENICILLAMINE *continued*

Primary biliary cirrhosis *(adults):*

Initial: 250 mg/24 hr PO; increase by 250 mg Q2 wk to a total of 1 g/24 hr (given as 250 mg QID).

Juvenile rheumatoid arthritis:

5 mg/kg/24 hr ÷ QD–BID PO × 2 mo, then 10 mg/kg/24 hr ÷ QD–BID PO × 4 mo

Dose should be given 1 hr before or 2 hr after meals. **AAP relegates this drug as a third-line agent for lead chelation indicated only after unacceptable reaction with oral succimer and calcium EDTA.** If used, must be in lead-free environment because it can increase absorption of lead if present in GI tract. **Avoid** use if patient's creatinine clearance is <50 mL/min. Follow CBC, LFTs, and urinalysis; monitor the patient's skin, lymph nodes, and body temperature. Can cause optic neuritis, fever, rash, nausea, altered taste, vomiting, lupus-like syndrome, nephrotic syndrome, peripheral neuropathy, leukopenia, eosinophilia, and thrombocytopenia. May reduce serum digoxin levels. **Avoid** concomitant administration with iron, antacids, and food.

Patients treated for Wilson disease, rheumatoid arthritis, or cystinuria should be treated with pyridoxine, 25–50 mg/24 hr. Titrate urinary copper excretion to >1 mg/24 hr for patients with Wilson disease. Patients with cystinuria should have doses titrated to maintain urinary cystine excretion at <100–200 mg/24 hr.

PENICILLIN G PREPARATIONS—AQUEOUS POTASSIUM AND SODIUM

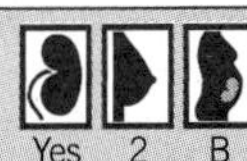

Pfizerpen and others

Antibiotic, aqueous penicillin

Injection (K^+): 1, 5, 20 million units (contains 1.7 mEq K and 0.3 mEq Na/ 1 million units Pen G)
Premixed frozen injection (K^+): 1 million units in 50 mL dextrose 4%; 2 million units in 50 mL dextrose 2.3%; 3 million units in 50 mL dextrose 0.7% (contains 1.7 mEq K and 0.3 mEq Na/1 million units Pen G)
Injection (Na^+): 5 million units (contains 2 mEq Na/1 million units Pen G)
Conversion: 250 mg = 400,000 U

Neonate: *IM/IV*

≤7 days:

- ***≤2 kg:*** 50,000–100,000 U/kg/24 hr ÷ Q12 hr
- ***>2 kg:*** 75,000–150,000 U/kg/24 hr ÷ Q8 hr

>7 days:

- ***<1.2 kg:*** 50,000–100,000 U/kg/24 hr ÷ Q12 hr
- ***1.2–2 kg:*** 75,000–150,000 U/kg/24 hr ÷ Q8 hr
- ***≥2 kg:*** 100,000–200,000 U/kg/24 hr ÷ Q6 hr

Group B streptococcal meningitis:

- ***≤7 days:*** 250,000–450,000 U/kg/24 hr ÷ Q8 hr
- ***>7 days:*** 450,000 U/kg/24 hr ÷ Q6 hr

Continued

For explanation of icons, see p. 680.

PENICILLIN G PREPARATIONS—AQUEOUS POTASSIUM AND SODIUM *continued*

Infant and child:

IM/IV: 100,000–400,000 U/kg/24 hr ÷ Q4–6 hr; **max. dose:** 24 million U/24 hr

Adult:

IM/IV: 4–24 million U/24 hr ÷ Q4–6 hr

Congenital syphilis, neurosyphilis: see Chapter 16.

Use penicillin V potassium for oral use. Side effects: anaphylaxis, urticaria, hemolytic anemia, interstitial nephritis, Jarisch-Herxheimer reaction (syphilis). $T_{1/2}$ = 30 min; may be prolonged by concurrent use of probenecid. For meningitis, use higher daily dose at shorter dosing intervals. For the treatment of anthrax (*Bacillus anthracis*), see www.bt.cdc.gov for additional information. May cause false-positive or negative urinary glucose (Clinitest method), false-positive direct Coombs test, and false-positive urinary and/or serum proteins. **Adjust dose in renal impairment (see Chapter 30).**

PENICILLIN G PREPARATIONS—BENZATHINE

Permapen, Bicillin L-A

Antibiotic, penicillin (very long-acting IM)

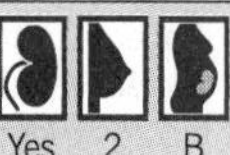

Injection: 600,000 U/mL (1, 2, 4 mL); contains parabens and povidone

Injection should be IM only.

Group A streptococci:

Infant and child: 25,000–50,000 U/kg/dose IM × 1. **Max. dose:** 1.2 million U/dose, **OR**

>1 mo and <27 kg: 600,000 U/dose IM × 1

≥27 kg and adult: 1.2 million U/dose IM × 1

Rheumatic fever prophylaxis:

Infant and child: 25,000–50,000 U/kg/dose IM Q3–4 wk. **Max. dose:** 1.2 million U/dose

Adult: 1.2 million U/dose IM Q3–4 wk or 600,000 U/dose IM Q2 wk

Syphilis: Early acquired and >1 yr duration: see Chapter 16.

Provides sustained levels for 2–4 wk. Side effects same as for Penicillin G Preparations—Aqueous Potassium and Sodium. **Use with caution in renal failure. Do not administer intravenously; cardiac arrest and death may occur.**

PENICILLIN G PREPARATIONS—PENICILLIN G BENZATHINE AND PENICILLIN G PROCAINE

Bicillin CR, Bicillin CR 900/300

Antibiotic, penicillin (very long acting)

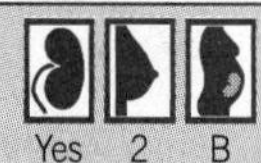

Bicillin CR: 300,000 U PenG procaine + 300,000 U PenG benzathine/mL to provide 600,000 U penicillin per 1 mL (1, 2 mL tubex, 4 mL syringe)

Continued

PENICILLIN G PREPARATIONS—PENICILLIN G BENZATHINE AND PENICILLIN G PROCAINE *continued*

Bicillin CR (900/300): 150,000 U PenG procaine + 450,000 U PenG benzathine/mL (2 mL tubex)
All preparations contain parabens and povidone.
Injection should be for IM use only.

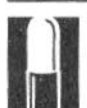

Dosage based on total amount of penicillin.
Group A streptococci:
Child <14 kg: 600,000 U/dose IM × 1
Child 14–27 kg: 900,000–1,200,000 U/dose IM × 1
Child >27 kg and adults: 2,400,000 U/dose IM × 1

This preparation provides early peak levels in addition to prolonged levels of penicillin in the blood. **Do not use this product to treat syphilis because of potential treatment failure. Use with caution in renal failure.** The addition of procaine penicillin has not been shown to be more efficacious than benzathine alone. However, it may reduce injection discomfort. **Do not administer IV.**

PENICILLIN G PREPARATIONS—PROCAINE

Wycillin and others
Antibiotic, penicillin (long-acting IM)

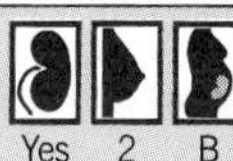

Injection: 600,000 U/ml (1, 2 mL); may contain parabens, phenol, povidone, and formaldehyde
Contains 120 mg procaine per 300,000 U penicillin.

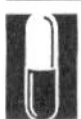

Newborn (see remarks): 50,000 U/kg/24 hr IM QD
Infant and child: 25,000–50,000 U/kg/24 hr ÷ Q12–24 hr IM. **Max. dose:** 4.8 million U/24 hr
Adult: 0.6–4.8 million U/24 hr ÷ Q12–24 hr IM
Congenital syphilis, syphilis, and neurosyphilis: see Chapter 16.

Provides sustained levels for 2–4 days. **Use with caution in renal failure and in neonates** (higher incidence of sterile abscess at injection site and risk for procaine toxicity). Side effects similar to *Penicillin G Preparations—Aqueous Potassium and Sodium*. In addition, may cause CNS stimulation and seizures. **Do not administer IV;** neurovascular damage may result. Large doses may be administered in two injection sites. No longer recommended for empiric treatment of gonorrhea due to resistant strains.

PENICILLIN V POTASSIUM

Veetids and others
Antibiotic, penicillin

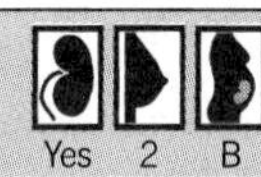

Tabs: 250, 500 mg
Oral solution: 125 mg/5 mL, 250 mg/5 mL (100, 200 mL); may contain saccharin
Contains 0.7 mEq potassium/250 mg drug
250 mg = 400,000 U

Continued

For explanation of icons, see p. 680.

PENICILLIN V POTASSIUM *continued*

Child: 25–50 mg/kg/24 hr ÷ Q6–8 hr PO. **Max. dose:** 3 g/24 hr
Adult: 250–500 mg/dose PO Q6–8 hr
Acute group A streptococcal pharyngitis:
Child: 250 mg PO BID–TID × 10 days
Adolescent and adult: 500 mg PO BID–TID × 10 days
Rheumatic fever/pneumococcal prophylaxis:
3–5 yr: 125 mg PO BID
>5 yr: 250 mg PO BID

See *Penicillin G Preparations—Aqueous Potassium and Sodium* for side effects and drug-lab interactions. GI absorption is better than penicillin G.
NOTE: Must be taken 1 hr before or 2 hr after meals. Penicillin will prevent rheumatic fever if started within 9 days of the acute illness. The BID regimen for streptococcal pharyngitis should be used **only** if good compliance is expected. **Adjust dose in renal failure (see Chapter 30).**

PENTAMIDINE ISETHIONATE

Pentam 300, NebuPent
Antibiotic, antiprotozoal

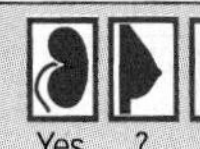
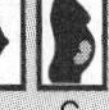
Yes ? C

Injection (Pentam 300): 300 mg
Inhalation (NebuPent): 300 mg

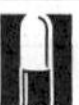

Treatment:
Pneumocystis carinii: 4 mg/kg/24 hr IM/IV QD × 14–21 days (IV is the preferred route)
Trypanosomiasis (T. gambiense, T. rhodesiense): 4 mg/kg/24 hr IM QD × 10 days
Leishmaniasis (L. donovani): 2–4 mg/kg/dose IM QD or QOD × 15 doses
Prophylaxis:
Pneumocystis carinii:
IM/IV: 4 mg/kg/dose Q2–4 wk
Inhalation (≥5 yr): 300 mg in 6 ml H_2O via inhalation Q month (Respigard II nebulizer). See also Chapter 16 for indications.
Trypanosomiasis (T. gambiense, T. rhodesiense): 4 mg/kg/24 hr IM Q3–6 mo.
Max. single dose: 300 mg

Use with caution in ventricular tachycardia, Stevens-Johnson syndrome, and daily doses >21 days. May cause hypoglycemia, hyperglycemia, hypotension (both IV and IM administration), nausea, vomiting, fever, mild hepatotoxicity, pancreatitis, megaloblastic anemia, nephrotoxicity, hypocalcemia, and granulocytopenia. Additive nephrotoxicity with aminoglycosides, amphotericin B, cisplatin, and vancomycin may occur. Aerosol administration may also cause bronchospasm, oxygen desaturation, dyspnea, and loss of appetite. Infuse IV over 1–2 hr to reduce the risk for hypotension. Sterile abscess may occur at IM injection site. **Adjust dose in renal impairment (see Chapter 30).**

PENTOBARBITAL

Nembutal and others

Barbiturate

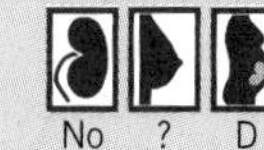

Caps: 100 mg
Injection: 50 mg/mL; contains propylene glycol and 10% alcohol
Elixir: 18.2 mg/5 mL; contains saccharin and 18% alcohol

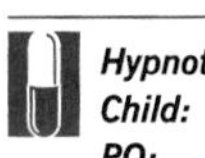

Hypnotic
Child:
PO:
<4 yr: 3–6 mg/kg/dose QHS
≥4 yr: 1.5–3 mg/kg/dose QHS
IM: 2–6 mg/kg/dose. **Max. dose:** 100 mg

Preprocedure sedation
Child:
PO/IM: 2–6 mg/kg/dose. **Max. dose:** 150 mg
IV: 1–3 mg/kg/dose. **Max. dose:** 150 mg

Barbiturate coma
Child and adult:
IV: Load: 10–15 mg/kg given slowly over 1–2 hr
Maintenance: Begin at 1 mg/kg/hr. Dose range: 1–3 mg/kg/hr as needed.

Contraindicated in liver failure, CHF, and hypotension. No advantage over phenobarbital for control of seizures. Adjunct in treatment of ICP. May cause drug-related isoelectric EEG. **Do not administer** for >2 wk in treatment of insomnia. May cause hypotension, arrhythmias, hypothermia, respiratory depression, and dependence.

Onset of action: PO: 15–60 min; IM: 10–15 min; IV: 1 min. Duration of action: PO: 1–4 hr; IV: 15 min.

Administer IV at a rate of <50 mg/min.

Therapeutic serum levels: Sedation: 1–5 mg/L; Hypnosis: 5–15 mg/L; Coma: 20–40 mg/L (steady state is achieved after 4–5 days of continuous IV dosing).

PERMETHRIN

Elimite, Acticin, Nix, and others

Scabicidal agent

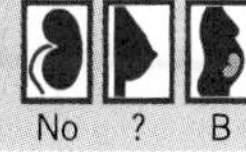

Cream (Elimite, Acticin): 5% (60 g); contains 0.1% formaldehyde
Liquid cream rinse (Nix-OTC): 1% (60 mL with comb); contains 20% isopropyl alcohol
Lotion (OTC): 1% (60 mL with comb)

Continued

For explanation of icons, see p. 680.

PERMETHRIN *continued*

Pediculus capitis, Phthirus pubis:
Head lice: Saturate hair and scalp with 1% cream rinse after shampooing, rinsing, and towel drying hair. Leave on for 10 min, then rinse. May repeat in 7–10 days. May be used for lice in other areas of the body (e.g., pubic lice) in same fashion.
Scabies *(see remarks):* Apply 5% cream from neck to toe (head to toe for infants and toddlers) wash off with water in 8–14 hr. May repeat in 7 days.

Ovicidal activity generally makes single-dose regimen adequate. However, resistance to permethrin has been reported. **Avoid** contact with eyes during application. Shake well before using. May cause pruritus, hypersensitivity, burning, stinging, erythema, and rash. For either lice or scabies, instruct patient to launder bedding and clothing. For lice, treat symptomatic contacts only. For scabies, treat all contacts even if asymptomatic. The 5% cream has been used safely in children <1 mo with neonatal scabies (a 6-hr application time was used). Topical cream dosage form contains formaldehyde. Dispense 60 g per adult or 2 small children.

PHENAZOPYRIDINE HCL

Pyridium, Azo-Standard (OTC), and others
Urinary analgesic

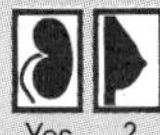
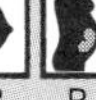
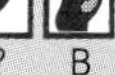

Yes ? B

Tabs: 95 mg (OTC), 97.2 mg, 100 mg (OTC/Rx), 150 mg, 200 mg
Oral suspension: 10 mg/mL

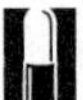

Child 6–12 yr: 12 mg/kg/24 hr ÷ TID PO until symptoms of lower urinary tract irritation are controlled or 2 days
Adult: 100–200 mg TID PO until symptoms are controlled or 2 days

May cause hepatitis, GI distress, vertigo, headache, renal insufficiency, methemoglobinemia, and hemolytic anemia. Colors urine orange; stains clothing. May also stain contact lenses and interfere with urinalysis tests based on spectrometry or color reactions. Give doses after meals. **Adjust dose in renal impairment (see Chapter 30).**

PHENOBARBITAL

Luminal and others
Barbiturate

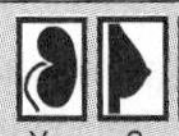
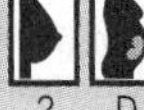
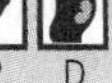

Yes 2 D

Tabs: 15, 16, 30, 60, 90, 100 mg
Caps: 16 mg
Elixir: 20 mg/5 mL; contains alcohol
Injection: 30, 60, 65, 130 mg/mL; may contain 10% alcohol, benzyl alcohol and propylene glycol

Continued

PHENOBARBITAL *continued*

Status epilepticus:
Loading dose, IV:
Neonate, infant, and child: 15–20 mg/kg/dose in a single or divided dose. May give additional 5 mg/kg doses Q15–30 min to a **max. total dose** of 30 mg/kg.

Maintenance dose, PO/IV: *Monitor levels.*
Neonate: 3–5 mg/kg/24 hr ÷ QD–BID
Infant: 5–6 mg/kg/24 hr ÷ QD–BID
Child 1–5 yr: 6–8 mg/kg/24 hr ÷ QD–BID
Child 6–12 yr: 4–6 mg/kg/24 hr ÷ QD–BID
>12 yr: 1–3 mg/kg/24 hr ÷ QD–BID

Hyperbilirubinemia: *<12 yr:* 3–8 mg/kg/24 hr PO ÷ BID–TID. Doses up to 12 mg/kg/24 hr have been used.

Preoperative sedation, child: 1–3 mg/kg/dose IM/IV/PO × 1. Give 60–90 min before procedure.

Contraindicated in porphyria, severe respiratory disease with dyspnea or obstruction. **Use with caution** in hepatic or renal disease (reduce dose). IV administration may cause respiratory arrest or hypotension. Side effects include drowsiness, cognitive impairment, ataxia, hypotension, hepatitis, skin rash, respiratory depression, apnea, megaloblastic anemia, and anticonvulsant hypersensitivity syndrome. Paradoxical reaction in children (not dose related) may cause hyperactivity, irritability, insomnia. Induces several liver enzyme (CYP450 1A2, 2B6, 2C8, 3A3/4, 3A5-7), thus decreases blood levels of many drugs (e.g., anticonvulsants). IV push **not to exceed** 1 mg/kg/min.

$T_{1/2}$ is variable with age: neonates, 45–100 hr; infants, 20–133 hr; children, 37–73 hr. Because of long half-life, consider other agents for sedation for procedures.

Therapeutic levels: 15–40 mg/L. Recommended serum sampling time at steady state: trough level obtained within 30 min before the next scheduled dose after 10–14 days of continuous dosing. **Adjust dose in renal failure (see Chapter 30).**

PHENTOLAMINE MESYLATE

Regitine and others

Adrenergic blocking agent (alpha); antidote, extravasation

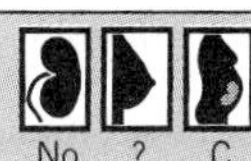

Injection: 5 mg vial; may contain mannitol

Treatment of alpha-adrenergic drug extravasation (most effective within 12 hr of extravasation):

Neonate: Make a solution of 0.25–0.5 mg/mL with preservative-free normal saline. Inject 1 mL (in 5 divided doses of 0.2 mL) SC around site of extravasation; **max. total dose:** 0.1 mg/kg or 2.5 mg total.

Infant, child, and adult: Make a solution of 0.5–1 mg/mL with preservative-free normal saline. Inject 1–5 mL (in 5 divided doses) SC around site of extravasation; **max. total dose:** 0.1–0.2 mg/kg or 5 mg total.

Continued

For explanation of icons, see p. 680.

PHENTOLAMINE MESYLATE *continued*

Diagnosis of pheochromocytoma, IM/IV:

Child: 0.05–0.1 mg/kg/dose up to a **max. dose** of 5 mg

Adult: 5 mg/dose

Hypertension, before surgery for pheochromocytoma, IM/IV:

Child: 0.05–0.1 mg/kg/dose up to a **max. dose** of 5 mg 1–2 hr before surgery, repeat Q2–4 hr PRN.

Adult: 5 mg/dose 1–2 hr before surgery, repeat Q2–4 hr PRN.

Contraindicated in MI, coronary insufficiency, and angina. **Use with caution** in hypotension, arrhythmias, and cerebral vascular spasm/occlusion.

For diagnosis of pheochromocytoma, patient should be resting in a supine position. A blood pressure reduction of more than 35 mmHg systolic and 24 mm Hg diastolic is considered a positive test for pheochromocytoma.

For treatment of extravasation, use 27- to 30-gauge needle with multiple small injections and monitor site closely as repeat doses may be necessary.

PHENYLEPHRINE HCL

Neo-Synephrine and others

Adrenergic agonist

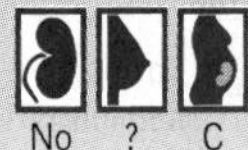

Nasal drops (OTC): 0.125, 0.25, 0.5, 1% (15, 30 mL)

Nasal spray (OTC): 0.25, 0.5, 1% (15, 30 mL)

NOTE: Neo-Synephrine 12 hours, see *Oxymetazoline.*

Ophthalmic drops: 0.12% (OTC) (0.3, 20 mL), 2.5% (2, 3, 5, 15 mL), 10% (2, 5 mL)

Injection: 10 mg/mL (1%) (1, 5 mL); may contain bisulfites

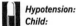

Hypotension:

Child:

IV bolus: 5–20 mcg/kg/dose Q10–15 min PRN

IV drip: 0.1–0.5 mcg/kg/min; titrate to effect

IM/SC: 0.1 mg/kg/dose Q1–2 hr PRN; **max. dose:** 5 mg

Adult:

IV bolus: 0.1–0.5 mg/dose Q10–15 min PRN

IV drip: Initial rate at 100–180 mcg/min; titrate to effect. Usual maintenance dose: 40–60 mcg/min.

IM/SC: 2–5 mg/dose Q1–2 hr PRN; **max. dose:** 5 mg

To prepare infusion: see inside front cover.

NOTE: The dosage units for adults are in mcg/min; compared with mcg/kg/min for children.

Nasal decongestant *(in each nostril; give up to 3 days):*

Infant (>6 mo): 1–2 drops of 0.16% sol (see remarks) Q3 hr PRN

<6 yr: 2–3 drops of 0.125% sol Q4 hr PRN

6–12 yr: 2–3 drops or 1–2 sprays of 0.25% sol Q4 hr PRN

>12 yr–adult: 2–3 drops or 1–2 sprays of 0.25% or 0.5% sol Q4 hr PRN

Pupillary dilation: 2.5% sol; 1 drop in each eye 15 min before exam

Continued

PHENYLEPHRINE HCL *continued*

Use with caution in presence of arrhythmias, hyperthyroidism, or hyperglycemia. May cause tremor, insomnia, palpitations. Metabolized by MAO. **Contraindicated** in pheochromocytoma and severe hypertension.

Nasal decongestants may cause rebound congestion with excessive use (>3 days). The 0.16% nasal drops are no longer available; may use the 0.125% solution or dilute the 0.25% or 0.5% concentrations with normal saline. The 1% nasal spray can be used in adults with extreme congestion.

Injectable product may contain sulfites. **NOTE:** Phenylephrine is found in a variety of combination cough and cold products.

PHENYTOIN

Dilantin, Dilantin Infatab, Phenytek, and others

Anticonvulsant, class Ib antiarrhythmic

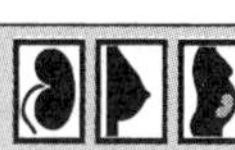

Chewable tabs (Infatab): 50 mg
Prompt-release caps: 100 mg
Extended-release caps: 30, 100, 200, 300 mg
Oral suspension: 125 mg/5 mL (240 mL); contains ≤0.6% alcohol
Injection: 50 mg/mL; contains alcohol and propylene glycol

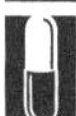

Status epilepticus: see Chapter 1
Loading dose (all ages): 15–20 mg/kg IV
Max. dose: 1500 mg/24 hr

Maintenance for seizure disorders:

Neonate: start with 5 mg/kg/24 hr PO/IV ÷ Q12 hr; usual range 5–8 mg/kg/24 hr PO/IV ÷ Q8–12 hr

Infant/child: start with 5 mg/kg/24 hr ÷ BID–TID PO/IV; usual dose range (doses divided BID–TID):

6 mo–3 yr: 8–10 mg/kg/24 hr
4–6 yr: 7.5–9 mg/kg/24 hr
7–9 yr: 7–8 mg/kg/24 hr
10–16 yr: 6–7 mg/kg/24 hr
NOTE: Use QD–BID dosing with extended-release caps.

Adult: Start with 100 mg/dose Q8 hr IV/PO, and carefully titrate (if needed) by 100 mg increments Q2–4 wk to 300–600 mg/24 hr (or 6–7 mg/kg/24 hr) ÷ Q8–24 hr IV/PO.

Antiarrhythmic *(secondary to digitalis intoxication):*

Load (all ages): 1.25 mg/kg IV Q5 min up to a total of 15 mg/kg

Maintenance:

Child: IV/PO: 5–10 mg/kg/24 hr ÷ Q8-12 hr
Adult: 250 mg PO QID × 1 day, then 250 mg PO Q12 hr × 2 days, then 300–400 mg/24 hr ÷ Q6–24 hr

Continued

FORMULARY
For explanation of icons, see p. 680.

PHENYTOIN *continued*

Contraindicated in patients with heart block or sinus bradycardia. IM administration is not recommended because of erratic absorption and pain at injection site. Side effects include gingival hyperplasia, hirsutism, dermatitis, blood dyscrasia, ataxia, lupus-like and Stevens-Johnson syndromes, lymphadenopathy, liver damage, and nystagmus. Many drug interactions: levels may be increased by cimetidine, chloramphenicol, INH, sulfonamides, trimethoprim, etc. Levels may be decreased by some antineoplastic agents. Phenytoin induces hepatic microsomal enzymes (CYP450 1A2, 2C8/9/19, and 3A3/4) leading to decreased effectiveness of oral contraceptives, quinidine, valproic acid, theophylline, and other substrates to the above CYP450 hepatic enzymes.

Suggested dosing intervals for specific oral dosage forms: extended-release caps (QD–BID); chewable and immediate-release tablets, and oral suspension (TID). Oral absorption reduced in neonates. $T_{1/2}$ is variable (7–42 hr) and dose dependent. Drug is highly protein bound; free fraction of drug will be increased in patients with hypoalbuminemia.

For seizure disorders, therapeutic levels: 10–20 mg/L (free and bound phenytoin) **OR** 1–2 mg/L (free only). **Monitor free phenytoin levels in hypoalbuminemia or renal insufficiency.** Recommended serum sampling times: trough level (PO/IV) within 30 min before the next scheduled dose; peak or post load level (IV) 1 hr after the end of IV infusion. Steady state is usually achieved after 5–10 days of continuous dosing. For routine monitoring, measure trough.

IV push/infusion rate: **Not to exceed** 0.5 mg/kg/min in neonates, or 1 mg/kg/min infants, children, and adults with **maximum** of 50 mg/min; may cause cardiovascular collapse. Consider fosphenytoin in situations of tenuous IV access and risk for extravasation.

PHOSPHORUS SUPPLEMENTS

Neutra-Phos, Neutra-Phos-K, K-PHOS Neutral, K-PHOS M.F., K-PHOS No.2, Uro-KP-Neutral, Sodium Phosphate, Potassium Phosphate

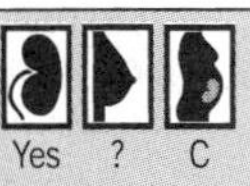

Oral: (reconstitute in 75 mL H_2O per capsule or packet)

Na and K phosphate:

Neutra-Phos; Caps, powder: 250 mg (8 mM) P, 7.125 mEq Na, 7.125 mEq K
Uro-KP-Neutral; Tabs: 250 mg (8 mM) P, 10.9 mEq Na, 1.27 mEq K
K-PHOS Neutral; Tabs: 250 mg (8 mM) P, 13 mEq Na, 1.1 mEq K
K-PHOS M.F.; Tabs: 125.6 mg (4 mM) P, 2.9 mEq Na, 1.1 mEq K
K-PHOS No.2; Tabs: 250 mg (8 mM) P, 5.5 mEq Na, 2.3 mEq K

K phosphate:

Neutra-Phos-K; Caps, powder: 250 mg (8 mM) P, 14.25 mEq K

Injection:

Na phosphate: 3 mM (94 mg) P, 4 mEq Na/mL
K phosphate: 3 mM (94 mg) P, 4.4 mEq K/mL

Conversion: 31 mg P = 1 mM P

Continued

PHOSPHORUS SUPPLEMENTS *continued*

Acute hypophosphatemia: 0.16–0.32 mM/kg/dose (or 5–10 mg/kg/dose) IV over 6 hr

Maintenance/replacement:

Child:

IV: 0.5–1.5 mM/kg (or 15–45 mg/kg) over 24 hr

PO: 30–90 mg/kg/24 hr (or 1–3 mM/kg/24 hr) ÷ TID–QID

Adult:

IV: 50–65 mM (or 1.5–2 g) over 24 hr

PO: 3–4.5 g/24 hr (or 100–150 mM/24 hr) ÷ TID–QID

Recommended infusion rate: ≤0.1 mM/kg/hr (or 3.1 mg/kg/hr) of phosphate. When potassium salt is used, the rate will be limited by the maximum potassium infusion rate. **Do not** coinfuse with calcium-containing products.

May cause tetany, hyperphosphatemia, hyperkalemia, hypocalcemia. **Use with caution** in patients with renal impairment. Be aware of sodium and/or potassium load when supplementing phosphate. IV administration may cause hypotension and renal failure, or arrhythmias, heart block, cardiac arrest with potassium salt. PO dosing may cause nausea, vomiting, abdominal pain, or diarrhea. See Chapter 20 for daily requirements and Chapter 10 additional information on hypophosphatemia and hyperphosphatemia.

PHYSOSTIGMINE SALICYLATE

Antilirium

Cholinergic agent

No ? C

Injection: 1 mg/mL (2 mL); contains 2% benzyl alcohol and 0.1% sodium bisulfite

For antihistamine overdose or anticholinergic poisoning, see Chapter 3.

Physostigmine antidote: Atropine always should be available. **Contraindicated** in asthma, gangrene, diabetes, cardiovascular disease, GI or GU tract obstruction, any vagotonic state, and patients receiving choline esters or depolarizing neuromuscular blocking agents (e.g., decamethonium, succinylcholine). May cause seizures, arrhythmias, bradycardia, GI symptoms, and other cholinergic effects.

PHYTONADIONE/VITAMIN K_1

Mephyton and others

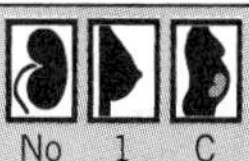

Tabs: 5 mg

Injection: 2 mg/mL (0.5 mL), 10 mg/mL (1 mL); contains 0.9% benzyl alcohol

Continued

For explanation of icons, see p. 680.

PHYTONADIONE/VITAMIN K_1 *continued*

Neonatal hemorrhagic disease:
Prophylaxis: 0.5–1 mg IM × 1 within 1 hr after birth
Treatment: 1–2 mg/24 hr IM/SC/IV
Oral anticoagulant overdose:
Infant and child: 0.5–5 mg/dose PO/IM/SC/IV
INR >8 (no bleeding or minor bleeding): 0.5–2.5 mg
Major bleeding: 5 mg
Adult: 2.5–10 mg/dose PO/IM/SC/IV
Dose may be repeated 12–48 hr after PO dose or 6–8 hr after parenteral dose.
Vitamin K deficiency:
Infant and child:
PO: 2.5–5 mg/24 hr
IM/SC/IV: 1–2 mg/dose × 1
Adult:
PO: 5–25 mg/24 hr
IM/SC//IV: 10 mg/dose × 1

Monitor PT/PTT. Large doses (10–20 mg) in newborns may cause hyperbilirubinemia and severe hemolytic anemia. Blood coagulation factors increase within 6–12 hr after oral doses and within 1–2 hr following parenteral administration.

IV injection rate **not to exceed** 3 mg/m²/min or 1 mg/min. IV or IM doses may cause flushing, dizziness, cardiac/respiratory arrest, hypotension, and anaphylaxis. IV or IM administration is indicated only when other routes of administration are not feasible (or in emergency situations).

Mineral oil may decrease GI absorption of vitamin K with concurrent oral administration. See Chapter 20 for multivitamin preparations.

PILOCARPINE HCL

Akarpine, Isopto Carpine, Pilocar, Ocusert Pilo, Salagen, and others
Cholinergic agent

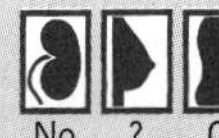

Ophthalmic solution: 0.25% (15 mL), 0.5% (15, 30 mL), 1% (1, 2, 15, 30 mL), 2% (2, 15, 30 mL), 3% (15, 30 mL), 4% (2, 15, 30 mL), 5% (15 mL), 6% (15, 30 mL), 8% (2, 15 mL), 10% (15 mL)
Ophthalmic gel: 4% (3.5 g)
Ocular therapeutic system (Ocusert Pilo): 20, 40 mcg/hr for 1 wk (8 units)
Tabs (Salagen): 5, 7.5 mg

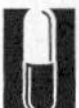

For elevated intraocular pressure:
Drops: 1–2 drops in each eye 4–6 times a day; adjust concentration and frequency as needed.
Gel: 0.5-inch ribbon applied to lower conjunctival sac QHS. Adjust dose as needed.

Continued

PILOCARPINE HCL *continued*

Xerostomia:

Adult: 5 mg/dose PO TID, dose may be titrated to 10 mg/dose PO TID in patients who do not respond to lower doses and who are able to tolerate the drug.

Contraindicated in acute iritis or anterior chamber inflammation and uncontrolled asthma. May cause stinging, burning, lacrimation, headache, and retinal detachment with ophthalmic use. **Use with caution** in patients with corneal abrasion or significant cardiovascular disease. Use with topical NSAIDs (e.g., ketorolac) may decrease topical pilocarpine effects. Sweating, nausea, rhinitis, chills, flushing, urinary frequency, dizziness, and headaches have also been reported with oral dosing. Reduce oral dosing in the presence of mild hepatic insufficiency (Child-Pugh score of 5–6); use in severe hepatic insufficiency is **not recommended.**

PIMECROLIMUS

Elidel

Topical immunosuppressant

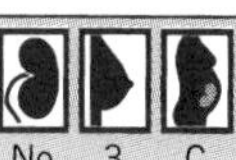

Cream: 1% (15, 30, 60, 100 g); contains benzyl alcohol and propylene glycol

---

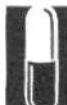

≥2 yr and adult: Apply a thin layer to affected area BID, and rub in gently and completely. Reevaluate patient in 6 wk if lesions are not healed.

Do not use in children <2 yr, immunecompromised patients, or with occlusive dressings (promotes systemic absorption). Approved as a second-line therapy for atopic dermatitis for patients who fail to respond, or do not tolerate, other approved therapies. Use medication for short periods of time by using the minimum amounts to control symptoms; long-term safety is unknown. **Avoid** contact with eyes, nose, mouth, and cut, infected, or scrapped skin. Minimize and **avoid** exposure to natural and artificial sunlight, respectively.

Most common side effects include burning at the application site, headache, viral infections, and pyrexia. Although the risk is uncertain, the FDA has issued an alert about the potential cancer risk with the use of this product. See www.fda.gov/medwatch for the latest information. Drug is a CYP450 3A3/4 substrate.

PIPERACILLIN

Pipracil and others

Antibiotic, penicillin (extended spectrum)

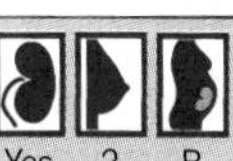

Injection: 2, 3, 40 g
Contains 1.85 mEq Na/g drug

Continued

For explanation of icons, see p. 680.

PIPERACILLIN *continued*

Neonates, IV:
≤7 days:
≤36 weeks' gestation: 150 mg/kg/24 hr ÷ Q12 hr
>36 weeks' gestation: 225 mg/kg/24 hr ÷ Q8 hr
>7 days:
≤36 weeks' gestation: 225 mg/kg/24 hr ÷ Q8 hr
>36 weeks' gestation: 300 mg/kg/24 hr ÷ Q6 hr
Infant and child:
200–300 mg/kg/24 hr IM/IV ÷ Q4–6 hr; **max. dose:** 24 g/24 hr
Cystic fibrosis:
350–600 mg/kg/24 hr IM/IV ÷ Q4–6 hr; **max. dose:** 24 g/24 hr
Adult: 2–4 g/dose IV Q4–6 hr or 1–2 g/dose IM Q6 hr; **max. dose:** 24 g/24 hr

Similar to penicillin. Like other penicillins, CSF penetration occurs only with inflamed meninges. May cause seizures, myoclonus, and fever. May falsely lower aminoglycoside serum levels if the drugs are infused close to one another; allow a minimum of 2 hr between infusions to prevent this interaction.

For IM use, drug may be diluted to 400 mg/mL with 0.5 or 1% lidocaine without epinephrine. **Adjust dose in renal impairment (see Chapter 30).**

PIPERACILLIN/TAZOBACTAM

Zosyn

Antibiotic, penicillin (extended spectrum with beta-lactamase inhibitor)

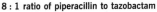

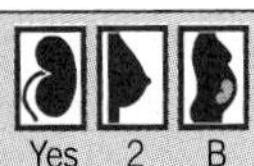

8 : 1 ratio of piperacillin to tazobactam
Injection, powder: 2 g piperacillin and 0.25 g tazobactam; 3 g piperacillin and 0.375 g tazobactam; 4 g piperacillin and 0.5 g tazobactam
Injection, premixed in iso-osmotic dextrose: 2 g piperacillin and 0.25 g tazobactam in 50 mL; 3 g piperacillin and 0.375 g tazobactam in 50 mL; 4 g piperacillin and 0.5 g tazobactam in 50 mL
Contains 2.35 mEq Na/g piperacillin

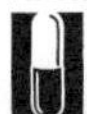

All doses based on piperacillin component
Infant <6 mo: 150–300 mg/kg/24 hr IV ÷ Q6–8 hr
Infant >6 mo and child: 300–400 mg/kg/24 hr IV ÷ Q6–8 hr
Adult:
Intra-abdominal or soft tissue infections: 3 g IV Q6 hr
Nosocomial pneumonia: 4g IV Q6hr
Cystic fibrosis: see *Piperacillin.*

Tazobactam is a beta-lactamase inhibitor, thus extending the spectrum of piperacillin. Like other penicillins, CSF penetration occurs only with inflamed meninges. See *Piperacillin* and *Penicillin Preparations—Aqueous Potassium*

Continued

PIPERACILLIN/TAZOBACTAM *continued*

and Sodium for additional comments. **Adjust dose in renal impairment (see Chapter 30).**

POLYCITRA

See *Citrate Mixtures*

POLYETHYLENE GLYCOL—ELECTROLYTE SOLUTION

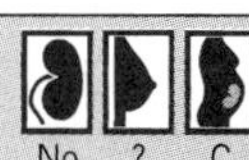

GoLYTELY, CoLyte, NuLYTELY, OCL, TriLyte, MiraLax
Bowel evacuant, osmotic laxative

Powder for oral solution:

GoLYTELY: polyethylene glycol 3350 236 g, Na sulfate 22.74 g, Na bicarbonate 6.74 g, NaCl 5.86 g, KCl 2.97 g. Contents vary somewhat. See package insert for contents of other products.
MiraLax: polyethylene glycol 3350 (255, 527 g)

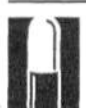

Bowel cleansing (patients should be NPO 3–4 hr before dosing):
Child:
Oral/nasogastric: 25–40 ml/kg/hr until rectal effluent is clear (usually in 4–10 hr)
Adult:
Oral: 240 ml PO Q10 min up to 4 L or until rectal effluent is clear
Nasogastric: 20–30 ml/min (1.2–1.8 L/hr) up to 4 L

Constipation (MiraLax):
Child (limited data in 20 children with chronic constipation, 18 mo–11 yr; see remarks): a mean effective dose of 0.84 g/kg/24 hr PO ÷ BID for 8 wk (range, 0.25–1.42 g/kg/24 hr) was used to yield two soft stools per day. If patient is >20 kg, use adult dose.
Adult: 17 g (one heaping tablespoonful) mixed in 240 mL of water, juice, soda, coffee, or tea PO QD

Contraindicated in polyethylene glycol hypersensitivity. Monitor electrolytes, BUN, serum glucose, and urine osmolality with prolonged administration.

BOWEL CLEANSING: Contraindicated in toxic megacolon, gastric retention, colitis, and bowel perforation. **Use with caution** in patients prone to aspiration or with impaired gag reflex. Effect should occur within 1–2 hr. Solution generally more palatable if chilled.

CONSTIPATION (MiraLax): Contraindicated in bowel obstruction.
Child: Dilute powder using the ratio of 17 g powder to 240 mL of water, juice, or milk. An onset of action within 1 wk in 12 of 20 patients, with the remaining 8 patients reporting improvement during the second wk of therapy. Side effects reported in this trial included diarrhea, flatulence, and mild abdominal pain. [See J Pediatr 2001;139(3):428–432 for additional information.]

Continued

For explanation of icons, see p. 680.

POLYETHYLENE GLYCOL—ELECTROLYTE SOLUTION *continued*

Adult: 2 to 4 days may be required to produce a bowel movement. Most common side effects include nausea, abdominal bloating, cramping, and flatulence. Use beyond 2 wk has not been studied.

POLYMYXIN B SULFATE AND BACITRACIN

See *Bacitracin ± Polymyxin B*

POLYMYXIN B SULFATE, NEOMYCIN SULFATE, HYDROCORTISONE

Cortisporin Otic, AK-Spore H.C. Otic, and others

Topical antibiotic (otic preparations listed)

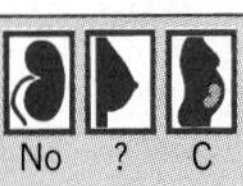

Otic solution or suspension: polymyxin B sulfate 10,000 U, neomycin sulfate 5 mg, hydrocortisone 10 mg/mL (10 mL)

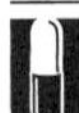

Otitis externa:

≥2 yr–adult: 3–4 drops TID–QID × 7–10 days. If preferred, a cotton wick may be saturated and inserted into ear canal. Moisten wick with antibiotic every 4 hr. Change wick Q24 hr.

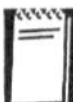

Shake suspension well before use. **Contraindicated** in patients with active varicella and herpes simplex. May cause cutaneous sensitization. **Do not use** in cases with perforated eardrum because of possible ototoxicity.

PORACTANT ALFA

See *Surfactant, pulmonary*

POTASSIUM IODIDE

Iostat, Pima, SSKI, and others

Antithyroid agent

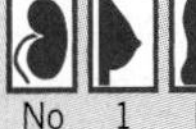

Tabs (Iostat): 65, 130 mg
Syrup (Pima): 325 mg/5 mL (473 mL, 4000 mL)
Saturated solution (SSKI): 1000 mg/mL (30, 240 mL); 10 drops = 500 mg potassium iodide
Lugol's (Strong Iodine) solution: iodine 50 mg and potassium iodide 100 mg per mL (15, 473 mL)

Neonatal Grave's disease: 1 drop strong iodine (Lugol's sol) PO Q8 hr

Thyrotoxicosis:

Child: 50–250 mg PO TID (about 1–5 drops of SSKI TID)
Adult: 50–500 mg PO TID (1–10 drops SSKI PO TID)

Continued

POTASSIUM IODIDE *continued*

Sporotrichosis:

Adult and child: 65–325 mg PO TID. Daily doses may be increased in increments of 150–250 mg/24 hr. **Max. dose:** increase to tolerance or 4.5–9 g/24 hr.

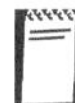

Contraindicated in pregnancy. GI disturbance, metallic taste, rash, salivary gland inflammation, headache, lacrimation, and rhinitis are symptoms of iodism. Give with milk or water after meals. Monitor thyroid function tests. Onset of antithyroid effects: 1–2 days.

Continue sporotrichosis treatment for 4–6 wk after lesions have completely healed. Increase dose until either **maximum dose** is achieved or signs of intolerance appear.

POTASSIUM SUPPLEMENTS

Many brand names

Electrolyte

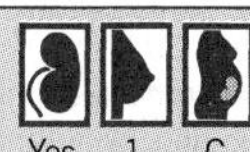

Potassium chloride:

40 mEq K = 3 g KCl
Sustained-release caps: 8, 10 mEq
Sustained-release tabs: 8, 10, 15, 20 mEq
Powder: 15, 20, 25 mEq/packet
Oral solution: 10% (6.7 mEq/5 mL), 15% (10 mEq/5 mL), 20% (13.3 mEq/5 mL)
Concentrated injection: 2 mEq/mL

Potassium gluconate:

40 mEq K = 9.4 g K gluconate
Tabs (OTC): 500 mg (2.15 mEq), 595 mg (2.56 mEq)
Oral liquid: 20 mEq/15 mL; may contain alcohol

Potassium acetate:

40 mEq K = 3.9 g K acetate
Concentrated injection: 2 mEq/mL

Potassium bicarbonate:

10 mEq K = 1 g K bicarbonate
Effervescent tab for oral solution: 25 mEq

Potassium phosphate:

See *Phosphorus Supplements.*

Normal daily requirements: see Chapter 20.
Replacement: Determine based on maintenance requirements, deficit, and ongoing losses. See Chapter 10.

Hypokalemia:

Oral:

Child: 1–4 mEq/kg/24 hr ÷ BID–QID. Monitor serum potassium.
Adult: 40–100 mEq/24 hr ÷ BID–QID
IV: **MONITOR SERUM K CLOSELY.**

Continued

For explanation of icons, see p. 680.

POTASSIUM SUPPLEMENTS *continued*

Child: 0.5–1 mEq/kg/dose given as an infusion of 0.5 mEq/kg/hr × 1–2 hr.
Max. IV infusion rate: 1 mEq/kg/hr. This may be used in critical situations (i.e., hypokalemia with arrhythmia).
Adult:
Serum K ≥2.5 mEq/L: Replete at rates up to 10 mEq/hr. Total dosage not to exceed 200 mEq/24 hr.
Serum K <2 mEq/L: Replete at rates up to 40 mEq/hr. Total dosage not to exceed 400 mEq/24 hr.
Maximum peripheral IV solution concentration: 40 mEq/L
Maximum concentration for central line administration: 150–200 mEq/L

PO administration may cause GI disturbance and ulceration. Oral liquid supplements should be diluted in water or fruit juice before administration. Sustained-release tablets must be swallowed whole and **NOT** dissolved in the mouth or chewed.

Do not administer IV potassium undiluted. IV administration may cause irritation, pain, and phlebitis at the infusion site. **Rapid or central IV infusion may cause cardiac arrhythmias.** Patients receiving infusion >0.5 mEq/kg/hr (>20 mEq/hr for adults) should be placed on an ECG monitor.

PRALIDOXIME CHLORIDE

Protopam, 2-PAM
Antidote: organophosphate poisoning

Yes ? C

Injection: 1000 mg

Use with atropine.
Child: 20–50 mg/kg/dose × 1 IM/IV/SC. May repeat in 1–2 hr if muscle weakness is not relieved, then at Q10-12 hr if cholinergic signs reappear.
Adult: 1–2 g/dose × 1 IM/IV/SC. May repeat in 1–2 hr if muscle weakness is not relieved, then at Q10–12 hr if cholinergic signs reappear.
Continuous infusions have also been recommended; see package insert.

Do not use as an antidote for carbamate classes of pesticides. Removal of secretions and maintaining a patent airway is critical. May cause muscle rigidity, laryngospasm, and tachycardia after rapid IV infusion. Drug is generally ineffective if administered 36–48 hr after exposure. Additional doses may be necessary.

For IV administration, dilute to 50 mg/mL or less and infuse over 15–30 min (**not to exceed** 200 mg/min). Reduce dosage in renal impairment because 80% to 90% of the drug is excreted unchanged in the urine 12 hr after administration.

PRAZIQUANTEL
Biltricide
Anthelmintic

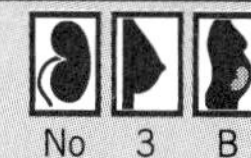

Tabs: 600 mg (tri-scored)

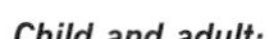

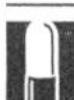

Child and adult:
Schistosomiasis: 20 mg/kg/dose PO BID–TID × 1 day
Flukes: 25 mg/kg/dose PO Q8 hr × 1 day (× 2 days for *P. westermani*)
Cysticercosis: 50–100 mg/kg/24 hr PO ÷ Q8 hr × 30 days (dexamethasone may be added to regimen for 2–3 days to minimize inflammatory response)
Tapeworms: 5–10 mg/kg/dose PO × 1 dose (25 mg/kg/dose × 1 dose for *H. nana*)

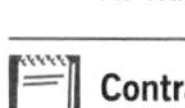

Contraindicated in ocular cysticercosis and spinal cysticercosis. **Use with caution** in patients with severe hepatic disease or history of seizures.

May cause dizziness and drowsiness. Headache, seizures, intracranial hypertension, increased CSF protein, and hyperthermia have occurred in patients treated for neurocysticercosis. Carbamazepine, phenytoin, and chloroquine may decrease praziquantel's effects. Cimetidine may increase praziquantel's effects. Take with food. **Do not** chew tablets due to bitter taste.

PREDNISOLONE
Orapred, Prelone, Pediapred, and others
Corticosteroid

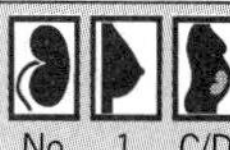

Tabs: 5 mg
Syrup (Prelone): 5 mg/5 mL (120 mL), 15 mg/5 mL (240 mL); contains alcohol and saccharin
Oral solution (as Na phosphate):
Pediapred: 5 mg/5 mL (120 mL); alcohol and dye free
Orapred: 15 mg /5 mL (237 mL); contains 2% alcohol and is dye free
Injection (as acetate): 25, 50 mg/mL (10, 30 mL); not for IV use and may contain benzyl alcohol
Injection (as Na phosphate): 20 mg/mL (2, 5, 10 mL); contains bisulfite
Injection (as tebutate): 20 mg/mL (10 mL); not for IV use
Ophthalmic suspension (as acetate): 0.12%, 0.125%, 1% (5, 10 mL)
Ophthalmic solution (as Na phosphate): 0.125%, 1% (5, 10, 15 mL)

See Prednisone (equivalent dosing).
Ophthalmic (consult ophthalmologist before use):
Child and adult: Start with 1–2 drops Q1 hr during the day and Q2 hr during the night until favorable response, then reduce dose to 1 drop Q4 hr. Dose may be further reduced to 1 drop TID–QID.

See *Prednisone* for remarks. See Chapter 29 for relative steroid potencies. Pregnancy category changes to D if used in the first trimester.
Orapred product should be stored in the refrigerator.

For explanation of icons, see p. 680.

PREDNISONE

Orasone, Deltasone, Liquid Pred, and others

Corticosteroid

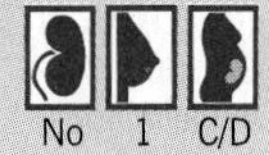

Tabs: 1, 2.5, 5, 10, 20, 50 mg

Oral syrup/solution: 1 mg/mL (120, 240, 500 mL); contains 5% alcohol and saccharin

Concentrated solution: 5 mg/mL (30 mL); contains 30% alcohol

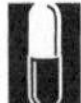

Child:

Antiinflammatory/immunosuppressive: 0.5–2 mg/kg/24 hr PO ÷ QD–BID

Acute asthma: 2 mg/kg/24 hr PO ÷ QD–BID × 5–7 days; **max. dose:** 80 mg/24 hr. Patients may benefit from tapering if therapy exceeds 5–7 days.

Nephrotic syndrome: Starting doses of 2 mg/kg/24 hr PO (**max. dose:** 80 mg/24 hr) are recommended. Further treatment plans are individualized. Consult a nephrologist.

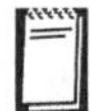

See Chapter 29 for physiologic replacement, relative steroid potencies, and doses based on body surface area. Methylprednisolone is preferable in hepatic disease because prednisone must be converted to methylprednisolone in the liver.

Side effects may include mood changes, seizures, hyperglycemia, diarrhea, nausea, abdominal distension, GI bleeding, HPA axis suppression, osteopenia, cushingoid effects, and cataracts with prolonged use. Prednisone is a cytochrome P-450 3A 3/4 substrate and inducer. Barbiturates, carbamazepine, phenytoin, rifampin, and isoniazid may reduce the effects of prednisone, whereas estrogens may enhance the effects. Pregnancy category changes to D if used in the first trimester.

PRIMAQUINE PHOSPHATE

Various generic brands

Antimalarial

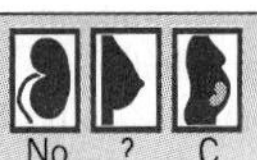

Tabs: 26.3 mg (15 mg base)

Doses expressed in mg of primaquine base.

Malaria:

Prevention of relapses for P. vivax or P. ovale only *(initiate therapy during the last 2 wk of, or following a course of, suppression with chloroquine or comparable drug):*

Child: 0.3 mg/kg/dose PO QD × 14 days

Adult: 15 mg PO QD × 14 days **OR** 45 mg PO Q7 days × 8 wk

Prevention of chloroquine-resistant strains *(initiate 1 day before departure, and continue until 7 days after leaving endemic area):*

Child: 0.5 mg/kg/dose PO QD

Adult: 30 mg PO QD

Pneumocystis carinii pneumonia (in combination with clindamycin):

Adult: 30 mg PO QD × 21 days

Continued

PRIMAQUINE PHOSPHATE *continued*

Contraindicated in granulocytopenia (e.g., rheumatoid arthritis, lupus erythematosus) and bone marrow suppression. **Avoid** use with quinacrine and with other drugs that can cause hemolysis or bone marrow suppression. **Use with caution** in G6PD and NADH methemoglobin-reductase deficient patients owing to increased risk for hemolytic anemia and leukopenia, respectively. Use in pregnancy is **not recommended** by the AAP *Redbook.*

May cause headache, visual disturbances, nausea, vomiting, and abdominal cramps. Administer all doses with food to mask bitter taste.

PRIMIDONE

Mysoline and others

Anticonvulsant, barbiturate

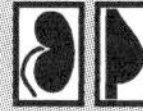
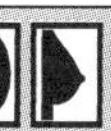
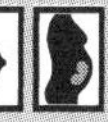

Yes 2 D

Tabs: 50, 250 mg

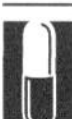

<8 yr	≥8 yr and Adults
DAY 1–3	
50 mg PO QHS	100–125 mg PO QHS
DAY 4–6	
50 mg PO BID	100–125 mg PO BID
DAY 7–9	
100 mg PO BID	100–125 mg PO TID
THEREAFTER	
125–250 mg PO TID or 10–25 mg/kg/24 hr ÷ TID–QID	250 mg PO TID–QID; max. dose: 2 g/24 hr

Use with caution in renal or hepatic disease and pulmonary insufficiency. Primidone is metabolized to phenobarbital and has the same drug interactions and toxicities (see *Phenobarbital*). Additionally, primidone may cause vertigo, nausea, leukopenia, malignant lymphoma-like syndrome, diplopia, nystagmus, systemic lupus-like syndrome. **Adjust dose in renal failure (see Chapter 30).**

Follow both primidone and phenobarbital levels. Therapeutic levels: 5–12 mg/L of primidone and 15–40 mg/L of phenobarbital. Recommended serum sampling time at steady state: trough level obtained within 30 min before the next scheduled dose after 1–4 days of continuous dosing.

PROBENECID

Various generic brands

Penicillin therapy adjuvant, uric acid lowering agent

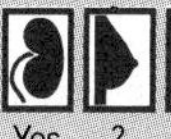

Yes ? C

Tabs: 500 mg

Continued

For explanation of icons, see p. 680.

PROBENECID *continued*

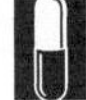

Use with penicillin.
Child (2–14 yr): 25 mg/kg PO × 1, then 40 mg/kg/24 hr ÷ QID; **max. dose:** 500 mg/dose. Use adult dose if >50 kg.
Adult: 500 mg PO QID

Hyperuricemia:
Adult: 250 mg PO BID × 1 wk, then 500 mg PO BID; may increase by 500 mg increments Q4 wk PRN up to a **max. dose** of 2–3 g/24 hr ÷ BID.

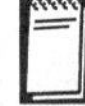

Use with caution in patients with peptic ulcer disease. **Contraindicated** in children <2 yr and in patients with renal insufficiency. **Do not use** if GFR <30 mL/min.

Increases uric acid excretion. Inhibits renal tubular secretion of acyclovir, ganciclovir, ciprofloxacin, gatifloxacin, nalidixic acid, moxifloxacin, organic acids, penicillins, cephalosporins, AZT, dapsone, methotrexate, nonsteroidal anti-inflammatory agents, and benzodiazepines. Salicylates may decrease probenecid's activity. Alkalinize urine in patients with gout. May cause headache, GI symptoms, rash, anemia, and hypersensitivity. False-positive glucosuria with Clinitest may occur.

PROCAINAMIDE

Procanbid and various generic brands
Antiarrhythmic, class Ia

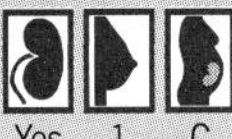

Sustained-release tabs (Procanbid): 250, 500, 750, 1000 mg
Caps: 250, 375, 500 mg
Injection: 500 mg/mL; contains methylparabens and bisulfites
Oral suspension: 5, 50, 100 mg/mL

Child:
V. tach with poor perfusion: Consider 15 mg/kg/dose IV × 1 over 30–60 min if cardioversion ineffective (see inside back cover); follow with continuous infusion if effective (see below).
IM: 20–30 mg/kg/24 hr ÷ Q4–6 hr; **max. dose:** 4 g/24 hr (peak effect in 1 hr).
IV: Load: 2–6 mg/kg/dose over 5 min (**max. dose:** 100 mg/dose); repeat dose. Q5–10 min PRN up to a **total max. dose** of 15 mg/kg. Do not exceed 500 mg in 30 min.
Maintenance: 20–80 mcg/kg/min by continuous infusion; **max. dose:** 2 g/24 hr.
To prepare infusion: See inside front cover.
PO: 15–50 mg/kg/24 hr ÷ Q3–6 hr; **max. dose:** 4 g/24 hr

Adult:
IM: 50 mg/kg/24 hr ÷ Q3–6 hr
IV: Load: 50–100 mg/dose; repeat dose Q5 min PRN to a **max. dose** of 1000–1500 mg.
Maintenance: 1–6 mg/min by continuous infusion

Continued

PROCAINAMIDE *continued*

NOTE: The IV infusion dosage units for adults are in mg/min; compared to mcg/kg/min for children.

PO: Usual dose: 50 mg/kg/24 hr

Immediate release: 250–500 mg/dose Q3–6 hr

Sustained release: 500–1000 mg/dose Q6 hr

Contraindicated in myasthenia gravis, complete heart block, SLE, and torsades de pointes. **Use with caution** in asymptomatic premature ventricular contractions, digitalis intoxication, CHF, and renal or hepatic dysfunction. **Adjust dose in renal failure (see Chapter 30).**

May cause lupus-like syndrome, positive Coombs test, thrombocytopenia, arrhythmias, GI complaints, and confusion. Increased LFTs and liver failure have been reported. Monitor BP and ECG when using IV. QRS widening by >0.02 sec suggests toxicity.

Cimetidine, ranitidine, amiodarone, beta-blockers, and trimethoprim may increase procainamide levels. Procainamide may enhance the effects of skeletal muscle relaxants and anticholinergic agents. Therapeutic levels: 4–10 mg/L of procainamide or 10–30 mg/L of procainamide and NAPA levels combined.

Recommended serum sampling times:

IM/PO intermittent dosing: Trough level within 30 min before the next scheduled dose after 2 days of continuous dosing (steady state).

IV continuous infusion: 2 and 12 hr after start of infusion and at 24-hr intervals thereafter.

PROCHLORPERAZINE

Compazine and others

Antiemetic, phenothiazine derivative

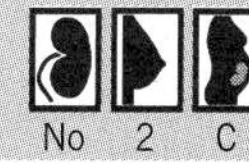

Tabs (as maleate): 5, 10, 25 mg
Slow-release caps (as maleate): 10, 15, 30 mg
Syrup (as edisylate): 5 mg/5 mL (120 mL)
Suppository: 2.5, 5, 25 mg (12s)
Injection (as edisylate): 5 mg/mL (2, 10 mL); may contain bisulfites and benzyl alcohol

Antiemetic doses:

Child (>10 kg or >2 yr):

PO or PR: 0.4 mg/kg/24 hr ÷ TID–QID or alternative dosing by weight:

10–14 kg: 2.5 mg QD–BID; **max. dose:** 7.5 mg/24 hr

15–18 kg: 2.5 mg BID–TID; **max. dose:** 10 mg/24 hr

19–39 kg: 2.5 mg TID or 5 mg BID; **max. dose:** 15 mg/24 hr

IM: 0.1–0.15 mg/kg/dose TID–QID; **max. dose:** 40 mg/24 hr

Adult:

PO:

Immediate release: 5–10 mg/dose TID–QID

Extended release: 10 mg/dose BID or 15 mg/dose QD

Continued

For explanation of icons, see p. 680.

PROCHLORPERAZINE *continued*

PR: 25 mg/dose BID
IM: 5–10 mg/dose Q3–4 hr
IV: 2.5–10 mg/dose; may repeat Q3–4 hr
Max. IM/IV dose: 40 mg/24 hr

Toxicity as for other phenothiazines (see *Chlorpromazine*). Extrapyramidal reactions (reversed by diphenhydramine) or orthostatic hypotension may occur. May cause false-positive test for phenylketonuria, urinary amylase, uroporphyrins, and urobilinogen. **Do not use** IV route in children. Use only in management of prolonged vomiting of known etiology.

0.15 mg/kg/dose IV over 10 min was effective in migraine headaches presenting in the emergency departments for children 5–18 yr [see Ann Emerg Med 2004;43:256–262].

PROMETHAZINE

Phenergan and others
Antihistamine, antiemetic, phenothiazine derivative

No ? C

Tabs: 12.5, 25, 50 mg
Syrup: 6.25 mg/5 mL (473 mL); contains alcohol
Suppository: 12.5, 25, 50 mg (12s)
Injection: 25, 50 mg/mL; may contain sulfites

Antihistaminic:
Child >2 yr: 0.1 mg/kg/dose (**max. dose:** 12.5 mg/dose) Q6 hr and 0.5 mg/kg/dose (**max. dose:** 25 mg/dose) QHS PO PRN
Adult: 12.5 mg PO TID and 25 mg QHS

Nausea and vomiting PO/IM/IV/PR:
Child >2 yr: 0.25–1 mg/kg/dose Q4–6 hr PRN; **max. dose:** 25 mg/dose
Adult: 12.5–25 mg Q4–6 hr PRN

Motion sickness: *(1st dose 0.5–1 hr before departure):*
Child >2 yr: 0.5 mg/kg/dose Q12 hr PO PRN; **max. dose:** 25 mg/dose
Adult: 25 mg PO Q8–12 hr PRN

Avoid use in children <2 yr because of risk for fatal respiratory depression. Toxicity similar to other phenothiazines (see *Chlorpromazine*). Administer oral doses with meals to decrease GI irritation. May cause profound sedation, blurred vision, respiratory depression (use lowest effective dose in children and **avoid** concomitant use of respiratory depressants), and dystonic reactions (reversed by diphenhydramine). Cholestatic jaundice and neuroleptic malignant syndrome have been reported. May interfere with pregnancy tests (immunologic reactions between hCG and anti-hCG). For nausea and vomiting, use only in management of prolonged vomiting of known etiology.

PROPRANOLOL
Inderal and others
Adrenergic blocking agent (beta), antiarrhythmic, class II

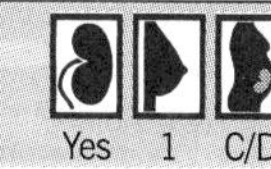

Tabs: 10, 20, 40, 60, 80, 90 mg
Extended-release caps: 60, 80, 120, 160 mg
Oral solution: 20, 40 mg/5 mL; contains parabens and saccharin
Concentrated solution: 80 mg/mL; alcohol and dye free
Injection: 1 mg/mL

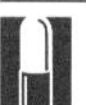

Arrhythmias:
Child:
IV: 0.01–0.1 mg/kg/dose IV push over 10 min, repeat Q6–8 hr PRN. **Max. dose:** 1 mg/dose for infants; **Max. dose:** 3 mg/dose for children.
PO: Start at 0.5–1 mg/kg/24 hr ÷ Q6–8 hr; increase dosage Q3–5 days PRN. Usual dosage range: 2–4 mg/kg/24 hr ÷ Q6–8 hr. **Max. dose:** 60 mg/24 hr or 16 mg/kg/24 hr.
Adult:
IV: 1 mg/dose Q5 min up to total 5 mg
PO: 10–20 mg/dose TID–QID. Increase PRN. Usual range 40–320 mg/24 hr ÷ TID–QID.
Hypertension:
Child:
PO: Initial: 0.5–1 mg/kg/24 hr ÷ Q6–12 hr. May increase dose Q3–5 days PRN; **max. dose:** 8 mg/kg/24 hr.
Adult:
PO: 40 mg/dose PO BID or 60–80 mg/dose (sustained-release capsule) PO QD. May increase 10–20 mg/dose Q3–5 days; **max. dose:** 640 mg/24 hr.
Migraine prophylaxis:
Child:
<35 kg: 10–20 mg PO TID
≥35 kg: 20–40 mg PO TID
Adult: 80 mg/24 hr ÷ Q6–8 hr PO; increase dose by 20–40 mg/dose Q3–4 wk PRN. Usual effective dose range: 160–240 mg/24 hr.
Tetralogy spells:
IV: 0.15–0.25 mg/kg/dose slow IV push. May repeat in 15 min × 1. See also Chapter 6.
PO: Start at 2–4 mg/kg/24 hr ÷ Q6 hr PRN. Usual dose range: 4–8 mg/kg/24 hr ÷ Q6 hr PRN. Doses as high as 15 mg/kg/24 hr have been used with careful monitoring.
Thyrotoxicosis:
Neonate: 2 mg/kg/24 hr PO ÷ Q6–12 hr
Adolescent and adult:
IV: 1–3 mg/dose over 10 min. May repeat in 4–6 hr.
PO: 10–40 mg/dose PO Q6 hr

Continued

For explanation of icons, see p. 680.

PROPRANOLOL *continued*

Contraindicated in asthma, Raynaud syndrome, heart failure, and heart block. **Use with caution** in presence of obstructive lung disease, diabetes mellitus, renal or hepatic disease. May cause hypoglycemia, hypotension, nausea, vomiting, depression, weakness, impotence, bronchospasm, and heart block. Cutaneous reactions, including Stevens-Johnson, TEN, exfoliative dermatitis, erythema multiforme, and urticaria have been reported. Acute hypertension has occurred after insulin-induced hypoglycemia in patients on propranolol.

Therapeutic levels: 30–100 ng/mL. Drug is metabolized by CYP450 1A2, 2C18, 2C19 and 2D6 isoenzymes.

Concurrent administration with barbiturates, indomethacin, or rifampin may cause decreased activity of propranolol. Concurrent administration with cimetidine, hydralazine, flecainide, quinidine, chlorpromazine, or verapamil may lead to increased activity of propranolol. **Avoid** IV use of propranolol with calcium-channel blockers; may increase effect of calcium-channel blocker.

Pregnancy category changes to D if used in second or third trimesters.

PROPYLTHIOURACIL
PTU
Antithyroid agent

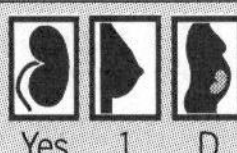

Tabs: 50 mg
Oral suspension: 5 mg/mL 
100 mg PTU = 10 mg Methimazole

Neonate: 5–10 mg/kg/24 hr ÷ Q8 hr PO
Child:
Initial: 5–7 mg/kg/24 hr ÷ Q8 hr PO, **OR** by age:
6–10 yr: 50–150 mg/24 hr ÷ Q8 hr PO
>10 yr: 150–300 mg/24 hr ÷ Q8 hr PO
Maintenance: Generally begins after 2 mo. Usually one third to two thirds the initial dose in divided doses (Q8–12 hr) when the patient is euthyroid.
Adult:
Initial: 300–450 mg/24 hr ÷ Q8 hr PO; some may require larger doses of 600–1200 mg/24 hr.
Maintenance: 100–150 mg/24 hr ÷ Q8–12 hr PO

May cause blood dyscrasias, fever, liver disease, dermatitis, urticaria, malaise, CNS stimulation or depression, and arthralgias. Glomerulonephritis, interstitial pneumonitis, exfoliative dermatitis, and erythema nodosum have also been reported. May decrease the effectiveness of warfarin. Monitor thyroid function. Dosages should be adjusted as required to achieve and maintain T_4, TSH levels in normal ranges. A dose reduction of beta-blocker may be necessary when the hyperthyroid patient becomes euthyroid.

For neonates, crush tablets, weigh appropriate dose, and mix in formula/breast milk. **Adjust dose in renal failure (see Chapter 30).**

PROSTAGLANDIN E_1

See *Alprostadil*

PROTAMINE SULFATE

Various generic brands
Antidote, heparin

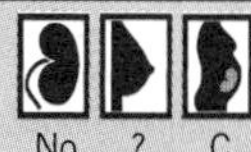
No ? C

Injection: 10 mg/mL (5, 25 mL); preservative free

Heparin antidote, IV:
1 mg protamine will neutralize 115 U porcine intestinal heparin or 90 U beef lung heparin.

Consider time since last heparin dose:

If <0.5 hr: give 100% of above dose.
If within 0.5–1 hr: give 50–75% of above dose.
If within 1–2 hr: give 37.5–50% of above dose.
If ≥2 hr: give 25–37.5% of above dose.
Max. dose: 50 mg IV
Max. infusion rate: 5 mg/min
Max. IV concentration: 10 mg/mL

If heparin was administered by deep SC injection, give 1–1.5 mg protamine per 100 U heparin as follows:

Load with 25–50 mg via slow IV infusion followed by the rest of the calculated dose via continuous infusion over 8–16 hr or the expected duration of heparin absorption.

Risk factors for protamine hypersensitivity include known hypersensitivity to fish and exposure to protamine-containing insulin or prior protamine therapy.

May cause hypotension, bradycardia, dyspnea, and anaphylaxis. Monitor aPTT or ACT. Heparin rebound with bleeding has been reported to occur 8–18 hr later. For neonates, reconstitute medication with preservative-free sterile water for injection.

PSEUDOEPHEDRINE

Sudafed, Efidac 24-Pseudoephedrine, and others
Sympathomimetic, nasal decongestant

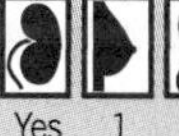
Yes 1 C

Tabs (OTC): 30, 60 mg
Chewable tabs (OTC): 15 mg; contains phenylalanine
Extended-release tabs (OTC): 120 mg, 240 mg (Efidac/24)
Caps (OTC): 30, 60 mg
Sustained-release caps (OTC): 120 mg
Liquid (OTC): 15, 30 mg/5 mL (120, 473 mL)
Drops (OTC): 7.5 mg/0.8 mL (15, 30 mL)

Continued

For explanation of icons, see p. 680.

PSEUDOEPHEDRINE *continued*

Child <12 yr: 4 mg/kg/24 hr ÷ Q6 hr PO or by age:
<2 yr: 4 mg/kg/24 hr ÷ Q6 hr PO
2–5 yr: 15 mg/dose Q6 hr PO; **max. dose:** 60 mg/24 hr
6–12 yr: 30 mg/dose Q6 hr PO; **max. dose:** 120 mg/24 hr
Child ≥12 yr and adult:
Immediate release: 30–60 mg/dose Q6 hr PO; **max. dose:** 240 mg/24 hr
Sustained release: 120 mg PO Q12 hr
Efidac/24: 240 mg PO Q24 hr

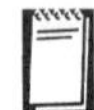

Contraindicated with MAO inhibitor drugs and in severe hypertension and severe coronary artery disease. **Use with caution** in mild/moderate hypertension, hyperglycemia, hyperthyroidism, and cardiac disease. May cause dizziness, nervousness, restlessness, insomnia, and arrhythmias. Pseudoephedrine is a common component of OTC cough and cold preparations and is combined with several antihistamines. Because drug and active metabolite are primarily excreted renally, doses should be adjusted in renal impairment. May cause false-positive test for amphetamines (EMIT assay).

PSYLLIUM

Metamucil, Fiberall, Serutan, Konsyl, Perdiem Fiber Therapy, and many others
Bulk-forming laxative

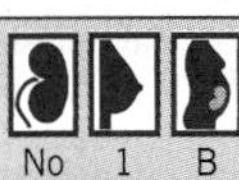

Granules (OTC): 2.5 g/rounded teaspoonful (480 g), 4.03 g/rounded teaspoonful (100, 170, 250, 540 g)
Powder (OTC): 50% psyllium, 50% dextrose (sugar-free version available) (Metamucil: 3.4 g/rounded teaspoon); 100% psyllium (Konsyl: 6 g/rounded teaspoon); for other products, check label for the amount of psyllium per unit of measurement.
Wafers (OTC): 3.4 g
Effervescent powder (OTC): 3.4 g/rounded teaspoonful (single-dose packet, 141 g, 261 g, 387 g, 621 g)
Chewable squares (OTC): 1.7 g, 3.4 g
Caps: 0.52 g

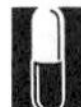

Child *(granules or powder must be mixed with a full glass of water or juice):*
<6 yr: 1.25–2.5 g/dose PO QD–TID; **max. dose:** 7.5 g/24 hr
6–11 yr: 2.5–3.75 g/dose PO QD–TID; **max. dose:** 15 g/24 hr
≥12 yr: 2.5–7.5 g/dose PO QD–TID; **max. dose:** 30 g/24 hr

Contraindicated in cases of fecal impaction or GI obstruction. **Use with caution** in patients with esophageal strictures and rectal bleeding. Phenylketonurics should be aware that certain preparations may contain aspartame. Should be taken with a full glass (240 mL) of liquid. Onset of action: 12–72 hr.

PYRANTEL PAMOATE

Antiminth, Reese's Pinworm, Pin-Rid, Pin-X
Antihelminthic

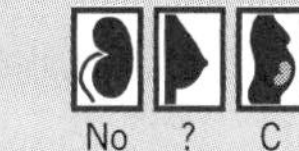
No ? C

Oral suspension (OTC): 50 mg/mL (60 mL)
Liquid (OTC): 50 mg/mL (30 mL); may contain parabens
Caps (OTC): 180 mg

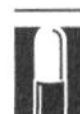

Adult and child:
Ascaris (roundworm) and Trichostrongylus: 11 mg/kg/dose PO × 1
Enterobius (pinworm): 11 mg/kg/dose PO × 1. Repeat same dose 2 wk later.
Hookworm or eosinophilic enterocolitis: 11 mg/kg/dose PO QD × 3 days
Max. dose (all indications): 1 g/dose

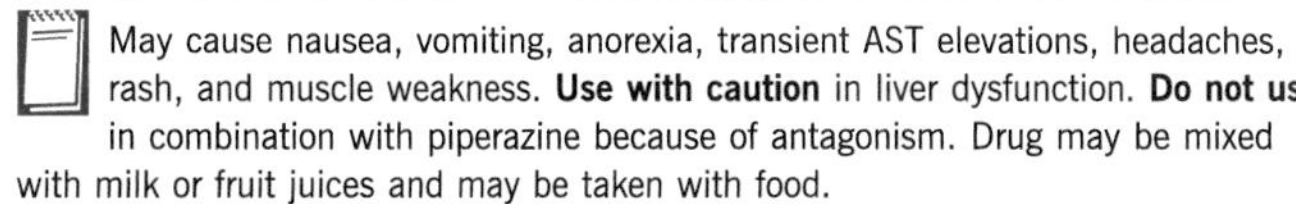

May cause nausea, vomiting, anorexia, transient AST elevations, headaches, rash, and muscle weakness. **Use with caution** in liver dysfunction. **Do not use** in combination with piperazine because of antagonism. Drug may be mixed with milk or fruit juices and may be taken with food.

PYRAZINAMIDE

Pyrazinoic acid amide
Antituberculous agent

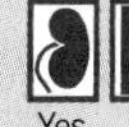
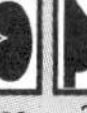
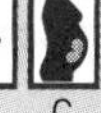
Yes ? C

Tabs: 500 mg
Oral suspension: 10, 100 mg/mL

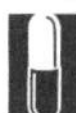

Use as part of a multi-drug regimen for tuberculosis.
See latest edition of the AAP *Red Book* for recommended treatment for tuberculosis.

Child:
Daily dose: 20–40 mg/kg/24 hr PO ÷ QD-BID; **max. dose:** 2 g/24 hr
Twice-weekly dose: 50 mg/kg/dose PO 2 ×/week; **max. dose:** 2 g/dose

Adult:
Daily dose: 15–30 mg/kg/24 hr PO ÷ QD-QID; **max. dose:** 2 g/24 hr
Twice-weekly dose: 50–70 mg/kg/dose PO 2 ×/week; **max. dose:** 4 g/dose

Contraindicated in severe hepatic damage. Hepatotoxicity is most common side effect. The CDC and ATS do not recommend the combination of pyrazinamide and rifampin for latent TB infections. Hyperuricemia, maculopapular rash, arthralgia, fever, acne, porphyria, dysuria, and photosensitivity may occur. **Use with caution** in patients with renal failure (dosage reduction has been recommended), gout, or diabetes mellitus.

For explanation of icons, see p. 680.

PYRETHRINS
Tisit, A-200, Pyrinyl, Pronto, RID, and others
Pediculicide

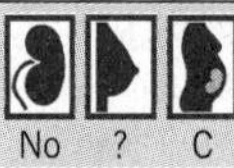

All products are available without a prescription.
Lotion: 0.3% pyrethrins and 2% piperonyl butoxide (59, 118 mL)
Gel: 0.3% pyrethrins and 3% piperonyl butoxide (30 mL)
Shampoo: 0.33% pyrethrins and 4% piperonyl butoxide (59, 118); may contain alcohol
Mousse: 0.33% pyrethrins and 4% piperonyl butoxide (165 mL); contains alcohol

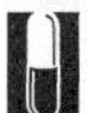

Pediculosis: Apply to hair or affected body area for 10 min, then wash thoroughly; repeat in 7–10 days.

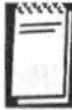

Contraindicated in ragweed hypersensitivity; drug is derived from the chrysanthemum flowers. For topical use only. **Avoid** eye or facial contact and PO intake. **Avoid** repeat applications in <24 hr. Low ovicidal activity requires repeat treatment. Dead nits require mechanical removal. Wash bedding and clothing to eradicate infestation.

PYRIDOSTIGMINE BROMIDE
Mestinon and others
Cholinergic agent

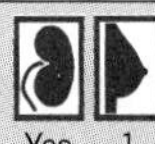
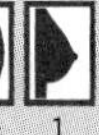
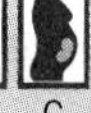

Syrup: 60 mg/5 mL (480 mL); contains 5% alcohol
Tabs: 60 mg
Sustained-release tab: 180 mg
Injection: 5 mg/mL; may contain parabens

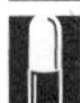

Myasthenia gravis:
Neonate:
PO: 5 mg/dose Q4–6 hr
IM/IV: 0.05–0.15 mg/kg/dose Q4–6 hr; **max. single IM/IV dose:** 10 mg

Child:
PO: 7 mg/kg/24 hr in 5–6 divided doses
IM/IV: 0.05–0.15 mg/kg/dose Q4–6 hr; **max. single IM/IV dose:** 10 mg

Adult:
PO (immediate release): 60 mg TID. Increase Q48 hr PRN. Usual effective dose: 60–1500 mg/24 hr.
PO (sustained release): 180–540 mg QD–BID
IM/IV: 2–5 mg/dose Q2–3 hr

Continued

PYRIDOSTIGMINE BROMIDE *continued*

Contraindicated in mechanical intestinal or urinary obstruction. **Use with caution** in patients with epilepsy, asthma, bradycardia, hyperthyroidism, arrhythmias, or peptic ulcer. May cause nausea, vomiting, diarrhea, rash, headache, and muscle cramps. Pyridostigmine is mainly excreted unchanged by the kidneys. Therefore, lower doses titrated to effect in renal disease may be necessary.

Changes in oral dosages may take several days to show results.

Atropine is the antidote.

PYRIDOXINE

Aminoxin, Vitamin B_6, and others

Vitamin, water soluble

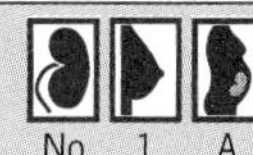

Tabs (OTC): 25, 50, 100, 250, 500 mg
Tabs, enteric-coated (Aminoxin) (OTC): 20 mg
Injection: 100 mg/mL (1 mL)

Deficiency, IM/IV/PO (PO preferred):
Child: 5–25 mg/24 hr × 3 wk, followed by 1.5–2.5 mg/24 hr as maintenance therapy (via multivitamin preparation)
Adult: 10–20 mg/24 hr × 3 wk, followed by 2–5 mg/24 hr as maintenance therapy (via multivitamin preparation)

Drug-induced neuritis, PO:
Prophylaxis:
Child: 1–2 mg/kg/24 hr
Adult: 25–100 mg/24 hr
Treatment:
Child: 10–50 mg/24 hr
Adult: 100–300 mg/24 hr

Sideroblastic anemia:
Adult: 200–600 mg/24 hr PO × 1–2 mo. If adequate response, dose may be reduced to 30–50 mg/24 hr.

Pyridoxine-dependent seizures:
Neonate/infant:
Initial: 50–100 mg/dose IM or rapid IV × 1
Maintenance: 50–100 mg/24 hr PO

Recommended daily allowance: see Chapter 20.

Use caution with concurrent levodopa therapy. Chronic administration has been associated with sensory neuropathy. Nausea, headache, increased AST, decreased serum folic acid level, and allergic reaction may occur. May lower phenytoin levels. See Chapter 19 for management of neonatal seizures.

For explanation of icons, see p. 680.

PYRIMETHAMINE ± SULFADOXINE

Daraprim; in combination with sulfadoxine- Fansidar

Antiparasitic agent ± sulfonamide antibiotic

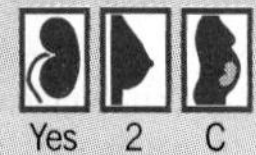

Tabs: 25 mg

Suspension: 2 mg/mL 

In combination with sulfadoxine:

Tabs: pyrimethamine 25 mg and sulfadoxine 500 mg

PYRIMETHAMINE:

Congenital toxoplasmosis *(administer with sulfadiazine; see remarks):*

Load: 2 mg/kg/24 hr PO ÷ Q12 hr × 2 days

Maintenance: 1 mg/kg/24 hr PO QD × 2–6 mo, then 1 mg/kg/24 hr 3 ×/week to complete total 12 mo of therapy.

Toxoplasmosis *(administer with sulfadiazine or trisulfapyrimidines)*

Child:

Load: 2 mg/kg/24 hr PO ÷ BID × 3 days; **max. dose:** 100 mg/24 hr

Maintenance: 1 mg/kg/24 hr PO ÷ QD-BID × 4 wk; **Max. dose:** 25 mg/24 hr

Adult: 50–75 mg/24 hr × 3–4 wk depending on response. After response, decrease dose by 50% and continue for an additional 4–5 wk.

PYRIMETHAMINE AND SULFADOXINE:

Malaria treatment *(single dose on the last day of quinine therapy):*

2–11 mo: one-fourth tab
1–3 yr: one-half tab
4–8 yr: 1 tab
9–14 yr: 2 tabs
>14 yr and adult: 3 tabs

Malaria prophylaxis *(for areas of chloroquine-resistant* P. falciparum *used as a single dose for self-treatment of febrile illness when medical care is not immediately available):*

2–11 mo: one-fourth tab
1–3 yr: one-half tab
4–8 yr: 1 tab
9–14 yr: 2 tabs
>14 yr and adults: 3 tabs

Pyrimethamine is a folate antagonist. Supplementation with folinic acid leucovorin at 5–15 mg/24 hr is recommended. **Contraindicated** in megaloblastic anemia secondary to folate deficiency. **Use with caution** in G6PD deficiency, malabsorption syndromes, alcoholism, pregnancy, and renal or hepatic impairment. Pyrimethamine can cause glossitis, bone marrow suppression, seizures, rash, and photosensitivity. [For congenital toxoplasmosis, see Clin Infect Dis 1994;18:38–72.] Administer doses with meals. Most cases of acquired toxoplasmosis **do not** require specific antimicrobial therapy.

PYRIMETHAMINE AND SULFADOXINE: Effective against certain strains of *P. falciparum* that are resistant to chloroquine. Resistance has been reported in Southeast Asia, the Amazon basin, sub-Saharan Africa, Bangladesh, and Oceania.

Continued

PYRIMETHAMINE ± SULFADOXINE *continued*

Contraindicated (in addition to above) in sulfa hypersensitivity, porphyria, severe renal or hepatic impairment, infants <2 mo, and pregnancy at term. May cause (in addition to above) erythema multiforme, Stevens-Johnson syndrome, toxic epidermal necrolysis, elevated ALT and AST, and renal impairment. Administer doses with meals.

QUINIDINE

Quinidex and various generic brands

Antiarrhythmic, class Ia

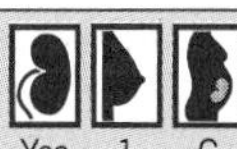

As gluconate (62% quinidine):

Slow-release tabs: 324 mg

Injection: 80 mg/mL; contains phenol

As sulfate (83% quinidine):

Tabs: 200, 300 mg

Slow-release tabs: 300 mg

Oral suspension: 10 mg/mL

Equivalents: 200 mg sulfate = 267 mg gluconate

All doses expressed as salt forms.

Antiarrhythmic:

Child *(Give PO as sulfate. Give IM/IV as gluconate):*

Test dose: 2 mg/kg × 1 IM/PO; **max. dose:** 200 mg

Therapeutic dose:

IV (as gluconate): 2–10 mg/kg/dose Q3–6 hr PRN

PO (as sulfate): 15–60 mg/kg/24 hr ÷ Q6 hr

Adult *(Give PO as sulfate. Give IM as gluconate):*

Test dose: 200 mg × 1 IM/PO

Therapeutic dose:

As sulfate:

PO, immediate release: 100–600 mg/dose Q4–6 hr. Begin at 200 mg/dose, and titrate to desired effect.

PO, sustained release: 300–600 mg/dose Q 8–12 hr

As gluconate:

IM: 400 mg/dose Q4–6 hr

IV: 200–400 mg/dose, infused at a rate of ≤10 mg/min

PO: 324–972 mg Q8–12 hr

Malaria:

Child and adult *(give IV as gluconate; see remarks):*

Loading dose: 10 mg/kg/dose (**max. dose:** 600 mg) IV over 1–2 hr followed by maintenance dose. Omit or decrease load if patient has received quinine or mefloquine.

Maintenance dose: 0.02 mg/kg/min IV as continuous infusion until oral therapy can be initiated. If more than 48 hr of IV therapy is required, reduce dose by one third to one half.

Continued

For explanation of icons, see p. 680.

QUINIDINE *continued*

Test dose is given to assess for idiosyncratic reaction to quinidine. Toxicity indicated by increase of QRS interval by ≥0.02 sec (skip dose or stop drug). May cause GI symptoms, hypotension, tinnitus, TTP, rash, heart block, and blood dyscrasias. When used alone, may cause 1:1 conduction in atrial flutter leading to ventricular fibrillation. May get idiosyncratic ventricular tachycardia with low levels, especially when initiating therapy.

Quinidine is an inhibitor of cytochrome P-450 3A 3/4 and 3A 5–7 enzymes, and inhibitor of P450 2D6 and 3A 3/4. Can cause increase in digoxin levels. Quinidine potentiates the effect of neuromuscular blocking agents, beta-blockers, anticholinergics, and warfarin. Amiodarone, antacids, delavirdine, diltiazem, grapefruit juice, saquinavir, ritonavir, verapamil, or cimetidine may enhance the drug's effect. Barbiturates, phenytoin, cholinergic drugs, nifedipine, sucralfate, or rifampin may reduce quinidine's effect. **Use with caution** in renal insufficiency (15%–25% of drug is eliminated unchanged in the urine).

Therapeutic levels: 3–7 mg/L. Recommended serum sampling times at steady state: trough level obtained within 30 min before the next scheduled dose after 1–2 days of continuous dosing (steady state).

MALARIA USE: Continuous monitoring of ECG, blood pressure, and serum glucose are recommended, especially in pregnant women and young children.

QUINUPRISTIN AND DALFOPRISTIN

Synercid

Antibiotic, streptogramin

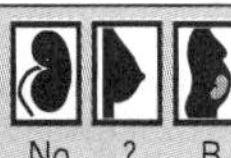

No ? B

Injection: 500 mg (150 mg quinupristin and 350 mg dalfopristin)

Doses expressed in mg of combined quinupristin and dalfopristin.

Child <16 yr (limited data), ≥16 yr and adult:

Vancomycin-resistant Enterococcus faecium (VREF): 7.5 mg/kg/dose IV Q8 hr

Complicated skin infections: 7.5 mg/kg/dose IV Q12 hr for at least 7 days

Peritonitis associated with peritoneal dialysis *(≥16 yr and adults):* 5–10 mg/kg/dose IV Q12 hr × 14 days

Not active against *Enterococcus faecalis*. **Use with caution** in hepatic impairment; dosage reduction may be necessary. Most common side effects include pain, burning, inflammation and edema at the IV infusion site, thrombophlebitis, and thrombosis. Nausea, diarrhea, vomiting, rash, arthralgia, myalgia, increased liver enzymes, hyperbilirubinemia, headache, pain, or pruritus may also occur.

Drug is an inhibitor to the cytochrome P-450 3A4 isoenzyme. **Avoid use** with cytochrome P-450 3A4 substrates, which can prolong QTc interval (e.g., cisapride). May increase the effects/toxicity of cyclosporine, tacrolimus, sirolimus, delavirdine, nevirapine, indinavir, ritonavir, diazepam, midazolam, carbamazepine, methylprednisolone, vinca alkaloids, docetaxel, paclitaxel, quinidine, and some calcium-channel blockers.

Continued

QUINUPRISTIN AND DALFOPRISTIN *continued*

Pediatric pharmacokinetic studies have not been completed. Reduce dose for patients with hepatic cirrhosis (Child-Pugh A or B).

Drug is compatible with D5W and incompatible with saline and heparin. Infuse each dose over 1 hr using the following **maximum** IV concentrations: peripheral line, 2 mg/mL; central line, 5 mg/mL. If injection site reaction occurs, dilute infusion to <1 mg/mL.

RANITIDINE HCL

Zantac, Zantac 75 (OTC), and others

Histamine-2 antagonist

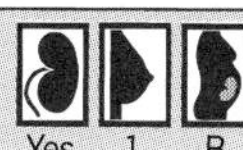

Tabs: 75 (OTC), 150, 300 mg
Effervescent tabs: 25, 150 mg
Syrup: 15 mg/mL; contains 7.5% alcohol and parabens
Effervescent granules: 150 mg; contains phenylalanine and povidone
Carbohydrate-free oral solution: 5, 10 mg/mL (dissolve 150 mg effervescent granules with 30 mL [5 mg/mL] or 15 mL [10 mg/mL] water; solution good for 24 hr)
Injection: 25 mg/mL (2, 6 mL); contains 0.5% phenol
Injection (premixed): 1 mg/mL (preservative-free in ½ normal saline, 50 mL)

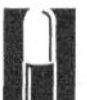

Neonate:
PO: 2–4 mg/kg/24 hr ÷ Q8–12 hr
IV: 2 mg/kg/24 hr ÷ Q6–8 hr

≥1 mo–16 yr:
Duodenal/gastric ulcer (see remarks):
PO:
Treatment: 2–4 mg/kg/24 hr ÷ Q12 hr; **max. dose:** 300 mg/24 hr
Maintenance: 2–4 mg/kg/24 hr ÷ Q12 hr; **max. dose:** 150 mg/24 hr
IV/IM: 2–4 mg/kg/24 hr ÷ Q6–8 hr; **max. dose:** 150 mg/24 hr
GERD/erosive esophagitis:
PO: 5–10 mg/kg/24 hr ÷ Q12 hr; GERD **max. dose:** 300 mg/24 hr, erosive esophagitis **max. dose:** 600 mg/24 hr
IV/IM: 2–4 mg/kg/24 hr ÷ Q6–8 hr; **max. dose:** 200 mg/24 hr

Adult:
PO: 150 mg/dose BID or 300 mg/dose QHS
IM/IV: 50 mg/dose Q6–8 hr; **max. dose:** 400 mg/24 hr

Continuous infusion, all ages: Administer daily IV dosage over 24 hr (may be added to parenteral nutrition solutions).

May cause headache and GI disturbance, malaise, insomnia, sedation, arthralgia, and hepatotoxicity. May increase levels of nifedipine. May decrease levels of ketoconazole, itraconazole, and delavirdine. May cause false-positive urine protein test (Multistix).

Duodenal/gastric ulcer doses for ≥1 mo–16 yr are extrapolated from clinical adult trials and pharmacokinetic data in children. Extemporaneously compounded carbohydrate-free oral solution dosage form useful for patients receiving the ketogenic diet. The syrup dosage form has a peppermint flavor and may not be tolerated. **Adjust dose in renal failure (see Chapter 30).**

For explanation of icons, see p. 680.

RASBURICASE
Elitek
Antihyperuricemic agent

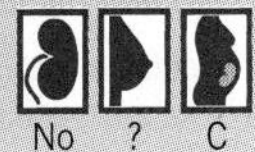

Injection: 1.5 mg

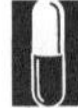

Hyperuricemia: 0.1–0.2 mg/kg/dose (rounded down to the nearest whole 1.5-mg multiple) IV over 30 min × 1. Patients generally respond to one dose, but if needed, dose may be repeated Q24 hr for up to 4 additional doses.

Contraindicated in G6PD deficiency or history of hypersensitivity, hemolytic reactions, or methemoglobinemia with rasburicase. **Use with caution** in asthma, allergies, hypersensitivity with other medications, and children <2 yr (decreased efficacy and increased risk for rash, vomiting, diarrhea, and fever).

Common side effects include nausea, vomiting, abdominal pain, discomfort, diarrhea, constipation, mucositis, fever, and rash.

During therapy, uric acid blood samples must be sent to the lab immediately. Blood should be collected in prechilled tubes containing heparin and placed in an ice-water bath to **avoid** potential falsely low uric acid levels (degradation of plasma uric acid occurs in the presence of rasburicase at room temperature). Centrifugation in a precooled centrifuge (4°C) is indicated.

RH_0 (D) IMMUNE GLOBULIN INTRAVENOUS (HUMAN)
WinRho-SDF
Immune globulin

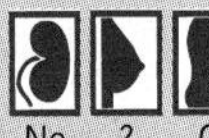

Injection: 600, 1500, 5000 IU
Conversion: 1 mcg = 5 IU

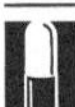

Immune thrombocytopenic purpura *(nonsplenectomized Rh_0 (D)–positive patients):*
Initial dose *(may given in two divided doses on separate days or as a single dose):*
- ***Hemoglobin ≥10 mg/dL:*** 250 IU/kg/dose IV × 1
- ***Hemoglobin <10 mg/dL:*** 125–200 IU/kg/dose IV × 1. See remarks.

Additional doses: 125–300 IU/kg/dose IV; actual dose and frequency of administration are determined by the patient's response and subsequent hemoglobin level.

WinRho SDF is currently the only Rh_0 (D) immune globulin product compatible with intravenous administration. **Contraindicated** in IgA deficiency. **Use with extreme caution in patients with a hemoglobin <8 mg/dL.** Adverse events associated with ITP include headache, chills, fever, and reduction in hemoglobin (due to the destruction of Rh_0 (D) antigen–positive red cells). Intravascular hemolysis resulting in anemia and renal insufficiency has been reported. May interfere with immune response to live virus vaccines (e.g., MMR, varicella). Rh_0 (D)–positive patients should be monitored for signs and symptoms of

Continued

RH$_0$ (D) IMMUNE GLOBULIN INTRAVENOUS (HUMAN) *continued*

intravascular hemolysis, anemia, and renal insufficiency. Administer IV doses over 3–5 min.

RIBAVIRIN

Rebetol, Copegus, Virazole

Antiviral agent

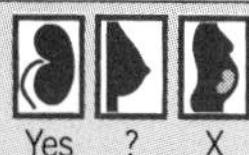

Oral solution (Rebetol): 200 mg/5 mL (100 mL); contains sodium benzoate
Oral caps (Rebetol): 200 mg
Tabs (Copegus): 200 mg
Aerosol (Virazole): 6 g

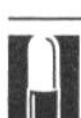

Hepatitis C *(PO, see remarks):*
Child *(≥3 yr, in combination with interferon alfa-2b at 3 million units 3× per week SC using Rebetol oral solution or capsule):*
25–36 kg: 200 mg BID
37–49 kg: 200 mg QAM and 400 mg QPM
50–61 kg: 400 mg BID
>61 kg: Use adult dose.

Dosage modification for toxicity: see remarks.

Adult:

Oral caps (Rebetol) in combination with interferon alfa-2b at 3 million units 3× per week SC:
≤75 kg: 400 mg QAM and 600 mg QPM
>75 kg: 600 mg BID

Oral caps (Rebetol) in combination with Peginterferon alfa-2b: 400 mg BID

Tabs (Copegus) in combination with Peginterferon alfa-2a for genotype 1, 4:
≤75 kg: 500 mg BID × 48 wk
>75 kg: 600 mg BID × 48 wk

Tabs (Copegus) in combination with Peginterferon alfa-2a for genotypes 2, 3: 400 mg BID × 24 wk

Dosage modification for toxicity: see remarks.

Inhalation:

Continuous: Administer 6 g by aerosol over 12–18 hr QD for 3–7 days. The 6-g ribavirin vial is diluted in 300 mL preservative-free sterile water to a final concentration of 20 mg/mL. Must be administered with Viratek Small Particle Aerosol Generator (SPAG-2).

Intermittent (for nonventilated patients): Administer 2 g by aerosol over 2 hours TID for 3–7 days. The 6-g ribavirin vial is diluted in 100 mL preservative-free sterile water to a final concentration of 60 mg/mL. The intermittent use is not recommended in patients with endotracheal tubes.

ORAL RIBAVIRIN: Contraindicated in pregnancy, significant or unstable cardiac disease, autoimmune hepatitis, hemoglobinopathies, and creatinine clearance <50 mL/min. Anemia (most common), insomnia, depression, irritability, and suicidal behavior have been reported with the oral route. Tinnitus, hearing loss, vertigo, and severe hypertriglyceridemia have been reported in combination with interferon. May decrease the effects of zidovudine, stavudine, and

Continued

For explanation of icons, see p. 680.

RIBAVIRIN *continued*

increase risk for lactic acidosis with nucleoside analogs. Reduce or discontinue dosage for toxicity as follows:

Patient with no cardiac disease:
Hgb <10 g/dL and ≥8.5 g/dL:
Child: 7.5 mg/kg/dose PO QD
Adult: 600 mg PO QD
Hgb <8.5 g/dL: Discontinue therapy permanently.
Patient with cardiac disease:
≥2 mg/dL decrease in Hgb during any 4 week period during therapy:
Child: 7.5 mg/kg/dose PO QD
Adult: 600 mg PO QD
Hgb <12 g/dL after 4 wk of reduced dose: Discontinue therapy permanently.

INHALED RIBAVIRIN: Use of ribavirin for RSV is controversial and **NOT** routinely indicated. Aerosol therapy may be considered for selected infants and young children at high risk for serious RSV disease [see recommendations in Pediatrics 1996;97: 137–140 and most recent edition of the AAP *Redbook*]. Most effective if begun early in course of RSV infection, generally in the first 3 days. May cause worsening respiratory distress, rash, conjunctivitis, mild bronchospasm, hypotension, anemia, and cardiac arrest. **Avoid** unnecessary occupational exposure to ribavirin due to its teratogenic effects. Drug can precipitate in the respiratory equipment.

RIBOFLAVIN

Vitamin B_2 and others
Water-soluble vitamin

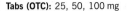

No 1 A/C

Tabs (OTC): 25, 50, 100 mg

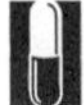

Riboflavin deficiency:
Child: 2.5–10 mg/24 hr ÷ QD–BID PO
Adult: 5–30 mg/24 hr ÷ QD–BID PO

RDA requirements: see Chapter 20.

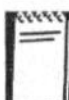

Hypersensitivity may occur. Administer with food. Causes yellow to orange discoloration of urine. For multivitamin information, see Chapter 20. Pregnancy category changes to C if used in doses above the RDA.

RIFABUTIN

Mycobutin
Antituberculous agent

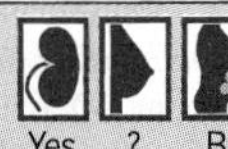

Yes ? B

Caps: 150 mg
Suspension: 10, 20 mg/mL

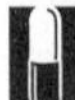

MAC prophylaxis for first episode and recurrence of opportunistic disease in HIV (may be in combination with a multidrug regimen that may include a macrolide antibiotic; see www.aidsinfo.nih.gov/guideline):
Infant and child: 5 mg/kg/24 hr PO QD; **max. dose:** 300 mg/24 hr
Adolescent and adult: 300 mg PO QD

Continued

RIFABUTIN *continued*

MAC treatment:

Child: 5–10 mg/kg/24 hr PO QD; **max. dose:** 300 mg/24 hr as part of a multidrug regimen

Adult: 300 mg PO QD; may be used in combination with azithromycin and ethambutol

In combination with nonnucleoside reverse transcriptase inhibitors:

With efavirenz: 450 mg PO QD or 600 mg PO 2× per week

With nevirapine: 300 mg PO 2× per week

In combination with protease inhibitors:

With amprenavir, indinavir, or nelfinavir: 150 mg PO QD or 300 mg PO 2× per week.

With ritonavir or lopinavir/ritonavir: 150 mg PO QOD

With saquinavir/ritonavir: 150 mg PO 2–3× per week or 300 mg PO Q week

May cause GI distress, discoloration of skin and body fluids (brown-orange color) and marrow suppression. **Use with caution** in renal failure. **Adjust dose in renal impairment (see Chapter 30)**. May permanently stain contact lenses. Uveitis can occur when using high doses (>300 mg/24 hr in adults) in combination with macrolide antibiotics.

Rifabutin is an inducer of cytochrome P450 3A enzyme and is structurally similar to rifampin (similar drug interactions, see Rifampin). Clarithromycin, fluconazole, itraconazole, nevirapine, and protease inhibitors increase rifabutin levels. Efavirenz may decrease rifabutin levels. May decrease effectiveness of dapsone, delavirdine, nevirapine, amprenavir, indinavir, nelfinavir, saquinavir, itraconazole, warfarin, oral contraceptives, digoxin, cyclosporin, ketoconazole, and narcotics.

Doses may be administered with food if patient experiences GI intolerance.

RIFAMPIN

Rimactane, Rifadin, and others

Antibiotic, antituberculous agent

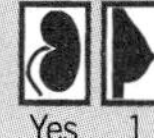
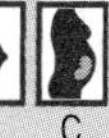

Yes 1 C

Caps: 150, 300 mg
Oral suspension: 10, 15, 25 mg/mL
Injection: 600 mg

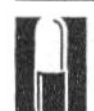

Tuberculosis: (see latest edition of the AAP *Red Book* for duration of therapy and combination therapy). Twice weekly therapy may be used after 1–2 mo of daily therapy.

Child:

Daily therapy: 10–20 mg/kg/24 hr ÷ Q12–24 hr IV/PO

Twice-weekly therapy: 10–20 mg/kg/24 hr PO twice weekly

Max. daily dose: 600 mg/24 hr

Adult:

Daily therapy: 10 mg/kg/24 hr QD PO

Twice-weekly therapy: 10 mg/kg/24 hr QD twice weekly

Max. daily dose: 600 mg/24 hr

Continued

For explanation of icons, see p. 680.

RIFAMPIN *continued*

Prophylaxis for N. meningitidis:

0–1 mo: 10 mg/kg/24 hr ÷ Q12 hr PO × 2 days
>1 mo: 20 mg/kg/24 hr ÷ Q12 hr PO × 2 days
Adult: 600 mg PO Q12 hr × 2 days
Max. dose *(all ages):* 1200 mg/24 hr

May cause GI irritation, allergy, headache, fatigue, ataxia, confusion, fever, hepatitis, blood dyscrasias, interstitial nephritis, and elevated BUN and uric acid. Causes red discoloration of body secretions such as urine, saliva, and tears (which can permanently stain contact lenses). Induces hepatic enzymes (CYP 450 2C9, 2C19, and 3A4), which may decrease plasma concentration of digoxin, corticosteroids, buspirone, benzodiazepines, fentanyl, calcium-channel blockers, beta-blockers, cyclosporine, tacrolimus, itraconazole, ketoconazole, oral anticoagulants, barbiturates, and theophylline. May reduce the effectiveness of oral contraceptives. Hepatotoxicity is a concern when used in combination with pyrazinamide or saquinavir/ritonavir combination therapy.

Adjust dose in renal failure (see Chapter 30). Reduce dose in hepatic impairment. Give 1 hr before or 2 hr after meals.

For *H. influenza* prophylaxis, see latest edition of the AAP *Red Book*.

RIMANTADINE

Flumadine
Antiviral agent

Yes 3 C

Syrup: 50 mg/5 mL (240 mL); contains saccharin and parabens
Tabs: 100 mg

Influenza A prophylaxis:
Child:
1–9 yr: 5 mg/kg/24 hr PO QD; **max. dose:** 150 mg/24 hr
≥10 yr:
<40 kg: 5 mg/kg/24 hr PO ÷ QD-BID; **max. dose:** 150 mg/24 hr
≥40 kg: 100 mg/dose PO BID
Adult: 100 mg PO BID

Influenza A treatment (within 48 hr of illness onset):
≥13 yr and adult: 100 mg PO BID × 5–7 days

During influenza season, use prophylaxis for 2–3 wk after influenza vaccination in order for patient to develop protective antibody response. Alternatively, may be used for 10 days after patient has been exposed. May cause GI disturbance, dizziness, headache, and urinary retention. CNS disturbances are less than with amantadine. **Contraindicated** in amantadine hypersensitivity. **Use with caution** in renal or hepatic insufficiency; dosage reduction may be necessary. A dosage reduction of 50% has been recommended in severe hepatic or renal impairment.

R

RISPERIDONE

Risperdal, Risperdal M-Tab, Risperdal Consta
Atypical antipsychotic, serotonin (5-HT$_2$) and dopamine (D$_2$) antagonist

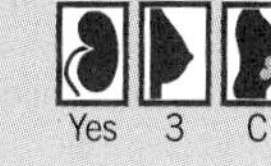

Tabs: 0.25, 0.5, 1, 2, 3, 4 mg
Oral solution: 1 mg/mL (30 mL)
Orally disintegrating tabs (Risperdal M-Tab): 0.5, 1, 2 mg; contains phenylalanine
Injection (Risperdal Consta): 25, 37.5, 50 mg (prefilled syringe with 2 mL diluent); for IM administration only

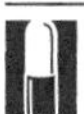

Child (PO):
Disruptive behavior in autism and other pervasive developmental disorders (limited data):
[Pediatrics 2004;114:e634–e641] (An 8-wk randomized placebo controlled trial in children 5–12 yr; mean, 7.6 yr): Start with 0.01 mg/kg/dose PO QD × 2 days and increase to 0.02 mg/kg/dose PO QD. At day 8, dose may be increased or decreased by a **maximum** of 0.02 mg/kg/24 hr at weekly intervals. **Max. dose:** 0.06 mg/kg/24 hr. 64% (N = 39) vs. 31% (N = 38) improvement in irritability with risperidone vs. placebo. Mean dose: 0.04 mg/kg/24 hr or 1.17 mg/24 hr.
[N Engl J Med 2002;347:314–321] (An 8-wk randomized placebo controlled trial in children 5–17 yr; mean, 8.8 ± 2.7 yr): If 20–45 kg, start with 0.5 mg PO QHS × 3 days followed by 0.5 mg PO BID. Dose was gradually increased by 0.5 mg to a **maximum** of 2.5 mg/24 hr (as 1 mg QAM and 1.5 mg QHS) by day 29. If >45 kg, a slightly accelerated dose schedule was used to achieve a **maximum** of 3.5 mg/24 hr (as 1.5 mg QAM and 2 mg QHS). 56.9% (N = 49) vs. 14.1% (N = 52) improvement in irritability with risperidone vs. placebo. Mean dose: 1.8 ± 0.7 mg/24 hr.
Aggressive behaviror in psychiatric disorders (limited data): See J Am Acad Child Adolesc Psychiatry 2000;39(4):509–516 and J Clin Pscyhiatry 2001; 62:239–248.

Adult:
Bipolar mania: Start with 2–3 mg PO QD. Dosage increases or decreases of 1 mg/24 hr can be made at 24-hr intervals. Dosage range: 1–6 mg/24 hr. Doses above 6 mg/24 hr have not been evaluated.
Schizophrenia:
PO: Start with 1 mg BID on day 1; if tolerated, increase to 2 mg BID on day 2 and to 3 mg BID thereafter. Dosage increases or decreases of 1–2 mg can be made on a weekly basis if needed. Usual effective dose: 4–8 mg/24 hr. Doses above 16 mg/24 hr have not been evaluated. In the presence of severe renal or hepatic impairment or risk for hypotension, start with 0.5 mg BID on days 1–2; if tolerated, increase to 1.5 mg BID. If needed, additional increases may be given at 1 week intervals at increments not to exceed 0.5 mg BID.
IM: Start with 25 mg Q2 wk; if no response, dose may be increased to 37.5 mg or 50 mg at 4-wk intervals. **Max. IM dose:** 50 mg Q2 wk.

Continued

For explanation of icons, see p. 680.

RISPERIDONE *continued*

Use with caution in cardiovascular disorders, diabetes, renal or hepatic impairment (dose reduction necessary), hypothermia or hyperthermia, seizures, breast cancer or other prolactin dependent tumors, and dysphagia. Common side effects include abdominal pain and other GI disturbances, arthralgia, anxiety, dizziness, headache, insomnia, somnolence (use QHS dosing), EPS, cough, fever, pharyngitis, rash, rhinitis, sexual dysfunction, tachycardia, and weight gain.

Pharmacokinetic data in children are incomplete. Limited studies in pediatric-related schizophrenia, Tourette syndrome, bipolar disorder, and aggressive behavior are reported. Weight gain, somnolence, and fatigue were common side effects reported in the autism studies.

Drug is a CYP450 2D6 and 3A4 isoenzyme substrate. Concurrent use of isoenzyme inhibitors (e.g., fluoxetine, paroxetine, sertraline, cimetidine) and inducers (e.g., carbamazepine, rifampin, phenobarbital, phenytoin) may increase and decrease the effects of risperidone, respectively. Alcohol, CNS depressants, and St. Johns wort may potentiate the drug's side effect. Risperidone may enhance the hypotensive effects of levodopa and dopamine agonists.

Oral dosage forms may be administered with or without food. Oral solution can be mixed in water, coffee, orange juice, or low-fat milk but is incompatible with cola or tea. Use IM suspension preparation within 6 hr after reconstitution.

ROCURONIUM

Zemuron

Nondepolarizing neuromuscular blocking agent

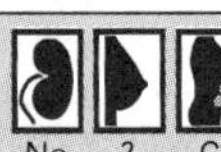

Injection: 10 mg/mL (5, 10 mL)

Infant:

IV: 0.5 mg/kg/dose; may repeat Q 20–30 min PRN

Child:

IV: 0.6 mg/kg/dose × 1; if needed, give maintenance doses of 0.075–0.125 mg/kg/dose Q 20–30 min.

Adolescent and adult:

IV: Start with 0.6–1.2 mg/kg/dose × 1, if needed, maintenance doses at 0.1–0.2 mg/kg/dose Q 20–30 min.

Continuous IV infusion: Start at 10–12 mcg/kg/min and titrate to effect. Maintenance infusion rates have ranged from 4–16 mcg/kg/min in adults.

To prepare infusion: see inside front cover.

Use with caution in hepatic impairment and history of anaphylaxis with other neuromuscular blocking agents. Hypertension, hypotension, arrhythmia, tachycardia, nausea, vomiting, bronchospasm, wheezing, hiccups, rash, and edema at the injection site may occur. Increased neuromuscular blockade may occur with concomitant use of aminoglycosides, clindamycin, tetracycline,

Continued

ROCURONIUM *continued*

magnesium sulfate, quinine, quinidine, succinylcholine, and inhalation anesthetics. Caffeine, calcium, carbamazepine, phenytoin, phenylephrine, azathioprine, and theophylline may reduce neuromuscular blocking effects.

Peak effects occur in 0.5–1 min for children and in 1–3.7 min for adults. Duration of action: 30–40 min in children and 20–94 min in adults (longer in geriatrics). Recovery time in children 3 mo to 1 yr is similar to adults. In obese patients, use actual body weight for dosage calculation.

SALMETEROL

Serevent Diskus

Beta-2-adrenergic agonist (long acting)

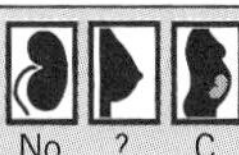

Aerosol metered dose inhaler (MDI): 21 mcg/actuation (6.5 g, 13 g; 6.5 g = 60 inhalations)

Dry-powder inhalation (DPI; Diskus): 50 mcg/inhalation (28, 60 inhalations)

In combination with fluticasone: *see Fluticasone propionate and Salmeterol.*

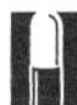

Persistent asthma *(see remarks):*

MDI:

Child: 1–2 puffs (21–42 mcg) Q12 hr

>12 yr and adult: 2 puffs (42 mcg) Q12 hr

DPI *(>4 yr and adult):* 1 inhalation (50 mcg) Q12 hr

Exercise-induced asthma *(>12 yr):*

MDI: 2 puffs 30–60 min before exercise. Additional doses should not be used for another 12 hr.

DPI: 1 inhalation 30–60 min before exercise. Additional does should not be used for another 12 hr.

Should not be used to relieve symptoms of acute asthma. It is long acting and has its onset of action in 10–20 min with a peak effect at 3 hr. May be used QHS (1–2 MDI puffs or 1 DPI) for nocturnal symptoms. Salmeterol is a chronic medication and is not used in similar fashion to short acting beta-agonists (e.g., albuterol). Patients already receiving salmeterol Q12 hr (MDI or DPI) should **NOT** use additional doses for prevention of exercise-induced bronchospasm; consider alternative therapy.

WARNING: Clinical safety data revealed a small but significant increase in asthma-related deaths when compared with placebo. A subgroup analysis suggested higher risk in African American patients compared to whites.

Use of spacers or chambers may enhance the efficacy of MDIs. Proper patient education is essential. Side effects are similar to albuterol. Hypertension and arrhythmias have been reported. See Chapter 22 for recommendations for asthma controller therapy.

For explanation of icons, see p. 680.

SCOPOLAMINE HYDROBROMIDE

Transderm Scop, Isopto Hyoscine, Scopace, and others

Anticholinergic agent

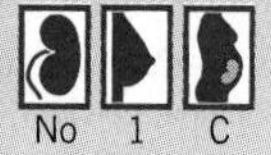

Injection: 0.3, 0.4, 0.86, 1 mg/mL
Transdermal: 1.5 mg/patch (4s); delivers ~1 mg over 3 days
Ophthalmic sol (Isopto Hyoscine): 0.25% (5, 15 mL)
Tab (Scopace): 0.4 mg

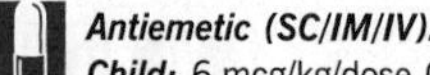

Antiemetic (SC/IM/IV):
- ***Child:*** 6 mcg/kg/dose Q6–8 hr PRN; **max. dose:** 300 mcg/dose
- ***Adult:*** 0.32–0.65 mg/dose Q6–8 hr PRN

Transdermal (≥12 yr) (see remarks):
- ***Motion sickness:*** Apply patch behind the ear at least 4 hr before exposure to motion; remove after 72 hr.
- ***Antiemetic before surgery:*** Apply patch behind the ear the evening before surgery.
- ***Antiemetic prior to cesarean section:*** Apply patch behind the ear 1 hr before to minimize infant exposure.

Ophthalmic:
- ***Child, refraction:*** 1 drop BID for 2 days before procedure
- ***Child, iridocyclitis:*** 1 drop up to TID

Toxicities similar to atropine. **Contraindicated** in urinary or GI obstruction and glaucoma. May cause dry mouth, drowsiness, and blurred vision. Transdermal route should **NOT** be used in children <12 yr. Drug withdrawal symptoms (nausea, vomiting, headache, and vertigo) have been reported following removal of transdermal patch in patients using the patch for >3 days. For perioperative use, the patch should be kept in place for 24 hr following surgery. Systemic effects have been reported with both transdermal and ophthalmic preparations. Compress nasolacrimal ducts to minimize systemic effects when using ophthalmic preparations.

SELENIUM SULFIDE

Selsun and Exsel (Rx)

Topical antiseborrheic agent

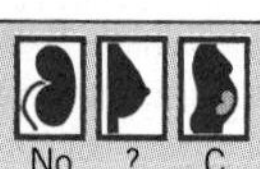

Lotion/shampoo: 1% (OTC) (210, 325, 400 mL)
Lotion: 2.5% (120 mL)

Seborrhea/dandruff: Massage 5–10 mL of 1% or 2.5% into wet scalp, and leave on scalp for 2–3 min. Rinse thoroughly and repeat. Shampoo twice weekly × 2 wk. Maintenance applications once every 1–4 wk.

Continued

SELENIUM SULFIDE *continued*

Tinea versicolor: Apply 2.5% lotion to affected areas of skin. Allow to remain on skin × 30 min. Rinse thoroughly. Repeat QD × 7 days. Follow with monthly applications for 3 mo to prevent recurrences.

Rinse hands and body well after treatment. May cause local irritation, hair loss, and hair discoloration. **Avoid** eyes and genital area. Shampoo may be used for tinea capitis to reduce risk for transmission to others (does not eradicate tinea infection).

For tinea versicolor, 15% to 25% sodium hyposulfite or thiosulfate (Tinver lotion) applied to affected areas BID × 2–4 wk is an alternative. Topical antifungals (e.g., clotrimazole, miconazole) may be used for small, focal infections.

SENNA

Senokot, Senna-Gen, Lax-Pills, and others

Laxative, stimulant

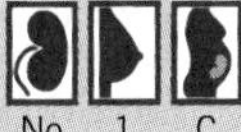

Granules [OTC]: 326 mg/tsp
Syrup [OTC]: 218 mg/5 mL (60, 240 mL)
Tab [OTC]: 187, 217, 374, 600 mg
Liquid [OTC]: 33.3 mg/mL (150 mL)

Child:

Oral: 10–20 mg/kg/dose PO QHS. **Max. doses** as shown below or

1 mo–1 yr: 55–109 mg PO QHS to **max. dose:** 218 mg/24 hr

1–5 yr: 109–218 mg PO QHS to **max. dose:** 436 mg/24 hr

5–15 yr: 218–436 mg PO QHS to **max. dose:** 872 mg/24 hr

Adult:

Granules: 326 mg (1 tsp) PO at bedtime; **max. dose:** 652 mg (2 tsp) BID

Syrup: 436–654 mg PO at bedtime; **max. dose:** 654 mg (15 mL) BID

Tabs: 374 mg (2 tabs) PO at bedtime; **max. dose:** 748 mg (4 tabs) BID

Effects occur within 6–24 hr after oral administration. May cause nausea, vomiting, diarrhea, abdominal cramps. Active metabolite stimulates the Auerbach plexus. Syrup may be administered with juice, milk, or mixed with ice cream. Granules may be sprinkled onto food or mixed with drinks.

SERTRALINE HCL

Zoloft

Antidepressant (selective serotonin reuptake inhibitor)

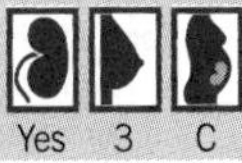

Tabs: 25, 50, 100 mg
Oral concentrate solution: 20 mg/mL (60 mL); contains 12% alcohol

Continued

For explanation of icons, see p. 680.

SERTRALINE HCL *continued*

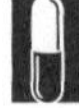

Depression:
Child ≥6–12 yr (data limited in this age group): Start at 25 mg PO QD. May increase dosage by 25 mg at 1-week intervals up to a **max. dose** of 200 mg/24 hr.
Child ≥13 yr and adult: Start at 50 mg PO QD. May increase dosage by 50 mg at 1-week intervals up to a **max. dose** of 200 mg/24 hr.
Obsessive-compulsive disorder:
Child ≥6–12 yr: Start at 25 mg PO QD. May increase dosage by 25 mg at 3–4 day intervals or by 50 mg at 7-day intervals up to a **max. dose** of 200 mg/24 hr.
Child ≥13 yr and adult: Start at 50 mg PO QD. May increase dosage by 50 mg at 1-wk intervals up to **max. dose** of 200 mg/24 hr.

This drug should **NOT** be used in combination with an MAO inhibitor (or within 14 days of discontinuing an MAO inhibitor) or pimozide. **Use with caution** in patients with hepatic or renal impairment. Adverse effects include nausea, diarrhea, tremor, and increased sweating. Hyponatremia and platelet dysfunction have been reported. Monitor for clinical worsening of depression and suicidal ideation/behavior following the initiation of therapy or after dose changes.

Use with drugs that interfere with hemostasis (e.g., NSAIDs, aspirin, and warfarin) may increase risk for GI bleeds. Use with warfarin may increase PT. Inhibits the CYP450 2D6 drug-metabolizing enzyme.

Mix oral concentrate solution with 4 oz. of water, ginger ale, lemon/lime soda, lemonade, or orange juice. After mixing, a slight haze may appear; this is normal. This dosage form should be **used cautiously** in patients with latex allergy because the dropper contains dry natural rubber.

SILVER SULFADIAZINE

Silvadene, Thermazene, SSD Cream, SSD AF Cream
Topical antibiotic

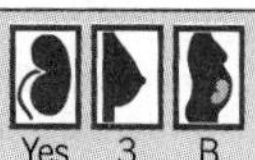

Cream: 1% (20, 25, 50, 85, 400, 1000 g); contains methylparabens and propylene glycol

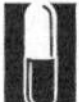

Cover affected areas completely QD–BID. Apply cream to a thickness of $\frac{1}{16}$-inch using sterile technique.

Contraindicated in premature infants and infant ≤2 mo of age due to concerns of kernicterus. **Use with caution** in G6PD and renal and hepatic impairment. Discard product if cream has darkened. Significant systemic absorption may occur in severe burns. Adverse effects include pruritus, rash, bone marrow suppression, hemolytic anemia, and interstitial nephritis. See Chapter 4 for more information.

SIMETHICONE

Mylicon, Phazyme, Mylanta Gas, Gas-X, and others

Antiflatulent

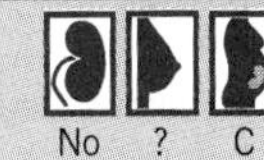

All dosage forms available OTC
Oral drops: 40 mg/0.6 mL (30 mL)
Caps: 125 mg
Tabs: 60, 95 mg
Chewable tabs: 80, 125, 150 mg

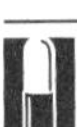

Infant and child <2 yr: 20 mg PO QID PRN; **max. dose:** 240 mg/24 hr
2–12 yr: 40 mg PO QID PRN
>12 yr: 40–125 mg PO QPC and QHS PRN; **max. dose:** 500 mg/24 hr

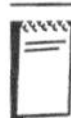

Efficacy has not been demonstrated for treating infant colic. **Avoid** carbonated beverages and gas-forming foods. Oral liquid may be mixed with water, infant formula, or other suitable liquids for ease of oral administration.

SODIUM BICARBONATE

Neut and others

Alkalinizing agent, electrolyte

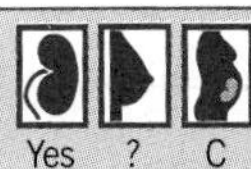

Injection: 4.2% (0.5 mEq/mL) (10 mL), 7.5% (0.89 mEq/mL), 8.4% (1 mEq/mL) (10, 50 mL)
Injection, premixed: 5% (0.6 mEq/mL) (500 mL)
Tabs: 325 mg (3.8 mEq), 650 mg (7.6 mEq)
Powder: 120, 480 g
Each 1 mEq bicarbonate provides 1 mEq Na^+

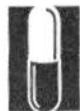

Cardiac arrest: see inside front cover.
Correction of metabolic acidosis: Calculate patient's dose with the following formulas.

Neonate, infant, and child:

HCO_3^- (mEq) = 0.3 × weight (kg) × base deficit (mEq/L), **OR**
HCO_3^- (mEq) = 0.5 × weight (kg) × [24 – serum HCO_3^- (mEq/L)]

Adult:

HCO_3^- (mEq) = 0.2 × weight (kg) × base deficit (mEq/L), **OR**
HCO_3^- (mEq) = 0.5 × weight (kg) × [24 – serum HCO_3^- (mEq/L)]

Urinary alkalinization (titrate dose accordingly to urine pH):

Child: 84–840 mg (1–10 mEq)/kg/24 hr PO ÷ QID
Adult: 4 g (48 mEq) × 1 followed by 1–2 g (12–24 mEq) PO Q4 hr. Doses up to 16 g (192 mEq)/24 hr have been used.

Continued

For explanation of icons, see p. 680.

SODIUM BICARBONATE *continued*

Contraindicated in respiratory alkalosis, hypochloremia, and inadequate ventilation during cardiac arrest. **Use with caution** in CHF, renal impairment, cirrhosis, hypocalcemia, hypertension, and concurrent corticosteroids. Maintain high urine output. Monitor acid-base balance and serum electrolytes. May cause hypernatremia (contains sodium), hypokalemia, hypomagnesemia, hypocalcemia, hyperreflexia, edema, and tissue necrosis (extravasation). Oral route of administration may cause GI discomfort and gastric rupture from gas production.

For direct IV administration (cardiac arrest) in neonates and infants, use the 0.5 mEq/mL (4.2%) concentration or dilute the 1 mEq/mL (8.4%) concentration 1 : 1 with sterile water for injection and infuse at a rate **no greater than** 10 mEq/min. The 1 mEq/mL (8.4%) concentration may be used in children and adults for direct IV administration.

For IV infusions (for all ages), dilute to a **maximum concentration** of 0.5 mEq/mL in dextrose or sterile water for injection and infuse over 2 hr using a **maximum rate** of 1 mEq/kg/hr.

Sodium bicarbonate should not be mixed with or be in contact with calcium, norepinephrine, or dobutamine.

SODIUM PHOSPHATE

Fleet, Fleet Phospho-Soda, Visicol

Laxative, enema/oral

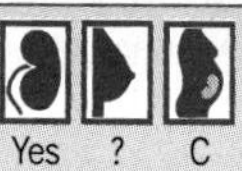

Enema (Fleet) (OTC): 6 g Na phos and 16 g Na biphosphate/100 mL
Pediatric size: 66 mL
Adult size: 133 mL

Oral solution (Fleet Phospho-Soda) (OTC): 18 g Na phos and 48 g Na biphosphate/100 mL (45, 90, 240 mL) contains 96.4 mEq Na per 20 mL

Oral tablets (Visicol): 1.5 g

Not to be used for phosphorus supplementation. See *Phosphorus* for supplementation.

Enema:

2–12 yr: 66 mL enema × 1. May repeat × 1.

>12 yr and adult: 133 mL enema × 1. May repeat × 1.

Oral laxative (mix with equal volume of water):

5–9 yr: 5 mL PO × 1

10–12 yr: 10 mL PO × 1

>12 yr: 20–30 mL PO × 1

Contraindicated in patients with severe renal failure, megacolon, bowel obstruction, and congestive heart failure. May cause hyperphosphatemia, hypernatremia, hypocalcemia, hypotension, dehydration, and acidosis. **Avoid** retention of enema solution, and **do not exceed** recommended doses because this may lead to severe electrolyte disturbances due to enhanced systemic absorption. Onset of action: PO, 3–6 hr; PR, 2–5 min.

SODIUM POLYSTYRENE SULFONATE

Kayexalate, SPS Suspension, Kionex, and others

Potassium-removing resin

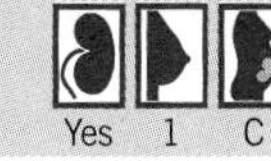

Yes 1 C

Powder: 454, 480 g

Suspension: 15 g/60 mL (contains 21.5 mL sorbitol/60 mL and 0.1%–0.3% alcohol) (60, 120, 200, 500 mL)

Contains 4.1 mEq Na^+/g drug

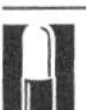

Child:

Usual dose: 1 g/kg/dose Q6 hr PO or Q2–6 hr PR

Adult:

PO: 15 g QD–QID

PR: 30–50 g Q6 hr

NOTE: Suspension may be given PO or PR. Practical exchange ratio is 1 mEq K per 1 g resin. May calculate dose according to desired exchange.

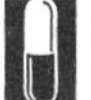

Contraindicated in obstructive bowel disease, neonates with reduced gut motility, and oral administration in neonates. **Use cautiously** in presence of renal failure, CHF, hypertension, or severe edema. May cause hypokalemia, hypernatremia, hypomagnesemia, and hypocalcemia.

1 mEq Na delivered for each mEq K removed. **Do not administer** with antacids or laxatives containing Mg^{2+} or Al^{3+}. Systemic alkalosis may result. Retain enema in colon for at least 30–60 min.

SPECTINOMYCIN

Trobicin

Antibiotic, aminoglycoside

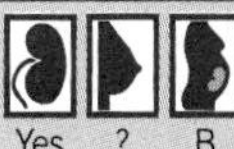

Yes ? B

Injection: 2 g with 3.2 mL diluent which contains 0.9% benzyl alcohol

Uncomplicated gonorrhea *(in combination with a macrolide):*

Child <45 kg: 40 mg/kg IM × 1; **max. dose:** 2 g/dose

≥45 kg and ≥8 yr old: 2 g IM × 1

Disseminated gonorrhea *(for patients allergic to beta-lactams and fluoroquinolones):*

≥45 kg and ≥8 yr old: 2 g IM Q12 hr × 7 days. Alternatively may treat × 24–48 hr and switch to oral alternative.

Not effective for syphilis. Drug is primarily used to treat gonorrhea in patients who cannot tolerate beta-lactams or fluoroquinolones. **Not recommended** for treatment of pharyngeal infections. Vertigo, malaise, nausea, anorexia, chills, fever, and urticaria may occur. Repeat dosing will cause accumuation in renal failure. IM use only. See latest edition of the AAP *Red Book.*

For explanation of icons, see p. 680.

SPIRONOLACTONE

Aldactone and others

Diuretic, potassium sparing

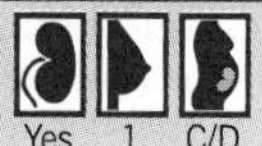

Tabs: 25, 50, 100 mg

Suspension: 1, 2, 2.5, 5, 25 mg/mL 

Diuretic:

Neonate: 1–3 mg/kg/24 hr ÷ QD–BID PO

Child: 1–3.3 mg/kg/24 hr ÷ QD–QID PO

Adult: 25–200 mg/24 hr ÷ QD–QID PO (see remarks)

Max. dose: 200 mg/24 hr

Diagnosis of primary aldosteronism:

Child: 125–375 mg/m²/24 hr ÷ BID–QID PO

Adult: 400 mg QD PO × 4 days (short test) or 3–4 wk (long test), then 100–400 mg QD maintenance.

Hirsutism in women:

Adult: 50–200 mg/24 hr ÷ QD–BID PO

Contraindicated in acute renal failure (see Chapter 30). May cause hyperkalemia, GI distress, rash, and gynecomastia. May potentiate ganglionic blocking agents and other antihypertensives. Monitor potassium levels and be aware of other K^+ sources, K^+-sparing diuretics, and angiotensin-converting enzyme inhibitors (all can increase K^+). May cause false elevation in serum digoxin levels measured by radioimmunoassay.

Although TID–QID regimens have been recommended, data suggest that QD–BID dosing is adequate. Pregnancy category changes to D if used in pregnancy-induced hypertension.

STREPTOKINASE

Streptase

Thrombolytic enzyme

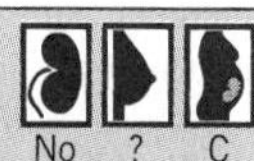

Injection: 250,000; 750,000; 1,500,000 IU

Thrombolytic: **Should be used in consultation with a hematologist.** Duration of therapy will depend on clinical response and generally does not exceed 3 days.

Child: 3500–4000 U/kg over 30 min, followed by 1000–1500 U/kg/hr; **OR** 2000 U/kg load over 30 min followed by 2000 U/kg/hr × 6–12 hr. Duration of infusion is individualized based on response.

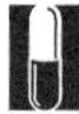

Pediatric safety and efficacy information is limited. **Contraindicated** with intracranial or intraspinal surgery, history of internal bleeding, recent streptococcal infection, or CVA within previous 2 mo. May cause hemorrhage, urticaria, itching, flushing, musculoskeletal pain, bronchospasm, and anaphylaxis.

Continued

STREPTOKINASE *continued*

Monitor fibrinogen, thrombin clotting time, PT, and APTT when used as a thrombolytic.

Newborns have reduced plasminogen levels (~50% of adult values), which decrease the thrombolytic effects of streptokinase. Plasminogen supplementation may be necessary.

Not recommended in restoring patency of intravenous catheters. Hypotension, hypersensitivity reactions, apnea, and bleeding, some of which were life threatening, have been reported when used in this manner.

STREPTOMYCIN SULFATE

Various brand names

Antibiotic, aminoglycoside; antituberculous agent

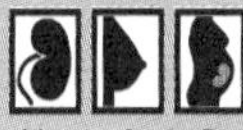

Injection: 400 mg/mL (2.5 mL)
Powder for injection: 1 g

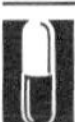

Tuberculosis: (use as part of multidrug regimen; see latest edition of AAP *Red Book*)

Infant, child, and adolescent:

Daily therapy: 20–40 mg/kg/24 hr IM QD
Max. daily dose: 1 g/24 hr
Twice-weekly therapy: 20–40 mg/kg/dose IM twice weekly
Max. daily dose: 1.5 g/24 hr

Adult:

Daily therapy: 15 mg/kg/24 hr IM QD
Max. daily dose: 1 g/24 hr
Twice-weekly therapy: 25–30 mg/kg/dose IM twice weekly
Max. daily dose: 1.5 g/24 hr

Brucellosis, tularemia, plague, and rat bite fever: see latest edition of the AAP *Red Book*.

Use with caution in preexisting vertigo, tinnitus, hearing loss, and neuromuscular disorders. Drug is administered via deep IM injection only.

Follow auditory status. May cause CNS depression, other neurologic problems, myocarditis, or serum sickness.

Therapeutic levels: peak, 15–40 mg/L; trough, <5 mg/L. Recommended serum sampling time at steady state: trough within 30 min before the third consecutive dose and peak 30–60 min after the administration of the third consecutive dose. Therapeutic levels are not achieved in CSF. **Adjust dose in renal insufficiency (see Chapter 30).**

For explanation of icons, see p. 680.

SUCCIMER

Chemet, DMSA (dimercaptosuccinic acid)
Chelating agent

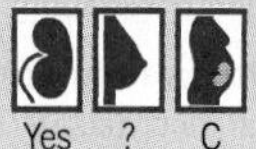

Caps: 100 mg

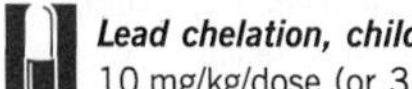

Lead chelation, child:
10 mg/kg/dose (or 350 mg/m^2/dose) PO Q8 hr × 5 days, then 10 mg/kg/dose (or 350 mg/m^2/dose) PO Q12 hr × 14 days.
Manufacturer recommends (see table below):

Weight (kg)	Dose (mg)
8–15	100
16–23	200
24–34	300
35–44	400
≥45	500

Give dose above every 8 hr for 5 days. Then the same dose Q12 hr for 14 days.

Use with caution in patients with compromised renal function. Repeated courses may be necessary. Follow serum lead levels. Allow minimum of 2 wk between courses, unless blood levels require more aggressive management. Side effects: GI symptoms, increased LFTs (10%), rash, headaches, and dizziness. **Coadministration with other chelating agents is not recommended.** Treatment of iron deficiency is recommended as well as environmental remediation. Contents of capsule may be sprinkled on food for those who are unable to swallow capsule.

SUCCINYLCHOLINE

Anectine, Quelicin, and others
Neuromuscular blocking agent

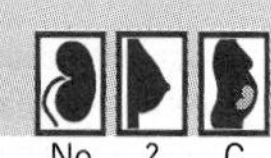

Injection: 20 mg/mL (5, 10 mL), 50 mg/mL (10 mL), 100 mg/mL (5, 10 mL); may contain parabens and/or benzyl alcohol
Powder for infusion: 500, 1000 mg

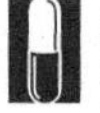

Paralysis for intubation:
Infant and child:
Initial:
- ***IV:*** 1–2 mg/kg/dose × 1
- ***IM:*** 2.5–4 mg/kg/dose × 1
- **Max. dose:** 150 mg/dose

Continued

SUCCINYLCHOLINE *continued*

Maintenance: 0.3–0.6 mg/kg/dose IV Q5–10 min PRN. **Continuous infusion not recommended**.

Adult:

Initial:

IV: 0.3–1.1 mg/kg/dose × 1

IM: 2.5–4 mg/kg/dose × 1

Max. dose: 150 mg/dose

Maintenance: 0.04–0.07 mg/kg/dose IV Q5–10 min PRN.

Continuous infusion not recommended.

Pretreatment with atropine is recommended to reduce incidence of bradycardia. For rapid sequence intubation, see Chapter 1.

Cardiac arrest has been reported in children and adolescents primarily with skeletal muscle myopathies (e.g., Duchenne muscular dystrophy). Identify developmental delays suggestive of a myopathy before use. Predose creatine kinase may be useful for identifying patients at risk. Monitoring of ECG for peaked T waves may be useful in detecting early signs of this adverse effect.

May cause malignant hyperthermia (use dantrolene to treat), bradycardia, hypotension, arrhythmia, and hyperkalemia. **Use with caution** in patients with severe burns, paraplegia, or crush injuries and in patients with preexisting hyperkalemia. Beware of prolonged depression in patients with liver disease, malnutrition, pseudocholinesterase deficiency, or hypothermia and in those receiving aminoglycosides, phenothiazines, quinidine, beta-blockers, amphotericin B, cyclophosphamide, diuretics, lithium, acetylcholine, and anticholinesterases. Diazepam may decrease neuromuscular blocking effects. Duration of action: 4–6 min IV, 10–30 min IM. Must be prepared to intubate within 1 min.

SUCRALFATE

Carafate and others

Oral antiulcer agent

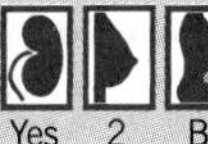

Tabs: 1 g

Suspension: 100 mg/mL (420 mL); contains sorbitol and parabens

Child: 40–80 mg/kg/24 hr ÷ Q6 hr PO

Adult: 1 g PO QID, 1 hr before meals and QHS

May cause vertigo, constipation, and dry mouth. Aluminum may accumulate in patients with renal failure. This may be augmented by the use of aluminum-containing antacids. Decreases absorption of phenytoin, digoxin, theophylline, cimetidine, fat-soluble vitamins, ketoconazole, omeprazole, quinolones, and oral anticoagulants. Administer these drugs at least 2 hr before or after sucralfate doses.

Drug requires an acidic environment to form a protective polymer coating for damaged GI tract mucosa. Doses as high as 1 g PO Q4 hr have been used in adults for stress ulcers.

For explanation of icons, see p. 680.

SULFACETAMIDE SODIUM

AK-Sulf, Bleph 10, Ocusulf-10, and others

Ophthalmic antibiotic, sulfonamide derivative

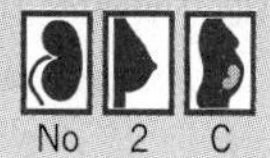

Ophthalmic solution: 10% (2, 2.5, 5, 15 mL), 30% (15 mL)
Ophthalmic ointment: 10% (3.5 g)

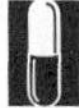

>2 mo and adult:
Ophthalmic ointment: Apply ribbon QID and QHS (5 × per 24 hr).
Drops: 1–2 drops Q2–3 hr to affected eye(s)

See *Sulfisoxazole.* 10% solution is used most frequently. May cause local irritation, stinging, burning, toxic epidermal necrolysis (rarely). Local irritation occurs more frequently with higher strength preparations. Usual duration of therapy for ophthalmic use is 7–10 days.

SULFADIAZINE

Various trade names

Antibiotic, sulfonamide derivative

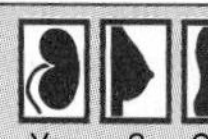

Tabs: 500 mg
Suspension: 100 mg/mL 

Congenital toxoplasmosis *(administer with pyrimethamine and folinic acid)* [From Clin Infect Dis 1994;18:38]:
Infant: 100 mg/kg/24 hr PO ÷ BID × 12 mo

Toxoplasmosis (administer with pyrimethamine and folinic acid):
Child: 100–200 mg/kg/24 hr ÷ Q6 hr PO × 3–4 wk
Adult: 4–6 g/24 hr PO ÷ Q6 hr × 3–4 wk

Rheumatic fever prophylaxis:
≤27 kg: 500 mg PO QD
>27 kg: 1000 mg PO QD

Most cases of acquired toxoplasmosis do not require specific antimicrobial therapy. **Contraindicated** in porphyria and hypersensitivity to sulfonamides. **Use with caution** in premature infants and infants <2 mo because of risk for hyperbilirubinemia and in hepatic or renal dysfunction (30%–44% eliminated in urine). Maintain hydration. May cause increased effects of warfarin, methotrexate, and sulfonylureas due to drug displacement from protein-binding sites. May cause fever, rash, hepatitis, SLE-like syndrome, vasculitis, bone marrow suppression and hemolysis (in patients with G6PD deficiency), and Stevens-Johnson syndrome. Pregnancy category changes from C to D if administered near term.

SULFASALAZINE

Salicylazosulfapyridine, SAS, Azulfidine, Azulfidine EN-tabs, and others

Anti-inflammatory agent

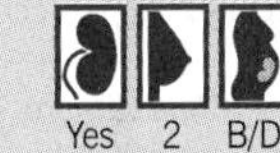

Tabs: 500 mg
Enteric-coated tabs (Azulfidine EN-tabs): 500 mg

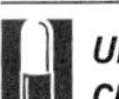

Ulcerative colitis:
Child >6 yr:
Initial dosing:
Moderate/severe: 50–75 mg/kg/24 hr ÷ Q4–6 hr PO; **max. dose:** 6 g/24 hr
Mild: *40–50 mg/kg/24 hr ÷ Q6 hr PO*
Maintenance: 30–50 mg/kg/24 hr ÷ Q4–8 hr PO; **max. dose:** 2 g/24 hr
Adult:
Initial: 3–4 g/24 hr ÷ Q4–6 hr PO
Maintenance: 2 g/24 hr ÷ Q6–12 hr PO
Max. dose: 6 g/24 hr
Juvenile rheumatoid arthritis:
Children >6 yr: Start with 10 mg/kg/24 hr ÷ BID PO and increase by 10 mg/kg/24 hr Q 7 days until planned maintenance dose is achieved. Usual maintenance dose is 30–50 mg/kg/24 hr ÷ BID PO up to a **maximum** of 2 g/24 hr.

Contraindicated in sulfa or salicylate hypersensitivity, porphyria, and GI or GU obstruction. **Use with caution** in renal impairment. Maintain hydration. May cause orange-yellow discoloration of urine and skin. May permanently stain contact lenses. May cause photosensitivity, hypersensitivity, blood dyscrasias, CNS changes, nausea, vomiting, anorexia, diarrhea, and renal damage. Hepatotoxicity has been reported. May cause hemolysis in patients with G6PD deficiency. Decreases folic acid absorption and reduces serum digoxin and cyclosporine levels. Slow acetylators may require lower dosage owing to accumulation of active sulfapyridine metabolite. Pregnancy category changes to D if administered near term.

SULFISOXAZOLE

Gantrisin and others

Antibiotic, sulfonamide derivative

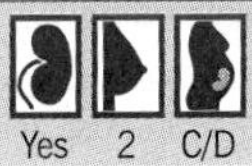

Tabs: 500 mg
Suspension: 500 mg/5 mL (480 mL); contains 0.3% alcohol and parabens
Ophthalmic solution: 4% (40 mg/mL) (15 mL)

Continued

For explanation of icons, see p. 680.

SULFISOXAZOLE *continued*

Child ≥2 mo: 75 mg/kg/dose PO × 1 followed by 120–150 mg/kg/24 hr OR 4 g/m^2/24 hr ÷ Q4–6 hr PO; **max. dose:** 6 g/24 hr
Adult: 2–4 g PO × 1 followed by 4–8 g/24 hr ÷ Q4–6 hr PO

Otitis media prophylaxis: 50 mg/kg/dose QHS PO

Rheumatic fever prophylaxis:
<27 kg: 500 mg PO QD
≥27 kg: 1000 mg PO QD

Ophthalmic solution:
Conjunctivitis or other superficial ocular infections: 1–2 drops Q1–4 hr; increase the time interval between doses as the condition improves.
Trachoma *(with systemic sulfonamide therapy):* 2 drops Q2 hr

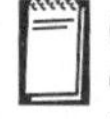

Contraindicated in urinary obstruction or near-term pregnant. **Use with caution** in infants <2 mo, the presence of renal or liver disease, or G6PD deficiency. Maintain adequate fluid intake. See *Sulfadiazine* for toxicities and drug interactions. Interferes with folate absorption. Usual duration of therapy for ophthalmic use is 7–10 days.

Adjust dose in renal impairment with systemic use (see Chapter 30). Pregnancy category changes to D if administered near term pregnancy. For combination with erythromycin, see *Erythromycin, Ethylsuccinate,* and *Acetylsulfisoxazole.*

SUMATRIPTAN SUCCINATE

Imitrex

Antimigraine agent, selective serotonin agonist

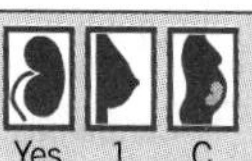

Injection: 12 mg/mL (0.5 mL)
Tabs: 25, 50, 100 mg
Oral suspension: 5 mg/mL
Nasal spray (as a unit-dose spray device): 5 mg dose in 100 microliters (6 units per pack); 20 mg dose in 100 microliters (6 units per pack)

Adolescent and adult *(see remarks):*
PO: 25 mg as soon as possible after onset of headache. If no relief in 2 hr, give 25–100 mg Q2 hr up to a **daily maximum** of 200 mg. **Max. single dose:** 100 mg/dose.
Max. daily dose: 200 mg/24 hr (with exclusive PO dosing or with an initial SC dose and subsequent PO dosing)
SC: 6 mg × 1 as soon as possible after onset of headache. If no response, may give an additional dose of ≤6 mg 1 hr later. **Max. daily dose:** 12 mg/24 hr.
Nasal: 5–20 mg/dose into one nostril or divided into each nostril after onset of headache. Dose may be repeated in 2 hr up to a **maximum** of 40 mg/24 hr.

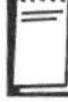

Contraindicated with concomitant administration of ergotamine derivatives, MAO inhibitors (and use within the past 2 wk), or other vasoconstrictive

Continued

SUMATRIPTAN SUCCINATE *continued*

drugs. Not for migraine prophylaxis. **Use with caution** in renal or hepatic impairment. A **maximum** single dose of 50 mg has been recommended in adults with hepatic dysfunction. Acts as selective agonist for serotonin receptor. Induration and swelling at the injection site, flushing, dizziness, and chest, jaw, and neck tightness may occur with SC administration. Weakness, hyper-reflexia, and incoordination have been reported with use in combination with selective serotonin reuptake inhibitors (e.g., fluoxetine, fluvoxamine, paroxetine, sertraline).

May cause coronary vasospasm if administered IV. **Use injectable form SC only!** Onset of action is 10–120 min SC, and 60–90 min PO. For nasal use, the safety of treating more than 4 headaches in a 30 day period has not been established.

Oral efficacy was not established in placebo-controlled trial in adolescents.

SURFACTANT, PULMONARY/BERACTANT

Survanta

Bovine lung surfactant

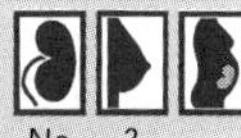

Suspension for inhalation: 25 mg/mL (4, 8 mL); contains 0.5–1.75 mg triglycerides, 1.4–3.5 mg free fatty acids and <1 mg protein/1 mL drug

Prophylactic therapy: 4 mL/kg/dose intratracheally as soon as possible; up to 4 doses may be given at intervals no shorter than Q6 hr during the first 48 hr of life.

Rescue therapy: 4 mL/kg/dose intratracheally, immediately following the diagnosis of respiratory distress syndrome (RDS). May repeat dose as needed Q6 hr to **maximum** of four total doses.

Method of administration for above therapies: Each dose is divided into four 1 mL/kg aliquots; administer 1 mL/kg in each of four different positions (slight downward inclination with head turned to the right, head turned to the left; slight upward inclination with the head turned to the right, head turned to the left).

Transient bradycardia, O_2 desaturation, pallor, vasoconstriction, hypotension, endotracheal tube blockage, hypercarbia, hypercapnia, apnea, and hypertension may occur during the administration process. Other side effects may include pulmonary interstitial emphysema, pulmonary air leak, and post-treatment nosocomial sepsis. Monitor heart rate and transcutaneous O_2 saturation during dose administration; monitor arterial blood gases for postdose hyperoxia and hypocarbia after administration.

All doses are administered intratracheally via a 5-French feeding catheter. If the suspension settles during storage, gently swirl the contents—**do not shake.** Drug is stored in the refrigerator, protected from light, and needs to be warmed by standing at room temperature for at least 20 min or warming in the hand for at least 8 min. Artificial warming methods should **NOT** be used.

For explanation of icons, see p. 680.

SURFACTANT, PULMONARY/CALFACTANT

Infasurf

Bovine lung surfactant

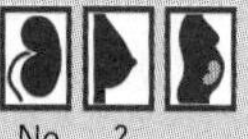

No ?

Intratracheal suspension: 35 mg/mL (3, 6 mL); contains 26 mg phosphatidylcholine and 0.26 mg surfactant protein B per 1 mL

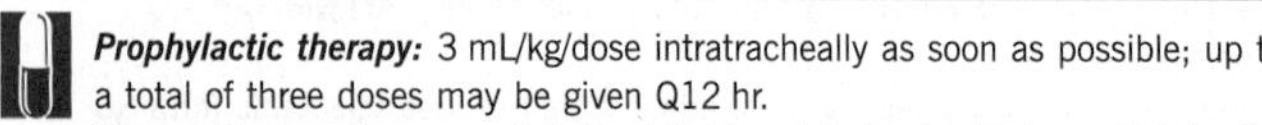

Prophylactic therapy: 3 mL/kg/dose intratracheally as soon as possible; up to a total of three doses may be given Q12 hr.

Rescue therapy *(see remarks):* 3 mL/kg/dose intratracheally immediately after the diagnosis of respiratory distress syndrome (RDS). May repeat dose as needed Q12 hr to **maximum** of three doses total.

Method of administration for above therapies: Manufacturer recommends administration through a side-port adapter into the endotracheal tube with two attendants (one to instill drug and another to monitor and position patient). Each dose is divided into two 1.5-mL/kg aliquots; administer 1.5 mL/kg in each of two different positions (infant positioned to the right or left side dependent). Drug in administered while ventilation is continued over 20–30 breaths for each aliquot, with small bursts timed only during the inspiratory cycles. A pause followed by evaluation of respiratory status and repositioning should separate the two aliquots.

Common adverse effects include cyanosis, airway obstruction, bradycardia, reflux of surfactant into the ET tube, requirement for manual ventilation, and reintubation. Monitor O_2 saturation and lung compliance after each dose such that oxygen therapy and ventilator pressure are adjusted as necessary.

All doses administered intratracheally via a 5-French feeding catheter. If suspension settles during storage, gently swirl the contents—**do not shake.** Drug is stored in the refrigerator, protected from light, and does not need to be warmed before administration. Unopened vials that have been warmed to room temperature (once only) may be refrigerated within 24 hr and stored for future use.

For **rescue therapy,** repeat doses may be administered as early as 6 hr after the previous dose for a total of up to four doses if the infant is still intubated and requires at least 30% inspired oxygen to maintain a PaO_2 ≥80 mmHg.

SURFACTANT, PULMONARY/PORACTANT ALFA

Curosurf

Porcine lung surfactant

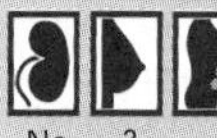

No ?

Intratracheal suspension: 80 mg/mL (1.5, 3 mL): contains 0.3 mg surfactant protein B per 1 mL drug

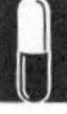

Prophylaxis therapy: 2.5 mL/kg/dose × 1 intratracheally as soon as possible; up to two subsequent 1.25 mL/kg/doses may be given at 12-hr intervals for a **max. total dose** of 5 mL/kg.

Continued

SURFACTANT, PULMONARY/PORACTANT ALFA *continued*

Rescue therapy: 2.5 mL/kg/dose × 1 intratracheally, immediately following the diagnosis of respiratory distress syndrome (RDS). May administer 1.25 mL/kg/dose Q12 hr × 2 doses as needed up to a **max. total dose** of 5 mL/kg.

Method of administration for above therapies: Each dose is divided into two aliquots, with each aliquot administered into one of the two main bronchi by positioning the infant with either the right or left side dependent. After the first aliquot is administered, remove the catheter from the ET tube and manually ventilate the infant with 100% oxygen at a rate of 40–60 breaths/min for 1 min. When the infant is stable, reposition the infant and administer the second dose. Then remove the catheter without flushing.

Transient episodes of bradycardia, decreased oxygen saturation, reflux of surfactant into the ET tube, and airway obstruction have occurred during dose administration. Monitor O_2 saturation and lung compliance after each dose, and adjust oxygen therapy and ventilator pressure as necessary.

All doses administered intratracheally via a 5-French feeding catheter. Suction infant before administration and 1 hr after surfactant instillation (unless signs of significant airway obstruction).

Drug is stored in the refrigerator and protected from light. Each vial of drug should be slowly warmed to room temperature and gently turned upside-down for uniform suspension (**do not shake**) before administration. Unopened vials that have been warmed to room temperature (once only) may be refrigerated within 24 hr and stored for future use.

TACROLIMUS

Prograf, FK506, Protopic

Immunosuppressant

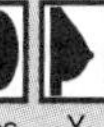
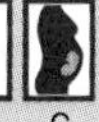

Yes X C

Caps: 0.5, 1, 5 mg

Suspension: 0.5 mg/mL

Injection: 5 mg/mL (1 mL); contains alcohol and polyoxyl 60 hydrogenated castor oil

Topical ointment (Protopic): 0.03%, 0.1% (30, 60, 100 g)

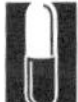

Child:

Liver transplantation without preexisting renal or hepatic dysfunction *(initial doses; titrate to therapeutic levels):*

IV: 0.03–0.15 mg/kg/24 hr by continuous infusion

PO: 0.15–0.2 mg/kg/24 hr ÷ Q12 hr

Adult (initial doses; titrate to therapeutic levels):

IV: 0.03–0.1 mg/kg/24 hr by continuous infusion

PO:

Liver transplantation: 0.1–0.15 mg/kg/24 hr ÷ Q12 hr

Kidney transplantation: 0.2 mg/kg/24 hr ÷ Q12 hr

Atopic dermatitis *(continue treatment for 1 wk after clearing of signs and symptoms; see remarks):*

Child ≥2 yr: Apply a thin layer of the 0.03% ointment to the affected skin areas BID and rub in gently and completely.

Continued

FORMULARY

For explanation of icons, see p. 680.

TACROLIMUS *continued*

Adult: Apply a thin layer of the 0.03% or 0.1% ointment to the affected skin areas BID and rub in gently and completely.

IV dosage form **contraindicated** in patients allergic to polyoxyl 60 hydrogenated castor oil. Experience in pediatric kidney transplantation is limited. Pediatric patients have required higher mg/kg doses than adults. For BMT use (beginning 1 day before BMT), dose and therapeutic levels similar to those in liver transplantation have been used.

Major adverse events include tremor, headache, insomnia, diarrhea, constipation, hypertension, nausea, and renal dysfunction. Hypokalemia, hypomagnesemia, hyperglycemia, confusion, depression, infections, lymphoma, liver enzyme elevation, and coagulation disorders may also occur. Tacrolimus is a substrate of the CYP450 3A4 drug-metabolizing enzyme. Calcium-channel blockers, imidazole antifungals (ketoconazole, itraconazole, fluconazole, clotrimazole), macrolide antibiotics (erythromycin, clarithromycin, troleandomycin), cisapride, cimetidine, cyclosporine, danazol, methylprednisolone, and grapefruit juice can increase tacrolimus serum levels. In contrast, carbamazepine, caspofungin, phenobarbital, phenytoin, rifampin, rifabutin, and sirolimus may decrease levels. Reduce dose in renal or hepatic insufficiency.

Monitor trough levels (just before a dose at steady state). Steady state is generally achieved after 2–5 days of continuous dosing. Interpretation will vary based on treatment protocol and assay methodology (whole-blood ELISA vs. MEIA vs. HPLC). Whole-blood trough concentrations of 5–20 ng/mL have been recommended in liver transplantation at 1–12 mo. Trough levels of 7–20 ng/mL (whole blood) for the first 3 mo and 5–15 ng/mL after 3 mo have been recommended in renal transplantation.

Tacrolimus therapy generally should be initiated 6 hr or more after transplantation. PO is the preferred route of administration and should be administered on an empty stomach. IV infusions should be administered at concentrations between 0.004 and 0.02 mg/mL diluted NS or D5W.

TOPICAL USE: Do not use in children <2yr, immunecompromised patients, or with occlusive dressings (promotes systemic absorption). Approved as a second-line therapy for short-term and intermittent treatment of atopic dermatitis for patients who fail to respond, or do not tolerate, other approved therapies. Long-term safety is unknown. Skin burn sensation, pruritus, flu-like symptoms, allergic reaction, skin erythema, headache, and skin infection are the most common side effects. Although the risk is uncertain, the FDA has issued an alert about the potential cancer risk with the use of this product. See www.fda.gov/medwatch for the latest information.

TERBUTALINE
Brethine and others
Beta-2-adrenergic agonist

Yes 1 B

Tabs: 2.5, 5 mg
Suspension: 1 mg/mL
Injection: 1 mg/mL (1 mL)

Continued

TEBRUTALINE *continued*

PO: ≤12 yr: Initial: 0.05 mg/kg/dose TID, increase as required. **Max. dose:** 0.15 mg/kg/dose TID or total of 5 mg/24 hr.
>12 yr and adult: 2.5–5 mg/dose PO TID
Max. dose:
12–15 yr: 7.5 mg/24 hr
>15 yr: 15 mg/24 hr

Nebulization:
<2 yr: 0.5 mg in 2.5 mL NS Q4–6 hr PRN
2–9 yr: 1 mg in 2.5 mL NS Q4–6 hr PRN
>9 yr: 1.5–2.5 mg in 2.5 mL NS Q4–6 hr PRN

SC:
≤12 yr: 0.005–0.01 mg/kg/dose Q15–20 min × 3 (**max. dose:** 0.4 mg/dose); if needed, Q2–6 hr PRN.
>12 yr and adult: 0.25 mg/dose Q15–30 min PRN ×3

Continuous infusion, IV: 2–10 mcg/kg loading dose followed by infusion of 0.1–0.4 mcg/kg/min. May titrate in increments of 0.1–0.2 mcg/kg/min Q30 min depending on clinical response. Doses as high as 10 mcg/kg/min have been used.
To prepare infusion: see inside front cover.

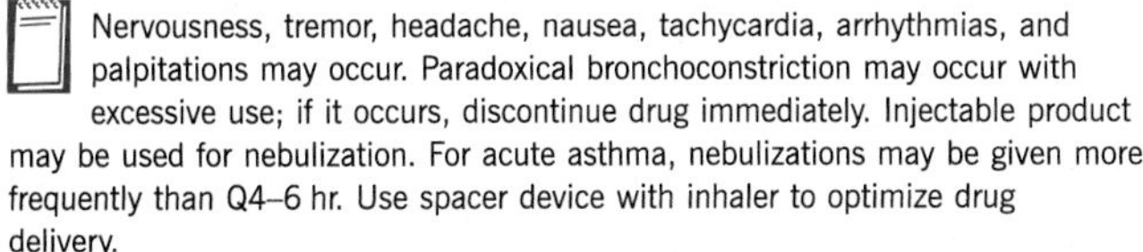

Nervousness, tremor, headache, nausea, tachycardia, arrhythmias, and palpitations may occur. Paradoxical bronchoconstriction may occur with excessive use; if it occurs, discontinue drug immediately. Injectable product may be used for nebulization. For acute asthma, nebulizations may be given more frequently than Q4–6 hr. Use spacer device with inhaler to optimize drug delivery.

Monitor heart rate, blood pressure, respiratory rate, and serum potassium when using the continuous IV infusion route of administration. **Adjust dose in renal failure (see Chapter 30).**

TETRACYCLINE HCL

Sumycin and others
Antibiotic

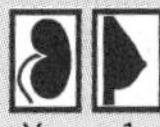
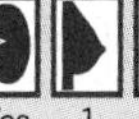

Yes 1 D

Caps: 250, 500 mg
Suspension: 125 mg/5 mL (480 mL); contains saccharin and sodium metabisulfite

Do not use in children <8 yr.
Child ≥8 yr: 25–50 mg/kg/24 hr PO ÷ Q6 hr.
Max. dose: 3 g/24 hr
Adult: 1–2 g/24 hr PO ÷ Q6–12 hr

Not recommended in patients <8 yr due to tooth staining and decreased bone growth. Also **not recommended** for use in pregnancy because these side effects may occur in the fetus. The risk for these adverse effects are

Continued

FORMULARY

For explanation of icons, see p. 680.

TETRACYCLINE HCL *continued*

highest with long-term use. May cause nausea, GI upset, hepatotoxicity, stomatitis, rash, fever, and superinfection. Photosensitivity reaction may occur. **Avoid** prolonged exposure to sunlight. May decrease the effectiveness of oral contraceptives and may increase serum digoxin levels.

Never use outdated tetracyclines because they may cause Fanconi-like syndrome. **Do not give** with dairy products or with any divalent cations (i.e., Fe^{2+}, Ca^{2+}, Mg^{2+}). Give 1 hr before or 2 hr after meals. **Adjust dose in renal failure (see Chapter 30).**

THEOPHYLLINE

Theo 24, Theobid Duracaps, Quibron-T/SR Dividose, Sustarie, and many others

Bronchodilator, methylxanthine

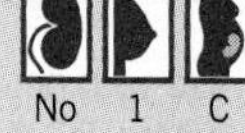

Other dosage forms may exist.

Immediate release:

Tabs: 100, 125, 200, 250, 300 mg

Caps: 100, 200 mg

Elixir/solution/syrup: 80 mg/15 mL. Some elixirs contain up to 20% alcohol. Some syrups and solutions are alcohol and dye free.

Injection: 0.8, 1.6, 2, 3.2, 4 mg/mL

Sustained release (see remarks):

Tabs: 100, 200, 250, 300, 400, 500, 600 mg

Caps: 60, 100, 125, 130, 200, 250, 260, 300, 400 mg

Sustained-release forms should **NOT** be chewed or crushed. Capsules may be opened and contents sprinkled on food.

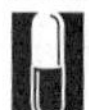

Dosing intervals are for immediate-release preparations.

For sustained-release preparations, divide daily dose >Q8–24 hr based on product.

Neonatal apnea:

Load: 5 mg/kg/dose PO × 1

Maintenance: 3–6 mg/kg/24 hr PO ÷ Q6–8 hr

Bronchospasm; PO:

Loading dose: 1 mg/kg/dose for each 2 mg/L desired increase in serum theophylline level.

Maintenance, infant (<1 yr):

Preterm:

<24 days old (postnatal): 1 mg/kg/dose PO Q12 hr

≥24 days old (postnatal): 1.5 mg/kg/dose PO Q12 hr

Full-term up to 1 yr: total daily dose (mg) = [(0.2 × age in wk) + 5] × (kg body weight)

≤6 mo: divide daily dose Q8 hr.

>6 mo: divide daily dose Q6 hr.

Maintenance, child >1 yr and adult without risk factors for altered clearance *(see remarks):*

Continued

THEOPHYLLINE *continued*

<45 kg: Begin therapy at 12–14 mg/kg/24 hr ÷ Q4–6 hr up to **max. dose** of 300 mg/24 hr. If needed based on serum levels, gradually increase to 16–20 mg/kg/24 hr ÷ Q4–6 hr. **Max. dose:** 600 mg/24 hr
≥45 kg: Begin therapy with 300 mg/24 hr ÷ Q6–8 hr. If needed based on serum levels, gradually increase to 400–600 mg/24 hr ÷ Q6–8 hr.

Drug metabolism varies widely with age, drug formulation, and route of administration. Most common side effects and toxicities are nausea, vomiting, anorexia, abdominal pain, gastroesophageal reflux, nervousness, tachycardia, seizures, and arrhythmias.

Serum levels should be monitored. **Therapeutic levels**—bronchospasm: 10–20 mg/L; apnea: 7–13 mg/L. Half-life is age dependent: 30 hr (newborns); 6.9 hr (infants); 3.4 hr (children); 8.1 hr (adults). See *Aminophylline* for guidelines for serum level determinations. Theophylline is a substrate for CYP450 1A2. Levels are increased with allopurinol, alcohol, ciprofloxacin, cimetidine, clarithromycin, disulfiram, erythromycin, estrogen, isoniazid, propranolol, thiabendazole, and verapamil. Levels are decreased with carbamazepine, isoproterenol, phenobarbital, phenytoin, and rifampin. May cause increased skeletal muscle activity, agitation, and hyperactivity when used with doxapram.

Use ideal body weight in obese patients when calculating dosage because of poor distribution into body fat. Risk factors for increased clearance include smoking, cystic fibrosis, hyperthyroidism, and high protein-carbohydrate diet. Factors for decreased clearance include CHF, correction of hyperthyroidism, fever, viral illness, and sepsis.

Suggested dosage intervals for sustained-release products (see table below):

THEOPHYLLINE SUSTAINED RELEASE PRODUCTS		
Trade Name	**Available Strengths**	**Dosage Interval**
CAPSULES		
Theo 24	100, 200, 300, 400 mg	Q24 hr
Theobid Duracaps	260 mg	Q12 hr
Theoclear-LA	130, 260 mg	Q12 hr
Theovent	125, 250 mg	Q12 hr
TABLETS		
Theophylline SR	100, 200, 300 mg	Q12–24 hr
Quibron-T/SR Dividose	300 mg	Q8–12 hr
Respbid	250, 500 mg	Q8–12 hr
Sustaire	100, 300 mg	Q8–12 hr
Theocron	100, 200, 300 mg	Q12–24 hr
Theolair SR	300 mg	Q8–12 hr
Theo-Sav	100, 200, 300 mg	Q8–24 hr
Theo X	100, 200, 300 mg	Q12–24 hr
T-phyl	200 mg	Q12 hr
Uniphyl	400, 600 mg	Q24 hr

For explanation of icons, see p. 680.

THIABENDAZOLE

Mintezol

Anthelmintic

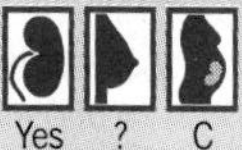

Suspension: 500 mg/5 mL
Chewable tabs: 500 mg; contains saccharin
Topical suspension: 10%–15%
Topical ointment: 10% in white petrolatum

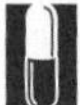

Child and adult: 50 mg/kg/24 hr PO ÷ BID; **max. dose:** 3 g/24 hr
Duration of therapy (consecutive days):
Strongyloides: × 2 days (5 days for disseminated disease)
Cutaneous larva migrans: × 2–5 days
Visceral larva migrans: × 5–7 days
Trichinosis: × 2–4 days
Angiostrongylosis: 75 mg/kg/24 hr PO ÷ TID × 3 days; **max. dose:** 3 g/24 hr

Topical therapy for cutaneous larva migrans: apply sparingly to all lesions 4–6× per 24 hr until lesions are inactivated. [See Arch Dermatol 1993;129:588 for additional information.]

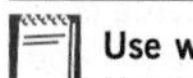

Use with caution in renal or hepatic impairment.

Nausea, vomiting, and vertigo are frequent side effects. May cause abnormal sensation in eyes, xanthopsia, blurred vision, dry mucous membranes, rash, hypersensitivity, erythema multiforme, leukopenia, and hallucinations. May increase serum levels of theophylline or caffeine. Clinical experience in children weighing <13.6 kg (30 lbs) is limited.

THIAMINE

Vitamin B_1, Thiomalate, and others

Water-soluble vitamin

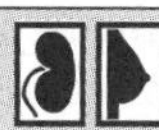
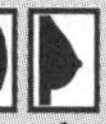
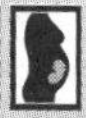

Tabs (OTC): 50, 100, 250, 500 mg
Enteric-coated tabs (OTC; Thiomalate): 20 mg
Injection: 100 mg/mL (2 mL); contains benzyl alcohol

For U.S. RDA, see Chapter 20.
Beriberi (thiamine deficiency):
Child: 10–25 mg/dose IM/IV QD (if critically ill) or 10–50 mg/dose PO QD × 2 wk, followed by 5–10 mg/dose QD × 1 mo.
Adult: 5–30 mg/dose IM/IV TID × 2 wk, followed by 5–30 mg/24 hr PO ÷ QD or TID × 1 mo.

Wernicke's encephalopathy syndrome: 100 mg IV × 1, then 50–100 mg IM/IV QD until patient resumes a normal diet. (Administer thiamine before starting glucose infusion.)

Continued

THIAMINE *continued*

Multivitamin preparations contain amounts meeting RDA requirements. Allergic reactions and anaphylaxis may occur, primarily with IV administration.

Therapeutic range: 1.6–4 mg/dL. High carbohydrate diets or IV dextrose solutions may increase thiamine requirements. Large doses may interfere with serum theophylline assay. Pregnancy category changes to C if used in doses above the RDA.

THIOPENTAL SODIUM

Pentothal and others

Barbiturate

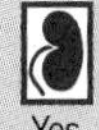
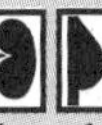
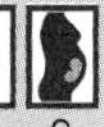

Yes 1 C

Injection: 250, 400, 500 mg, 1, 2.5, 5 g (reconstituted to 20 mg/mL or 25 mg/mL)
Rectal solution: 100 mg/mL (3.6 mL sterile water for injection in 400 mg of the injectable powder)

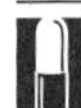

Cerebral edema: 1.5–5 mg/kg/dose IV. Repeat PRN for increased ICP.
Anesthesia induction, child and adult:
IV: 2–6 mg/kg: Use lower doses in patients with hemodynamic instability. See Chapter 1 for rapid sequence intubation.
Deep sedation:
Child: 30 mg/kg PR × 1; **max. dose:** 1 g/dose

Contraindicated in acute intermittent porphyria. May cause respiratory depression, hypotension, anaphylaxis, and decreased cardiac output. The injectable dosage form is alkaline and **cannot** be mixed with acidic drugs (e.g., vecuronium).

Onset of action: 30–60 sec for IV; 7–10 min for PR. Duration of action: 5–30 min for IV; 90 min for PR. **Adjust dose in renal failure (see Chapter 30).**

THIORIDAZINE

Various generics

Antipsychotic, phenothiazine derivative

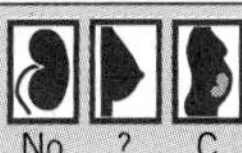

No ? C

Tabs: 10, 15, 25, 50, 100, 150, 200 mg
Oral concentrate solution: 30, 100 mg/mL (120 mL); may contain alcohol

Child 2–12 yr: 0.5–3 mg/kg/24 hr PO ÷ BID–TID. **Max. dose:** 3 mg/kg/24 hr
>12 yr and adult: Start with 75–300 mg/24 hr PO ÷ TID. Then gradually increase PRN to **max. dose** 800 mg/24 hr ÷ BID–QID.

Continued

For explanation of icons, see p. 680.

THIORIDAZINE *continued*

Indicated for schizophrenia unresponsive to standard therapy. **Contraindicated** in severe CNS depression, brain damage, narrow-angle glaucoma, blood dyscrasias, and severe liver or cardiovascular disease. **DO NOT** coadminister with drugs that may inhibit the CYP450 2D6 isoenzymes (e.g., SSRIs such as fluoxetine, fluvoxamine, paroxetine; and beta-blockers such as propranolol and pindolol); with drugs that may widen the QTc interval (e.g., disopyramide, procainamide, quinidine); and in patients with known reduced activity of CYP450 2D6.

May cause drowsiness, extrapyramidal reactions, autonomic symptoms, ECG changes (QTc prolongation in a dose-dependent manner), arrhythmias, paradoxical reactions, and endocrine disturbances. Long-term use may cause tardive dyskinesia. Pigmentary retinopathy may occur with higher doses; a periodic eye exam is recommended. More autonomic symptoms and less extrapyramidal effects than chlorpromazine. Concurrent use with epinephrine can cause hypotension. Increased cardiac arrhythmias may occur with tricyclic antidepressants. **Do not** simultaneously administer oral liquid dosage form with carbamazepine oral suspension because an orange rubbery precipitate may form.

In an overdose situation, monitor ECG and **avoid** drugs that can widen QTc interval.

TIAGABINE
Gabitril
Anticonvulsant

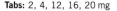

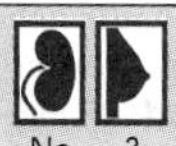
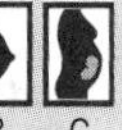
No ? C

Tabs: 2, 4, 12, 16, 20 mg

Adjunctive therapy for refractory seizures:
Child ≥2 yr (limited data from a safety and tolerability study in 52 children 2–17 yr; mean, 9.3 ± 4.1): Initial dose of 0.25 mg/kg/24 hr PO ÷ TID × 4 wk. Dosage was increased at 4-wk intervals to 0.5, 1, and 1.5 mg/kg/24 hr until an effective and well-tolerated dose was established. Criteria for dose increase required tolerance of the current dosage level and <50% reduction in seizures.

Adjunctive therapy for partial seizures:
≥12 yr and adult: Start at 4 mg PO QD ×7 days. If needed, increase dose to 8 mg/24 hr PO ÷ BID. Dosage may be increased further by 4–8 mg/24 hr at weekly intervals (daily doses may be divided BID–QID) until a clinical response is achieved or up to specified **maximum** dose.

Max. dose:
12–18 yr: 32 mg/24 hr
Adult: 56 mg/24 hr

Use with caution in hepatic insufficiency (may need to reduce dose and/or increase dosing interval). Most common side effects include dizziness, asthenia, nausea, nervousness, tremor, abdominal pain, confusion, and difficulty in concentrating. Cognitive/neuropsychiatric symptoms resulting in

Continued

TIAGABINE *continued*

nonconvulsive status epilepticus requiring subsequent dose reduction or drug discontinuation have been reported.

Tiagabine's clearance is increased by concurrent hepatic enzyme-inducing antiepileptic drugs (e.g., phenytoin, carbamazepine, and barbiturates). Lower doses or a slower titration for clinical response may be necessary for patients receiving non–enzyme-inducing drugs (e.g., valproate, gabapentin, and lamotrigine). **Avoid** abrupt discontinuation of drug.

TID dosing schedule may be preferred since BID schedule may not be well tolerated. Doses should be administered with food.

TICARCILLIN

Ticar

Antibiotic, penicillin (extended spectrum)

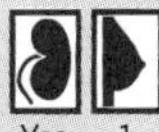
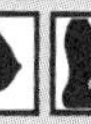
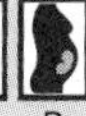

Yes 1 B

Injection: 3, 20 g

Each gram contains 5.2–6.5 mEq Na.

Neonate, IM/IV:

≤7 days:

<2 kg: 150 mg/kg/24 hr ÷ Q12 hr

≥2 kg: 225 mg/kg/24 hr ÷ Q8 hr

>7 days:

<1.2 kg: 150 mg/kg/24 hr ÷ Q12 hr

1.2–2 kg: 225 mg/kg/24 hr ÷ Q8 hr

>2 kg: 300 mg/kg/24 hr ÷ Q6–8 hr

Infant and child (IM/IV): 200–300 mg/kg/24 hr ÷ Q4–6 hr; **max. dose:** 24 g/24 hr

Cystic fibrosis (IM/IV): 300–600 mg/kg/24 hr ÷ Q4–6 hr; **max. dose:** 24 g/24 hr

Adult (IM/IV): 1–4 g/dose Q4–6 hr; **max. dose:** 24 g/24 hr

May cause decreased platelet aggregation, bleeding diathesis, hypernatremia, hematuria, hypokalemia, hypocalcemia, allergy, rash, and increased AST. Like other penicillins, CSF penetration occurs only with inflamed meninges. **Do not** mix with aminoglycoside in same solution. May cause false-positive tests for urine protein and serum Coombs tests. **Adjust dose in renal failure (see Chapter 30).**

TICARCILLIN/CLAVULANATE

Timentin

Antibiotic, penicillin (extended spectrum with beta-lactamase inhibitor)

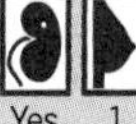
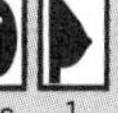
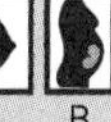

Yes 1 B

Injection: 3.1 g (3 g ticarcillin and 0.1 g clavulanate); contains 4.75 mEq Na^+ and 0.15 mEq K^+ per 1 g drug

Premixed injection: 3.1 g (3 g ticarcillin and 0.1 g clavulanate) in 100 mL; contains 18.7 mEq Na^+ and 0.5 mEq K^+ per 100 mL

Continued

For explanation of icons, see p. 680.

TICARCILLIN/CLAVULANATE *continued*

Doses should be based on ticarcillin component; see *Ticarcillin*.
Max. dose: 18–24 g/24 hr

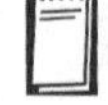

Activity similar to ticarcillin except that beta-lactamase inhibitor broadens spectrum to include *S. aureus* and *H. influenzae*. See *Ticarcillin* for side effects. Like other penicillins, CSF penetration occurs only with inflamed meninges. May cause false-positive tests for urine protein and serum Coombs tests. **Adjust dosage in renal impairment (see Chapter 30).**

TOBRAMYCIN

Nebcin, Tobrex, AKTob, TOBI and others
Antibiotic, aminoglycoside

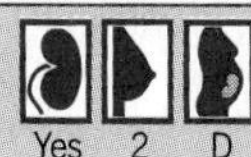

Injection: 10, 40 mg/mL; may contain phenol and bisulfites
Powder for injection: 1.2 g
Ophthalmic ointment (Tobrex, AKTob): 0.3% (3.5 g)
Ophthalmic solution (Tobrex): 0.3% (5 mL)
Nebulizer solution (TOBI): 300 mg/5 mL (preservative free) (56s)

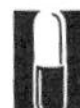

Neonate, IM/IV *(see table below):*

Postconceptional Age (wk)	Postnatal Age (days)	Dose (mg/kg/dose)	Interval (hr)
≤29*	0–7	5	48
	8–28	4	36
	>28	4	24
30–33	0–7	4.5	36
	>7	4	24
≥34	0–7	4	24
	>7	4	12–18

*Or significant asphyxia, PDA, indomethacin use, poor cardiac output, reduced renal function.

Child: 7.5 mg/kg/24 hr ÷ Q8 hr IV/IM
Cystic fibrosis: 7.5–10.5 mg/kg/24 hr ÷ Q8 hr IV
Adult: 3–6 mg/kg/24 hr ÷ Q8 hr IV/IM
Ophthalmic:

Child and adult: Apply thin ribbon of ointment to affected eye BID–TID; or 1–2 drops of solution to affected eye Q4 hr.

Inhalation:

Cystic fibrosis prophylaxis therapy (TOBI):

≥6 yr and adult: 300 mg Q12 hr administered in repeated cycles of 28 days on drug followed by 28 days off drug.

Continued

TOBRAMYCIN *continued*

Use with caution in patients receiving anesthetics or neuromuscular blocking agents and in patients with neuromuscular disorders. May cause ototoxicity, nephrotoxicity, and myelotoxicity. Serious allergic reactions including anaphylaxis and dermatologic reactions including exfoliative dermatitis, toxic epidermal necrolysis, erythema multiforme, and Stevens-Johnson syndrome have been reported rarely. **Ototoxic effects synergistic with furosemide.**

Higher doses are recommended in patients with cystic fibrosis, neutropenia, or burns. **Adjust dose in renal failure (see Chapter 30).** Monitor peak and trough levels.

Therapeutic peak levels:

6–10 mg/L in general

8–10 mg/L in pulmonary infections, neutropenia, osteomyelitis, and severe sepsis

Therapeutic trough levels: <2 mg/L. Recommended serum sampling time at steady state: trough within 30 min before the third consecutive dose and peak 30–60 min after the administration of the third consecutive dose.

For inhalation use with other medications in cystic fibrosis, use the following order of administration: bronchodilator first, chest physiotherapy, other inhaled medications (if indicated), and tobramycin last.

TOLNAFTATE

Tinactin, Aftate, and many others

Antifungal agent

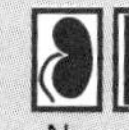 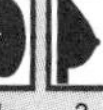 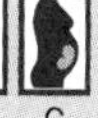

No ? C

Topical aerosol liquid (OTC): 1% (90, 120 mL)
Aerosol powder (OTC): 1% (90, 100, 150 g)
Cream (OTC): 1% (15, 30 g)
Gel (OTC): 1% (21 g)
Topical powder (OTC): 1% (45 g)
Topical solution (OTC): 1% (10, 60 mL)
Topical liquid (OTC): 1% (30, 55 mL)

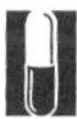

Topical:

Apply 1–3 drops of solution or small amount of gel, liquid, cream, or powder to affected areas BID–TID for 2–4 wk.

May cause mild irritation and sensitivity. **Avoid** contact with eyes. **Do not use** for nail or scalp infections.

For explanation of icons, see p. 680.

TOPIRAMATE

Topamax

Anticonvulsant

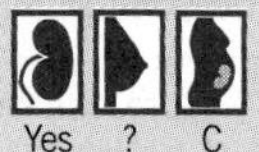

Caps, sprinkle: 15, 25 mg
Tabs: 25, 50, 100, 200 mg

Child 2–16 yr: Start with 1–3 mg/kg/dose (**max. dose:** 25 mg/dose) PO QHS × 7 days, then increase by 1–3 mg/kg/24-hr increments at 1- to 2-wk intervals (divided daily dose BID) to response. Usual maintenance dose is 5–9 mg/kg/24 hr PO ÷ BID.

≥17 yr and adult: Start with 25–50 mg PO QHS ×7 days, then increase by 25–50 mg/24 hr increments at 1-wk intervals until adequate response. Doses >50 mg should be divided BID. Consult with neurologist.

Usual maintenance dose: 200–400 mg/24 hr.

Doses above 1600 mg/24 hr have not been studied.

Used as adjunctive therapy for primary generalized tonic-clonic or partial seizures and Lennox-Gastaut syndrome. **Use with caution** in renal and hepatic dysfunction (decreased clearance) and sulfa hypersensitivity. **Reduce dose by 50% when creatinine clearance is <70 mL/min.** Common side effects (incidence lower in children) include ataxia, cognitive dysfunction, dizziness, nystagmus, paresthesia, sedation, visual disturbances, nausea, dyspepsia, and kidney stones. Secondary angle-closure glaucoma characterized by ocular pain, acute myopia, and increased intraocular pressure has been reported and may lead to blindness if left untreated. Patients should be instructed to seek immediate medical attention if they experience blurred vision or periorbital pain. Oligohidrosis and hyperthermia have been reported primarily in children and should be monitored especially during hot weather and with use of drugs that predispose patients to heat-related disorders (e.g., carbonic anhydrase inhibitors and anticholinergics). Hyperchloremic, non–anion gap metabolic acidosis has also been reported.

Drug is metabolized by and inhibits the cytochrome P-450 system. Phenytoin, valproic acid, and carbamazepine may decrease topiramate levels. Topiramate may decrease valproic acid, digoxin, and ethinyl estradiol (to decrease oral contraceptive efficacy) but may increase phenytoin levels. Alcohol and CNS depressants may increase CNS side effects. Carbonic anhydrase inhibitors (e.g., acetazolamide) may increase risk for metabolic acidosis, nephrolithiasis, or paresthesia.

Doses may be administered with or without food. Sprinkle capsule may be opened and sprinkled on small amount of food (e.g., 1 teaspoonful of applesauce) and swallowed whole (**do not chew**). Maintain adequate hydration to prevent kidney stone formation.

TRAZODONE

Desyrel and many others

Antidepressant, triazolopyridine derivative

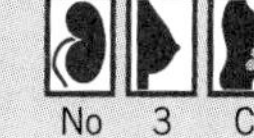

No 3 C

Tabs: 50, 100, 150, 300 mg

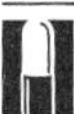

Depression *(titrate to lowest effective dose):*

Child (6–18 yr): Start at 1.5–2 mg/kg/24 hr PO ÷ BID–TID; if needed, gradually increase dose Q3–4 days up to a **maximum** of 6 mg/kg/24 hr ÷ TID.

Adult: Start at 150 mg/24 hr PO ÷ TID; if needed, increase by 50 mg/24 hr Q 3–4 days up a **maximum** of 600 mg/24 hr for hospitalized patients (400 mg/24 hr for ambulatory patients).

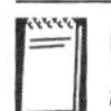

Use with caution in preexisting cardiac disease, initial recovery phase of MI, and electroconvulsive therapy. Common side effects include dizziness, drowsiness, dry mouth, and diarrhea. Seizures, tardive dyskinesia, EPS, arrhythmias, priapism, blurred vision, neuromuscular weakness, anemia, orthostatic hypotension, and rash have been reported.

Trazodone is a CYP450 3A4 isoenzyme substrate (may interact with inhibitors and inducers) and may increase digoxin levels and increase CNS effects of alcohol, barbiturates, and other CNS depressants. **Maximum** antidepressant effect is seen at 2–6 wk.

TRETINOIN

Retin-A, Retin-A Micro, Avita, Renova

Retinoic acid derivative, topical acne product

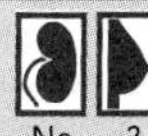
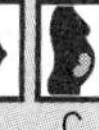
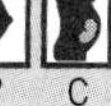

No ? C

Cream: 0.02% (40 g), 0.025% (20, 45 g), 0.05% (20, 40, 45, 60 g), 0.1% (20, 45 g)
Topical gel: 0.01% (15, 45 g), 0.025% (15, 45 g), 0.04% (20, 40 g); may contain 90% alcohol
Topical gel (Retin-A Micro): 0.1%; contains glycerin, propylene glycol, benzyl alcohol (20, 45 g)
Topical liquid: 0.05%; contains 55% alcohol (28 mL)

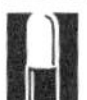

Topical:

Child >12 yr and adult: Gently wash face with a mild soap, pat the skin dry, and wait 20 to 30 min before use. Initiate therapy with either 0.025% cream or 0.01% gel, and apply a small pea-sized amount to the affected areas of the face QHS. See remarks.

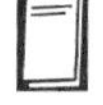

Contraindicated in sunburns. **Avoid** excessive sun exposure. If stinging or irritation occurs, decrease frequency of administration to QOD. **Avoid** contact with eyes, ears, nostrils, mouth, or open wounds. Local adverse effects include irritation, erythema, excessive dryness, blistering, crusting, hyperpigmentation or

Continued

For explanation of icons, see p. 680.

TRETINOIN *continued*

hypopigmentation, and acne flare-ups. Concomitant use of other topical acne products may lead to significant skin irritation. Onset of therapeutic benefits may be experienced within 2–3 wk with optimal effects in 6 wk. The gel dosage form is flammable and should **not** be exposed to heat or temperatures >120°F.

TRIAMCINOLONE

Azmacort, Tri-Nasal, Nasacort AQ, Kenalog, Aristocort, and others

Corticosteroid

No ? C/D

Nasal spray:

Tri-Nasal: 50 mcg/actuation (120 actuations per 15 mL)

Nasacort AQ: 55 mcg/actuation (30 actuations per 6.5 g, 120 actuations per 16.5 g)

Oral inhaler: 100 mcg/actuation (240 actuations per 20 g)

Tabs: 4, 8 mg

Oral syrup: 4 mg/5 mL (120 mL)

Cream: 0.025%, 0.1%, 0.5%

Ointment: 0.025%, 0.1%

Lotion: 0.025%, 0.1% (60 mL)

Topical aerosol: 0.2 mg/2-second spray (63 g); contains 10.3% alcohol

Dental paste: 0.1% (5 g)

See Chapter 29 for potency rankings and sizes of topical preparations.

Injection as acetonide: 10, 40 mg/mL; contains benzyl alcohol

Injection as diacetate: 25, 40 mg/mL; contains polyethylene glycol and benzyl alcohol; for IM injection use only

Injection as hexacetonide: 5, 20 mg/mL; contains benzyl alcohol

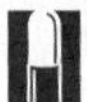

Oral inhalation:

Child 6–12 yr: 1–2 puffs TID–QID or 2–4 puffs BID; **max. dose:** 12 puffs/24 hr

≥12 yr and adult: 2 puffs TID–QID or 4 puffs BID; **max. dose:** 16 puffs/24 hr

NIH–National Heart Lung and Blood Institute recommendations (divide daily doses BID–QID): see Chapter 22.

Intranasal *(always titrate to lowest effective dose after symptoms are controlled):*

Nasacort:

Child 6–11 yr: 2 sprays in each nostril QD

≥12 yr and adult: 2 sprays in each nostril QD. After 4–7 days, may increase to 4 sprays/nostril/24 hr ÷ QD–QID.

Nasacort AQ:

Child 6–11 yr: Start with 1 spray in each nostril QD. If no benefit in 1 week, dose may be increased to 2 sprays in each nostril QD.

≥12 yr and adult: 2 sprays in each nostril QD

Continued

TRIAMCINOLONE *continued*

Topical: Apply to affected areas BID–TID.
Systemic use: Use one sixth of cortisone dose. See Chapter 29.
Intralesional, ≥12 yr and adult (as diacetate or acetonide): 1 mg/site at intervals of 1 wk or more. May give separate doses in sites >1 cm apart, **not to exceed** 30 mg.

Rinse mouth thoroughly with water after each use of the oral inhalation dosage form. Nasal preparations may cause epistaxis, cough, fever, nausea, throat irritation, and dyspepsia. Topical preparations may cause dermal atrophy, telangiectasias, and hypopigmentation. Topical steroids should be **used with caution** on the face and in intertriginous areas. See Chapter 7.

Dosage adjustment for hepatic failure with systemic use may be necessary. Pregnancy category changes to D if used in the first trimester.

TRIAMTERENE
Dyrenium
Diuretic, potassium sparing

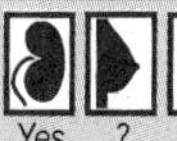
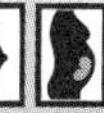

Caps: 50, 100 mg

Child: 2–4 mg/kg/24 hr ÷ QD–BID PO. May increase up to a **maximum** of 6 mg/kg/24 hr or 300 mg/24 hr.
Adult: 50–100 mg/24 hr ÷ QD–BID PO; **max. dose:** 300 mg/24 hr

Do not use if GFR <10 mL/hr. **Adjust dose in renal impairment (see Chapter 30).** Monitor serum electrolytes. May cause hyperkalemia, hyponatremia, hypomagnesemia, and metabolic acidosis. Interstitial nephritis, thrombocytopenia, and anaphylaxis have been reported.

Concurrent use of ACE inhibitors may increase serum potassium. **Use with caution** when administering medications with high potassium load (e.g., some penicillins), and in patients with hepatic impairment or on high-potassium diets. Cimetidine may increase effects. This drug is also available as a combination product with hydrochlorothiazide. Administer doses with food to minimize GI upset. Pregnancy category changes to D if used in pregnancy-induced hypertension.

TRIETHANOLAMINE POLYPEPTIDE OLEATE
Cerumenex
Otic ceruminolytic

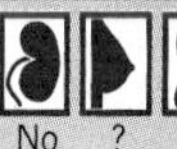

Otic solution: 10% (6, 12 mL)

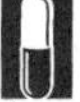

Child and adult: Fill ear canal and insert cotton plug. After 15–30 min, flush ear with warm water. May repeat dose in the presence of unusually hard impactions.

Contraindicated with perforated tympanic membrane. **Avoid** undue exposure to the periaural skin. Hypersensitivity and localized dermatitis may occur.

For explanation of icons, see p. 680.

TRIMETHOBENZAMIDE HCL

Tigan and others

Antiemetic

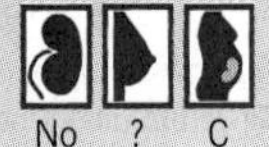

Caps: 100, 250, 300 mg

Suppository: 100 mg (10s), 200 mg (10s, 50s); contains 2% benzocaine

Injection: 100 mg/mL (2, 20 mL); may contain phenol or parabens

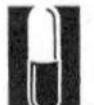

Child:

<13.6 kg *(excluding premature and newborn infants):*

PR: 100 mg/dose TID–QID

13.6–40.9 kg:

PO/PR: 100–200 mg/dose TID–QID

Adult:

PO: 250–300 mg/dose TID–QID

PR/IM: 200 mg/dose TID–QID

Do not use in premature or newborn infants. **Avoid** use in patients with hepatotoxicity, acute vomiting, or allergic reaction. CNS disturbances are common in children (extrapyramidal symptoms, drowsiness, confusion, dizziness). Hypotension, especially with IM use, may occur. Suppository contains 2% benzocaine. IM **not recommended** in children.

TRIMETHOPRIM-SULFAMETHOXAZOLE

See *Co-Trimoxazole*

UROKINASE

Abbokinase

Thrombolytic enzyme

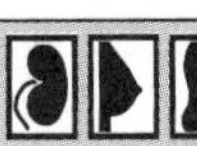

Injection: 250,000 U; preservative-free and contains 250 mg albumin, 25 mg mannitol, and 50 mg sodium chloride

Deep vein thromboses and pulmonary emboli: Should be used in consultation with a hematologist. 4400 U/kg over 10 min, followed by 4400 U/kg/hr for 6–12 hr; some patients may require 12–72 hr of therapy. Titrate to effect.

Occluded IV catheter:

Aspiration method: Use 5,000 U/mL concentration. Instill into catheter a volume equal to the internal volume of catheter over 1–2 min, leave in place for 1–4 hr, then aspirate. May repeat with 10,000 U/mL in each lumen if no response. **DO NOT** infuse into patient.

IV infusion method: 150–200 U/kg/hr in each lumen for 8–48 hr at a rate of at least 20 mL/hr.

For dialysis patients: 5,000 U in each lumen administered over 1–2 min; leave drug in for 1–2 days, then aspirate.

Continued

UROKINASE *continued*

Contraindicated for patients with active internal bleeding, bacterial endocarditis, intracranial neoplasm, arteriovenous malformation, aneurysm, bleeding diathesis, DIC, history of cerebrovascular accident within the past 2 mo, or recent trauma/surgery. Monitor fibrinogen, thrombin clotting time, PT, and APTT when used as a thrombolytic (before and during continuous infusion therapy).

Discontinue administration if signs of bleeding occur. Side effects include allergic reactions, fever, rash, and bronchospasm.

Newborns have reduced plasminogen levels (~50% of adult values), which decrease the thrombolytic effects of urokinase. Plasminogen supplementation may be necessary.

URSODIOL

Actigall, Urso

Gallstone-solubilizing agent, cholelitholytic agent

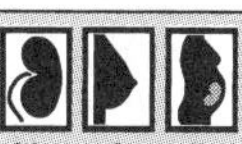

Suspension: 20, 25, 50, 60 mg/mL
Caps (Actigall): 300 mg
Tabs (Urso): 250 mg

Child: 10–15 mg/kg/24 hr QD PO
Adult: 8–10 mg/kg/24 hr ÷ BID–TID PO
Cystic fibrosis *(to improve fatty acid metabolism in liver disease):* 15–30 mg/kg/24 hr ÷ QD–TID PO

Contraindicated in calcified cholesterol stones, radiopaque stones, bile pigment stones, or stones >20 mm in diameter. May cause GI disturbance, rash, arthralgias, anxiety, headache, and elevated liver enzymes. Aluminum-containing antacids, cholestyramine, and oral contraceptives decrease ursodiol effectiveness. Dissolution of stones may take several months. Stone recurrence occurs in 30%–50% of patients within 5 yr.

Limited data for use in TPN-induced cholestasis at 30 mg/kg/24 hr ÷ TID PO [Gastroenterology 1996;111(3):716–719].

VALACYCLOVIR

Valtrex

Antiviral agent

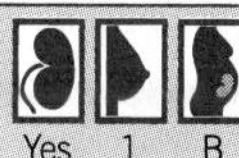

Tabs: 500, 1000 mg
Oral suspension: 50 mg/mL 

Child: Recommended dosages based on steady-state pharmacokinetic data in immunocompromised children. Efficacy data are incomplete.

To mimic an IV acyclovir regimen of 250 mg/m²/dose or 10 mg/kg/dose TID: 30 mg/kg/dose PO TID or alternatively by weight:

4–12 kg: 250 mg PO TID
13–21 kg: 500 mg PO TID

Continued

For explanation of icons, see p. 680.

VALACYCLOVIR *continued*

22–29 kg: 750 mg PO TID
≥30 kg: 1000 mg PO TID

To mimic a PO acyclovir regimen of 20 mg/kg/dose 4 or 5 times a day:
20 mg/kg/dose PO TID or alternatively by weight:

6–19 kg: 250 mg PO TID
20–31 kg: 500 mg PO TID
≥32 kg: 750 mg PO TID

Herpes zoster *(see remarks):*

Adult *(immunocompetent):* 1 g/dose PO TID × 7 days within 48–72 hr of onset of rash.

Genital herpes:

Adolescent and adult:
Initial episodes: 1 g/dose PO BID × 10 days
Recurrent episodes: 500 mg/dose PO BID × 3 days
Suppressive therapy: 500–1000 mg/dose PO QD × 1 year, then reassess for recurrences.

Herpes labialis (cold sores):

Adolescent and adult: 2 g/dose PO Q12 hr × 1 day

This prodrug is metabolized to acyclovir and L-valine with better oral absorption than acyclovir. **Use with caution** in hepatic or renal insufficiency. **Adjust dose in renal insufficiency (see Chapter 30).** Thrombotic thrombocytopenic purpura/hemolytic-uremic syndrome (TTP/HUS) has been reported in patients with advanced HIV infection and in bone marrow and renal transplant recipients. Probenecid or cimetidine can reduce the rate of conversion to acyclovir. See acyclovir for additional drug interactions and adverse effects.

For initial episodes of genital herpes, therapy is most effective when initiated within 48 hr of symptom onset. Therapy should be initiated immediately after the onset of symptoms in recurrent episodes (no efficacy data when initiating therapy >24 hr after onset of symptoms). Data are not available for use as suppressive therapy for periods >1 yr.

Valacyclovir **CANNOT** be substituted for acyclovir on a one-to-one basis. Doses may be administered with or without food.

VALGANCICLOVIR

Valcyte
Antiviral agent

Yes 3 C

Tabs: 450 mg
Oral suspension: 90 mg/mL

Child:
CMV prophylaxis in liver transplantation (limited data based on a retrospective review in 10 patients, mean age 4.9 ± 5.6 yr): 15–18 mg/kg/dose PO QD × 100 days following transplantation resulted in one case of asymptomatic CMV infection detected by CMV antigenemia at day 7 of therapy. This patient then received a higher dose of 15 mg/kg/dose BID until three

Continued

VALGANCICLOVIR *continued*

consecutive negative CMV antigenemia were achieved. The dose was switched back to a prophylactic regimen at day 46 posttransplant.

Adult:

CMV retinitis:

Induction therapy: 900 mg PO BID × 21 days with food

Maintenance therapy: 900 mg PO QD with food

CMV prophylaxis in heart, kidney, and kidney-pancreas transplantation: 900 mg PO QD starting within 10 days of transplantation until 100 days post-transplantation

This prodrug is metabolized to ganciclovir with better oral absorption than ganciclovir. **Use with caution** in renal insufficiency. **Adjust dose in renal insufficiency (see Chapter 30).** May cause headache, insomnia, peripheral neuropathy, diarrhea, vomiting, neutropenia, anemia, and thrombocytopenia. See *Ganciclovir* for drug interactions and additional adverse effects.

Valganciclovir **CANNOT** be substituted for ganciclovir on a one-to-one basis. All doses are administered with food.

VALPROIC ACID

Depakene, Depacon, and others
(Depakote: See Divalproex Sodium)
Anticonvulsant

No 1 D

Caps: 250 mg
Syrup: 250 mg/5 mL (473 mL); may contain parabens
Injection (Depacon): 100 mg/mL (5 mL)

Oral:

Initial: 10–15 mg/kg/24 hr ÷ QD–TID

Increment: 5–10 mg/kg/24 hr at weekly intervals to **max. dose** of 60 mg/kg/24 hr

Maintenance: 30–60 mg/kg/24 hr ÷ BID–TID. Due to drug interactions, higher doses may be required in children on other anticonvulsants.

Intravenous *(use only when PO is not possible):*

Use same PO daily dose ÷ Q6 hr. Convert back to PO as soon as possible.

Rectal *(Use syrup, diluted 1 : 1 with water, given PR as a retention enema):*

Load: 20 mg/kg/dose

Maintenance: 10–15 mg/kg/dose Q8 hr

Migraine prophylaxis:

Child: 15–30 mg/kg/24 hr PO ÷ BID

Adult: Start with 500 mg/24 hr ÷ PO BID. Dose may be increased to a **maximum** of 1000 mg/24 hr ÷ PO BID. If using divalproex sodium extended-release tablets, administer daily dose QD.

Contraindicated in hepatic disease. May cause GI, liver, blood, and CNS toxicity; weight gain; transient alopecia; pancreatitis (potentially life threatening); nausea; sedation; vomiting; headache; thrombocytopenia; platelet dysfunction; rash (especially with lamotrigine); and hyperammonemia.

Continued

For explanation of icons, see p. 680.

VALPROIC ACID *continued*

Hepatic failure has occurred, especially in children <2 yr. Idiosyncratic life-threatening pancreatitis has been reported in children and adults. Hyperammonemic encephalopathy has been reported in patients with urea cycle disorders.

Valproic acid is a substrate for CYP450 2C19 isoenzyme and an inhibitor of CYP450 2C9, 2D6, and 3A3/4 (weak). It increases amitriptyline/nortriptyline, phenytoin, diazepam, and phenobarbital levels. Concomitant phenytoin, phenobarbital, topiramate, meropenem, and carbamazepine may decrease valproic acid levels. Amitriptyline or nortriptyline may increase valproic acid levels. May interfere with urine ketone and thyroid tests.

Do not give syrup with carbonated beverages. Use of IV route has not been evaluated for >14 days of continuous use. Infuse IV over 1 hr up to a **max. rate** of 20 mg/min. Depakote and Depakote ER are **NOT** bioequivalent; see package insert for dose conversion.

Therapeutic levels: 50–100 mg/L. Recommendations for serum sampling at steady state: obtain trough level within 30 min before the next scheduled dose after 2–3 days of continuous dosing. Levels of 50–60 mg/L and as high as 85 mg/L have been recommended for bipolar disorders. Monitor CBC and LFTs before and during therapy.

VANCOMYCIN

Vancocin and others

Antibiotic

Yes ? C/B

Injection: 0.5, 1, 5, 10 g
Caps: 125, 250 mg
Solution: 1 g (reconstitute to 250 mg/5 mL), 10 g (reconstitute to 500 mg/6 mL)

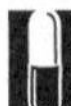

Neonate, IV *(see table below):*

	Postnatal Age	
Weight (kg)	*<7 Days*	*≥7 Days*
<1.2	15 mg/kg/dose Q24 hr	15 mg/kg/dose Q24 hr
1.2–2	10–15 mg/kg/dose Q12–18 hr	10–15 mg/kg/dose Q8–12 hr
>2	10–15 mg/kg/dose Q8–12 hr	15–20 mg/kg/dose Q8 hr

Infant and child, IV:

CNS and serious infections: 60 mg/kg/24 hr ÷ Q6 hr
Other infections: 40 mg/kg/24 hr ÷ Q6–8 hr
Max. dose: 1 g/dose

Adult: 2 g/24 hr ÷ Q6–12 hr IV; **max. dose:** 4 g/24 hr

C. difficile colitis:

Child: 40–50 mg/kg/24 hr ÷ Q6 hr PO × 7–10 days
Max. dose: 500 mg/24 hr
Adult: 125 mg/dose PO Q6 hr × 7–10 days

Endocarditis prophylaxis: see Chapter 6.

Continued

VANCOMYCIN *continued*

Ototoxicity and nephrotoxicity may occur and may be exacerbated with concurrent aminoglycoside use. **Adjust dose in renal failure (see Chapter 30).** Low concentrations of the drug may appear in CSF with inflamed meninges. "Red man syndrome" associated with rapid IV infusion may occur. Infuse over 60 min (may infuse over 120 min if 60-min infusion is not tolerated). **NOTE:** Diphenhydramine is used to reverse red man syndrome. Allergic reactions have been reported.

Measuring serum levels is primarily indicated for enhancing efficacy. Toxicity has not been correlated with serum levels. Although the monitoring of serum levels is controversial, the following guidelines are recommended. Therapeutic levels: peak, 25–40 mg/L (for CNS infections, ≥35 mg/L); trough, 5–10 mg/L. Recommended serum sampling time at steady state: trough within 30 min before the third consecutive dose and peak 60 min after the administration of the third consecutive dose.

Metronidazole (PO) is the drug of choice for *C. difficile* colitis; vancomycin should be **avoided** because of the emergence of vancomycin-resistant enterococcus. Pregnancy category B is assigned with the oral route of administration.

VARICELLA-ZOSTER IMMUNEGLOBULIN (HUMAN)

VZIG

Hyperimmune globulin

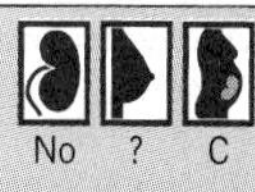

1 vial = 125 U (~1.25 mL), 625 U (~6.25 mL); contains 10%–18% globulin and may contain thimerosal

≤10 kg: 125 U IM
10.1–20 kg: 250 U IM
20.1–30 kg: 375 U IM
30.1–40 kg: 500 U IM
>40 kg: 625 U IM (**maximum** 2.5 mL per injection site)
Max. dose: 625 U/dose

Contraindicated in severe thrombocytopenia due to IM injection. See Chapter 15 for indications. Dose should be given within 48 hr of exposure and no later than 96 hr postexposure. Local discomfort, redness, and swelling at the injection site may occur. May induce anaphylactic reactions in immunoglobulin A–deficient individuals. Interferes with immune response to live virus vaccines such as measles, mumps, and rubella; defer administration of live vaccines 5 mo or longer after VZIG dose. See latest AAP *Red Book* for additional information.

For explanation of icons, see p. 680.

VASOPRESSIN
Pitressin and others
Antidiuretic hormone analog

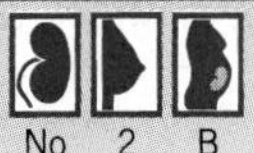

Injection: 20 U/mL (aqueous) (0.5, 1, 10 mL)

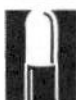

Diabetes insipidus: Titrate dose to effect.
SC/IM:
Child: 2.5–10 U BID–QID
Adult: 5–10 U BID–QID
Continuous infusion (adult and child): Start at 0.5 milliunit/kg/hr (0.0005 U/kg/hr). Double dosage every 30 min PRN up to **max. dose** of 10 milliunit/kg/hr (0.01 U/kg/hr).

Growth hormone and corticotropin provocative tests:
Child: 0.3 U/kg IM; **max. dose:** 10 U
Adult: 10 U IM

GI hemorrhage (IV):
Child: Start at 0.002–0.005 U/kg/min. Increase dose as needed to **max. dose** of 0.01 U/kg/min.
Adult: Start at 0.2–0.4 U/min. Increase dose as needed to **max. dose** of 0.9 U/min.

Cardiac arrest, ventricular fibrillation and pulseless ventricular tachycardia:
Adult: 40 U IV × 1

Use with caution in seizures, migraine, asthma, and vascular disease. Side effects include tremor, sweating, vertigo, abdominal discomfort, nausea, vomiting, urticaria, anaphylaxis, hypertension, and bradycardia. May cause vasoconstriction, water intoxication, and bronchoconstriction. Drug interactions: lithium, demeclocycline, heparin, and alcohol reduce activity; carbamazepine, tricyclic antidepressants, fludrocortisone, and chlorpropamide increase activity.

Do not abruptly discontinue IV infusion (taper dose). Patients with variceal hemorrhage and hepatic insufficiency may respond to lower dosages. Monitor fluid intake and output, urine specific gravity, urine and serum osmolality, and sodium.

VECURONIUM BROMIDE
Norcuron
Nondepolarizing neuromuscular blocking agent

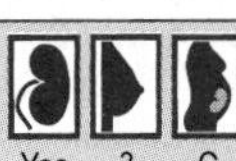

Injection: 10, 20 mg; may contain benzyl alcohol

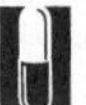

Neonate:
Initial: 0.1 mg/kg/dose IV
Maintenance: 0.03–0.15 mg/kg/dose IV Q1–2 hr PRN

>7 wk–1 yr:
Initial: 0.08–0.1 mg/kg/dose IV
Maintenance: 0.05–0.1 mg/kg/dose IV Q1 hr PRN

Continued

VECURONIUM BROMIDE *continued*

>1 yr–adult *(see remarks):*

Initial: 0.08–0.1 mg/kg/dose IV

Maintenance: 0.05–0.1 mg/kg/dose IV Q1 hr PRN; may administer via continuous infusion at 0.05–0.07 mg/kg/hr IV

Use with caution in patients with renal or hepatic impairment or neuromuscular disease. Dose reduction may be necessary in hepatic insufficiency. Infants (7 wk to 1 yr) are more sensitive to the drug and may have a longer recovery time. Children (1–10 yr) may require higher doses and more frequent supplementation than adults. Enflurane, isoflurane, aminoglycosides, beta-blockers, calcium-channel blockers, clindamycin, furosemide, magnesium salts, quinidine, procainamide, and cyclosporine may increase the potency and duration of neuromuscular blockade. Calcium, caffeine, carbamazepine, phenytoin, steroids (chronic use), acetylcholinesterases, and azathioprine may decrease effects. May cause arrhythmias, rash, and bronchospasm.

Neostigmine, pyridostigmine, and edrophonium are antidotes. Onset of action within 1–3 min. Duration is 30–40 min. See Chapter 1 for rapid sequence intubation.

VERAPAMIL

Isoptin, Isoptin SR, Calan, Calan SR, Verelan, Verelan PM, Covera-HS, and others

Calcium-channel blocker

Yes 1 C

Tabs: 40, 80, 120 mg
Extended/sustained-release tabs: 120, 180, 240 mg
Extended/sustained-release caps: 100, 120, 180, 200, 240, 300, 360 mg
Injection: 2.5 mg/mL (2, 4 mL)
Suspension: 50 mg/mL

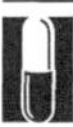

IV for dysrhythmias: Give over 2–3 min. May repeat once after 30 min.

1–16 yr, for PSVT: 0.1–0.3 mg/kg/dose × 1 may repeat dose in 30 min; **max. dose:** 5 mg first dose, 10 mg second dose.

Adult, for SVT: 5–10 mg (0.075–0.15 mg/kg) × 1; may administer second dose of 10 mg 15–30 min later.

PO for hypertension:

Child: 4–8 mg/kg/24 hr ÷ TID

Adult: 240–480 mg/24 hr ÷ TID–QID or divide QD–BID for sustained-release preparations

Contraindications include hypersensitivity, cardiogenic shock, severe CHF, sick-sinus syndrome, or AV block. **Because of negative inotropic effects, verapamil should not be used to treat SVT in an emergency setting in infants. Avoid IV use** in neonates and young infants due to apnea, bradycardia, and hypotension. Monitor ECG. **Have calcium and isoproterenol available to reverse myocardial depression.** May decrease neuromuscular transmission in patients with Duchenne muscular dystrophy and may worsen myasthenia gravis.

Continued

For explanation of icons, see p. 680.

VERAPAMIL *continued*

Drug is a substrate of CYP450 1A2 and 3A3/4 and an inhibitor of CYP3A4. Barbiturates, sulfinpyrazone, phenytoin, vitamin D, and rifampin may decrease serum levels/effects of verapamil; quinidine and grapefruit juice may increase serum levels/effects. Verapamil may increase effects of beta-blockers (severe myocardial depression), carbamazepine, cyclosporine, digoxin, ethanol, fentanyl, lithium, nondepolarizing muscle relaxants, and prazosin. **Reduce dose in renal insufficiency (see Chapter 30).**

VIDARABINE

Adenine arabinoside, ara-A, Vira-A

Antiviral agent

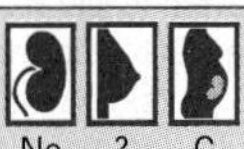

Ophthalmic ointment: 3% monohydrate (2.8% vidarabine base) (3.5 g)

Keratoconjunctivitis (HSV, VZV): Apply ½-inch ribbon of ointment to lower conjunctival sac Q3 hr, 5× per 24 hr until complete reepithelialization has occurred, then decrease dose to BID for an additional 7 days. If there are no signs of improvement after 7 days or if complete re-epithelialization has not occurred in 21 days, consider other forms of therapy.

Ophthalmic product may cause burning, lacrimation, keratitis, photophobia, and blurred vision. Ophthalmic steroids are **contraindicated** in suspected herpetic keratoconjunctivitis.

VITAMIN A

Aquasol A and others

Vitamin, fat soluble

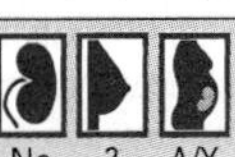

Caps: 10,000 IU (OTC), 15,000 IU (OTC), 25,000 IU
Tabs: 5000 IU (OTC), 15,000 IU
Injection: 50,000 IU/mL (2 mL); contains polysorbate 80

U.S. RDA: see Chapter 20

Supplementation in measles (6 mo to 2 yr)

6 mo–1 yr: 100,000 IU/dose QD PO ×2 days. Repeat 1 dose at 4 wk.

1–2 yr: 200,000 IU/dose QD PO ×2 days. Repeat 1 dose at 4 wk.

Malabsorption syndrome prophylaxis:

Child >8 yr and adult: 10,000–50,000 IU/dose QD PO of water-miscible product.

High doses above the U.S. RDA are teratogenic (category X). The use of vitamin A in measles is recommended in children 6 mo to 2 yr who are either hospitalized or have any of the following risk factors: immunodeficiency, ophthalmologic evidence of vitamin A deficiency, impaired GI absorption, moderate

Continued

VITAMIN A *continued*

to severe malnutrition, or recent immigration from areas with high measles mortality. May cause GI disturbance, rash, headache, increased ICP (pseudotumor cerebri), papilledema, and irritability. Large doses may increase the effects of warfarin. Mineral oil, cholestyramine, and neomycin will reduce vitamin A absorption. See Chapter 20 for multivitamin preparations.

VITAMIN B_1

See *Thiamine*

VITAMIN B_2

See *Riboflavin*

VITAMIN B_3

See *Niacin*

VITAMIN B_6

See *Pyridoxine*

VITAMIN B_{12}

See *Cyanocobalamin*

VITAMIN C

See *Ascorbic Acid*

VITAMIN D_2

See *Ergocalciferol*

VITAMIN E/ALPHA-TOCOPHEROL

Aquavit-E, Nutr-E-sol, and others

Vitamin, fat soluble

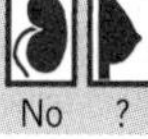
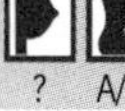
No ? A/C

Tabs (OTC): 100, 200, 400, 500, 800 IU
Caps (OTC): 100, 200, 400, 1000 IU
Drops (OTC): 50 IU/mL
Liquid (OTC): 400 IU/15 mL

Continued

For explanation of icons, see p. 680.

VITAMIN E/ALPHA-TOCOPHEROL *continued*

U.S. RDA: see Chapter 20.
Vitamin E deficiency, PO: Follow levels.
Use water-miscible form with malabsorption.
Neonate: 25–50 IU/24 hr
Child: 1 IU/kg/24 hr
Adult: 60–75 IU/24 hr

Cystic fibrosis *(use water-miscible form):* 5–10 IU/kg/24 hr PO QD; **max. dose:** 400 IU/24 hr.

Adverse reactions include GI distress, rash, headache, gonadal dysfunction, decreased serum thyroxine and tri-iodothyronine, and blurred vision.

Necrotizing enterocolitis has been associated with large doses (>200 units/24 hr). May increase hypoprothrombinemic response of oral anticoagulants (e.g., warfarin), especially in doses >400 IU/24 hr.

One unit of vitamin E = 1 mg of DL-alpha tocopherol acetate. In malabsorption, water-miscible preparations are better absorbed. Therapeutic levels: 6–14 mg/L.

Pregnancy category changes to C if used in doses above the U.S. RDA. See Chapter 20 for multivitamin preparations.

VITAMIN K_1

See *Phytonadione*

VORICONAZOLE

VFEND

Antifungal, triazole

Yes ? D

Tabs: 50, 200 mg; contains povidone
Oral suspension: 40 mg/mL (75 mL); contains sodium benzoate
Injection: 200 mg; contains 3200 mg sulfobutyl ether beta-cyclodextrin

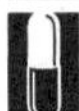

IV *(Pediatric dosing not well established, also see remarks):*
Loading dose: 6 mg/kg/dose Q12 hr × 2 doses.
Maintenance dose: 4 mg/kg/dose Q12 hr; may be increased to 5 mg/kg/dose Q12 hr if needed or reduced to 3 mg/kg/dose Q12 hr if patient unable to tolerate.

PO >12 yr (see remarks):

Invasive aspergillosis/Fusarium/Scedosporium/and other serious infections:

<40 kg:
Loading dose: 200 mg PO Q12 hr × 2 doses
Maintenance dose: 100 mg PO Q12 hr; dose may be increased to 150 mg PO Q12 hr if response is inadequate

≥40 kg:
Loading dose: 400 mg PO Q12 hr × 2 doses
Maintenance dose: 200 mg PO Q12 hr; dose may be increased to 300 mg PO Q12 hr if response is inadequate.

Continued

W
FORMULARY

VORICONAZOLE *continued*

Esophageal candidiasis (treat for a minimum 14 days and until 7 days after resolution of symptoms):

<40 kg: 100 mg PO Q12 hr
≥40 kg: 200 mg PO Q12 hr

Contraindicated with concomitant administration with CYP450 3A4 substrates that can lead to prolonged QTc interval (e.g., cisapride, pimozide, and quinidine); concomitant administration with rifampin, carbamazepine, barbiturates, ritonavir, efavirenz, and rifabutin (decreases voriconazole levels); concomitant administration with sirolimus, efavirenz, rifabutin, and ergot alkaloids (voriconazole increases levels of these drugs). Drug is a substrate and inhibitor for CYP450 2C9, 2C19 (major substrate), and 3A4 isoenzymes.

Currently approved for use in invasive aspergillosis, candidal esophagitis, and *Fusarium* and *Scedosporium apiospermum* infections. Common side effects include GI disturbances, fever, headache, hepatic abnormalities, photosensitivity, rash (6%), and visual disturbances (30%). Serious but rare side effects include anaphylaxis, liver or renal failure, and Stevens-Johnson syndrome.

Adjust dose in hepatic impairment by decreasing only the maintenance dose by 50% for patients with a Child-Pugh class A or B. **Do not use** IV dosage form for patients with GFR <50 mL/min because of accumulation of the cyclodextrin excipient; switch to oral therapy if possible. Patients receiving concurrent phenytoin should increase their maintenance doses (IV, 5 mg/kg/dose Q 12 hr; PO, double the usual dose).

Administer IV over 1–2 hr with a **maximum** rate of 3 mg/kg/hr at a concentration ≤5 mg/mL. Administer oral doses 1 hr before and after meals.

WARFARIN
Coumadin, Sofarin
Anticoagulant

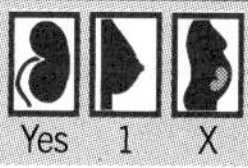

Tabs: 1, 2, 2.5, 3, 4, 5, 6, 7.5, 10 mg
Injection: 5 mg

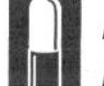

Infant and child: to achieve an INR between 2 and 3.
Loading dose on day 1:

Baseline INR 1–1.3: 0.2 mg/kg/dose PO; **max. dose:** 10 mg/dose
Liver dysfunction: 0.1 mg/kg/dose PO; **max. dose:** 5 mg/dose

Loading dose on days 2–4:

If INR 1.1–1.3: Repeat day 1 loading dose.
If INR 1.4–1.9: 50% of day 1 loading dose
If INR 2-3: 50% of day 1 loading dose
If INR 3.1–3.5: 25% of day 1 loading dose
If INR >3.5: Hold doses until INR <3.5, and restart according to the maintenance dose guidelines below.

Continued

For explanation of icons, see p. 680.

WARFARIN *continued*

Maintenance dose:

If INR 1.1–1.4: Increase previous dose by 20%.
If INR 1.5–1.9: Increase previous dose by 10%.
If INR 2-3: No change
If INR 3.1–3.5: Decrease previous dose by 10%.
If INR >3.5: Hold doses until INR <3.5, and restart at 20% less than the last dose.

Usual maintenance dose: ~0.1 mg/kg/24 hr PO QD; range, 0.05–0.34 mg/kg/24 hr. See remarks.

Adult: 5–15 mg PO QD × 2–5 days. Adjust dose to achieve the desired INR or PT. Maintenance dose range: 2–10 mg/24 hr PO QD.

Contraindicated in severe liver or kidney disease, uncontrolled bleeding, GI ulcers, and malignant hypertension. Acts on vitamin K–dependent coagulation factors II, VII, IX, and X. Side effects include fever, skin lesions, skin necrosis (especially in protein C deficiency), anorexia, nausea, vomiting, diarrhea, hemorrhage, and hemoptysis.

Warfarin is a substrate for CYP450 1A2, 2C8, 2C9, 2C18, 2C19, and 3A3/4. Chloramphenicol, chloral hydrate, cimetidine, delavirdine, fluconazole, fluoxetine, metronidazole, indomethacin, large doses of vitamins A or E, nonsteroidal antiinflammatory agents, omeprazole, quinidine, salicylates, SSRIs (e.g., fluoxetine, paroxetine, sertraline), sulfonamides, and zafirlukast may increase warfarin's effect. Ascorbic acid, barbiturates, carbamazepine, cholestyramine, dicloxacillin, griseofulvin, oral contraceptives, rifampin, spironolactone, sucralfate, and vitamin K (including foods with high content) may decrease warfarin's effect.

Younger children generally require higher doses to achieve desired effect. A cohort study of 319 children found that infants <1 yr required an average daily dose of 0.33 mg/kg and teenagers 11–18 yr required 0.09 mg/kg to maintain a target INR of 2–3. Children receiving Fontan cardiac surgery may require smaller doses than children with either congenital heart disease (without Fontan) or no congenital heart disease. [See Chest 2004;126:645-687S and Blood 1999;94(9):3007–3014 for additional information.]

The INR (international ratio) is the recommended test to monitor warfarin anticoagulant effect. Monitor INR after 5–7 days of new dosage. The particular INR desired is based on the indication and has been extrapolated from adults. An INR of 2–3 has been recommended for prophylaxis and treatment of DVT, pulmonary emboli, and bioprosthetic heart valves. An INR of 2.5–3.5 has been recommended for mechanical prosthetic heart valves and the prevention of recurrent systemic emboli. If PT is monitored, it should be 1.5–2 times the control.

Onset of action occurs within 36–72 hr, and peak effects occur within 5–7 days. IV dosing is equivalent to PO doses and is used in situations in which oral dosing is not possible. **The antidote is vitamin K and fresh-frozen plasma.**

ZAFIRLUKAST

Accolate

Antiasthmatic, leukotriene receptor antagonist

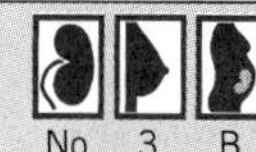

Tabs: 10, 20 mg

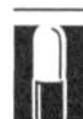

Asthma:

Child 5–11 yr: 10 mg PO BID

Child ≥12 yr and adult: 20 mg PO BID

Use with caution in hepatic insufficiency; 50%–60% reduction in clearance occurs in alcoholic cirrhosis. May cause headache, dizziness, nausea, diarrhea, abdominal pain, vomiting, generalized pain, asthenia, myalgia, fever, LFT elevation, and dyspepsia. Eosinophilia, vasculitic rash, worsening pulmonary symptoms, cardiac complications, and/or neuropathy have been reported primarily in patients with oral steroid dose reduction. Hepatitis, hyperbilirubinemia, hepatic failure, and hypersensitivity reactions (e.g., urticaria, angioedema, and rashes) have also been reported.

Drug is a substrate for CYP450 2C9 and inhibits CYP450 2C9 and 3A4 isoenzymes. Erythromycin, terfenadine, and theophylline decrease zafirlukast levels; aspirin increases levels. Zafirlukast may increase the effects of warfarin. Administer doses on an empty stomach, at least 1 hr before or 2 hr after eating.

ZANAMIVIR

Relenza

Antiviral

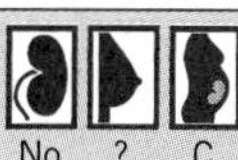

Powder for inhalation: 5 mg/inhalation (5 Rotodisks [4 inhalations/Rotadisk] with Diskhaler); each 5-mg drug contains 20 mg lactose (which contains milk proteins).

Treatment of uncomplicated influenza *(initiate therapy within 2 days of onset of symptoms):*

≥7 yr and adult:

Day 1: 10 mg inhaled (as two 5 mg inhalations) BID (2–12 hr between the two doses) × 2 doses

Day 2–5: 10 mg inhaled (as two 5 mg inhalations) Q12 hr × 4 days

Currently indicated for the treatment of influenza A and B strains. **Not recommended** for patients with underlying respiratory diseases (e.g., asthma or COPD) because bronchospasm may occur, and efficacy could not be demonstrated. May cause nasal discomfort, cough, and throat/tonsil discomfort and pain. Allergic reactions involving oropharyngeal edema and serious skin rashes have been reported; **discontinue** therapy if this occurs.

See package insert for specific instructions for using the Rotodisk/Diskhaler system. If patient is concurrently using a bronchodilator, use the bronchodilator before taking zanamivir.

For explanation of icons, see p. 680.

ZIDOVUDINE

Retrovir, AZT

Antiviral agent, nucleoside analog reverse transcriptase inhibitor

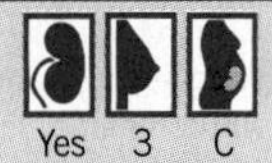

Caps: 100 mg
Tabs: 300 mg
Liquid: 50 mg/5 mL (240 mL); contains 0.2% sodium benzoate
Injection: 10 mg/mL (20 mL)
In combination with lamivudine (3TC) as Combivir:
Tabs: 300 mg zidovudine + 150 mg lamivudine
In combination with abacavir and lamivudine (3TC) as Trizivir:
Tabs: 300 mg zidovudine + 300 mg abacavir + 150 mg lamivudine

HIV: See www.aidsinfo.nih.gov/guidelines.
Prevention of vertical transmission:
14–34 wk of pregnancy:
Until labor: 100 mg PO 5× per 24 hr or 600 mg/24 hr PO ÷ BID–TID
During labor: 2 mg/kg/dose IV over 1 hr followed by 1 mg/kg/hr IV infusion until umbilical cord clamped.
Neonate: 2 mg/kg/dose Q6 hr PO or 1.5 mg/kg/dose Q6 hr IV over 60 min. Begin within 12 hr of birth, and continue until 6 wk of age.
Premature infant:
<30 weeks' gestation: 2 mg/kg/dose PO Q12 hr or 1.5 mg/kg/dose IV Q12 hr for first 4 wk of life, then increase dosing interval to Q8 hr thereafter.
≥30 weeks' gestation: 2 mg/kg/dose PO Q12 hr or 1.5 mg/kg/dose IV Q12 hr for first 2 wk of life, then increase dosing interval to Q8 hr thereafter. Dosage interval may be further reduced to Q6 hr when the child reaches full term (40 wk postconceptional age [PCA]).
Needle-stick prophylaxis: 200 mg/dose PO TID or 300 mg/dose PO BID × 28 days. Use in combination with lamivudine, 150 mg/dose PO BID, and indinavir, 800 mg/dose PO TID × 28 days.

See www. aidsinfo.nih.gov/guidelines for additional remarks.
Use with caution in patients with impaired renal or hepatic function.
Dosage reduction is recommended in severe renal impairment and may be necessary in hepatic dysfunction. Drug penetrates well into the CNS. Most common side effects include anemia, granulocytopenia, nausea, and headache (dosage reduction, erythropoietin, filgrastim/GCSF, or discontinuance may be required depending on event). Seizures, confusion, rash, myositis, myopathy (use >1 yr), hepatitis, and elevated liver enzymes have been reported. Macrocytosis is noted after 4 wk of therapy and can be used as an indicator of compliance. Lactic acidosis and severe hepatomegaly with steatosis, including fatal cases, have been reported.

Do not use in combination with stavudine because of poor antiretroviral effect. Effects of interacting drugs include increased toxicity (acyclovir, trimethoprim-sulfamethoxazole); increased hematologic toxicity (ganciclovir, interferon alfa, marrow-suppressive drugs); and granulocytopenia (drugs that affect glucuronidation). Methadone, atovaquone, cimetidine, valproic acid, probenecid,

Continued

ZIDOVUDINE *continued*

and fluconazole may increase levels of zidovudine; rifampin, rifabutin, and clarithromycin may decrease levels.

Do not administer IM. IV form is incompatible with blood product infusions and should be infused over 1 hr (intermittent IV dosing). Despite manufacturer recommendations of administering oral doses 30 min before or 1 hr after meals, doses may be administered with food.

ZINC SALTS

Galzin, Orazinc, Zincate, and others

Trace mineral

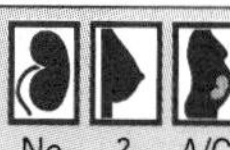

No ? A/C

Tabs as sulfate (Orazinc; OTC), 23% elemental: 66, 110, 200 mg
Caps as sulfate (Orazinc, Zincate; OTC), 23% elemental: 220 mg
Tabs as gluconate, 14.3% elemental (OTC): 10, 15, 50 mg
Caps as acetate (Galzin): 25, 50 mg elemental per capsule
Liquid as acetate: 5 mg elemental Zn/mL
Liquid as sulfate: 10 mg elemental Zn/mL
Injection as sulfate: 1 mg, 5 mg elemental Zn/mL; may contain benzyl alcohol
Injection as chloride: 1 mg elemental Zn/mL

Zinc deficiency:
Infant and child: 0.5–1 mg elemental Zn/kg/24 hr PO ÷ QD–TID
Adult: 25–50 mg elemental Zn/dose (100–220 mg Zn sulfate/dose) PO TID
U.S. RDA: see Chapter 20.
For supplementation in parenteral nutrition, see Chapter 20.

Nausea, vomiting, GI disturbances, leukopenia, and diaphoresis may occur. Gastric ulcers, hypotension, and tachycardia may occur at high doses.

Patients with excessive losses (burns) or impaired absorption require higher doses. Therapeutic levels: 70–130 mcg/dL. May decrease the absorption of penicillamine, tetracycline, and fluoroquinolones (e.g., ciprofloxacin). Drugs that increase gastric pH (e.g., H_2 antagonists and proton pump inhibitors) can reduce the absorption of zinc.

About 20%–30% of oral dose is absorbed. Oral doses may be administered with food if GI upset occurs. Pregnancy category is A for zinc acetate.

ZONISAMIDE

Zonegran

Anticonvulsant

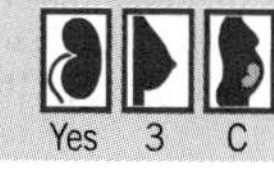

Yes 3 C

Caps: 25, 50, 100 mg

Infant and child (data are incomplete):
Suggested dosing from a review of Japanese open-labeled studies for partial and generalized seizures: Start with 1–2 mg/kg/24 hr PO ÷ BID. Increase

Continued

For explanation of icons, see p. 680.

ZONISAMIDE *continued*

dosage by 0.5–1 mg/kg/24 hr Q2 wk to the usual dosage range of 5–8 mg/kg/24 hr PO ÷ BID

Recommended higher alternative dosing: Start with 2–4 mg/kg/24 hr PO ÷ BID–TID. Gradually increase dosage at 1- to 2-wk intervals to 4–8 mg/kg/24 hr; **max. dose:** 12 mg/kg/24 hr.

>16 yr–adult:

Adjunctive therapy for partial seizures: 100 mg PO QD × 2 wk. Dose may be increased to 200 mg PO QD × 2 wk. Additional dosage increments of 100 mg/24 hr can be made at 2-wk intervals to allow attainment of steady-state levels. Effective doses have ranged from 100–600 mg/24 hr ÷ QD–BID; no additional benefit has been shown for doses >400 mg/24 hr.

Because zonisamide is a sulfonamide, it is **contraindicated** in patients allergic to sulfonamides (may result in Stevens-Johnson syndrome or TEN). Common side effects of drowsiness, ataxia, anorexia, gastrointestinal discomfort, headache, rash, and pruritus usually occur early in therapy and can be minimized with slow dose titration. Urolithiasis has been reported. Children are at increased risk for hyperthermia and oligohydrosis, especially in warm or hot weather.

Although not fully delineated, therapeutic serum levels of 20–30 mg/L have been suggested because higher rates of adverse reactions have been seen at levels >30 mg/L.

Zonisamide is a CYP450 3A4 substrate. Phenytoin, carbamazepine, and phenobarbital can decrease levels of zonisamide.

Use with caution in renal or hepatic impairment; slower dose titration and more frequent monitoring are recommended. **Do not use** if GFR is <50 mL/min. **Avoid** abrupt discontinuation or radical dose reductions. Swallow capsules whole and do **not** crush or chew.

VII. REFERENCES

1. Package inserts of medications.
2. Committee on Drugs: The transfer of drugs and other chemicals into human milk. Pediatrics 2001;108(3):776–789.
3. Briggs GG, Freeman RK, Yaffe SJ: A Reference Guide to Fetal and Neonatal Risk: Drugs in Pregnancy and Lactation, 6th ed. Baltimore, Williams & Wilkins, 2002.
4. Pickering LK (ed): Red Book: 2003 Report of the Committee on Infectious Diseases, 26th ed. Elk Grove Village, IL, American Academy of Pediatrics, 2003.
5. Gilbert DN, Moellering RE, Sande MA: The Sanford Guide to Antimicrobial Therapy, 33rd ed. Vienna, VA, Antimicrobial Therapy, Inc, 2003.
6. Nelson JD, Bradley JS: 2002–2003 Nelson's Pocket Book of Pediatric Antimicrobial Therapy, 15th ed. Philadelphia, Lippincott Williams & Wilkins, 2002.
7. Bartlett JG, Gallant JE: 2003 Medical Management of HIV Infection. Sterling, VA, PMR Printing, 2003.
8. Young TE, Mangum OB: Neofax: A Manual of Drugs used in Neonatal Care, 16th ed. Raleigh, NC, Acorn Publishing, 2003.
9. McEvoy GK, et al: AHFS 2004 Drug Information. Bethesda, MD, American Society of Health-System Pharmacists, 2004.
10. Facts and Comparisons: E Facts, online drug information service. Available: www.efacts.com. Philadelphia, JB Lippincott.

11. Micromedex, Inc: Micromedex Healthcare Series, vol. 111 [Online].
12. Takemoto CK, Hodding JH, Kraus DM: Pediatric Dosage Handbook, 10th ed. Hudson, OH, Lexi-Comp, 2003.
13. Ellsworth AJ, Witt DM, Dugdale DC, Oliver LM: 2004 Mosby's Medical Drug Reference. St. Louis, Mosby, 2004.
14. U.S. Department of Health and Human Services. AIDS Info [Online]. Available: www.aidsinfo.nih.gov.
15. National Institutes of Health: National Heart, Lung and Blood Institute: Expert Panel Report 2. Clinical practice guidelines: Guidelines for the diagnosis and management of asthma. NIH Publ. No. 97-4051; April 1997.
16. National High Blood Pressure Education Program Working Group on High Blood Pressure in Children and Adolescents: The Fourth Report on the Diagnosis, Evaluation, and Treatment of High Blood Pressure in Children and Adolescents. Pediatrics 2004;114:555–576.
17. Hazinski MF, Cummins RO, Field JM: 2000 Handbook of Emergency Cardiovascular Care for Healthcare Providers. American Heart Association, 2000.
18. Monagle P, Chan A, Massicotte P, et al: Antithrombotic therapy in children. Seventh ACCP Conference on Antithrombotic and Thrombolytic Therapy. Chest 2004;126:645–687S.
19. American Thoracic Society: Targeted tuberculin testing and treatment of latent tuberculosis infection. Am J Respir Crit Care Med 2000;161:1376–1395.
20. Burg FD, Ingelfinger JR, Polin RA, Gershon, AA: Gellis and Kagan's Current Pediatric Therapy, 17th ed. Philadelphia, WB Saunders, 2002.
21. Physicians' Desk Reference, vol. 58. Montvale, NJ, Thomson PDR, 2004.
22. Food and Drug Administration Safety Information and Adverse Event Reporting Program [Online]. Available: www.fda.gov/medwatch/.
23. Jew RK, Mullen RJ, Soo-Hoo W: The Children's Hospital of Philadelphia Extemporaneous Formulations. Bethesda, MD, American Society of Health-System Pharmacists, 2003.

For explanation of icons, see p. 680.

Analgesia and Sedation

Kamie Yang, MD

28

I. PAIN ASSESSMENT (Table 28-1)

A. INFANT[1]

1. **Physiologic response:** Seen primarily in acute pain; subsides with continuing pain. Is unreliable as an indicator of chronic pain. Increases in blood pressure, heart rate, and respiratory rate; oxygen desaturation; crying; diaphoresis; flushing; pallor.
2. **Behavioral response:** Observe characteristics and duration of cry, facial expressions, visual tracking, body movements, and response to stimuli. Is an excellent indicator for continuing pain.

B. PRESCHOOLER

In addition to physiologic and behavioral responses, use the "FACES" pain rating scale to assess pain intensity in children as young as 3 years.

C. SCHOOL-AGE AND ADOLESCENT

Evaluate physiologic and behavioral responses; ask about description, location, and character of pain. Children 7–8 years old can use the standard pain rating scale (0 is no pain and 10 is the worst pain ever experienced).

II. ANALGESICS[1,2]

A. NONOPIOID ANALGESICS

Weak analgesics with antipyretic activity are commonly used to manage mild to moderate pain of nonvisceral origin. Administer alone or in combination with opiates (Table 28-2).

1. **Acetaminophen:** Weak analgesic with no anti-inflammatory activity; does not affect platelets.
2. **Nonsteroidal anti-inflammatory drugs (NSAIDs):** Especially useful for sickle cell, bony, rheumatic, and inflammatory pain. Recommend H_2-receptor blocker concurrently with prolonged use. Primary adverse effects are gastrointestinal (epigastric pain, gastritis, and bleeding), interference with platelet aggregation, bronchoconstriction, hypersensitivity reactions, and azotemia. May interfere with bone healing. Should be avoided in patients with several renal disease, dehydration, or heart failure. Cyclooxygenase-2 inhibitors (COX-2) should be used only in postpubertal children.

B. OPIOIDS (Table 28-3)

1. Opiods produce analgesia by binding mu receptors in the brain and spinal cord.

TABLE 28-1

DEVELOPMENTAL RESPONSES TO PAIN

Age	Response	
Infant	Younger than 6 mo	**No expression of anticipatory fear.** Level of anxiety reflects that of the parent.
	6 to 18 mo	**Anticipatory fear** of painful experiences begins to develop.
Preschooler	18 to 24 mo	**Verbalization.** Children express pain with words such as "hurt" and "boo-boo."
	3 yr	**Localization and identification of external causes.** Children more reliably assess their pain but continue to depend on visual cues for localization and are unable to understand a reason for pain.
School-age child	5 to 7 yr	**Cooperation.** Children have improved understanding of pain and ability to localize it and cooperate.

Data from Hsu DC: Pain Control and Sedation in Children. Uptodate Online 113, www.utdol.com.

TABLE 28-2

NONOPIOID ANALGESICS

Drug	Route	GI Irritation	Platelet Inhibition	Comments
Acetaminophen	PO/PR	No	No	Weak analgesic with excellent antipyretic activity. No anti-inflammatory properties
Aspirin	PO/PR	Yes	Yes	Avoid owing to Reye syndrome
NSAID				
Ibuprofen	PO	Yes	Yes	
Ketorolac	IV/IM PO	Yes	Yes	Potent analgesic, 1 mg/kg IV is comparable to 0.1 mg/kg morphine. Only parenteral NSAID.
Naproxen	PO	Yes	Yes	
Rofecoxib	PO	Yes	Yes	
Choline MG trisalicylate	PO	Yes	No	Avoid owing to Reye syndrome No antiplatelet effect. Useful in patients with leukemia.

TABLE 28-3
COMMONLY USED OPIATES

Drug	Equi-analgesic Doses (mg/kg/dose)	Routes	Onset (min)	Duration (hr)	Notable Side Effects	Comments
Codeine	1.2	PO	30–60	3–4	• Can cause severe nausea and vomiting • Histamine release	Converted in liver to morphine (10%) Newborns and 10% of U.S. population cannot make this conversion.
Meperidine (Demerol)	1.0 1.5–2.0	IV PO	5–10 30–60	3–4 2–4	• Catastrophic interaction with **MAO inhibitors** • Tachycardia, histamine release • Metabolite can cause **seizures;** avoid in predisposed patients	Euphoric effects are greater than with morphine. Low doses stop shivering (0.1–0.25 mg/kg). Not recommended for prolonged use or patient-controlled analgesia.
Oxycodone	0.1	PO	30–60	3–4		Available in sustained-release form for chronic pain. Much less nauseating than codeine.
Methadone	0.1 0.1	IV PO	5–10 30–60	4–24 4–24		Initial dose may produce analgesia for 3–4 hr; duration of action is increased with repeated dosing.

continued

TABLE 28-3

COMMONLY USED OPIATES—*cont'd*

Drug	Equi-analgesic Doses (mg/kg/dose)	Routes	Onset (min)	Duration (hr)	Notable Side Effects	Comments
Morphine	0.1	IV	5–10	3–4	• Seizures in neonates	The "gold standard" against which all other opioids are compared.
	0.1–0.2	IM/SC	10–30	4–5	• Can cause significant **histamine release**	Available in sustained-release form for chronic pain.
	0.3–0.5	PO	30–60	4–5		
Hydromorphone	0.015	IV/SC	5–10	3–4		Less sedation, nausea, pruritus than morphine.
	0.02–0.1	PO	30–60			
Fentanyl	0.001	IV	1–2	0.5–1	• **Pruritus**	Rarely causes cardiovascular instability (relatively safer in hypovolemia, congenital heart disease, or head trauma vs other opioids).
	0.001	Transdermal	12	2–3	• Bradycardia	Respiratory depressant effect much longer (4 hr) than analgesic effect.
	0.01	Transmucosal	15		• **Chest wall rigidity** with doses >5 µg/kg (but can occur at all doses). Treat with naloxone or neuromuscular blockade	Levels of unbound drug are higher in newborns. Most commonly used opioid for short painful procedures.

Data from Yaster M, et al: Pediatric Pain Management and Sedation Handbook. St. Louis, Mosby, 1997.

2. Most flexible and widely used analgesics. Side effects include pruritus, nausea, vomiting, constipation, urinary retention, and rarely respiratory depression and hypotension.
3. Morphine is the gold (unit) standard of this drug class.

C. LOCAL ANESTHETICS

Local anesthetics are used primarily to anesthetize areas for minor procedures. They are administered topically, subcutaneously, into peripheral nerves (e.g., digital nerve, penile nerve block), or centrally (epidural/spinal). They act by blocking nerve conduction at the sodium channel.

1. For all local anesthetics, 1% solution = 10 mg/mL.

2. Topical local anesthetics (Table 28-4):

a. EMLA (eutectic mixture of local anesthetics).
b. LET (lidocaine, epinephrine, tetracaine).
c. TAC (tetracaine, adrenaline [epinephrine], cocaine).
d. Viscous lidocaine.

3. Injectable local anesthetics (Table 28-5):

a. *Infiltration of the skin at the site:* Used for painful procedures such as wound closure, blood drawing, intravenous (IV) line placement, or lumbar puncture.
b. *To reduce stinging from injection:* Use a small needle (27–30 gauge). Alkalinize anesthetic: Add 1 mL (1 mEq) sodium bicarbonate to 9 mL lidocaine (or 29 mL bupivacaine), use lowest concentration of anesthetic available, warm solution (between 37° and 42°C), inject anesthetic slowly, and rub skin at injection site first.
c. *To enhance efficacy and duration:* Add epinephrine to decrease vascular uptake. **Never use local anesthetics with epinephrine in areas supplied by end arteries** (e.g., pinna, digits, nasal tip, and penis).
d. *Local anesthetic toxicity:* CNS and cardiac toxicity are of greatest concern. CNS symptoms are seen before cardiovascular collapse. Progression of symptoms: Perioral numbness, dizziness, auditory disturbances, muscular twitching, unconsciousness, seizures, coma, respiratory arrest, cardiovascular collapse.

Note: *Bupivicaine is associated with more severe cardiac toxicity than lidocaine.*

III. SEDATION[1,3,4]

A. DEFINITIONS

1. **Mild sedation (anxiolysis):** Intent is anxiolysis with maintenance of consciousness. Practically, obtained when a single drug is given once at a low dose (not chloral hydrate).
2. **Moderate sedation:** Formerly known as *conscious sedation*. A controlled state of depressed consciousness during which airway

TABLE 28-4
COMMONLY USED TOPICAL LOCAL ANESTHETICS

	Components (1% of any anesthetic = 10 mg/mL)	Site		Directions for Use	Peak Effect (min)	Approximate Duration (min)	Cautions
		Intact skin	Nonintact skin				
EMLA (eutectic mixture of local anesthetics)	• Lidocaine 2.5% • Prilocaine 2.5%	✓		Good for: venipuncture, circumcision, lumbar puncture, and bone marrow aspiration. Apply to intact skin. Cover with occlusive dressing at least 90 min.	90	60	**Nonsterile:** Use only on intact skin. **Methemoglobinemia:** Do not use in patients with methemoglobinemia-predisposing conditions (G6PD deficiency, use of methemoglobin-inducing medications). Infants <3 mo have low levels of methemoglobin reductase. Use sparingly; up to 1 g is safe. **Maximum dose:** Maximum lidocaine dose, 5 mg/kg.
LET	• Lidocaine 4% • Epinephrine 0.1% • Tetracaine 0.5%	✓	✓	Good for: scalp and facial wounds. Available in gel or liquid form. Apply 1–3 mL of liquid-saturated cotton ball or gel to wound for 20–30 min.	30	45	**Vasoconstriction:** Contraindicated in areas supplied by end-arteries (e.g., pinna, nose, penis, and digits). Avoid contact to mucous membranes. **Maximum dose:** Maximum lidocaine dose, 5 mg/kg.

TAC	• Tetracaine 0.25%–0.5% • Adrenaline 0.025%–0.05% (epinephrine) • Cocaine 4%–11.8%	✓	✓	Available in gel or liquid form. Apply 1–3 mL of liquid-saturated cotton ball or gel to wound for 15 minutes.	15	?	**Vasoconstriction:** Contraindicated in areas supplied by end-arteries (e.g., pinna, nose, penis, and digits). **Cocaine toxicity:** Avoid contact to mucous membranes and in patients taking monoamine oxidase (MAO) inhibitors. Reapplication contraindicated. Seizures can occur even with appropriate dosing. **Maximum dose:** Maximum cocaine dose, 3 mg/kg.
Viscous lidocaine	• 2% lidocaine	✓	✓	Good for: superficial mouth and throat ulcerations (ex: herpetic stomatitis, mucositis). Do not use for teething.	10	30	**Maximum dose:** Maximum lidocaine dose, 5 mg/kg. *Note:* May combine with Maalox and benadryl elixir in a 1 : 1 : 1 fashion to make formula more palatable. 3 mg/kg/dose no more often than q2 hr.

TABLE 28-5
COMMONLY USED INJECTABLE LOCAL ANESTHETICS

Agent	Concentration (%) (1% solution = 10 mg/mL)	Max dose (mg/kg)	Onset (min)	Duration (hr)
Lidocaine	0.5–2	5	3	0.5–2
Lidocaine with epinephrine	0.5–2	7	3	1–3
Bupivicaine	0.25–0.75	2.5	15	2–4
Bupivicaine with epinephrine	0.25–0.75	3	15	4–8

Data from St. Germaine Brent A: Pediatr Clin North Am 2000;47(3):651–679; Yaster, et al: Pediatric Pain Management and Sedation Handbook. St Louis, Mosby, 1997.

TABLE 28-6
FASTING RECOMMENDATIONS

Food Type	Minimum Fasting Period (hr)
Clear liquids	2
Breast milk	4
Nonhuman milk, formula	6
Solids	8

Data from Practice guidelines for preoperative fasting and the use of pharmacologic agents to reduce the risk of pulmonary aspiration: Application to healthy patients undergoing elective procedures. A report by the American Society of Anesthesiologists Task Force on Preoperative Fasting and Use of Pharmacologic Agents to Reduce the Risk of Pulmonary Aspiration [Online]. Available: http://www.asahq.org/publicationsAndServices/NPO.pdf.

reflexes and airway patency ***are maintained***. Patient responds appropriately to age-appropriate commands ("open your eyes") and light touch. Practically, obtained any time a combination of sedative-hypnotic and analgesic are used.

3. **Deep sedation:** A controlled state of depressed consciousness during which airway reflexes and airway patency ***may not be maintained*** and the child is unable to respond to physical or verbal stimuli. Practically, required for most painful procedures in children. The following IV drugs always produce deep sedation: ketamine, propofol, etomidate, thiopental, methohexital.
4. **Mild and moderate sedation can easily progress to deep sedation.**

B. PREPARATION

1. **Patient must be NPO for solids and clear liquids** (Table 28-6 shows current American Society of Anesthesiologists [ASA] recommendations).
2. **Obtain written informed consent.**

3. **Obtain a focused patient history:**
a. Allergies and medications.
b. Airway (asthma, acute respiratory disease, reactive airway disease), airway obstruction (mediastinal mass, history of noisy breathing, obstructive sleep apnea), craniofacial abnormalities (e.g., Pfeiffer, Crouzon, Apert, Pierre-Robin syndromes), recent upper respiratory infection (suggests increased risk of laryngospasm).
c. Aspiration risk (neuromuscular disease, gastroesophageal reflux disease [GERD], altered mental status, obesity, pregnancy).
d. Prematurity, comorbidities, and adverse reactions to sedatives and anesthesia.
4. **Physical examination** with specific attention to head, ears, eyes, nose, and throat (HEENT); lungs; cardiac examination; and neuromuscular function. Assess ability to open mouth and extend neck. If risk for moderate sedation is too high, consider an anesthesia consultation and general anesthesia.
5. **Have an emergency plan ready.** Make sure qualified backup personnel and equipment are close by.
6. **Personnel.** At least two individuals must be available: Physician (to administer sedation and perform procedure) and an assistant (e.g., to monitor patient and document vital signs, drug administration).
7. **Intravenous access.**
8. **Airway equipment** (SOAP mnemonic):
a. **S**uction.
b. **O**xygen.
c. **A**irway equipment: Appropriately sized oral and nasal airways, laryngoscope with blades (Table 28-7), endotracheal tubes (ETT) with stylet (ETT size = AGE/4 + 4), bag-valve with mask, and tape.
d. **P**harmacy:
   (1) Intubation medications: Atropine, paralytic, induction agent (i.e. sedative-hypnotic).
   (2) Emergency medications: Epinephrine, atropine, glucose.
   (3) Antagonist ("reversal") agents: Naloxone, flumazenil.

TABLE 28-7
LARYNGOSCOPE SIZES

Age	Blade
Premature	Miller 00 or 0
Term	Miller 0
0–6 mo	Miller 1
6–24 mo	Miller 2
>24 mo	Miller 2 or Mac 2

Data from Fisher QA: Pediatric Anesthesia Pearls, Baltimore, MD. Johns Hopkins Department of Anesthesiology and Critical Care Medicine, 2000.

C. MONITORING

1. **Vital signs:** Obtain baseline vital signs (including pulse oximetry). Continuously monitor heart rate and oxygen saturation; intermittently monitor blood pressure and respiratory rate. Record vital signs at least every 5 minutes until the patient returns to the presedation level of consciousness. ***Note***: Complications most often occur 5 to 10 minutes after administration of IV medication and immediately after a procedure is completed (when stimuli associated with the procedure are removed).[5]
2. **Airway:** Assess airway patency and adequacy of ventilation through capnography, auscultation, or direct visualization frequently.

D. PHARMACOLOGIC AGENTS

1. **Goal of sedation:** To tailor drug combination to provide levels of analgesia, sedation-hypnosis, and anxiolysis deep enough to facilitate the procedure but shallow enough to avoid loss of airway reflexes.
2. **Central nervous system (CNS), cardiovascular, and respiratory depression are potentiated by combining sedative drugs and/or opioids and by rapid drug infusion.** Titrate to effect.
3. **Common sedative agents (**Table 28-8**):**
   a. Sedating antihistamines (diphenhydramine, hydroxyzine): Mild sedative hypnotics used for sedation and treatment of opiate-induced pruritus. See Formulary for dosing.
   b. Chloral hydrate: Oral sedative agent often used to produce immobilization for non-painful procedures. Associated with a high risk for failure and airway obstruction. Not recommended for routine use.
   c. Barbiturates: See Table 28-9.
   d. Benzodiazepines: See Table 28-9.
   e. Opiates: See Table 28-3.
   f. Ketamine: A phencyclidine derivative that causes potent dissociative anesthesia, analgesia, and amnesia. Causes bronchodilation, maintains ventilatory response to hypoxia, and allows relative maintenance of airway reflexes (Table 28-10).
4. **Reversal agents (**Table 28-11**):**
   a. Naloxone: Opioid antagonist. See Table 28-12 for Narcan administration protocol.
   b. Flumazenil: Benzodiazepine antagonist.

E. DISCHARGE CRITERIA[6]

1. Airway patency and stable cardiovascular function.
2. Easy arousability with intact protective reflexes (swallows and coughs, gag reflex).
3. Ability to talk and sit up unaided (if age appropriate).
4. Adequate hydration.

Text continues on p. 1025

TABLE 28-8
PROPERTIES OF COMMON SEDATIVE AGENTS

	Anxiolysis	Analgesia	Sedation/ Hypnosis	Reversible	Comments
Sedating antihistamines Diphenhydramine Hydroxyzine	No	No	Yes	No	• Antiemetic and antipruritic often used to treat opioid side effects
Chloral hydrate*	No	No	Yes	No	• May cause severe airway obstruction in children with OSA • 30%–40% failure rate • Long and unpredictable onset/duration of action
Barbiturates	No	No	Yes	No	• Contraindicated in patients with porphyria
Benzodiazepines	Yes	No	Yes	Yes	
Opiates	No	Yes	Yes	Yes	
Ketamine	Yes	Yes	Yes	No	• Dissociative agent • Increases heart rate, blood pressure, intraocular pressure, intracranial pressure • Administer with benzodiazepine (to counter emergence delirium) + antisialagogue

*High rate of failure of chloral hydrate combined with its adverse effects increase the risk/benefit profile of this agent. We recommend considering alternative sedatives whenever possible. See Formulary for dosing recommendations.

TABLE 28-9

COMMONLY USED BENZODIAZEPINES* AND BARBITURATES

Drug Class	Duration of Action	Drug	Route	Onset (min)	Duration (hr)	Comments
Benzodiazepines	Short	Midazolam (Versed)	IV	1–3	1–2	• Has rapid and predictable onset of action, a short recovery time
			IM/IN	5–10		• Causes amnesia
			PO/PR	10–30		• Results in mild depression of hypoxic ventilatory drive
	Intermediate	Diazepam (Valium)	IV (painful)	1–3	0.25–1	• Poor choice for procedural sedation
			PR	7–15	2–3	• Excellent for muscle relaxation or prolonged sedation
			PO	30–60	2–3	• Painful on IV injection • Faster onset than midazolam
	Long	Lorzepam (Ativan)	IV	1–5	3–4	• Poor choice for procedural sedation
			IM	10–20	3–6	• Ideal for prolonged anxiolysis, seizure treatment
			PO	30–60	3–6	
Barbiturates	Short	Methohexital	PR†	5–10	1–1.5	• PR form used as sedative for nonpainful procedures
		Thiopental	PR†	5–10	1–1.5	• IV form induces general anesthesia, do not use for sedation
	Intermediate	Pentobarbital	IV	1–10	1–4	• Predictable sedation and immobility for nonpainful procedures
			IM	5–15	2–4	
			PO/PR	15–60	2–4	• Minimal respiratory depression when used alone • Associated with slow wake up and agitation

*Use IV solution for PO, PR, and IN administration. Rectal diazepam gel (Diastat) is also available.

†IV administration produces general anesthesia; only PR should be used for sedation.

Data from Yaster M, et al: Pediatric Pain Management and Sedation Handbook. St. Louis, Mosby, 1997; St Germaine Brent A: Pediatr Clin North Am 2000;47(3):651–679; and Cote CJ, et al: A Practice of Anesthesia for Infants and Children. Philadelphia, WB Saunders, 2001.

TABLE 28-10

KETAMINE DOSING AND PHARMACOKINETICS

Route	Onset (min)	Duration (min)	Effects	Contraindications	Comments
IV	0.5–2	20–60*	• ***CNS effects:*** Increased ICP, emergence delirium with auditory, visual, and tactile hallucinations • ***Cardiovascular effects:*** Inhibits catecholamine reuptake, causing increased HR, BP, SVR, PVR, direct myocardial depression • ***Respiratory effects:*** Bronchodilation, increased secretions (can result in laryngospasm), maintenance of ventilatory response to hypoxia, relative maintenance of airway reflexes • ***Other effects:*** Increased muscle tone, myoclonic jerks, increased IOP, nausea, emesis	• Increased ICP • Increased IOP • Hypertension • Pre-existing psychotic disorders	• Causes bronchodilation, useful in asthmatics • Nystagmus indicates likely therapeutic effect • Vocalizations/movement may occur even with adequate sedation • Results in "deep sedation" by any route
IM (painful)	5–10	30–90			
PO/PR	20–45	60–120+			

*IV ketamine has a high risk for inducing general anesthesia; this should only be used by providers highly skilled in airway management.

ICP, intracranial pressure; IOP, intraocular pressure; HR, heart rate; BP, blood pressure; SVR, systemic vascular resistance; PVR, pulmonary vascular resistance.

Data from Yaster M, et al: Pediatric Pain Management and Sedation Handbook. St. Louis, Mosby, 1997; St Germaine Brent A: Pediatr Clin North Am 2000;47(3):651–679; and Cote CJ, et al: A Practice of Anesthesia for Infants and Children. Philadelphia, WB Saunders, 2001.

TABLE 28-11
REVERSAL AGENTS

	IV Dose	Routes	Onset (min)	Duration (min)	Indications	Cautions
Naloxone (opioid antagonist)	Nonarrest scenario: 1–2 μg/kg If no effect in 1–2 min, repeat dose every 2 min until the child responds or a total of 10 μg/kg is given. Arrest scenario: 0.1 mg/kg/dose (<20 kg) 2 mg/kg/dose (>20 kg)	IV IM IO/via ETT	1–2 (IV) 2–5 2–5	45	• Respiratory depression • Newborn with **acute** maternal opiate exposure • Pruritus • Urinary retention • Biliary spasm	Duration of action may be shorter than the duration of action of the opiate. May require repeated doses. **Monitor for the return of respiratory depression for at least 2 h.** Use lowest effective dose to reverse respiratory depression and not analgesia.
Flumazenil (benzodiazepine antagonist)	10 μg/kg (max dose 0.2 mg) If no effect in 1–2 min, repeat dose every 2 min until the child responds or a total of 1 mg is given	IV	1–3	45–60	• Respiratory depression • Excessive sedation	Duration of action may be shorter than the duration of benzodiazepine. May require repeated doses. **Monitor for the return of respiratory depression for at least 2 h.** May precipitate seizures in patients with an underlying seizure disorder, tricyclic antidepressant overdose, or chronic benzodiazepine use.

Data from Yaster M, et al: Pediatric Pain Management and Sedation Handbook. St. Louis, Mosby, 1997.

TABLE 28-12

NALOXONE (NARCAN) ADMINISTRATION
INDICATIONS: PATIENTS REQUIRING NALOXONE (NARCAN) USUALLY MEET ALL OF THE FOLLOWING CRITERIA*
• Unresponsive to physical stimulation • Shallow respirations or respiratory rate <8 breaths/min† • Pinpoint pupils
PROCEDURE
1. **Stop opioid administration** (as well as other sedative drugs), start the **ABCs** (**A**irway, **B**reathing, **C**irculation), and call for **HELP**. 2. **Dilute naloxone:** Mix 0.4 mg (1 ampule) of naloxone with 9 mL of normal saline (final concentration 0.04 mg/mL = 40 μg/mL). (If child <40 kg, dilute 0.1 mg (one-fourth ampule) in 9 mL of normal saline to make 0.01 mg/mL solution = 10 μg/mL.) 3. **Administer and observe response:** Administer dilute naloxone slowly (1–2 μg/kg/dose IV over 2 min). Observe patient response. 4. **Titrate to effect:** Within 1–2 min, patient should open eyes and respond. If not, continue until a total dose of 10 μg/kg is given. If no response is obtained, evaluate for other cause of sedation/respiratory depression. 5. **Discontinue naloxone administration:** Discontinue naloxone as soon as patient responds (e.g., takes deep breaths when directed). 6. **Caution:** Another dose of naloxone may be required within 30 min of first dose (duration of action of naloxone <most opioids). 7. **Monitor patient:** Assign a staff member to monitor sedation/respiratory status and to remind the patient to take deep breaths as necessary. 8. **Alternative analgesia:** Provide nonopioids for pain relief. Resume opioid administration at half the original dose when the patient is easily aroused and respiratory rate is >9 breaths/min.

*Patients with significant opiate exposure (sickle cell, cancer) should be carefully evaluated for the need for naloxone. The reversal of analgesia could produce hypertension, tachycardia, ventricular arrhythmias, and pulmonary edema. If necessary, give at the lowest dose possible and titrate carefully.

†Respiratory rates that require naloxone vary according to infant's/child's usual rate.

Modified from McCaffery M, Pasero C: Pain: Clinical Manual. St Louis, Mosby, 1999.

5. Recovery after sedation protocols varies but typically ranges from 60 to 120 minutes.

F. EXAMPLES OF SEDATION PROTOCOLS (Tables 28-13 and 28-14)

G. SEDATIVE-HYPNOTIC AND ANALGESICS QUICK REFERENCE GUIDE (Table 28-15)

IV. PATIENT-CONTROLLED ANALGESIA (PCA)

A. DEFINITION

PCA is a device that enables a patient to receive continuous ("basal") opioids and/or self-administer small supplemental doses ("bolus") of analgesics on an as-needed basis. In children younger than 6 years, a family member, caregiver, or nurse may administer doses.

TABLE 28-13

EXAMPLES OF SEDATION PROTOCOLS*

	Dosage		Comments
Midazolam + fentanyl	Midazolam	0.1 mg/kg IV × 3 doses PRN	• High likelihood of respiratory depression
	Fentanyl	1 mcg/kg IV × 3 doses PRN	• Infuse fentanyl no faster than at 3 min intervals
Ketamine + midazolam + atropine "ketodazzline"	**PO route:** combine		• Atropine = antisialogogue
	Ketamine	5 mg/kg	• Midazolam = counter emergence delirium
	Midazolam	0.5 mg/kg	
	Atropine	0.02 mg/kg	
	IV route:		
	Ketamine	0.25 mg/kg × 1 dose†	
	Midazolam	0.1 mg/kg × 3 doses PRN	
	Atropine	0.02 mg/kg × 1 dose	
	IM route: combine (use smallest volume possible)		
	Ketamine	1.5–2.0 mg/kg	
	Midazolam	0.15–0.2 mg/kg	
	Atropine	0.02 mg/kg	

*These examples reflect commonly used current protocols at the Johns Hopkins Children's Center; variations of the above are common at other institutions.

†Ketamine can be given intravenously, but the risk for inducing general anesthesia is very high; this should only be used by providers skilled in airway management.

Data from Yaster M, et al: Pediatric Pain Management and Sedation Handbook. St. Louis, Mosby, 1997.

TABLE 28-14
SUGGESTED SEDATION PROTOCOLS

Pain Threshold	Procedure	Suggested Drug Choices
Nonpainful	CT scan/EEG/ECHO	Midazolam
Mild	Phlebotomy, LP, IV access	EMLA
	BM aspiration	EMLA + midazolam
	Pelvic exam	Midazolam
	Minor laceration, well vascularized	TAC/LET
	Minor laceration, not well vascularized	Lidocaine
Moderate	Arthrocentesis	Midazolam + fentanyl
	Dislocation repair	Midazolam + fentanyl
	I & D abscess	Midazolam + fentanyl
	Fracture reduction	Midazolam + morphine
	Major laceration	Ketamine + atropine + midazolam
	Burn débridement	Ketamine + atropine + midazolam
Severe	Consider anesthesia consultation and general anesthesia	

CT, computed tomography; EEG, electroencephalogram; BM, bone marrow; I&D, incision and drainage; TAC/LET, Tetracaine, Adrenaline, Cocaine/Lidocaine, epinephrine, tetracaine.
Data from Yaster M, et al: Pediatric Pain Management and Sedation Handbook. St. Louis, Mosby, 1997.

B. INDICATIONS
Moderate to severe pain of acute or chronic nature. Commonly used in sickle cell disease, post-surgery, post-trauma, burns, and cancer. Also for pre-emptive pain management (e.g., to facilitate dressing changes).

C. ROUTES OF ADMINISTRATION
IV, subcutaneous (SC), or epidural.

D. AGENTS (Table 28-16)
E. COMPLICATIONS
Pruritus, nausea, constipation, urinary retention, excessive drowsiness, and respiratory depression (see Table 28-12)

V. OPIOID TAPERING[2]
A. INDICATION
Tapering schedule is required if the patient has received frequent opioid analgesics for more than 5 to 10 days.

B. GUIDELINES
1. **Conversion:** Convert all drugs to a single equi-analgesic member of that group (Table 28-17).
2. **PCA wean:** Change drug dosing from continuous/intermittent IV infusion to oral (PO) bolus therapy around the clock. If on PCA,

TABLE 28-15

ANALGESICS AND SEDATIVE-HYPNOTIC DRUGS QUICK REFERENCE (ALPHABETICAL)

Drug	Route	Dose
SEDATIVE-HYPNOTIC		
Diazepam	PO	0.25–0.3 mg/kg
	IV (painful)	0.1 mg/kg
Diphenhydramine	PO, IV, IM	5 mg/kg/day divided q6hr
Hydroxyzine	PO	2 mg/kg/day divided q6–8 hr
	IM	0.5–1 mg/kg/dose q4–6 hr
Lorazapam	PO, IV, IM	0.05 mg/kg
Midazolam	PO	0.5–0.8 mg/kg
	PR	0.5–1.0 mg/kg
	IN	0.2–0.3 mg/kg
	IM	0.15–0.2 mg/kg
	IV sedation	0.1 mg/kg up to 0.25 mg/kg
ANALGESIC		
Fentanyl	IV	1 μg/kg
	IV infusion	1–5 μg/kg/hr
	PO oralet	10–15 μg/kg, max 400 μg
Hydromorphone	IV	0.015 mg/kg
	IV infusion	2–4 μg/kg/hr
Ketorolac	IV, IM	0.5 mg/kg q6 hr
Methadone	PO, IV, IM, SC	0.1 mg/kg q8–12 hr
Morphine	IV	0.05–0.1 mg/kg
	IV infusion	10–40 μg/kg/hr
Oxycodone	PO	0.1 mg/kg q4–6 hr
OTHER		
Ketamine	PO	5 mg/kg
	IV	0.25–0.5 mg/kg
	IM	1.5–2.0 mg/kg

Data from Fisher QA: Pediatric Anesthesia Pearls, Baltimore, MD. Johns Hopkins Department of Anesthesia and Critical Care Medicine, 2000.

TABLE 28-16

ORDERS FOR PATIENT-CONTROLLED ANAGESIA

Drug	Basal Rate (μg/kg/hr)	Bolus Dose (μg/kg)	Lockout Period (min)	Boluses (hr)	Max Dose (hr) (μg/kg)
Morphine	10–30	10–30	6–10	4–6	100–150
Hydromorphone	3–5	3–5	6–10	4–6	15–20
Fentanyl	0.5–1	0.5–10	6–10	2–3	2–4

Data from Yaster M, et al: Pediatric Pain Management and Sedation Handbook. St. Louis, Mosby, 1997.

TABLE 28-17

RELATIVE POTENCIES AND EQUIVALENCE OF OPIOIDS

	Morphine Equivalence Ratio	IV Dose (mg/kg)	Equivalent PO Dose (mg/kg)
Meperidine	0.1	1	1.5–2
Methadone	0.25–1	0.1	0.1
Morphine	1	0.1	0.3–0.5
Hydromorphone	5–7	0.015	0.02–0.1
Fentanyl	80–100*	0.001	NA

Note: Removing a transdermal fentanyl patch does not stop opioid uptake from the skin, and fentanyl will continue to be absorbed for 12–24 hours after patch removal; fentanyl, 25-μg patch administers 25 μg/hr of fentanyl.

From Yaster M, et al: Pediatric Pain Management and Sedation Handbook. St. Louis, Mosby, 1997.

TABLE 28-18

EXAMPLES OF OPIOID TAPERING

EXAMPLE 1

Patient on morphine PCA to be converted to PO morphine with home weaning. For example: morphine PCA basal rate = 2 mg/hr, average bolus rate = 0.5 mg/hr.

Step 1: Calculate daily dose: Basal + bolus = (2 mg/hr × 24 hr) + (0.5 mg/hr × 24 hr) = 60 mg IV morphine.

Step 2: Convert according to drug potency: Morphine IV/morphine oral = approx 3 : 1 potency. 3 × 60 mg = 180 mg PO morphine.

Step 3: Prescribe 90 mg bid or 60 mg tid; wean 10%–20% of original dose (30 mg) every 1–2 days.

EXAMPLE 2

Patient on morphine PCA to be converted to transdermal fentanyl. Morphine PCA basal rate = 2 mg/hr. No boluses.

Step 1: Convert according to drug potency: Fentanyl/Morphine = approx 100 : 1 potency; 2 mg/hr morphine = 2000 μg/hr morphine = 20 μg/hr fentanyl.

Step 2: Prescribe 25 μg fentanyl patch (delivers 25 μg/hr fentanyl).

Step 3: Stop IV morphine 8 h after patch is applied; prescribe second patch at 72 h.

Step 4: Prescribe PRN IV morphine with caution.

Data from Yaster M, et al: Pediatric Pain Management and Sedation Handbook. St. Louis, Mosby, 1997.

administer first PO dose, then stop basal infusion 30 to 60 minutes later. Keep bolus doses, but reduce by 25% to 50%. Discontinue PCA if no boluses are required in next 6 hours, or increase PO dose, or add adjuvant analgesic (e.g., NSAID).

3. **Slow dose decrease:** During an intermittent IV/PO wean, decrease total daily dose by 10% to 20% every 1 to 2 days (e.g., to taper a morphine dose of 40 mg/day, decrease the daily dose by 4–8 mg every 1–2 days).

4. **Oral regimen:** If not done previously, convert IV dosing to equivalent PO administration 1 to 2 days before discharge, and continue titration as outlined previously.

C. EXAMPLES

See Table 28-18.

REFERENCES

1. Yaster M, et al: Pediatric Pain Management and Sedation Handbook. St. Louis, Mosby, 1997.
2. Yaster M, Maxwell LG: Pediatric regional anesthesia. Anesthesiology 1989;70:324–338.
3. St. Germain Brent A: The management of pain in the emergency department. Pediatr Clin North Am 2000;47(3):651–679.
4. Cote CJ, et al: A Practice of Anesthesia for Infants and Children. Philadelphia, WB Saunders, 2001.
5. Krauss B, Green SM: Sedation and analgesia for procedures in children. N Engl J Med 2000;342:938.
6. American Academy of Pediatrics Committee on Drugs: Guidelines for monitoring and management of pediatric patients during and after sedation for diagnostic and therapeutic procedures. Pediatrics 1992;89:1110.

Formulary Adjunct

Jason Robertson, MD

29

I. TOPICAL CORTICOSTEROIDS

A. POTENCY

Table 29-1 provides a listing of topical steroids from the most potent (group I) to the least potent (group VII). Use intermediate- and low-potency steroids (groups IV–VII) for pediatric patients. Topical steroid use is contraindicated in the treatment of varicella.

B. OCCLUSIVE DRESSINGS

Occlusive dressings (including waterproof diapers) increase systemic absorption of topical steroids and should not be used with high-potency preparations. Topical steroids should be used with caution in intertriginous areas and on the face.

C. APPLICATION

Apply once or twice daily. Penetration of the skin is greatest with ointments, with decreasing effectiveness in gels, creams, and lotions. Prolonged use may result in cutaneous and systemic side effects.

D. COVERAGE

A gram of topical cream or ointment should cover a 10 × 10 cm area. A 30- to 60-g tube will cover the entire body of an adult once.

II. COMMON INDICATIONS AND DOSES OF SYSTEMIC CORTICOSTEROIDS

A. ENDOCRINE[1]

1. Physiologic replacement:

a. Hydrocortisore: PO: 12–24 mg/m^2/24 hr ÷ q8hr; IM: 6–12 mg/m^2/dose daily.

b. PO: 12–24 mg/m^2/24 hr ÷ q8hr; IM: 6–12 mg/m^2/24 hr a day.

c. Prednisolone: PO: 1.75–3.5 mg/m^2/24 hr ÷ q12 hr.

2. Stress dosing: Consider for patients on glucocorticoid therapy >1 month:

a. PO/IM: Two to three times the physiologic replacement dose. Give preoperatively and postoperatively, with gradual decrease to a maintenance dose.

b. Stress with vomiting: IV: Hydrocortisone sodium succinate (Solu-Cortef): 25–100 mg/m^2/24 hr (give as a continuous infusion). If IV access is not available, administer 25 mg/m^2/dose IM q8hr.

3. Adrenal insufficiency:

a. Chronic: See section II.A.1.

b. Acute:

(1) Fluids: Start hydration with 20 mL/kg D_5 NS, then 60 mL/kg D_5 NS administered over 24 hours.

TABLE 29-1
TOPICAL STEROID POTENCY RANKING

Group	Brand	Generic Name	Sizes (in grams unless otherwise specified)
I (MOST POTENT)	Temovate cr, ot 0.05%	Clobetasol propionate	15, 30, 45
	Diprolene ot 0.05%, cr 0.05%	Betamethasone dipropionate	15, 45
	Diprolence AF		15, 45
	Psorcon ot 0.05%	Diflorasone diacetate	15, 30, 60
	Ultravate cr, ot 0.05%	Halobetasol dipropionate	15, 45
II	Cyclocort ot 0.1%	Amcinonide	15, 30, 60
	Diprosone ot 0.05%	Betamethasone dipropionate	15, 45
	Elocon ot 0.1%	Mometasone furoate	15, 45
	Florone ot 0.05%	Diflorasone diacetate	15, 30, 60
	Halog cr, ot, sl 0.1%	Halcinonide	15, 30, 60, 240 sl: 20, 60 mL
	Lidex cr, gl, ot, sl 0.05%	Fluocinonide	15, 30, 60, 120 sl: 20, 60 mL
	Maxiflor ot 0.05%	Diflorasone diacetate	15, 30, 60
	Maxivate cr, ot 0.05%	Betamethasone dipropionate	15, 45
	Topicort cr, ot 0.25%	Desoximetasone	15, 60, 120
	Topicort gl 0.05%		15, 60
III	Aristocort A ot 0.1%	Triamcinolone acetonide	15, 60
	Cyclocort cr, lt 0.1%	Amcinonide	15, 30, 60 lt: 20, 60 mL
	Diprosone cr 0.05%	Betamethasone dipropionate	15, 45
	Florone cr 0.05%	Diflorasone diacetate	15, 30, 60
	Lidex E cr 0.05%	Fluocinonide	15, 30, 60, 120
	Maxiflor cr 0.05%	Diflorasone diacetate	15, 30, 60
	Maxivate lt 0.05%	Betamethasone dipropionate	60 mL
	Valisone ot 0.1%	Betamethasone valerate	14, 45
IV	Aristocort ot 0.1%	Triamcinolone acetonide	15, 60 240, 454
	Cordran ot 0.05%	Flurandrenolide	15, 30, 60, 225
	Elocon cr, lt 0.1%	Mometasone furoate	15, 45 lt: 30, 60 mL
	Kenalog cr, ot 0.1%	Triamcinolone acetonide	15, 60, 80, 240
	Kenalog aerosol 0.2%	Triamcinolone acetonide	63

TABLE 29-1
TOPICAL STEROID POTENCY RANKING—*cont'd*

Group	Brand	Generic Name	Sizes (in grams unless otherwise specified)
	Dermatop cr, ot 0.1%	Prednicarbate	15, 60
	Synalar ot 0.025%	Fluocinolone acetonide	15, 30, 60, 120 425
	Topicort LP cr 0.05%	Desoximetasone	15, 60
V	Cordran cr 0.05%	Flurandrenolide	15, 30, 60, 225
	Kenalog lt 0.1%	Triamcinolone acetonide	15, 60 mL
	Kenalog ot 0.025%		15, 60, 80, 240
	Locoid cr, ot 0.1%	Hydrocortisone butyrate	15, 45
	Synalar cr 0.025%	Fluocinolone acetonide	15, 30, 60, 425
	Tridesilon ot 0.05%	Desonide	15, 60
	Valisone cr, lt 0.1%	Betamethasone valerate	15, 45, 110, 430 lt: 20, 60 mL
	Westcort cr, ot 0.2%	Hydrocortisone valerate	15, 45, 60 cr only: 120
VI	Aclovate cr, ot 0.05%	Alclometasone dipropionate	15, 45
	Aristocort cr 0.1%	Triamcinolone acetonide	15, 60, 240, 2520
	Kenalog cr, lt 0.025%	Triamcinolone acetonide	15, 60, 80, 240, 2520 lt: 60 mL
	Locoid sl 0.1%	Hydrocortisone butyrate	20, 60 mL
	Locorten cr 0.03%	Flumethasone pivalate	15, 60
	Synalar cr, sl 0.01%	Fluocinolone	15, 45, 60, 425 sl: 20, 60 mL
	Tridesilon cr 0.05%	Desonide	15, 60
VII (LEAST POTENT)	Hytone cr, ot, lt 1%	Hydrocortisone	cr, ot: 30 cr, lt: 120 mL
	Hytone cr, ot, lt 2.5%		cr, ot: 30 cr, lt: 60 mL

Note: There are other topical steroid preparations containing dexamethasone, flumethasone, prednisolone, and methylprednisolone.

cr, cream; *gl,* gel; *lt,* lotion; *ot,* ointment; *sl,* solution.

From Ferndale Laboratories, Ferndale, MI.

(2) Steroids: Hydrocortisone sodium succinate (Solu-Cortef), 50 mg/m^2 IV bolus, then begin continuous infusion over 24 hours as per "stress dosing" protocol above.

4. Congenital adrenal hyperplasia:

a. Non–salt losing: See section II.A.1.

b. Salt losing: Fludrocortisone acetate (Florinef): PO: Usually 0.1 mg/m^2/24 hours, with a range of 0.05–0.15 mg/24 hours in addition to physiologic glucocorticoid replacement. Dose is adjusted for blood pressure and plasma rennin activity.[1,2]

B. PULMONARY

1. Airway edema:

a. Dexamethasone: PO/IV/IM: 0.5–2 mg/kg/24 hr ÷ q6hr. Begin 24 hours before extubation, and continue for 4 to 6 doses after extubation.

b. Croup: Dexamethasone, 0.6 mg/kg/dose PO/IM/IV.[3,4] Recent studies suggest benefit of 0.6 mg/kg even in mild croup.[5] Inhaled budesonide, 2 mg q12hr (maximum: four doses).[6]

2. Acute asthma:

a. Prednisone/prednisolone:

(1) PO: 2 mg/kg/24 hr ÷ q12–24hr × 3 to 7 days.

(2) Maximum dose: 80 mg/24 hr.

b. Methylprednisolone:

(1) IV/IM: Load (optional) 2 mg/kg/dose × 1.

(2) Maintenance: 2 mg/kg/24 hr ÷ q6–8hr.

c. Hydrocortisone:

(1) IV: Load (optional) 4–8 mg/kg/dose; maximum dose: 250 mg.

(2) Maintenance: 8 mg/kg/24 hr ÷ q6hr.

C. MISCELLANEOUS

1. Antiemetic (chemotherapy induced): Dexamethasone.

a. IV: Initial: 10 mg/m^2/dose (maximum dose: 20 mg).

b. Subsequent: 5 mg/m^2/dose q6hr.

2. Cerebral edema: Dexamethasone.

a. PO/IM/IV: Loading dose: 1–2 mg/kg/dose × 1.

b. Maintenance: 1–1.5 mg/kg/24 hr ÷ q4–6hr (maximum dose: 16 mg/24 hours).

3. Spinal cord injury: Methylprednisolone.

a. 30 mg/kg bolus dose over 15 minutes, followed 45 minutes later by a continuous infusion of 5.4 mg/kg/hr × 23 hours.[7,8] Should be administered within 8 hours of injury for efficacy.

b. Methylprednisolone does not appear to be of benefit in acute head injury.

4. Bacterial meningitis[9]:

a. Indications:

(1) Dexamethasone is recommended for children >6 weeks old with Hib meningitis.

(2) Dexamethasone could be considered for children >6 weeks old with pneumococcal meningitis, but this is still controversial.

b. Dose: Dexamethasone: 0.15 mg/kg/dose IV q6hr × 48 hours. Ideally given with or just before first parenteral antibiotic dose. Initiation >4 hours after parenteral antibiotics is unlikely to be effective. Do not delay antibiotic therapy because of steroid administration.

5. Idiopathic thrombocytic purpura[10]:

a. Indications: Clinical bleeding.

b. Dose: Pulse steroid therapy with dexamethasone, 20–25 mg/m^2 IV × 4 days.[9]

6. Transfusion reactions: Methylprednisolone:

a. IV: 0.5–1 mg/kg before initiation of blood product transfusion in patients with known transfusion reaction.[11]

b. If hives and/or itching is present during transfusion, curtail transfusion and administer methylprednisolone.

III. INHALED CORTICOSTEROIDS FOR AIRWAY INFLAMMATION (Table 29-2)

IV. DOSE EQUIVALENCE OF COMMONLY USED STEROIDS (Table 29-3)

V. INSULIN (Table 29-4)

All preparations except Lantus are available as human, purified pork, pork/beef, and beef. The human and more purified preparations produce less subcutaneous atrophy and less insulin resistance. For the management of diabetic ketoacidosis, see Chapter 9.

VI. PANCREATIC ENZYME SUPPLEMENTS (Table 29-5)

VII. COMMON INDUCERS AND INHIBITORS OF THE CYTOCHROME P450 SYSTEM (Table 29-6)

VIII. OPHTHALMIC DRUGS (Table 29-7)

IX. OXIDIZING AGENTS AND GLUCOSE-6-PHOSPHATE DEHYDROGENASE (G6PD) DEFICIENCY (Box 29-1)

XI. PSYCHIATRY DRUG FORMULARY (Table 29-8)

XII. CHEMOTHERAPEUTIC AGENTS (Table 29-9)

Text continues on p. 1052

TABLE 29-2

ESTIMATED COMPARATIVE DAILY DOSAGES FOR INHALED CORTICOSTEROIDS

Drug	Low Dose	Medium Dose	High Dose
CHILDREN			
Beclomethasone dipropionate	84–336 μg	336–672 μg	>672 μg
42 μg/puff	(2–8 puffs)	(8–16 puffs)	(>16 puffs)
84 μg/puff	(1–4 puffs)	(4–8 puffs)	(>8 puffs)
Budesonide	100–200 μg	200–400 μg	>400 μg
DPI: 200 μg/dose		(1–2 inhalations)	(>2 inhalations)
Respules: 0.25 mg/2 mL, 0.5 mg/2 mL	0.25 mg	0.5 mg	1 mg
Flunisolide	500–750 μg	1000–1250 μg	>1250 μg
250 μg/puff	(2–3 puffs)	(4–5 puffs)	(>5 puffs)
Fluticasone	88–176 μg	176–440 μg	>440 μg
MDI: 44 μg/puff	(2–4 puffs)	(4–10 puffs)	—
110 μg/puff	—	(2–4 puffs)	(>4 puffs)
220 μg/puff	—	(1–2 puffs)	(>2 puffs)
DPI (Rotadisk): 50, 100, 250 μg/ dose	(2–4 inhalations, 50 μg)	(2–4 inhalations, 100 μg)	(>4 inhalations, 100 μg) (>2 inhalations, 250 μg)
Triamcinolone acetonide	400–800 μg	800–1200 μg	>1200 μg
100 μg/puff	(4–8 puffs)	(8–12 puffs)	(>12 puffs)
ADULTS			
Beclomethasone dipropionate	168–504 μg	504–840 μg	>840 μg
42 μg/puff	(4–12 puffs)	(12–20 puffs)	(>20 puffs)
84 μg/puff	(2–6 puffs)	(6–10 puffs)	(>10 puffs)
Budesonide	200–400 μg	400–600 μg	>600 μg
DPI: 200 μg/dose	(1–2 inhalations)	(2–3 inhalations)	(>3 inhalations)
Respules: 0.25 mg/2 mL, 0.5 mg/2 mL	0.25 mg	0.5 mg	1 mg
Flunisolide	500–100 μg	1000–2000 μg	>2000 μg
250 μg/puff	(2–4 puffs)	(4–8 puffs)	(>8 puffs)

TABLE 29-2

ESTIMATED COMPARATIVE DAILY DOSAGES FOR INHALED CORTICOSTEROIDS—*cont'd*

Drug	Low Dose	Medium Dose	High Dose
Fluticasone	—	264–660 μg	>660 μg
MDI:	(2–6 puffs)	—	—
44 μg/puff			
110 μg/puff	(2 puffs)	(2–6 puffs)	(>6 puffs)
220 μg/puff	—	—	(>3 puffs)
DPI (Rotadisk): 50, 100, 250 μg/ dose	(2–6 inhalations, 50 μg)	(3–6 inhalations, 100 μg)	(>6 inhalations, 100 μg; or >2 inhalations, 250 μg)
Triamcinolone acetonide 100 μg/puff	400–1000 μg (4–10 puffs)	1000–2000 μg (10–20 puffs)	>2000 μg (>20 puffs)

Note: **The most important determinant of appropriate dosing is the clinician's judgment of the patient's response to therapy. The clinician must monitor the patient's response on several clinical parameters and adjust the dose accordingly.** The stepwise approach to therapy emphasizes that once control of asthma is achieved, the dose of medication should be carefully titrated to the minimum dose required to maintain control, thus reducing the potential for adverse effect. The reference point for the range of doses in children is data on the safety of inhaled corticosteroids in children, which in general, suggest that the dose ranges are equivalent to those of beclomethasone dipropionate 200–400 μg/day (low dose), 400–800 μg/day (medium dose), and >800 μg/day (high dose). Metered-dose inhaler (MDI) dosages are expressed as the activator dose (the amount of drug leaving the activator and delivered to the patient), which is the labeling required in the United States. Dry-powder inhaler (DPI) doses are expressed as the amount of drug in the inhaler after activation.

From Expert Panel Report II. Guidelines for the Diagnosis and Management of Asthma. National Institutes of Health Pub. No. 97-4051. Bethesda, MD, National Asthma Education and Prevention Program, 1997.

TABLE 29-3

DOSE EQUIVALENCE OF COMMONLY USED STEROIDS*

Drug	Glucocorticoid Effect Equivalent to 100 mg Cortisol PO	Mineralocorticoid (mg): Na Retention Effect Equivalent to 0.1 mg Florinef†
Cortisone	125	20
Cortisol (hydrocortisone)	100	20
Prednisone	20	50
Prednisolone	15	50
Methylprednisolone	15–20	No effect
Triamcinolone	10–20	No effect
9α-Fluorocortisol	6.5	0.1
Dexamethasone	1.5–3.75	No effect

*The doses give approximately equivalent clinical effects. When using this table, select equipotent doses based on glucocorticoid or mineralocorticoid effects, because this is different for each drug.

†Total physiologic replacement for salt retention is usually 0.1 mg Florinef, regardless of size.

Modified from Kappy MS, Blizzard RM, Migeon CJ, editors. The Diagnosis and Treatment of Endocrine Disorders in Childhood and Adolescence, 4th ed. Springfield, Ill: Charles C Thomas; 1994, p 769.

TABLE 29-4
CURRENTLY AVAILABLE INSULIN PRODUCTS

Insulin*	Onset	Peak	Effective Duration, hr
Rapid acting	5–15 min	30–90 min	5
Lispro (Humalog)			
Aspart (NovoLog)			
Short acting	30–60 min	2–3 hr	5–8
Regular U100			
Regular U500 (concentrated)			
Buffered regular (Velosulin)			
Intermediate acting			
Isophane insulin (NPH, Humulin N/Novolin N)	2–4 hr	4–10 hr	10–16
Insulin zinc (Lente, Humulin L/Novolin L)	2–4 hr	4–12 hr	12–18
Long acting			
Insulin zinc extended (Ultralente, Humulin U)	6–10 hr	10–16 hr	18–24
Glargine (Lantus)	2–4 hr†	No peak	20–24
Premixed			
70% NPH/30% regular (Humulin 70/30)	30–60 min	Dual	10–16
50% NPH/50% regular (Humulin 50/50)	30–60 min	Dual	10–16
75% NPL/25% lispro (Humalog Mix 75/25)	5–15 min	Dual	10–16
70% NP/30% aspart (NovoLog Mix)	5–15 min	Dual	10–16

*Assuming 0.1–0.2 U/kg per injection. Onset and duration vary significantly by injection site.
†Time to steady state.
L, lente; NPH, neutral protamine Hagedom; NPL, insulin lispro protamine (neutral protamine lispro).
Adapted with permission from Practical Insulin: A Handbook for Prescribing Providers. The American Diabetes Association, 2002.

TABLE 29-5
PANCRELIPASE*

Product	Dosage Form	Lipase (USP) Units	Amylase (USP) Units	Protease (USP) Units
Cotazym	Capsule	8000	30,000	30,000
Cotazym-S	Capsule, enteric-coated sphere	5000	20,000	20,000
Creon 5	Capsule, delayed release with enteric-coated microsphere	5000	16,600	18,750
Creon 10	Same as Creon 5	10,000	33,200	37,500
Creon 20	Same as Creon 5	20,000	66,400	75,000
Pancrease	Capsule, delayed release	4500	20,000	25,000
Pancrease MT	Capsule, enteric-coated microtabs			
4		4000	12,000	12,000
10		10,000	30,000	30,000
16		16,000	48,000	48,000
20		20,000	56,000	44,000
Pancreacarb MS	Delayed-release capsule, enteric-coated, microsphere			
4		4000	25,000	25,000
8		8000	40,000	45,000
16		16,000	52,000	52,000
Ultrase	Capsule, enteric-coated, microsphere	4500	20,000	25,000
Ultrase MT	Capsule, enteric-coated minitab			
12		12,000	39,000	39,000
18		18,000	58,500	58,500
20		20,000	65,000	65,000
Viokase	Powder ¼ tsp = 0.7 g	16,800/0.7 g	70,000/0.7 g	70,000/0.7 g
	Tablet	8000	30,000	30,000
Zymase	Capsule	12,000	24,000	24,000

*See Formulary for side effects associated with administration.

Modified from Taketomo CK, Hodding JH, Kraus DM: American Pharmaceutical Association Pediatric Dosage Handbook. Hudson, OH, Lexi-Comp, 1998; and Solvay Pharmaceuticals, Inc. 1994; Fact and Comparisons: September, 1998; Scandipharm Product Information: July 1994 and May 1995.

TABLE 29-6
INDUCERS AND INHIBITORS OF THE CYTOCHROME P450 SYSTEM

Isoenzyme	Substrate (drug metabolized by isoenzyme)	Inhibitors	Inducers
CYP1A2	Caffeine, tacrine, theophylline, lidocaine, R-warfarin	Cimetidine, ciprofloxacin, erythromycin, tacrine	Omeprazole, smoking, phenobarbital
CYP2B6	Cocaine, ifosphamide, cyclophosphamide	Chloramphenicol	Phenobarbital
CYP2C9/10	S-Warfarin, phenytoin, tolbutamide, diclofenac, piroxicam	Amiodarone, fluconazole, lovastatin	Rifampin, phenobarbital
CYP2C19	Diazepam, omeprazole, mephenytoin	Fluvoxamine, fluoxetine, omeprazole, felbamate	Rifampin, phenobarbital
CYP2D6	Codeine, haloperidol, dextromethorphan, tricyclic antidepressants, phenothiazines, metoprolol, propranolol (4-OH), venlafaxine, risperidone, encainide, paroxetine, sertraline	Quinidine, fluoxetine, sertraline, amiodarone, propoxyphene	None known
CYP2E1	Acetaminophen, alcohol	Disulfiram	Isoniazid, alcohol
CYP3A3/4	Nifedipine, verapamil, cyclosporine, carbamazepine, terfenadine, cisapride, astemizole, tacrolimus, midazolam, alfentanil, diazepam, loratadine, ifosphamide, cyclophosphamide, ritonavir, indinavir	Erythromycin, cimetidine, clarithromycin, fluvoxamine, fluoxetine, ketoconazole, itraconazole, grapefruit juice, metronidazole, ritonavir, indinavir, mibefradil	Rifampin, phenytoin, phenobarbital, carbamazepine

Note: The cytochrome P450 enzyme system is composed of different isoenzymes. Each isoenzyme metabolizes a unique group of drugs or substrates. When an ***inhibitor*** of a particular isoenzyme is introduced, the serum concentration of any drug of ***substrate*** metabolized by that particular isoenzyme will ***increase***. When an ***inducer*** of a particular isoenzyme is introduced, the serum concentration of drugs or ***substrates*** metabolized by that particular isoenzyme will ***decrease***.
CYP, cytochrome P-450.
Modified from Hansten PD, Horn JR: Hansten and Horn's Drug Interaction Analysis and Management. Vancouver, BC, Canada, Applied Therapeutics, 1997.

BOX 29-1
OXIDIZING AGENTS AND G6PD DEFICIENCY
p-Aminosalicylic acid
Acetaminophen (Phenacetin)*
Acetylsalicylic acid
Aniline dyes
Antipyrine
Ascorbic acid†
Chloramphenicol‡
Dapsone (diaminodiphenylsulfone)
Fava beans
Furazolidone (Furoxone)
Henna
Methylene blue*
Naphthalene*
Nitrofurantoin (Furadantin)
Primaquine
Probenecid
Salicylazosulfapyridine (Azulfidine)
Sulfacetamide (Sulamyd)
Sulfanilamide
Sulfisoxazole (Gantrisin)*
Sulfoxone*
Trisulfapyrimidine (Sultrin)
Vitamin K, water-soluble analogs only

Note: These drugs and chemicals may cause hemolysis of "reacting" (primaquine-sensitive) red blood cells (e.g., in patients with glucose-6-phosphate dehydrogenase [G6PD] deficiency).
*Only slightly hemolytic to G6PD A patients in very large doses.
†Hemolytic in G6PD Mediterranean but not in G6PD A or Canton.
‡In massive doses.

TABLE 29-7
OPHTHALMIC DRUGS

Brand Name	Ingredient	Indication	Dose
Bleph-10 (>2 mo) (Soln: 2.5 mL, 5 mL, 15 mL; Oint 3.5 g)	Sulfacetamide sodium 10% Oph soln contains benzalkonium chloride Oph oint contains phenylmercuric acetate	Conjunctivitis Oph soln used as adjunct in trachoma	1–2 gtt q2–3 hr or small amount of oint q3–4 hr for 7–10 days Trachoma: 2 gtt q2 hr with systemic therapy
Garamycin Oph Soln and Oint (Soln: 5 mL; Oint: 35 g)	Gentamicin as sulfate	Conjunctivitis	Severe infections: 2 gtt q1 hr. Mild-moderate infections: 1–2 gtt q4 hr, or oint: bid–tid
Ilotycin (Oint: ⅛ oz)	Erythromycin (5 mg/g)	Conjunctivitis Prophylaxis of ophthalmia neonatorum	Small amount of oint ≥ qd 0.5–1 cm to each conjunctival sac
Neosporin (Oint: 3.75 g; Soln: 10 mL)	Oint (per g): Polymyxin B sulfate (10,000 units), bacitracin Zn (400 units), neomycin sulfate (3.5 mg) Soln (per mL): Polymyxin B sulfate (10,000 U), neomycin sulfate (1.75 mg), gramicidin (0.025 mg), 0.5% alcohol	Conjunctivitis	1–2 gtt or small amount of oint 2–4 times daily for 7–10 days For acute infections, use 1–2 gtt 2–4 times q1 hr initially
Ocuflox (>1 yr) (Soln: 5 mL, 10 mL)	Ofloxacin 0.3% , benzalkonium chloride	Conjunctivitis Corneal ulcer	1–2 gtt q2–4 hr × 2 days, then qid × 5 days 1–2 gtt q30 min while awake; at 4 hr and 6 hr during sleep × 2 days; then 1–2 gtt q1 hr while awake for 5–7 days, then qid until treatment completion
Polysporin (Oint: 3.75 g)	Polymyxin B sulfate (10,000 U), bacitracin zinc (500 U) per g of oint	Conjunctivitis	q3–4 hr; do not use >7 days
Polytrim (>2 mo) (Soln: 10 mL)	Trimethoprim sulfate (1 mg), polymyxin B sulfate (10,000 U/mL), benzalkonium chloride	Conjunctivitis	1 gtt q3 hr × 7–10 days

Tobrex (Soln: 5 mL; Oint: 3.5 g)	Soln: Tobramycin 0.3%, benzalkonium chloride Oint: Tobramycin 0.3%, chlorobutanol	Conjunctivitis	Severe infections: 2 gtt q1 hr or 0.5 inch of ointment q3–4 hr Mild-moderate infections: 1–2 gtt q4 hr or 0.5 inch of oint bid–tid
Vira-A (>2 yr) (Oint: 3.5 g)	Vidarabine 3%	Acute keratoconjunctivitis, recurrent epithelial keratitis caused by HSV 1 and 2	0.5 inch in lower conjunctival sac five times daily (q3 hr); continue for 7 more days (bid) after re-epithelialization
Viroptic (>6 yr) (Soln: 7.5 mL)	Trifluridine 1%, contains thimerosal	Primary keratoconjunctivitis, recurrent epithelial keratitis caused by HSV 1 and 2	1 gtt q2 hr while awake (maximum 9 gtt/day) 1 gtt q4 hr × 7 days after re-epithelialization (maximum 21 days)
Alocril (≥3 yr) (Soln: 5 mL)	Nedocromil sodium 2% (mast cell stabilizer), benzalkonium chloride	Allergic conjunctivitis	1–2 gtt several times a day; remove contact lenses during therapy
Alomide (>2 yr) (Soln: 10 mL)	Lodoxamide tromethamine 0.1% (mast cell stabilizer)	Vernal conjunctivitis and keratitis, keratoconjunctivitis	1–2 gtt qid up to 3 mo
Corticosporin (Oph Susp: 7.5 mL; Oph oint: 3.5 g)	Susp (per mL): Polymyxin B sulfate (10,000 U), neomycin sulfate (0.35%), hydrocortisone (1%). Oint (per g): Polymyxin B sulfate (10,000 U), neomycin sulfate (0.35%), bacitracin zinc (400 U), hydrocortisone (1%)	Ocular inflammation associated with infection **Contraindicated in fungal, viral, or mycobacterial infection** Use with caution in glaucoma, corneal or scleral thinning	1–2 gtt or small amount of oint 3–4 times daily
Poly-Pred (Susp: 5 mL, 10 mL)	Susp (per mL): Prednisolone acetate (0.5%), neomycin sulfate (0.35%), polymyxin B sulfate (10,000 U)	Ocular inflammation associated with infection **Contraindicated in fungal, viral, or mycobacterial infections** Use with caution in glaucoma, corneal or scleral thinning	1–2 gtt q3–4 hr

From Prescribing reference for pediatricians. Spring–Summer 2001.

TABLE 29-8

PSYCHIATRY DRUG FORMULARY

Agent	Suggested Dose	Side Effects/Comments
STIMULANTS (ADHD TREATMENT)		
See Formulary for methylphenidate and amphetamine preparations.		
NONPSYCHOSTIMULANTS (ADHD TREATMENT)		
See Formulary for clonidine.		
ANTIPSYCHOTICS		
Clozapine (Clozaril)	Starting dose: 6.25 mg/day Titrate upward by 6.25 mg/wk in divided doses Max Dose: Prepubescent: 300 mg/day Adolescent: 400 mg/day	Obtain baseline EEG. Repeat EEG prn for sudden behavioral deterioration. Monitor CBC. Because of potentially lethal hematologic changes, use is reserved for patients resistant to treatment.
Haloperidol (Haldol)	See Formulary	Obtain baseline ECG, HR, BP, LFTs. Check q3 mo, with dose changes. In general, anticholinergic effects include orthostatic hypotension, sedation, weight gain, dystonic reactions; tardive dyskinesia, akathisia, neuroleptic malignant syndrome.
Olanzapine (Zyprexa)	Prepubescent: 2.5 mg qd Adolescent: 5 mg qd Increase q3–4 days to maximum of 20 mg/day	See comments for haloperidol.
Risperidone (Risperdal)	Prepubescent: 2.5 mg qd Adolescent: 0.5 mg/day qd–bid Adult: 1 mg bid Increase q wk 1 mg bid as needed Max dose: 3 mg bid	Renal/hepatic dosing. See comments for haloperidol; hyperprolactinemia, amenorrhea, galactorrhea.
Quetiapine (Seroquel)	Prepubescent: 12.5–750 mg/day Adolescent: 25–750 mg/day Adult: 150–750 mg/day	See comments for haloperidol. Baseline and semiannual ophthalmologic examination recommended because cataracts occurred in drug studies in canines.
Ziprasidone	120 mg/day	Dyspepsia, constipation, nausea, abdominal pain. Low incidence of extrapyramidal side effects.
ANXIOLYTICS		
Buspirone (BuSpar) Please see SSRI and venlafaxine	Prepubescent: 2.5–5 mg/day Increase by 2.5 mg/day q3–4 d Max dose: 20 mg/day ÷ q12 hr Adolescent: 5–10 mg/day Increase by 5 mg/day q3–4 days Max dose: 60 mg/day ÷ q12 hr	Tachycardia, central nervous system (CNS) effects (headache, insomnia, confusion, dizziness); gastrointestinal (GI) effects.

TABLE 29-8

PSYCHIATRY DRUG FORMULARY—*cont'd*

Agent	Suggested Dose	Side Effects/Comments
MOOD STABILIZERS		
See Formulary for lithium, divalproex sodium, and carbamazepine.		
ANTIDEPRESSANTS/ANXIOLYTICS		
Selective Serotonin Reuptake Inhibitors (SSRIs)		
Fluoxetine (Prozac)	Starting dose <12 yr: 5–10 mg/day Maintenance: 10–30 mg/day Starting dose ≥12 yr: 10 mg/day Maintenance: 20–40 mg/day Max dose: 60 mg/day	Do not use if MAOIs have been used in previous 14 days. Can cause GI upset, CNS side effects (headaches, nervousness, sedation), activate bipolar switchbacks.
Fluvoxamine (Luvox)	Starting dose <12 yr: 25 mg qhs Maintenance: 100–200 mg/day Starting dose ≥12 yr: 25–50 mg qhs Maintenance: 150–300 mg/day	Contraindications: MAOIs, cisapride, terfenadine, astemizole. Smoking increases levels.
Paroxetine (Paxil)	Starting dose <12 yr: 5–10 mg/day Maintenance: 10–20 mg/day Starting dose ≥12 yr: 10–20 mg/day Maintenance: 20–40 mg/day	Purpura, hyponatremia, cytochrome p450 system (multiple drug interactions). Also see comments for fluoxetine.
Sertraline (Zoloft)	Starting dose <12 yr: 25 mg/day Maintenance: 100–150 mg/day Starting dose ≥12 yr: 25–50 mg/day Maintenance: 150–200 mg/day	See comments for fluoxetine.
Citalopram (Celexa)	<12 yr: 10–20 mg/day ≥12 yr: 10–40 mg/day	See comments for fluoxetine; multiple drug interactions.
TRICYCLICS (TCAs)		
See Formulary for nortriptyline and imipramine.		
Serotonin Norepinephrine Reuptake Inhibitors		
Venlafaxine (Effexor)	Starting dose prepubescent: 37.5 mg/day Maintenance: 75–150 mg/day Starting dose adolescent: 37.5–75 mg/day Maintenance: 150–300 mg/day	Nausea, dizziness, somnolence, constipation, xerostomia.

continued

TABLE 29-8

PSYCHIATRY DRUG FORMULARY—*cont'd*

Agent	Suggested Dose	Side Effects/Comments
5-HT Blockers		
Nefazodone (Serzone)	Start 50 mg bid. Titrate to effectiveness by 50 mg q3 days Max dose Children: 300 mg/day >12 yr: 600 mg/day	Nausea, dizziness, priapism, agitation, dry mouth, vision changes. Contraindications: MAOIs, astemizole, cisapride, terfenadine.
Other		
Bupropion Sustained Release (Wellbutrin SR)	≥18 yr: 100 mg bid × 3 days. If tolerated, increase by 100 mg TID (minimum q6 hr) Max dose: 450 mg/day, 150 mg/dose/hr	CNS stimulation, weight change, dry mouth, headache, GI effects, insomnia. Contraindications: Seizures, eating disorders, MAOIs.
Mirtazapine (Remeron)	≥18 yr: Initially 15 mg qhs Increase q1–2 wk	Obtain baseline CBC, LFTs, and monitor periodically. Side effects: Increased appetite, weight gain, dizziness, nausea dry mouth, constipation, CNS effects (somnolence), hypotension/hypertension, elevated triglycerides, cholesterol.

From Physician's Desk Reference, 54th ed. Montvale, NJ, Medical Economics, 2000; Riddle MA, et al: J Am Acad Child Adolesc Psychiatry. 1999;38:546–556; Findling RL, Blumer JL, (eds): Child and adolescent psychopharmacology. Pediatr Clin North Am 1998;45(5); Shoaf TL, Emslie GJ, Mayes TL: Pediatr Ann 2001;30(3):130–171; Emslie GJ, Mayes TL, Hughes CW. Updates in the Pharmacologic Treatment of Childhood Depression. In: Dunner DL, Rosenbaum JF, editors. The Psychiatric Clinics of North America Annual of Drug Therapy. Philadelphia: WB Saunders; 2000;235–256; and Velosa JF, Riddle MA: Child Adolesc Psychiatr Clin N Am 2000;9:119–133.

TABLE 29-9

CHARACTERISTICS OF CHEMOTHERAPEUTIC AGENTS

Drug Name (drug class in italics)	Acute Toxicity (DLT*)	Long-Term Toxicity
Asparaginase (L-ASP, Elspar, PEG-ASP) *Enzyme*	DLT: Pancreatitis, seizures, hypersensitivity reactions (both acute and delayed; less with PEG modified), encephalopathy Other: Nausea, pancreatitis, hyperglycemia, azotemia, fever, coagulopathy, sagittal sinus thrombosis and other venous thromboses, hyperammonemia	Neurologic deficits secondary to stroke
Bleomycin (Blenoxane) *DNA strand breaker*	DLT†: Anaphylaxis, pneumonitis Other: Pain, fever, chills, mucositis, skin reactions	Pulmonary fibrosis related to cumulative dose
Busulfan (Myleran) *Alkylator*	DLT: Myelosuppression, mucositis, seizures, hepatic veno-occlusive disease Other: Hyperpigmentation, hypotension	Infertility, endocardial fibrosis, secondary malignancy
Carboplatin (CBDCA, Paraplatin) *DNA cross-linker*	DLT†: Thrombocytopenia, nephrotoxicity Other: Severe emesis, ototoxicity, peripheral neuropathy, optic neuritis (rare)	Renal insufficiency (less than cisplatin), hearing loss
Carmustine (bis-chloronitrosourea, BCNU, BiCNU) *Alkylator*	DLT: Myelosuppression (prolonged cumulative) Other: Vesicant, brownish discoloration of skin, hepatic and renal toxicity, severe emesis	Pulmonary fibrosis, infertility, secondary malignancy
Cisplatin (Platinol, *cis*-platinum, CDDP) *DNA cross-linker*	DLT†: Tubular and glomerular nephrotoxicity (related to cumulative dose), peripheral neuropathy Other: Severe emesis, myelosuppression, ototoxicity, SIADH (rare), papilledema and retrobulbar neuritis (rare)	Renal insufficiency, hearing loss, peripheral neuropathy
Cladribine (2-CdA, Leustatin) *Antimetabolite or nucleotide analog*	Myelosuppression, nausea and vomiting, headache, fever, chills, fatigue	
Cyclophosphamide (CTX, Cytoxan) *Alkylator prodrug*	DLT: Leukopenia, cardiomyopathy Other: Hemorrhagic cystitis (improved by mesna), emesis, direct ADH effect	Infertility, cardiomyopathy, secondary malignancy, leukoencephalopathy Leukoencephalopathy

continued

TABLE 29-9
CHARACTERISTICS OF CHEMOTHERAPEUTIC AGENTS—*cont'd*

Drug Name (drug class in italics)	Acute Toxicity (DLT*)	Long-Term Toxicity
Cytarabine (Ara-C) *Antimetabolite or nucleotide analog*	DLT†: Myelosuppression, cerebellar toxicity Other: Nausea and vomiting, anorexia, diarrhea, metallic taste, severe gastrointestinal ulceration, conjunctivitis, lethargy, ataxia, nystagmus, slurred speech, respiratory distress rapidly progressing to pulmonary edema, influenza-like syndrome, fever	
Dacarbazine (DIC, DTIC, imidazole carboxamide) *Alkylator*	DLT: Myelosuppression Other: Severe emesis, transaminitis, facial paresthesias (rare), rash	Infertility
Dactinomycin (actinomycin-D) *Antibiotic*	DLT: Myelosuppression, severe diarrhea Other: Vesicant, nausea, acne, erythema, radiation recall, hepatic veno-occlusive disease	Secondary malignancy
Daunorubicin (daunomycin) *Anthracycline*	DLT‡: Leukopenia, arrhythmia, congestive heart failure (related to cumulative dose) Other: Stomatitis, emesis, vesicant, red urine, radiation recall	Cardiomyopathy
Doxorubicin (Adriamycin) *Anthracycline*	Refer to daunorubicin	Cardiomyopathy
Etoposide (VP-16, VePesid) *Topoisomerase inhibitor*	DLT: Leukopenia, anaphylaxis (rare), transient cortical blindness Other: Hyperbilirubinemia transaminitis, peripheral neuropathy (rare), hypotension	Secondary malignancy (AML)
Fludarabine (Fludara) *Purine antimetabolite or nucleotide analog*	Myelosuppression†, anorexia, increased SGOT, somnolence, fatigue	Peripheral neuropathy, immune suppression
Fluorouracil (5-FU, Adrucil) *Nucleotide analog*	DLT: Myelosuppression (reversible with urdine), mucositis, severe diarrhea Other: Hand-foot syndrome, tear duct stenosis, hyperpigmentation, loss of nails; cerebellar syndrome (rare), and anaphylaxis	—

Hydroxyurea (Hydrea) *Ribonucleotide reductase inhibitor*	DLT: Leukopenia, pulmonary edema (rare) Other: Megaloblastic erythropoiesis, hyperpigmentation, azotemia, transaminitis, radiation recall	—
Idarubicin (Idamycin) *Anthracycline*	DLT: Arrhythmia, cardiomyopathy (cumulative) Other: Vesicant, diarrhea, mucositis, enterocolitis	Cardiomyopathy
Ifosfamide (isophosphamide, Ifex) *Alkylator prodrug*	DLT†: Myelosuppression, encephalopathy (rarely progressing to death), renal tubular damage Other: Emesis, hemorrhagic cystitis (improved with Mesna), direct ADH effect	Secondary malignancy, infertility
Liposomal doxorubicin (Doxil) *Anthracycline*	Refer to Daunorubicin	Refer to Daunorubicin
Lomustine (CCNU) *Alkylating agent*	Myelosuppression, nausea and vomiting, disorientation, fatigue	Secondary malignancy (leukemia)
Mechlorethamine (nitrogen mustard, HN_2 [mustine], Mustargen) *Alkylator*	DLT: Leukopenia, thrombocytopenia Other: Severe emesis, vesicant (antidote sodium thiosulfate), peptic ulcer (rare)	Secondary malignancy, infertility
Melphalan (L-PAM, Alkeran) *Alkylator*	DLT: Prolonged leukopenia (6–8 wk), mucositis, diarrhea Other: Pruritus, emesis	Pulmonary fibrosis, secondary malignancy, infertility, cataracts
Mercaptopurine (6-MP) *Nucleotide analog*	DLT: Hepatic necrosis and encephalopathy (especially doses >2.5 mg/kg/day Other: Vesicant, headache, diarrhea, nausea	Cirrhosis
Methotrexate (MTX, Folex, Mexate, amethopterin) *Folate antagonist*	DLT§: Stomatitis, diarrhea, renal dysfunction, encephalopathy, cortical blindness, ventriculitis (intrathecal) Other: Photosensitivity, erythema, excessive lacrimation, transaminitis	Leukoencephalopathy, cirrhosis, pulmonary fibrosis, aseptic necrosis of bone, osteoporosis
Mitoxantrone (Novantrone, DHAD, DHAQ, dihydroxyanthracenedione) *DNA intercalator*	DLT: Myelosuppression, cumulative cardiomyopathy Other: Stomatitis, blue-green urine and serum	Cardiomyopathy

continued

TABLE 29-9

CHARACTERISTICS OF CHEMOTHERAPEUTIC AGENTS—*cont'd*

Drug Name (drug class in italics)	Acute Toxicity (DLT*)	Long-Term Toxicity
Paclitaxel (Taxol) *Tubulin inhibitor*	DLT: Neutropenia, anaphylaxis, ventricular tachycardia and myocardial infarction (rare) Other: Mucositis, peripheral neuropathy, bradycardia, hypertriglyceridemia	Too soon to know
Procarbazine (Matulane) *Alkylator*	DLT: Encephalopathy; pancytopenia, especially thrombocytopenia Other: Emesis, paresthesias, dizziness, ataxia, hypotension; adverse effects with tyramine-rich foods, ethanol, MAOIs, meperidine, and many other drugs	Secondary malignancy, infertility
Teniposide (VM-26) *Topoisomerase inhibitor*	DLT: Leukopenia, anaphylaxis (rare) Other: Hyperbilirubinemia, transaminitis	Secondary malignancy (AML)
Thioguanine (6-TG, 6-thioguanine) *Nucleotide analog*	DLT: Myelosuppression, bronchospasm and shock with rapid IV infusion, stomatitis, diarrhea Other: Hyperbilirubinemia, transaminitis, decreased vibratory sensation, ataxia, dermatitis	—
Thiotepa *Alkylating agent*	DLT: Cognitive impairment, leukopenia Other: Increased SGOT, headache, dizziness, rash, desquamation	Secondary malignancy (leukemia) impaired fertility, weakness of lower extremities
Topotecan (Hycamptamine) *Topoisomerase inhibitor*	DLT: Leukopenia, peripheral neuropathy (rare), Horner syndrome Other: Nausea, diarrhea, transaminitis, headache	Too soon to know
Vinblastine (Velban, VBL, vincaleukoblastine)	DLT‡: Leukopenia Other: Vesicant (improved by hyaluronidase and applied heat),	—

Microtubule inhibitor	constipation, bone pain (especially in the jaw), peripheral and autonomic neuropathy, rarely SIADH	
Vincristine (VCR, Oncovin) *Microtubule inhibitor*	DLT‡: Peripheral and autonomic neuropathy, encephalopathy Other: Vesicant, bone pain, constipation, SIADH (rare)	—
Amifostine	Reduces the toxicity of radiation and alkylating agents	Hypotension (62%), severe nausea and vomiting, flushing, chills, dizziness, somnolence, hiccups, sneezing, hypocalcemia in susceptible patients (<1%), short-term reversible loss of consciousness (rare), rigors (<1%), mild skin rash
Dexrazoxane	Protective agent for doxorubicin-induced cardiotoxicity	Myelosuppression
Leucovorin	Reduces methotrexate toxicity	Allergic sensitization (rare)
Mesna	Reduces risk of hemorrhagic cystitis	Headache, limb pain, abdominal pain, diarrhea, rash

ADH, antidiuretic hormone; AML, acute myeloid leukemia; MAOI, monoamine oxidase inhibitors; SGOT, serum glutamic-oxaloacetic transaminase; SIADH, syndrome of inappropriate antidiuretic hormone.

*The dose-limiting toxicity (DLT) is the toxicity most likely to require adjustment or withholding of drug.

†Dose must be adjusted in renal insufficiency.

‡Dose must be adjusted in hyperbilirubinemia.

§Dose must be adjusted in renal insufficiency and in patients with third spacing.

REFERENCES

1. Kappy MS, Blizzard RM, Migeon CJ (eds): Diagnosis and Treatment of Endocrine Disorders in Childhood and Adolescence, 4th ed. Springfield, IL, Charles C Thomas, 1994.
2. Migeon CJ, Wisniewski AB: Congenital adrenal hyperplasia owing to 21-hydroxylase deficiency: Growth, development, and therapeutic considerations. Endocrinol Metab Clin North Am 2001;30(1):193–206.
3. Geelhoed GC, Turner F, Macdonald WGG: Efficacy of a small dose of oral dexamethasone for outpatient croup: A double blind placebo controlled trial. BMJ 1996;313:140–142.
4. Rittichier KK, Ledwith CA: Outpatient treatment of moderate croup with dexamethasone: Intramuscular versus oral dosing. Pediatrics 2000;106:1344–1348.
5. Bjornson CL, Klassen TP, Williamson J, et al: A randomized trial of a single dose of oral dexamethasone for mild croup. N Engl J Med 2004;351(13):1306–1313.
6. Roberts GW: Repeated dose inhaled budesonide versus placebo in the treatment of croup. J Pediatr Child Health 1999;35(2):170–174.
7. Bracken MB, et al: A randomized controlled trial of methylprednisolone or naloxone in the treatment of acute spinal cord injury: Results of the Second National Acute Spinal Cord Injury Study. N Engl J Med 1990;322(20):1405–1411.
8. Bracken MB: Pharmacological treatment of acute spinal cord injury: Current status and future projects. J Emerg Med 1993;11:43.
9. Pickering LK (ed): 2003 Red Book: Report of the Committee on Infectious Diseases, 25th ed. Elk Grove Village, IL, American Academy of Pediatrics, 2003.
10. Adams DM, et al: High dose oral dexamethasone therapy for chronic childhood idiopathic thrombocytopenic purpura. J Pediatr 1996;128.
11. Taketomo CK, Hodding JH, Kraus DM: American Pharmaceutical Association Pediatric Dosage Handbook. Hudson, OH, Lexi-Comp, 1998.

Drugs in Renal Failure

Jason Robertson, MD, and Nicole Shilkofski, MD

30

I. DOSE ADJUSTMENT METHODS

A. MAINTENANCE DOSE

In patients with renal insufficiency, the dose may be adjusted using the following methods:

1. **Interval extension (I):** Lengthen the intervals between individual doses, keeping the dose size normal. For this method, the suggested interval is shown.
2. **Dose reduction (D):** Reduce the amount of individual doses, keeping the interval between the doses normal. This method is particularly recommended for drugs in which a relatively constant blood level is desired. For this method, the percentage of the usual dose is shown.
3. **Interval and dose reduction (DI):** Lengthen the interval and reduce the dose.
4. **Interval or dose reduction (D, I):** In some instances, either the dose or the interval can be changed.

Note *These dose adjustments are for beyond the neonatal period. These dose modifications are only approximations. Each patient must be monitored closely for signs of drug toxicity, and serum levels must be measured when available. Drug dose and interval should be monitored accordingly.*

B. DIALYSIS

The quantitative effects of hemodialysis (He) and peritoneal dialysis (P) on drug removal are shown. "Y" indicates the need for a supplemental dose with dialysis. "N" indicates no need for adjustment. The designation "No" does not preclude the use of dialysis or hemoperfusion for drug overdose.

II. ANTIMICROBIALS REQUIRING ADJUSTMENT IN RENAL FAILURE (Table 30-1)

III. NONANTIMICROBIALS REQUIRING ADJUSTMENT IN RENAL FAILURE (Table 30-2)

TABLE 30-1

ANTIMICROBIALS REQUIRING ADJUSTMENT IN RENAL FAILURE

Drug	Pharmacokinetics			Adjustments in Renal Failure				
					Creatinine Clearance (mL/min)			
	Route of Excretion[a]	Normal $t_{1/2}$ (hr)	Normal Dose Interval	Method	Mild (>50)	Moderate (10–50)	Severe (<10)	Supplemental Dose for Dialysis
Acyclovir (IV)	Renal	2–4	Q8 hr	DI	Q8 hr	Q12–24 hr	50% and Q24 hr	Y (He) N (P)
Amantidine	Renal	10–28	Q12–24 hr	I	Q12–24 hr	Q48–72 hr	Q7 days	N (He) N (P)
Amikacin[b]	Renal	1.5–3	Q8–12 hr	I	Q8–12 hr	Q12–18 hr	Q24–48 hr	Y (He) Y (P)
Amoxicillin	Renal	1–3.7	Q8–12 hr	I	Q8–12 hr	Q12 hr	Q24 hr	Y (He) N (P)
Amoxicillin-clavulanate	Renal	1	Q8–12 hr	I	Q8–12 hr	Q12 hr	Q24 hr	Y (He) Y (P)
Amphotericin B	Renal 40% up to 7 days	Up to 15 days	QD	I	Dosage adjustments are unnecessary with preexisting renal impairment; if decreased renal function is due to amphotericin B, the daily dose can be decreased by 50% or the dose given QOD			N (He) N (P)
Amphotericin B cholesteryl sulfate (Amphotec)	?	28–29	QD	I	No guidelines established			N (He)

Amphotericin B lipid complex (Abelcet)	Renal 1%	170	QD	I	No guidelines			?
Amphotericin B liposomal (AmBisome)	Renal ≤10%	100–173	QD	I	No guidelines established			?
Ampicillin	Renal	1–4	Q6 hr	I	Q6 hr	Q6–12 hr	Q12–16 hr	Y (He) N (P)
Ampicillin/ sulbactam	Renal	1–1.8	Q4–6 hr	I	Q4–6 hr	Q12 hr	Q24 hr	Y (He) N (P)
Aztreonam	Renal (hepatic)	1.3–2.2	Q6–12 hr	D	75%–100%	50%	25%	Y (He)
Carbenicillin[c]	Renal (hepatic)	0.8–1.8	Q6 hr	I	Q8–12 hr	Q12–24 hr	Q24–48 hr	Y (He)
Cefaclor	Renal	0.5–1	Q8–12 hr	D	100%	100%	50%	Y (He) Y (P)
Cefadroxil	Renal	1–2	Q12 hr	I	Q12 hr	Q12–24 hr	Q24–48 hr	Y (He) N (P)
Cefazolin	Renal	1.5–25	Q8 hr	I	Q8 hr	Q12 hr	Q24 hr	Y (He) N (P)
Cefdinir	Renal	1.1–2.3	Q12–24 hr	I	Q12–24 hr	7 mg/kg/dose Q24 hr or 300 mg Q24 hr for adults (CrCl < 30)		Y (H)

CrCl, creatinine clearance; GFR, glomerular filtration rate; He, hemodialysis; P, peritoneal dialysis.
[a]Route in parentheses indicates secondary route of excretion.
[b]Subsequent doses are best determined by measurement of serum levels and assessment of renal insufficiency.
[c]May inactivate aminoglycosides in patients with renal impairment.

TABLE 30-1

ANTIMICROBIALS REQUIRING ADJUSTMENT IN RENAL FAILURE—*cont'd*

	Pharmacokinetics			Adjustments in Renal Failure				
					Creatinine Clearance (mL/min)			
Drug	Route of Excretion[a]	Normal $t_{1/2}$ (hr)	Normal Dose Interval	Method	Mild (>50)	Moderate (10–50)	Severe (<10)	Supplemental Dose for Dialysis
Cefepime	Renal	1.8–2	Q8–12 hr	DI	Q12 hr regimens: *Est CrCl (mL/Min)*			Y (He) N (P)
					30–60	50 mg/kg/dose Q24 hr		
					11–29	25 mg/kg/dose Q24 hr		
					≤10	12.5 mg/kg/dose Q24 hr		
					Q8 hr regimens: *Est CrCl (mL/min)*			
					30–50	50 mg/kg/dose Q12 hr		
					10–30	50 mg/kg/dose Q24 hr		
					<10	50 mg/kg/dose Q24–48 hr		
Ceflxime	Renal (hepatic)	3–4	Q12–24 hr	D	100%	75% (CrCl 21–50)	50% (CrCl < 20)	N (He, P)
Cefotaxime	Renal	1–3.5	Q6–12 hr	D	100%	CrCl < 20 = ↓ dose by 50%		Y (He) N (P)
Cefotetan	Renal (hepatic)	3.5	Q12 hr	I	Q12 hr	CrCl 10–30 = Q24 hr	Q48	Y (He, P)
Cefoxitin	Renal	0.75–1.5	Q4–8 hr	I	Normal interval	CrCl 30–50 = Q8–12 hr CrCl 10–30 = Q12–24 hr	Q24–48 hr	Y (He) N (P)

Cefpodoxime proxetil	Renal	2.2	Q12 hr	I	Q12 hr	CrCl < 30 = Q24 hr	Q24 hr	Y (He) N (P)
Cefprozil	Renal	1.3	Q12 hr	D	100%	CrCl < 30 = 50%	50%	Y (He)
Ceftazidime	Renal	1–2	Q8–12 hr	I	Q8–12 hr	CrCl 30–50 = Q12 hr CrCl 10–30 = Q24 hr	Q24–48 hr	Y (He, P)
Ceftibuten	Renal	1.5–2.5	Q24 hr	D	100%	50% (CrCl 30–49)	25% (CrCl 5–29)	Y (He) N (P)
Ceftizoxime	Renal	1.6	Q6–12 hr	I	Q8–12 hr	Q36–48 hr	Q48–72 hr	Y (He)
Cefuroxime (IV)	Renal	1.6–2.2	Q8–12 hr	I	Q8–12 hr	CrCl 10–20 = Q12 hr	Q24 hr	Y (He) N (P)
Cephalexin	Renal	0.5–1.2	Q6 hr	I	Q6 hr	Q8–12 hr	Q12–24 hr	Y (He) N (P)
Cephradine	Renal	0.7–2	Q6–12 hr	D, I	100%	50% or Q12–24 hr	25% or Q36 hr	Y (He)
Ciprofloxacin	Renal (hepatic)	1.2–5	Q8–12 hr	D, I	100%	50%–75% (or Q18–24 hr for CrCl < 30)	50% (or Q18–24 hr for CrCl < 30)	Y (He, P)
Clarithromycin	Renal/hepatic	3–7	Q12 hr	DI	No change	CrCl < 30 = ↓ dose by 50% and administer BID–QD		?

TABLE 30-1
ANTIMICROBIALS REQUIRING ADJUSTMENT IN RENAL FAILURE—*cont'd*

	Pharmacokinetics			Adjustments in Renal Failure				
					Creatinine Clearance (mL/min)			
Drug	Route of Excretion[a]	Normal $t_{1/2}$ (hr)	Normal Dose Interval	Method	Mild (>50)	Moderate (10–50)	Severe (<10)	Supplemental Dose for Dialysis
Co-trimoxazole (sulfa-methoxazole/trimethoprim)	Sulfameth-oxazole: Hepatic (renal) Trimethoprim: Renal (hepatic)	Sulfamethox-azole: 9–11 Trimethoprim: 8–15	Q12 hr	D	No change	CrCl 15–30 = 50%	CrCl < 15 = not recommended	Y (He) N (P)
Erythromycin	Hepatic (renal)	1.5–2	Q6–8 hr	D	100%	100%	50%–75%	N (He, P)
Ethambutol	Renal (hepatic)	2.5–3.6	Q24 hr	I	Q24 hr	Q24–36 hr	Q48 hr = ↓ dose	Y (He) N (P)
Famciclovir	Renal (hepatic)	2–3	500 mg Q8 hr	DI	CrCl 40–59 = 500 mg Q12 hr CrCl 20–39 = 500 mg Q24 hr <20 = 250 mg Q48 hr			Y (He)
Fluconazole[d]	Renal	19–25	Q24 hr	D	100%	25–50%	25%	Y (He, P)
Flucytosine[b]	Renal	3–8	Q 6hr	I	Q6 hr	Q12 hr	Q24 hr	Y (He, P)
Foscamet	Renal	3–4.5	Q8–12	D	See package insert			Y (He)
Ganciclovir	Renal	2.5–3.6	IV: Q12 hr	IV: DI	IV: 50%–100% and Q12 hr	25%–50% and Q24 hr	25% and Q24 hr	Y (He)
			PO: TID	PO: DI	PO: 50%–100% and TID	50% and BID–QD	50% and QD	

Gatifloxacin	Renal (hepatic)	7–14 hr	Q24 hr	D	*EstCrCl (mL/min)* ≥40: 100% <40: 50%			N (He, P)
Gentamicin[b,d]	Renal	1.5–3	Q8–12 hr	I	Q8–12 hr	Q12–18 hr	Q24–48 hr	Y (He, P)
Imipenem/ cilastatin	Renal	1–1.4	Q6–8 hr	DI	50%–100% and Q6–8 hr	25%–50% and Q8 hr	25% and Q12 hr	Y (He)
Isoniazid	Hepatic (renal)	2–4 (slow)[e] 0.5–1.5 (fast)	Q24 hr	D	100%	100%	50%	Y (He, P)
Kanamycin	Renal	2–3	Q8 hr	I	Q8–12 hr	Q12 hr	Q24 hr	Y (He, P)
Lamivudine[f]	Renal	1.7–2.5	Q12 hr	DI	CrCl 30–49 = 100% and Q24 hr 15–29 = 66% and Q24 hr 5–14 = 33% and Q24 hr <5 = 17% and Q24 hr			?
Levofloxacin	Renal (hepatic)	6–8 hr	Q24 hr	DI	500 mg Q24 hr regimen: *Est CrCl (mL/min)* ≥50: 100% 20–49: 50% ≤19: 50% Q48 hr 750 mg Q24 hr regimen: *Est CrCl (mL/min)* ≥50: 100% 20–49: 100% Q48 hr ≤19: 66% Q48 hr 250 mg Q24 hr regimen: *Est CrCl (mL/min)* ≥20: 100% ≤19: 100% Q48 hr			N (He, P)

[d]May add to peritoneal dialysate to obtain adequate serum levels.

[e]Rate of acetylation of isoniazid.

[f]GFR ≥5 mL/min, give full dose as first dose; for GFR <5 mL/min, give 33% of full dose as first dose.

TABLE 30-1
ANTIMICROBIALS REQUIRING ADJUSTMENT IN RENAL FAILURE—*cont'd*

	Pharmacokinetics			Adjustments in Renal Failure				
					Creatinine Clearance (mL/min)			
Drug	Route of Excretion[a]	Normal $t_{1/2}$ (hr)	Normal Dose Interval	Method	Mild (>50)	Moderate (10–50)	Severe (<10)	Supplemental Dose for Dialysis
Loracarbef	Renal	0.78–1	Q12 hr	D, I	Q12 hr	Q24 hr or 50%	Q72–120 hr	Y (He)
Meropenem	Renal	1–1.4	Q8 hr	DI	100% and Q8 hr	50%–100% and Q12 hr	50% and Q24 hr	Y (He)
Methicillin	Renal	0.5–1.2	Q4–6 hr	I	Q4–6 hr	Q6–8 hr	Q8–12 hr	N (He, P)
Metronidazole	Hepatic (renal)	6–12	Q6–12 hr	D	100%	100%	50%	Y (He) N (P)
Mezlocillin	Renal (hepatic)	0.5–1	Q4–6 hr	I	Q4–6 hr	Q6–8 hr (CrCl 10–30)	Q8–12 hr	Y (He) N (P)
Norfloxacin	Hepatic (renal)	2–4	BID	I	BID	QD–BID	QD	N (He)
Oseltamivir	Renal	1–10	Q12–24 hr	I	Normal	Q24 hr (CrCl 10–30)	?	?
Oxacillin	Renal (liver)	0.3–1.8	Q4–12 hr	D	100%	100%	Use lower range of normal dose	N (P)
Penicillin G–potassium/ Na⁺ (IV)	Renal (hepatic)	0.5–3.4	Q4–6 hr	D	100%	75%	20%–50%	Y (He) N (P)

Penicillin VK (PO)	Renal (hepatic)	30–40 min	Q6 hr	I	Q6 hr	Q6 hr	Q8 hr	Y (He) N (P)
Pentamidine	Renal	6.4–9.4	Q24 hr	I	Q24 hr	CrCl 10–30 = Q36 h	Q48 hr	N (He, P)
Piperacillin	Renal (hepatic)	0.39–1	Q4–6 hr	I	Q4–6 hr	CrCl 20–40 = Q8 hr	CrCl < 20 = Q12 hr	Y (He) N (P)
Piperacillin/ tazobactam	Renal	Piperacillin: 0.39–1 Tazobactam: 0.7–0.9	Q6–8 hr	DI	100% and Q6–8 hr	70% and Q6 hr (CrCl 20–40)	70% and Q8 hr (CrCl < 20)	Y (He) N (P)
Rifabutin	Renal (hepatic)	16–69	Q12–24 hr	D	Normal	50% (CrCl < 30)		?
Rifampin	Hepatic (renal)	3–4	Q12–24 hr	D	100%	50%–100%	50%	N (He, P)
Streptomycin sulfate	Renal	2–4.7	Q24 hr	I	Q24 hr	Q24–72 hr	Q72–96 hr	Y (He)
Sulfamethoxazole	Renal	7–12	Q12 hr	D	100%	50% (CrCl 10–30)	25%	Avoid
Sulfisoxazole	Renal	4–8	Q6 hr	I	Q6 hr	Q8–12 hr	Q12–24 hr	Y (He, P)
Tetracycline	Renal (hepatic)	6–12	Q6 hr	I	Q8–12 hr	Q12–24 hr	**AVOID**	?
Ticarcillin[c]	Renal	0.9–1.3	Q4–6 hr	I	Q4–6 hr	Q8 hr (CrCl 10–30)	Q12 hr	Y (He) N (P)
Ticarcillin-clavulanate[c]	Renal	Ticarcillin: 0.9–1.3 Clavulanate: 1–1.5	Q4–6 hr	I	Q4–6 hr	Q8 hr (CrCl 10–30)	Q12 hr (Q24 hr if comorbid hepatic impairment)	Y (He) N (P)

TABLE 30-1
ANTIMICROBIALS REQUIRING ADJUSTMENT IN RENAL FAILURE—*cont'd*

	Pharmacokinetics			Adjustments in Renal Failure				
					Creatinine Clearance (mL/min)			
Drug	Route of Excretion[a]	Normal $t_{1/2}$ (hr)	Normal Dose Interval	Method	Mild (>50)	Moderate (10–50)	Severe (<10)	Supplemental Dose for Dialysis
Tobramycin[b,d]	Renal	1.5–3	Q8–12 hr	I	Q8–12 hr	Q12–18 hr	Q24–48 hr	Y (He, P)
Valacyclovir	Valacyclovir: Hepatic	Valacyclovir: 2.5–3.6	Q12–24 hr	DI	Herpes zoster: 100% and Q8 hr	100% and Q12–24 hr	50% and Q24 hr	Y (He) N (P)
					Genital herpes (initial): 100% and Q12 hr	100% and Q12–24 hr	50% and Q24 hr	
					Genital herpes (recurrent): 100% and Q12 hr	100% and Q12–24 hr	100% and Q24 hr	
					Genital herpes (suppressive): 100% and Q24 hr	50%–100% and Q24 hr	50% and Q24 hr	
Valgancyclovir (see gancyclovir)								
Vancomycin[b]	Renal	2.2–8	Q6–12 hr	I	Q6–12 hr	Q18–48 hr	Q48–96 hr	Y/N (He)[g] N (P)

[g]If using high-flux hemodialysis (polysulfone polyamide and polyacrylonitrile), give supplemental dose after dialysis.

TABLE 30-2

NONANTIMICROBIALS REQUIRING ADJUSTMENT IN RENAL FAILURE

	Pharmacokinetics			Adjustments in Renal Failure				
					Creatinine Clearance (mL/min)			
Drug	Route of Excretion[a]	Normal $t_{1/2}$ (hr)	Normal Dose Interval	Method	Mild (>50)	Moderate (10–50)	Severe (<10)	Supplemental Dose for Dialysis
Acetaminophen	Hepatic	2–4	Q4 hr	I	Q4 hr	Q6 hr	Q8 hr	Y (He) N (P)
Acetazolamide	Renal	2.4–5.8	Q6–24 hr	I	Q6–8 hr	Q12 hr	**AVOID**	N (He, P)
Allopurinol	Renal	1–3	Q6–12 hr	D, I	100% or Q8 hr	50% or Q12–24 hr	10%–25% or Q48–72 hr	?
Amantadine	Renal	10–14	Q12–24 hr	I	Q12–24 hr	Q48–72 hr	Q168 hr (7 days)	N (He, P)
Aminocaproic acid	Renal	1–2	Q4–6 hr	D	Reduce dose to 15%–25% in patients with renal disease or oliguria. No specific recommendations available			Y (He)
Aspirin[b]	Hepatic (renal)	2–19	Q4 hr	I	Q4 hr	Q4–6 hr	**AVOID**	Y (He) Y (P)
Atenolol	Renal (GI)	3.5–7	QD	D, I	100% or Q24 hr	50% or Q48 hr	25% or Q96 hr	Y (He)
Azathioprine[c]	Hepatic (renal)	0.7–3	QD	D, I	100% or Q24 hr	75% or Q36 hr	50% or Q48 hr	Y (He)
Bismuth subsalicylate	Hepatic (renal)	Salicylate: 2–5 Bismuth: 21–72 days	Q30 min–4 hr	D	**AVOID**	**AVOID**	**AVOID**	NA

TABLE 30-2

NONANTIMICROBIALS REQUIRING ADJUSTMENT IN RENAL FAILURE—*cont'd*

	Pharmacokinetics			Adjustments in Renal Failure				
					Creatinine Clearance (mL/min)			
Drug	Route of Excretion[a]	Normal $t_{1/2}$ (hr)	Normal Dose Interval	Method	Mild (>50)	Moderate (10–50)	Severe (<10)	Supplemental Dose for Dialysis
Captopril	Renal (hepatic)	0.98–2.3	Q6–24 hr	D, I	100% or Q8–12 hr	75% or Q12–18 hr	50% or Q24 hr	Y (He) N (P)
Carbamazepine	Hepatic (renal)	Initial: 25–65 Subsequent: 8–17	Q6–24 hr	D	100%	100%	75% (monitor serum levels)	N (He, P)
Cetirizine	Renal (hepatic)	6.2–9	BID–QD	D	100%	50%–100%	50%	N (He)
Chloroquine	Renal (hepatic)	3–5 days	Q6 hr–7 days	D	100%	100%	50%	?
Cimetidine	Renal (hepatic)	1.4–2	Q6–12 hr	D, I	100% or Q6 hr	75% or Q8 hr	50% or Q12 hr	N (He, P)
Codeine	Hepatic (renal)	2.5–3.5	Q6–12 hr Q4–6 hr	D	100%	75%	50%	?
Digoxin[d]	Renal	35–48	Q12–24 hr	D, I	100% or Q24 hr	25%–75% or Q36 hr	10%–25% or Q48 hr	N (He, P)
Diphenhydramine	Hepatic	4–7	Q6–8 hr	I	Q6 hr	Q6–12 hr	Q12–18 hr	?
Disopyramide	Renal (GI)	4–10	Q6 hr	I	Q6 hr	Q8–12 hr	Q24 hr	Y (He)
Enalapril (IV: Enalaprilat)	Renal (hepatic)	1.3–6	Q8–24 hr	D	100%	75%–100%	50%	?

Famotidine	Renal (hepatic)	2.5–4	Q8–12 hr	D, I	100% or Q8–12 hr	50% or Q24 hr	25% or Q36–48 hr	N (He, P)
Fentanyl	Renal (hepatic)	2–4	Q30 min–1 hr	D	100%	75%	50%	N (He)
Flecainide	Renal/hepatic	8–12	Q8–12 hr	D	CrCl < 20: 25–50%			N (He, P)
Gabapentin	Renal (hepatic)	5–9	TID	I	TID	BID–QD	QOD	Y (He)
Hydralazine[e]	Hepatic (renal)	2–8	IV: Q4–6 hr	I	Normal dosing	Q8 hr	Q8–16 hr (fast acetylator) Q12–24 hr (slow acetylator)	N (He, P)
Insulin (regular)[f]	Hepatic (renal)	5–15 min	Variable	D	100%	75%	25% –50%	N (He, P)
Lisinopril	Renal	12 hr	Q24 hr	D	*Est CrCl (mL/min)* >30: 100% 10–30: 50% <10: 25%			Y (He) N (P)
Lithium	Renal	18–24	BID–QID	D	100%	50% –75%	25% –50%	Y (He, P)
Loratidine	Renal/hepatic	8–15 hr	QD	I	Normal	CrCl < 30: QOD		N (He, P)
Meperidine	Renal (hepatic) (nor-meperidine: renal)	2.3–4	Q3–4 hr	D	100%	75%	50%	?

TABLE 30-2
NONANTIMICROBIALS REQUIRING ADJUSTMENT IN RENAL FAILURE—*cont'd*

	Pharmacokinetics			Adjustments in Renal Failure				
					Creatinine Clearance (mL/min)			
Drug	Route of Excretion[a]	Normal $t_{1/2}$ (hr)	Normal Dose Interval	Method	Mild (>50)	Moderate (10–50)	Severe (<10)	Supplemental Dose for Dialysis
Methadone	Hepatic (renal)	4–62	Q3–6 hr	D	100%	100%	50%–75%	?
Methyldopa	Hepatic (renal)	1–3	PO: Q6–12 hr IV: Q6–8 hr	I	Q8 hr	Q8–12 hr	Q12–24 hr	Y (He)
Metoclopramide	Renal	2.5–6	PO: Q6 hr IV: Q6–8 hr	D	100%	50%–75%	25%–50%	N (He)
Midazolam	Hepatic (renal)	2.9–4.5	Variable	D	100%	100%	50%	?
Morphine	Hepatic (renal)	1–6.2	Variable	D	100%	75%	50%	N (He)
Neostigmine	Hepatic (renal)	0.5–2.1	Single dose	D	100%	50%	25%	?
Phenazopyridine	Renal (hepatic)	?	TID for 2 days	I	Q8–16 hr	**AVOID**	**AVOID**	NA
Phenobarbital	Hepatic (renal 30%)	65–150	Q8–12 hr	I	Q8–12 hr	Q8–12 hr	Q12–16 hr	Y (He, P)

Primidone	Hepatic (renal, 20%)	10–16	Q6–12	I	Q8 hr	Q8–12 hr	Q12–24 hr	Y (He)
Procainamide	Hepatic (renal)	Procainamide: 1.7–4.7 NAPA: 6–8	PO: Q3–6 hr IM: Q4–6 hr	I	Normal interval	Q6–12 hr	Q8–24 hr	Y (He) N (P)
Propylthiouracil	Hepatic (renal)	1.5–5	Q8 hr	D	100%	75%	50%	?
Ranitidine	Renal (hepatic)	1.8–2.5	Q8–12 hr	D	100%	75%	50%	N (He, P)
Spironolactone	Renal (hepatic)	78–84 min	Q6–12 hr	I	Q6–12 hr	Q12–24 hr[g]	**AVOID**	?
Terbutaline (IV/PO)	Renal (hepatic)	11–26	Variable	D	100%	50%	**AVOID**	?
Thiopental	Hepatic (renal)	3–11.5	One-time dose	D	100%	100%	75%	?
Triamterene	Hepatic (renal)	1.5–2.5	Q12–24 hr	I	Q12 hr	Q12 hr[g]	**AVOID**	N (He)
Verapamil	Renal (hepatic)	2–8	Variable	D	100%	100%	50%–75%	N (He)

CrCl, creatinine clearance; GFR, glomerular filtration rate; He, hemodialysis; P, peritoneal dialysis; NA, not applicable.

[a]Route in parentheses indicates secondary route of excretion.

[b]With large doses, the $t_{1/2}$ is prolonged up to 30 hr.

[c]Azathioprine rapidly converted to mercaptopurine ($t_{1/2}$ = 0.5–4 hr).

[d]Decrease loading dose by 50% in end-stage renal disease because of decreased volume of distribution.

[e]Dose interval varies for rapid and slow acetylators with normal and impaired renal function.

[f]Renal failure may cause hyposensitivity or hypersensitivity to insulin; adjust to clinical response and blood glucose.

[g]Hyperkalemia common with GFR < 30 mL/min.

REFERENCES

1. Taketomo C, Hodding JH, Kraus DM: Pediatric Dosage Handbook, 8th ed. Hudson, OH, Lexi-Comp, 2001–2002.
2. American Society of Health-System Pharmacists: American Hospital Formulary Service. Bethesda, MD, The Society, 1998.
3. Johnson C, Simmons W: Dialysis of drugs. Pharm Practice News Dec 1988;(Dec):30–33.
4. Micromedex, Inc. Vol. 111. 1974–2002.

INDEX

Page numbers followed by b indicate boxed material; those followed by f indicate figures; those followed by t indicate tables.

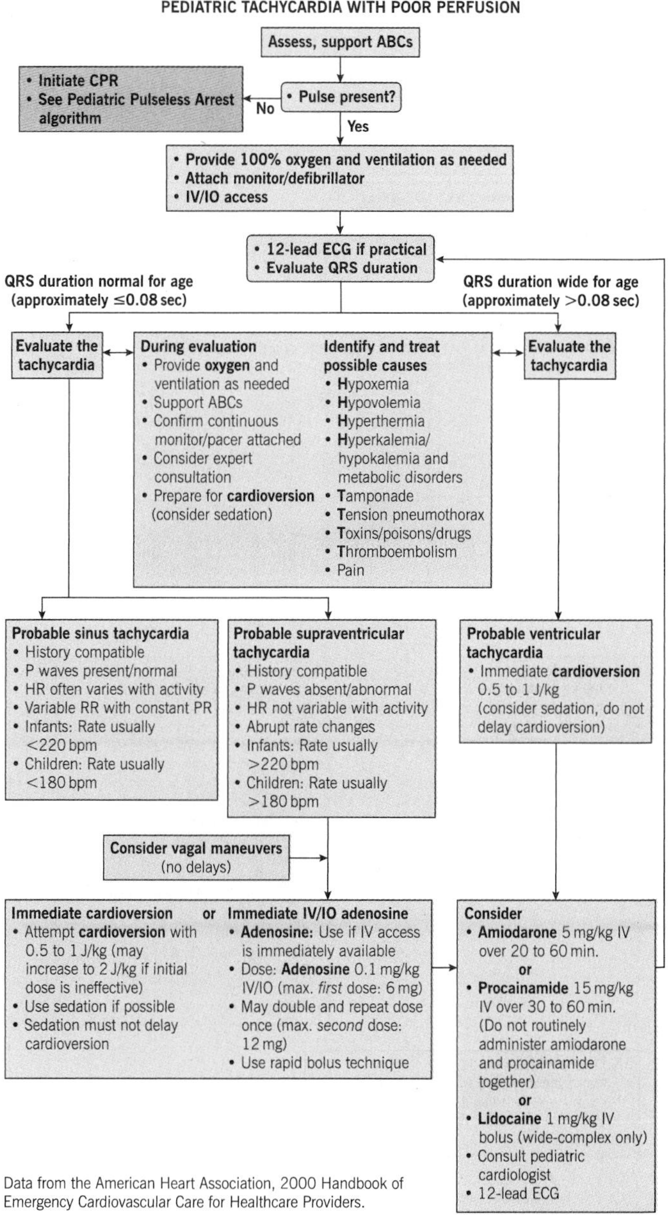

PEDIATRIC TACHYCARDIA WITH POOR PERFUSION
Assess, support ABCs
• Pulse present?
No
• Initiate CPR
• See Pediatric Pulseless Arrest algorithm
Yes
• Provide 100% oxygen and ventilation as needed
• Attach monitor/defibrillator
• IV/IO access
• 12-lead ECG if practical
• Evaluate QRS duration
QRS duration normal for age (approximately ≤0.08 sec)
QRS duration wide for age (approximately >0.08 sec)
Evaluate the tachycardia
During evaluation
• Provide oxygen and ventilation as needed
• Support ABCs
• Confirm continuous monitor/pacer attached
• Consider expert consultation
• Prepare for cardioversion (consider sedation)
Identify and treat possible causes
• Hypoxemia
• Hypovolemia
• Hyperthermia
• Hyperkalemia/hypokalemia and metabolic disorders
• Tamponade
• Tension pneumothorax
• Toxins/poisons/drugs
• Thromboembolism
• Pain
Evaluate the tachycardia
Probable sinus tachycardia
• History compatible
• P waves present/normal
• HR often varies with activity
• Variable RR with constant PR
• Infants: Rate usually <220 bpm
• Children: Rate usually <180 bpm
Probable supraventricular tachycardia
• History compatible
• P waves absent/abnormal
• HR not variable with activity
• Abrupt rate changes
• Infants: Rate usually >220 bpm
• Children: Rate usually >180 bpm
Probable ventricular tachycardia
• Immediate cardioversion 0.5 to 1 J/kg (consider sedation, do not delay cardioversion)
Consider vagal maneuvers (no delays)
Immediate cardioversion
• Attempt cardioversion with 0.5 to 1 J/kg (may increase to 2 J/kg if initial dose is ineffective)
• Use sedation if possible
• Sedation must not delay cardioversion
or
Immediate IV/IO adenosine
• Adenosine: Use if IV access is immediately available
• Dose: Adenosine 0.1 mg/kg IV/IO (max. first dose: 6 mg)
• May double and repeat dose once (max. second dose: 12 mg)
• Use rapid bolus technique
Consider
• Amiodarone 5 mg/kg IV over 20 to 60 min.
or
• Procainamide 15 mg/kg IV over 30 to 60 min. (Do not routinely administer amiodarone and procainamide together)
or
• Lidocaine 1 mg/kg IV bolus (wide-complex only)
• Consult pediatric cardiologist
• 12-lead ECG

Data from the American Heart Association, 2000 Handbook of Emergency Cardiovascular Care for Healthcare Providers.

PEDIATRIC TACHYCARDIA WITH ADEQUATE PERFUSION

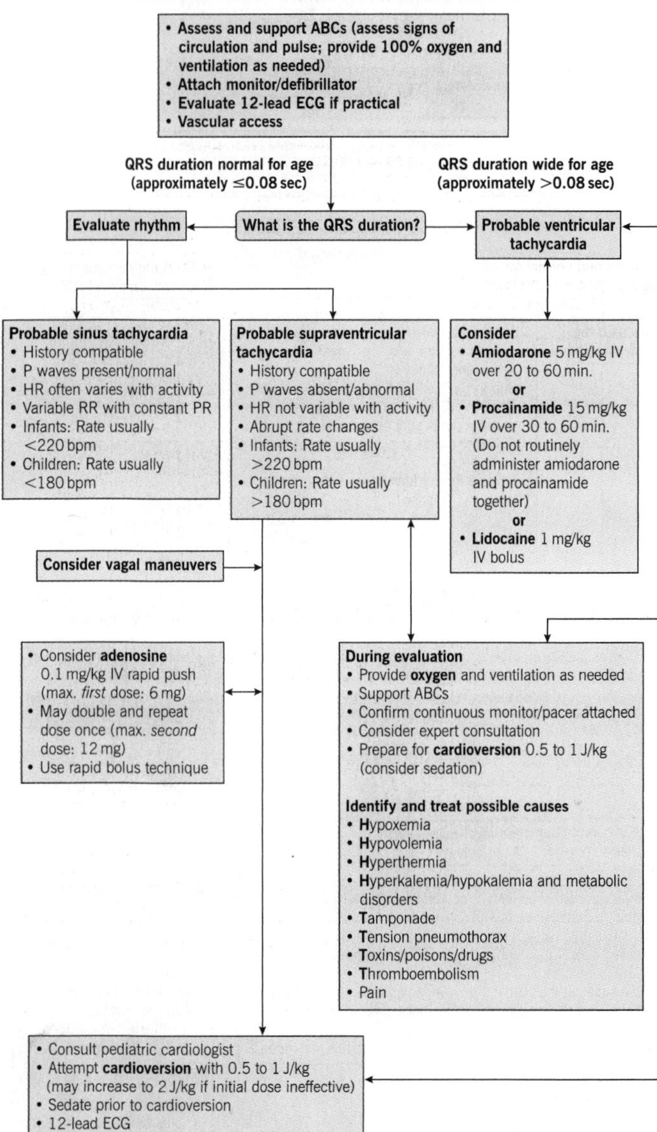

• Assess and support ABCs (assess signs of circulation and pulse; provide 100% oxygen and ventilation as needed)
• Attach monitor/defibrillator
• Evaluate 12-lead ECG if practical
• Vascular access
QRS duration normal for age (approximately ≤0.08 sec)
QRS duration wide for age (approximately >0.08 sec)
Evaluate rhythm
What is the QRS duration?
Probable ventricular tachycardia
Probable sinus tachycardia
• History compatible
• P waves present/normal
• HR often varies with activity
• Variable RR with constant PR
• Infants: Rate usually <220 bpm
• Children: Rate usually <180 bpm
Probable supraventricular tachycardia
• History compatible
• P waves absent/abnormal
• HR not variable with activity
• Abrupt rate changes
• Infants: Rate usually >220 bpm
• Children: Rate usually >180 bpm
Consider
• Amiodarone 5 mg/kg IV over 20 to 60 min.
or
• Procainamide 15 mg/kg IV over 30 to 60 min. (Do not routinely administer amiodarone and procainamide together)
or
• Lidocaine 1 mg/kg IV bolus
Consider vagal maneuvers
• Consider adenosine 0.1 mg/kg IV rapid push (max. first dose: 6 mg)
• May double and repeat dose once (max. second dose: 12 mg)
• Use rapid bolus technique
During evaluation
• Provide oxygen and ventilation as needed
• Support ABCs
• Confirm continuous monitor/pacer attached
• Consider expert consultation
• Prepare for cardioversion 0.5 to 1 J/kg (consider sedation)
Identify and treat possible causes
• Hypoxemia
• Hypovolemia
• Hyperthermia
• Hyperkalemia/hypokalemia and metabolic disorders
• Tamponade
• Tension pneumothorax
• Toxins/poisons/drugs
• Thromboembolism
• Pain
• Consult pediatric cardiologist
• Attempt cardioversion with 0.5 to 1 J/kg (may increase to 2 J/kg if initial dose ineffective)
• Sedate prior to cardioversion
• 12-lead ECG

Data from the American Heart Association, 2000 Handbook of Emergency Cardiovascular Care for Healthcare Providers.

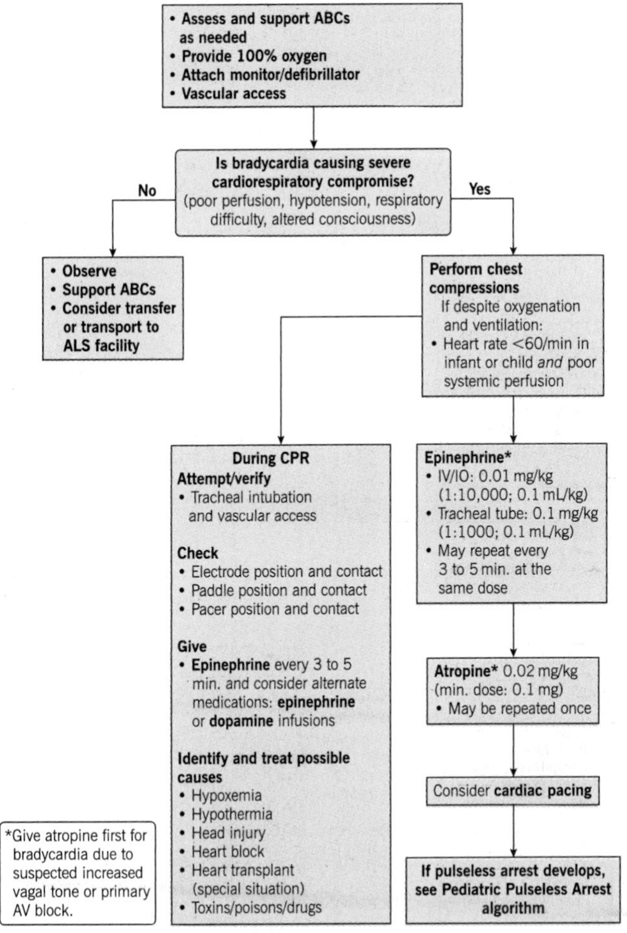

PEDIATRIC BRADYCARDIA
• Assess and support ABCs as needed
• Provide 100% oxygen
• Attach monitor/defibrillator
• Vascular access
Is bradycardia causing severe cardiorespiratory compromise?
(poor perfusion, hypotension, respiratory difficulty, altered consciousness)
No
Yes
• Observe
• Support ABCs
• Consider transfer or transport to ALS facility
Perform chest compressions
If despite oxygenation and ventilation:
• Heart rate <60/min in infant or child and poor systemic perfusion
During CPR
Attempt/verify
• Tracheal intubation and vascular access
Check
• Electrode position and contact
• Paddle position and contact
• Pacer position and contact
Give
• Epinephrine every 3 to 5 min. and consider alternate medications: epinephrine or dopamine infusions
Identify and treat possible causes
• Hypoxemia
• Hypothermia
• Head injury
• Heart block
• Heart transplant (special situation)
• Toxins/poisons/drugs
Epinephrine*
• IV/IO: 0.01 mg/kg (1:10,000; 0.1 mL/kg)
• Tracheal tube: 0.1 mg/kg (1:1000; 0.1 mL/kg)
• May repeat every 3 to 5 min. at the same dose
Atropine* 0.02 mg/kg (min. dose: 0.1 mg)
• May be repeated once
Consider cardiac pacing
If pulseless arrest develops, see Pediatric Pulseless Arrest algorithm
*Give atropine first for bradycardia due to suspected increased vagal tone or primary AV block.

Data from the American Heart Association, 2000 Handbook of Emergency Cardiovascular Care for Healthcare Providers.

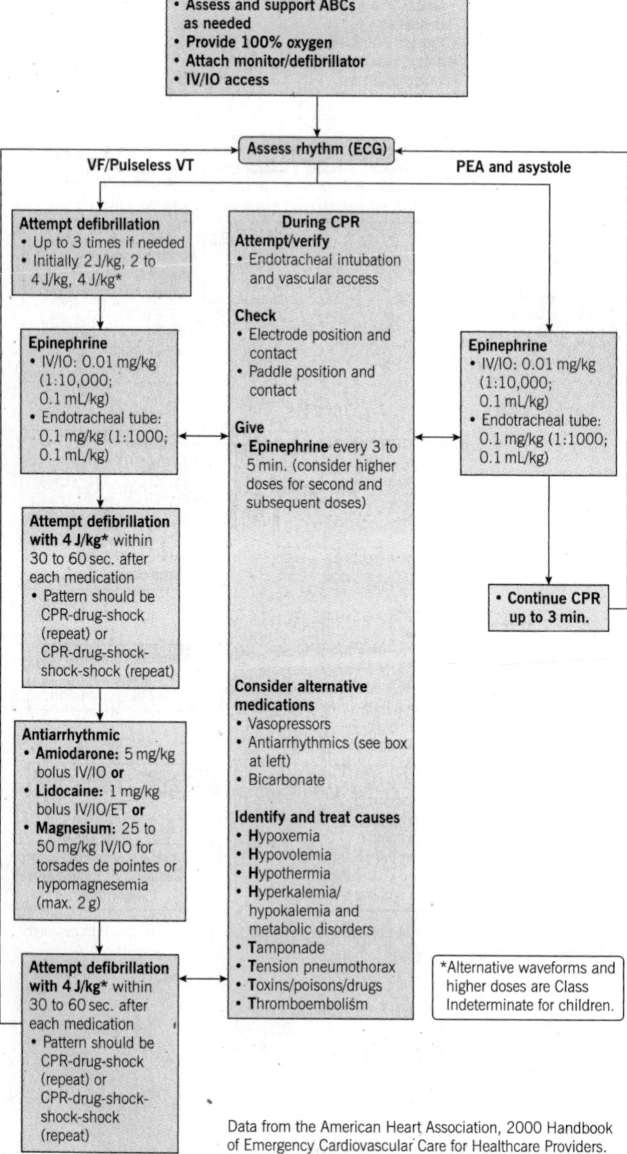
PEDIATRIC PULSELESS ARREST
• Assess and support ABCs as needed
• Provide 100% oxygen
• Attach monitor/defibrillator
• IV/IO access
Assess rhythm (ECG)
VF/Pulseless VT
PEA and asystole
Attempt defibrillation
• Up to 3 times if needed
• Initially 2 J/kg, 2 to 4 J/kg, 4 J/kg*
Epinephrine
• IV/IO: 0.01 mg/kg (1:10,000; 0.1 mL/kg)
• Endotracheal tube: 0.1 mg/kg (1:1000; 0.1 mL/kg)
Attempt defibrillation with 4 J/kg* within 30 to 60 sec. after each medication
• Pattern should be CPR-drug-shock (repeat) or CPR-drug-shock-shock-shock (repeat)
Antiarrhythmic
• Amiodarone: 5 mg/kg bolus IV/IO or
• Lidocaine: 1 mg/kg bolus IV/IO/ET or
• Magnesium: 25 to 50 mg/kg IV/IO for torsades de pointes or hypomagnesemia (max. 2 g)
Attempt defibrillation with 4 J/kg* within 30 to 60 sec. after each medication
• Pattern should be CPR-drug-shock (repeat) or CPR-drug-shock-shock-shock (repeat)
During CPR
Attempt/verify
• Endotracheal intubation and vascular access
Check
• Electrode position and contact
• Paddle position and contact
Give
• Epinephrine every 3 to 5 min. (consider higher doses for second and subsequent doses)
Consider alternative medications
• Vasopressors
• Antiarrhythmics (see box at left)
• Bicarbonate
Identify and treat causes
• Hypoxemia
• Hypovolemia
• Hypothermia
• Hyperkalemia/hypokalemia and metabolic disorders
• Tamponade
• Tension pneumothorax
• Toxins/poisons/drugs
• Thromboembolism
Epinephrine
• IV/IO: 0.01 mg/kg (1:10,000; 0.1 mL/kg)
• Endotracheal tube: 0.1 mg/kg (1:1000; 0.1 mL/kg)
• Continue CPR up to 3 min.
*Alternative waveforms and higher doses are Class Indeterminate for children.
Data from the American Heart Association, 2000 Handbook of Emergency Cardiovascular Care for Healthcare Providers.